Methods of Hormone Radioimmunoassay

Second Edition

Edited by

Bernard M. Jaffe

Department of Surgery
Washington University
School of Medicine
St. Louis, Missouri

Harold R. Behrman

Reproductive Biology Section
Department of Obstetrics and Gynecology
and Pharmacology
Yale University
School of Medicine
New Haven, Connecticut

Academic Press
New York   San Francisco   London   1979
A Subsidiary of Harcourt Brace Jovanovich, Publishers

ACADEMIC PRESS, INC.
111 Fifth Avenue, New York, New York 10003

United Kingdom Edition published by
ACADEMIC PRESS, INC. (LONDON) LTD.
24/28 Oval Road, London NW1 7DX

Library of Congress Cataloging in Publication Data

Jaffe, Bernard M., Date
    Methods of hormone radioimmunoassay.

    Includes bibliographies and index.
    1. Hormones--Analysis. 2. Radioimmunoassay.
I. Behrman, Harold R. II. Title. [DNLM: 1. Hormones
--Analysis. 2. Radioimmunoassay. QY330 M593]
QP571.J33   1978   612'.405'0154582   78-3340
ISBN 0-12-379260-6

JOHN P. WIEBE

Methods of Hormone Radioimmunoassay

Second Edition

Contributors

Josephine Arendt
Glen Arth
Frederick J. Auletta
Rahim M. Bassiri
Harold R. Behrman
Muriel H. Blanchard
S. R. Bloom
Guenther Boden
John C. Brown
Maire T. Buckman
Burton V. Caldwell
Robert E. Carraway
Ronald E. Chance
Ernest S. Chang
Ronald H. Chochinov
William H. Daughaday
Leonard J. Deftos
Laurence M. Demers
Jill R. Dryburgh
Josef Dvorak
Gerald R. Faloona
Arthur E. Freedlender
Henry G. Friesen
Joseph F. Garcia
Seymour M. Glick
Theodore L. Goodfriend
Harry Gregory
John G. Haddad, Jr.

Gerald L. Hamilton
Ray Haning
Akira Harada
Virginia Harris
Richard F. Harvey
Jerome M. Hershman
Martin Hichens
Charles S. Hollander
Jennifer E. Holmes
D. L. Horwitz
Laurence S. Jacobs
Bernard M. Jaffe
Melvin G. Johnson
Avir Kagan
Susan E. Leeman
M. E. Mako
Nancy E. Moon
Josephine Morris
N. R. Moudgal
Edmund A. Mroz
K. Muralidhar
T. M. Nett
Wendell E. Nicholson
Gordon D. Niswender
John D. O'Connor
Charles E. Odya
Gayle P. Orczyk
David N. Orth

Kent Painter
Yogesh C. Patel
Glenn T. Peake
Jeereddi A. Prasad
H. G. Madhwa Raj
Seymour Reichlin
Bernard A. Roos
Buddha P. Roy
A. H. Rubenstein
Judith D. Saide
O. David Sherwood
J. I. Starr
Alton L. Steiner
Koshi Tanaka
Armen H. Tashjian, Jr.
Richard H. Underwood
Roger H. Unger
Robert D. Utiger
Judith L. Vaitukaitis
P. Vecsei
Edward F. Voelkel
John H. Walsh
Michael Wilkinson
Gordon H. Williams
Ian R. Willshire
Robert M. Wilson
Helen C. Wong
Michael Young

*To our wives
Marlene
and Jo*

Contents

INTRACELLULAR MESSENGERS

1   Cyclic AMP and Cyclic GMP

ALTON L. STEINER

2   Prostaglandins and Prostaglandin Metabolites

BERNARD M. JAFFE AND HAROLD R. BEHRMAN

HYPOTHALAMIC AND PINEAL HORMONES

PITUITARY HORMONES

16 Vasopressin

SEYMOUR M. GLICK AND AVIR KAGAN

THYROID AND PARATHYROID HORMONES

17 Human Calcitonin: Application of Affinity Chromatography

ARMEN H. TASHJIAN, JR., AND EDWARD F. VOELKEL

18 Thyroxine and Triiodothyronine

JEEREDDI A. PRASAD AND CHARLES S. HOLLANDER

32   Glucagon

VIRGINIA HARRIS, GERALD R. FALOONA, AND ROGER H. UNGER

33   Human Pancreatic Polypeptide (HPP) and Bovine Pancreatic Polypeptide (BPP)

RONALD E. CHANCE, NANCY E. MOON, AND MELVIN G. JOHNSON

STEROID HORMONES

34   Plasma Estradiol, Estrone, Estriol, and Urinary Estriol Glucuronide

RAY HANING, GAYLE P. ORCZYK, BURTON V. CALDWELL, AND HAROLD R. BEHRMAN

35   Progesterone and 20α-Dihydroprogesterone

GAYLE P. ORCZYK, MARTIN HICHENS, GLEN ARTH, AND HAROLD R. BEHRMAN

UTERINE AND PLACENTAL HORMONES

VASOACTIVE PEPTIDE HORMONES

List of Contributors

Numbers in parentheses indicate the pages on which the authors' contributions begin.

JOSEPHINE ARENDT* (101), Department of Pediatrics and Genetics, University of Geneva, Geneva, Switzerland

GLEN ARTH† (701), Merck Institute for Therapeutic Research, Merck Sharp & Dohme Research Laboratories, Rahway, New Jersey

FREDERICK J. AULETTA (715), Dreyfus Research Laboratories, Laboratory of Gynecologic Endocrinology, Michael Reese Medical Center, Chicago, Illinois

RAHIM M. BASSIRI (45), Endocrine Section, Department of Medicine, University of Pennsylvania School of Medicine, Philadelphia, Pennsylvania

HAROLD R. BEHRMAN (19, 675, 701), Reproductive Biology Section, Departments of Obstetrics and Gynecology and Pharmacology, Yale University School of Medicine, New Haven, Connecticut

MURIEL H. BLANCHARD (941), Laboratory of Physical Biochemistry, Department of Medicine, Massachusetts General Hospital, Boston, Massachusetts

S. R. BLOOM (553), Department of Medicine, Hammersmith Hospital, Royal Postgraduate Medical School, University of London, London, United Kingdom

GUENTHER BODEN (479), Department of Medicine, and General Clinical Research Center, Temple University Health Sciences Center, Philadelphia, Pennsylvania

JOHN C. BROWN (541, 567), Department of Physiology, Faculty of Medicine, The University of British Columbia, Vancouver, British Columbia, Canada

* Present address: Department of Biochemistry, University of Surrey, Guildford, Surrey, United Kingdom.

† Deceased.

MAIRE T. BUCKMAN (223), Medicine and Research Services, Veterans Administration Hospital, and Department of Medicine, School of Medicine, The University of New Mexico, Albuquerque, New Mexico

BURTON V. CALDWELL (675, 715), Departments of Obstetrics and Gynecology and Medicine, Yale University School of Medicine, New Haven, Connecticut

ROBERT E. CARRAWAY (139), Department of Physiology, and Laboratory of Human Reproduction and Reproductive Biology, Harvard Medical School, Boston, Massachusetts

RONALD E. CHANCE (657), Lilly Research Laboratories, Indianapolis, Indiana

ERNEST S. CHANG* (797), Department of Biology, University of California, Los Angeles, California

RONALD H. CHOCHINOV (959), Departments of Medicine and Physiology, Faculty of Medicine, The University of Manitoba, Winnipeg, Manitoba, Canada

WILLIAM H. DAUGHADAY (959), Metabolism Division, Department of Medicine, Washington University School of Medicine, St. Louis, Missouri

LEONARD J. DEFTOS (401), Endocrine Section, Department of Medicine, Veterans Administration Hospital, and Department of Medicine, School of Medicine, University of California, San Diego, La Jolla, California

LAURENCE M. DEMERS (595), Department of Clinical Pathology, The Milton S. Hershey Medical Center, The Pennsylvania State University, Hershey, Pennsylvania

JILL R. DRYBURGH† (541, 567), Department of Physiology, Faculty of Medicine, The University of British Columbia, Vancouver, British Columbia, Canada

JOSEF DVORAK (45), Endocrine Section, Department of Medicine, University of Pennsylvania School of Medicine, Philadelphia, Pennsylvania

GERALD R. FALOONA (643), Department of Life Sciences, Bishop College, Dallas, Texas

ARTHUR E. FREEDLANDER‡ (889), William S. Middleton Memorial Veterans Hospital, and Departments of Internal Medicine and Pharmacology, Center for Health Sciences, University of Wisconsin, Madison, Wisconsin

HENRY G. FRIESEN (831), Department of Physiology, Faculty of Medicine, The University of Manitoba, Winnipeg, Manitoba, Canada

JOSEPH F. GARCIA (421), Lawrence Berkeley Laboratory, University of California, Berkeley, California

SEYMOUR M. GLICK (327, 341), Department of Medicine, Downstate Medical Center, State University of New York, Brooklyn, New York

* Present address: Department of Biochemistry, University of Chicago, Chicago, Illinois.

† Present address: Department of Histochemistry, Hammersmith Hospital, Royal Postgraduate Medical School, University of London, London, United Kingdom.

‡ Present address: Departments of Pharmacology and Medicine, Medical College of Virginia, and Veterans Administration Hospital, Richmond, Virginia.

THEODORE L. GOODFRIEND (889, 909), William S. Middleton Memorial Veterans Hospital, and Departments of Internal Medicine and Pharmacology, Center for Health Sciences, University of Wisconsin, Madison, Wisconsin

HARRY GREGORY (927), Pharmaceuticals Division, Imperial Chemical Industries, Limited, Mereside, Alderley Park, Macclesfield, Cheshire, United Kingdom

JOHN G. HADDAD, JR. (437), Department of Medicine, The Jewish Hospital of St. Louis, Washington University School of Medicine, St. Louis, Missouri

GERALD L. HAMILTON (715), Laboratory of Gynecologic Endocrinology, Department of Obstetrics and Gynecology, Yale University School of Medicine, New Haven, Connecticut

RAY HANING (675), Department of Gynecology and Obstetrics, University of Wisconsin Center for Health Sciences, Madison, Wisconsin

AKIRA HARADA (867), Medical and Research Services, Veterans Administration–Wadsworth Hospital Center, Los Angeles, California

VIRGINIA HARRIS (643), Veterans Administration Hospital, Dallas, Texas

RICHARD F. HARVEY (495), Department of Medicine, Bristol Royal Infirmary, Department of Medicine and Gastroenterology Unit, Frenchay Hospital, Bristol, United Kingdom

JEROME M. HERSHMAN (867), Medical and Research Services, Veterans Administration–Wadsworth Hospital Center, Los Angeles, California

MARTIN HICHENS (701), Department of Reproductive Biology, Merck Institute for Therapeutic Research, Merck Sharp & Dohme Research Laboratories, Rahway, New Jersey

CHARLES S. HOLLANDER (375), Endocrine Division, Department of Medicine, New York University School of Medicine, New York, New York

JENNIFER E. HOLMES (927), Pharmaceuticals Division, Imperial Chemical Industries, Limited, Mereside, Alderley Park, Macclesfield, Cheshire, United Kingdom

D. L. HORWITZ (613), Section of Endocrinology, Department of Medicine, The University of Chicago, Chicago, Illinois

LAURENCE S. JACOBS (199), Clinical Research Center, and Department of Medicine, The University of Rochester Medical Center, Rochester, New York

BERNARD M. JAFFE (19, 455, 527), Department of Surgery, Washington University School of Medicine, St. Louis, Missouri

MELVIN G. JOHNSON (657), Lilly Research Laboratories, Indianapolis, Indiana

AVIR KAGAN (327, 341), Department of Nuclear Medicine, Coney Island Hospital, New York City Health and Hospitals Corporation, Brooklyn, New York

SUSAN E. LEEMAN (121), Department of Physiology, and Laboratory of Human Reproduction and Reproductive Biology, Harvard Medical School, Boston, Massachusetts

M. E. MAKO (613), Section of Endocrinology, Department of Medicine, The University of Chicago, Chicago, Illinois

NANCY E. MOON (657), Lilly Research Laboratories, Indianapolis, Indiana

JOSEPHINE MORRIS (223), Department of Medicine, School of Medicine, The University of New Mexico, Albuquerque, New Mexico

N. R. MOUDGAL (173), Department of Biochemistry, Indian Institute of Science, Bangalore, India

EDMUND A. MROZ (121), Biotechnology Resource in Electron Probe Microanalysis, Laboratory of Human Reproduction and Reproductive Biology, Harvard Medical School, Boston, Massachusetts

K. MURALIDHAR (173), Department of Biochemistry, Indian Institute of Science, Bangalore, India

T. M. NETT (57), Department of Physiology and Biophysics, Colorado State University, Fort Collins, Colorado

WENDELL E. NICHOLSON (285), Division of Endocrinology, Department of Medicine, School of Medicine, Vanderbilt University, Nashville, Tennessee

GORDON D. NISWENDER (57), Department of Physiology and Biophysics, Colorado State University, Fort Collins, Colorado

JOHN D. O'CONNOR (797), Department of Biology, University of California, Los Angeles, California

CHARLES E. ODYA* (909), William S. Middleton Memorial Veterans Hospital, and Departments of Internal Medicine and Pharmacology, Center for Health Sciences, University of Wisconsin, Madison, Wisconsin

GAYLE P. ORCZYK (675, 701), Department of Obstetrics and Gynecology, Yale University School of Medicine, New Haven, Connecticut

DAVID N. ORTH (245, 285), Division of Endocrinology, Department of Medicine, School of Medicine, Vanderbilt University, Nashville, Tennessee

KENT PAINTER (727), Department of Radiology and Radiation Biology, Colorado State University, Fort Collins, Colorado

YOGESH C. PATEL (77), Department of Medicine, Royal Victoria Hospital, McGill University, Montreal, Quebec, Canada

GLENN T. PEAKE (223), Department of Medicine, School of Medicine, The University of New Mexico, Albuquerque, New Mexico

JEEREDDI A. PRASAD (375), Endocrine Division, Department of Medicine, New York University School of Medicine, New York, New York

H. G. MADHWA RAJ (173), Departments of Obstetrics and Gynecology, and Pharmacology, School of Medicine, The University of North Carolina at Chapel Hill, Chapel Hill, North Carolina

SEYMOUR REICHLIN (77), Endocrinology Division, New England Medical Center Hospital, Tufts University School of Medicine, Boston, Massachusetts

BERNARD A. ROOS (401), Endocrinology and Mineral Metabolism, Department of Medicine, Veterans Administration Hospital, and Department of

* Present address: Laboratory of Cellular Metabolism, National Institutes of Health, Bethesda, Maryland.

Medicine, School of Medicine, Case Western Reserve University, Cleveland, Ohio

BUDDHA P. ROY (831), Department of Physiology, Faculty of Medicine, The University of Manitoba, Winnipeg, Manitoba, Canada

A. H. RUBENSTEIN (613), Section of Endocrinology, Department of Medicine, The University of Chicago, Chicago, Illinois

JUDITH D. SAIDE* (941), Laboratory of Physical Biochemistry and Department of Medicine, Massachusetts General Hospital, Boston, Massachusetts

O. DAVID SHERWOOD (875), School of Basic Medical Sciences and Department of Physiology and Biophysics, University of Illinois, Urbana, Illinois

J. I. STARR (613), Division of Biological Science, Department of Medicine, The University of Chicago, Chicago, Illinois

ALTON L. STEINER (3), Division of Endocrinology, Department of Medicine, School of Medicine, The University of North Carolina at Chapel Hill, Chapel Hill, North Carolina

KOSHI TANAKA† (285), Department of Medicine, School of Medicine, Vanderbilt University Nashville, Tennessee

ARMEN H. TASHJIAN, JR. (355), Laboratory of Pharmacology, Harvard School of Dental Medicine, Boston, Massachusetts

RICHARD H. UNDERWOOD (743), Endocrinology–Hypertension Unit, Peter Bent Brigham Hospital, and Department of Medicine, Harvard Medical School, Boston, Massachusetts

ROGER H. UNGER (643), Veterans Administration Hospital and The University of Texas Southwestern Medical School, Health Science Center at Dallas, Dallas, Texas

ROBERT D. UTIGER (45, 315), Endocrine Section, Department of Medicine, University of Pennsylvania School of Medicine, Philadelphia, Pennsylvania

JUDITH L. VAITUKAITIS (817), Thorndike Memorial Laboratory, Section of Endocrinology and Metabolism, Boston City Hospital, and Departments of Medicine and Physiology, Boston University School of Medicine, Boston, Massachusetts

P. VECSEI (767), Pharmakologisches Institut der Universität, Heidelberg, Heidelberg, Federal Republic of Germany

EDWARD F. VOELKEL (355), Laboratory of Pharmacology, Harvard School of Dental Medicine, Boston, Massachusetts

JOHN H. WALSH (455, 581), Department of Medicine, School of Medicine, The Center for the Health Sciences, University of California, Los Angeles, California

* Present address: Department of Physiology, Boston University School of Medicine, Boston, Massachusetts.

† Present address: First Department of Medicine, Faculty of Medicine, University of Tokyo, Tokyo, Japan.

‡ Present address: Department of Physiology, Royal Free Hospital School of Medicine, London, United Kingdom.

MICHAEL WILKINSON‡ (101), Department of Physiology, University of Geneva, Geneva, Switzerland

GORDON H. WILLIAMS (743), Endocrinology–Hypertension Unit, Peter Bent Brigham Hospital, and the Department of Medicine, Harvard Medical School, Boston, Massachusetts

IAN R. WILLSHIRE (927), ICI Pharmaceuticals Division, Mereside, Alderley Park, Macclesfield, Cheshire, United Kingdom

ROBERT M. WILSON (479), Department of Medicine, School of Medicine, The Center for the Health Sciences, University of California, Los Angeles, California

HELEN C. WONG (581) Department of Medicine, School of Medicine, The Center for the Health Sciences, University of California, Los Angeles, California

MICHAEL YOUNG (941), Laboratory of Physical Biochemistry, and Department of Medicine, Massachusetts General Hospital, Boston, Massachusetts

Preface

Since the publication of the first edition of "Methods of Hormone Radioimmunoassay," there has been a virtual explosion in the number of hormones recognized and characterized. With the current state of the art, there is little lag in time between purification of hormone and development of a procedure for its quantification by radioimmunoassay. This edition is a current compilation of such methodology.

In assessing recent developments, interesting trends have developed. It is no longer feasible to ascribe necessarily the origin of a hormone to a single cell or organ. The close association between the humoral mediators of the brain and the gastrointestinal tract provides ample evidence that the same biologically active compounds can be synthesized by widely divergent tissues. As a result of this complication, we have had to make arbitrary decisions on the sequence and categorization of chapters. Equally difficult to classify were the growth factors, the importance of which have only recently been recognized.

In addition to the development of new assays, there have been substantial improvements in the existing radioimmunoassay techniques. Recognition of the complexity of antigenic determinants on hormones and the heterogeneity of the forms in which they circulate has stimulated the production of highly specific antibodies and careful characterization of the ligands they measure. As a result, several radioimmunoassays may be needed to evaluate fully a single hormone.

Recognizing these advances, both in number and quality of radioassays, the second edition of "Methods of Hormone Radioimmunoassay" has been prepared for both clinicians and investigators.

BERNARD M. JAFFE
HAROLD R. BEHRMAN

Preface to the First Edition

Radioimmunoassay systems have been developed to quantitate virtually every hormone available in pure form. Utilizing the potent tools of radioactivity and immunology, these exquisitely sensitive techniques have revolutionized the fields of endocrine physiology and clinical endocrinology. It is therefore remarkable that despite their widespread use, there has been, until now, no one volume available which describes all of the current techniques. This book is comprised of chapters in which methods for measuring hormones by radioimmunoassay are described. Each paper was written by an authority chosen particularly because of his contribution to the radioimmunoassay method.

Although the absence of such a book might alone serve to justify its need at this time, it was the expanded use of radioimmunoassays that prompted its preparation. For example, it is now becoming increasingly obvious that measuring single hormone responses to stimuli is gross oversimplification. Endocrine responses are coordinated activities of multiple hormones and must be studied as such. Thus, there is a tendency now for the utilization of multiple radioimmunoassay systems for the simultaneous evaluation of several hormones. In addition, diagnostic techniques are being refined to the degree that clinical laboratories are starting to use radioimmunoassays. By describing what we think are the best techniques for each hormone, we hope to direct such interests to effective completion.

Although specific problems are associated with specific immunoassays, it must be obvious that there is some overlap. By compiling a series of discussions of the successful management of a variety of problems, we hope to present a wealth of information which might be utilized to solve problems in related areas.

We do not anticipate nor would we recommend that a description of methodology, no matter how detailed, replace laboratory experience. We hope, however, that this volume will point out the problems and advantages of each system, aid in selection of techniques, and serve as a source of reference material.

BERNARD M. JAFFE
HAROLD R. BEHRMAN

INTRACELLULAR MESSENGERS

1

Cyclic AMP and Cyclic GMP

ALTON L. STEINER

I. INTRODUCTION

The ubiquitous roles of cyclic adenosine-3',5-monophosphate (cAMP) and cyclic guanosine-3,5'-monophosphate (cGMP) in cellular metabolism have made it increasingly desirable to measure these nucleotides in tissues and body fluids with ease and dependability. Both of these cyclic nucleotides are present in extremely low concentrations in tissues, and methods developed for measurement of these

3

Methods of Hormone Radioimmunoassay, Second Edition
Copyright © 1979 by Academic Press, Inc.
All rights of reproduction in any form reserved. ISBN 0-12-379260-6

cyclic nucleotides must contend with high concentrations of interfering noncyclic nucleotides.

Radioimmunoassay is a relatively simple, sensitive, and specific method for measuring cyclic AMP and cyclic GMP in tissues and body fluids. Antibodies to the cyclic nucleotides were developed in rabbits after immunization with an antigen in which a 2′-O-succinyl derivative of the cyclic nucleotide had been conjugated to protein (Steiner et al., 1969, 1972). The label is an iodinated derivative of the cyclic nucleotide. Because of the specificity of the antibodies, chromatographic separation of tissue extracts prior to assay is not required, and, in addition, both nucleotides can be measured simultaneously by radioimmunoassay (Wehmann et al., 1972). All of the ingredients for the cyclic nucleotide radioimmunoassays can be obtained commercially.

An important advance in increasing the sensitivity of the cyclic nucleotide radioimmunoassays has been described recently (Cailla et al., 1973). Steiner et al. (1972) showed that the cyclic nucleotides substituted at the 2′-O position had a higher affinity for the antibody and displaced the ^{125}I-labeled cyclic nucleotide derivatives employed in the assays far better than the unsubstituted cyclic nucleotides. Cailla et al. (1973) showed that 2′-O-succinylation of cAMP in tissue extracts could be achieved rapidly in 100% yield in a reaction carried out in water. This procedure increased assay sensitivity for cAMP approximately 100 times. This advance has been applied to the measurement of cGMP (Cailla et al., 1976) and has been particularly helpful, since cGMP is present in most tissues at significantly lower concentrations than cAMP. A number of laboratories have confirmed the findings of Cailla et al. (1973) and described succinylation procedures for cyclic nucleotide radioimmunoassay (Zimmerman et al., 1976; Frandsen and Krishna, 1976). Harper and Brooker (1975) as well as Frandsen and Krishna (1976) have shown that acetylation of tissue samples prior to assay also dramatically increases the sensitivity of the nucleotide radioimmunoassays. Harper and Brooker (1975) have emphasized the advantage of acetylation versus succinylation of both cyclic nucleotides prior to radioimmunoassay.

In this update on cyclic nucleotide radioimmunoassay, I shall review the procedures employed for developing and performing both the standard radioimmunoassay and the acylated nucleotide assays. It should be noted that the synthesis of 2′-O-succinyl cyclic nucleotides has been greatly simplified by the method described by Cailla et al. (1973).

II. METHOD OF RADIOIMMUNOASSAY

A. Synthesis of Succinyl Cyclic Nucleotides

The cyclic nucleotides were rendered immunogenic by conjugating the nucleotide to a high molecular weight protein. In order to increase the possibility of obtaining specific antibody, conjugates were prepared in which neither the purine rings nor the diester 3',5'-bonds of cAMP or cGMP were altered. Consequently, the cyclic nucleotides were succinylated at the 2'-O position by modification of the method of Falbriard et al. (1967), and the free carboxyl group of these derivatives conjugated to protein. This method of synthesis of 2'-O-succinyl cAMP (ScAMP) and 2'-O-succinyl cGMP (ScGMP) (Steiner et al., 1972) was hindered by the low solubility of the cyclic nucleotides in organic solvents. Yields were usually less than 50%.

The currently preferred method for preparing 2'-O-succinyl cyclic nucleotides is to react cAMP or cGMP with succinic anhydride in water in the presence of triethylamine (Cailla et al., 1973, 1976). The product (ScAMP or ScGMP) forms instantaneously in 100% yield.

Either cyclic nucleotide (0.03 M maximum) was dissolved in 100 μl H$_2$O. To this volume was added 10 μl triethylamine, followed by 5 mg succinic anhydride. The mixture was vortexed intermittently for 20 minutes. Thin layer chromatography of the reaction mixture on cellulose with butanol–glacial acetic acid–H$_2$O [12 : 3 : 5 (v/v)] demonstrated 2'-O-succinyl cAMP, which ran ahead (R_f 0.42) of cAMP (R_f 0.30). The R_f values for 2'-O-succinyl cAMP and cGMP are 0.42 and 0.31, respectively. Separation of unreacted succinic acid was achieved by preparative chromatography in the solvent system described above. Alternatively, chromatography over anion exchange resins can be utilized. Harper and Brooker (1975) diluted the incubation mixtures to 2.1 ml in water and applied them to 0.5 × 4 cm columns of AG1X2 (Bio-Rad) Cl$^-$ form, 50–200 mesh. The columns were serially eluted with 40 ml HCl, pH 2.0, 20 ml HCl, pH 1.3, and 40 ml HCl, pH 1.0. The pure 2'-O-succinyl derivatives were contained in the final 30 ml. Cailla et al. (1973) utilized 2.5 × 10 cm columns of Sephadex QAE A-25. They eluted purified succinylated nucleotides in the final peak, utilizing a linear gradient 0.01 M phosphate, pH 6.0 (600 ml)/0.4 ml NaCl 0.01 M phosphate, pH 6.0 (600 ml), flow rate 66 ml/hour, 4°C. Column peaks should be monitored by ultraviolet absorption at 258 nm for ScAMP and 255 nm for ScGMP. On brief treatment with 0.1 N NaOH, both ScAMP and ScGMP reverted to cAMP and cGMP, confirming that the succinyl substitution was exclusively at the $2'$-O position (Falbriard *et al.*, 1967).

B. Preparation of Antigen

Succinylated cyclic nucleotides were coupled to protein [human serum albumin (HSA), keyhole limpet hemocyanin, or poly-L-lysine polymers]. ScAMP (10 mg) was reacted with 20 mg HSA and 10 mg 1-ethyl-3-(3-diethylaminopropyl) carbodiimide-HCl (EDC) in aqueous solution at pH 5.5. After incubation of this mixture at 24°C for 16 hours in the dark, the conjugate was dialyzed against phosphosaline buffer (0.01 M sodium phosphate, 0.15 M sodium chloride, pH 7.4) for 48 hours. The dialyzed conjugate, ScAMP–albumin, exhibited an absorption maximum at 260 nm. On the basis of the spectrum of ScAMP–albumin and unconjugated HSA, and assuming a molar extinction coefficient of 15,000 for ScAMP, the conjugate was estimated to contain an average of five to six cyclic AMP residues per albumin molecule. ScAMP was also coupled to poly-L-lysine and keyhole limpet hemocyanin using the same method with similar results. Using essentially identical conditions, Weinryb (1972) found four to five residues of nucleotide per albumin molecule.

C. Immunization and Bleeding Schedule

Randomly bred rabbits were immunized with 0.25 mg protein conjugate emulsified in Freund's complete adjuvant (FCA) and injected into each foot pad. Booster injections totaling 0.25 to 0.30 mg were injected subcutaneously either into the foot pads or the back at four- to six-week intervals, and the animals were bled ten days later. Serum was separated by centrifugation, diluted 1 : 100 with 0.05 acetate buffer (pH 6.2), and stored in small aliquots at -20°C.

Weinryb (1972) has immunized goats with an initial injection of 0.1 mg nucleotide–HSA conjugate in FCA into each of four surgically exposed lymph nodes in the posterior cervical and high inguinal regions. They were boosted six weeks later with a total of 1.0 mg conjugate in FCA subcutaneously in the regions of the initial incisions. Subsequent booster injections were given subcutaneously every six weeks, each with a total of 1.0 mg of conjugate in saline, and the animals were bled ten days to two weeks after each booster injection. High antibody titers were found as early as after the second boost.

D. Synthesis of Tyrosine Methyl Ester Derivatives of 2'-O-Succinyl Cyclic Nucleotides: ScAMP-TME and ScGMP-TME

Tritiated hydrogen or iodinated derivatives of the cyclic nucleotides serve as labeled compounds in the cyclic nucleotide radioimmunoassays. While good sensitivity can be achieved with ^{3}H-cAMP and ^{3}H-cGMP, sensitivity is enhanced when iodinated derivatives are used, since the specific activity achieved is more than an order of magnitude greater. In addition, significantly reduced amounts of antibody are required when iodinated derivatives are employed in the radioassays.

Radioactive derivatives of the cyclic nucleotides of high specific activity were synthesized by tyrosination of the succinylated compounds and subsequent iodination of the tyrosine moiety. The synthesis of these compounds by the mixed carboxylic–carbonic acid reaction using ethyl chloroformate is recommended (Greenstein and Winitz, 1961). This reaction is run in two steps and can be easily controlled. This method of synthesis achieves significantly higher yields of ScAMP–TME than synthesis with N,N'-dicyclohexylcarbodiimide as described in our initial publication (Steiner *et al.*, 1969). Cailla and Delaage (1972) also prefer the mixed carboxylic–carbonic acid reaction and have described the reaction conditions and products in detail.

The synthesis of succinyl cyclic nucleotide tyrosine methyl ester was performed in two steps: (1) One equivalent (5 moles) of the succinylated cyclic nucleotide was dissolved in 0.1 ml dimethylformamide at 0°C with three equivalents of trioctylamine. ScGMP remained as a fine suspension, while ScAMP readily dissolved. One equivalent of ethyl chloroformate in dimethylformamide was added, and the reaction carried out at 0°C for 15 minutes. (2) Two equivalents of both tyrosine methyl ester hydrochloride and trioctylamine were added in 0.1 ml of dimethylformamide, and the reaction continued at room temperature for an additional 2 to 3 hours with continuous stirring. The tyrosinated product was isolated by thin layer chromatography on cellulose with butanol–glacial acetic acid–H_2O [12:3:5 (v/v)]. The new nitrosonaphthol-positive derivative (R_f 0.65) migrated ahead of the succinylated methyl ester hydrochloride (R_f 0.57). The tyrosinated derivatives exhibited an absorption maximum in water identical with that of the parent cyclic nucleotide. About 20% of the succinylated cyclic nucleotide was converted to the parent cyclic nucleotide during the course of this reaction but was completely separated from the tyrosinated derivative by thin-layer chromatography.

The yield of the tyrosine methyl ester derivatives of cAMP and cGMP ranged from 40 to 55% on repeated synthesis.

E. Preparation of Radioactive ^{125}I- or ^{131}I-Succinyl Cyclic Nucleotide Tyrosine Methyl Ester

The procedure employed has not been modified from the conditions described previously (Steiner *et al.*, 1972). Succinyl cyclic nucleotide tyrosine methyl ester was iodinated with ^{125}I or ^{131}I by the method of Hunter and Greenwood (1962). Approximately 1 to 3 μg of the derivative (in 50 μl water) was added to 40 μl of 0.5 M phosphate buffer, pH 7.5. After the addition of 0.5 to 1.0 mCi ^{125}I or ^{131}I, 50 μl of a solution of chloramine-T (35 mg per 10 ml 0.05 M phosphate buffer) was added and the reaction run for 45 seconds. The iodine was then reduced by the addition of 100 μl of a sodium metabisulfite solution (24 mg per 10 ml 0.05 M phosphate buffer).

The iodinated cyclic nucleotide derivatives were purified either by column chromatography on Sephadex G-10 or by thin-layer chromatography on cellulose. The reaction mixture was applied to a 0.9 × 9 cm Sephadex G-10 albumin in phosphosaline buffer, pH 7.5, and eluted with phosphosaline buffer (flow rate 40 ml/hr). Three distinct peaks of radioactivity were found: peak 1 (void volume) has not been identified, peak 2 (9 to 12 ml) was free iodide, and peak 3 (22 to 32 ml) was ^{125}I-succinyl cyclic nucleotide. The iodinated tyrosine methyl ester derivatives isolated in peak 3 cochromatographed with their respective uniodinated compounds on thin layer chromatography using the previously described solvent system. All iodinated compounds had a specific activity of >150 Ci/mmole. The iodinated ligands were diluted in 0.05 M acetate buffer, pH 6.2 (3 × 10⁶ to 4 × 10⁶ cpm/ml) and stored as small aliquots at -20°C. The ^{125}I material retained full immunoreactivity for periods up to two months or longer, provided it was stored at -20°C in small aliquots and not subjected to repeated freezing and thawing. The ^{131}I derivatives were stable for three to four weeks.

F. Preparation of Tissues, Blood, and Urine

Frozen tissue samples are homogenized at 4°C in 1.0 ml of cold 6% trichloroacetic acid (TCA). TCA supernatants are extracted three times with 5 ml of ethyl ether saturated under a stream of air, and the residue is dissolved in 0.05 M sodium acetate buffer, pH 6.2, and used directly in the immunoassay.

While tissue extracts are only rarely purified prior to immunoassay in our laboratory, others continue to utilize column purification. Ion exchange resin column chromatography, using either Dowex 50 (0.6 × 30 cm column AG 50W-X8, 100–200 mesh, eluant 0.1 N HCl, 0.36 ml/min) or QAE Sephadex A-25, is well suited for purification of tissue extracts of both cyclic nucleotides (Schultz $et\ al.$, 1974).

Blood is collected in heparinized tubes and centrifuged immediately at 2500 g for 5 minutes at 4°C. Because of an unidentified substance(s) in plasma which occasionally interferes in the cAMP but not in the cGMP radioimmunoassay, we routinely separate plasma cAMP from interfering substances by Dowex column chromatography. Extracts of plasma are divided into two fractions: To 0.5 ml of plasma (for cAMP assay), an equal volume of 0.6 N perchloric acid is added. The supernatant fraction is applied to a column of Dowex 50W-X8 (100–200 mesh) 4 × 8 mm, and the column eluted with water. Cyclic AMP elutes in the fourth to eighth milliliters. This fraction is dried at 60°C under a stream of air and resuspended in 0.05 M sodium acetate buffer, pH 6.2. For cGMP assay, 0.5 ml 10% TCA is added to an equal volume of plasma. The TCA supernatant is treated in a manner identical to that of tissue extracts. Urine samples 2–10 μl are added directly into the immunoassay.

G. Immunoassay Procedure

1. Standard Immunoassay

cAMP and cGMP immunoassays are performed in 0.05 M sodium acetate buffer, pH 6.2. Each tube contains (in order of addition) 50 to 100 μl of cyclic nucleotide standard (0.025 to 5.0 pmoles/tube) or unknown solution, 100 μl of antibody in appropriate buffer at a dilution sufficient to bind 40 to 55% of the labeled marker, 100 μl of the ^{125}I-labeled marker (approximately 15,000 cpm and representing <0.01 pmole of ligand), and 100 μl containing 500 μg of rabbit γ-globulin as carrier, in a final volume of 600 μl. The most commonly employed method for separating bound and free ^{125}I ligand used in our laboratory is ammonium sulfate precipitation. After 2 to 18 hr of incubation, 2.5 ml of 60% $(NH_4)_2SO_4$ solution is added. The tubes are centrifuged at 4°C for 15 minutes, and the precipitates are counted in a gamma spectrometer. All analyses are carried out in triplicate.

In the simultaneous assays of cAMP and cGMP, the immunoassay procedure is identical, except that specific cAMP and cGMP antibodies are added in the 100 μl antibody aliquot. ^{131}I-ScAMP-TME and ^{125}I-ScGMP-TME (approximately 15,000 cpm each) are added in the 100-μl aliquot. The precipitates are then counted in a dual channel spectrometer equipped with a punched paper tape printout. A computer program for use on a NCR Century 200 system using intermediate FORTRAN has been written for analysis for both the single and simultaneous radioimmunoassays.

Tritiated cyclic nucleotide can be used instead of the iodinated labeled compounds in either the cAMP or cGMP assay (Weinryb, 1972). Significantly more antibody is required since tritiated cyclic nucleotide binds 200 times less avidly than succinyl cyclic nucleotide tyrosine methyl ester (Steiner *et al.*, 1972). If ^{3}H-succinyl cyclic nucleotide were available, it would be anticipated that significantly reduced amounts of antibody could be used.

The separation of bound from free labeled compounds can also be performed by the second antibody method (Steiner *et al.*, 1969), precipitation with polyethylene glycol (Desbuquois and Aurbach, 1971), filtration on cellulose ester (Millipore) filters (Weinryb, 1972), alcohol precipitation (Frandsen and Krishna, 1976), or by charcoal adsorption (Harper and Brooker, 1975).

2. *Immunoassay of Acylated Cyclic Nucleotides*

Succinylation or acetylation of the cyclic nucleotides isolated from tissue extracts is performed in our laboratory by a one-step addition of premixed succinylation or acetylation reagent, as described by Frandsen and Krishna (1976).

The succinylation reagent is made by mixing 25 volumes of a solution of succinic anhydride (200 mg/ml) in acetone with nine volumes of triethylamine. The acetylation reagent is made by mixing two volumes of acetic anhydride with five volumes of triethylamine. Both reagents are made up immediately before use. The cyclic nucleotides are derivatized by adding 10 μl of the premixed reagent to the lyophilized samples dissolved in 50 μl of 0.05 M acetate buffer, pH 6.2. It is essential to mix the sample immediately after addition of the reagents, since hydrolysis of the anhydrides occurs in less than 30 seconds. Standards containing 1–10,000 fmole of cyclic nucleotides in 50 μl of acetate buffer are also acylated along with the samples. The assay is then carried out as described in the standard immunoassay procedure.

H. Cyclic Nucleotide Immunoassays

The selection of appropriate antisera is most important for successful cyclic nucleotide immunoassay. While almost all animals make antibody to either cAMP or cGMP conjugates, certain antibodies are definitely superior. We screen antibodies after each booster injection, both for sensitivity and specificity, checking in particular cross-reactivity with ATP. Since tissue concentrations of ATP are approximately 10,000- and 100,000-fold greater than cAMP and cGMP, respectively, it is necessary to select antisera which cross-react <0.02% with ATP in the cAMP immunoassay and <0.002% in the cGMP immunoassay to avoid chromatographic preparation of tissues. We initially immunized a group of ten rabbits for each cyclic nucleotide immunoassay and found several antisera in each group which met these cross-reactivity requirements. Since tissue concentrations of cGMP are usually an order of magnitude less than cAMP, the cross-reactivity of cGMP in the cAMP immunoassay can be 1.0% or higher and yet chromatographic steps will be unnecessary. For the cGMP immunoassay, the cross-reactivity of the antisera with cAMP should be minimal. Several cGMP antibodies require at least 10,000-fold greater concentrations of cAMP to produce displacement of marker equal to that of cGMP.

A standard immunoassay curve for cAMP is shown in Figure 1. The antiserum currently used was made at Schwartz-Mann Bioresearch, Orangeburgh, New York, and shows a linear displacement of ^{125}I-ScAMP–TME by unlabeled cAMP, plotted as a semilogarithmic function from 0.025 to 5.0 pmole. When the reaction volume is reduced to 150 μl, a fourfold increase in sensitivity is achieved. Since this degree of sensitivity is rarely necessary, the 600 μl reaction volume is routinely used. The cross-reactivity of this antibody with ATP,

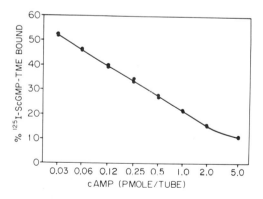

Figure 1.   Standard immunoassay curve for cAMP. Reaction conditions described in text. Reaction volume was 600 μl. Antibody was kindly supplied by Schwartz-Mann Bioresearch, Orangeburgh, N.Y. (Reproduced from Steiner, 1973, with permission of the publisher.)

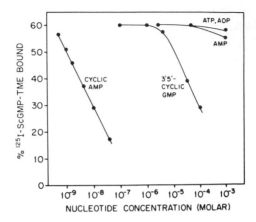

Figure 2. The inhibition of ^{125}I-ScAMP-TME binding to cAMP antibody by various nucleotides. (Reproduced from Steiner, 1973, with permission of the publisher.)

5′-AMP and cyclic GMP is shown in Figure 2. ATP, in a several millionfold higher concentration, failed to cause significant cross-reactivity with the cAMP antibody. The cross-reactivity of cGMP is 0.01%. The sensitivity and specificity of several cAMP antisera are shown in Table I.

A standard immunoassay curve for cGMP is shown in Figure 3. The

Table I   Sensitivity and Specificity of Various cAMP Antisera[a]

	Maximal sensitivity		Relative binding affinity	
Antisera	Serum dilution	cAMP (pmoles/tube)	ATP (%)	cGMP (%)
RC A-1	1:5,000	1.0	0.002	0.01
RC A-3	1:5,000	1.0	0.0001	0.005
RC A-7	1:5,000	0.25	0.002	0.01
SM-381[b]	1:5,000	0.025	0.00001	0.01
SM-291[b]	1:4,000	0.05	0.01	0.10
LCA-1[c]	1:40,000	0.25	0.0001	1.0
LCA-2[c]	1:40,000	0.25	0.0001	1.0

[a] Expressed as the minimal concentration of cAMP that causes linear displacement in the immunoassay.

[b] cAMP Antisera obtained from rabbits after four boosts of ScAMP-albumin at monthly invervals kindly supplied by Schwartz-Mann Bioresearch, Orangeburgh, NY.

[c] cAMP Antisera obtained from rabbits after three boosts of ScAMP-albumin at monthly intervals kindly supplied by Drs. G. Little and N. Kaminsky of Vanderbilt University.

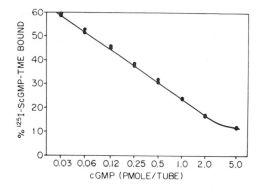

Figure 3.   Standard immunoassay curve for cGMP. Reaction conditions described in text. Reaction volume was 600 μl.

assay is sensitive to 0.03 pmoles cGMP. This degree of sensitivity allows measurement of cGMP in triplicate on 10–20 mg of most tissues. Cross-reactivity of the cGMP antibody with all purine and pyrimidine nucleotides is minimal (<0.002%) except for cyclic IMP which reacts at the 1.0% level.

I. Acylated Cyclic Nucleotide Immunoassay

Acylation of tissue extracts increases the sensitivity of the cAMP and cGMP immunoassays approximately 100 and 40 times, respectively. The acylated assay is particularly helpful for measuring cGMP in tissues, since the tissue concentration of the nucleotide is generally so low (Table II).

Table II   Concentrations of cAMP and cGMP in Various Rat Tissues[a]

	cAMP	cGMP
Liver	960 ± 98	15 ± 2.0
Kidney cortex	980 ± 92	38 ± 4.0
Skeletal muscle	360 ± 52	18 ± 1.6
Lung	1,250 ± 110	56 ± 6.0
Jejunum	1,010 ± 97	120 ± 11
Pituitary[b]	880 ± 105	9.0 ± 1.1

[a] Concentration in pmole per gm wet weight of tissue.
[b] Hemipituitaries were incubated for 2 hours at 37°C in TC 199.

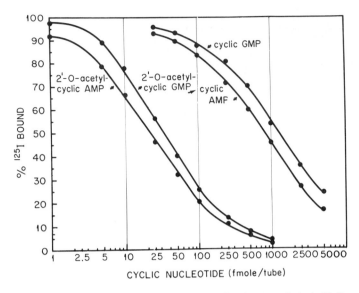

Figure 4. Standard curves for cyclic AMP and cyclic GMP and their 2′-O-acetylated derivatives. (Reproduced from Harper and Brooker, 1975, with permission of the publisher.)

The sensitivity of the acylated immunoassay is in the femtomolar range (Figure 4). Succinylation or acetylation of the cyclic nucleotides appears to produce equally sensitive immunoassays. With certain antibodies, succinylation causes problems in specificity which are avoided in the acetylation procedure (Zimmerman *et al.*, 1976; Harper and Brooker, 1975). Since both cyclic nucleotides will be acylated in unpurified tissue extracts, it is important to determine the relative cross-reactivity of cAMP in the cGMP acylated immunoassay. In general, specificity does not decrease in the acylated immunoassay. Tissue levels of the cyclic nucleotides, as measured after acylation, are the same as those obtained by standard immunoassay.

J. Tissue Measurement of Cyclic Nucleotide by Single and Simultaneous cAMP and cGMP Radioimmunoassay

The concentrations of cAMP and cGMP in various rat tissues are shown in Table II. The values are in the same range as those reported by others using enzymatic techniques or competitive protein binding radioassay (Goldberg *et al.*, 1969b; Ishikawa *et al.*, 1969; Gilman, 1970). The intraassay coefficient of variation for a number of tissues in both the cAMP and cGMP immunoassays is 5–8%, while the interassay coefficient of variation is 14% for cAMP and 17% for cGMP. These results indicate that the precision of the immunoassay technique for the cyclic nucleotides allows the discrimination of differences of approximately 20% for small groups of samples when measured in the same assay and approximately 50% when analyzed in separate assays.

Tissue values for cAMP and cGMP when measured by simultaneous immunoassay are identical to those found by individual radioassay. Since the tissue concentration of cAMP relative to cGMP is, in general, an order of magnitude greater, it is important to select a cGMP antibody that shows minimal cross-reactivity with cAMP. With certain antibodies, even a 1000-fold increase in cAMP relative to cGMP causes no significant change in the amount of cGMP measured.

A convenient verification of the reliability of a cyclic nucleotide determination is measurement of the amount of immunologically reactive cyclic nucleotide before and after hydrolysis by cyclic nucleotide phosphodiesterase. After such treatment, greater than 90% of the immunologically reactive cAMP is hydrolyzed in various rat tissues and human urine and plasma. In certain rat tissues (liver, kidney, cortex, skeletal muscle) a blank of 15–40% is found. The cause of the blank in these tissues has not been determined, but most likely represents interference in the cyclic nucleotide phosphodiesterase reaction since values for cGMP in these unpurified tissue extracts are identical to those for cGMP purified by anion exchange chromatography.

III. PROBLEMS RELATED TO MEASURING cAMP AND cGMP

A. Hydrolysis of Sample during Processing

Since the cyclic nucleotides can be hydrolyzed by cyclic nucleotide phosphodiesterase in the course of obtaining tissue and body fluid samples, it is important to freeze tissue quickly and not allow thawing during homogenization. When such precautions are taken, recovery of added cyclic nucleotide is greater than 90%.

B. Interfering Substances

Certain substances, particularly high salt concentrations, can affect binding in both the cAMP and cGMP assays. EDTA (10^{-3}–$10^{-4}M$) will interfere with certain antisera in the cAMP, but not with the cGMP immunoassay. As noted above, occasional human plasma samples will give a falsely high value for cAMP; consequently, chromatography of plasma extracts is recommended before measurement of cAMP by radioimmunoassay. Weinryb (1972) has noticed that extracts of rat cerebral cortex and lipocytes can enhance binding in the cAMP radioimmunoassay by 10–20%. This "antibody binding enhancing factor" was removed by Dowex 50 H$^+$ column chromatography, but not by 12% TCA or heating to 90°C. This phenomenon apparently occurs with only certain cAMP antibodies, since this author has not observed enhancement of binding with extracts of rat cerebral cortex or lipocytes.

ACKNOWLEDGMENTS

This work was supported by Research Grant AM-17438 from the United States Public Health Service.

REFERENCES

Cailla, H., and Delaage, M. (1972). Succinyl derivatives of adenosine 3',5'-cyclic monophosphate: Synthesis and purification. *Anal. Biochem.* **48**, 62–72.

Cailla, H. L. Racine-Weisbuch, M. S., and Delaage, M. A. (1973). Adenosine 3',5'-cyclic monophosphate assay at 10–15 mole level. *Anal. Biochem.* **56**, 394–407.

Cailla, H., Vannier, C. J., and Delaage, M. A., (1976). Guanosine 3',5'-cyclic monophosphate assay at 10–15 mole level. *Anal. Biochem.* **70**, 195–202.

Desbuquois, B., and Aurbach, G. D. (1971). Use of polyethylene gylcol to separate free and antibody-bound peptide hormones in radioimmunoassays. *J. Clin. Endocrinol. Metab.* **33**, 732–737.

Falbriard, J. G., Posternak, T., and Sutherland, E. W. (1967). Preparation of derivatives of adenosine 3',5'-phosphate. *Biochim. Biophys. Acta* **148**, 99–105.

Frandsen, E. K. and Krishna, G. (1976). A simple ultrasensitive method for the assay of cyclic AMP and cyclic GMP in tissues. *Life Sci.* **19**, 529–542.

Gilman, A. G. (1970). A protein binding assay for adenosine 3',5'-cyclic monophosphate. *Proc. Natl. Acad. Sci. U.S.A.* **67**, 305–312.

Goldberg, N. D., Dietz, S. B., and O'Toole, A. G. (1969a). Cyclic guanosine 3'5'-monophosphate in mammalian tissue and urine. *J. Biol. Chem.* **244**, 4458–4466.

Goldberg, N. D., Larner, J., Sasko, H., and O'Toole, A. G. (1969b). Enzymatic analysis of cyclic 3',5'-AMP in mammalian tissues and urine. *Anal. Biochem.* **28**, 523–544.

Greenstein, J. P., and Winitz, M. A. (1961). *In* "Chemistry of the Amino Acids," Vol. 2, p. 978. Wiley, New York.

Harper, J. F., and Brooker, G. (1975). Femtomole sensitive radioimmunoassay for cyclic AMP and cyclic GMP after 2'-O-acetylation by acetic anhydride in aqeous solution. *J. Cyclic Nucleotide Res.* **1**, 207–218.

Hunter, W. M., and Greenwood, F. C. (1962). Preparation of iodine-131 labeled human growth hormone of high specific activity. *Nature (London)* **194**, 495–496.

Ishikawa, E., Ishikawa, S., Davis, J. W., and Sutherland, E. W. (1969). Determination of guanosine 3′,5′-monophosphate in tissues and guanyl cyclase in rat intestine. *J. Biol. Chem.* **244**, 6371–6376.

Schultz, G., Bohme, E., and Hardman, J. G. (1974). Separation and purification of cyclic nucleotides by ion-exchange resin column chromatography. *In* "Methods in Enzymology" (J. G. Hardman and B. W. O'Malley, eds.), Vol. 38, Part C, pp. 9–19. Academic Press, New York.

Steiner, A. L., Kipnis, D. M., Utiger, R., and Parker, C. W. (1969). Radioimmunoassay for the measurement of adenosine 3′,5′-cyclic phosphate. *Proc. Natl. Acad. Sci. U.S.A.* **64**, 367–373.

Steiner, A. L., Parker, C. W., and Kipnis, D. M. (1972). Radioimmunoassay for cyclic nucleotides. I. Preparation of antibodies and iodinated cyclic nucleotides. *J. Biol. Chem.* **247**, 1106–1113.

Steiner, A. L. (1973). Cyclic AMP and cyclic GMP. *In* "Methods of Hormone Radioimmunoassay" (B. M. Jaffe and H. R. Behrman, eds.), pp. 3–17. Academic Press, New York.

Wehmann, R. E., Blonde, L., and Steiner, A. L., (1972). Simultaneous radioimmunoassay for the measurement of adenosine 3′,5′-monophosphate and guanosine 3′-5′-monophosphate. *Endocrinology* **90**, 330–335.

Weinryb, I. (1972). Protein binding assays for cyclic AMP: Radioimmunoassay and cyclic AMP-dependent protein kinase binding assay. *Methods Mol. Biol.* **3**, 29–79.

Zimmerman, T. P., Winston, M. S., and Chu, L. C. (1976). A more sensitive radioimmunoassay (RIA) for guanosine 3′,5′-cyclic monophosphate (cGMP) involving prior 2′-O-succinylation of samples. *Anal. Biochem.* **71**, 79–95.

2

Prostaglandins and Prostaglandin Metabolites

BERNARD M. JAFFE AND HAROLD R. BEHRMAN

I. INTRODUCTION

Although prostaglandins were initially described in 1935, it is only recently that their significance has been recognized. Many experiments have documented a wide range of pharmacologic activities, but studies evaluating the physiologic importance of prostaglandins depend on the ability to measure these compounds *in vivo*. Bioassay

Methods of Hormone Radioimmunoassay, Second Edition

systems (Ferreira and Vane, 1967; Kannegeisser and Lee, 1971; Eakins *et al.*, 1970), gas chromatography–mass spectroscopy (Thompson *et al.*, 1970; Axen *et al.*, 1971), and absorption spectrophotometry (Shaw and Ramwell, 1969) are either not specific or not sensitive enough or both. Radioimmunoassay systems have been developed which have the required sensitivity; specificity is accomplished by separating the major prostaglandin groups on silicic acid columns. These techniques and their application to the measurement of prostaglandins in plasma and tissues are described in this chapter.

II. METHOD OF RADIOIMMUNOASSAY

A. Antibodies

1. Preparation of Immunogens

Antibodies to prostaglandins have been produced by immunizing animals with prostaglandins conjugated to serum proteins (Jaffe *et al.*, 1971) or to poly-L-lysine (Levine and Van Vunakis, 1970). As judged by the number of investigators who have had success producing antibodies to PGF compounds (Orczyk and Behrman, 1972; Kirton *et al.*, 1972; Caldwell *et al.*, 1971; Dray *et al.*, 1972), PGF–protein conjugates are relatively immunogenic. Similarly, antibodies specific for PGA compounds have been produced (Jaffe *et al.*, 1971; Stylos and Rivetz, 1972; Zusman *et al.*, 1972). Production of antibodies to PGE compounds has been slightly more difficult. Levine and co-workers (1971) have demonstrated that animals immunized with PGE conjugates produced antibodies which reacted better with PGB and PGA than with PGE. Yu and Burke (1972) reported that although five out of six anti-PGE antibodies cross-reacted completely with PGA and/or PGB compounds, one specific anti-PGE antiserum was produced. In our experience, the use of carbodiimides to conjugate PGE_1 and PGE_2 to protein carriers results in antisera with a great deal of PGA cross-reactivity. On the other hand, conjugates produced using ethyl chloroformate induce PGE-specific antisera.

The conjugates we have utilized to produce anti-prostaglandin antibodies are listed in Table I.

In a typical carbodiimide conjugation reaction, 4 mg (12 μmole) of PGA_1 (1.0 mg/ml in 10% 0.1 M Na_2CO_3), 8 mg of HSA (0.1 μmole), and 4 mg of 1-ethyl-3-(3-dimethylaminopropyl) carbodiimide-HCl (EDC) (20 μmole) were incubated together in the presence of nitrogen at

Table I   Prostaglandin Immunogens Utilized

Prosta-glandin	Conjugating agent	Protein carrier	Moles PG/mole carrier
PGE$_1$	EDC^a	Human serum albumin	1.5
PGE$_1$	Ethyl chloroformate	Keyhole limpet hemocyanin	—
PGE$_2$	CMC^b	Bovine serum albumin	3.8
PGF$_{1\alpha}$	CMC	Bovine serum albumin	—
PGF$_{2\alpha}$	EDC	Bovine serum albumin	—
PGA$_1$	EDC	Human serum albumin	3.3
PGA$_2$	EDC	Human serum albumin	2.2

^{a} 1-Ethyl-3-(3-dimethylaminopropyl) carbodiimide-HCl.
^{b} 1-Cyclohexyl-3-morpholinyl-(4)ethyl carbodiimide metho-p-toluenesulfonate.

20°C, pH 5.5, for 24 hours. The reaction mixture was then dialyzed thoroughly against several liters of 0.15 M NaCl, 0.01 M phosphate, pH 7.4 (PBS). The degree of conjugation (moles PG/mole of albumin) was determined by the increase in absorption at 278 nm in alkali as compared to control protein solutions [E_m for PGA$_1$ is 27,700 (Shaw and Ramwell, 1969)]. An alternative approach to evaluating the degree of conjugation is to include trace amounts of tritiated PGA$_1$ in the original reaction mixture and to evaluate the amount of label included in the product as an index of the efficiency of conjugation.

In a typical ethyl chloroformate conjugation reaction, 2.0 mg of PGE$_1$ was incubated with equimolar amounts of ethyl chloroformate and triethylamine in dioxane at 4°C for 15 minutes. Keyhole limpet hemocyanin (5.5 mg) was added in 0.45 ml of 0.1 M NaHCO$_3$ and the reaction mixture stirred at 4°C for another hour. The product was extensively dialyzed against 2.0 liters of PBS.

2. Immunization

Solutions of PG–protein conjugates were emulsified with equal volumes of complete Freund's adjuvant and administered to rabbits subcutaneously in the foot pads (0.25 ml/foot pad). The initial immunizing dose was 1.0 mg. At 2- to 4-month intervals, rabbits were reimmunized with 50 to 150 μg of conjugate in complete adjuvant. Ten days after each immunization, rabbits were bled from the ear arteries; the sera were separated and either frozen in aliquots or lyophilized.

3. Binding and Cross-Reactivity

Serial dilutions of antisera were examined for their ability to bind tritiated prostaglandins (see below). In the radioimmunoassay system

Table II Binding and Cross-Reactivity of Anti-Prostaglandins

Antiserum	Final dilution	Percentage of ^{3}H-PG bound	Cross-reactivity					
			PGA_1	PGA_2	PGE_1	PGE_2	$PGF_{1\alpha}$	$PGF_{2\alpha}$
Anti-PGE$_1$-KLH	1:9000	52	0.11	0.09	1.00	0.11	<0.001	<0.001
Anti-PGA$_1$-HSA	1:600,000	35	1.00	0.14	0.03	0.01	0.002	—
Anti-PGF$_{2\alpha}$-BSA	1:9000	40	<0.001	<0.001	<0.001	<0.001	0.45	1.00

anti-PGA$_1$-HSA, anti-PGE$_1$-KLH, and anti-PGF$_{2\alpha}$-BSA are utilized. These antibodies demonstrate specificity for both the cyclopentane ring (which distinguishes between PGF and PGE, etc.) and for the number of unsaturated bonds in the aliphatic side chains (which distinguishes PGE$_1$ from PGE$_2$, etc.). The binding characteristics as well as the degree of prostaglandin cross-reactivity for each of these antibodies is outlined in Table II.

Insignificant cross-reactivity has been demonstrated for the homologous 15-keto derivatives (the major immediate metabolites of PGE and PGF inactivation) (Anggard and Samuelsson, 1964) as well as for steroids, fat-soluble vitamins, and unsaturated fatty acids (Jaffe, 1974; Orczyk and Behrman 1972).

B. Preparation of Samples for Radioimmunoassay

1. Extraction

Since antibody specificity is not sufficient to entirely eliminate interference by other prostaglandins, we have found it necessary to extract prostaglandins from the samples and separate the major groups on silicic acid columns prior to radioimmunoassay (Jaffe et al., 1973; Caldwell et al., 1971). Gutierrez-Cernocek and co-workers (1972) use 2.0 ml of a methylal : ethanol mixture to extract prostaglandins from 5.0 ml of serum and measure samples obtained by equilibrium dialysis. We have carefully studied several extraction techniques (Jaffe and Parker, 1972) and suggest the technique described below.

a. Blood. Smith and Willis (1970) and Smith and co-workers (1973) have suggested that in the presence of thrombin, platelets release prostaglandins. Although we have not noted any differences in concentrations of prostaglandins in human serum and plasma (Jaffe et al., 1973), we draw blood in siliconized plastic syringes, transfer it to heparinized, siliconized tubes, and separate off the cells within 1 hour. If samples are not to be extracted immediately, they are frozen at $-20°C$. Since samples that have been frozen for prolonged periods of time yield spurious radioimmunoassay results, we routinely extract all samples within one week after they are collected.

To 1.0-ml aliquots of plasma in graduated conical glass centrifuge tubes we add 13 pg (4000 cpm) of ^{3}H-PGE$_1$ (New England Nuclear- 87 Ci/mM) in 50 μl to follow recovery. Plasma is extracted with 3.0 ml of petroleum ether to remove neutral lipids. After aspiration of the organic phase, we add to the aqueous phase 3.0 ml of a solvent consisting of ethyl acetate, isopropanol, and 0.1 M HCl, 3:3:1 by volume. The mixture is vortexed for 15 seconds twice, and then 2.0 ml of ethyl acetate and 3.0 ml of water are added. After mixing, the phases are separated by centrifugation. The organic phase (3.0 ml of 3.5 ml) is transferred to a polypropylene test tube and dried at 55°C in air.

b. Tissue. Tissue samples are processed immediately after removal by adding the samples directly to 1.0 ml of PBS and 3.0 ml of the extraction solution (see above) in a homogenizing tube and mechanically homogenizing with a Virtis homogenizer. Fifty microliters containing 13 pg of ^{3}H-PGE$_1$, 2.0 ml of ethyl acetate, and 3.0 ml of water is added and the samples processed exactly like plasma (Jaffe *et al.*, 1972a).

c. Biologic Fluids. Samples of biologic fluids containing small amounts of protein can be measured directly without extraction. These include aqueous humor (Podos *et al.*, 1972), tissue culture medium with up to 25% fetal calf serum (Jaffe *et al.*, 1972b), urine, and cerebrospinal fluid. Fretland (1974) used Amberlite CG-50 to extract prostaglandins from human urine. One gram of resin was mixed with 5 ml urine, shaken for 5 minutes, allowed to stand 10 minutes, and centrifuged at 5°C and 2000 g for 10 minutes. Ten milliliters methanol was used to extract the prostaglandins from the ion exchange resin.

Extraction is required particularly for samples containing high concentrations of albumin. Albumin binds prostaglandins with association constants of 0.9 to 4.8×10^4 liters/M (Raz, 1972). We have found in equilibrium dialysis that 30% of PGE$_1$ (0.1 to 10 mg/ml) is bound to HSA (10 mg/ml). Thus, albumin and antibodies compete for prostaglandins. The technique we have described eliminates albumin by precipitation, while the prostaglandins remain in the organic solvent.

2. Silicic Acid Chromatography

The required solvents are tabulated below:

1.	Benzene:ethyl acetate	60:40
2.	Benzene:ethyl acetate:methanol	60:40:20
3.	Benzene:ethyl acetate:methanol	60:40:10
4.	Benzene:ethyl acetate:methanol	60:40:2

Silicic acid, 100 mesh (Sigma Chemical Company, St. Louis, Missouri), is made up to a slurry using 0.25 gm/ml of solvent 1. Two milliliters of slurry are poured into 10-ml disposable pipettes with glass wool inserted at their tips. The resin is washed with 5.0 ml of solvent 2 and 1.5 ml of solvent 1. Sample residues are dissolved in 0.2 ml of solvent 3, vortexed, and 0.8 ml of solvent 1 added. The samples are applied to the columns which are allowed to run dry. Major prostaglandin groups are eluted serially using solvents with increasing concentrations of methanol:

Fraction I: 6 ml of solvent 1, PGA and PGB
Fraction II: 12 ml of solvent 4, PGE
Fraction III: 3 ml of solvent 2, PGF

The individual chromatographic fractions are dried at 55°C in air and dissolved in 1.0 ml of PBS containing gelatin, 1.0 mg/ml (GPBS).

3. Calculation of Recovery

Duplicate 50-μl aliquots of fraction II (or the appropriate fraction for the ^{3}H-PG added) are dissolved in 0.5 ml of Nuclear Chicago Solubilizer and 10 ml of toluene scintillation solution are added for scintillation counting.

When added to plasma, ^{3}H-PGA$_1$, ^{3}H-PGE$_1$, and ^{3}H-PGF$_{1\alpha}$ are recovered in the individual fractions with the same efficiency, i.e., $64.3 \pm 2.6\%$ ($n = 3$), $68.1 \pm 13.7\%$ ($n = 255$), and $68.9 \pm 6.6\%$ ($n = 12$), respectively. Therefore, we ordinarily follow recovery of just ^{3}H-PGE$_1$ and correct radioimmunoassay determinations of all three prostaglandin groups by this figure. If we are particularly interested in determinations of PGA or PGF, we find it appropriate to add that particular label to plasma for recovery correction.

The chromatographic separation technique completely separates the major groups of prostaglandins (Figure 1). When ^{3}H-PGF$_{1\alpha}$ and ^{3}H-PGA$_1$ are extracted from serum and chromatographed, 98% of the recovered radioactivity is in fractions III and I, respectively. Conversion of PGE to PGA compounds occurs readily at acid pH and is a potentially serious problem. With the technique described less than 5% of PGE is converted to PGA, and when ^{3}H-PGE$_1$ is extracted from serum, more than 93% of the recovered radioactivity is in fraction II.

C. Assay Incubation

For each sample, separate radioimmunoassays are set up for PGA$_1$, PGE$_1$, and PGF$_{2\alpha}$ using in each specific antisera homologous tritiated marker, homologous prostaglandin standards, and the chromatographic fraction containing that prostaglandin.

Levine and Van Vunakis (1970) initially described a radioiodinated

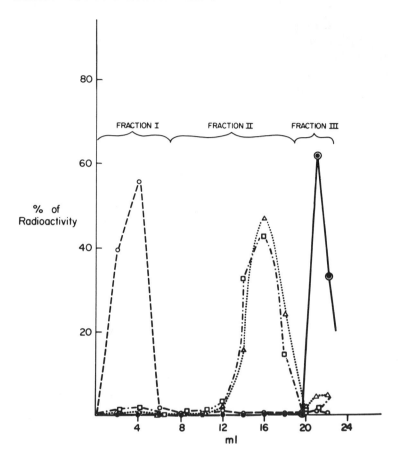

Figure 1. Silicic acid chromatographic separation of the prostaglandins, ³H-PGA₁ 100,000 cpm (O—O), ³H-PGE₁ 100,000 cpm (□—□), and ³H-PGF₁ₐ 60,000 cpm (●—●) were added to serum and extracted and chromatographed as described in the text, except that rather than collecting entire fractions, for this experiment we collected 2.0-ml samples of fractions I and II and 1.0-ml samples of fraction III. To evaluate the degree of PGE–PGA conversion, ³H-PGE₁ was chromatographed directly as supplied by the New England Nuclear Corporation (△—△). [Reprinted from Jaffe *et al.* (1973) with permission of the publisher.]

marker consisting of PGE₁ conjugated to a random copolymer of glutamic acid, lysine, alanine, and tyrosine, 36 : 24 : 35 : 5 mole ratios, respectively. In our experience, this marker does not yield satisfactory sensitivity. Tritiated prostaglandins are available (New England Nuclear Corp., Cambridge, Massachusetts) in pure form and high specific activity: PGE₁ at 87 Ci/m*M*, PGA₁ at 81 Ci/m*M*, PGF₁ₐ at 73 Ci/m*M*, and $PGF_{2\alpha}$ at 20 Ci/mM. We suggest the use of these markers in the prostaglandin radioimmunoassays. Delivered in ethanol, we seal aliquots under nitrogen and keep them at $-20°C$.

Purified prostaglandin standards have been generously given to us by the Upjohn Corporation. These compounds are dissolved at 1.0 mg/ml in 10% ethanol: 90% 0.1 M Na_2CO_3, and maintained as a stock solution of 1.0 μl/ml diluted in GPBS.

For each radioimmunoassay, we incubate for 1 to 2 hours at 4°C,

Stock solution	Amount (μl)
Diluted antiserum	50
8–10,000 cpm of ^{3}H-prostaglandin	50
1 mM EDTA	50
Homologous PG standards (1, 3, 8, 15, 30, 75, 150, 300, and 800 pg)	
or	100
Silicic acid chromatographic fraction	

D. Separation of Antibody-Bound from Free Prostaglandins

A variety of techniques have been utilized, including nitrocellulose membranes (Gershman *et al.*, 1972), ammonium sulfate precipitation (Brummer, 1972), and immunoprecipitation by the double antibody technique (Yu *et al.*, 1972). We have found dextran-coated charcoal (Herbert *et al.*, 1965) to be rapid and effective. Because of the problem of stripping, prolonged contact of the reaction mixture with the charcoal is avoided by processing no more than 20 samples at a time.

Before separation of antibody bound from free ^{3}H-PG, 0.1 ml of PBS containing gelatin, 5 mg/ml, is added to each tube to minimize stripping by charcoal and nonspecific binding. Dextran-coated charcoal is prepared by thoroughly mixing 500 mg of activated Norit A charcoal and 50 mg of dextran T70 (Pharmacia) into 200 ml of PBS. Of this mixture 1.0 ml is added to each reaction tube. Tubes are vortexed and immediately centrifuged at 3000 rpm, 4°C, for 10 minutes. The supernatants are rapidly decanted into scintillation vials containing 10 ml of Triton-toluene scintillation solution [7 gm PPO, 0.3 gm POPOP, 333 ml of Triton X (Sigma), and 667 ml of toluene] and counted.

E. Calculation of Results

Typical calibration curves for PGA_1, PGE_1, and $PGE_{2\alpha}$, radioimmunoassay are illustrated in Figure 2. Over the range of standards

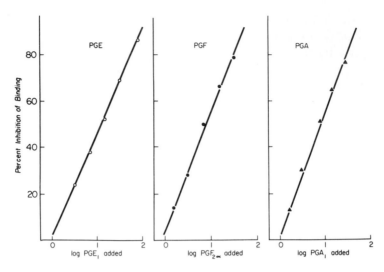

Figure 2. Typical calibration curves for PGA$_1$, PGE$_2$, and PGF$_{1\alpha}$ radioimmunoassay.

utilized, plots of the percentage inhibition of binding versus the log of the amount of unlabeled prostaglandin added are linear. Consequently, PG concentrations in the samples measured are calculated using a computer program for the best fit of data to a straight line. These raw data are corrected first for dilution (we measure 0.1-ml aliquots of 1.0 ml of GPBS in each chromatographic fraction) and then for the percentage recovery of labeled prostaglandin.

III. EVALUATION OF THE RADIOIMMUNOASSAY

A. Sensitivity

As the radioimmunoassays are currently used, 1.0 pg of PGA$_1$, PGE$_1$, and PGF$_{1\alpha}$ can be detected. The addition of 1.5 pg each of PGA$_1$, PGE$_1$, and PGF$_{1\alpha}$ inhibits antibody binding of the homologous labeled prostaglandins by more than 15%. Since ordinarily 0.1-ml samples are measured, the radioimmunoassays can detect 10 pg of each prostaglandin per milliliter of plasma. Samples containing lower prostaglandin concentrations can be measured only by concentration. Tenfold larger amounts of sample can be extracted and dried; the residues are then taken up in the chromatography solvent system and processed identically as for 1.0-ml initial samples.

B. Specificity

Using silicic acid chromatography, prostaglandin group specificity (PGA versus PGE versus PGF) is achieved, but the technique does not separate individual prostaglandins within these groups (i.e., PGE_1 versus PGE_2). Thus total PGA (PGA_1 + PGA_2), PGE (PGE_1 + PGE_2), and PGF ($PGF_{1\alpha}$ + $PGF_{2\alpha}$) immunoreactivity is measured and data should be expressed as such. Using two antisera to PGE with differential affinity for PGE_1 and PGE_2, Raz et al. (1975) and Ritzi and Stylos (1974) have described a technique for independently measuring PGE_1 and PGE_2.

PGE and PGF compounds are rapidly inactivated in the lungs (Piper et al., 1970) by conversion to 15-keto derivatives (Anggard and Samuelsson, 1964). Although these compounds circulate in concentrations thirty times those of the parent compounds (Green et al., 1972), they cross-react to such a minor degree (<0.004) that they do not interfere with the radioimmunoassay measurement of active prostaglandins. PGA compounds, on the other hand, pass through the lungs without being oxidized (McGiff et al., 1969) and are converted to PGB derivatives in the serum by the action of a specific isomerase (Polet and Levine, 1971). Since PGA and PGB compounds are eluted in the same silicic acid fraction (fraction I), it is possible, depending on the antibody, that some PGB is measured with PGA.

Arachidonic acid, the immediate precursor of PGE_2 and $PGF_{2\alpha}$, circulates in serum at approximately 7 μg/ml (Schrade et al., 1961). Since only 2–3% of ^{3}H-arachidonic acid is recovered in any silicic acid fraction, and the relative degree of cross-reactivity is between 10^{-5} and 10^{-6}, even at this high concentration, the long-chain fatty acid precursors do not interfere with the prostaglandin radioimmunoassay.

C. Comparison of Radioimmunoassay Data with Data Derived with Other Techniques

1. Bioassays

We have found excellent agreement between radioimmunoassay data and PGE data obtained using the cat blood pressure bioassay (Kannegeisser and Lee, 1971; Jaffe et al., 1972b) and using the superperfused organ bioassay system (Ferreira and Vane, 1967; Douglas et al., 1973).

2. Mass Spectroscopy

In a program organized by Dr. Bengt Samuelsson of the Karolinska Institutet, Stockholm, identical samples were measured by mass spectroscopy and radioimmunoassay by a number of investigators. Although radioimmunoassay tended to overestimate prostaglandin concentrations in this particular study, agreement between mass spectroscopy and radioimmunoassay data was generally good (Samuelsson, 1973b).

3. Urinary Excretion of Metabolites

After the injection of tritium-labeled marker, Samuelsson (1973a) determined the daily urinary excretion of PGE and PGF metabolites in men of 46 to 333 and 42 to 120 μg/day, respectively, and in women of 18 to 38 and 36 to 61 μg/day, respectively. Calculating back from this data, he has suggested that PGE and PGF levels in blood should be less than 20 pg/ml. This discrepancy between measured levels and values estimated from the urinary excretion of by-products remains unexplained.

4. Other Techniques

Radioreceptor assays (Kuehl and Humes, 1972) and viroimmunoassays (Andrieu et al., 1974; Mitani and Shoji, 1974) have been developed, and in general have corroborated findings made using radioimmunoassay.

D. Values of Prostaglandins in Plasma

Normal plasma levels of prostaglandins E and F from our laboratory are listed in Table III. In contrast to these values, Dray et al. (1975) reported average immunoreactive PGE levels of 40 pg/ml. A number of investigators have reported mean basal levels of PGF ranging from 10 to 710 pg/ml (Dray et al., 1975; Wilks et al., 1973; Challis and Tulchinsky, 1974; Yousefnejadian et al., 1974; Hennan et al., 1974; Van Orden and Farley, 1973).

Elevated levels of plasma PGE have been demonstrated in pa-

Table III   Normal Plasma Levels of Prostaglandins

	PGE (pg/ml)	PGF (pg/ml)
Females	316 ± 36	154 ± 35
Females on oral contraceptives	478 ± 55	162 ± 19
Males	378 ± 73	84 ± 15
Range	139–1011	50–359
Mean ± S.E.M.	385 ± 30	141 ± 15

tients with medullary carcinoma of the thyroid, the carcinoid syndrome (Jaffe *et al.*, 1973; Jaffe and Condon, 1976), and the Verner-Morrison syndrome (Jaffe *et al.*, 1977). In addition, levels of PGE and $PGF_{2\alpha}$ have been found to be high in women in labor (Caldwell *et al.*, 1971; Brummer, 1972; Hertelendy *et al.*, 1973), in patients rejecting renal allografts (Anderson *et al.*, 1975), and in hypercalcemic patients with a variety of carcinomas (Brereton *et al.*, 1974; Demers *et al.*, 1977; Robertson *et al.*, 1975).

Aspirin and indomethacin have been shown to inhibit prostaglandin synthesis (Smith and Willis, 1971; Vane, 1971). This inhibition has been confirmed in radioimmunoassay studies (Zusman *et al.*, 1972; Orczyk and Behrman, 1972; Jaffe and Parker, 1973; Jaffe *et al.*, 1973). Kantrowitz *et al.* (1975) and Tashjian and co-workers (1975) have similarly demonstrated that hydrocortisone inhibits biosynthesis of PGE; this too has been confirmed in radioimmunoassay studies (Santoro *et al.*, 1976).

IV. PROSTAGLANDIN METABOLITES

A. Metabolism

As shown in Figure 3, PGE_2 and $PGF_{2\alpha}$ are initially oxidized at the 15-position, producing 15-keto derivatives which are virtually inactive. The first step occurs predominantly in the lung and renal cortex. Enzymatic reduction at the 13–14 bond results in the major circulating metabolites, 13,14-dihydro-15-keto derivatives. These molecular

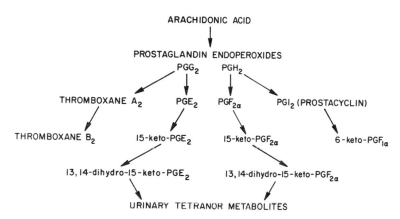

Figure 3. The metabolism of the prostaglandins, thromboxane, and prostacyclin.

forms should theoretically predominate in the plasma, because they have relatively long half-lives. The final steps in the metabolism of the native prostaglandins is further oxidation to 16-carbon dicarboxylic acids usually considered as tetranor derivatives.

In addition to the major groups of prostaglandins, Hamberg *et al.* (1975) described a potent vasoconstrictor and platelet aggregator derived from the endoperoxides. This compound, thromboxane A_2, has a half-life of less than one minute, and it is metabolized to an inactive acetal derivative, thromboxane B_2 (TXB_2); measurement of TXB_2 activity is an accurate estimation of TXA_2 activity and, thus, allows for evaluation of the physiologic role of this compound.

Bunting and co-workers (1976) recently described another product of the endoperoxides, PGI_2 or prostacyclin. This potent vasodilator and inhibitor of platelet aggregation is enzymatically converted to 6-keto-$PGF_{1\alpha}$ in less than one minute. Although estimation of this latter product should permit accurate quantitation of prostacyclin, there have been no 6-keto-$PGF_{1\alpha}$ radioimmunoassays described as yet.

B. Circulating Prostaglandin Metabolites

1. Antibodies

a. **15-Keto-$PGF_{2\alpha}$.** For immunization, Levine and Gutierrez-Cernosek (1972) conjugated 15-keto-$PGF_{2\alpha}$ (5.16 mg in 0.25 ml of N,N-dimethylformamide) to poly-L-lysine HBr (6.2 mg in 0.25 ml of water) using 1-ethyl-3-(3-diethylaminopropyl)carbodiimide (6.3 mg). Of the dialyzed conjugate, 2.4 mg was mixed with an equal amount of succinylated hemocyanin, made up to 2.0 ml in 0.14 M NaCl, emulsified with 2.0 ml of complete Freund's adjuvant, and administered subcutaneously to monkeys (1.0 mg/animal). Immunizations were repeated at four and eight weeks, and animals were bled seven days later. All four immunized animals made antibodies which bound [3]H-15-keto-$PGF_{2\alpha}$; the specificity of one of these antisera is summarized in Table IV (Pong and Levine, 1977). Cornette *et al.* (1974) utilized a similar technique to elicit anti-15-keto-$PGF_{2\alpha}$ antibodies in rabbits and goats (Table IV).

b. **13,14-Dihydro-15-keto-$PGF_{2\alpha}$.** Granström and Samuelsson (1972) conjugated 10 mg of 13,14-dihydro-15-keto-$PGF_{2\alpha}$ to 40 mg of BSA using 10 mg of EDC. Rabbits were immunized with conjugate in complete Freund's adjuvant at weekly intervals for 4 weeks. The re-

Table IV   Cross-Reactivity of Anti-PG Metabolite Antibodies

Antiserum	15-Keto-PGF$_{2\alpha}$	13,14-Dihydro-15-keto-PGF$_{2\alpha}$	15-Keto-PGE$_2$	13,14-Dihydro-15-keto-PGE$_2$	PGF$_{2\alpha}$	PGE$_2$	Reference
Anti-15-keto-PGF$_2$	1.00	0.04	0.69	<0.01	<0.01	—	Levine and Gutierrez-Cernosek (1972)
Anti-13,14-dihydro-15-keto-PGF$_{2\alpha}$	1.00	0.10	—	—	<0.01	—	Cornette et al. (1974)
	0.10	1.00	—	—	<0.01	—	Cornette et al. (1974)
	0.04	1.00	—	—	<0.01	<0.01	Granström and Samuelsson (1973)
	0.06	1.00	<0.01	—	<0.01	—	Levine and Gutierrez-Cernosek (1973)
Anti-13,14-dihydro-15-keto-PGE$_2$	—	1.00	—	0.40	<0.01	—	Haning et al. (1977)
	<0.01	0.05	0.07	1.00	<0.01	<0.01	Levine (1977)
	<0.01	<0.01	0.04	1.00	<0.01	<0.01	Peskar et al. (1974)
Anti-15-keto-PGE$_2$	0.04	0.01	1.00	0.07	<0.01	<0.01	Gordon et al. (1977)

sultant antiserum had good specificity for the homologous ligand and cross-reacted only minimally with $PGF_{2\alpha}$ and 15-keto-$PGF_{2\alpha}$ (Table IV). Since that time, a number of investigators, using the same technique, have described antibodies to 13,14 dihydro-15-keto-$PGF_{2\alpha}$ (Cornette *et al.*, 1974; Haning *et al.*, 1977; Stylos *et al.*, 1973; Levine and Gutierrez-Cernosek, 1973); in general, there have been no problems with cross-reactivity by metabolites of either PGF or PGE.

c. 13,14-Dihydro-15-keto-PGE_2. Levine (1977) elicited antibodies to 13,14-dihydro-15-keto-PGE_2 by immunizing rabbits with an HSA–PG conjugate. Five milligrams of 13,14-dihydro-15-keto-PGE_2 in 0.1 ml N,N-dimethylformamide, 3.0 mg dicyclohexylcarbodiimide, and 3.5 mg N-hydroxysuccinimide was incubated at 20°C for 30 minutes. The precipitate that formed was removed by centrifugation and the supernatant was incubated for 4°C for 2 hours with 12 mg HSA in 0.5 ml 0.1 N $NaHCO_3$. The product was dialyzed at 4°C against 10 liters of 0.005 M phosphate, 0.15 M NaCl, pH 7.5, emulsified with an equal volume of complete Freund's adjuvant, and injected i.m. and s.c. to rabbits, 2.0 mg/animal. The specificity of the elicited antisera, as well as that of Peskar *et al.* (1974), are outlined in Table IV.

d. 15-Keto-PGE_2. Using the same carbodiimide condensation technique, 15-keto-PGE_2 was conjugated to BSA at a mole ratio of PG : HSA of 2 : 1. Antisera raised in sheep bound ^{3}H-15-keto-PGE_2; this binding was similarly specific for 15-keto-PGE_2 (Table IV).

2. Tritiated Labels

Tritiated 13,14-dihydro-15-keto-$PGF_{2\alpha}$ and 13,14-dihydro-15-keto-PGE_2, at specific activities of 60–100 Ci/mmole, are commercially available from the Amersham Corporation, Arlington Heights, Illinois.

Tritiated 15-keto-PGE_2 was prepared by incubating ^{3}H-PGE_2 with a swine lung homogenate (Granström, 1971). Swine kidneys were homogenized in three volumes of Bucher medium, centrifuged at 8500 g for 15 minutes and the supernatant centrifuged at 105,000 g for one hour. The supernatant from the higher speed spin was incubated with ^{3}H-PGE, specific activity 0.2 mCi/mmole, and NAD^+ at a concentration of 0.1 mM for 60 minutes at 37°C. The reaction was terminated by adding five volumes of ethanol; the metabolite was extracted with ether and purified by thin-layer chromatography in chloroform–tetrahydrofuran–acetic acid, 100 : 10 : 5. The final product had a specific activity of 87 Ci/mmole (Gordon *et al.*, 1977).

Tritiated 15-keto-PGF$_{2\alpha}$ was synthesized by selective oxidation at the 15-position (Cornette *et al.*, 1974; Levine and Gutierrez-Cernosek, 1972). Twenty-five microliters of ^{3}H-PGF$_{2\alpha}$ (25 μCi) was reacted with 125 mg 2,3-dichloro-5,6-dicyano-1,4-benzoquinone (DDQ) in 0.5 ml dioxane overnight at 20°C. After evaporation of the dioxane in N$_2$, 0.25 ml methylene chloride was added and the insoluble DDQ removed by centrifugation. The ^{3}H-15-keto-PGF$_{2\alpha}$ was purified by silica gel thin-layer chromatography using chloroform : methanol : water, 80 : 20 : 2 and chloroform : methanol : acetic acid, 80 : 5 : 10. The purified product was eluted in 6.0 ml acetone containing 0.3 ml methanol, dried under N$_2$ at 4°C, and redissolved in assay buffer.

3. Handling of Plasma Samples

a. Metabolites of PGF. There has been significant variation in the techniques used for preparation of plasma samples for radioimmunoassay. Cornette *et al.* (1974) measured plasma samples directly. Granström and Samuelsson (1972) extracted mildly acidified samples with two volumes of ethyl acetate, whereas Fairclough and Payne (1975) and Mitchell *et al.* (1976) utilized four to five volumes of ether for extraction of samples titrated to pH 3. Finally, Haning *et al.* (1977) and Stylos *et al.* (1973) extracted samples (with 0.1 volume 1.0 N HCl, two volumes ethyl acetate, and four volumes acetate buffer, pH 4.5, plus 7.5 volumes ethyl acetate, respectively) and chromatographically separated the major groups of prostaglandins on silicic acid using the technique described above.

b. Metabolites of PGE. Both Levine (1977) and Gordon *et al.* (1977) measured plasma samples directly without prior extraction.

4. Results of Metabolite Radioimmunoassays

Normal levels of prostaglandin metabolites are summarized in Table V; there is considerable variation in the reported levels. Although not all the assays have been thoroughly validated, Granström and Samuelsson (1972) reported equivalent levels of 13,14-dihydro-15-keto-PGF$_{2\alpha}$ measured by radioimmunoassay and gas chromatography–mass spectroscopy. Infusion of PGF$_{2\alpha}$ in monkeys (4.0 μg/minute) did not significantly elevate levels of immunoreactive PGF$_{2\alpha}$ levels, but did increase plasma concentrations of both 15-keto-PGF$_{2\alpha}$ and 13,14-dihydro-15-keto-PGF$_{2\alpha}$ by 4 and 17 times, respectively.

Table V   Plasma Levels of Prostaglandin Metabolites

15-Keto-PGF$_{2\alpha}$	13,14-Di-hydro-15-keto-PGF$_{2\alpha}$	15-Keto-PGE$_2$	13,14-Di-hydro-15-keto-PGE$_2$	Reference
0.5 ng/ml	4.8 ng/ml			Levine and Gutierrez-Cernosek (1973)
	1.4 ng/ml			Cornette *et al.* (1974)
	<0.24 ng/ml			Granström and Samuelsson (1972)
	63 pg/ml			Stylos *et al.* (1973)
	100 pg/ml			Haning *et al.* (1977)
		<50 pg/ml		Gordon *et al.* (1977)
			28 pg/ml	Levine (1977)

C. Urinary Tetranor Metabolites of Prostaglandins

Granström and Kindahl (1976) and Ohki *et al.* (1974, 1975) have developed radioimmunoassays for the main urinary metabolite (MUM), i.e., the tetranor derivative of PGF$_{2\alpha}$–MUM. Both groups conjugated the dicarboxylic acid to albumin, and this served as the immunogen for rabbits. The antibodies elicited were quite specific and did not cross-react significantly with any other derivative of the prostaglandins.

Granström and Kindahl (1976) purified ^{3}H-PGF$_{2\alpha}$–MUM from the urine of a patient who received 17,18-^{3}H-PGF$_{2\alpha}$, at 50 Ci/mmole, intravenously. Ohki *et al.* (1974) prepared radioiodinated ligand by conjugating the metabolite to tyrosine methyl ester; 1.5 mmoles of PGF$_{2\alpha}$–MUM and of tyrosine methyl ester were reacted overnight at 4°C with 1.5 mmole of N,N-dicyolohexylcarbodiimide in tetrahydrofuran : dioxane, 1 : 1 (v/v). The precipitate was removed by filtration and the mixture was dried by evaporation. The residue was dissolved in a minimal volume of ethyl acetate and chromatographed on silica gel columns in ethyl acetate : cyclohexane, 3 : 2 (v/v). Five micrograms of the tyrosinated metabolite in 20 μl of 0.2 M phosphate buffer, pH 7.2, 1.5 mCi ^{125}I, and 25 μg chloramine-T in 10 μl phosphate were incubated for 30 seconds. The reaction was terminated by the addition of 75 μg sodium metabisulfate in 15 μl phosphate. The ^{125}I-tyrosine–PGF$_{2\alpha}$–MUM, 256 mCi/mg, was purified on a silica gel plate using benzene : dioxane : acetic acid, 20 : 20 : 1.

Both assays reported equivalent data. Normal levels ranged from 5.0–14 μg/day for females and 11–53 μg/day for males (Granström and Kindahl, 1976; Ohki *et al.*, 1976; Kitamura *et al.*, 1977).

D. Thromboxane B_2

Thromboxane B_2 (TXB_2) has recently been made available in limited supply from the Upjohn Company. The preparation of this compound and ^3H-TXB_2 has been reported by Granström et al. (1976a). Platelet-rich plasma was prepared by centrifugation of 970 ml blood plus 30 ml 77 mM NaEDTA for 15 minutes at 275 g and then for 25 minutes at 650 g. The platelet pellet was washed in 100 ml 0.012 M Tris, 0.14 M NaCl, pH 7.4, containing 1.5 mM EDTA, and after centrifugation at 650 g for 15 minutes, the pellet was suspended in 50 ml Krebs–Henseleit medium at 37°C for two minutes. Arachidonic acid, 3.5 mg in 100 μl ethanol, was added (in the preparation of ^3H-TXB_2, 0.25 mCi ^3H-arachidonic acid, 69 Ci/mmole, in 15 μl ethanol was added to 1.5 ml suspension of washed platelets) for 10 minutes at 37°C. The reaction was terminated by the addition of four volumes of cold ethanol. After the ethanol was removed by evaporation, TXB_2 was extracted with ether at pH 3 and chromatographed on a 5-gm silicic acid column in ether:hexane, 20:8 (v/v). The column was washed with 400 ml ether–hexane, and TXB_2 was eluted with 400 ml ethyl acetate. The product was purified by reverse phase partition chromatography on a 4.5-gm column of hydrophobic Hyflo Super Cel in methanol:water:acetic acid, 135:165:2 for the moving and chloroform:isooctanol, 15:15, for the stationary phase and collecting from 65–85 ml (Hamberg, 1968); this was followed by thin-layer chromatography in chloroform:methanol:water:acetic acid, 90:8:1:0.8 ($R_f = 0.30$). The purified product was eluted with methanol.

Antibodies were elicited in rabbits immunized with a conjugate of TXB_2–HSA (Granström et al., 1976a). 2.8 mg TXB_2 in 0.5 ml N,N-dimethylformamide, 1.5 mg N,N-carbonyldiimidazole, and 10 mg BSA in 0.75 ml water were incubated for five hours and then diluted with 5 ml N,N-dimethylformamide:water, 3:2. The dialyzed product was emulsified with complete Freund's adjuvant, and used for immunization. The resulting antisera cross-reacted no more than 0.1% with any PGE or PGF compound or metabolite and, in a radioimmunoassay in which antibody-bound ^3H-TXB_2 was separated from free labeled ligand by polyethylene glycol, permitted a maximal sensitivity of 10 pg TXB_2. Collagen-induced platelet aggregation caused a significant increase in immunoreactive TXB_2 levels.

In a recent modification, Granström et al. (1976b) have developed a radioimmunoassay for the mono-O-methyl derivative of TXB_2, since this metabolite more accurately reflects the activity of the biologically active thromboxane A_2.

REFERENCES

Anderson, C. B., Newton, W. T., and Jaffe, B. M. (1975). Circulating prostaglandin E and allograft rejection. *Transplantation* 19, 527–528.

Andrieu, J. M., Mamas, S., and Dray, F. (1974). Viroimmunoassay of prostaglandin $F_{2\alpha}$ at the program level. *Prostaglandins* 6, 15–22.

Anggard, E., and Samuelsson, B. (1964). Prostaglandins and related factors. Metabolism of prostaglandin E in guinea pig lung: The structure of two metabolites. *J. Biol. Chem.* 239, 4097–4102.

Axen, U., Green, K., Hörlin, D., and Samuelsson, B. (1971). Mass spectrometric determination of picomole amounts of prostaglandins E_2 and $F_{2\alpha}$ using synthetic deuterium labeled carriers. *Biochem. Biophys. Res. Commun.* 45, 519–525.

Brereton, H. D., Halushka, P. V., Alexander, R. W., Mason, D. M., Keiser, H. R., and DeVita, V. T., Jr. (1974) Indomethacin-responsive hypercalcemia in a patient with renal-cell adenocarcinoma. *N. Engl. J. Med.* 291, 83–85.

Brummer, H. C. (1972). Serum $PGF_{2\alpha}$ levels during late pregnancy, labour, and the puerperium. *Prostaglandins* 2, 185–194.

Bunting, S., Gryglewski, R., Moncada, S., and Vane, J. R. (1976). Arterial walls generate from prostaglandin endopenoxides a substance (Prostaglandin X) which relaxes strips of mesenteric and coeliac arteries and inhibits platelet aggregation. *Prostaglandins* 12, 897–913.

Caldwell, B. V., Burstein, S., Brock, W. A., and Speroff, L. (1971). Radioimmunoassay of the F prostaglandins. *J. Clin. Endocrinol. Metab.* 33, 171–175.

Challis, J. R. G., and Tulchinsky, D. (1974). A comparison between the concentration of prostaglandin F in human plasma and serum. *Prostaglandins* 5, 27–31.

Cornette, J. C., Harrison, K. L., and Kirton, K. T. (1974). Measurement of prostaglandin $F_{2\alpha}$ metabolites by radioimmunoassay. *Prostaglandins* 5, 155–164.

Demers, L. M., Allegra, J. C., Harvey, H. A., Lipton, A., Luderer, J. R., Mortel, R., and Brenner, D. E. (1977). Plasma prostaglandins in hypercalcemic patients with neoplastic disease. *Cancer* 39, 1559–1562.

Douglas, J. R., Jr., Johnson, E. M., Marshall, G. R., Jaffe, B. M., and Needleman, P. (1973). Stimulation of splenic prostaglandin release by angiotensin and specific inhibition by cysteine[8] A II. *Prostaglandins* 3, 67–74.

Dray, F., Maron, E., Tillson, S. A., and Sela, M. (1972). Immunochemical detection of prostaglandins with prostaglandin-coated bacteriophage T4 and by radioimmunoassay. *Anal. Biochem.* 50, 399–408.

Dray, F., Charbonnel, B., and Maclouf, J. (1975). Radioimmunoassay of prostaglandins $F\alpha$, E_1 and E_2 in human plasma. *Eur. J. Clin. Invest.* 5, 311–318.

Eakins, K. E., Karim, S. M. M., and Miller, J. D. (1970). Antagonism of some smooth muscle actions of prostaglandins by polyphloretin phosphate. *Br. J. Pharmacol.* 39, 556–563.

Fairclough, R. J., and Payne, E. (1975). Radioimmunoassay of 13,14-dihydro-15-keto prostaglandin F in bovine peripheral plasma. *Prostaglandins* 10, 266–272.

Ferreira, S. H., and Vane, J. R. (1967). Prostaglandins: Their disappearance from and release into the circulation. *Nature (London)* 216, 868–873.

Fretland, D. (1974). Use of ion-exchange resins for removing prostaglandins from human urine prior to radioimmunoassay. *Prostaglandins* 6, 421–425.

Gershman, H., Powers, E., Levine, L., and Van Vunakis, H. (1972) Radioimmunoassay of prostaglandins, angiotensin, digoxin, morphine, and adenosin-3′,5-cyclic monophosphate with nitrocellulose membranes. *Prostaglandins* 1, 407–423.

Gordon, D., Myatt, L., Gordon-Wright, A., Hanson, J., and Elder, M. G. (1977). Radioimmunoassay of 15-keto-prostaglandin E_2 in peripheral plasma after administration of prostaglandin E_2 tablets used for induction of labor. *Prostaglandins* 13, 399–408.

Granström, E. (1971). Metabolism of prostaglandin $F_{2\alpha}$ in swine kidney. *Biochim. Biophys. Acta* 239, 120–125.

Granström, E., and Samuelsson, B. (1972). Development and mass spectrometric evaluation of a radioimmunoassay for 9α, 11α, dihydroxy-15-ketoprost-5-enoic acid. *FEBS Lett.* 26, 211–214.

Granström, E., and Kindahl, H. (1976). Radioimmunoassays for prostaglandin metabolites. *Adv. Prostaglandin Thromboxane Res.* 1, 81–92.

Granström, E., Kindahl, H., and Samuelsson, B. (1976a). Radioimmunoassay for thromboxane B_2. *Anal. Lett.* 9, 611–627.

Granström, E., Kindahl, H., and Samuelsson, R. (1976b). A method for measuring the unstable thromboxane A_2: Radioimmunoassay of the derived mono-O-methylthromboxane B_2. *Prostaglandins* 12, 929–941.

Green, K., Beguin, F., Bygdeman, M., Toppozada, M., and Wiqvist, N. (1972) Analysis of prostaglandin $F_{2\alpha}$ and metabolites following intravenous, intraamniotic, and intravaginal administration of prostaglandin $F_{2\alpha}$. *In* "Third Conference on Prostaglandins in Fertility Control" (S. Bergström, K. Green, and B. Samuelsson, eds.), pp. 189–200. Karolinska Institutet, Stockholm.

Gutierrez-Cernosek, R. M., Morrill, L. M., and Levine, L. (1972). Prostaglandin $F_{2\alpha}$ levels in peripheral sera of man. *Prostaglandins* 1, 71–80.

Hamberg, M. (1968). Metabolism of prostaglandins in rat liver mitochrondria. *Eur. J. Biochem.* 6, 135–146.

Hamberg, M., Svensson, J., and Samuelsson, B. (1975) Thromboxanes: A new group of biologically active compounds derived from prostaglandin endoperoxides. *Proc. Natl. Acad. Sci. U.S.A.* 72, 2994–2998.

Haning, R. V., Jr., Kieliszek, F. X., Alberino, S. P., and Speroff, L. (1977). A radioimmunoassay for 13,14-dihydro-15-keto prostaglandin $F_{2\alpha}$ with chromatography and internal recovery standard. *Prostaglandins* 13, 455–477.

Hannam, J. F., Johnson, D. A., Newton, J. R., and Collins, W. P. (1974). Radioimmunoassay of prostaglandin $F_{2\alpha}$ in peripheral venous plasma from men and women. *Prostaglandins* 5, 531–542.

Herbert, V., Lau, K., Gottlieb, C. W., and Bleicher, S. J. (1965). Coated charcoal immunoassay of insulin. *J. Clin. Endocrinol. Metab.* 25, 1375–1384.

Hertelendy, F., Woods, R., and Jaffe, B. M. (1973) Prostaglandin E levels in peripheral blood during labor. *Prostaglandins* 3, 223–227.

Jaffe, B. M. and Parker, C. W. (1974). Radioimmunoassay for prostaglandins. *In* "Radioassays in Clinical Medicine" (R. Donati and W. T. Newton, eds.), pp. 33–48. Thomas, Springfield, Illinois.

Jaffe, B. M., and Condon, S. (1976). Prostaglandins E and F in endocrine diarrheagenic syndromes. *Ann. Surg.* 184, 516–524.

Jaffe, B. M., and Parker, C. W. (1972). Extraction of PGE from human serum for radioimmunoassay. *In* "Third Conference on Prostaglandins in Fertility Control" (S. Bergström, K. Green, and B. Samuelsson, eds.), pp. 69–82. Karolinska Institutet, Stockholm.

Jaffe, B. M., and Parker, C. W. (1973). Physiologic implications of prostaglandin radioimmunoassay. *Metab., Clin. Exp.* 22, 1129–1137.

Jaffe, B. M., Smith, J. W., Newton, W. T., and Parker, C. W. (1971). Radioimmunoassay for prostaglandins. *Science* **171**, 494–496.

Jaffe, B. M., Parker, C. W., Marshall, G. R., and Needleman, P. (1972a). Renal concentrations of prostaglandin E in acute and chronic renal ischemia. *Biochem. Biophys. Res. Commun.* **49**, 799–805.

Jaffe, B. M., Parker, C. W., and Philpott, G. W. (1972b). Prostaglandin release by human cells *in vitro. In* "Prostaglandins in Cellular Biology and the Inflammatory Process" (P. Ramwell and B. P. Phariss, eds.), pp. 207–226. Plenum, New York.

Jaffe, B. M., Behrman, H. R., and Parker, C. W. (1973). Radioimmunoassay measurement of prostaglandins E, A, and F in human plasma. *J. Clin. Invest.* **52**, 398–405.

Jaffe, B. M., Kopen, D. F., DeSchryver-Kecskmeti, K., Gingerich, R. L., and Greider, M. (1977). Indomethacin-responsive pancreatic cholera. *N. Engl. J. Med.* **297**, 817–821.

Kannegeisser, H., and Lee, J. B. (1971). Difference in hemodynamic response to prostaglandins A and E. *Nature (London)* **229**, 498–500.

Kantrowitz, F., Robinson, D. R., McGuire, M. B., and Levine, L. (1975) Corticosteroids inhibit prostaglandin production by rheumatoid synovia. *Nature (London)* **258**, 737–739.

Kirton, K. T., Cornette, J. C., and Barr, K. L. (1972). Characterization of antibody to prostaglandin $F_{2\alpha}$. *Biochem. Biophys. Res. Commun.* **47**, 903–909.

Kitamura, S., Ishihara, Y., and Kosaka, K. (1977). Radioimmunoassay of main urinary metabolite of prostaglandin $F_{2\alpha}$ in normal subjects. *Prostaglandins* **14**, 961–965.

Kuehl, F. A., Jr., and Humes, J. L. (1972). Direct evidence for a prostaglandin receptor and its application to prostaglandin measurements. *Proc. Natl. Acad. Sci. U.S.A.* **69**, 480–484.

Levine, L. (1977). Levels of 13,14-dihydro-15-keto-PGE_2 in some biological fluids as measured by radioimmunoassay. *Prostaglandins* **14**, 1125–1139.

Levine, L., and Gutierrez-Cernosek, R. M. (1972). Preparation and specificity of antibodies to 15-keto prostaglandin $F_{2\alpha}$. *Prostaglandins* **2**, 281–294.

Levine, L., and Gutierrez-Cernosek, R. M. (1973). Levels of 13,14-dihydro-15-keto-$PGF_{2\alpha}$ in biological fluids as measured by radioimmunoassay. *Prostaglandins* **3**, 785–804.

Levine, L., and Van Vunakis, H. (1970). Antigenic activity of prostaglandins. *Biochem. Biophys. Res. Commun.* **41**, 1171–1177.

Levine, L., Gutierrez-Cernosek, R. M., and Van Vunakis, H. (1971). Sepectificities of prostaglandins B_1, $F_{1\alpha}$ and $F_{2\alpha}$ antigen–antibody reactions. *J. Biol. Chem.* **246**, 6782–6785.

McGiff, J. C., Terragno, N. A., Strand, J. C., Lee, J. B., Lonigro, A. J., and Ng, K. K. F. (1969). Selective passage of prostaglandins across the lungs. *Nature (London)* **223**, 742–745.

Mitani, M., and Shoji, S. (1974). Determination of prostaglandin F in blood plasma using chemically modified bacteriophage technique. *Prostaglandins* **8**, 67–77.

Mitchell, M. D., Flint, A. P. F., and Turnbull, A. C. (1976). Plasma concentrations of 13,14-dihydro-15-keto-prostaglandin F during pregnancy in sheep. *Prostaglandins* **11**, 319–325.

Ohki, S., Hanyu, T., Imaki, K., Nakazawa, N., and Hirata, F. (1974). Radioimmunoassays of prostaglandin $F_{2\alpha}$ and prostaglandin $F_{2\alpha}$-main urinary metabolite with prostaglandin-^{125}I-tyrosine methylester amide. *Prostaglandins* **6**, 137–148.

Ohki, S., Imaki, K., and Hirata, F. (1975). Radioimmunoassay of main urinary metabolite of prostaglandin $F_{2\alpha}$. *Prostaglandins* **10**, 549–555.

Ohki, S., Nishigaki, Y., Imaki, K., Kurono, M., and Hirata, F. (1976). The levels of main urinary metabolite of prostaglandin $F_{1\alpha}$ and $F_{2\alpha}$ in human subjects measured by radioimmunoassay. *Prostaglandins* **12**, 181–186.

Orcyzk, G. P., and Behrman, H. R. (1972). Ovulation blockade by aspirin or indomethacin-*in vivo* evidence for a role of prostaglandin in gonadotrophin secretion. *Prostaglandins* **1**, 3–20.

Peskar, B. A., Holland, A., and Peskar, B. M. (1974). Antisera against 13,14-dihydro-15-keto-prostaglandin E_2. *FEBS Lett.* **43**, 45–48.

Piper, P. J., Vane, J. R., and Wyllie, J. H. (1970). Inactivation of prostaglandins by the lungs. *Nature (London)* **225**, 600–604.

Podos, S. M., Jaffe, B. M., and Becker, B. (1972). Prostaglandins and glaucoma. *Br. Med. J.* **4**, 432.

Polet, H., and Levine, L. (1971). Serum prostaglandin A_1 isomerase. *Biochem. Biophys. Res. Commun.* **45**, 1169–1176.

Pong, S.-S., and Levine, L. (1977). Prostaglandin biosynthesis and metabolism measured by radioimmunoassay. In "The Prostaglandins," Vol. 3, (P. W. Ramwell, ed.), pp. 41–76, Plenum Press, New York.

Raz, A. (1972). Interaction of prostaglandins with blood plasma proteins. *Biochem. J.* **130**, 631–636.

Raz, A., Schwartzman, M., Kenig-Wakshal, R., and Perl, E. (1975). The specificity of antisera to conjugates of prostaglandins E with bovine serum albumin and thyroglobumin. *Eur. J. Biochem.* **53**, 145–150.

Ritzi, E. M., and Stylos, W. A. (1974). The simultaneous use of two prostaglandin E radioimmunoassays employing two antisera of differing specificity. *Prostaglandins* **8**, 55–66.

Robertson, R. P., Baylink, D. J., Marini, J. J., and Adkinson, H. W. (1975). Elevated prostaglandins and suppressed parathyroid hormone associated with hypercalcemia and renal cell carcinoma. *J. Clin. Endocrinol. Metab.* **41**, 164–167.

Samuelsson, B. (1973a). Quantitative aspects of prostaglandin synthesis in man. *Adv. Biosci.* **9**, 7–14.

Samuelsson, B. (1973b). Round table discussion on analytical methods. *Adv. Biosci.* **9**, 121–123.

Santoro, M. G., Philpott, and Jaffe, B. M. (1976). Inhibition of tumor growth *in vivo* and *in vitro* by prostaglandin E. *Nature (London)* **263**, 777–779.

Schrade, W., Biegler, R., and Bohle, E. (1961). Fatty acid distribution in the lipid fractions of healthy persons of different age, patients with atherosclerosis, and patients with idiopathic hyperlipidemia. *J. Atheroscler. Res.* **1**, 47–61.

Shaw, J. E., and Ramwell, P. W. (1969). Separation, identification, and estimation of prostaglandins. *Methods Biochem. Anal.* **17**, 325–371.

Smith, J. B., and Willis, A. L. (1970). Formation and release of prostaglandins by platelets in response to thrombin. *Br. J. Pharmacol.* **40**, 545 P.

Smith, J. B., and Willis, A. L. (1971). Aspirin selectively inhibits prostaglandin production in human platelets. *Nature (London), New Biol.* **231**, 235–237.

Smith, J. B., Ingerman, C., Kocsis, J. J., and Silver, M. J. (1973). Formation of prostaglandins during the aggregation of human blood platelets. *J. Clin. Invest.* **52**, 965–969.

Stylos, W. A., and Rivetz, B. (1972). Preparation of specific antiserum to prostaglandin A. *Prostaglandins* **2**, 103–113.

Stylos, W. A., Burstein, S., Rosenfeld, J., Ritzi, E. M., and Watson, D. J. (1973). A radioimmunoassay for the initial metabolites of the F prostaglandins. *Prostaglandins* **4**, 553–565.

Tashjian, A. H., Jr., Voelkel, E. F., McDonough, J., and Levine, L. (1975). Hydrocortisone inhibits prostaglandin production by mouse fibrosarcoma cells. *Nature (London)* **258**, 739–741.

Thompson, S., Los, M., and Horton, E. W. (1970). The separation, identification, and estimation of prostaglandins in nanogram quantities by combined gas chromatography–mass spectroscopy. *Life Sci.* **9**, 983–988.

Vane, J. R. (1971). Inhibition of prostaglandin synthesis as a mechanism of action for aspirin-like drugs. *Nature (London), New Biol.* **231**, 232–235.

Van Orden, D. E., and Farley, D. B. (1973). Prostaglandin $F_{2\alpha}$ radioimmunoassay utilizing polyethylene gylcol separation technique. *Prostaglandins* **4**, 215–233.

Wilks, J. W., Wentz, A. C., and Jones, G. S. (1973). Prostaglandin $F_{2\alpha}$ concentrations in the blood of women during normal menstrual cycles and dysmenorrhea. *J. Clin. Endocrinol Metab.* **37**, 469–471.

Youssefnejadian, E., Walker, E., Sommerville, I. F., and Craft, I. (1974). Simple direct radioimmunoassay of the F prostaglandins. *Prostaglandins* **6**, 23–35.

Yu, S.-C. and Burke, G. (1972). Antigenic activity of the prostaglandins: Specificities of prostaglandins E_1, A_1, and $F_{2\alpha}$ antigen–antibody reactions. *Prostaglandins* **2**, 11–22.

Yu, S.-C., Chang, L., and Burke, G. (1972). Thyrotropin increases prostaglandin levels in isolated thyroid cells. *J. Clin. Invest.* **51**, 1038–1042.

Zusman, R. M., Caldwell, B. V., Speroff, L., and Behrman, H. R. (1972). Radioimmunoassay of the A prostaglandins. *Prostaglandins* **2**, 41–53.

HYPOTHALAMIC AND PINEAL HORMONES

3

Thyrotropin-Releasing Hormone

RAHIM M. BASSIRI, JOSEF DVORAK, AND
ROBERT D. UTIGER

I. INTRODUCTION

Thyrotropin-releasing hormone (TRH) was first characterized in extracts of hypothalamic tissue in 1969 and its total synthesis achieved soon thereafter (Boler *et al.*, 1969; Burgus *et al.*, 1969). A number of quantitative systems for TRH assay have been devised that use as indices of response increases in the thyrotropin (TSH) concentration of incubation media following exposure of anterior pituitary tissue to TRH *in vitro* or increases in plasma TSH concentrations following *in vivo* administration of TRH (Bowers and Schally, 1970). These methods are all relatively insensitive and cumbersome and cannot be used for the measurement of TRH in biologic fluids or tissue. Another

Methods of Hormone Radioimmunoassay, Second Edition
Copyright © 1979 by Academic Press, Inc.
All rights of reproduction in any form reserved. ISBN 0-12-379260-6

problem limiting the measurement of TRH in plasma or tissue is the presence of an enzyme(s) which rapidly destroys the biologic activity of TRH (Redding and Schally, 1969; Nair *et al.*, 1971; Vale *et al.*, 1971b; Bassiri and Utiger, 1972a). Subsequent studies have shown that TRH immunoreactivity is equally readily destroyed by plasma or tissue homogenates (see below).

The availability of synthetic TRH made possible the application of radioimmunoassay methodology to its measurement. Since TRH is a tripeptide, L-(pyro)Glu-L-His-L-prolineamide, and therefore, was considered unlikely to be immunogenic per se, TRH was coupled to bovine serum albumin. Using this material as immunogen, highly specific and sensitive anti-TRH sera have been prepared. The following is a description of the TRH radioimmunoassay developed in this laboratory (Bassiri and Utiger, 1972a).

II. METHOD OF RADIOIMMUNOASSAY

A. Source of Hormone

Synthetic TRH and ^{3}H-TRH of high specific activity are commercially available.

B. Preparation of TRH–Bovine Serum Albumin

TRH is conjugated to bovine serum ablumin (BSA) with bis-diazotized benzidine (BDB). The BDB is prepared by dissolving 0.23 gm benzidine hydrochloride in 45 ml 0.2 N HCl and then adding 0.175 gm NaNO$_2$ in 5.0 ml distilled water (Likhite and Sehon, 1967). The reaction mixture, which immediately becomes orange, is stirred intermittently at 4°C for 60 minutes. One-milliliter aliquots are then quickly frozen in a dry ice–acetone bath and stored at −60°C. BDB stored beyond six months has not been used, although deterioration after prolonged storage has not been documented.

Coupling of TRH to BSA is accomplished by addition of 8.0 mg BDB to 50 mg BSA and 5.0 mg TRH in 10 ml 0.16 M borate, 0.13 M NaCl, pH 9.0. Tracer quantities of ^{3}H-TRH are included in the reaction mixture to allow determination of the quantity of TRH conjugated to BSA. The mixture turns brown immediately after addition of BDB. The reaction is allowed to continue for 2 hours at 5°C and is then dialyzed against 1000 ml water for seven days and 0.15 M NaCl for one day. The final product is analyzed for protein by the method of Lowry *et al.* (1951) and, if ^{3}H-TRH is included, by liquid scintillation counting. Recovery of ^{3}H radioactivity varies from 15 to 25%, indicating that the conjugates contain 29 to 49 μg TRH/mg BSA. The TRH–BSA conjugate does not have thyrotropin-releasing hormone biologic activity (Bassiri and Utiger, 1972a).

C. Preparation of Anti-TRH Serum

For immunization, rabbits are injected in the foot pads (0.5 ml/foot pad) with a total of 0.4 to 0.8 mg TRH–BSA conjugate emulsified in complete Freund's adjuvant. These injections are continued at monthly or bimonthly intervals, and the animals are bled one to two weeks after administration of the immunogen. Detectable antibody may be found after the first or second immunization, but antisera of sufficient potency to allow detection of picogram quantities of TRH have usually been obtained only after six to eight injections and then not regularly.

D. Preparation of ^{125}I-TRH

While ^{3}H-TRH is available, ^{125}I-TRH is preferred for use in the assay because of its higher specific activity, the ease in preparation of samples for counting, and the fact that plasma or tissue does not destroy the immunoreactivity of ^{125}I-TRH (see below). ^{125}I-TRH is prepared by the method of Greenwood *et al.*, (1963) using 1.0 mCi ^{125}I, 5.0 μg TRH, and 175 μg chloramine-T in a final volume of 0.17 ml 0.5 M phosphate, pH 7.5. After reaction for 30 seconds, 240 μg sodium metabisulfite is added and the reaction product purified by gel filtration on a 1.0 × 12 cm column of Sephadex G-10 in 0.05 M phosphate, pH 7.5. The column is prewashed with 0.25% BSA before use. One-milliliter fractions are collected. The ^{125}I-TRH emerges in fractions 5 to 10, whereas unreacted ^{125}I- appears in fractions 15 to 20. The ^{125}I-TRH is diluted four to fivefold with 0.25% BSA, 0.01 M phosphate, 0.15 M NaCl, pH 7.5, and stored at $-5°$C in small aliquots. Calculated specific activity values have ranged from 10 to 100 μCi/μg. Attempts to increase the specific activity by altering the quantity of chloramine-T or TRH used have been unsuccessful. The TRH is iodinated on its histidyl residue, and the product undoubtedly contains TRH with both mono- and diiodohistidyl residues. It is unlikely to contain significant quantities of unlabeled TRH, since incubation with plasma does not increase the proportion of ^{125}I-TRH that binds to anti-TRH serum.

For each radioimmunoassay, ^{125}I-TRH is repurified by gel filtration

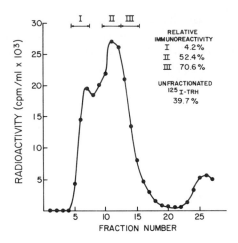

Figure 1.   The pattern of elution of radioactivity after gel filtration (Sephadex G-10) of ^{125}I-TRH. The fractions (1.0 ml) were pooled as indicated. Similar quantities of radioactivity from each fraction and unpurified ^{125}I-TRH were reacted with diluted anti-TRH serum. (Reproduced from Bassiri and Utiger, 1972a, with permission of the publisher.)

on a 1.0×15 cm column of Sephadex G-10 in $0.01\ M$ phosphate, $0.15\ M$ NaCl, pH 7.5 (Figure 1). Two peaks of radioactivity are obtained. The radioactivity of the descending limb of the first peak is the most immunoreactive (Bassiri and Utiger, 1972a). The early fractions of this peak probably contain aggregated ^{125}I-TRH and are clearly less immunoreactive. Only fresh material from the descending limb of this peak is used in the radioimmunoassay, thus allowing greater dilution of the anti-TRH serum and, therefore, enhanced assay sensitivity.

E. Assay Procedure

For the TRH assay, reaction mixtures containing 100 μl repurified ^{125}I-TRH (4–8000 cpm), 100 μl of unlabeled TRH (2.0–200 pg) or other substances to be assayed, 100 μl anti-TRH serum (diluted so that 40–50% of ^{125}I-TRH is bound in the absence of unlabeled TRH) and 100 μl buffer are prepared. The assay buffer is 0.25% BSA, $0.01\ M$ phosphate, $0.15\ M$ NaCl, pH 7.5. After 24 hours at 5°C, goat anti-rabbit IgG is added. Twenty-four hours later, 1.5 ml $0.01\ M$ phosphate, $0.15\ M$ NaCl, pH 7.5, is added, the tubes centrifuged for 45 minutes at 2000 rpm, and the precipitate radioactivity determined. With some anti-TRH sera, longer reaction times result in greater ^{125}I-TRH binding; the optimal incubation time must be determined for each anti-TRH serum. The sensitivity of the assay is currently 5 pg TRH.

F. Specificity of the TRH Radioimmunoassay

Anti-TRH sera prepared in this and other laboratories by immunization with TRH–BSA conjugates have proved to be quite specific, most TRH analogs, TRH constituent amino acids, or other hypothalamic peptides being minimally (<1.0%) or not at all reactive (Bassiri and Utiger, 1972a,b; Jackson and Reichlin, 1974b; Saito *et al.*, 1975; Eskay *et al.*, 1976). L-(Pyro)Glu-D-His-L-prolineamide (LDL-TRH) had 1.08% of the reactivity of TRH; this analog cross-reacted to the extent of 25% with an anti-TRH serum prepared by Eskay *et al.* (1976). They also found substantial cross-reaction with L-(pyro)Glu-L-His-hyp-NH$_2$ (40%) and L-(pyro)Glu-L-His-azetidine carboxamide (24%) as well. These synthetic materials have not been tested in this laboratory. Recently we have found that L-(pyro)Glu-L-(N-^{3im}methyl)His-L-prolineamide (3-methyl-TRH) had 25 to 60% of the reactivity of TRH in tests with several anti-TRH sera. This compound is remarkable in that it is the only presently known TRH analog that has greater biologic potency, both *in vivo* and *in vitro*, than TRH (Vale *et al.*, 1971a). Antisera which react with TRH can also be prepared by conjugation of L-(pyro)Glu-L-His-proline to BSA, but such antisera are less specific and do not react well with ^{125}I-TRH (Visser *et al.*, 1974). Anti-TRH sera do contain antibody to BSA, a fact which can easily be demonstrated by immunodiffusion techniques, but BSA does not inhibit binding of ^{125}I-TRH in such sera.

III. ASSAY AND INACTIVATION OF TRH IN BIOLOGIC FLUIDS AND TISSUE

As experience with TRH radioimmunoassays has increased, it has become apparent that their applicability to the measurement of TRH in biologic fluids or tissue is limited. There are several reasons for this. First, the concentration of TRH in plasma, urine, and cerebrospinal fluid appears to be near or below the sensitivity of the assays. Second, these materials often nonspecifically inhibit the binding of ^{125}I-TRH to anti-TRH serum. Finally, plasma and tissue rapidly destroy TRH immunologic, as well as biologic, activity. Destruction of TRH by urine is much slower, and cerebrospinal fluid is only minimally active in this regard. Since each of these materials poses different problems in the TRH radioimmunoassay, they will be considered separately.

A. Plasma or Serum

Inactivation of TRH immunoreactivity by plasma or serum at 37°C is rapid, occurring at rate of 5.0% or more per minute *in vitro* (Figure 2) (Bassiri and Utiger, 1972b; Utiger and Bassiri, 1973). Similar results have been obtained by other investigators (May and Donabedian, 1973; Jeffcoate and White, 1974; Eskay *et al.*, 1976). This reaction has been extensively studied and has the characteristics outlined in Table I (Bassiri and Utiger, 1972b; Utiger and Bassiri, 1973). It has been

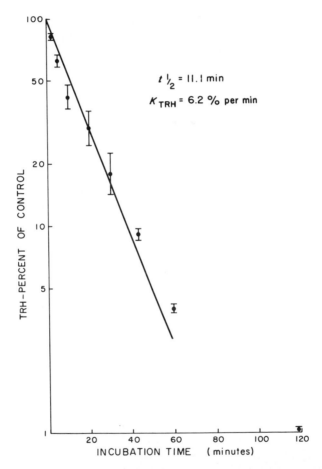

$t\,\tfrac{1}{2}$ = 11.1 min

K_{TRH} = 6.2 % per min

Figure 2.   Destruction of TRH by incubation with plasma. TRH (2 μg) was incubated in 1.0 ml plasma and aliquots removed for TRH assay at the times indicated. Note the log scale on the vertical axis. The vertical bars indicate ± SEM. Similar rates of TRH destruction have been found with TRH concentrations of 40 and 2.0 ng/ml.

Table I   Some Characteristics of the Human Plasma TRH
Inactivator(s)

1. Disappears during prolonged storage of plasma
2. Destroyed by heating at 60°C
3. Destroyed by exposure to acid (pH 3.0) or alkali (pH 10.0)
4. Nondialyzable
5. Excluded from Sephadex G-100
6. Retained by XM-3000 ultrafilter
7. Not dependent on endogenous serum T4 or T3 concentrations

proposed that the inactivation of TRH results from its deamidation (Nair *et al.*, 1971), but this could not be confirmed by Visser *et al.* (1975). Destruction of TRH by plasma can be inhibited by 2,3-dimercaptopropanol (BAL), benzamidine, 8-hydroxyquinoline, some poorly immunoreactive TRH analogs, and ethyl-*p*-(6-guanidino-hexanoyloxy)benzoate methanesulfonate (May and Donabedian, 1973; Jeffcoate and White, 1974; Utiger and Bassiri, 1973; Saito *et al.*, 1975; Eskay *et al.*, 1976). However, none of these compounds is fully effective, their inhibitory effect may be transient, and, in the concentrations required, several nonspecifically inhibit ^{125}I-TRH binding to anti-TRH serum (Bassiri and Utiger, 1973; Eskay *et al.*, 1976). TRH is not destroyed by blood which has been frozen and thawed (Eskay *et al.*, 1976). Agents which more effectively inhibit TRH degradation by plasma are clearly needed, since it is apparent that anything less than immediate inhibition of TRH destruction by blood or plasma *in vitro* is likely to result in underestimation of endogenous plasma TRH concentrations.

Several methods for the extraction and concentration of TRH from plasma have been described. Simple extraction with 1.5 to 3.0 volumes of methanol or ethanol results in recovery of about 70 to 80% of added TRH in the dried extracts, but little concentration can be achieved. TRH has been found in some human and rat plasma samples using such methods (Jackson and Reichlin, 1974a; Saito *et al.*, 1975; Eskay *et al.*, 1976). A procedure whereby TRH in plasma is adsorbed to charcoal and then eluted with ethanol was described by Oliver *et al.* (1974a). Recovery of TRH added *in vitro* was 59.7%, and endogenous human plasma TRH concentrations ranging from 7.0 to 33 pg/ml were reported. There is reason to doubt, however, that the immunoreactivity in these several types of extracts is indeed TRH, since it is not clear in these reports what steps were taken to prevent *in vitro* TRH destruction before extraction, and data further confirming that the immunoreactivity is indeed TRH are lacking (see below). Affinity chromatography has also been used to extract and concentrate TRH from immediately prepared blood or plasma extracts (Montoya *et al.*, 1975; Emerson and Utiger, 1975). These methods result in substantial purification and concentration of TRH, but they are cumbersome and recovery is incomplete. Using such methods, Montoya *et al.* (1975) reported normal rat blood TRH concentrations of 40 pg/ml; Emerson and Utiger (1975) found normal rat plasma TRH concentrations of 7.0 to 30 pg/ml. Similar concentrations were found in hypo- and hyperthyroid rats. These methods have not as yet been applied to the measurement of plasma TRH in the human.

Preparation of anti-TRH-Sepharose conjugates was done by the following method. Fifty-six mg of anti-TRH IgG dissolved in 2.0 ml 0.2 *M* NaHCO$_3$, pH 9.0 was incubated with 200 ml 0.2 *M* sodium citrate, pH 6.5 and 20 ml activated Sepharose 4B (activated with 6.0 gm cyanogen bromide and washed with 1500 ml 0.2 *M* sodium citrate, pH 6.5) overnight at 5°C. The material was transferred to a 2 × 10 cm column and the buffer collected in 10 ml fractions. Since the buffer contained no material absorbing at 280 nm and bound no labeled ^{125}I-TRH, it was concluded that the conjugation of anti-TRH to Sepharose was complete. Rat plasma samples (20–30 ml) were extracted with two volumes of methanol. After centrifugation, the supernatants were dried in air at 60°C overnight. The extracts were dissolved in half the initial volume of 0.01 *M* phosphate, 0.15 *M* NaCl, pH 7.5, and applied to the 1.0 ml anti-TRH-sepharose columns at 20°C. The columns were washed with 5.0 ml buffer, and TRH was eluted with 8.0 ml 1.5 *M* acetic acid into vials containing 1.0 ml 0.25% BSA. The samples were lyophilized and dissolved in 1.0 ml water for radioimmunoassay. The affinity columns can be regenerated by washing with 20 ml 1.5 *M* acetic acid and a large volume of buffer (Emerson and Utiger, 1975).

B. Urine

Unlike plasma, urine destroys TRH much more slowly (Bassiri and Utiger, 1973; Saito *et al.*, 1975). Occasional reports have described the detection of endogenous TRH in untreated urine (Jackson and Reichlin, 1974a), but there is reason to doubt that the material being measured is indeed TRH. In our experience, urine nonspecifically inhibits ^{125}I-TRH binding to anti-TRH serum, since the effect of individual urine samples in the TRH radioimmunoassay varies greatly and markedly different apparent TRH values in the same urine samples are obtained when different anti-TRH sera are used in the assay. Furthermore, urine TRH immunoreactivity is not abolished by incubation of urine with plasma using conditions in which synthetic TRH immunoreactivity is readily destroyed, its chromatographic behavior differs from that of TRH, and its effect in the radioimmunoassay is abolished by incubation with urease (Jeffcoate and White, 1975; Vagenakis *et al.*, 1975). Charcoal–ethanol extracts of urine have also been reported to contain TRH (Oliver *et al.*, 1974a; Saito *et al.*, 1975), but the TRH immunoreactivity in similar extracts could not be destroyed by incubation with plasma (Vagenakis *et al.*, 1975). Thus, there is reason to doubt the validity of the reported measurements of endogenous urinary TRH concentrations.

C. Cerebrospinal Fluid

Cerebrospinal fluid only slowly inactivates TRH immunologic activity, even at 37°C (Shambaugh *et al.*, 1975). Several reports have described the detection of TRH immunoreactivity in spinal fluid or extracts of spinal fluid (Oliver *et al.*, 1974b; Shambaugh *et al.*, 1975). In neither of these reports were data included establishing that the immunoreactivity found was indeed TRH (see below).

D. Tissue

Homogenates of many tissues destroy TRH biologic and immunoreactivity (Redding and Schally, 1969; Bassiri and Utiger, 1974; Griffiths *et al.*, 1975), and the rate of TRH destruction by such homogenates is comparable to that occurring in plasma.

When brain tissue is quickly frozen and/or extracted with methanol (homogenization in 0.01 M phosphate, 0.15 M NaCl, pH 7.5, and extracted with 5 volumes of methanol), the extracts dried and then redissolved in aqueous buffer for radioimmunoassay, TRH can be readily detected in the hypothalamus and many other regions of the brain (Winokur and Utiger, 1974; Jackson and Reichlin, 1974b; Oliver *et al.*, 1974c). Recovery of TRH added to neural tissue homogenates subsequently extracted in this way is excellent (89.0 to 103.8%) (Winokur and Utiger, 1974). That the material in these extracts is indeed TRH is indicated by its immunologic similarity to TRH, its chromatographic similarity to TRH, its susceptibility to destruction by incubation with plasma, and by biologic assay studies. Methanol extracts of neural tissue do not destroy TRH. TRH has also been identified in nonneural tissue, i.e. gut. Subcellular fractionation studies indicate that TRH in neural tissue is concentrated in synaptosomes (Barnea *et al.*, 1975; Winokur *et al.*, 1976). It is of interest that incubation of brain homoge-

Table II   Criteria for the Recovery and Identification of TRH in Biologic Fluids and Tissue

---
1.   Dose responsiveness in the TRH radioimmunoassay
2.   Recovery of synthetic TRH by the extraction–concentration method used
3.   Physiochemical similarity to synthetic TRH
4.   Destruction by plasma
5.   Biologic activity
6.   Physiologic validation (?)

---

nates at 37°C results in little loss of endogenous TRH, whereas TRH added *in vitro* is rapidly destroyed (Winokur *et al.*, 1976). These results indicate that the synaptosomal localization of endogenous TRH protects it from destruction. All of these data have suggested a neurotransmitter, as well as releasing hormone, function for TRH.

IV. CONCLUSIONS

These data indicate that there are many problems in the determination of TRH concentrations in biologic fluids. A variety of methods have been devised to circumvent these problems, but their validity has not been rigorously defined. Some criteria that should be met to establish that the material in biologic materials and extracts and/or concentrates of them are listed in Table II. These criteria, except that of physiologic validation, have been adequately fulfilled only in regard to the TRH immunoreactivity in extracts of homogenates and subcellular fractions of neural tissue. What data may constitute physiologic validation of TRH results is unclear at this time.

REFERENCES

Barnea, A., Ben-Jonathan, N., Colston, C., Johnston, J., and Porter, J. C. (1975). Differential subcellular compartmentalization of thyrotropin releasing hormone (TRH) and gonadotropin releasing hormone (LRH) in hypothalamic tissue. *Proc. Natl. Acad. Sci. U.S.A.* **72**, 3153–3157.

Bassiri, R. M., and Utiger, R. D. (1972a). The preparation and specificity of antibody to thyrotropin releasing hormone. *Endocrinology* **90**, 722–727.

Bassiri, R. M., and Utiger, R. D. (1972b). Serum inactivation of the immunological and biological activity of thyrotropin-releasing hormone (TRH). *Endocrinology* **91**, 657–664.

Bassiri, R. M., and Utiger, R. D. (1973). Metabolism and excretion of exogenous thyrotropin-releasing hormone in humans. *J. Clin. Invest.* **52**, 1616–1619.

Bassiri, R. M., and Utiger, R. D. (1974). Thyrotropin-releasing hormone in the hypothalamus of the rat. *Endocrinology* **94**, 188–197.

Boler, J., Enzmann, F., Folkers, K., Bowers, C. Y., and Schally, A. V. (1969). The identity of chemical and hormonal properties of the thyrotropin releasing hormone and pyroglutamyl-histidyl-proline amide. *Biochem. Biophys. Res. Commun.* **37**, 705–710.

Bowers, C. Y., and Schally, A. V. (1970). Assay of thyrotropin-releasing hormone. In "Hypothalamic Hypophysiotropic Hormones" (J. Meites, ed.), pp. 74–89. Williams & Wilkins, Baltimore, Maryland.

Burgus, R., Dunn, T., Desiderio, D., and Guillemin, R. (1969). Structure moléculaire du facteur hypothalamique hypophysiotrope TRH d'origine ovine: Mise en évidence par spectometrie de masse de la sequence PCA-His-Pro-NH$_2$. *C. R. Hebd. Seances Acad. Sci., Ser. D* **269**, 1870–1874.

Emerson, C. H., and Utiger, R. D. (1975). Plasma thyrotropin-releasing hormone concentration in the rat: Effect of thyroid excess and deficiency and cold exposure. *J. Clin. Invest.* **56**, 1564–1570.

Eskay, R. L., Oliver, C., Warberg, J., and Porter, J. C. (1976). Inhibition of degradation and measurement of immunoreactive thyrotropin-releasing hormone in rat blood and plasma. *Endocrinology* **98**, 269–277.

Greenwood, F. C., Hunter, W. L., and Glover, J. J. (1963). The preparation of ^{131}I-labeled growth hormone of high specific activity. *Biochem. J.* **89**, 114–123.

Griffiths, E. C., Hooper, K. C., Jeffcoate, S. L., and White, N. (1975). Peptidases in the rat hypothalamus inactivating thyrotropin-releasing hormone (TRH). *Acta Endocrinol. (Copenhagen)* **79**, 209–216.

Jackson, I. M. D., and Reichlin, S. (1974a). Thyrotropin releasing hormone (TRH): Distribution in the brain, blood and urine of the rat. *Life Sci.* **14**, 2259–2266.

Jackson, I. M. D., and Reichlin, S. (1974b). Thyrotropin releasing hormone (TRH): Distribution in hypothalamic and extrahypothalamic brain tissues of mammalian and submammalian chordates. *Endocrinology* **95**, 854–859.

Jeffcoate, S. L., and White, N. (1974). Use of benzamidine to prevent the destruction of thyrotropin-releasing hormone (TRH) by blood. *J. Clin. Endocrinol. Metab.* **38**, 155–157.

Jeffcoate, S. L., and White, N. (1975). Clearance and identification of thyrotropin releasing hormone in human urine after intravenous injections. *Clin. Endocrinol.* **4**, 421–426.

Likhite, V., and Sehon, A. (1967). Protein–protein conjugation. *Methods Immunol. Immunochem.* **1**, 150–165.

Lowry, D. H., Roseborough, N. J., Farr, A. L., and Randall, R. J. (1951). Protein measurement with Folin phenol reagent. *J. Biol. Chem.* **193**, 265–271.

May, P., and Donabedian, R. K. (1973). Factors in blood influencing the determination of thyrotropin-releasing hormone. *Clin. Chim. Acta* **46**, 377–382.

Montoya, E., Seibel, M. J., and Wilber, J. F. (1975). Thyrotropin-releasing hormone secretory physiology: Studies by radioimmunoassay and affinity chromatography. *Endocrinology* **96**, 1413–1418.

Nair, R. M. G., Redding, T. W., and Schally, A. V. (1971). Site of inactivation of thyrotropin-releasing hormone by human plasma. *Biochemistry* **4**, 3621–3624.

Oliver, C., Charvet, J. P., Codaccioni, J. L., and Vague, J. (1974a). Radioimmunoassay of thyrotropin-releasing hormone (TRH) in human plasma and urine. *J. Clin. Endocrinol. Metab.* **39**, 406–409.

Oliver, C., Charvet, J. P., Codaccioni, J. L., Vague, J., and Porter, J. C. (1974b). TRH in human CSF. *Lancet* **1**, 873.

Oliver, C., Eskay, R. L., Ben-Jonathan, N., and Porter, J. C. (1974c). Distribution and concentration of TRH in the rat brain. *Endocrinology* **96**, 540–546.

Redding, T. W., and Schally, A. V. (1969). Studies on the inactivation of thyrotropin-releasing hormone (TRH). *Proc. Soc. Exp. Biol. Med.* **131**, 415–420.

Saito, S., Musa, K., Yamamoto, S., Oshima, S., and Funato, T. (1975). Radioimmunoassay of thyrotropin releasing hormone. *Endocrinol. Jpn.* **22**, 303–309.

Shaumbaugh, G. E., III, Wilber, J. F., Montoya, E., Ruder, H., and Blonsky, E. R. (1975). Thyrotropin releasing hormone (TRH): Measurements in human spinal fluid. *J. Clin. Endocrinol. Metab.* **41**, 131–134.

Utiger, R. D., and Bassiri, R. M. (1973). Thyrotropin-releasing hormone (TRH) radioimmunoassay. *In* "Hypothalamic Hypophysiotropic Hormones" (C. Gual and E. Rosemberg, eds.), Int. Congr. Ser. No. 263, pp. 146–150. Excerpta Med Found., Amsterdam.

Vagenakis, A. G., Roti, E., Mannix, J., and Braverman, L. E. (1975). Problems in the measurement of urinary TRH. *J. Clin. Endocrinol. Metab.* **41**, 801–804.

Vale, W., Rivier, J., and Burgus, R. (1971a). Synthetic TRF (thyrotropin-releasing factor) analogues. II. pGlu-N^{3im}Me-His-Pro-NH_2: A synthetic analogue with specific activity greater than that of TRF. *Endocrinology* **89**, 1485–1488.

Vale, W. W., Burgus, R., Dunn, T. F., and Guillemin (1971b). In vitro plasma inactivation of thyrotropin releasing factor (TRF) and related peptides. Its inhibition by various means and by the synthetic dipeptide PCA-His-OMe. *Hormones* **2**, 193–203.

Visser, T. J., Docter, R., and Henneman, G. (1974). Radioimmunoassay of thyrotropin releasing hormone. *Acta Endocrinol. (Copenhagen)* **77**, 417–421.

Visser, T. J., Klootwijk, W., Docter, R., and Henneman, G. (1975). A radioimmunoassay for the measurement of pyroglutamyl-histidyl-proline, proposed thyrotropin releasing hormone metabolite. *J. Clin. Endocrinol. Metab.* **40**, 742–745.

Winokur, A., and Utiger, R. D. (1974). Thyrotropin releasing hormone: Regional distribution in rat brain. *Science* **185**, 265–267.

Winokur, A., Davis, R., and Utiger, R. D. (1976). Subcellular distribution of thyrotropin-releasing hormone (TRH) in rat brain and hypothalamus. *Brain Res.* **120**, 423–434.

4

Gonadotropin-Releasing Hormone

T. M. NETT AND GORDON D. NISWENDER

I. INTRODUCTION

It has been well established that the hypothalamus is responsible for the control of gonadotropin secretion from the anterior pituitary gland. Over the past several years, gonadotropin-releasing activity in hypothalamic extracts has been quantified by bioassay or bioimmunoassay. Only after the chemical characterization as a decapeptide (pyro-Glu-His-Try-Ser-Tyr-Gly-Leu-Arg-Pro-Gly-NH$_2$) and subsequent synthesis of gonadotropin-releasing hormone (GnRH) by Matsuo and co-workers (1971a,b) were sufficient quantities of this substance available for the preparation of conjugates and subsequent immunization of animals necessary for the development of specific antiserum. In recent years, a myriad of radioimmunoassays have been reported for the

57

Methods of Hormone Radioimmunoassay, Second Edition

quantitative analysis of GnRH in tissue extracts and body fluids. Although most investigators utilizing these procedures have reported similar concentrations of GnRH in extracts of hypothalami, wide discrepancies have been observed when radioimmunoassays have been used for quantification of GnRH in serum or plasma.

This chapter describes methodologies for the conjugation of GnRH to bovine serum albumin, the production of antiserum, and for preparation and purification of radioiodinated GnRH. Methods to evaluate specificity of antisera developed for radioimmunoassay and a discussion of some of the problems involved in the measurement of GnRH in tissue extracts and body fluids will also be presented.

II. RADIOIMMUNOASSAY

A. Preparation of GnRH Conjugates

Although some research workers have generated antisera by immunizing animals with native GnRH (Arimura *et al.*, 1973; Kerdelhué *et al.*, 1973; Dermody *et al.*, 1975) most investigators have opted to covalently link this compound to a large carrier molecule for the immunogen. GnRH has been conjugated to carrier molecules via its C-terminal amino acid residue (Nett *et al.*, 1973; Arimura *et al.*, 1975), via its N-terminal amino acid residue (Arimura *et al.*, 1975), via internal amino acid residues (Koch *et al.*, 1973; Nett *et al.*, 1973; Bryce, 1974; Shin and Kracier, 1974; Saito *et al.*, 1975), or to fragments of GnRH (Jeffcoate *et al.*, 1974). When the C-terminal amino acid of GnRH is to be conjugated to a carrier molecule, [Gly^{10}]-GnRH has been used as the starting compound. This compound may be covalently linked to the carrier molecule [usually bovine serum albumin (BSA)] via the mixed anhydride or carbodiimide reactions using procedures similar to those described by Erlanger *et al.* (1957) for conjugation of steroid derivatives to proteins. The conjugation of GnRH to human serum albumin via its N-terminus was recently reported by Arimura *et al.* (1975). In this procedure [Glu^1]-GnRH was coupled to human serum albumin as described by Goodfriend *et al.* (1964).

When GnRH has been coupled to BSA (or other carrier molecules) via internal amino acid residues, the bisdiazotized benzidine reaction is used most commonly (Nett *et al.*, 1973; Bryce, 1974; Shin and Kracier, 1974; Saito *et al.*, 1975). This technique is described in detail in relation to conjugation of TRH (Chapter 3). Although antisera have

been produced successfully when the GnRH-BSA conjugate is produced, as described by these investigators [originally described by
Bassiri and Utiger (1972) for conjugation of TRH to BSA], a brown
insoluble precipitate which cannot be characterized is also produced.
In all probability this conjugate contains GnRH–GnRH and BSA–BSA
linkages as well as GnRH–BSA linkages. Koch *et al.* (1973) improved
this procedure by conjugating *p*-aminophenylacetic acid to GnRH
using the bisdiazotized benzidine reaction which provided derivatives of GnRH (azohistidyl-GnRH-phenylacetic acid and azotyrosyl-
GnRH-phenylacetic acid) that could be conjugated to BSA by the carbodiimide or mixed anhydride reaction. In this technique, 10 μmole
each *p*-aminophenyl acid in 25 μl cold 2 N HCl and sodium nitrate in
25 μl cold water were incubated at 4°C for eight minutes, after which
75 μmole $NaHCO_3$ in 150 μl water and 11.8 mg (10 μmole) GnRH in
90 μl 60% aqueous N,N'-dimethylformamide containing 20 μmole
$NaHCO_3$ are added. The reaction is allowed to proceed for 12 hours at
4°C, during which time an orange-brown color develops. The product
is purified by acidification to pH 2 with 2 N HCl and extracted several
times with two volumes of ether. The aqueous phase is neutralized by
addition of 0.5 M $NaHCO_3$ for conjugation to BSA. This procedure
yields a more soluble product, and there is less likelihood that
GnRH–GnRH and BSA–BSA linkages will be formed. In addition,
antisera formed against GnRH conjugated to BSA through internal
amino acid residues are less likely to cross-react with fragments of
GnRH than antisera produced in response to GnRH conjugated to
BSA through terminal amino acid residues (Koch *et al.*, 1973; Nett *et
al.*, 1973).

B. Immunization

In general, classical immunization techniques have been used to
produce antisera to GnRH. That is, GnRH, or a GnRH–protein conjugate, is emulsified in complete Freund's adjuvant and injected into
rabbits, rats, or sheep. Most investigators have boosted the immunized
animals at approximately monthly intervals and obtained antibodies
to GnRH in two to six months. Continued immunizations have resulted in increased titers in most instances. Antisera to GnRH usable
at final dilutions in excess of 1 : 100,000 have been obtained in some
laboratories. At present there is no good evidence that a particular
species or immunization scheme provides superior antisera, since usable antibodies have been obtained using a number of different procedures. Our antisera were raised in rabbits immunized intradermally

on the back with 0.2 to 1.0 mg of conjugate in complete Freund's adjuvant; the animals were boosted at monthly intervals by subcutaneous administration of the conjugate in incomplete adjuvant.

C. Radioiodination of GnRH

Most investigators have employed a modification of the chloramine-T procedure (Greenwood *et al.*, 1963) to radioiodinate GnRH. This procedure results in an efficient radioiodination, but can destroy both the biologic and immunologic activity of the GnRH molecule. To overcome this difficulty, concentrations of chloramine-T and reaction times have been decreased (2.5 μg GnRH, 1.0 mCi ^{125}I; 20 μg chloramine-T in 0.5 M phosphate, pH 7.0 for 15 seconds followed by 40 μg sodium metabisulfite) (Nett *et al.*, 1973). These modifications have resulted in preparations of radioiodinated GnRH retaining very high levels of immunoreactivity (i.e., more than 90% of the radioactivity in GnRH can be precipitated in the presence of excess antiserum). However, few investigators have prepared radioiodinated GnRH by the chloramine-T procedure that is biologically active. In fact, radioiodination procedures that employ high oxidative potential can oxidize the tryptophanyl residues of protein molecules (Alexander, 1973), and this may lead to the loss of biologic and immunologic activity of GnRH. Therefore, methods to radioiodinate GnRH that employ a low oxidation potential have been developed. Miyachi *et al.* (1973) radioiodinated GnRH using the lactoperoxidase–glucose oxidase technique. This technique resulted in a radioiodinated GnRH which retained a high degree of biologic activity and which was capable of binding to membrane fractions of adenohypophyseal cells (Spona, 1973). In our laboratory, 3.0 μg GnRH in 50 μl 0.1 M phosphate buffer, pH 7.1, 1.0 μl (1.0 mg/ml) lactoperoxidase (Sigma Chemical Co., 46 U/mg), and 1.5–2.0 mCi ^{125}I are added to a stoppered reaction vial. Hydrogen peroxide (20 ng) is added via a 25-gauge needle, and the reaction is allowed to proceed for five minutes at 0°C. The reaction is terminated by addition of 200 μl 0.1 M borate buffer, pH 9.2, containing 0.1% gelatin.

Most investigators have separated free radioiodide from radioiodinated GnRH using columns of Sephadex G-10 or G-25. When Sephadex G-10 is used to purify radioiodinated GnRH, the radioactive hormone is eluted prior to the salt peak. However, if a 0.6 × 20 cm column of Sephadex G-25 in 0.01 M phosphate-buffered saline containing 0.1% gelatin is used for purification, radioiodinated GnRH is eluted from the column (15–19 ml) after the salt peak (10–13 ml), due to absorption of GnRH to the beads of Sephadex G-25. Neither of these methods are capable of routinely separating nonradioactive GnRH from monoiodinated or diiodinated GnRH. Therefore, the specific activity of the radioiodinated preparation is dependent upon the quantity of nonradioiodinated GnRH eluted from the Sephadex column coincident with radioiodinated GnRH. Arimura *et al.* (1973) have utilized columns of carboxymethyl cellulose and eluted with buffers of different ionic strengths to purify radioiodinated GnRH. Using this procedure, free radioiodide was eluted from the column in the void volume using 0.002 *M* ammonium acetate buffer (pH 4.6). An unidentified peak of radioactivity was observed in the initial fractions after the column was eluted with 0.1 *N* ammonium acetate buffer (pH 4.6). This was followed by the elution of a broad peak of radioactivity which contained the radioiodinated GnRH (specific activity $\simeq$ 325 μCi/μg). Miyachi *et al.* (1973) utilized electrophoresis on polyacrylamide gels to purify products after the enzymatic radioiodination of GnRH. These investigators showed that radioiodinated GnRH was separated from nonradioactive GnRH by electrophoresis. It seems equally important to separate monoiodo-GnRH from diiodo-GnRH, since it has been reported that diiodination of tyrosyl residues may induce a structural disorganization in small peptides resulting in reduced sensitivity in radioimmunoassays (Gondolfi *et al.*, 1971).

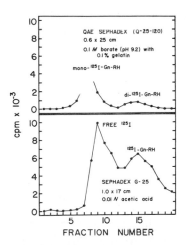

Figure 1.   Purification of radioiodinated GnRH by chromatography on columns of QAE Sephadex (upper panel) or Sephadex G-25 (lower panel). Nonradioactive GnRH elutes in fractions 3–5 on the QAE Sephadex column and free ^{125}I is retained on the column. Monoiodo-GnRH, diiodo-GnRH, and nonradioactive GnRH elute coincidentally from the Sephadex G-25 column under the conditions shown in the figure.

We have recently developed a method to purify radioiodinated GnRH which is very simple and efficient. The radioiodinated GnRH is layered onto a column of QAE Sephadex Q-25 (0.6 × 25 cm) which has been equilibrated with 0.1 M borate buffer (pH 9.2) containing 0.1% gelatin. The column is eluted with 1.0-ml fractions of the same buffer (Figure 1). Nonradioiodinated GnRH passes through the column in the void volume; monoiodinated GnRH is eluted from the column next, followed by diiodinated GnRH. Free iodide is not eluted from the column in the first 50 ml. This procedure allows preparation of radioiodinated GnRH with maximal specific activity (1380 μCi/μg for monoiodo-GnRH and 2760 μCi/μg for diiodo-GnRH). However, some antisera do not bind diiodo-GnRH as readily as monoiodo-GnRH. Therefore, this form of radioiodinated GnRH may not necessarily be useful for increasing the sensitivity of a radioimmunoassay (Table I).

D. Specificity of Antisera to GnRH

Essentially all antisera produced in response to an immunogenic challenge against GnRH (or conjugates of GnRH) are specific with respect to other substances produced within the hypothalamus. However, different antisera exhibit variable degrees of reactivities with analogs or fragments of GnRH. In general, the degree of cross-reaction appears to depend upon (1) the site through which GnRH is conjugated to carrier proteins, (2) whether intact GnRH or a fragment of the molecule is used as immunogen, and (3) the response of individual

Table I   Binding of Radioiodinated GnRH to Antisera, Effect of Monoiodo-GnRH and Diiodo-GnRH on Sensitivity

	Antiserum R-31[a]		Antiserum R-42[b]	
	Monoiodo-GnRH[c]	Diiodo-GnRH[d]	Monoiodo-GnRH	Diiodo-GnRH
GnRH Bound (pg)	1.99	0.53	2.13	0.39
Sensitivity[e]	24.5	28.4	5.3	5.8

[a] Antiserum R-31 was used at a final dilution of 1:4000.
[b] Antiserum R-42 was used at a final dilution of 1:500,000.
[c] 6.8 pg monoiodinated GnRH was added to each tube.
[d] 6.8 pg diiodinated GnRH was added to each tube.
[e] Sensitivity was defined as the quantity (pg) of GnRH necessary to decrease the binding of radioiodinated GnRH to antibody by 50%.

animals to the immunogenic challenge. Table II summarizes available data concerning cross-reactivities of antisera to GnRH. It is apparent that if one wants to produce antisera having specificity for the C-terminal end of GnRH, then GnRH conjugated to a carrier molecule via internal amino acid residues or via the N-terminus should be used as the immunogen. Conversely, if antisera having specificity for the N-terminus of GnRH are desired, then GnRH conjugated to a carrier molecule via internal amino acids or via the C-terminal end should be used as the immunogen. Antisera possessing the highest specificity, with respect to fragments of GnRH, have been produced when GnRH conjugated to a carrier molecule via internal amino acid residues was used as the immunogen.

E. Assay Procedures

The procedures used for quantification of GnRH in serum and tissue extracts are as numerous as the laboratories that have developed radioimmunoassays for this substance. The following is a description of the procedure used routinely in our laboratory and which should be adaptable to all antisera. Standards, tissue extracts, or serum extracts are added to 12×75 mm assay tubes and diluted to $500\ \mu l$ with $0.01\ M$ phosphate-buffered saline ($0.14\ M$, pH 7.0) containing 0.1% gelatin (gel-PBS). Two hundred microliters of antibody (1 : 100,000) diluted appropriately with 1 : 400 normal rabbit serum in $0.05\ M$ EDTA–PBS is added to each assay tube in conjunction with approximately 6.0 pg monoiodo-GnRH. The reactants are incubated at 4°C for 24 hours and $200\ \mu l$ of appropriately diluted anti-rabbit γ-globulin are added to each tube. After 72 hours of incubation at 4°C, GnRH–antibody complexes are separated from free GnRH by centrifugation. The supernatants are decanted and the precipitates are counted in an automatic gamma spectrometer. We have found this method to be satisfactory for analysis of GnRH using six different antisera. However, it has been possible to improve the sensitivity of the GnRH assay approximately fourfold by incubating samples or standard with the antisera for 24 hours prior to the addition of radioiodinated GnRH (Figure 2). The increased sensitivity has been necessary only when trying to quantify samples containing less than 20 pg of GnRH. Arimura et al. (1973) developed an extremely sensitive radioimmunoassay for GnRH utilizing an antiserum which demonstrated paradoxical binding. In this assay, the addition of small amounts of unlabeled antigen enhanced (rather than inhibited) the binding of radioiodinated antigen to the antiserum (Matsukura et al., 1971). However, most antisera do not

Table II   Specificity of Antisera to GnRH

Compound	1^a	2^b	3^c
pGlu-His-Trp-Ser-Tyr-Gly-Leu-Arg-Pro- Gly-NH$_2$	1.000	1.000	1.000
pGlu ——————————— Gly-COOH	0.006	1.000	
pGlu ——————————— Gly-OCH$_3$	0.003	0.833	
ZPro ——————————— Gly-NH$_2$	<0.001	0.026	
ZSer ——————————— Gly-NH$_2$	0.700		0.557
pGlu ——————————— Gly-NHCH$_3$	0.005	0.998	
dpGlu ——————————— Gly-NH$_2$	0.015	0.042	
pGlu ——————————— Gly-Tyr-OH	<0.001	0.754	
pGlu ——————————— Pro-β-Ala-NH$_2$	0.100	0.738	
pGlu —— Phe ——————————— Gly-NH$_2$	0.011	0.025	
pGlu-Arg ——————————— Gly-NH$_2$	0.016	0.021	
pGlu ——————— Ser ——————————— Gly-NH$_2$	0.005	0.181	
pGlu ——————————— Pro-ethylamide	<0.001		<0.001
pGlu ——————— Ala ——————————— Gly-NH$_2$	0.710		0.979
pGlu ——————————— Leu —— Gly-NH$_2$	0.690		0.110
pGlu ——————————— Orn —— Gly-NH$_2$	0.533		0.120
homo			
pGlu ——————————— Arg —— Gly-NH$_2$	0.507		0.049
pGlu-Trp-His ——————————— Gly-NH$_2$			
pGlu —— Pro-Trp-Ser-Tyr-Gly-Leu-Arg-Pro-Gly-NH$_2$			
pGlu ——————————— Ser ——————————— Gly-NH$_2$			
pGlu ——————————— Gln —— Gly-NH$_2$			
pGlu ——————————— Pro-Arg-Gly-NH$_2$			
pGlu ——————— Thr ——————————— Gly-NH$_2$			
pGlu ——————— Phe ——————————— Gly-NH$_2$			
pGlu ——————— Ile ——————————— Gly-NH$_2$			
pGlu ——————————— Lys —— Gly-NH$_2$			
pGlu( ) ——————————— Gly-NH$_2$	0.002	0.008	
pGlu ——————————— Pro-OH			
pGlu ——————————— Leu-OH			
pGlu ——————————— Gly-OH	<0.001	0.002	<0.001
pGlu —— Trp-OH	<0.001		<0.001
His ——————————— Gly-NH$_2$	0.038		0.544
Trp ——————————— Gly-NH$_2$	<0.001		0.747
Ser ——————————— Gly-NH$_2$	<0.001		0.511
Try ——————————— Gly-NH$_2$	<0.001		0.486
Gly ——————————— Gly-NH$_2$	<0.001	<0.001	
Leu ——————————— Gly-NH$_2$			
Arg —— Gly-NH$_2$	<0.001		0.200
His ——————————— Leu-OH			
Trp ——————————— Pro-NH$_2$			
Trp ——————————— Pro-OH			
Trp ——————————— Arg-NH$_2$			
Trp ——————————— Leu-OH			
Trp ——————— Gly-OH			
Ser ——————— Leu-OH	<0.001		<0.001

[a] Antiserum produced in response to GnRH conjugated to BSA via tyrosyl or histidyl residues (Nett *et al.*, 1973).

[b] Antiserum produced in response to GnRH conjugated to BSA via Gly^{10} residue (Nett *et al.*, 1973).

[c] Antiserum produced in response to the 3–10-octapeptide of GnRH conjugated to BSA via tryptophanyl residue (Jeffcoate *et al.*, 1974).

[d] Antiserum produced in response to GnRH adsorbed to polyvinylpyrrolidone (Arimura *et al.*, 1973).

[e] Antiserum produced in response to GnRH conjugated to BSA via Gly^{10} residue (Arimura *et al.*, 1975).

			Antisera			
4[d]	5[e]	6[f]	7[g]	8[h]	9[i]	10[j]
1.000	1.000	1.000	1.000	1.000	1.000	1.000
0.600	1.000		<0.001		<0.001	0.002
					0.622	
		0.800				
					0.064	
		<0.001				
		0.140			0.360	
		0.546			<0.001	
		0.585				
		0.565				
					0.120	
					0.840	
					0.071	
					<0.001	
					<0.001	
						0.012
						0.070
						0.064
						0.012
0.104	<0.001		1.000			
0.730	1.000		<0.001			
<0.001	<0.001		<0.001			
<0.001	<0.001	<0.001	<0.001			
<0.001	<0.001	<0.001	<0.001	<0.001		<0.001
0.168	0.150	0.037	1.000		0.833	0.200
0.730	<0.001	<0.001	1.000			0.024
<0.001	<0.001	<0.001	1.000	<0.001		
		<0.001				
						0.018
		<0.001				
<0.001	<0.001		<0.001			
0.130	<0.001		<0.001			
0.008	<0.001		<0.001			
<0.001	<0.001		<0.001			<0.001
<0.001	<0.001		<0.001			
						<0.001
<0.001	<0.001	<0.001	<0.001			

[f] Nature of conjugate unknown (Dahlén et al., 1976).
[g] Antiserum produced in response to GnRH conjugated to BSA via Glu[1] residue (Arimura et al., 1975).
[h] Antiserum produced in response to native GnRH (Kerdelhué et al., 1973).
[i] Antiserum produced in response to GnRH conjugated to BSA via tyrosyl or histidyl residues (Saito et al., 1975).
[j] Antiserum produced in response to GnRH conjugated to BSA via tyrosyl or histidyl residues (Koch et al., 1973).

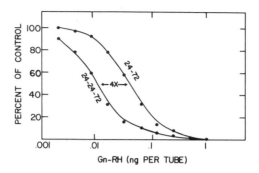

Figure 2.   Standard curves for the radioimmunoassay of GnRH utilizing antiserum R-42. One curve (24–72) was generated by incubating antiserum, radioiodinated GnRH, and the GnRH standard together for 24 hours and then adding precipitating antibody and allowing the incubation to continue for an additional 72 hours. The other curve (24–24–72) was generated by allowing the antiserum and standard GnRH to react for 24 hours, after which radioiodinated GnRH was added and incubation was continued for an additional 24 hours. After the second incubation, precipitating antibody was added and allowed to react for 72 hours. The antibody–antigen complexes were separated from free antigen by centrifugation. The fourfold increase in sensitivity achieved by nonequilibrium assay conditions (24–24–72) approaches the maximum theoretical increase attainable when the dilution of antiserum used for the assay is capable of binding 50% of the radioiodinated GnRH added to the assay tube and the binding of GnRH is irreversible.

demonstrate paradoxical binding, and the utility of such an assay remains to be established.

F. Effects of Serum and Tissue Extracts

Measurement of GnRH in extracts of hypothalamic tissue has been possible with all assays developed to date, and most investigators have observed excellent agreement between levels of GnRH measured by bioassay and those determined by radioimmunoassay. However, this same relationship has not held true for measurements of GnRH in serum. Levels of GnRH in systemic blood, as reported from various laboratories, have ranged from nondetectable or a few picograms per milliliter to several nanograms per milliliter (Table III). Furthermore, most investigators have failed to demonstrate a high degree of correlation between levels of immunoassayable GnRH in systemic blood and release of LH. This has cast doubt on the validity of these assay systems for the measurement of GnRH in systemic blood. In fact, measurement of GnRH in the hypothalamohypophyseal portal circulation of rats and monkeys indicated that levels of GnRH are in the range of 50 to 500 pg/ml. Using radioactive microspheres we have estimated

Table III   Levels of Immunoassayable GnRH-Like Activity in
Peripheral Serum (or Plasma)

Species	Concentration	Reference
Humans	<1.0–9.5 pg/ml	Jeffcoate et al., 1974
	<1.0–17 pg/ml	Arimura et al., 1974
	6.0–27 pg/ml	Clemens et al., 1975
	<10–30 pg/ml	Jonas et al., 1975
	<3.0–50 pg/ml	Saito et al., 1975
	<5.0–40 pg/ml	Rosenblum and Schlaff, 1976
	<20–80 pg/ml	Keye et al., 1973
	<0.1–1.0 ng/ml	Jutisz and Kerdehué, 1974
Rats	<3.0 pg/ml	Dahlén et al., 1976
	<2.0–10 pg/ml	Ojeda et al., 1975
	5.0–18 pg/ml	Arimura et al., 1973
	5.0–20 pg/ml	Park et al., 1976
	20–50 pg/ml	Eskay et al., 1975
	5.0–59 pg/ml	Jeffcoate et al., 1974
	5.0–150 pg/ml	Meyer et al., 1974
	0.3–0.6 ng/ml	Shin et al., 1974
	<0.1–0.8 ng/ml	Jutisz and Kerkehué, 1974
	<10–900 pg/ml	Fraser et al., 1973
	0.2–3.2 ng/ml	Shin and Kracier, 1974
	<0.5–4.5 ng/ml	Kerdehué et al., 1973
Sheep	<10–45 pg/ml	Jonas et al., 1975
	5.0–350 pg/ml	Jeffcoate et al., 1974
	<5.0–365 pg/ml	Nett et al., 1974
	<1.0–6 ng/ml	Jutisz and Kerdehué, 1974
	<0.5–12 ng/ml	Kerdehué et al., 1973
	<10–14,000 pg/ml	Crighton et al., 1973
	<10–16,000 pg/ml	Foster et al., 1976

that portal blood in sheep is diluted approximately 500-fold by the
time it enters the external jugular vein (Nett et al., 1974). Therefore,
maximum levels in the peripheral circulation would not be expected
to exceed 1.0 pg/ml, a level which would test even the most sensitive
assays. Thus, it is unlikely that most reports of measurements of GnRH
in systemic blood are meaningful.

If measurements of GnRH in portal blood are indeed correct, then it
seems clear that levels of GnRH in systemic blood are probably not
measurable using current methodology, unless the GnRH is concentrated prior to analysis. This prompts the question as to the nature of
the factors in serum quantified previously by radioimmunoassay.
Arimura et al. (1973) first reported that plasma from which GnRH has
been removed by treatment with charcoal decreased the binding of

radioiodinated GnRH to antibody. Subsequently, Jonas *et al.* (1975) reported that serum obtained from some sheep contained high levels of immunoassayable GnRH-like activity, but that inhibition curves produced by variable quantities of this serum were not parallel to the standard curve. Furthermore, the factor causing the high degree of inhibition could not be extracted from serum using methanol, whereas synthetic GnRH was readily extractable. More recently de la Cruz and Arimura (1975) fractionated serum by gel filtration chromatography and found that factors eluting in the void volume appeared to prevent the binding of radioiodinated GnRH to antibody. In addition, Barnea and Porter (1975) reported that a macromolecular component present in saline extracts of the hypothalamus, liver, kidney, spleen, and skeletal muscle inhibited the binding of radioiodinated GnRH to antisera. The nature of this macromolecule was not determined.

We have since completed a more detailed study to determine how the method of radioiodination (including the procedures used to purify radioiodinated GnRH), differences between sera, and the affinity of the antiserum used for quantification influence immunoassayable levels of GnRH in unextracted serum (Nett and Adams, 1977). Results from these studies indicate that each of the variables studied had a significant effect on levels of immunoassayable GnRH-like activity in unextracted serum. Radioiodinated GnRH prepared by the chloramine-T and lactoperoxidase procedures were used to measure GnRH in unextracted sera. Levels of immunoassayable GnRH-like activity were lower ($p < 0.05$) when the radioiodinated GnRH prepared by the lactoperoxidase procedure was used for quantification. Furthermore, levels of GnRH-like activity in sera were lower ($p < 0.05$) when monoiodo-GnRH from a lactoperoxidase radioiodination was used for quantification than when diiodo-GnRH was used. Secondly, levels of immunoassayable GnRH-like activity in sera were lower ($p < 0.01$) when a high affinity antiserum was used for quantification than when a low affinity antiserum was used, independent of the method used to prepare radioiodinated GnRH.

Regardless of the affinity of the antiserum and the nature of the radioiodinated preparation, many of the serum samples produced inhibition curves which were not parallel to the standard. The nature of the nonparallelism led us to hypothesize that a binding protein in serum was competing with the antiserum for radioiodinated GnRH and that serum samples having high levels of immunoassayable levels of GnRH-like activity contained more binding protein than samples with low levels of GnRH-like activity. To test this hypothesis, different preparations of radioiodinated GnRH were incubated with 1.0-ml aliquots of pools of sera having high, or low, levels of immunoassayable GnRH-like activity for 30 minutes at room temperature. The sera and GnRH were then fractionated on a 0.8 × 20 cm column of Sephadex G-25. More radioiodinated GnRH appeared in the void volume after incubation with the serum having high levels of immunoassayable GnRH-like activity independent of the radioiodinated preparation. In addition, a greater percentage of the radioactivity eluted in the void volume when GnRH radioiodinated by the chloramine-T procedure (compared to radioiodination by the lactoperoxidase procedure) was incubated with serum. The association of nonradioiodinated GnRH with macromolecular components of serum could not be demonstrated, indicating that a binding protein specific for GnRH is not present in serum.

From these data, we inferred that if the GnRH molecule is exposed to a high oxidation potential during radioiodination, i.e., during radioiodination by the chloramine-T procedure or by the addition of a second atom of radioiodine into the tyrosyl residue (approximately 56 times more energy is required for the formation of diiodotyrosine than monoiodotyrosine) (Mayberry and Hockert, 1970), it appears to develop a stickiness and binds nonspecifically to macromolecular components of serum. When GnRH that was damaged during the radioiodination procedure is used to quantify levels of GnRH in serum by radioimmunoassay, it is likely that an overestimation will be made, since macromolecular components of serum can compete with the antiserum for radioiodinated GnRH. Thus, the binding of radioiodinated GnRH to the antiserum is decreased and may be interpreted falsely as an inhibition produced by endogenous GnRH present in the sample. This may account for the presence of GnRH-like immunoreactivity in macromolecular components of serum reported by de la Cruz and Arimura (1975). In addition, it seems likely that the macromolecular components in tissue extracts reported to cross-react with antisera to GnRH (Barnea and Porter, 1975; Shin and Howitt, 1976) may also be the result of a nonspecific association between radioiodinated GnRH and tissue proteins. Similar problems have been described for direct analysis of steroid hormones in unextracted serum (Niswender and Midgley, 1970).

The actual level of GnRH in serum is more grossly overestimated when an antiserum of low affinity is used for quantification than when an antiserum of high affinity is used. This is due to the fact that the high affinity antiserum can compete more favorably with macromolecular components of serum for the radioiodinated GnRH.

An additional problem has also become apparent. When GnRH is incubated with serum, it loses both its biologic (Sandow *et al.*, 1973) and immunologic activity (Clemens *et al.*, 1975; Jonas *et al.*, 1975; Nett and Adams, 1977). The loss of activity appears to be the result of degradation of GnRH by proteolytic enzymes. That is, it occurs in a time- and temperature-dependent manner, being most rapid at 37°C and least rapid at 0°C (Nett and Adams, 1977). The rate of degradation can be reduced dramatically, but not inhibited totally, by the addition of EDTA, benzamidine or bacitracin to the serum samples.

Proteolytic enzymes in serum or tissue extracts can have at least two effects on the radioimmunoassay of GnRH: (1) Degradation of GnRH in the sample would lead to an underestimation of the actual level of GnRH in the unknown if the antiserum recognizes the entire GnRH molecule, or possibly to an overestimation of the actual quantity of GnRH in the sample if the degraded fragments retain immunologic activity. (2) Degradation of the radioiodinated GnRH would prevent binding of the radioiodinated GnRH to antiserum and would be interpreted falsely as an inhibition of binding of the radioiodinated GnRH (i.e., an overestimation of GnRH in the sample). To overcome these problems with the measurement of GnRH in serum or tissue extracts, it is recommended that GnRH be extracted from the biologic sample in which it is to be measured using a system which eliminates macromolecules (i.e., proteins which bind radioiodinated GnRH nonspecifically and enzymes which degrade GnRH). Recently, systems to extract GnRH from serum have been described; similar systems should be employed for accurate quantification of GnRH in tissue extracts.

G. Extraction of GnRH from Tissue or Serum

In general, acidic extracts of hypothalamic tissue have been made prior to quantification of GnRH by radioimmunoassay. Most investigators have employed 0.1 N hydrochloric acid or 0.1 N acetic acid to extract GnRH from the hypothalamus and other tissues in the central nervous system. This results in a very efficient extraction of GnRH, but many other peptides and proteins are also extracted by this procedure. As discussed above, it seems likely that some of the other proteins may nonspecifically bind the radioiodinated GnRH and result in false high estimates of GnRH in the tissues extract. Therefore, these proteins should be removed prior to final quantification of GnRH in the extract. This may be accomplished by treatment of the extract with ammonium sulfate (to 50% saturation), solvent partitioning, or gel filtration. In fact, one or more of these procedures should be used to purify GnRH for analysis during the validation of the radioimmunoassay. We have found direct extraction of tissue with ethanol or methanol to provide adequate purification of GnRH prior to final quantification utilizing our antisera. It is likely that the degree to which GnRH in tissue extracts will need to be purified prior to final quantification will depend on the affinity of the antiserum and the method used to radioiodinate GnRH. Therefore, individual investigators should determine the reliability of their own antisera with respect to interference by macromolecular components of tissue extracts.

Nonspecific interference in the radioimmunoassay for GnRH in peripheral blood is a particularly difficult problem. It is imperative that macromolecular components of serum (or plasma) that may nonspecifically bind radioiodinated GnRH or degrade GnRH be removed prior to quantification. Once again, the degree of purification required to achieve accurate quantification of GnRH will likely depend upon the specificity and affinity of the antiserum and the method used to prepare radioiodinated GnRH. Some investigators have used methanol (Jonas *et al.*, 1975; Schmidt-Gollwitzer *et al.*, 1977) or acid–ethanol (Arimura *et al.*, 1973) extraction to remove interfering substances. Such treatment appears to provide an adequate purification for analysis of GnRH utilizing some, but not all, antisera to GnRH (de la Cruz and Arimura, 1975). Thus, depending on the antisera and method of radioiodination, it may be necessary to extract GnRH from serum (or plasma) and to further purify the extract by gel filtration or isoelectric focusing before accurate quantification can be achieved. De la Cruz *et al.* (1977) have used Florisil adsorption to remove GnRH from plasma and subsequently extracted GnRH from the Florisil with methanol. This procedure was found to eliminate nonspecific interference by components of plasma even when antisera of low specificity and affinity are used for quantification; it has also been used to concentrate the GnRH from several milliliters of plasma into a small volume so that a more accurate analysis could be achieved. We have found that extraction of serum with methanol removes interfering substances when an antiserum of high affinity is used in conjunction with radioiodinated GnRH prepared by the lactoperoxidase procedure. Serum (1.0 ml) was extracted with ten volumes of methanol. After vortexing 30 seconds and centrifuging at 2300 g for ten minutes, the supernatant was dried at 50°C and reconstituted in 1.0 ml assay buffer. Recovery of labeled GnRH averaged 89.4 ± 2.1%

Once, again we advise individual investigators to determine the sources of nonspecific interference in their radioimmunoassay systems and to take the necessary steps to remove these sources of interference.

III. SUMMARY

The availability of synthetic GnRH has led to the development of radioimmunoassays for GnRH in several laboratories. Antisera have been produced in response to direct immunization with GnRH or after immunization with GnRH (or derivatives) covalently linked to a large carrier molecule. Essentially none of the antisera to GnRH cross-reacts with other hypothalamic or pituitary hormones; however, many antisera to GnRH exhibit some degree of cross-reactivity with fragments of GnRH. The most specific antisera have been produced in response to conjugates in which GnRH is covalently linked to the carrier molecule via internal amino acid residues. Antisera produced in response to such conjugates cross-react minimally with fragments of GnRH.

The procedure used to radioiodinate GnRH should be as mild as possible, and only monoiodo-GnRH should be used for radioimmunoassay. Antisera having a high affinity for GnRH should be used wherever possible. This will improve the sensitivity of the radioimmunoassay and help reduce nonspecific interference by proteins present in serum or tissue extracts.

For accurate quantification of GnRH in biologic samples the following steps must be taken: (1) Degradation of endogenous GnRH during handling and storage of the sample must be prevented. (2) Degradation of endogenous GnRH and of radioiodinated GnRH during the incubation steps of the assay should be avoided. (3) Nonspecific binding of the radioiodinated GnRH by macromolecular components of the sample must be eliminated. Deproteination of samples of whole blood or tissue immediately after collection are recommended.

ACKNOWLEDGMENTS

Some of the studies described herein were supported by NIH Grant HD-07841. The authors are indebted to Abbott Laboratories, North Chicago, Illinois, for supplying the synthetic GnRH used in these studies.

REFERENCES

Alexander, N. M. (1973). Oxidation and oxidative cleavage of tryptophanyl peptide bonds during iodination. *Biochem. Biophys. Res. Commun.* **54**, 614–621.

Arimura, A., Sato, H., Kumasaka, T., Worobec, R. B., Debeljuk, L., Dunn, J., and Schally, A. V. (1973). Production of antiserum to LH-releasing hormone (LH-RH) associated with gonadal atrophy in rabbits: Development of radioimmunoassays for LH-RH. *Endocrinology* **93**, 1092–1103.

Arimura, A., Kastin, A. J., and Schally, A. V. (1974). Immunoreactive LH-releasing hormone in plasma: Mid-cycle elevation in women. *J. Clin. Endocrinol. Metab.* **38**, 510–513.

Arimura, A., Sato, H., Coy, D. H., Worobec, R. B., Schally, A. V., Yanihara, H., Hashimoto, T., Yanihara, C., and Sukura, N. (1975). The antigenic determinant of the LH-releasing hormone for three different antisera. *Acta Endocrinol. (Copenhagen)* **78**, 222–231.

Barnea, A., and Porter, J. C. (1975). Demonstration of a macromolecule cross-reacting with antibodies to luteinizing hormone releasing hormone and its tissue distribution. *Biochem. Biophys. Res. Commun.* **67**, 1346–1352.

Bassiri, R. M., and Utiger, R. D. (1972). The preparation and specificity of antibody to thyrotropin releasing hormone. *Endocrinology* **90**, 722–727.

Bryce, G. F. (1974). Development of a radioimmunoassay for luteotropin releasing hormone (LRH) and thyrotropin releasing hormone (TRH). *Immunochemistry* **11**, 507–511.

Clemens, L. E., Kelch, R. P., Markovs, M., Westhoff, M. H., and Dermody, W. C. (1975). Analysis of the radioimmunoassay for gonadotropin-releasing hormone (GnRH): Studies on the effect of radioiodinated GnRH. *J. Clin. Endocrinol. Metab.* **41**, 1058–1064.

Crighton, D. B., Foster, J. P., Holland, D. T., and Jeffcoate, S. L. (1973). Simultaneous determination of luteinizing hormone and luteinizing hormone releasing hormone in the jugular venous blood of sheep at oestrus. *J. Endocrinol.* **59**, 373–374.

Dahlen, H. G., Voigt, K. H., and Schneider, H. P. G. (1976). C- and N-terminal specific LH-releasing hormone (LRH) radioimmunoassay. *Horm. Metab. Res.* **8**, 61–66.

de la Cruz, K. G., and Arimura, A. (1975). Evidence for the presence of immunoreactive plasma LH-RH which is unrelated to LH-RH decapeptide. *Program 57th Annu. Meet., Am. Endocr. Soc.* Abstract, p. 103.

de la Cruz, K. G., Arimura, A., and Bettendorf, G. (1977). Radioimmunoassay (RIA) for luteinizing hormone releasing hormone (LHRH): Plasma LHRH levels in normal ovarian cycles of women. *Endocrinol., Proc. Vth Int. Congr. Endocrinol., 5th, 1976* Excerpta Med. Found. Int. Congr. Ser. No. 402, Vol. 1Abstract, p. 128.

Dermody, W. C., Becvar, E. A., Windsor, B. L., Wong, A., Vaitkus, J. W., Caple, J. E., and Sakowski, R. (1975). Radioimmunoassay of hypothalamic peptide hormones: Emphasis on validation of a luteinizing hormone-releasing hormone (LH-RH) radioimmunoassay. *In* "Hypothalamic Hormones" (E. S. E. Hafez and J. R. Reel, eds.), pp. 71–82. Ann Arbor Sci. Publ., Ann Arbor, Michigan.

Erlanger, B. F., Borek, F., Beiser, S. M., and Lieberman, S. (1957). Steroid-protein conjugates. I. Preparation and characterization of conjugates of bovine serum albumin with testosterone and with cortisone. *J. Biol. Chem.* **228**, 713–727.

Eskay, R. L., Warberg, J., Mical, R. S., and Porter, J. C. (1975). Prostaglandin E_2-induced release of LHRH into hypophysial portal blood. *Endocrinology* **97**, 816–824.

Foster, J. P., Jeffcoate, S. L., Crighton, D. B., and Holland, D. T. (1976). Luteinizing hormone and luteinizing hormone-releasing hormone-like immunoreactivity in the jugular venous blood of sheep at various stages of the oestrous cycle. *J. Endocrinol.* **68**, 409–417.

Fraser, H. M., Jeffcoate, S. L., Holland, D. T., and Gunn, A. (1973). Detection of luteinizing hormone releasing hormone in the peripheral blood of the rat on the afternoon of pro-oestrus. *J. Endocrinol.* **59**, 375–376.

Gondolfi, C., Malvano, R., and Rosa, U. (1971). Preparation and immunoreactive properties of monoiodinated angiotensin labelled at high specific activity. *Biochim. Biophys. Acta* **251**, 254–261.

Goodfriend, T. L., Levine, L., and Fasman, G. D. (1964). Antibodies to bradykinin and angiotensin: A use of carbodiimides in immunology. *Science* **144**, 1344–1346.

Greenwood, F. C., Hunter, W. M., and Glover, J. S. (1963). The preparation of ^{131}I-labelled human growth hormone of high specific activity. *Biochem. J.* **89**, 114–123.

Jeffcoate, S. L., Fraser, H. M., Holland, D. T., and Gunn, A. (1974). Radioimmunoassay of luteinizing hormone-releasing hormone (LH-RH) in serum from man, sheep and rat. *Acta Endocrinol. (Copenhagen)* **75**, 625–635.

Jonas, H. A., Burger, H. G., Cumming, I. A., Findlay, J. K., and de Kretser, D. M. (1975). Radioimmunoassay for luteinizing hormone-releasing hormone (LH-RH): Its application to the measurement of LH-RH in ovine and human plasma. *Endocrinology* **96**, 384–393.

Jutisz, M., and Kerdelhué, B. (1974). Immunological and biological specificity of luteinizing hormone releasing hormone (LH-RH) and its pattern through the estrous cycle in two species and in the menstrual cycle in women. *In* "Recent Progress in Reproductive Endocrinology" (P. G. Crosignani and V. H. T. James, eds.), pp. 323–343. Academic Press, New York.

Kerdelhué, B., Jutisz, M., Gillessen, D., and Studer, R. D. (1973). Obtention of antisera against a hypothalamic decapeptide (luteinizing hormone/follicle stimulating hormone releasing hormone) which stimulates the release of pituitary gonadotropins and development of its radioimmunoassay. *Biochim. Biophys. Acta* **297**, 540–548.

Keye, W. R., Jr., Kelch, R. P., Niswender, G. D., and Jaffe, R. B. (1973). Quantitation of endogenous and exogenous gonadotropin releasing hormone by radioimmunoassay. *J. Clin. Endocrinol. Metab.* **36**, 1263–1267.

Koch, Y., Wilchek, M., Fridkin, M., Chobsieng, P., Zor, U., and Lindner, H. R. (1973). Production and characterization of an antiserum to synthetic gonadotropin-releasing hormone. *Biochem. Biophys. Res. Commun.* **55**, 616–622.

Matsukura, S., West, C. D., Ichikawa, Y., Jubiz, W., Harada, G., and Tyler, F. H. (1971). A new phenomenon of usefulness in the radioimmunoassay of plasma adrenocorticotropic hormone. *Biochemistry* **77**, 490–500.

Matsuo, H., Baba, Y., Nair, R. M. G., Arimura, A., and Schally, A. V. (1971a). Structure of the porcine LH- and FSH-releasing hormone. I. The proposed amino acid sequence. *Biochem. Biophys. Res. Commun.* **43**, 1334–1339.

Matsuo, H., Arimura, A., Nair, R. M. G., and Schally, A. V. (1971b). Synthesis of the porcine LH- and FSH-releasing hormone by the solid-phase method. *Biochem. Biophys. Res. Commun.* **45**, 822–827.

Mayberry, W. E., and Hockert, T. J. (1970). Kinetics of iodination. VI. Effect of solvent on hydroxyl ionization and iodination of L-tyrosine and 3-iodo-L-tyrosine. *J. Biol. Chem.* **245**, 697–700.

Meyer, M. H., Masken, J. F., Nett, T. M., and Niswender, G. D. (1974). Serum levels of gonadotropin-releasing hormone (Gn-RH) during the estrous cycle and in pentobarbital-treated rats. *Neuroendocrinology* **15**, 32–37.

Miyachi, Y., Chrambach, A., Mecklenburg, R., and Lipsett, M. B. (1973). Preparation and properties of ^{125}I-LH-RH. *Endocrinology* **92**, 1725–1730.

Nett, T. M., and Adams, T. E. (1977). Further studies on the radioimmunoassay of gonadotropin-releasing hormone: Effect of radioiodination, antiserum and unextracted serum on levels of immunoreactivity in serum. *Endocrinology* **101**, 1135–1144.

Nett, T. M., Akbar, A. M., Niswender, G. D., Hedlund, M. T., and White, W. F. (1973). A radioimmunoassay for gonadotropin-releasing hormone (Gn-RH) in serum. *J. Clin. Endocrinol. Metab.* **36**, 880–885.

Nett, T. M., Akbar, A. M., and Niswender, G. D. (1974). Serum levels of luteinizing hormone and gonadotropin-releasing hormone in cycling, castrated and anestrous ewes. *Endocrinology* **94**, 713–718.

Niswender, G. D., and Midgley, A. R., Jr. (1970). Hapten-radioimmunoassay for steroid hormones. *In* "Immunologic Methods in Steroid Determination" (F. G. Perón and B. V. Caldwell, eds.), pp. 149–173. Appleton, New York.

Ojeda, S. R., Wheaton, J. E., and McCann, S. M. (1975). Prostaglandin E_2-induced release of luteinizing hormone-releasing factor (LRF). *Neuroendocrinology* **17**, 283–287.

Park, K. R., Saxena, B. B., and Gandy, H. M. (1976). Specific binding of LH-RH to the anterior pituitary gland during the oestrous cycle in the rat. *Acta Endocrinol. (Copenhagen)* **82**, 62–70.

Rosenblum, N. G., and Schlaff, S. (1976). Gonadotropin-releasing hormone radioimmunoassay and its measurement in normal human plasma, secondary amenorrhea, and postmenopausal syndrome. *Am. J. Obstet. Gynecol.* **124**, 340–347.

Saito, S., Kimitaka, M., Oshima, I., Yamamoto, S., and Funato, T. (1975). Radioimmunoassay for luteinizing hormone releasing hormone in plasma. *Endocrinol. Jpn.* **22**, 247–253.

Sandow, J., Heptner, W., and Vogel, H. G. (1973). Studies on *in vivo* inactivation of synthetic LH-RH. *In* "Hypothalamic Hypophysiotropic Hormones" (C. Gual and E. Rosemberg, eds.), Int. Congr. Ser. No. 263, pp. 64–67. Excerpta Med. Found., Amsterdam.

Schmidt-Gollwitzer, M., Pollow, K., Müller, E., and Nevinny-Stickel, J. (1977). Proof for measurement of endogenous gonadotropin-releasing hormone (Gn-RH) in peripheral serum. *Endocrinol., Proc. Int. Congr. Endocrinol., 5th, 1976* Excerpta Med. Found. Int. Congr. Ser. No. 402, Vol. 1, Abstract, p. 304.

Shin, S. H., and Howitt, C. (1976). Evidence for the presence of a hypothalamic LH-RH binding protein. *Program 58th Annu. Meet., Am. Endocr. Soc.* Abstract, p. 156.

Shin, S. H., and Kracier, J. (1974). LH-RH radioimmunoassay and its applications; evidence of antigenically distinct FSH-RH and a diurnal study of LH-RH and gonadotropins. *Life Sci.* **14**, 281–288.

Shin, S. H., Howitt, C., and Milligan, J. V. (1974). A paradoxical castration effect on LH-RH levels in male rat hypothalamus and serum. *Life Sci.* **14**, 2491–2496.

Spona, J. (1973). LH-RH interaction with the pituitary plasma membrane. *FEBS Lett.* **34**, 24–26.

5

Somatostatin

YOGESH C. PATEL AND SEYMOUR REICHLIN

I. INTRODUCTION

The existence of a growth hormone-inhibiting factor [somatotropin release-inhibiting factor (SRIF)] in fractions of hypothalamic extract was suggested by the studies of Krulich *et al.* (1972). Subsequent studies by Guillemin and colleagues (Rivier *et al.*, 1973; Brazeau *et al.*, 1973; Burgus *et al.*, 1973) led to the isolation and characterization of a cyclic tetradecapeptide from ovine hypothalamic fragments that inhibits the spontaneous secretion of growth hormone (GH) by cul-

77

Methods of Hormone Radioimmunoassay, Second Edition
Copyright © 1979 by Academic Press, Inc.
All rights of reproduction in any form reserved. ISBN 0-12-379260-6

tures of enzymatically dissociated rat anterior pituitary cells and GH secretion in a number of species of animals, including man (see Reichlin *et al.*, 1976, for review). This substance, to which the name somatostatin has been applied, has been shown to possess a wide range of biologic activities which include the inhibition of multiple endocrine and exocrine secretions, e.g., GH, TSH, prolactin, insulin, glucagon, gastrin, secretin, gastric acid, and pancreatic exocrine secretion (Reichlin *et al.*, 1976; Boden *et al.*, 1975). In addition, the peptide has been reported to induce behavioral changes in the rat and to possess an inhibitory action on single neuron units in many parts of the brain (Cohn and Cohn, 1975; Renaud *et al.*, 1975).

The anatomic distribution of SRIF was studied initially by bioassay, with the surprising demonstration of high concentrations of bioactive SRIF not only in the hypothalamus but throughout the extrahypothalamic brain, spinal cord, and in the pancreas (Vale *et al.*, 1975). The availability of specific antibodies led to the development of radioimmunoassays (RIA's) (Arimura *et al.*, 1975a; Patel *et al.*, 1975; Kronheim *et al.*, 1976) and immunohistochemical localization techniques (Pelletier *et al.*, 1975; Dubois, 1975; Polak *et al.*, 1975; Rufener *et al.*, 1975; Hökfelt *et al.*, 1975; Alpert *et al.*, 1976) and confirmed the presence of SRIF-like material throughout the brain and spinal cord, in cerebrospinal fluid, in pancreatic islets, and, in addition, in the gastrointestinal tract (Dubois, 1975; Polak *et al.*, 1975; Rufener *et al.*, 1975; Hökfelt *et al.*, 1975; Brownstein *et al.*, 1975; Arimura *et al.*, 1975a,b; Patel *et al.*, 1977a). These localizations correspond surprisingly well to regions known to be responsive to injected SRIF, suggesting that the hormone may have important physiologic effects in these sites. A physiologic role of circulating SRIF on GH and TSH regulation has already been demonstrated by means of passive immunization studies with anti-SRIF serum in rats (Terry *et al.*, 1976; Arimura *et al.*, 1976; Arimura and Schally, 1976). Furthermore, within the pancreatic islets, striking changes in the immunoassayable SRIF content and in the number of SRIF-producing cells have been observed in experimental diabetes and in human juvenile diabetes, suggesting a possible role of SRIF in the pathogenesis of these disorders (Patel and Weir, 1976; Orci, *et al.*, 1976; Patel *et al.*, 1976; Patel *et al.*, 1977b; Patel *et al.*, 1978).

These reports highlight the growing interest in SRIF and for the need for specific and reliable RIA's for studying its physiology. To date, only a few such assay procedures have been described, a fact which may be related in part to a number of special problems inherent in the assay: (1) Since native somatostatin cannot be satisfactorily iodinated, analogs such as Tyr_1-SRIF must be used for radioiodination. (2) Since SRIF and Tyr_1-SRIF are highly labile in plasma and tissue extracts, precautions must be taken to prevent the proteolytic degradation of the peptides during extraction and in assay.

In this chapter, we present details of a method we have developed for the radioimmunoassay of somatostatin (Patel and Reichlin, 1978) with special emphasis on methodologic studies of SRIF and ^{125}I-Tyr_1-SRIF stability. The technique has been successfully utilized to study tissue concentrations of somatostatin and cerebrospinal fluid somatostatin. The presence of somatostatin in blood and in urine has been suggested by recent studies. However, because of major technical problems, particularly with blood, methods for the assay of blood and urine somatostatin are still in a preliminary stage.

II. MATERIALS

A. Somatostatin and Analogs

Synthetic cyclic somatostatin was obtained from Ayerst Laboratories, Montreal, through the courtesy of Dr. Manfred Götz. Dihydrosomatostatin (linear SRIF) was obtained through the courtesy of Beckman Instruments Inc., California (Dr. Lynnor Marshall). The analog Tyr_1-SRIF was obtained as a gift from Dr. Roger Guillemin, Salk Institute, La Jolla, California, and from Dr. Monroe Glitzer, Merck Research Laboratories, Rahway, New Jersey. All other SRIF analogs were supplied by Dr. Guillemin. Somatostatin, dihydrosomatostatin, and Tyr_1-SRIF may now be purchased commercially also (e.g., Bachem Fine Chemicals, Marina del Rey, California).

H-Ala-Gly-Cys-Lys-Asn-Phe-Phe-Trp-Lys-Thr-Phe-Thr-Ser-Cys-OH
|_____ S — S _____|

B. Hormones Used in Specificity Studies

The peptide hormones used for specificity studies were obtained as follows: synthetic TRH, LHRH, oxytocin, angiotensin I, and angiotensin II from Bachem Fine Chemicals; crystalline porcine glucagon and insulin (mixed porcine and bovine) from Eli Lilly Co., Indianapolis, Indiana; bovine pancreatic polypeptide (BPP) from Dr. R. Chance, Lilly Research Laboratories, Indianapolis, Indiana; gastrin (synthetic human gastrin I) from ICI, Cheshire, England; cholecysto-kinin–pancreozymin (CCK–PKZ) (purified extract of porcine intestinal wall) from Professor J. E. Jorpes, Karolinska Institute, Sweden; synthetic secretin from Schwarz-Mann, Orangeburg, New Jersey; vaso-active intestinal peptide (VIP) (highly purified extract of porcine intestinal wall) from Dr. S. I. Said, Dallas, Texas; synthetic human calcitonin from Dr. Armen Tashjian, Jr., Harvard School of Dental Medicine, Boston, Massachusetts; synthetic substance P and neuro-tensin from Dr. Susan Leeman, Harvard Medical School, Boston, Massachusetts; synthetic 1–24-ACTH (cortrosyn) from Organon Laboratories.

III. METHODS

A. Production of Anti-somatostatin Serum

1. Preparation of Immunogen

Because SRIF is a small molecule which is immunologically indistinguishable among different animal species, and because it is subject to rapid enzymatic destruction both in blood and in tissues, it is necessary to covalently conjugate the peptide to a larger protein for immunization. A satisfactory immunogen can be prepared by conjugating cyclic SRIF to bovine thyroglobulin (TG) (Sigma Chemical Co.) using the coupling agent carbodiimide, which produces a condensation reaction between the free amino and carboxyl groups of proteins (Abraham and Grover, 1971). Thyroglobulin has been found to be a particularly good carrier protein (Skowsky and Fisher, 1972), although other proteins, such as bovine serum albumin (BSA) and human serum globulin, can also be used.

To 50 mg TG in 2.0 ml distilled water add 30 mg CMC [1-cyclohexyl-3-(2-morpholinoethyl)carbodiimide metho-p-toluene sulfonate] (Aldrich Chemical Co.) dissolved in 1.0 ml distilled water; 5.45 mg SRIF in 1.0 ml distilled water containing a trace quantity of ^{125}I-Tyr$_1$-SRIF (see below for details of preparation) is then added dropwise while stirring. The pH of the reaction mixture is adjusted to 5.5 with dilute HCl or NaOH. The solution is kept at room temperature with constant stirring for 24 hours and at the end of this time it will be found to be cloudy. The reaction mixture is dialyzed for 48 hours at room temperature against four liters of distilled water with several changes of the dialysis bath. The dialyzed material is lyophilized and stored at $-20°C$. Under these conditions, the coupling of SRIF to Tg is presumed to occur via the free amino groups on alanine (position 1) or lysine (position 4 or 9) or the free carboxyl group of cystine at the carboxyl-terminus. Assuming that Tyr_1-SRIF and SRIF react identically, the molar ratio of SRIF : TG in the conjugate can be calculated by determining the percent (of total counts added) of ^{125}I-Tyr_1-SRIF remaining in the dialysis bag. We have generally achieved molar ratios of SRIF : TG of the order of 30 : 1.

2. Immunization Procedure

Ten milligrams of the SRIF–TG complex and 30 mg dried tubercle bacilli (Difco) are suspended in 6.0 ml saline, thoroughly emulsified with 6.0 ml complete Freund's adjuvant, and injected into the toepads of six 3.0 -kg male rabbits (1.7 mg conjugate per animal). Each animal also receives 0.5 ml pertussis vaccine subcutaneously with the primary immunization. A series of four booster injections, each consisting of 1.0 mg conjugate per animal, are then administered subcutaneously at two-week intervals. Antibody to somatostatin can be detected by reaction of 10–20 pg ^{125}I-Tyr_1-SRIF with varying quantities of rabbit serum (e.g., 1/100, 1/1000, 1/5000 final dilution) for 24 hours followed by the addition of a potent goat anti-rabbit γ-globulin (for preparation of the incubation mixture see Section III,C). It is important to titrate the second antibody against each dilution of rabbit serum to ensure maximal precipitation of antibody-bound counts. Two of our six rabbits showed detectable antibody within two months following the initial immunization, the titer rising steadily to reach a peak at 12–15 months. Most of the studies reported here were performed with serum obtained from one of these rabbits at a final dilution of 1 : 7000 to 1 : 10,000.

B. Preparation of ^{125}I-Tyr_1-SRIF and Assessment of Stability

Somatostatin cannot be labeled by iodine substitution because it contains neither a tyrosine nor a histidine moiety. For this reason, tyrosinated analogs of somatostatin are used as antigens for iodination. We have obtained maximal binding to our antibody and optimal sensitivity with radioiodinated Tyr_1-SRIF (more recent studies have shown that radioiodinated N-Tyr-SRIF is equivalent in our system). Radioiodinated Tyr_{11}-SRIF can also be used as tracer, although our antibody does not bind this antigen as well as it binds Tyr_1-SRIF or N-Tyr-SRIF (see also Table II).

1. Iodination Procedure

a. Reagents
Tyr$_1$-SRIF
Chloramine-T
Carrier-free ^{125}I (Amersham-Searle or New England Nuclear)
0.5 M PO$_4$ buffer, pH 7.5
BSA
Sephadex G-25 (fine)
Acetic acid

b. Chromatoelectrophoresis. This technique can be used for assessing the degree of iodination of ^{125}I-Tyr$_1$-SRIF and for determining the extent of damage or degradation of ^{125}I-Tyr$_1$-SRIF. Chromatoelectrophoresis can be performed in a variety of ways. For details of the underlying principles, the reader is referred to appropriate publications (e.g., Berson et al., 1956; Landon et al., 1967). We have employed Beckman paper electrophoresis strips (type 5 and S2043 A mgl), a Beckman Model R Spinco paper electrophoresis cell, and 0.05 M PO$_4$ buffer, pH 7.5. Samples (20 μl) are applied along a line 5.0 cm from the cathodal end of the strip. A constant voltage (340 V) is applied, and separation is carried out at 4°C for 90 minutes. At the end of the run, strips are air-dried, cut into 1.0 -cm lengths toward the anode, and the radioactivity counted. Under these conditions, intact ^{125}I-Tyr$_1$-SRIF remains within 1.0 cm of the point of application of the sample, whereas damaged ^{125}I-Tyr$_1$-SRIF migrates as a second peak 5.0–6.0 cm in advance of this. Free ^{125}I moves toward the anode.

Iodination is carried out in 10 × 75 mm (or smaller) disposable glass tubes. To 2.0 μg Tyr$_1$-SRIF dissolved in 5.0 μl 0.05 M PO$_4$ buffer, pH 7.5, is added 10 μl 0.5 M PO$_4$ buffer, pH 7.5, 1.0 mCi ^{125}I (2.0–10 μl depending on concentration), and 2.0 μg chloramine-T (in 2.0 μl water). After agitating for 30 seconds by gentle tapping, the iodination reaction is interrupted by the addition of 100 μl 10% BSA in 0.1 M acetic acid. Sodium metabisulfite is not added in order to avoid the reduction of the disulfide bound of Tyr$_1$-SRIF.

The iodination mixture is fractionated at 4°C on a Sephadex G-25 column (1.0 × 26 cm) equilibrated with 0.1 M acetic acid 0.1% BSA. Twenty drops per fraction (approx. 0.5 ml) are collected and counted for radioactivity in a well-type gamma counter. Three main peaks of radioactivity are obtained, as shown in Figure 1. The first, or void volume, peak (fractions 13–18) consists of iodinated albumin and aggregated ^{125}I-Tyr$_1$-SRIF with poor immunoreactivity. Radioactivity

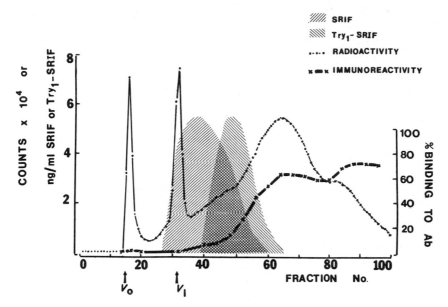

Figure 1.   Elution pattern following purification of iodinated Tyr$_1$-SRIF on Sephadex G-25 and comparison of immunoreactivity of the radioactive peaks. ^{125}I-Tyr$_1$-SRIF elutes as a broad peak in fractions 40–100. The elution profiles of SRIF and uniodinated Tyr$_1$-SRIF measured by radioimmunoassay are shown for comparison. Column conditions: a 1.0 × 26 cm column was eluted with 0.1 M acetic acid–0.1% BSA; 20-drop fractions were collected. [Reproduced from *Endocrinology* (1978), **102**; 523–530.]

from this peak remains either at the origin or migrates with serum albumin on chromatoelectrophoresis. The second sharp peak (fractions 30–35) represents unreated iodide as judged by the migration on chromatoelectrophoresis. ^{125}I-Tyr$_1$-SRIF is retarded by Sephadex (see Section III,B,2) and elutes after the iodide as a broad peak (fractions 40–100) with frequently a small shoulder along the descending slope. From this peak 93–96% of radioactivity remains at the point of application on chromatoelectrophoresis. Excess anti-SRIF antibody binds 80–95% of counts from tubes in this peak. Tubes 82–90 comprising the shoulder (probably diido-Tyr$_1$-SRIF) exhibit the highest antibody binding (Figure 1). However, any of the fractions from the peak along the descending slope of the ^{125}I-Tyr$_1$-SRIF peak (e.g., fractions 65–90) is suitable for use in the assay. These fractions are stored at $-20°$C and used as required for six to eight weeks. ^{125}I-Tyr$_1$-SRIF shows some loss of immunoreactivity with time, but this is small and accompanied by only slight loss of assay sensitivity. When maximal sensitivity is required, however, it is advisable to use freshly prepared ^{125}I-Tyr$_1$-SRIF.

2. Specific Activity of ^{125}I-Tyr$_1$-SRIF

The extent of incorporation of ^{125}I-Tyr$_1$-SRIF is assessed by chromatoelectrophoresis of the iodination mixture and in our hands has ranged from 80–90% for ten consecutive iodinations (Patel and Reichlin, 1978). The mean specific activity calculated by this method was 425 μCi/μg. However, the actual specific activity attained is much higher than this due to the separation of labeled and unlabeled peptide during Sephadex gel filtration. Figure 1 shows the elution profile of ^{125}I-Tyr$_1$-SRIF with respect to Tyr$_1$-SRIF (as measured by RIA) following separate passage through a Sephadex G-25 column. The elution pattern of cyclic SRIF is also shown for comparison. It is clear from this figure that both SRIF and Tyr$_1$-SRIF are retarded by Sephadex and elute after the iodide. Furthermore, cold Tyr$_1$-SRIF elutes in advance of its iodinated counterpart, resulting in marked enhancement of the specific activity of the label.

The reason for the retardation of some peptides (e.g., vasopressin, LHRH, SRIF, Tyr$_1$-SRIF) on Sephadex and other gels is not completely understood but appears to be related to charge (a positive charge favors retardation on the weakly acidic Sephadex matrix) and the presence of certain aromatic amino acids especially tyrosine. Because of the separation of labeled and unlabeled Tyr$_1$-SRIF, specific activities of the order of 1000 μCi/μg have been achieved, which is close to the maximum theoretical specific activity for substitution of one atom of ^{125}I per mole of peptide (~1050 μCi/μg).

3. Stability of ^{125}I-Tyr$_1$-SRIF in BSA, Gelatin, Serum, and Tissue Extracts

One of the major problems attending the use of ^{125}I-Tyr$_1$-SRIF in the radioimmunoassay of SRIF is the marked susceptibility of the label to incubation damage in the presence of serum and tissue extracts. Destruction of the label during incubation results in a reduction in the binding and spuriously high values due to the apparent "displacement." Most iodinated hormones undergo a certain amount of incubation damage which is usually proportional to the concentration of serum in the reaction mixture. In the case of the polypeptide hormones, e.g., hTSH, such damage is generally small and can be corrected to a large extent by the inclusion of hormone-free serum in standard tubes in order to equalize the serum content of standard and unknown tubes. In assay systems in which the labeled hormone is capable of undergoing extensive incubation damage (e.g., ACTH, glucagon), it is necessary to use inhibitors of proteolysis (e.g., Trasylol, benzamidine) and/or to correct for damage by chromatoelectrophoresis. In the experiments that follow, we demonstrate the marked instability of ^{125}I-Tyr$_1$-SRIF in serum and tissue extracts and the measures employed to overcome it.

a. Effect of BSA, Gelatin, and Serum. In this experiment, the stability of ^{125}I-Tyr$_1$-SRIF incubated in 0.1 M PO$_4$ buffer, pH 7.5, and 0.1% crystalline BSA was compared with the stability in gelatin, fraction V–BSA, and dilutions of normal rabbit serum (NRS) in the same buffer at 4°C for 24 hours. Normal rabbit serum was chosen because the radioimmunoassay incubation mixture routinely contains a small quantity of NRS (1/2100 final concentration) as a source of carrier rabbit γ-globulin for optimal precipitation by the second antibody (see Section III,C). Freshly labeled ^{125}I-Tyr$_1$-SRIF (0.1–0.5 mg) was incubated in 1.0 ml of the appropriate solution. Aliquots of the reaction mixture were then diluted, and the concentration of immunoreactive ^{125}I-Tyr$_1$-SRIF was determined by immunoprecipitation (Table I). The

Table I   Immunoreactivity of ^{125}I-Tyr$_1$-SRIF following Incubation in BSA, Gelatin, or NRS[a]

Medium	Immunoreactivity (% buffer control)
Incubation	
0.1 M PO$_4$–0.1% cBSA (buffer)	100
0.1 M PO$_4$–0.1% BSA (fraction V)	86
0.1 M PO$_4$–0.1% gelatin	99
1/10 NRS	4
1/100 NRS	47
1/1000 NRS	86
1/2100 NRS	88
With Trasylol 500 KIU/ml	
1/10 NRS	0
1/100 NRS	57
1/1000 NRS	100
1/2100 NRS	100
After boiling	
1/10 NRS	100
1/100 NRS	95
1/1000 NRS	98
1/2100 NRS	95

[a] Freshly prepared ^{125}I-Tyr$_1$-SRIF was incubated with the above solutions at 4°C for 24 hours. The solutions were diluted 100- to 1000-fold, reacted with anti-SRIF serum, and the counts bound precipitated with an anti-rabbit γ-globulin.

immunoreactivity of ^{125}I-Tyr$_1$-SRIF decreased slightly after a 24-hour incubation with fraction V–BSA compared to crystalline BSA or gelatin. This suggests that fraction V–BSA may be contaminated by traces of serum enzymes capable of degrading ^{125}I-Tyr$_1$-SRIF. Incubation of ^{125}I-Tyr$_1$-SRIF for 24 hours at 4°C in NRS diluted 1/100, 1/1000, and 1/2100 led to 53, 14, and 12% loss of immunoreactivity, respectively, even in the presence of EDTA (Table I). In the presence of Trasylol (Aprotinin, FBA Pharmaceuticals, Inc.), 500 KIU/ml, the immunoreactivity of ^{125}I-Tyr$_1$-SRIF was completely preserved after incubation in 1/1000 and 1/2100 NRS. Trasylol is, thus, of value if antisera of only low titers are available and in double antibody assays such as the present one in which a small quantity of NRS is routinely included in all assay tubes. In the presence of 1/100 dilution of NRS, the use of Trasylol still resulted in 43% loss of ^{125}I-Tyr$_1$-SRIF immunoreactivity (Table I). Boiling the NRS solutions prior to incubation of ^{125}I-Tyr$_1$-SRIF prevented loss of immunoreactivity, suggesting that heat inactivates the enzymes responsible for degrading the label. Additional studies using different concentrations of EDTA (0.01–0.25 M) with and without Trasylol have shown that complete protection against degradation by serum diluted $> 1/1000$ is afforded by incubation in the presence of 0.25 M EDTA; in this concentration Trasylol affords no further protective benefit. Trasylol alone is not as effective in protecting against degradation as it is in combination with low concentrations of EDTA (0.01 M). The combination is as effective as 0.25 M EDTA.

   b. Effect of Tissue Extracts. Rat cerebral cortical extracts were prepared by homogenizing tissue (~150 mg/ml) in PO$_4$ buffer pH 7.5 or 1.0 M acetic acid. ^{125}I-Tyr$_1$-SRIF was incubated with the homogenates at 4°C for 24 hours, and aliquots of the incubation mixture were studied by chromatoelectrophoresis at different times to determine the concentration of intact labeled peptide.

   As shown in Figure 2, ^{125}I-Tyr$_1$-SRIF is rapidly destroyed by cortical extracts at pH 7.5, approximately 50% of the label being lost in five minutes. The label is, however, completely stable in boiled extract (pH 7.5) or in an unboiled acetic acid extract.

   On the basis of the preceding observations, we recommend the use of Trasylol (with 0.01 M EDTA) or 0.25 M EDTA to prevent damage to ^{125}I-Tyr$_1$-SRIF resulting from the normal constituents of the radioimmunoassay incubation mixture, such as BSA and carrier NRS. Neither Trasylol nor EDTA may be required when carrier serum is not used, e.g., in charcoal separation methods (Arimura *et al.*, 1975a).

   During assay of SRIF in tissue extracts, the damaging effect of tissue

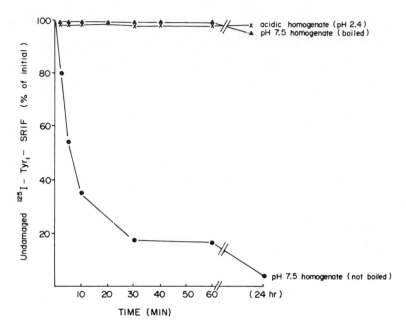

Figure 2. Stability of ^{125}I-Tyr$_1$-SRIF in tissue extracts with and without boiling at pH 7.5 and pH 2.4. The concentration of undamaged and damaged (not shown) ^{125}I-Tyr$_1$-SRIF was assessed by chromatoelectrophoresis.

enzymes on ^{125}I-Tyr$_1$-SRIF can be prevented by prior boiling of tissue extracts. As discussed above, although ^{125}I-Tyr$_1$-SRIF is stable in acidified cortical tissue, it tends to be degraded even at a pH of 2–3 by extracts containing a high concentration of acid proteases, e.g., stomach. Furthermore, the acidic extracts have to be neutralized before assay. For these and other considerations (see also Section V,A,2) we feel it is important to boil all tissue extracts prior to assay. Under these conditions, ^{125}I-Tyr$_1$-SRIF remains stable in the incubation mixture for at least 24 hours showing <10% damage on chromatoelectrophoresis.

C. Assay Procedure

1. Basic Reagents

Assay buffer: 0.1 M PO$_4$, 0.1% BSA (fraction V), 0.1% sodium azide, pH 7.5

NRS diluted 1/300 in 0.05 M EDTA–0.1 M PO$_4$ buffer, pH 7.0 con-

taining   5000   KIU   Trasylol/ml   (NRS–EDTA–PO$_4$–Trasylol)
0.1 M acetic acid, 0.1% BSA

2. Preparation of Standard Solutions

Weigh out approximately 100 μg cyclic somatostatin accurately using an electronic balance. Dissolve in 0.1 M acetic acid, 0.1% BSA to give a stock solution containing 10 μg/ml. Prepare suitable aliquots of this solution (e.g., 0.2 ml), snap-freeze, and store at -20°C. Under these conditions, the stock solution will remain stable for a minimum of six months. Standard solutions for use in the assay are prepared by subdiluting the stock solution in assay buffer to give solutions containing 0–5000 pg/ml.

3. Pipetting of Reagents

Reagents are added to duplicate disposable 10 × 75 mm glass tubes as follows:

1. 100 μl test samples or standard solutions
2. 100 μl anti-SRIF serum diluted 1:1000 in 1/300 NRS–EDTA–PO$_4$–Trasylol solution
3. 100 μl ^{125}I-Tyr$_1$-SRIF diluted in assay buffer to give 5000 cpm or 5.0–10 pg
4. 400 μl assay buffer

Following a period of incubation of 24 hours at 4°C, ^{125}I-Tyr$_1$-SRIF bound to antibody is precipitated by addition of 0.1 ml of an appropriate dilution (in buffer) of a potent goat or sheep anti-rabbit γ-globulin. Each batch of second antibody should be titered for maximal precipitation. The precipitation step requires a further period of incubation of 24 hours at 4°C. At the end of this time, the incubation mixture is diluted by the addition of 2.0 ml of assay buffer. The tubes are then centrifuged at 2000 rpm for 30 minutes at 4°C, the supernatants aspirated, and the precipitated counts measured in an automatic gamma spectrometer. Counts bound in the absence of somatostatin antibody are determined in duplicate tubes containing 0.1 ml 1/300 NRS-EDTA-PO$_4$-Trasylol without the antibody.

The double antibody method of separation of bound from free ^{125}I-Tyr$_1$-SRIF outlined above has been used in the studies described in this chapter. Equivalent results can be obtained using BSA-coated charcoal (0.7 ml 0.5% charcoal and 0.2% BSA). Results are calculated manually or using a standard RIA computer program (eg. Rodbard, 1974; Burger *et al.*, 1972).

IV. CHARACTERISTICS OF SRIF RADIOIMMUNOASSAY

A. Binding of ^{125}I-Tyr$_1$-SRIF, Standard Curve, and Sensitivity

The specific binding ($\%B$) of ^{125}I-Tyr$_1$-SRIF at final antibody dilutions of 1 : 7000 and 1 : 10,000 in our assay is 50 and 35%, respectively. Nonspecific binding in the absence of antibody ranges from 2–4%. Typical standard curves obtained with cyclic and linear (dihydrosomatostatin) are depicted in Figure 3. Linear SRIF cross-reacts 32.7% in this system. The minimum detectable dose of SRIF calculated according to the method of Burger *et al.* (1972) is 1.6 ± 0.4 (standard deviation) pg with a range from 0.8–2.1 pg for ten assays.

B. Hormonal Specificity

The immunoreactivity of a number of SRIF analogs is shown in Table II. The extent of cross-reactivity varies from 100% for Tyr$_1$-SRIF to <1% for Ala$_3$-SRIF and Ala$_3$-acetamido-methyl-Cys$_{14}$-SRIF, neither of which can cyclize. Tyrosine substitution in position 11 retains 34% immunoreactivity, whereas Ala$_6$-SRIF shows limited (1.7%) reactivity.

It appears likely that antibody specificity is directed toward the C-terminal end of SRIF in view of the equal reactivity between Tyr$_1$-SRIF and SRIF. Furthermore, the disulfide bond appears important for antibody recognition, since dihydrosomatostatin shows only 32.7% cross-reactivity in this system. In view of the tendency for dihydrosomatostatin to cyclize spontaneously in dilute solutions, the actual cross-reactivity may be much less than this. The difference in immunoreactivity contrasts with the reported biologic activity of the two forms of SRIF, both of which appear to be equipotent in a variety of *in*

Table II   Relative Activity of SRIF Analogs in SRIF Radioimmunoassay

Analog	Cross-reactivity (%)
Tyr$_1$-SRIF	100
Tyr$_{11}$-SRIF	34
H-Ala$_3$-SRIF	0.7
Ala$_3$-Acetamido-methyl-Cys$_{14}$-SRIF	0.8
Ala$_6$-SRIF	1.7

vitro and *in vivo* systems (Reichlin *et al.*, 1976). The importance of the disulfide bond is further suggested by the finding that analogs which cannot cyclize owing to substitutions or modifications in positions 3 or 14 have minimal (<1%) biologic activity. Alternative explanations, however, are also possible, since these analogs differ from SRIF in other respects apart from their inability to cyclize.

The cross-reactivity of the anti-SRIF serum with other peptide hormones was also checked. As shown in Figure 3 there was no inhibition by 1.0 μg TRH, LHRH, oxytocin, vasopressin, substance P, neurotensin, glucagon, bovine pancreatic polypeptide, gastrin, secretin, VIP, CCK–PKZ, calcitonin, angiotensins I and II, 1-24-ACTH, 50 mU insulin, or 1.0 mg bovine thyroglobulin.

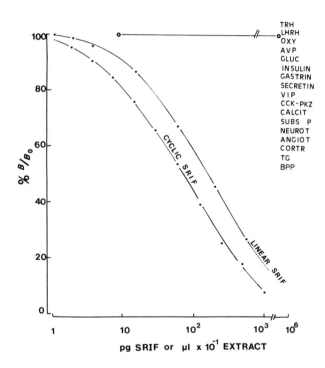

Figure 3.   Comparison of inhibition curves produced by cyclic and linear SRIF. 1.0 μg of a wide range of peptide hormones produced no inhibition. Oxy, oxytocin; VIP, vasoactive intestinal peptide; CCK–PKZ, cholecystokinin–pancreozymin; Calcit, human calcitonin. Subs P, substance P; Neurot, neurotensin; Angiot, angiotensin; Cortr, 1,24-ACTH; Tg, bovine thyroglobulin (1.0 mg); BPP, bovine pancreatic polypeptide. $B_0 = 37\%$.

C. Precision

Intraassay precision can be calculated by using replicate determinations ($n = 10$) at different levels over the range 10–100 pg/tube. The intraassay coefficient of variation for this assay is ±5.4% at 31 pg/tube and <10% over the range 10–100 pg/tube ($n = 6$). The interassay coefficient of variation is ±10% at 21.8 pg/tube ($n = 10$) and ±9% at 53 pg/tube ($n = 10$).

V. MEASUREMENT OF SRIF

The assay has found wide application for measurement of SRIF-like material in tissues and in biologic fluids, e.g., CSF. Technical problems have limited the usefulness of the method for studying circulating concentrations of the peptide. In this section, we present details of techniques that we have employed for studying tissue somatostatin concentrations in the rat. The method is applicable to other tissues as well.

A. Measurement of Tissue Concentrations of SRIF

1. Preparation of Tissue Extracts

Male Sprague–Dawley rats are killed by rapid decapitation and the following organs removed by gross dissection: portions of the brain and spinal cord; anterior and posterior pituitary glands; stomach (body, fundus, and pyloric antrum); duodenum; jejunum (proximal 10 cm); whole pancreas; whole adrenal glands; and portions (~300–400 mg) of the lungs, liver, kidneys, and salivary glands. Pancreatic islets (approximately 20–100 islets/animal) can be isolated from additional animals using the collagenase technique (Lacy and Kostianovsky, 1967). Individual tissue fragments and pools of islets are collected at 0°C in 1.0 M acetic acid (1.0–5.0 ml, depending on weight of tissue sample). All tissues (except brain and islets) are homogenized initially in a Sorvall Omnimix blender in iced 1.0 M acetic acid followed by further homogenization by means of sonication (Branson Sonifier Model B-30). For softer tissues, such as brain and pancreatic islets, the Sorvall step can be omitted. The extracts are immersed in a boiling water bath for five minutes and quickly chilled at 0°C. A small aliquot is removed for total protein determination (Lowry et al., 1951) following which the homogenates are centrifuged (60 min, 700 g), the supernatant removed, neutralized with 1.0 N NaOH or diluted, and assayed for somatostatin.

2. Stability of Endogenous SRIF during Extraction

Like ^{125}I-Tyr$_1$-SRIF, endogenous SRIF is highly susceptible to proteolytic digestion from tissue proteases during extraction. Our method for extracting SRIF from tissues as outlined above includes steps such as homogenization in acid, heating, and neutralization prior to assay. These conditions were selected following a series of experiments (described below) which demonstrated that extracted SRIF is stable during the procedure. Rat cerebral cortex was found to contain a high concentration of SRIF (see Table IV) and was the tissue chosen for these particular studies.

a. Stability of Synthetic SRIF in Boiling Acetic Acid. Synthetic SRIF was added to a solution of 1.0 M acetic acid which was then divided into eight aliquots, four of which were kept at 4°C and the remaining four boiled five minutes before being assayed. The SRIF content of the boiled tubes 67.3 ± 6.7 ng/100 ml was 12% lower than the control tubes 76 ± 7.4 ng/100 ml, but the difference was not significant, suggesting that SRIF is stable in boiling acetic acid.

b. Stability of Endogenous SRIF during Extraction Procedure. Rat cerebral cortical tissue (~450 mg) was homogenized in 3.0 ml 1.0 M acetic acid or PO$_4$ buffer, pH 7.5. The pH 7.5 extract was divided into two aliquots which were incubated for 60 minutes at 4° or at 25°C, respectively. The acidic extract was likewise divided into two aliquots, one of which was boiled for five minutes and then kept at 25°C for 60 minutes, the other kept at 4°C for 60 minutes without boiling. At different times, aliquots were removed from each of the four homogenates, boiled (except for the homogenate which had previously been boiled), and assayed for SRIF. At pH 7.5, there was a progressive loss of SRIF from the extract both at 4° and at 25°C, although the rate of decay was lower at the lower temperature (Figure 4). By contrast, SRIF was stable in the acidic extracts for at least one hour both at 4° and 25°C with and without boiling.

This experiment demonstrates that acidification alone will prevent SRIF degradation by rat cerebral cortical enzymes. For other tissues, however, which contain a high concentration of acid proteases, e.g., stomach, we consider it necessary to heat-inactivate these enzymes. Since somatostatin is stable to boiling, we have retained this step for all our extractions in order to keep the procedure uniform.

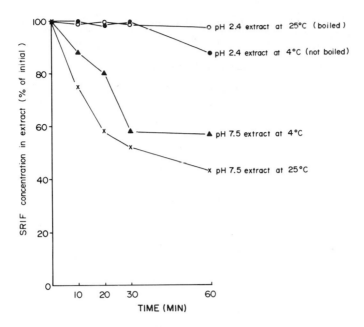

Figure 4. Stability of endogenous SRIF in pH 7.5 and pH 2.4 rat cortical extract at 4° and 25°C. SRIF in the extracts was measured by radioimmunoassay.

c. Effect of Lyophilization on SRIF Content of Extracts. In order to determine the effect of lyophilization on immunoreactive SRIF, equal aliquots of a rat cortical extract were assayed following lyophilization or after neutralization. Lyophilization resulted in a 48% loss of SRIF compared to neutralization (12.1 ± 0.4 ng/ml versus 23.2 ± 1.9 ng/ml). We, thus, advise against lyophilizing extracts.

3. *Recovery of Exogenous SRIF*

For recovery studies, an extract of cerebral cortex low in SRIF was used. This was prepared by homogenizing cortical tissue in PO_4 buffer, pH 7.5, and incubating the extract at 25°C for six hours followed by boiling. Synthetic SRIF in amounts ranging from 1.0–100 ng/ml was satisfactorily recovered from the extract (Table III). Recovery was quantitative at levels of 10 and 100 ng/ml (99–104%), although it was low at 1.0 ng/ml (69%). Since most tissue extracts contain endogenous SRIF far in excess of 1.0 ng/ml and usually in the range 10–100 ng/ml, recovery is considered satisfactory.

Table III   *In Vitro* Recovery of SRIF from Cortical Extract

SRIF added (ng/ml)	No. of experiments	Percent recovery (mean ± SEM)
1.0	5	69.0 ± 1.7
10.0	5	98.8 ± 2.2
100.0	5	104 ± 2.1
Total	15	90.5 ± 4.9

Table IV   Distribution of Somatostatin in Rat CNS, Pituitary, and Peripheral Organs

	SRIF[a] pg/μg protein (mean ± SEM)[b]
CNS structures	
Hypothalamus	26.1 ± 1.7
SME[c]	248 ± 26
VMN[d]	17.5 ± 2.5
Brain stem	5.1 ± 0.7
Spinal cord	10.4 ± 1.9
Olfactory lobe	1.07 ± 0.15
Cerebral cortex	6.7 ± 1.7
Cerebellum	0.43 ± 0.07
Pineal gland	0.14 ± 0.2
Pituitary	
Anterior	<0.001
Posterior	5.63 ± 1.9
Gut, pancreas, and other structures	
Stomach	2.4 ± 0.22
Pylorus	6.4 ± 0.92
Duodenum	1.94 ± 0.2
Jejunum	1.94 ± 0.2
Whole pancreas	1.8 ± 0.13
Pancreatic islets	786 ± 85
Liver	<0.001
Lungs	<0.001
Kidneys	<0.001
Submandibular glands	<0.001

[a] Denotes SRIF-like immunoreactive material expressed as picogram equivalents of synthetic SRIF.

[b] $n = 6$.

[c] SME, stalk median eminence.

[d] VMN, ventromedial nucleus.

4. Tissue Distribution of Somatostatin

a. Somatostatin in Hypothalamic and Extrahypothalamic Rat Brain.
The values obtained for the concentration of SRIF in various tissues
studied with our assay are depicted in Table IV. The upper half of this
table shows a comparison of SRIF in different regions of the brain. It is
clear that significant quantities of immunoreactive SRIF are present
not only in the hypothalamus but throughout the extrahypothalamic
brain and spinal cord. For neural tissue, the highest concentration is
found in the stalk median eminence (SME) region of the
hypothalamus followed by the ventromedial nucleus (VMN). The
whole hypothalamus contains 26.1 ± 1.7 pg/μg protein. Of extrahypothalamic brain structures, the spinal cord contains the highest
concentration, 10.4 ± 1.9 pg/μg, a value similar to that for the whole
hypothalamus. SRIF concentration in the cerebral cortex and brain
stem is approximately one-quarter to one-fifth that of the
hypothalamus, whereas the olfactory lobe, cerebellum, and pineal
gland contain less than 5% of the hypothalamic level. SRIF has been
repeatedly found in high concentration in the posterior pituitary, but is
undetectable in the anterior pituitary.

Within the CNS, cerebral cortex accounts for 50%, the spinal cord
31%, and the brain stem 13% of the total somatostatin (Table V). The
hypothalamus contains only 7% of the total amount, and the cerebellum and olfactory lobes less than 1% each.

b. SRIF in Peripheral Organs. Immunoreactive SRIF is present in
high concentration in the rat stomach, pylorus, duodenum, jejunum,
and pancreas (Table IV, lower half). Isolated pancreatic islets contain
between 500–720 pg per islet, which when expressed per microgram
of islet protein gives a concentration 786 pg/μg protein, exceeding that
in SME (248 pg/μg protein). In the gut, the pyloric antrum contains the
highest SRIF concentration (6.4 pg/μg protein). No SRIF-like material
is detected in lungs, liver, kidney, salivary glands, or adrenal glands.

5. Immunologic Identity of Tissue Somatostatin

One way to study the immunologic properties of the SRIF-like ma-
terial(s) present in tissues is to assay serial dilutions of extracts and
compare them with a standard SRIF curve. As shown in Figure 5, all
SRIF-containing tissue extracts produced parallel inhibition curves to
synthetic SRIF, suggesting immunologic identity between the tissue
SRIF-like material and SRIF. This finding also excludes nonspecific
interference by the extracts in the radioimmunoassay and provides

Table V   Total SRIF Content of Brain and Peripheral Organs[a]

	Mean wet wt. (mg)	SRIF[b] (ng/mg wet wt.)	SRIF[b] (ng/region)
Central nervous system			
Hypothalamus	33.4	2.3 ± 0.2	76.9 ± 5.3
Brain stem (including midbrain and thalamus)	289	0.44 ± 0.06	128 ± 18
Olfactory lobes	90	0.08 ± 0.01	7.4 ± 1.0
Cerebellum	234	0.03 ± 0.01	7.7 ± 1.3
Cerebral cortex	996	0.52 ± 0.03	516 ± 34
Spinal cord	476	0.67 ± 0.03	317 ± 16.5
			Total 1015
Gut and pancreas			
Stomach	834	0.37 ± 0.04	306 ± 32
Pylorus	222	0.52 ± 0.07	116 ± 15.7
Duodenum	282	0.15 ± 0.03	42 ± 9.6
Jejunum (10 cm)	751	0.07 ± 0.003	50 ± 2.3
Pancreas	790	0.17 ± 0.004	137 ± 3
			Total 651

[a] Mean ± SEM; $n = 6$.
[b] Denotes SRIF-like immunoreactivity expressed as nanogram equivalents of synthetic SRIF.

further evidence for the immunologic specificity of tissue SRIF measurements. By Sephadex gel filtration, the bulk of immunoreactive SRIF-like material in tissues has been shown to have a molecular weight similar to that of synthetic SRIF. In addition, however, there is material(s) with a molecular weight greater than that of SRIF (Patel and Reichlin, 1978; Arimura et al., 1975b).

B. Measurement of SRIF in Cerebrospinal Fluid (CSF)

For the measurement of SRIF in human CSF, the assay needs to be optimally sensitive. By using freshly prepared ^{125}I-Tyr$_1$-SRIF and nonequilibrium conditions (addition of tracer delayed by 16–24 hours), we have been able to achieve a sensitivity of 0.7–1.0 pg SRIF per tube. Human CSF is collected by lumbar puncture into iced tubes, and 0.1–0.2 ml assayed directly. SRIF is stable in CSF both at room temperature and 0°C for at least two hours (Patel et al., 1976b). Synthetic SRIF added to CSF can be adequately recovered by this method. Detectable levels of CSF SRIF ranging from 15–55 pg/ml were found in seven neurologically normal individuals. The values

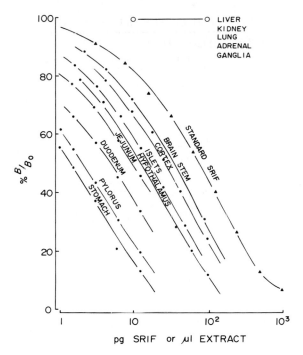

Figure 5. Comparison of inhibition curves produced by cyclic SRIF and serial dilutions of tissue extracts. All extracts showed parallelism with standard SRIF. $B_0 = 42\%$. [Reproduced from *Endocrinology* (1978) **102**, 523–530.]

were considerably elevated in 30 patients with a wide range of neurological diseases, including inflammatory, metabolic, and neoplastic disorders, suggesting that brain damage may result in nonspecific leakage of SRIF into the CSF (Patel *et al.*, 1976b).

ACKNOWLEDGMENT

Supported by the C. J. Martin Fellowship of the National Health and Medical Research Council, Australia (Yogesh C. Patel) and in part by United States Public Health Service Grant No. 16684.

REFERENCES

Abraham, G. E., and Grover, P. K. (1971). Covalent linkages of hormonal haptens to protein carriers for use in radioimmunoassay. *In* "Principles of Competitive Protein-Binding Assays" (W. D. Odell and W. H. Daughaday, eds.), pp. 134–139. Lippincott, Philadelphia, Pennsylvania.

Alpert, L. C., Brawer, J. R., Patel, Y. C., and Reichlin, S. (1976). Somatostatinergic neurons in anterior hypothalamus: Immunohistochemical localization. *Endocrinology* **98,** 255–258.

Arimura, A., and Schally, A. V. (1976). Increase in basal and thyrotropin-releasing hormone-stimulated secretion of thyrotropin by passive immunization with antiserum to somatostatin in rats. *Endocrinology* **98,** 1069–1072.

Arimura, S., Sato, H., Coy, D. H., and Schally, A. V. (1975a). Radioimmunoassay for GH-release inhibiting hormone. *Proc. Soc. Exp. Biol. Med.* **148,** 784–789.

Arimura, A., Sato, H., Dupont, A., Nishi, N., and Schally, A. V. (1975b). Somatostatin: Abundance of immunoreactive hormone in rat stomach and pancreas. *Science* **189,** 1007–1009.

Arimura, S., Smith, W. D., and Schally, A. V. (1976). Blockade of the stress-induced decrease in blood GH by anti-somatostatin serum in rats. *Endocrinology* **98,** 540–543.

Berson, S. A., Yalow, R. S., Bauman, S., Rothschild, M. A., and Newerly, K. (1956). Insulin-^{131}I metabolism in human subjects: Demonstration of insulin binding globulin in the circulation of insulin treated subjects. *J. Clin. Invest* **35,** 170–190.

Boden, G., Sivitz, M. C., Owen, O. E., Essa-Koumar, N., and Landor, J. H. (1975). Somatostatin suppresses secretin and pancreatic exocrine secretion. *Science* **190,** 163–165.

Brazeau, P., Vale, W., Burgus, R., Ling, N., Butcher, M., Rivier, J., and Guillemin, R. (1973). Hypothalamic polypeptide that inhibits the secretion of immunoreactive pituitary growth hormone. *Science* **179,** 77–79.

Brownstein, M., Arimura, A., Sato, H., Schally, A. V., and Kizer, J. S. (1975). The regional distribution of somatostatin in the rat brain. *Endocrinology* **96,** 1456–1461.

Burger, H. G., Lee, V. W. K., and Rennie, G. C. (1972). A generalized computer program for the treatment of data from competitive protein-binding assays including radioimmunoassays. *J. Lab. Clin. Med.* **80,** 302–312.

Burgus, R., Ling, N., Butcher, M., and Guillemin, R. (1973). Primary structure of somatostatin, a hypothalamic peptide that inhibits the secretion of pituitary growth hormone. *Proc. Natl. Acad. Sci. U.S.A.* **70,** 684–688.

Cohn, L., and Cohn, M. (1975). 'Barrel rotation' induced by somatostatin in the nonlesioned rat. *Brain Res.* **96,** 138–141.

Dubois, M. P. (1975). Immunoreactive somatostatin is present in discrete cells of the endocrine pancreas. *Proc. Natl. Acad. Sci. U.S.A.* **72,** 1340–1343.

Hökfelt, T., Effendic, S., Hellerström, C., Johansson, O., Luft, R., and Arimura, A. (1975). Cellular localization of somatostatin in endocrine-like cells and neurons of the rat with special reference to the A_1 cells of the pancreatic islets and to the hypothalamus. *Acta Endocrinol. (Copenhagen)* **80,** 5–41.

Kronheim, S., Berelowitz, M., and Pimstone, B. L. (1976). A radioimmunoassay for growth hormone release-inhibiting hormone: method and quantitative tissue distribution. *Clin Endocrinol.* **5,** 619–630.

Krulich, L., Illner, P., Fawcett, C. P., Quijada, M., and McCann, S. M. (1972). Dual hypothalamic regulation of growth hormone secretion. *Growth Horm., Proc. Int. Symp., 2nd, 1971* Excerpta Med. Found. Int. Congr. Ser. No. 244, pp. 306–316.

Lacy, P. E., and Kostianovsky, M. (1967). Method for the isolation of intact islets of Langerhans from the rat pancreas. *Diabetes* **16,** 35–39.

Landon, J., Livanou, T., and Greenwood, F. C. (1967). The preparation and immunological properties of ^{131}I-labelled adrenocorticotrophin. *Biochem. J.* **105,** 1075–1083.

Lowry, O. H., Rosebrough, N. J., Ferrell, A. L., and Randall, R. (1951). Protein measurement with Folin phenol reagent. *J. Biol. Chem.* **193,** 265–271.

Orci, L., Baetens, D., Rufener, C., Amherdt, M., Ravazzola, M., Studer, P., Malaisse-Lagae, F., and Unger, R. H. (1976). Hypertrophy and hyperplasia of somtatostatin containing D-cells in diabetes. *Proc. Natl. Acad. Sci. U.S.A.* **73**, 1338–1342.

Patel, Y. C., and Reichlin, S. (1978). Somatostatin in hypothalamus, extrahypothalamic brain and peripheral tissues of the rat. *Endocrinology* **102**, 523–530.

Patel, Y. C., Cameron, D. P., Bankier, A., Malaisse-Lagae, F., Ravazzola, M., Studer, P., and Orci, L. (1978). Changes in somatostatin concentration in pancreas and other tissues of streptozotocin diabetic rats. *Endocrinology* (in press).

Patel, Y. C., and Weir, G. C. (1976). Increased somatostatin content of islets from streptozotocin diabetic rats. *Clin. Endocrinol.* **5**, 191–197.

Patel, Y. C., Weir, G. C., and Reichlin, S. (1975). Anatomic distribution of somatostatin (SRIF) in brain and pancreatic islets as studied by radioimmunoassay. *Program 57th Annu. Meet., Am. Endocr. Soc.* Abstract No. 154, p. 127.

Patel, Y. C., Orci, L., Bankier, A., and Cameron, D. (1976). Decreased pancreatic somatostatin concentration in spontaneously diabetic mice. *Endocrinology* **99**, 1415–1418.

Patel, Y. C., Rao, K., and Reichlin, S. (1977a). Somatostatin in human cerebrospinal fluid. *N. Engl. J. Med.* **296**, 524–533.

Patel, Y. C., Cameron, D. P., Stefan, Y., Malaisse-Lagae, F., and Orci, L. (1977b). Somatostatin: widespread abnormality in tissues of spontaneously diabetic mice. *Science* **198**, 930–931.

Pelletier, G., Le Clerc, R., Dube, D., Labrie, F., Duviani, R., Arimura, A., and Schally, A. V. (1975). Localization of growth hormone-release-inhibiting hormone (Somatostatin) in the rat brain. *Am. J. Anat.* **142**, 397–400.

Polak, J. M., Pearse, A. G. E., Grimelius, L., Bloom, S. R., and Arimura, S. (1975). Growth-hormone release inhibiting hormone in gastrointestinal and pancreatic D-cells. *Lancet* **1**, 1220–1222.

Reichlin, S., Saperstein, R., Jackson, I. M. D., Boyd, A. E., III, and Patel, Y. C. (1976). Hypothalamic hormones. *Annu. Rev. Physiol.* **38**, 389–424.

Renaud, L. P., Martin, J. B., and Brazeau, P. (1975). Depressant action of TRH, LHRH and somatostatin on activity of central neurones. *Nature (London)* **255**, 233–235.

Rivier, J., Brazeau, P., Vale, W., Ling, N., Burgus, R., Gilon, C., Yardley, J., and Guillemin, R. (1973). Synthèse totale par phase solide d'un tétradécapeptide ayant les propriétés chimiques et biologiques de la somatostatine. *C.R. Hebd. Seances Acad. Sci.* **276**, 2737–2740.

Rodbard, D. (1974). Statistical quality control and routine data processing for radioimmunoassays (RIA) and immunoradiometric assays (IRMA). *Clinical Chemistry* **20**, 1255–1270.

Rufener, C., Dubois, M. P., Malaisse-Lagae, F., and Orci, L. (1975). Immunofluorescent reactivity to anti-somatostatin in the gastrointestinal mucosa of the dog. *Diabetologia* **11**, 321–324.

Skowsky, W. R., and Fisher, D. A. (1972). The use of thyroglobulin to induce antigenicity to small molecules. *J. Lab. Clin. Med.* **80**, 134–144.

Terry, L. C., Willoughby, J. O., Brazeau, P., Martin, J. B., and Patel, Y. C. (1976). Antiserum to somatostatin prevents stress-induced inhibition of growth hormone secretion in the rat. *Science* **192**, 565.

Vale, W., Brazeau, P., Rivier, C., Brown. M., Boss, B., Rivier, J., Burgus, R., Ling, N., and Guillemin, R. (1975). Somatostatin. *Recent Progress Hormone Research* **31**, 365–397.

6

Melatonin

JOSEPHINE ARENDT AND MICHAEL WILKINSON

I. INTRODUCTION

The isolation in 1958 of the amphibian skin-lightening agent of beef pineal gland by A. B. Lerner (Lerner *et al.*, 1958), and its characterization as the indoleamine, melatonin (MT) have led to a vast body of work (Axelrod, 1974), which, in addition to clarifying the nature of the gland, is designed, in a more general manner, to study its β-receptor-mediated activation. Most of this work has been performed using the activity of enzymes involved in the biosynthesis of melatonin as parameters.

The quantitation of melatonin itself has been accomplished by bioassay (Mori and Lerner, 1960; Ralph and Lynch, 1970), fluorimetry (Maickel and Miller, 1968), gas chromatography–mass spectrometry

101

(GCMS) (Pelham *et al.*, 1972; Smith *et al.*, 1977), and, recently, radioimmunoassay (RIA) (Arendt *et al.*, 1975, 1977; Pang *et al.*, 1976; Levine and Riceberg, 1975; Rollag and Niswender, 1976; Ozaki *et al.*, 1976; Wurzburger *et al.*, 1976). Bioassay measurements, while apparently specific (Quay and Bagnara, 1964), suffer from two disadvantages, namely, requiring animal breeding facilities and being tedious to perform. Furthermore, while the sensitivity is adequate for the studies of the gland itself, large amounts of serum must be extracted in order to determine concentrations of circulating melatonin (Vaughan *et al.*, 1976). Fluorimetric measurements necessitate lengthy separation techniques in view of their lack of specificity and, because of sensitivity considerations, are absolutely restricted to estimations of pineal content.

The vast potential of GCMS measurements, not only of melatonin but of related indoles as well, has remained largely unexploited until recently (Smith *et al.*, 1977). Clearly, radioimmunoassay measurements and GCMS are most useful in both clinical and research situations. The recent publication of six radioimmunoassays for melatonin (Arendt *et al.*, 1975, 1977; Pang *et al.*, 1976; Levine and Riceberg, 1975; Rollag and Niswender, 1976; Wurzburger *et al.*, 1976; Kennaway *et al.*, 1977) testifies to the current upsurge of interest in this compound. Each of these assays fulfills the basic requisites of a workable radioimmunoassay system, i.e., sensitivity, specificity, and precision. A short review of these assays followed by a more detailed description of that used in our laboratory follows.

II. METHODS OF RADIOIMMUNOASSAY

Five different antigenic preparations have been used thus far to raise specific antibodies to melatonin (MT), as shown in Table I. All these structurally different antigens have produced relatively specific high-titer antisera of sufficient sensitivity to be used in serum determinations of MT. The type of protein carrier and mode of injection do not appear to influence greatly the formation of antibodies; further, integrity of the *N*-acetyl group does not appear to be necessary for specificity. All investigators have used rabbits as experimental animals, and it is, thus, not yet possible to discuss interspecies variations in antibody production. Iodinated hapten, iodinated antigen, and tritiated melatonin (^{3}H-MT) have all been used as tracers. A notable advantage of the iodinated hapten assay system (Rollag and Niswender, 1976) is the high sensitivity of the standard curve (2.0–3.0 pg/

Table I Methods of Producing Anti-melatonin Serum in Rabbits

Indole derivative	Protein carrier[a]	Conjugation reaction	Hapten/ protein molar ratio	Tracer	Titer	Reference
Melatonin	BSA	Formaldehyde condensation (Mannich reaction)	3.0–50	³H-Melatonin	1 : 20,000	Pang et al., 1976
N-Acetyl-5-methoxytryptophan	TG, BSA	Carbodiimide coupling	10–47	³H-Melatonin		Arendt et al., 1975
Indomethacin	HSA	Carbodiimide coupling	?	³H-Melatonin	1 : 13,000	Levine and Riceberg, 1975
N-Succinyl-5-methoxytryptamine	BSA	Mixed anhydride	30	¹²⁵I-N-3-(4-hydroxy-phenyl)-propionyl-5-methoxy-tryptamine	1 : 256,000	Rollag and Niswender, 1976
Melatonin	BSA	Coupled to p-amino-benzoic acid (diazotiza-tion), then mixed anhydride conjugation with BSA		³H-Melatonin	1 : 4,000	Wurzburger et al., 1976

[a] BSA, bovine serum albumin; TG, thyroglobulin; HSA, human serum albumin.

tube). The availability of very high specific activity tritiated tracer would obviate the recurring problem of preparing iodinated tracer. Some investigators have used double antibody precipitation to separate bound and free hormone. In our hands, ammonium sulfate precipitation is equally effective and considerably cheaper. All assays require prior extraction procedures, together with, in one case, column chromatography (Kennaway *et al.*, 1977).

A direct comparison of absolute MT values obtained with different assays has now been published (Wetterberg, 1977). Investigators have variously used sheep, rats, and man for physiologic studies, and reported values have all been in the same range, both for pineal gland (rat) and serum (rat and human) as those found previously by tadpole bioassay (Arendt *et al.*, 1977; Pang *et al.*, 1976; Ozaki *et al.*, 1976; Kennaway *et al.*, 1977). A description now follows of the radioimmunoassay for MT developed and used routinely in our laboratory.

III. RADIOIMMUNOASSAY TECHNIQUE

A. Materials

Solvents were obtained from commercial sources as analytical grade reagents and redistilled before use. Glassware was siliconized and acid-washed before use. All other reagents were obtained from commercial sources and used without further purification. Thin layer chromatography plates (Merck), cellulose F, and silica gel G, were washed twice with the solvents used for migration. Chromatography solvents routinely used were as follows: (a) chloroform:methanol:glacial acetic acid, 93:7:1, (b) chloroform:methanol, 9:1, (c) isopropanol:ammonia (5%), 4:2, (d) *n*-butanol. Stock potassium phosphate buffer (TPG) for radioimmunoassay, pH 7.1, was made up at 0.2 M and 0.2% sodium azide included. This solution was diluted 1:1 before use and 0.9% NaCl and 0.1% gelatin incorporated. Potassium phosphate buffer for extraction was made at 2.0 M, pH 10, and saturated with KCl.

Antibody was stored in 100-μl aliquots at $-20°C$. Sufficient antibody for one week's work was diluted 1:5000 with TPG and stored at $-20°C$.

Standard MT (Fluka 1.0 mg/ml) was made up by dissolving 10 mg MT in 0.5 ml absolute ethanol and adjusting the volume to 10 ml with H_2O. This solution was stored at $-20°C$ and freshly diluted for each assay. ^{3}H-MT, 26 Ci/mM (New England Nuclear Corp.) was diluted to 2.0 μCi/ml in absolute ethanol and stored at $-20°C$. Intermittent chromatography of this solution in solvent systems (a) (R_f = 0.9) and (b) (R_f = 0.5) indicated that the product is stable for at least six months under these conditions. The stock solution was freshly diluted with TPG for each assay.

Scintisol liquid scintillation solvent was obtained from Biolab AG, as were polyethylene radioactivity counting vials.

Serum or plasma was decanted rapidly and stored at −20°C. Rat pineal glands were rapidly dissected (<30 seconds after decapitation) and stored at −20°C. Human pineal glands were obtained at autopsy within 12 hours of death and stored at −20°C.

B. Preparation of Antiserum

D,L-5-Methoxytryptophan was acetylated by the method of Berg *et al.* (1929–1930) to give D,L-5-methoxy-N-acetyltryptophan (MNAT). In this preparation, D,L-5-methoxytryptophan is dissolved in 1.0 N NaOH (100 mg/ml). Acetic anhydride is added in three successive 1.0-ml aliquots, shaking vigorously after each addition. After being treated at 35°–40°C for two to three hours, the white precipitate is collected, washed successively with water, 1.0 N HCl, and water, and dried at 80°C. The identity of the product is confirmed by infrared spectroscopy, elementary analysis, and thin-layer chromatography (Pasini *et al.*, 1963). Elementary analysis indicated D,L-5-methoxy-N-acetyltryptophan, with one molecule of water of crystallization—calculated: C, 57.20%; H, 6.13% N, 9.51%; found: C, 57.29%; H, 6.06%; N 9.49%. MNAT (50 mg) was dissolved in 5.0 ml dioxane. Fifty milligrams of bovine serum albumin (BSA) or thyroglobulin (TG) in 3.5 ml of 0.05 M phosphate buffer, pH 7.8, was added, followed by 67 mg of 1-ethyl-3-(3-dimethylaminopropyl) carbodiimide in 2.5 ml H_2O. After mixing, the reaction was allowed to proceed for 24 hours at 22°C in the dark. The reaction products were then dialyzed for three days against six changes of distilled water. The amount of MNAT coupled to protein was determined by estimating fluorimetrically the amount of free MNAT removed by dialysis. It was calculated that 47.5 moles of hapten were conjugated per mole of protein. Rabbits were injected subcutaneously with 1.0 mg conjugate emulsified in 0.5 ml physiologic saline and 0.5 ml complete Freund's adjuvant at three sites. After three weeks, booster injections were given at monthly intervals and bleedings taken ten to 15 days after each injection. After 16 weeks and four booster injections, specific and sensitive but low titer antibodies were demonstrated (rabbit 8) and characterized (Arendt *et al.*, 1975).

Preliminary physiologic studies have been reported with this antibody (Wetterberg *et al.*, 1976). In collaboration with L. Wetterberg and Kabi-Diagnostica, a less substituted, more soluble MNAT–protein conjugate (approximately 10 moles per mole) was synthesized. This conjugate, when emulsified with Freund's adjuvant and injected intracutaneously at multiple sites, according to Vaitukaitis *et al.* (1971), produced a high titer MT antiserum in four and detectable titer in four of eight rabbits after 14 weeks with no booster injections. The evolution of anti-MT titer is shown in Figure 1. The studies described in this chapter were performed using the best characterized of the latter antibodies, i.e., K 244.

C. Characterization of Antibody

1. *Tracer*

Of paramount importance in the characterization of an antibody is the availability of high specific activity tracer. ^{3}H-MT was obtained from the New England Nuclear Corp. with a specific activity of 26

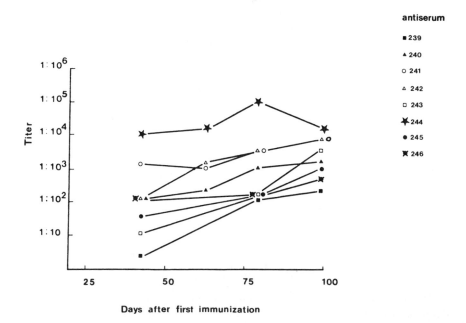

Figure 1. Evolution of titer of melatonin-binding antibodies as a function of time in eight rabbits, immunized as described in the text. Tracer, ^{3}H-MT, 26 Ci/mM, 2000 cpm.

Ci/mM. Chromatographic purity was established in solvent systems (a) and (b) on silica gel G plates. All the studies described in this chapter were performed using this tracer.

2. Titer and Affinity

All bleedings were tested for their ability to bind ³H-MT. Serial dilutions of serum were set up and tested using the assay system described in Section III,D. In order to test sensitivity and titer simultaneously, a parallel series of serum dilutions was set up incorporating a known amount of unlabeled hormone (100 pg). It was, thus, possible to judge the displacement of ³H-MT by 100 pg MT at a number of antibody dilutions (Figure 2). Optimal sensitivity was found for K-244 at a final dilution of 1:20,000 resulting in 50% maximum binding. The affinity constant for this antibody, calculated as $K = [HB]/[H][B]$ where $[HB]$ is the concentration of antibody-bound hapten and $[H]$ and $[B]$ are the concentrations of free hapten and antibody at half-

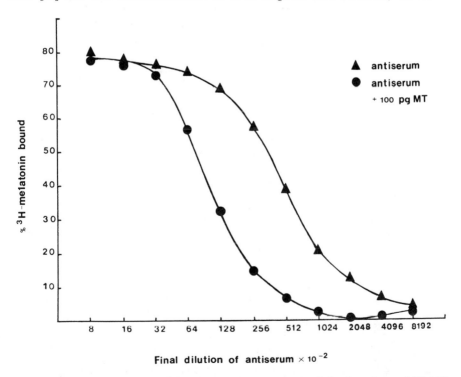

Figure 2. Simultaneous evaluation of antiserum titer and displacement of ³H-MT bound by 100 pg of unlabeled melatonin at each dilution. Tracer, ³H-MT, 26 Ci/mM, 2000 cpm. Antiserum, K-244.

Table II   Cross-Reactions of Anti-melatonin Antibody K-244[a]

Product	Picograms for 50% displacement
Melatonin	42
6-Hydroxymelatonin	7,000
N-Acetyltryptophan	8,000
N-Acetyltryptamine	13,000
5-Methoxytryptophan	48,000
5-Methoxytryptamine	200,000
N-Acetylserotonin	>1,000,000
5-Methoxytryptophol	>1,000,000
5-Methoxyindoleacetic acid	>1,000,000
5-Hydroxytryptamine	>1,000,000
5-Hydroxytryptophan	>1,000,000
5-Hydroxyindoleacetic acid	>1,000,000
Tryptophan	>10,000,000
Tryptamine	>10,000,000

[a] Final dilution 1:20,000; Tracer ^{3}H-MT, 26 Ci/mM, 2000 cpm.

saturation of antibody binding sites, i.e. [HB] = [B], was found to be 3.4×10^{10} liter/mole.

3. Cross-Reactions

Thirteen indolic analogs were tested for the potency of their binding to the antiserum, i.e., the quantity required to displace 50% of antibody-bound ^{3}H-MT. Relative cross-reactivities are shown in Table II. The only potential important interfering compounds are 6-hydroxymelatonin, and N-acetyltryptamine, whose serum concentrations are unknown. However, 6-hydroxymelatonin has been excluded by a chromatographic method described in Section III,E,3. The structurally unrelated steroids, testosterone, progesterone, and β-estradiol, have also been found to produce negligible cross-reaction in this antibody system.

D. Preparation of Samples and Assay Procedure

1. Extraction of Plasma or Serum

To 1.0–2.0 ml of plasma or serum in 50-ml centrifuge tubes are added 1.5 ml phosphate buffer, 2.0 M, pH 10, and 24 ml CHCl₃. The tubes are shaken for ten minutes and centrifuged at 2000 rpm for 15 minutes. The aqueous phase is aspirated and 20 ml of the organic phase is transferred to a clean tube and evaporated at 37°C under N_2. The residue is taken up in 2.0 ml of absolute ethanol and transferred to 10-ml centrifuge tubes. The solvent is evaporated at 37°C under N_2 and the residue taken up in 0.6 ml TPG. This solution is further extracted with 3.0 ml petroleum ether and the organic phase aspirated and discarded. The aqueous phase is then used directly for radioimmunoassay. The efficiency of each extraction is monitored by adding 100,000 cpm of ^{3}H-MT, 5.94 Ci/mM, synthesized in our laboratory (Arendt *et al.*, 1975) to one serum and counting the final extract in duplicate. Recoveries are absolutely reproducible (65.5 ± 1.1%) and are not corrected for. It is possible to perform this extraction using half the quantities of solvent indicated, but with some loss of recovery.

2. Pineal Glands

Human or rat pineal glands, after being weighed, are homogenized in TPG centrifuged at 2000 rpm for ten minutes and suitably diluted aliquots of the supernatant used for radioimmunoassay.

3. Assay Protocol

All solutions and tubes are kept on ice throughout.

  i. Pipette 0.2 ml of antibody diluted 1:5000.
 ii. Pipette unlabeled MT and test solutions (Standard curve of K-244 is 10, 20, 50, 100, 200, 500 pg MT).
iii. Pipette TPG to make each tube up a final volume of 0.8 ml.
 iv. Mix five seconds, wait 10 minutes.
  v. Pipette tracer, 1.25 nCi, 11 pg, in 0.1 ml.
 vi. Mix.
vii. Incubate 15–17 hours at 0°–4°C.
viii. Pipette 0.8 ml saturated $(NH_4)_2 SO_4$. This must not take more than ten minutes.
 ix. Mix gently without foaming.
  x. Wait ten minutes.
 xi. Spin 30 minutes at 3000 rpm.
xii. Pipette 1.0 ml supernatant into plastic scintillation vials.
xiii. Add 5 ml Scintisol. Shake five seconds. Wait five hours and count to ±2% S.D.

Calculations are performed either manually or by computer (Wang 600).

E. Evaluation of the Assay

1. Sensitivity

The mean least detectable concentration of MT, defined as twice the standard deviation of maximum binding, is 10 pg. Extraction blanks approach this value and, in combination with the various aliquoting procedures employed, give a detection limit for 2.0 ml and 1.0 ml extracted plasma or serum of 14 and 28 pg/ml, respectively.

2. Precision

For each assay, three standard sera are put through the entire procedure. To two of the three sera are added known amounts of unlabeled MT (100 and 300 pg/ml) calculated to read at approximately 30, 50, and 80% of maximum binding. This procedure simultaneously provides a measure of the cold recovery of melatonin and interassay variability. Interassay variability of pineal homogenates was performed at four different dose levels. Coefficient of variation was defined as (one standard deviation/mean value) × 100. Five replicates of each of three sera of known MT concentration were put through the same assay to provide a measure of intraassay variability. Results are shown in Table III.

Table III   Specifications of Anti-melatonin Antibody K-244[a]

Recovery of added melatonin: mean ± SEM
100 pg (91 ± 5)% $n = 10$
300 pg (102 ± 4.2)% $n = 10$
Interassay variability (extracted plasma)
18 pg 39.0% $n = 15$
49 pg 15.0% $n = 15$
134 pg 19.0% $n = 15$
Interassay variability (extracted pineal glands)
13 pg 18.0% $n = 7$
27 pg 19.0% $n = 8$
67 pg 6.8% $n = 5$
157 pg 10.4% $n = 5$
Intraassay variability (extracted plasma)
10 pg 21.5% $n = 5$
40 pg 4.4% $n = 5$
90 pg 9.9% $n = 5$

[a] Final dilution 1 : 20,000; tracer ^{3}H-MT, 26 Ci/mM, 2000 cpm; sensitivity (standard curve) 10 pg; blank, mean ± SEM = 8.8 ± 0.9 pg; $n = 15$.

3. Validation and Specificity

Validation of the assay is performed by measurements of parallelism, evaluation of cross-reactivity, chromatographic identity of extracted immunoreactivity and known hormone, and comparison with bioassay measurements. Parallelism of aliquots of extracted serum and aliquots of pineal homogenate is shown in Figure 3. Cross-reactivity estimates indicated that 6-hydroxy-MT was a potentially interfering compound (Table II). Pooled extracted sera were thus chromatographed on cellulose F plates in system (c) which clearly separates 6-hydroxy-MT and MT. ^{3}H-MT was used to localize the hormone. Chromatograms were eluted with TPG and immunoreactivity determined using two antibodies, rabbit 8 and K-244 (Figure 4). All immunoreactivity was found in the spot corresponding to MT. Cross-reactivity measurements would appear to eliminate the possibility of interference of the other indoles migrating with MT in this chromatographic system, in view of known pineal or serum levels. Furthermore, chromatography of extracted plasma on silica gel G plates in solvent systems (b) and (d) gives only one immunoreactive peak, corresponding to authentic melatonin. Rabbit 8, however, consistently gives values approximately 2.0 times higher than K-244. This may conceivably be due to a 1%

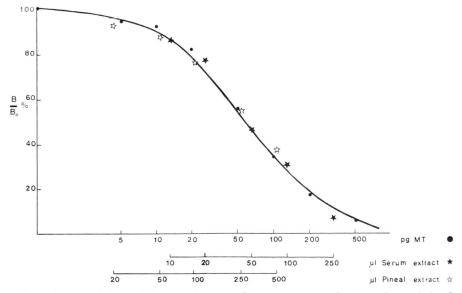

Figure 3. Parallelism of aliquots of extracted human serum and extracted pineal gland with the standard curve. Tracer, ^{3}H-MT, 26 Ci/mM, 2000 cpm. Antiserum, K-244. Extractions and assay were performed as described in the text. (Reprinted from Arendt *et al.*, 1977, with permission of the publisher.)

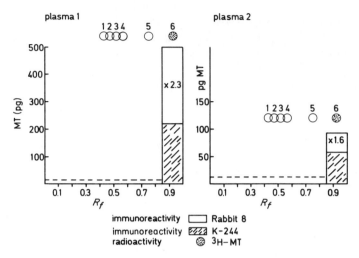

Figure 4. Chromatographic localization of immunoreactivity of extracted human plasma as determined by two different antisera to melatonin, rabbit 8 and K-244. Tracer, ³H-MT, 26 Ci/mM, 2000 cpm, final dilution of rabbit 8, 1 : 500, otherwise assay conditions are as described in text. (1) 5-Hydroxytryptophan; 5-hydroxyindoleacetic acid; (2) 5-methoxyindoleacetic acid; (3) tryptophan; (4) 5-methoxytryptophan; (5) 5-hydroxytryptamine, 6-hydroxymelatonin (6) 5-methoxytryptophol, 5-methoxytryptamine, N-acetylserotonin, tryptamine, N-acetyltryptamine, melatonin. (Reprinted from Arendt *et al.*, 1977, with permission of the publisher).

cross-reaction with N-acetyltryptamine, whose plasma levels are, however, unknown.

Rigorous comparison of MT levels as determined by bioassay and radioimmunoassay using antiserum K-244 has not been performed. This has, however, been done for the antiserum derived from rabbit 8. A series of 17 human pineal glands assayed for MT using the tadpole bioassay technique of Ralph and Lynch (1970) (*Xenopus laevis* larvae)

TABLE IV   Bioassay and Radioimmunoassay of Melatonin (MT) in Human Pineal Glands

Number of gland	MT (pg/mg gland)			
	Bioassay (*Xenopus laevis*)	RIA rabbit 8	RIA K-244	RIA rabbit 8 / RIA K-244
13	317	407	165	2.46
18	7879	6514	2572	2.53
25	850	703	218	3.22
26	1176	1354	521	2.59

and antiserum from rabbit 8 gave a good correlation $-r = 0.965$, p <0.001. Four of these glands have also been assayed by radioimmunoassay using antiserum K-244. The results are shown in Table IV. Antibody K-244 gives immunoreactive MT values 2.5 times lower than both radioimmunoassay with antiserum rabbit 8 and bioassay. Lack of specificity has not been shown for any of these methods, except for the possible interference of N-acetyltryptamine with antiserum from rabbit 8; the reason for this discrepancy is unclear.

IV. APPLICATIONS AND IMPORTANCE OF MELATONIN RADIOIMMUNOASSAY

A. Human Studies

Normal values (X ± SEM) for serum immunoreactive (K244) melatonin were: women, January to November 1977, 12 hours, 13.9 ± 0.5 pg/ml, 24 hours 66.1 ± 5.3 pg/ml $n = 50$; men, January to November 1977, 12 hours, 14.6 ± 0.9 pg/ml, $n = 45$, 24 hours, 49.1 ± 3.8 pg/ml, $n = 47$. Midnight samples were taken after three hours of dim red light.

Clear circadian variations in circulating human serum MT have been shown at short time intervals in both men and women (Arendt, *et al.*, 1977) with a maximum in darkness at 2 AM and a minimum during daylight. We have also been able to demonstrate a seasonal rhythm in human serum melatonin sampled at 8 AM in six healthy males, (Arendt *et al.*, 1978), peak values being found in January and July with nadirs in May and October, and a menstrual cycle variation with peak values during the luteal phase, at 8 AM in five healthy women (Arendt, 1978). Studies are currently being performed to compare different radioimmunoassay systems and compare these data with GCMS measurements.

B. Animal Studies

It has long been maintained that the biosynthesis of MT in the rat pineal is controlled in a rate-limiting fashion by the activity of N-acetyltransferase (NAT) (Klein and Weller, 1970). It is known, for example, that during the night-induced increase in pineal function, leading to elevated blood levels of MT, the activity of hydroxyindole-O-methyltransferase (HIOMT) changes very little in comparison with the large rise in NAT. Thus, more MT is formed after a rise in NAT by a simple process of mass action (Klein *et al.*, 1970).

In a recent study (Wilkinson *et al.*, 1976a), we have demonstrated
that the endogenous rise and fall of NAT during the dark phase are
indeed paralleled very closely by variations in pineal and serum
melatonin content (Figure 5). These results appear to confirm the idea
of a NAT-dependent increase in MT biosynthesis.

On the other hand, and also under physiologic conditions, the activity of HIOMT appears to vary significantly during the estrous cycle of
the rat and could, therefore, be controlled not just by NAT but by
gonadal steroids as well, (Wallen and Yochim, 1974). Clearly, the direct assay of MT is likely to be a more valid index of the secretion of
this hormone than estimates of biosynthetic activity. Preliminary evidence has been obtained for the divergence of NAT activity and MT
secretion under particular *in vitro* conditions (Wilkinson and Arendt,
1978); progesterone acutely reduces the output of MT from female rat

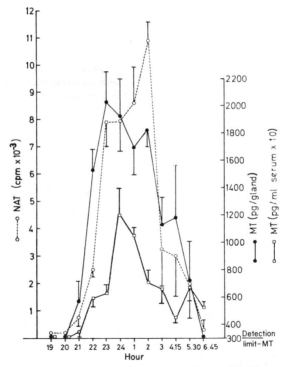

Figure 5. Parallel changes in pineal *N*-acetyltransferase (NAT) activity with pineal
and serum melatonin through a dark cycle. Each point is the mean from at least six
animals ± S.E.M. NAT, O----O; pineal MT, ●——●; serum MT, □——□. (Reprinted from
Wilkinson *et al.*, 1977, with permission of the publisher.)

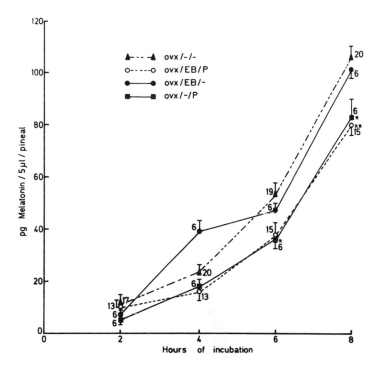

Figure 6.   Melatonin content of incubation media after stimulation of rat pineal glands with $5.0 \times 10^{-9}\, M$ L-isoproterenol (8 hr); effects of (i) priming ovariectomized animals with estrogen and (ii) progesterone *in vitro* (10 μg/ml). Numbers refer to the number of pineals; each point $\pm$ S.E.M. $**p < 0.01$; $*p \leq 0.05$. Groups OVX/P and OVX/EB/P are compared with OVX/EB.

pineals stimulated *in vitro* with isoproterenol (Figure 6), presumably by inhibiting HIOMT. In this work, the concentration of progesterone (10 μg/ml) is highly nonphysiologic, and further studies are required to investigate the effect of the steroid in more detail, as well as its interaction with estrogen. However, it is possible to suggest that progesterone may exert some control on MT output quite independent of NAT activation. This view is reinforced by the observation that in the presence of progesterone, a large increase in NAT activity is associated with an inhibition of MT secretion, i.e., the activity of NAT in the OVX/P group (Figure 6) is 2194 $\pm$ 174 pmoles/gland/hour ($n = 7$), while for the other three groups, the activity is approximately 1000 pmoles/gland/hour ($p < 0.001$).

It should be clear from the *in vitro* studies in which MT concentrations in the culture media are assayed, that a decrease in MT concentration may not always reflect a decrease in HIOMT activity, but could be accounted for by a change in secretion rate. The mode of secretion of MT is an aspect of pineal physiology that has been seriously neglected in view of the sophisticated techniques used to elucidate secretory mechanisms in other neuroendocrine tissues (Quay, 1974).

We have begun studies on the role of calcium, a cation known to be intimately concerned with secretory mechanisms, in the control of pineal biosynthetic activity. Calcium appears to have a profound effect on the sensitivity of the pineal to stimulation with β-agonists (Wilkinson, 1976; Wilkinson *et al.*, 1976b). During the course of this work, we have observed that MT secretion can be inhibited at the same time as NAT activity is increased. Thus, repeated stimulation of pineals with β-agonists *in vitro* leads to large increases in NAT, even in the absence of calcium, although the secretion of MT is inhibited in calcium-free medium (M. Wilkinson and J. Arendt, unpublished observations). Changes in intracellular calcium could, therefore, be a further mechanism controlling pineal MT output independent of NAT activity.

In conclusion, it may be said that the direct assay of MT by such a sensitive and precise technique as radioimmunoassay is essential for the elucidation of pineal function, particularly in man and that it may serve to distinguish between the various control mechanisms acting on the pineal gland in experimental studies.

V. RADIOIODINATED MELATONIN ANALOG

Rollag and Niswender (1976) have described the use of an iodinated analog, N-[3-^{125}I](4-hydroxyphenyl)-3-propionyl-5-methoxytryptamine, in a melatonin radioimmunoassay. This approach warrants description, although it may be neither necessary nor appropriate for every MT immunoassay. A general description of the use of iodinated derivatives for steroid radioimmunoassays is presented in Chapter 37.

The hydroxyphenylpropionyl derivative of methoxytryptamine which is radiodinated must be synthesized from methoxytryptamine. In this reaction, 1.0 mmole each of methoxytryptamine (190 mg), tri-n-butylamine (238 μl), and N-succinimidyl-3-(4-hydroxyphenyl)propionate (263 mg) are shaken in 10 ml dioxane at room temperature for 60 minutes. After discarding the precipitate collected by centrifugation at 2000 g for 30 minutes, 10 ml 0.1 M aqueous $NaHCO_3$ (pH 8.0) is added to the dioxane solution, and one hour later, 10 ml ethyl acetate is added. N-3-(4-Hydroxyphenyl)-propionyl-5-methoxytryptamine is contained in the upper organic phase. The organic phase is washed with $0.1 M$ NaHCO$_3$, pH 8.9 and then $0.1 N$ HCl to remove unreacted 5-methyoxytryptamine and dried *in vacuo*. The analog, a white oil, is made up to 1.0 mg/ml in methanol and stored at $-20°C$.

For radioiodination, 1.0 μg analog is transferred to a vial and the methanol allowed to evaporate. Iodination is performed by serially adding 50 μl $0.1 M$ phosphate buffer, pH 7.1, 1.0 μg (21.4 mU) lactoperoxidase in 1.0 μl water, 2.0 mCi ^{125}I, and 1.2 nmoles (40 ng) H$_2$O$_2$ in 10 μl water. After five minutes at 4°C, 100 μl 16% sucrose in buffer containing 22 mM boric acid, 6.4 mM EDTA, 14 mM Tris, pH 8.9, are added. Purification of label is accomplished on polyacrylamide gel electrophoresis. Aliquots (50 μl) of the reaction mixtures are transferred to the cathodal surface of 5.0×75 mm gel columns and anodal electrophoresis is performed for 75 minutes at 4 mA, in a continuous buffer of 11 mM boric acid, 3.2 mM EDTA, and 7 mM Tris, pH 8.9. Segments which migrate 30 mm into the gel contain the radioiodinated analog. The   N-[3-^{125}I](4-hydroxyphenyl)-3-propionyl-5-methoxytryptamine is eluted overnight into 1.0 ml assay buffer.

REFERENCES

Arendt, J., Sizonenko, P. C., and Paunier, L. (1975). Melatonin radioimmunoassay. *J. Clin. Endocrinol. Metab.* **40**, 347–350.

Arendt, J., Wetterberg, L., Heyden, T., Sizonenko, P. C. and Paunier, L. (1977). Radioimmunoassay of melatonin: Human serum and cerebrospinal fluid. *Hormone Res.* **8**, 65–75.

Arendt, J., Wirz-Justice, A. and Bradtke, J. (1978). Annual rhythm of serum melatonin in man. *Neuroscience Letters*, in press.

Arendt, J. (1978). Melatonin assays in body fluids. Proceedings of the International Symposium on the Pineal Gland. *J. Neural Transmission*, in press.

Axelrod, J. (1974). The pineal gland: A neurochemical transducer. *Science* **184**, 1341–1348.

Berg, C. P., Rose, W. C., and Marvel, C. S. (1929–1930). Tryptophan and growth. *J. Biol. Chem.* **85**, 207–218.

Kennaway, D. J., Frith, E. G., Phillipou, G., Matthews, C., and Seamark, R. F. (1977). A specific radioimmunoassay for melatonin in biological tissues and its validation by gas chromatography–mass spectrometry. *Endocrinology* **101**, 119–123.

Klein, D. C., and Weller, J. L. (1970). Indole metabolism in the pineal gland: A circadian rhythm in N acetyltransferase. *Science* **169**, 1093–1095.

Klein, D. C., Berg, G. R., and Weller, J. L. (1970). Melatonin synthesis: Adenosine 3, 5-monophosphate and norepinephrine stimulate N-acetyltransferase. *Science* **168**, 979–980.

Lerner, A. B., Case, J. D., Takahashi, Y., Lee, T. H., and Mori, W. (1958). Isolation of melatonin, the pineal gland factor that lightens melanocytes. *J. Am. Chem. Soc.* **80**, 2587.

Levine, L., and Riceberg, L. J. (1975). Radioimmunoassay for melatonin. *Res. Commun. Chem. Pathol. Pharmacol.* **10**, 693–702.

Maickel, R. P., and Miller, F. P. (1968). The fluorometric determination of indole alkylamines in brain and pineal gland. *Adv. Pharmacol.* **6**, 71–77.

Mori, W., and Lerner, A. B. (1960). A microscopic bioassay for melatonin. *Endocrinology* **67**, 443–450.

Ozaki, Y., Lynch, H. J., and Wurtman, R. J. (1976). Melatonin in rat pineal, plasma and urine: 24 hour rhythmicity and effect of chlorpromazine. *Endocrinology* **98**, 1418–1424.

Pang, S. F., Brown, G. M., Grota, L. J., and Rodman, R. L. (1976). Radioimmunoassay of melatonin in pineal glands, harderian glands, retinas and sera of rats or chickens. *Fed. Proc., Fed. Am. Soc. Exp. Biol.* **35**, 691.

Pasini, C., Colo, V., and Coda, S. (1963). Sintesi di alcuni derivati idrossi-sostituti del tryptofanos. *Gazz. Chim. Ital.* **93**, 1066.

Pelham, R. W., Ralph, C. L., and Campbell, I. M. (1972). Mass spectral identification of melatonin in blood. *Biochem. Biophys. Res. Commun.* **46**, 1236–1241.

Quay, W. B. (1974). "Pineal Chemistry." Thomas, Springfield, Illinois.

Quay, W. B., and Bagnara, J. T. (1964). Relative potencies of indolic and related compounds in the body-lightening reaction of larval Xenopus. *Arch. Int. Pharmacodyn. Ther.* **150**, 137–143.

Ralph, C. L., and Lynch, H. J. (1970). A quantitative melatonin bioassay. *Gen. Comp. Endocrinol.* **15**, 334–338.

Rollag, M. D., and Niswender, G. D. (1976). Radioimmunoassay of serum concentrations of melatonin in sheep exposed to different lighting regimes. *Endocrinology* **98**, 482–489.

Smith, I., Landon, J., Mullen, P. E., Silman, R. E., Sneddon, W., and Wilson, B. (1977). The absolute identification of melatonin in human plasma by GCMS. *Endocrinol., Proc. Int. Congr. Endocrinol., 5th, 1976* Abstracts, p. 13.

Vaitukaitis, J., Robbins, J. B., Mieschlag, E., and Ross, G. Y. (1971). A method for producing specific antisera with small doses of immunogen. *J. Clin. Endocrinol. Metab.* **33**, 988–991.

Vaughan, G. M., Pelham, R. W., Pang, S. F., Loughlin, L. L., Wilson, K. M., Sandock, K. L., Vaughan, M. K., Koslow, S. H., and Reiter, R. J. (1976). Nocturnal elevation of plasma melatonin and urinary 5-hydroxy indole acetic acid in young men: Attempts at modification by brief changes in environmental lighting and sleep and by autonomic drugs. *J. Clin. Endocrinol. Metab.* **42**, 752–764.

Wallen, E. P., and Yochim, J. M. (1974). Rhythmic function of pineal hydroxyindole-O-methyl transferase during the estrous cycle: An analysis. *Biol. Reprod.* **10**, 461–466.

Wetterberg, L., Arendt, J., Paunier, L., Sizonenko, P. C., Van Donselaar, W., and Heyden, T. (1976). Human serum melatonin changes during the menstrual cycle. *J. Clin. Endocrinol. Metab.* **42**, 185–188.

Wetterberg, L., Arendt, J., and Heyden, T. (1977). Melatonin in serum and cerebrospinal fluid in the human. *Endocrinol., Proc. Int. Congr. Endocrinol., 5th, 1976* Abstracts, p. 8.

Wetterberg, L., (1977). Melatonin in serum. *Nature,* **269**, 646.

Wilkinson, M. (1976). Inhibition of the noradrenergic induction of pineal N-acetyltransferase by dibutyryl cyclic guanosine monophosphate and by ionophore X-537A. *Neurosci. Lett.* **2**, 29–33.

Wilkinson, M., and Arendt, J. (1978). Stimulatory and inhibitory effects of estrogen and progesterone on rat pineal N-acetyl transferase activity and melatonin production. *Experientiu*, in press.

Wilkinson, M., de Ziegler, D., and Ruf, K. B. (1976a). The role of Ca^{++} in development of hyposensitivity of pineal β-receptors. *Experientia* **32**, 764.

Wilkinson, M., Arendt, J., Bradtke, J., and de Ziegler, D. (1977). Determination of dark-induced elevation of pineal N-acetyltransferase activity with simultaneous radioimmunoassay of melatonin in pineal, serum and pituitary of the male rat. *J. Endocrinol.* **72**, 243–244.

Wurzburger, R. J., Kawashima, K., Miller, R. L., and Spector, S. (1976). Determination of rat pineal gland melotonin content by a radioimmunoassay. *Life Sci.* **18**, 867–877.

7

Substance P

EDMUND A. MROZ AND SUSAN E. LEEMAN

I. INTRODUCTION

Substance P is a hypotensive and smooth muscle-contracting peptide which was first detected in crude extracts of intestine and brain by von Euler and Gaddum (1931). Early attempts to purify substance P were only partially successful (Lembeck and Zetler, 1971). Chang and Leeman (1970) reported the purification of a sialagogic peptide from bovine hypothalamic extracts, and showed that their isolated material had the chemical and biologic properties of the substance P of von Euler and Gaddum. Since then, Studer and co-workers (1973), beginning with the more traditional starting material of equine intestine and using the contraction of guinea pig ileum as the bioassay, have isolated the same peptide and confirmed both Chang and

121

Methods of Hormone Radioimmunoassay, Second Edition
Copyright © 1979 by Academic Press, Inc.

Leeman's isolation of substance P and the amino acid sequence determined by Chang *et al.* (1971). The amino acid sequence determined by both groups for substance P is H-Arg-Pro-Lys-Pro-Gln-Gln-Phe-Phe-Gly-Leu-Met-NH$_2$. Synthetic material prepared according to this structure has chemical and biologic properties identical with those of native substance P (Tregear *et al.*, 1971).

Since the purification, the determination of the structure, and the chemical synthesis of substance P, large quantities of pure material have been available for study. On a molar basis, substance P is one of the most potent hypotensive agents yet discovered, with an intravenous infusion of 2.0 pmole kg^{-1}min^{-1} producing detectable hypotension in dogs (Hallberg and Pernow, 1975). Substance P has also been shown to be pharmacologically active within the nervous system. Several groups have demonstrated effects of exogenously applied substance P upon the activity of neurons in the central nervous system (Otsuka and Konishi, 1976; Henry *et al.*, 1975; Phillis and Limacher, 1974; Davies and Dray, 1976). Following an earlier suggestion of Lembeck (1953), Otsuka and Konishi (1976) have now produced much evidence that substance P may be a transmitter of primary sensory neurons.

Investigation of the possible neural or hormonal roles of substance P requires an assay capable of measuring its levels in tissue extracts, in blood, and in physiologic salt solutions used for perfusing organs or for superfusing isolated tissues. The assay described here is a modification of our initially reported assay (Powell *et al.*, 1973), using a different antiserum, different incubation conditions, and a better defined tracer. The present assay is about 100 times more sensitive than our earlier assay and has been used successfully for all three of the above sample types.

Although the following reflects our experience with our own substance P assay, the optimal conditions for, and the specificity of any other radioimmunoassay for this peptide of course must be determined anew for each antiserum.

II. ASSAY TECHNIQUES

A. Potential Problems in the Radioimmunoassay of Substance P

There are three facts about substance P that deserve special comment with regard to the development and performance of its radioimmunoassay. First, it is a relatively small molecule. Thus, the best results in the preparation of antisera would be expected from coupling substance P to a larger carrier molecule and using this conjugate as the immunogen. Second, substance P lacks a tyrosine, so it cannot be iodinated directly. However, substitution of a tyrosine for the phenylalanine in position 8 [as occurs in the related peptide physalaemin (Erspamer *et al.*, 1964)] has little effect on the biologic activity of the molecule (G. W. Tregear and S. E. Leeman, unpublished results; Fisher *et al.*, 1976). This 8-Tyr substance P, which is commercially available, can be radioiodinated to produce tracer for the assay. Third, substance P has a pronounced tendency to adhere to glass (Cleugh and Gaddum, 1963), plastic, and metal surfaces (S. E. Leeman, E. A. Mroz, J. Losay, and W. J. Gamble, unpublished). This tendency is especially pronounced in protein-free solutions, but the addition of protein to substance P-containing solutions does not completely solve the problem. Although such behavior is not uncommon among polypeptides, substance P seems much worse in this regard than neurotensin (Carraway and Leeman, 1973), another peptide recently discovered in this laboratory.

B. Antiserum Production

1. Preparation of Immunogen

In the first report of a radioimmunoassay for substance P (Powell *et al.*, 1973), synthetic substance P (Tregear *et al.*, 1971) was coupled to bovine γ-globulin by 1-ethyl-3-(3-dimethylaminopropyl) carbodiimide. More recently, we have prepared immunogen by coupling substance P to succinylated thyroglobulin. Thyroglobulin is succinylated at room temperature by the method of Klapper and Klotz (1972). One hundred milligrams of bovine thyroglobulin (Sigma Chemical Co.) is stirred in 20 ml 0.15 M NaCl, and 200 mg solid succinic anhydride is added in small aliquots to the stirring solution over the course of 30 to 60 minutes. The pH of the solution is monitored and kept in the range of 7 to 9 by addition of a concentrated solution of NaOH. The solution is allowed to stand for two hours after addition of the succinic anhydride, after which the product is dialyzed exhaustively against distilled water and lyophilized. A solution of succinylated thyroglobulin, 10 mg/ml, is made in a phosphate-buffered saline containing 0.01 M sodium phosphate buffer, pH 7.4, and 0.15 M NaCl. Fifty milligrams of 1-ethyl-3-(3-dimethylaminopropyl) carbodiimide is added to 2.0 ml of this solution in a stoppered conical centrifuge tube. Then, 1.0

ml of a 10 mg/ml solution of substance P in the same phosphate-buffered saline is added with mixing; flocculation occurs almost immediately. The mixture is kept at 4°C for 16 hours, with vortexing every four hours. Finally, the mixture is dialyzed against ten liters of the phosphate buffered saline for 24 hours at room temperature, with two changes of buffer.

In our hands, this leads to a suspension of conjugate containing about 25% substance P by weight with 60% of the added substance P recovered in the conjugate (determined by amino acid analysis of an acid hydrolysate). The scale of the above preparation may be a bit large for researchers who depend on commercial sources (e.g., Beckman or Bachem) of substance P, but it should be possible to reduce the scale significantly if required.

2. Immunization Procedure

We have followed the procedure of Vaitukaitis *et al.* (1971) with only slight modification. Two days before immunization, young female New Zealand white rabbits are injected subcutaneously with 0.5 ml crude pertussis vaccine. For immunization with substance P, an emulsion of 1.0 ml complete Freund's adjuvant, 1.0 ml saline containing the appropriate amount of substance P coupled to thyroglobulin, and 5.0 mg dried tubercle bacilli per animal is made with a Virtis homogenizer. As little as 10 μg of conjugate has produced measurable anti-substance P activity in the serum, although 50 to 200 μg give more consistent production. This emulsion is injected in 30 to 50 sites intradermally on the back, close to the spinal column. Titer is checked eight weeks later (Section II,B,3), and animals are boosted with one-half the initial amount of immunogen in incomplete Freund's adjuvant without added tubercle bacilli if an insufficient response is seen at that time. A rabbit is also boosted if the titer of its antiserum begins to fall appreciably.

3. Screening of Antisera

Antisera useful for radioimmunoassay are those which have antibodies with high affinity; their titers are relatively unimportant. Thus, we check antisera both for their ability to bind tracer and for the ability of small amounts of unlabeled substance P to displace the tracer, under the conditions of our radioimmunoassay (Section II,E). A range of antiserum dilutions is incubated with 5000 cpm tracer (corresponding to 2.5 fmole), both with and without an additional 50 fmole of unlabeled substance P. At antiserum dilutions where about 30% of the label is bound in the absence of unlabeled substance P (corresponding to our assay conditions), 50 fmole of unlabeled substance P will displace 80–90% of the bound tracer from the most useful anti-sera. Other antisera can be used, but assays employing them will be less sensitive.

C. Preparation of Tracer

We have attempted to produce a highly purified moniodinated tracer molecule under reasonably gentle conditions, so that the tracer might be useful both in radioimmunoassay and in biologic studies. Iodination of 8-Tyr substance P is performed with limiting amounts of chloramine-T, and the iodinated molecule is separated from the un-iodinated by ion-exchange chromatography.

1. Preparation of the Ion-Exchange Column

Sulfopropyl (SP) Sephadex (Pharmacia) C-25 is swollen in 0.2 M sodium carbonate buffer, pH 9.9, and is then washed repeatedly in the same buffer diluted to 5.0 mM. An 11-ml column of this SP Sephadex is prepared in a disposable 10-ml glass pipette, and at least 200 ml of the 5.0 mM buffer is washed through to ensure equilibration. The column is poured and run in a cold room at 4°C.

2. Iodination Conditions

The reagents and amounts typically used for iodination are indi-cated in Table I. If the iodine is supplied in a conical vial covered by a rubber septum, the reaction can be performed conveniently in the vial by injecting reagents through the septum; alternatively, reagents can be mixed in a tapered tube formed from a Pasteur pipette. The reac-tion mixture is buffered with 0.3 M sodium phosphate buffer, pH 7.4; to terminate the reaction, 0.5 ml 5 mM carbonate buffer, pH 9.9, con-taining 1.0 mg/ml bovine serum albumin is added.

Table I   Reagents for Iodination of 8-Tyr Substance P

Solution	Volume added (μl)	Moles added
Sodium phosphate buffer, 0.3 M pH, 7.4	10	—
Na^{125}I, carrier-free, 500 mCi/ml in 0.1 M NaOH	10	2×10^{-9}
8-Tyr substance P,[a] 1.0 mg/ml in 0.1M acetic acid	10	7×10^{-9}
Chloramine-T,[b] 100 μg/ml in phosphate buffer	10	4×10^{-9}

[a] Available from Beckman Instruments, Spinco Division, Bioproducts Department, Palo Alto, California.

[b] Chloramine-T is added in two 5.0-μl aliquots delivered about 15 seconds apart.

3. *Separation of the Reaction Mixture*

The reaction mixture is applied to the top of the column; the reaction vial is washed once with 5.0 mM carbonate buffer with 1.0 mg/ml bovine serum albumin and the wash is applied to the column after the reaction mixture has entered. Twenty milliliter of 5.0 mM carbonate buffer (without albumin) is run through the column at about 10 ml/hr to remove free iodide, iodine bound to albumin, and the very small amount of diiodinated tyrosyl substance P that is produced under the above iodination conditions. The buffer is then changed to 20 mM carbonate buffer at the same pH; this is run at no more than 6.0 ml/hr, and 2.0 ml fractions are collected into 13 × 100 mm glass tubes containing 40 μl 100 mg/ml bovine serum albumin in water. As shown in Figure 1, this buffer change elutes a peak of coincident radioactivity and immunoactivity, but the uniodinated peptide is retained on the column.

4. *Yield, Properties, and Storage of Tracer*

Although the separated peak of labeled peptide may not be completely homogeneous, it has an initial specific activity (determined by

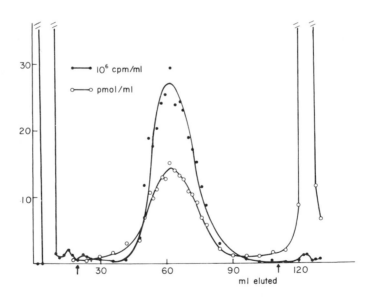

Figure 1.   Profile of radioactivity and immunoreactivity in the eluate of a column used to separate the iodination mixture, as described in the text. At the first arrow, buffer was changed to 20 mM carbonate buffer; at the second arrow, NaCl was added to the buffer reservoir to produce a concentration of 2.0 M.

radioimmunoassay) of 2000 Ci/mmole consistent with moniodination. About one-third of the iodine is recovered in the peak of moniodinated product, while 10% of the original 8-Tyr substance P is labeled. The peak of monoiodinated product is diluted two-fold with ethanol, aliquoted in appropriate amounts, and stored at −20°C until use. "Damage" under the assay conditions described below is about 2% after preparation, and gradually increases to 5% in six to eight weeks.

Nilsson and colleagues (1977) have described additional methods of purification of tracer, including absorption to QUSO G32 (also used by O'Connell *et al.*, 1976) and Whatman CF1 cellulose and starch gel vertical electrophoresis.

D. Sample Preparation

Slight differences in sample preparation are called for depending upon the type of sample to be assayed.

1. Tissue Extracts

Tissue extracts have been the samples most frequently assayed by this laboratory. Although it is possible to use the acid–acetone extraction method of Chang and Leeman (1970), it is more convenient to use 2.0 *M* acetic acid as an extraction medium, and we have not found substantial differences in the amounts of substance P detected. Samples are homogenized in about ten volumes of 2.0 *M* acetic acid, extracted overnight at 4°C, spun, and the supernatant is saved. The pellet is resuspended in acetic acid, respun, and this wash is pooled with the original supernatant. The combined extract is then shell-frozen and lyophilized. The sample is resuspended in an appropriate volume of assay buffer (Section II,E,1) immediately before assay, and, if necessary, spun to remove sediment. The recovery of substance P added to the original homogenate in this procedure is quantitative.

2. Physiologic Salt Solutions

These are acidified with glacial acetic acid to about 2.0 *M* final concentration, spun if necessary to remove denatured protein, and the supernatant is lyophilized. Protein-containing salt solutions retain some acetic acid upon lyophilization, and must be neutralized before assay. Phenol red (often present in tissue culture media) is a useful acid–base indicator for this purpose, and does not interfere with our assay. Recovery of added substance P is quantitative.

Table II   Measurements of Substance P in Plasma[a]

Sample treatment	Animal	Number of samples	fmole/ml (mean ± SD)
Unextracted	Rat	12	423 ± 75
Extracted[b]	Rat	7	9.0 ± 2.0
Unextracted	Calf	1	165 ± 23
Extracted	Calf	4	18.0 ± 5.4

[a] Table from Leeman and Carraway (1977).
[b] Extraction procedure as in Section II,D,3.

3. Plasma

In our assay for substance P, the assay of unextracted plasma apparently leads to spuriously high results. Plasma was extracted with five volumes of acetone: 1.0 M HCl (100 : 3), followed by reextraction of the precipitate with acetone: 0.01 M HCl (80 : 20). The supernatants were pooled and organic solvents removed by extraction of the pooled extracts with petroleum ether. The aqueous residue was dried by rotary evaporation and lyophilization. As shown in Table II, this extraction recovered only a small fraction of the apparent immunoactivity seen in the direct assay of unextracted plasma. Recovery of added substance P under these conditions is quantitative. We have observed similar results with cold ethanol extraction of plasma, but recoveries using that technique were only 60–70%.

E. Performing the Assay

1. Buffer

The assay buffer is phosphate-buffered saline, with added gelatin to minimize the loss of substance P to the surface of the incubation tubes. It contains 50 mM sodium phosphate buffer, pH 7.4, 8.5 gm/liter NaCl, 1.0 gm/liter gelatin, and 0.2 gm/liter NaN$_3$ as a preservative.

2. Standard Substance P

A concentrated solution of synthetic substance P (about 1.5 mg/ml, or, equivalently, 1.0 mM) is made in 0.1 M acetic acid, and the precise concentration of substance P is determined by amino acid analysis following acid hydrolysis. Further dilutions of this solution to produce working stock solutions are made into assay buffer and frozen. So long as such solutions remain cool, freezing and thawing do not seem to affect their immunoactivity, although exposure of such solutions to room temperature overnight leads to considerable loss. We have found a 100 nM stock solution of substance P to give consistent standard values over a period of several months.

The tendency of substance P to adhere to surfaces makes serial dilutions inaccurate. Rather, standards are delivered in the form of different volumes of two standard solutions made from the stock solution. For our present assay, we make standards of 240 and 80 fmole/ml for each assay from the 100 nM stock solution, and then deliver 200, 100, 50, and 25 μl of each of these solutions as standards. This spans a range of 48 to 2.0 fmole per assay tube, which is sufficient for most purposes. However, reasonably precise standard values can be obtained with 1.0 fmole or less if necessary.

3. Choice of Antiserum Dilution and Tracer Concentration

The conditions for optimum assay sensitivity depend on the affinity of the antibody, the specific activity of the tracer, the volume of incubate counted, the time available for counting, and the various experimental errors in pipetting, separating bound from free, and so on. In general, for assays in which only the bound fractions are counted after separation of bound from free, the antibody sites and the tracer should be in concentrations on the order of magnitude of the antibody–tracer dissociation constant, with an excess of tracer such that 20–30% of tracer is bound (Ekins, 1970).

We estimate that the dissociation constant for our present antiserum is 2.0×10^{-12} mole liter^{-1}. In our incubation volume of 0.5 ml we use 5000 cpm of tracer (2.5 fmole, final concentration $5.0 \times 10^{-12} M$) and an estimated 1.25 fmole of antibody sites (concentration $2.5 \times 10^{-12} M$).

4. Setting up the Assay

As a precaution, the assay is set up on ice. A standard curve is set up both at the beginning and at the end of the assay, using the concentrations as outlined above. Eight tubes without sample or standard are set aside at both the beginning and the end of the assay for the determination of maximum binding and nonspecific apparent binding or "damage." Samples of approximately known concentration are prepared as above and are usually assayed in duplicate at three different doses delivered in the form of three different volumes of a single sample solution. A completely unknown sample is taken up in 1.0 ml buffer, 200, 100, and 50 μl are assayed directly, then, the same volumes of a fivefold dilution of the sample are also assayed. Under our conditions, this will allow an estimation of the content of a completely unknown sample provided it has anywhere from 10 fmole to 4.8 pmole substance P. Both standard and sample solutions are drawn up and down in the pipette tip four or five times before delivery to ensure equilibration of the solution with the surface of the pipette tip.

The volume in each incubation tube is 0.5 ml, added in the order: sample plus buffer to make a total of 200 μl 100 μl diluted antibody (or 100 μl buffer for "damage" tube) 100 μl tracer containing 4000 to 5000 cpm and a final 100 μl buffer. The tubes are vortexed briefly and placed in the cold room for three to four days, so that the binding comes close to equilibrium.

Powell and his colleagues continue to use delayed addition of tracer (Rodbard *et al.*, 1971; Powell *et al.*, 1973), but with only a few hours separating addition of antibody from addition of tracer and with a shorter total incubation time (O'Connell *et al.*, 1976). In their hands, this leads to somewhat higher sensitivity than an equilibrium assay. However, we are more comfortable with the equilibrium assay, since we feel it is less prone to nonspecific effects. In any event, those who choose to use such a nonequilibrium assay must empirically determine the appropriate conditions for the available antiserum.

5. *Separation of Bound Tracer from Free Tracer*

A charcoal suspension is prepared from 10 gm charcoal (carbon, decolorizing, neutral, "Norit") and 1.0 gm dextran T-20 (Pharmacia) in a total of 400 ml of the assay buffer as described above (Section II,E,1) but without the gelatin. To ensure even coating of the charcoal with dextran, the dextran is first dissolved in half of the total buffer volume, and then added slowly to the charcoal which is being stirred in the remainder of the buffer. This suspension can be stored at 4°C.

After the assay has incubated, 200 μl of this suspension is added to each incubation tube, and after ten minutes, the tubes are spun for 20 to 25 minutes at 2000 cpm in an IEC model PR-J centrifuge refrigerated to 4°C. The supernatants containing the antibody-bound tracer are decanted into clean tubes and are counted for five minutes each along with the charcoal pellets from the standard curve tubes in order to determine the total counts in the original incubation tubes.

6. *Calculation of Assay Results*

We use a truncated but otherwise unweighted logit–log linearization method (Rodbard and Frazier, 1975). Only those values of bound counts which are between 12 and 88% of the maximum counts bound in the absence of cold substance P (appropriately corrected for nonspecific apparent binding) are considered to lie on the curve. Since we have eight different standard values spaced around the half-

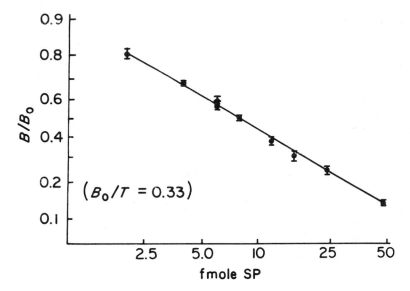

Figure 2. A typical standard curve for our substance P radioimmunoassay. B/B_0, ratio of counts bound with a given amount of substance P to counts bound in absence of added substance P, plotted on a logit scale. Bars indicate ± one S.D. from mean of triplicate determinations. B_0/T, fraction of counts bound specifically in the absence of added substance P.

displacement point, this method of analysis is adequate (Chang *et al.*, 1975). Most recently, calculations have been performed with a program written in this laboratory for the HP-67 programmable calculator (Hewlett-Packard, Cupertino, California). This program calculates slopes, standard errors of slopes, and intercepts for both sample and standard dose–response curves, and interpolates substance P values for samples from the raw bound counts. A typical dose–response curve is shown in Figure 2.

III. SOME CHARACTERISTICS AND RESULTS OF THE ASSAY

A. Nonspecific Interference

We have found that common inorganic ions in concentrations in excess of those anticipated in samples have no influence on our assay. Values of pH below 6 inhibit binding, but the assay is unaffected by pH values between 6 and 8.

B. Cross-Reactivity with Other Peptides and with Fragments of Substance P

Table III lists for a variety of peptides the amount that displaces 15% of bound tracer under the conditions of the assay. The table includes the amino acid sequences of several peptides related structurally to substance P. Of these, physalaemin and eledoisin cross-react appreciably in the assay, but they have so far been reported present only in nonmammalian species. The eledoisin-related peptide is a synthetic peptide often used in pharmacologic studies. Bombesin, which, like substance P, has a Leu-Met-NH$_2$ carboxy terminus, does not cross-react in the assay reported here, but this peptide cross-reacts strongly in assays using another antiserum we have obtained (data not shown). Bombesin, thus, should be checked to test the specificity of antisera to substance P. Cross-reaction of peptides not related to substance P should not pose problems in assays of most biologic samples, but the slight cross-reactions of methionine–enkephalin, somatostatin,

Table III   Cross-Reaction of Other Peptides in Substance P Radioimmunoassay

Peptide		15% Displacement (fmole)
Substance P:	H-Arg-Pro-Lys-Pro-Gln-Gln-Phe-Phe-Gly-Leu-Met-NH$_2$	1.5
Peptides[a] structurally related to substance P		
Physalaemin:	<Glu-Ala-Asp-Pro-Asn-Lys-Phe-Tyr-Gly-Leu-Met-NH$_2$	240
Eledoisin:	<Glu-Pro-Ser-Lys-Asp-Ala-Phe-Ile-Gly-Leu-Met-NH$_2$	1.4×10^3
Eledoisin-related peptide:	H-Lys-Phe-Ile-Gly-Leu-Met-NH$_2$	5×10^4
Bombesin: <Glu-Gln-Arg-Leu-Gly-Asn-Gln-Trp-Ala-Val-Gly-His-Leu-Met-NH$_2$		$>1.0 \times 10^6$
Other peptides		
Methionine–enkephalin		5.0×10^4
Somatostatin		5.0×10^4
ACTH		5.0×10^4
Bradykinin		3.5×10^5
Angiotensin II		3.5×10^5
Oxytocin		1.0×10^6
LH-RH		1.0×10^6
Pancreatic polypeptide		$>2.0 \times 10^5$
Glucagon		$>2.6 \times 10^5$
TRH		$>1.0 \times 10^6$
Neurotensin		$>1.0 \times 10^6$
Bacitracin		$>1.0 \times 10^6$
Insulin		$>1.0 \times 10^6$

[a] <Glu = pyroglutamyl.

Table IV   Relative Activities of Some Carboxy-Terminal Fragments of Substance P[a]

	Percent sialagogic activity[b]	Percent immunologic activity[c]
H-Arg-Pro-Lys-Pro-Gln-Gln-Phe-Phe-Gly-Leu-Met-NH$_2$ (Substance P)	100	100
H-Pro-Gln-Gln-Phe-Phe-Gly-Leu-Met-NH$_2$	12	47
<Glu-Phe-Phe-Gly-Leu-Met-NH$_2$	15	0.01
H-Phe-Gly-Leu-Met-NH$_2$	≈1.0	<0.00004
H-Leu-Met-NH$_2$	<0.04	<0.00004

[a] Table from Leeman et al. (1977).
[b] Sialagogic activity based on i.v. dose needed to elicit 50 μl saliva from a 100-gm rat anesthetized with Nembutal. 100% = 40 pmole.
[c] Immunologic activity based on dose needed to displace 50% of bound counts under conditions described in text. 100% = 8.0 fmole.

and ACTH must be considered in studies in which pharmacologic doses of these peptides are used.

Table IV presents a comparison of the relative immunologic and biologic activities of various carboxy-terminal fragments of substance P. The octapeptide (which is biologically active) is the smallest of those which are recognized appreciably by our assay.

Parallelism between standard and sample dose–response curves can be checked as a crude indication of cross-reaction with materials not identical to substance P. The linearization afforded by the logit–log analysis makes such comparisons objective. If a type of sample is measured in several different assays, paired comparisons of sample and standard dose–response curves can be made, increasing the ability to detect sample-dependent lack of parallelism. We estimate that in recent studies we could have detected a 15% difference in slope from that of substance P. Calculations based on simple mass action assumptions indicate that a ligand with one-tenth the affinity of substance P for the antibody would demonstrate a slope 19% less than that of substance P.

C. Chemical Characterization of Cross-Reacting Material

The sensitivity of the assay permits partial chemical characterization of relatively small amounts of material. For example, the immunoreactivity recovered from Sephadex G-25 fractionation of an extract of rat substantia nigra containing 3.0 pmole substance P activity eluted

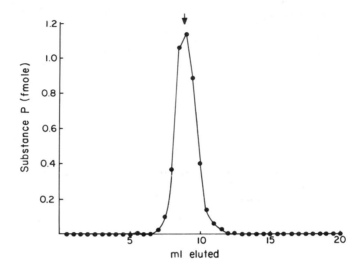

Figure 3. Immunoreactivity profile of the eluate from a Sephadex G-25 column after application of an extract of rat substantia nigra containing 3.0 pmole of substance P immunoreactivity. Column volume, 11.5 ml; the column was run in assay buffer. The arrow indicates the elution volume of synthetic substance P applied separately to the same column.

identically as synthetic substance P (Figure 3). A relatively minor side peak could have been observed, despite the small content of the sample.

The chemical nature of the immunoreactivity extracted from calf plasma by acid–acetone (Section II,D,3) has been followed through gel filtration and two ion-exchange steps. It has behaved identically with synthetic substance P in these procedures. However, it must be emphasized that this assay gives erroneously high values when used to assay unextracted plasma.

D. Sensitivity and Reproducibility

In this assay, the counts bound in the absence of substance P can usually be distinguished statistically ($p < 0.05$, one-tailed t test) from the counts bound in the presence of a sample, assayed in duplicate, that displaces 6% of the maximum binding; this displacement corresponds to 0.5 to 0.6 fmole in the incubation volume of 0.5 ml. In practice, this sensitivity has not often been needed. To allow for possible nonspecific displacement of bound tracer by relatively uncharacterized samples, we require at least 10% displacement (equivalent to

1.0 to 1.2 fmole) by such samples before considering the immunoactivity as substance P-like.

The intraassay coefficient of variation is 4% for samples containing 40 fmole substance P in the incubation volume, and increases to 8% for samples containing 2.0 fmole. The interassay coefficient of variation is 12%. This variability can be compared to the 19% interanimal coefficient of variation of the concentration of substance P in extracts of rat substantia nigra. The precision of the assay thus has not been a limiting factor in our biologic studies.

E. Assays of Blood, Tissue Extracts, and Perfusates

1. Blood

We feel that the substance P values indicated above for extracted plasma (Table II) reflect an actual level of substance P in the blood, although this material may be biologically inactive due to some subtle alteration not detected by our chemical characterization to this point. These values are in line with recently reported values given by Powell and his co-workers (1977), although they are considerably lower than the values first reported by Nilsson *et al.* (1975).

2. Tissue Extracts

The distribution of substance P in the central nervous system has been determined both from grossly dissected and from microdissected samples of rat brain (Brownstein *et al.*, 1976). It is found to have a widespread but differential distribution, with relatively little in cortically organized structures, such as the olfactory bulb or the cerebral and cerebellar cortices. Even within regions such as the mesencephalon, the assay has detected tenfold differences in substance P concentration among different microdissected nuclei. The highest concentration yet found (about 10 pmole/mg protein) is in the reticular part of the substantia nigra. Subsequent experimental studies (Mroz *et al.*, 1976, 1977), examining by radioimmunoassay the effects of various lesions of the nervous system, have determined the nerve tracts supplying most of the substance P in the interpeduncular nucleus and in the reticular part of the substantia nigra.

3. Perfusates

The assay has been used to show a calcium-dependent release of substance P from superfused synaptosomes in response to depolarization by high potassium concentrations (Schenker *et al.*, 1976). The sensitivity of the assay allowed the use of relatively small amounts of tissue, minimizing logistical problems in these studies. As little as 1.0 pmole of substance P in the bed of synaptosomes allowed for precise analysis of the substance P released into the salt solution superfusing the preparation.

ACKNOWLEDGMENTS

This research has been supported by grants from the National Institutes of Health. Edmund A. Mroz is a Hoechst-Roussel predoctoral fellow in the Department of Physiology, Harvard Medical School.

REFERENCES

Brownstein, M. J., Mroz, E. A., Kizer, J. S., Palkovits, M., and Leeman, S. E. (1976). Regional distribution of substance P in the brain of the rat. *Brain Res.* **116**, 299–305.

Carraway, R. E., and Leeman, S. E. (1973). The isolation of a new hypotensive peptide, neurotensin, from bovine hypothalami. *J. Biol. Chem.* **248**, 6854–6861.

Chang, M. M., and Leeman, S. E. (1970). Isolation of a sialogogic peptide from bovine hypothalamic tissue and its characterization as substance P. *J. Biol. Chem.* **245**, 4784–4790.

Chang, M. M., Leeman, S. E., and Niall, H. D. (1971). Amino-acid sequence of substance P. *Nature (London), New Biol.* **232**, 86–87.

Chang, P. C., Rubin, R. T., and Yu, M. (1975). Optimal statistical design of radioimmunoassays and competitive protein-binding assays. *Endocrinology* **96**, 973–981.

Cleugh, J., and Gaddum, J. H. (1963). The stability of purified preparations of substance P. *Experientia* **19**, 72–73.

Davies, J., and Dray, A. (1976). Substance P in the substantia nigra. *Brain Res.* **107**, 623–627.

Ekins, R. P. (1970). Theoretical aspects of saturation analysis. *In* "*In Vitro* Procedures with Radioisotopes in Medicine," pp. 325–353. IAEA, Vienna.

Erspamer, V., Anastasi, A., Bertaccini, G., and Cei, J. M. (1964). Structure and pharmacological actions of physalaemin, the main active polypeptide of the skin of *Physalaemus fuscumaculatus*. *Experientia* **20**, 489–490.

Fisher, G. H., Folkers, K., Pernow, B., and Bowers, C. Y. (1976). Synthesis and some biological activities of the tyrosine-8 analog of substance P. *J. Med. Chem.* **19**, 325–328.

Hallberg, D., and Pernow, B. (1975). Effect of substance P on various vascular beds in the dog. *Acta Physiol. Scand.* **93**, 277–285.

Henry, J. L., Krnjevic, K., and Morris, M. E. (1975). Substance P and spinal neurons. *Can. J. Physiol. Pharmacol.* **53**, 423–432.

Klapper, M. H., and Klotz, I. M. (1972). Acylation with dicarboxylic acid anhydrides. *In* "Methods in Enzymology" (C. H. W. Hirs and S. N. Timasheff, eds.), Vol. 25, pp. 531–536. Academic Press, New York.

Leeman, S. E., and Carraway, R. E. (1977). Discovery of a sialogogic peptide in bovine hypothalamic extracts: Its isolation, characterization as substance P, structure, and synthesis. *In* "Substance P" (U. S. von Euler and B. Pernow, eds.), pp. 5–14. Raven Press, New York.

Leeman, S. E., Mroz, E. A., and Carraway, R. E. (1977). Substance P and neurotensin. *In* "Peptides in Neurobiology" (H. Gainer, ed.), pp. 99–144. Plenum, New York.

Lembeck, F. (1953). Zur Frage der zentralen Übertragung afferenter Impulse. III. Das Vorkommen und die Bedeutung der Substanz P in den dorsalen Wurzeln des Rückenmarks. *Naunyn-Schmiedebergs Arch. Exp. Pathol. Pharmakol.* **219**, 197–213.

Lembeck, F., and Zetler, G. (1971). Substance P. *Int. Encyl. Pharmacol. Ther.* **1**, Sect. 72, 29–71.

Mroz, E. A., Brownstein, M. J., and Leeman, S. E. (1976). Evidence for substance P in the habenulo-interpeduncular tract. *Brain Res.* **113**, 597–599.

Mroz, E. A., Brownstein, M. J., and Leeman, S. E. (1977). Evidence for substance P in the striato-nigral tract. *Brain Res.* **125**, 305–311.

Nilsson, G., Pernow, B., Fischer, G. H., and Folkers, K. (1975). Presence of substance P-like immunoreactivity in plasma from man and dog. *Acta Physiol. Scand.* **94**, 542–544.

Nilsson, G., Pernow, B., Fisher, G. H., and Folkers, K. (1977). Radioimmunological determination of substance P. *In* "Substance P" (U. S. von Euler and B. Pernow, eds.), pp. 41–48. Raven Press, New York.

O'Connell, R. O., Skrabanek, P., Cannon, D., and Powell, D. (1976). High-sensitivity radioimmunoassay for substance P. *Ir. J. Med. Sci.* **145**, 392–398.

Otsuka, M., and Konishi, S. (1976). Substance P and excitatory transmitter of primary sensory neurons. *Cold Spring Harbor Symp. Quant. Biol.* **40**, 135–143.

Phillis, J. W., and Limacher, J. J. (1974). Substance P excitation of cerebral cortical Betz cells. *Brain Res.* **69**, 158–163.

Powell, D., Leeman, S. E., Tregear, G. W., Niall, H. D., and Potts, J. T., Jr. (1973). Radioimmunoassay for substance P. *Nature (London), New Biol.* **241**, 252–254.

Powell, D., Skrabanek, P., and Cannon, D. (1977). Substance P: Radioimmunoassay studies. *In* "Substance P" (U. S. von Euler and B. Pernow, eds.), pp. 35–40. Raven Press, New York.

Rodbard, D., and Frazier, G. R. (1975). Statistical analysis of radioligand assay data. *In* "Methods in Enzymology" (B. W. O'Malley and J. G. Hardman, eds.), Vol. 37, pp. 3–22. Academic Press, New York.

Rodbard, D., Ruder, H. J., Vaitukaitis, J., and Jacobs, H. S. (1971). Mathematical analysis of kinetics of radioligand assays: Improved sensitivity obtained by delayed addition of labelled ligand. *J. Clin. Endocrinol. Metab.* **33**, 343–355.

Schenker, C., Mroz, E. A., and Leeman, S. E. (1976). Release of substance P from isolated nerve endings. *Nature (London)* **264**, 790–792.

Studer, R. O., Trzeciak, H., and Lergier, W. (1973). Isolierung und Aminosäuresequenz von Substanz P aus Pferdedarm. *Helv. Chim. Acta* **56**, 860–866.

Tregear, G. W., Niall, H. D., Potts, J. T., Jr., Leeman, S. E., and Chang, M. M. (1971). Synthesis of substance P. *Nature (London), New Biol.* **232**, 87–88.

Vaitukaitis, J., Robbins, J. B., Nieschlag, E., and Ross, G. T. (1971). A method for producing specific antisera with small doses of immunogen. *J. Clin. Endocrinol. Metab.* **33**, 988–991.

von Euler, U. S., and Gaddum, J. H. (1931). An unidentified depressor substance in certain tissue extracts. *J. Physiol. (London)* **72**, 74–87.

8

Neurotensin and Related Substances

ROBERT E. CARRAWAY

I. INTRODUCTION

Neurotensin (NT) is a hypotensive peptide, the biologic activity of which was first detected by Susan Leeman in acid–acetone extracts of

139

Methods of Hormone Radioimmunoassay, Second Edition
Copyright © 1979 by Academic Press, Inc.

hypothalamic tissue. After its isolation from extracts of bovine hypothalami (Carraway and Leeman, 1973), the structure of NT (see Table I) was determined (Carraway and Leeman, 1975a), and synthetic material was prepared and shown to be biologically and chemically indistinguishable from the native substance (Carraway and Leeman, 1975b). Among its several biologic properties, NT has been found to contract the gut and to produce hypotension, increased vascular permeability, and cyanosis when injected intravenously into anesthetized rats. NT also promotes an elevation in the blood levels of ACTH (Leeman et al., 1977), LH, FSH (Makino et al., 1973), and glucose (Carraway et al., 1976).

An investigation of the structural requirements for the biologic activity of NT has indicated that the participants in the biologic action of the peptide reside primarily in its COOH-terminal region; the COOH-terminal pentapeptide, H-Arg-Pro-Tyr-Ile-Leu-OH, appeared to have reduced binding ability but full intrinsic biologic activity (Carraway and Leeman, 1975c). In keeping with these results is the finding that an antiserum directed exclusively toward the COOH-terminal region of NT neutralized its biologic action.

Recently, a radioimmunoassay for NT has been described that employs synthetic bovine NT and rabbit antisera raised against various NT–protein conjugates (Carraway and Leeman, 1976a). Using this assay and several antisera shown to have different specificities, the distribution and character of radioimmunoassayable NT have been investigated in the rat (Carraway and Leeman, 1976b). The results of this study suggested the presence of NT in other regions of brain, as well as in small intestinal tissue, and further work led to the isolation of a tridecapeptide with the same amino acid composition as NT from acid–acetone extracts of bovine jejuno-ileum (Kitabgi et al., 1976).

Immunoreactivity, behaving chromatographically as NT, has been measured in rat and bovine plasma, and its normal concentration estimated to be about 50 fmole/ml (Carraway and Leeman, 1976b). The detection of immunoreactive NT in plasma suggests a hormonal role for NT. This notion is supported by the recent demonstration of NT immunoreactivity in endocrinelike cells in the ileum of the dog (Orci et al., 1976), and in the jejunum–ileum of the rat, rabbit, cat, dog, pig, and human (Sunder et al., 1977a) using immunohistochemical techniques. The NT-staining cells, which were found in both the crypt epithelium and in the villi, appeared to make luminal contact via a narrow apical process. Ultrastructural work (Sundler et al., 1977b) has shown that these cells contain numerous electron-dense cytoplasmic granules (260–290 nm diameter) which appear to be storage sites for NT.

Using radioimmunoassay, NT-like substances of differing structure have been detected in a variety of tissues, such as rat and rabbit stomach, rat and bovine plasma (Carraway and Leeman, 1976b), and human synovial fluid (Carraway et al., 1974). We are presently investigating the immunochemical character of these various substances, which appear to share some common structural features with NT, primarily at their COOH-termini. The purpose of this chapter is to provide the reader with a basis for the design and performance of radioimmunoassay for NT. Rather than limit the reader to a particular method, it is the author's intention to offer some understanding of the many options available to the radioimmunoassayist. It is also hoped that in pointing out some of the shortcomings of radioimmunoassay, the author will stimulate the reader to experiment with novel approaches in attempting to extend the value of this wonderful technique.

II. GENERAL CONSIDERATIONS FOR INTERMEDIATE-SIZED PEPTIDES

Unique specificity, great sensitivity, and high precision of measurement are all desirable characteristics for any assay. It is unfortunate that in the performance of radioimmunoassay these attributes usually depend primarily upon properties of the antiserum of which we presently seem to have little control. The generation of useful antisera for radioimmunoassay should realistically be viewed largely as a matter of chance. Particularly troublesome to the radioimmunoassayist are peptides of intermediate size, such as NT, because it is unusually difficult to obtain "specific" antisera directed against them. Since peptides of this size seem to present a special set of problems, it might be helpful to describe briefly some of these difficulties and to outline several approaches which might allow one to solve or circumvent these problems. Unfortunately, some of these ideas have not yet been widely tested.

A. The Specificity Problem

Most desirable for radioimmunoassay, as it is commonly performed, is an antiserum which interacts equally well with all areas on the peptide–antigen and, thus, is highly sensitive to alterations at any point in the molecule. However, since the binding site of an antibody can accommodate only six to ten amino acids, no single antibody molecule can make close contact with the entire surface of a peptide larger than this. An ideal antiserum is heterogeneous, composed of a full complement of site-directed antibodies, each of which is directed against a different antigenic site in the peptide. Unfortunately, this ideal is extremely difficult to realize, because in practice one often finds that particular regions of a peptide are highly immunogenic, while other areas do not elicit antibody formation. For larger peptides with a number of these highly antigenic regions, this is not a major obstacle to the development of a useful radioimmunoassay; however, in the case of intermediate-sized peptides (10–30 amino acids) which may contain only one or two highly antigenic sites, this problem can be especially troublesome. Figure 1 illustrates these concepts. Whereas the entirety of the small peptide shown can be contained within an antibody-binding site, only small portions of the intermediate and larger peptides usually serve as major antigenic determinants. With five highly antigenic regions, the large peptide shown is likely to produce relatively heterogeneous antisera, a capacity which would require the presence of each region of the molecule for the full integrated response in a radioimmunoassay. In contrast, the

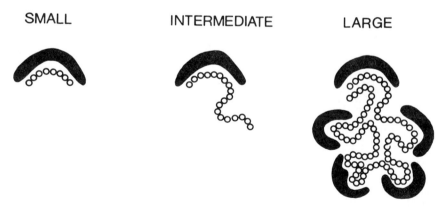

SMALL   INTERMEDIATE   LARGE

Figure 1.   Diagrammatic representation of antibody-binding sites on three hypothetical peptides of small, intermediate, and large size. The open circles represent amino acid units in each peptide, and the solid arclike structures represent major species of antibody binding sites. The small peptide (eight amino acids) is fully contained within the binding site. The intermediate-sized peptide (20 amino acids) is pictured with one highly antigenic region. The large peptide (100 amino acids) is pictured, with five highly antigenic regions.

intermediate-sized peptide shown has but one highly antigenic region, and partial sequences containing this region may interact fully with antisera raised against the whole molecule. For this reason (and possibly others), antisera against peptides of intermediate size are seldom "specific" and display considerable cross-reactivity toward related substances, such as precursors, breakdown products, and congeners of the peptide.

B. Directed Specificity

Antisera toward intermediate-sized peptides have been obtained in a number of ways. In general, peptides of this size are not very immunogenic unless administered in a "bound" form, covalently attached to or tightly associated with a carrier substance. One approach, used with some success for intermediate-sized peptides, such as glucagon (Assan *et al.*, 1965) and oxytocin (Chard *et al.*, 1970), calls for physical adsorption of the peptide to carbon microparticles or to polyvinylpyrrolidone. Although it is simply performed and probably does not alter the chemical structure of the peptide, the adsorption technique allows no command over antibody specificity. An alternative method, which has been used more frequently, involves the chemical attachment of the hapten to a carrier protein of large molecular weight. A feature of the hapten approach is the ability to influence antibody specificity by determining the orientation of coupling to carrier, since antisera raised against hapten–protein conjugates are often found to be directed primarily toward the region(s) of the hapten furthest from the site of attachment (Parker, 1971). This property suggests that heterogeneous antisera might best be obtained by immunization using heterogeneous conjugates made with the peptide in many different orientations on the carrier. Some benefit might also be gained by insertion of a spacer between the peptide and its carrier substance in order to permit the antibody-generating system to see more of the peptide.

The ability to direct specificity might be employed in a number of ways to facilitate the task of obtaining useful antisera against difficult peptides. In cases when one particular region of a peptide is found to be highly antigenic, one might attempt to encourage antibody formation toward weakly antigenic regions by proper orientation of the peptide itself or by the use of fragments of the peptide. Thus, one might immunize with conjugates in which the hapten is oriented predominantly with the weakly antigenic regions outward. Since antisera raised toward partial sequences of a peptide sometimes also bind to that portion of the entire molecule, an alternative suggestion is to use partial peptides as haptens in order to promote antibody formation toward particular sites. This is particularly useful if only one portion of the molecule is biologically active. Heterogeneous antisera could then be concocted by mixing many of the resulting site-directed antisera. This approach has the added advantage of providing one with region-specific antisera which can be quite useful in other ways.

C. Mixed Antisera

Even though it seems to be quite a reasonable approach, it has not been a common practice to mix antisera obtained from different animals. The fact that only a small percentage of immunized animals produce highly heterogeneous or specific antisera might possibly be due to a genetic inability (for most animals) to make more than just a few sorts of antibody toward a given substance. If different animals are limited to different sets of antibodies, then it would seem that by mixing antisera from several selected animals one might be able to greatly enhance the heterogeneity of the antibody population. This approach might be very useful for radioimmunoassay, provided that one is careful to select antisera with similar average affinities for antigen and to combine proportionate amounts of each according to titer.

Despite efforts such as these, which should enable one to obtain rather heterogeneous antisera directed toward multiple regions of the peptide (which should be less susceptible to major cross-reactions), no antiserum should be expected to display absolute specificity for a single substance. At best, the recognition of related substances is only relatively weak. Thus, work with a single antiserum deemed to be highly specific can be misleading if proper experimentation is not performed to substantiate its specificity in each instance.

D. Equal Immunologic Potency

As an adjunct to the single heterogeneous antiserum approach to radioimmunoassay, the additional use of multiple site-directed antisera and the application of the equal immunologic potency criterion for identity of the unknown and standard are recommended. This approach involves the use of several antisera, each directed primarily toward a different portion of the peptide. Specificity derives from the requirement that radioimmunoassays using each antiserum give similar results, indicating that each region of the peptide is present in the same concentration. The utility of this method depends upon the generation of antisera with well-defined specificities which can be shown to differ; these are best obtained using various hapten–protein conjugates.

The demonstration of equal immunologic potency using several site-directed antisera should greatly bolster one's confidence in measurements obtained with heterogeneous antisera. Furthermore, armed with a battery of site-directed antisera, one can quickly characterize cross-reacting substances, such as precursors, breakdown products, and related peptides. Antisera directed toward the region(s) of the peptide most necessary for biologic activity could be especially interesting, since they might be used to search for biologically active variants, such as isohormones or phylogenetically related substances. Such antisera might also neutralize the biologic actions of the peptide and be useful to induce and study a deficiency syndrome.

III. SPECIFIC CONSIDERATIONS FOR NEUROTENSIN

A. Approach

Choosing from among the various possible approaches to radioimmunoassay is the first important decision in the formulation of an assay for NT. This decision should depend predominantly on the proposed research application. With sufficient manpower and facilities available, several different programs might be undertaken; otherwise, a more modest approach is suggested. Work with a single heterogeneous antiserum might be adequate for measurements of immunoreactive NT in systems in which immunoreactivity has already been well-characterized e.g., hypothalamus and small intestine. On the other hand, for measurements in other tissues and for characterization of NT-like substances, it would be advisable to employ multiple "heterogeneous" as well as site-directed antisera.

In developing a radioimmunoassay for NT, we set out to obtain multiple antisera with different specificities, some of which would preferentially bind to the biologically active carboxy-terminal region of NT (Carraway and Leeman, 1976a). Reasoning that linkage through a central amino acid might direct antibody specificity toward both terminal regions, we prepared several immunogens in which NT was coupled specifically through its lysine side chain as shown in Figure 2. Using conjugates with NT oriented in this manner, several interesting antisera were obtained, three of which displayed very different specificities toward NT (Figure 2). While two of the antisera (PGL-4

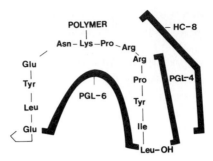

Figure 2. Diagram illustrating the orientation of NT in immunogens used and the average binding sites determined for some antisera obtained. Polymer refers to carrier; PGL, antisera obtained with NT-poly(Glu⁶⁰, Lys⁴⁰) conjugate; HC, antisera obtained with NT-succinylated hemocyanin conjugate.

and HC-8) were site-directed, giving close to 100% cross-reactivity with COOH-terminal partial sequences of NT, another (PGL-6) was more heterogeneous, requiring determinants from both the NH_2- and COOH-terminal region for full recognition. All three antisera, however, were highly sensitive to alterations in the region most necessary for biologic activity, the COOH-terminus. Although antiserum PGL-6 appeared to be relatively "specific" for NT, measurements were performed with all three antisera and equal immunologic potency was used as the criterion for acceptance of the unknown as NT. This approach greatly facilitated the immunochemical characterization of immunoreactive NT in extracts of various regions of the central nervous system and the gastrointestinal tract (Carraway and Leeman, 1976b) and led to the discovery of NT-like substances of different size in human synovial fluid (Carraway *et al.*, 1974) and in extracts of stomach and plasma (Carraway and Leeman, 1976b).

B. Preparation of Immunogen

1. Carrier

At the present time, very little information is available concerning the ability of various immunogens to elicit formation of antibodies toward NT. We have reported on our work with four different NT–protein conjugates made by coupling NT (with the same procedure) to polyglutamic acid, polyglutamic acid:lysine (60:40), succinylated thyroglobulin, and succinylated hemocyanin (Carraway and Leeman, 1976a). The results of this study indicated that, in general, the larger and more immunogenic the carrier substance, the higher the success rate and the antibody titer. For example, the hemocyanin complex (MW ca. 2×10^6) gave 100% success rate (four animals) with titers near 1 : 150,000, while the NT–polyglutamic acid complex (MW ca. 9×10^4) gave only 16% success rate (six animals) with titers <1 : 10, even though the NT content of the complexes were similar (20%). Judging from these findings and the comments of others (Odell *et al.*, 1971), it would seem that thyroglobulin and hemocyanin are certainly two carriers which deserve further consideration.

2. *Hapten*

An important consideration in the design of immunogens is whether to use the native or synthetic peptide. Even though synthetic NT is much more easily obtained than native NT, it is preferable to raise some antisera against the native substance, since the latter is less likely to be contaminated with very similar peptides, such as the failure sequences often found in synthetic preparations. Fragments of NT for generation of site-directed antisera are most easily obtained by digestion of synthetic NT with various specific enzymes (Table I).

3. *Method of Coupling*

Neurotensin contains multiple reactive groupings suitable for coupling to carrier proteins (e.g., one amino and two carboxyl groups and two tyrosyl residues) and any one of a number of procedures could be employed to react these sites with various carriers or modified carriers (Table II). Great care, however, should be exercised in the choice and performance of coupling reactions so as to avoid or minimize side reactions which might alter the structure of the coupled product. For example, carbodiimide-mediated coupling of amino and carboxyl groups of NT to corresponding groups on a protein might also lead to dimerization of NT as well as intramolecular cross-linking. Administration of an immunogen containing such altered forms of NT could lead to the production of undesirable antibodies. In some instances, removable blocking groups could be employed to disallow certain side reactions. For example, trifluoroacetylation might be used to reversibly block the amino function in NT so as to permit a cleaner coupling of carbodiimide-activated NT carboxyl groups to protein amino groups. Alternatively, one could choose to block the NT carboxyl groups by esterification with methanol in order to avoid side reactions when conjugating neurotensin (via its amino groups) to the protein carrier. In addition to minimizing side reactions, manipulations such as these might also be employed to anchor NT or one of its

Table I Useful Fragments of Neurotensin Obtained by Enzymic Cleavage[a]

Enzyme	Fragment	Structure
—	NT	<Glu-Leu-Tyr-Glu-Asn-Lys-Pro-Arg-Arg-Pro-Tyr-Ile-Leu-OH
Trypsin	T-1	<Glu-Leu-Tyr-Glu-Asn-Lys-Pro-Arg-OH
	T-2	H-Arg-Pro-Tyr-Ile-Leu-OH
Chymotrypsin	C-1	<Glu-Leu-Tyr-OH
	C-2	H-Glu-Asn-Lys-Pro-Arg-Arg-Pro-Tyr-OH
	C-3	H-Ile-Leu-OH
Papain	P-1	<Glu-Leu-Tyr-Glu-OH
	P-2	H-Asn-Lys-Pro-Arg-OH
	P-3	H-Arg-Pro-Tyr-Ile-Leu-OH
Carboxypeptidase A	CPA-1	<Glu-Leu-Tyr-Glu-Asn-Lys-Pro-Arg-Arg-Pro-OH
Pyroglutamyl peptidase	PCA-1	H-Leu-Tyr-Glu-Asn-Lys-Pro-Arg-Arg-Pro-Tyr-Ile-Leu-OH

[a] Conditions for enzymic treatments and isolation of peptides described by Carraway and Leeman (1975a).

Table II Suggested Reactions for Carrier and Hapten Modification and Coupling

Carrier modification
1. Enrich COOH content by succinylation
2. Enrich NH_2 content by carbodiimide-mediated coupling of COOH groups with excess 1,6-diaminohexane
3. Add spacer group such as diglycine via mixed anhydride or carbodiimide reaction

Hapten modification (reversible)
1. Trifluoracetylation of NH_2 groups
2. Maleation of NH_2 groups
3. Esterification of COOH groups

Coupling reagents	Group involved
1. Carbodiimide	—COOH
2. Alkylchloroformate	—COOH
3. Diisocyanates	—NH_2
4. Glutaraldehyde	—NH_2
5. Diazonium salts	Tyr, —NH_2

fragments in a single orientation so as to favor the production of site-directed antisera.

In coupling NT specifically through its lysine side chain, we have employed the procedure outlined in Figure 3. NT was initially esterified with methanol to render its carboxyl groups unreactive to carbodiimide; the resulting NT diester was then reacted with a carbodiimide-activated, carboxyl-enriched protein; finally, the conjugate was deesterified and dialyzed. Using carboxypeptidase A, we demonstrated that the carboxyl-terminus of coupled neurotensin was indeed free (Carraway and Leeman, 1976a).

4. Degree of Substitution

Although as a general rule, the larger the degree of incorporation of hapten into carrier, the more pronounced the antibody response, a maximal incorporation is not always found to be optimal (Marks *et al.*, 1974). In fact, there are several reasons to believe that a high hapten : carrier ratio might be disadvantageous: (a) Whereas reaction of hapten with highly available sites on the surface of the carrier might be expected to result in highly available derivatives, reaction with sterically hindered groups might give rise to partially buried forms. These partially buried forms could initiate production of antibodies directed partly toward the hapten and partly toward the carrier. (b) Overcrowding the surface of the carrier might also conceivably result in the formation of antigenic determinants made from parts of several hapten molecules. With these considerations in mind, we thought it

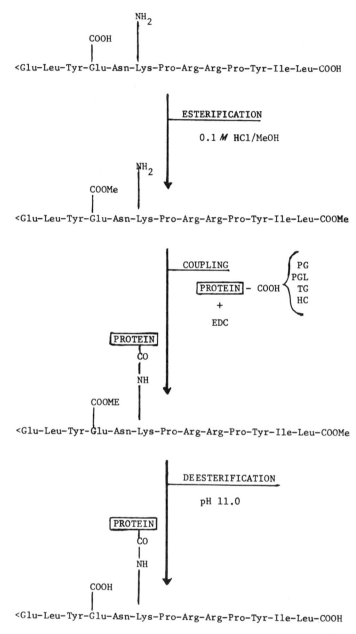

Figure 3. Synthetic route employed for preparation of immunogen by coupling NT specifically through its lysine side chain to COOH-groups on proteins. PG, polyglutamic acid; PGL, poly(Glu[60], Lys[40]); TG, succinylated thyroglobulin; HC, succinylated hemocyanin; EDC, 1-ethyl-3-(3-dimethylaminopropyl)carbodiimide-HCl; MeOH, methanol.

advisable to (1) modify the carrier prior to coupling so as to insert a suitable spacer between it and the hapten, (2) carry out the coupling reaction under conditions which do not unfold the carrier, and (3) allow a moderately high but less than maximal degree of coupling to occur. It also seemed reasonable to consider the size of the hapten and the surface area available on the carrier. For peptides close to the size of NT, one might best utilize conjugates containing 10–20% hapten by weight.

As yet, few experiments have been performed with NT-containing conjugates. Our studies indicate that a high degree of incorporation is not essential to obtain useful antisera toward NT, since several avid antisera were produced (although in low titer) using a conjugate having only three moles of NT per mole carrier (12% by weight). We have also shown that by using a succinyl moiety as a spacer, high affinity antisera can be obtained (in much higher titer) using NT–hemocyanin conjugates with greater than 200 moles of NT per mole carrier (22% by weight).

5. Administration of Immunogen

Antisera are commonly raised in rabbits and guinea pigs, not because they are exceptional producers, but rather because they are readily available, simply housed, and easily bled. It is quite possible that a different species of animal in which the bovine NT sequence is more foreign might more readily produce an avid antibody to NT. Whatever species are used, however, one should avoid inbred strains which might exhibit a genetically limited antibody response, each animal producing antisera with much the same character. While the adjuvant used, the route of injection, and the precise immunization schedule all seem to be of lesser importance, the dose and character of the immunogen are highly critical for the successful production of useful antisera against peptides. An immunogen which is absorbed too quickly or given in too high a dose can produce tolerance or can result in the production of low affinity antisera. It has been suggested that low doses favor the selective stimulation of high affinity antibody-producing lymphocytes (Parker, 1971).

Using Freund's adjuvant and the intradermal injection method described by Vaitukaitis et al. (1971), we have found that several NT conjugates, when given to rabbits in doses totaling about one mg, promoted the formation of high affinity antisera (K_a, ca. 10^{10} M^{-1}) in high titers (usable dilution, ca. 1 : 10^5). Based on these findings, we suggest that each immunogen be tested at several doses ranging from about 0.1 mg to 1.0 mg per animal.

C. Characterization of Antisera

If one intends to do extensive work with well-characterized antisera, it is advisable to select those with titers >1 : 500. Sensitivity requirements for the assay depend primarily upon which tissues are to be examined. For reliable measurements, a sensible rule is that the amount of NT giving 50% displacement in the assay should be no greater than the concentration of immunoreactive NT in the tissue times a typical sample size. Brain and intestinal tissues have concentrations of about 1.0–50 pmole/gm, while plasma concentrations are near 0.05 pmole/ml. If necessary, the sensitivity of the assay can usually be increased by a factor of three to five by using lower antibody concentrations and longer incubation times (three to four days). Using antiserum HC-8, the 50% displacement point in our assay for an overnight incubation is 12–15 fmole, while that obtained for a three-day incubation is 4.0–5.0 fmole.

Although the titer of an antiserum and the assay sensitivity it allows are important considerations, its specificity is clearly of paramount importance. Insensitive antisera in low titer can be very useful, but antisera which are not selective are useless. A simple means of assessing specificity involves the determination of the relative cross-reactivity of the antiserum toward partial sequences of NT. Several fragments of NT are easily obtained by treatment of the molecule with specific proteolytic enzymes (Table I); COOH-terminal sequences can be generated during the solid phase synthesis of NT (Carraway and Leeman, 1975b). The average recognition sites depicted in Figure 2 were defined by measuring the extent to which partial sequences of NT reacted in the assay with each antiserum (Table III).

Another rapid measure of the selectivity of an antiserum toward NT can be obtained by determining the profile of immunoreactivity observed when a 2.0 N acetic acid extract of hypothalamic or intestinal tissue is chromatographed on Sephadex G-25. Although extracts of this sort contain multiple substances resembling NT, a discriminating antiserum should give a single peak of immunoreactivity eluting at about 1.4 void volumes. Note, however, that antisera giving multiple peaks may still be useful, provided that they can be shown to be directed solely toward one region of NT.

D. Radioiodination

Since it contains two tyrosyl residues and no functional groups which are sensitive to mild oxidizing and reducing agents, NT is par-

Table III Comparative Immunoreactivity and Biologic Activity of Neurotensin and Its Partial Sequences

Peptide	Immunoreactivity[a] (%)			Biologic[b] activity (%)
	PGL-6	HC-8	PGL-4	
<Glu-Leu-Tyr-Glu-Asn-Lys-Pro-Arg-Arg-Pro-Tyr-Ile-Leu-OH	100	100	100	100
H-Leu-Tyr-Glu-Asn-Lys-Pro-Arg-Arg-Pro-Tyr-Ile-Leu-OH	9	100	100	100
H-Glu-Asn-Lys-Pro-Arg-Arg-Pro-Tyr-Ile-Leu-OH	8	100	100	25
H-Lys-Pro-Arg-Arg-Pro-Tyr-Ile-Leu-OH	8	100	100	20
H-Arg-Arg-Pro-Tyr-Ile-Leu-OH	5	50	100	55
H-Arg-Pro-Tyr-Ile-Leu-OH	3	2	75	1
H-Pro-Tyr-Ile-Leu-OH	<0.01	0.04	440	<0.1
H-Tyr-Ile-Leu-OH	<0.01	0.02	5	<0.1
H-Ile-Leu-OH	<0.01	<0.01	<0.01	<0.1
<Glu-Leu-Tyr-Glu-Asn-Lys-Pro-Arg-Arg-Pro-OH	<0.01	<0.01	<0.01	<0.2
<Glu-Leu-Tyr-OH	<0.01	<0.01	<0.01	<0.01

[a] As determined by the amount of peptide needed to inhibit by 50% the binding of ^{125}I-NT to antiserum indicated.

[b] As determined by the hyperglycemic response in rat.

ticularly well suited for the iodination reaction mediated by chloramine-T (Greenwood *et al.*, 1963). In addition, this reaction can be simply and safely performed using large amounts of radioactivity, and the iodinated NT can be easily separated from the reagents by gel filtration on Sephadex G-10. However, since iodination can lead to at least eight different iodinated derivatives of NT, some of which may not be highly immunoreactive, a means of selectively purifying those derivatives with high affinity for antibody would be most desirable. In our laboratory, the approach used for obtaining an iodinated preparation of NT with high radiologic specific activity as well as high immunologic reactivity has been to iodinate strongly so as to minimize the amount of uniodinated NT present and then to select by affinity chromatography those iodinated derivatives with the highest affinity for antibody. An optional next step is to subject this material to ion-exchange chromatography in order to separate any remaining uniodinated NT and to define better the chemical nature of the selected product(s).

This approach offers a number of distinct advantages over the more commonly used method of iodinating lightly and then purifying the monoiodinated product(s) from the unreacted material by ion-exchange chromatography: (a) The affinity method has universal applicability, requiring only that the iodinated product be stable to some condition which dissociates it from the Sepharose-bound antibody. (b) The affinity method selects for the desired property, the ability to associate with antibody; therefore, it automatically rejects iodinated derivatives with impaired binding ability (which is especially important when more than one tyrosine is present in the molecule). (c) The radiologic specific activity of the product is primarily a function of the ratio of ^{125}I and peptide reacted, rather than a function of the efficiency of a separation procedure. (d) The affinity method is rapid (one day), easily performed, and not costly. The antibody–Sepharose resins can be reused; one preparation in our laboratory has been used successfully for three years.

The results of a simple experiment aptly demonstrate the utility of the affinity method. An iodinated NT preparation (post-Sephadex G-10) was divided in half and each half was purified on an anti-NT–Sepharose made with one of two antisera (PGL-4 and PGL-6) known to have different specificities. The iodinated products obtained were examined for their ability to interact with the two antisera giving the dose–response curves shown in Figure 4. It is clear that each antiserum preferred the iodinated product(s) obtained from its own antibody–Sepharose. Thus, the two antisera selected different popula-

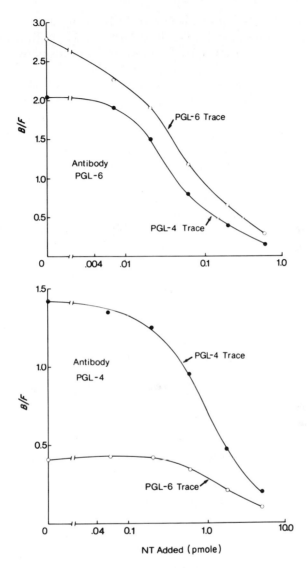

Figure 4. Dose–response curves in the radioimmunoassay using antiserum PGL-6 (upper) and antiserum PGL-4 (lower) with tracer purified on PGL-6 Sepharose (○) and with tracer purified on PGL-4 Sepharose (●).

tions of iodinated NT, possibly having the iodine atom(s) at different ends of the molecule. It would be extremely difficult, if not impossible, to separate the various possible iodinated forms of neutrotensin by any means other than affinity chromatography.

The technique recently described by Bolton and Hunter (1972) is an alternative method of iodination that might be used for antisera sensitive to alterations at the tyrosyl residues in neurotensin. This approach involves reaction of NT with a radioiodinated acylating agent, 3-(4-hydroxyphenyl)propionic acid hydroxysuccinimide ester, which should react exclusively with the lysine amino group in NT. Besides placing the iodine at a different site in NT, this labeling method has several other features: (a) Assuming one uses a homogeneous reagent, only one labeled derivative of NT can be expected. (b) Since the labeling reaction modifies the lysine amino group, abolishing its charge property, labeled and unlabeled NT should be easily separated by ion-exchange chromatography.

E. Performing Measurements

Great care should be exercised in the validation of measurements obtained by radioimmunoassay, since multiple artifacts can lead to false positives in the assay. Any substance which alters the binding constant between antigen and antibody (such as protein denaturants, acids, bases, and salts) might register as NT. Plasma proteins are notorious for producing various nonspecific effects which are not well understood. It is conceivable that high concentrations of some proteins might interact with antibody to occlude binding sites or alter binding site structures. Another possible artifact, which is often overlooked, stems from the ability of proteolytic enzymes in tissue extracts to alter the form of the tracer, making it less attractive to the antibody.

Since these nonspecific effects could exhibit dose–response curves which resemble that of the standard, they are sometimes difficult to distinguish from genuine measurements. The likelihood of obtaining these kinds of false measurements can be greatly reduced by using extraction methods which destroy proteolytic enzymes and by employing volatile buffers for chromatography. When other reagents are employed, appropriate controls must be included in the assays.

In performing radioimmunoassay for NT, we have chosen to extract plasma and tissue samples with acid–acetone, which solubilizes NT while precipitating most larger proteins. Extraction with $2.0 N$ acetic acid has also been used to measure immunoreactive NT in samples of brain; however, this method also solubilizes other larger substance(s) which cross-react with some of the antisera toward NT. Chromatography of extracts is usually performed using acetic acid and pyridine buffers.

At present, measurements obtained by direct addition of plasma to the assay are unreliable and difficult to interpret. Since neurotensin-deficient plasma is not yet available, nonspecific effects are difficult to rule out. Not only is the source of immunoreactive NT in plasma not known, but experiments in our laboratory indicate that neither prolonged incubation at 37°C nor charcoal treatment of plasma removes endogenous NT (measured by extraction). Measurements of unextracted plasma obtained without addition of control plasma to standards are higher by a factor of two to five than those obtained after extraction. This discrepancy might be due to nonspecific effects of plasma proteins or to the presence of NT-like substances which are insoluble in acid–acetone. Until an appropriate control plasma is found, it is advisable to extract plasma prior to measurement. The concentration of radioimmunoassayable NT in extracted plasma is usually in the range 25–75 fmole/ml.

F. Interpretation

One must be cautious and open-minded when interpreting measurements obtained by radioimmunoassay, since the precise nature of an immunoreactive substance cannot be known until its isolation and chemical characterization are performed. It is possible, for example, that NT is merely one member of a class of related hormones, the NT family, all of whose members may share certain immunoreactive determinants; an analogous situation has been shown for the gastrin family (Jaffe and Walsh, 1974). Structural variants of NT may react in the assay and could even display dose–response curves parallel to that of NT, making it extremely difficult to distinguish them from genuine NT. Other NT-like substances which might register in the assay are precursor forms and degradation products.

A certain degree of confidence in interpretation of radioimmunoassay results can be acquired from information concerning the immunochemical, physiochemical, and biologic character of the immunoreactive material. A careful examination of the behavior of the test material in the radioimmunoassay can be extremely informative. If the test substance exhibits (a) displacement curves which are parallel to those of NT in the assay and (b) equipotency when assayed using several different antisera, it is likely to possess the structural features of NT. Discrepant results indicate the presence of immunologically related substance(s) of different structure. Rapid comparisons of physicochemical properties might be based on chromatographic and electrophoretic behavior, while more detailed studies could involve determinations of stability to various chemical and enzymic treatments. Information concerning the biologic activity of the immunoreactive material is of utmost interest since bioassays are potentially very discriminating. It would seem that the ultimate test of similarity to NT would involve chemical sequencing performed on the isolated immunoreactive substance(s). Such studies, if performed in at least one animal species for the tissue under examination, could provide valuable information for the proper interpretation of all measurements obtained by radioimmunoassay.

Results obtained in our laboratory nicely illustrate how work with multiple antisera can provide a rapid indicator of the character of immunoreactive substances. We routinely obtain measurements on each sample using two or three different antisera; estimates of the concentration of immunoreactive NT in crude extracts of various rat tissues obtained with antisera PGL-6, HC-8, and PGL-4 are given in Table IV. Note that some of the tissues gave nearly equivalent results with the three different antisera (i.e., activity ratios near 1.0), suggesting that these measurements reflect the presence of NT in hypothalamus and regions of small intestine. In contrast to these results, a 500-fold discrepancy was observed for extracts of stomach tissue, indicating the detection of NT-like substance(s) of differing structure. These preliminary conclusions were indeed borne out when

Table IV   Distribution and Concentration of Immunoreactive NT in Tissues of Adult Rats[a]

Tissue[b]	NT[c] (pmole/gm)			Ratio of PGL-4/PGL-6
	PGL-6	HC-8	PGL-4	
Hypothalamus	62	63	160	3
Ileum	56	50	97	2
Jejunum	46	48	91	2
Postduodenum	6.3	5.6	30	5
Duodenum	2.0	1.4	107	54
Stomach	0.7	0.6	383	547
Esophagus	2.0	1.1	46	23

[a] Data obtained from Carraway and Leeman (1976a,b).

[b] Tissues were extracted with acid–acetone.

[c] Given is the mean concentration obtained for three to five measurements using the three antisera previously described.

these extracts were analyzed chromatographically. Figure 5 shows the chromatographic patterns obtained when extracts of rat jejuno-ileum and stomach were chromatographed on a column of Sephadex G-25. Using PGL-6, the most heterogeneous antiserum, the extract of jejuno-ileum gave a main peak of immunoreactivity that eluted in the region of NT and displayed equipotency with the other antisera. Other smaller peaks tended to react more with PGL-4, the carboxyl-terminal site-directed antiserum, thus explaining the small discrepancy (twofold) observed for the crude extract (Table IV, jejunum and ileum). The stomach extract reacted poorly with antisera PGL-6 and HC-8, but gave a major peak of activity with antiserum PGL-4 that eluted after NT.

Since immunoreactive NT from the stomach gave a displacement curve parallel to that of the standard peptide with antiserum PGL-4,

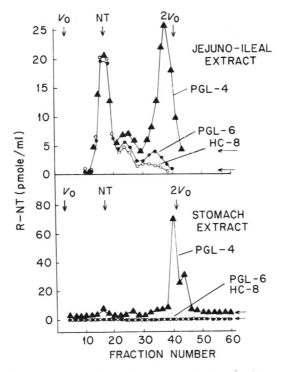

Figure 5. Gel chromatography of extracts of rat gastrointestinal tissues on Sephadex G-25. On the ordinate, immunoreactivity as measured with the antiserum indicated. On the abscissa, the fraction number, the void volume (V_0), and the elution position for synthetic neurotensin (NT) are indicated. (From Carraway and Leeman, 1976b, with permission of the publisher.)

and since this antiserum was shown to be directed exclusively toward the carboxyl-terminal region of NT, this substance is likely to resemble NT, at least at its carboxyl terminus. Supporting this notion is the finding that the immunoreactivity was labile to treatments with carboxypeptidase A and chymotrypsin. Although an estimate of its molecular size indicated that it was similar to the NT-(9–13)-pentapeptide, the pattern of cross-reactivity of stomach immunoreactive NT with the three different antisera was not consistent with it being a carboxyl-terminal breakdown product of NT. One possibility is that this substance is a variant of NT that has its biologically active carboxyl-terminal portion in common with NT.

We have also reported on the detection of NT-like substance(s) of large molecular weight in synovial fluids and in extracts of synovial tissue obtained from arthritic patients (Carraway et al., 1974). Dose–response curves, generated in the radioimmunoassay using antiserum PGL-4, indicated that synovial fluids from a variety of patients exhibited parallel displacement (Figure 6). However, when these samples were examined with other antisera (PGL-6 and HC-8), discrepant measurements were obtained which were less than 1% of those with

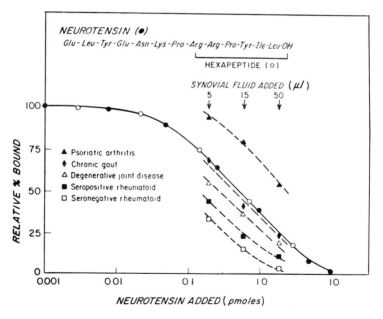

Figure 6. Dose–response curves in the radioimmunoassay using antiserum PGL-4 with synthetic NT (●), synthetic NT-(8–13)-hexapeptide (○), and synovial fluid samples from patients with various arthritic diseases.

the carboxyl-terminal directed antiserum, PGL-4. This discrepancy suggested that the immunoreactive substance(s) were different from NT, and further studies indicated that a number of the physicochemical properties of this material differed from those of NT, i.e., the activity was insoluble in acid–acetone, precipitable with 50% ammonium sulfate, and exhibited a molecular weight near 70,000.

The immunoreactivity of synovial fluid was rapidly destroyed by treatment with carboxypeptidase A, suggesting that the NT-like sequence also is located at the carboxyl-terminus of the protein. It is also interesting that highly purified immunoreactivity of synovial fluid, like NT, was found to exhibit chemotactic activity toward human leukocytes and that this activity was also labile to treatment with carboxypeptidase A (Carraway *et al.*, 1975). These data support the notion that this material represents a large molecular weight variant of NT that is likely to have the biologically active portion of NT at its carboxyl-terminus; it is possible that this substance(s) serves as a precursor to NT or another peptide in the NT family.

Bovine tissues have recently been used in order to define precisely the chemical character of immunoreactive NT in extracts of hypothalami (Carraway and Leeman, 1976a) and in extracts of small intestine (Kitabgi *et al.*, 1976). The immunoreactivity in extracts of both tissues displayed the chemical, biologic, and immunologic properties of NT and was shown to be attributable to a peptide having the amino acid composition of NT. These results greatly strengthen our belief that our radioimmunoassay gives a valid measure of NT in these tissues and support the continued use of these antisera for the immunohistochemical localization of NT in brain and gut.

IV. METHODS

The following procedures serve to describe the approach used to formulate the radioimmunoassay for NT in our laboratory. After consideration of the many possible alternatives one has in constructing the assay, it may be possible to deal with some of the limitations inherent in radioimmunoassay and to improve upon the methodology presented here.

A. Preparation of Immunogen

Esterification of NT is carried out in a dry, stoppered conical tube, to which is added synthetic NT (50 mg, Beckman Instruments) and

5.0–10 ml of 0.1 M methanolic HCl, prepared by bubbling dry HCl gas through methanol. While the tube sits with occasional mixing at about 20°C, the course of the esterification is monitored by high voltage paper electrophoresis of 5.0-μl aliquots at pH 6.5. The electrophoretic mobilities relative to lysine are NT, 0.2; NT monoester, 0.4; NT diester, 0.6. The reaction is usually complete in 24–48 hours, at which time the contents of the tube are washed into a round bottom flask with methanol and flash evaporated to dryness at 20°–30°C, dissolved in methanol, and reevaporated. The dry flask is then capped and stored at −20°C until the NT diester is used. Since the ester tends to hydrolyze to form NT, it might be wise to examine the preparation electrophoretically if it is stored longer than one week.

Succinylation of the carrier protein is performed in a 50-ml beaker in which bovine thyroglobulin (50 mg, Sigma Chemical Co.) or keyhole limpet hemocyanin (50 mg, Calbiochem) is dissolved in 10 ml 0.15 M NaCl. A total of 100 mg succinic anhydride is added over 30 minutes while the solution is stirred and the pH is maintained between 7 and 9 for one to two hours with addition of 1.0 M NaOH. When a constant pH is achieved, the preparation is dialyzed exhaustively against distilled water and lyophilized.

Coupling of the NT diester and protein is performed as follows: Five milliliters of a solution of the succinylated protein (8.0 mg/ml) dissolved in 0.01 M sodium phosphate, 0.15 M NaCl, pH 7 is placed in a stoppered tube and 1.0 ml of a freshly prepared solution of 1-ethyl-3(3-dimethylaminopropyl) carbodiimide (50 mg/ml) in the same buffer is added. After gentle mixing for five to ten minutes, 2.0 ml of a freshly prepared solution of NT diester (20 mg/ml) in the same buffer is added rapidly and the reaction mixture, shielded from light with aluminum foil, is kept at 20°C for 30 minutes with occasional vortexing. After sitting overnight in the refrigerator at 4°C, the reaction mixture is transferred to a dialysis bag and diluted with an equal volume of distilled water. The conjugates are dialyzed successively for 24 hours, each against multiple changes of (a) distilled water, (b) 0.05 M sodium carbonate, pH 11, and (c) 0.85% NaCl and then stored at −20°C until used.

B. Administration of Immunogen

One or two days prior to immunization, a single intramuscular injection of *Bordetella pertussis* vaccine (Difco, 0.5 ml) is given to New Zealand white rabbits weighing 2.0–4.0 kg. The conjugates, dissolved or suspended in 0.85% saline (1.0 mg/ml), are emulsified with an equal volume of complete Freund's adjuvant supplemented with killed tubercle bacilli (5.0 mg/ml, Difco) using a Virtis tissue homogenizer at high speed. The frothy white mixture is injected intradermally at 40–50 sites across the shaved backs of the rabbits at a total dose of about 1.0 mg conjugate per animal. Three months later, the animals are boosted using one-fifth the initial dose of conjugate in incomplete Freund's adjuvant and bled from the ear vein 10–15 days afterward. After the blood is allowed to clot at 20°C for several hours and left overnight in the refrigerator, sera are isolated by centrifugation at 5000 g. In order to minimize repeated freezing and thawing, some of each antiserum is diluted 1 : 100 with PBS-gel (0.05 M Na phosphate, 0.15 M NaCl, pH 7.4, 0.02% NaN$_3$, 0.1% gelatin) and the dilutions are aliquoted into sets of tubes which are kept at −20°C; each tube can be used several times.

C. Characterization of Antisera

An antiserum is titered by incubating overnight at 4°C 100 μl of various dilutions (1 : 100 to 1 : 100,000) with about 10,000 cpm of ^{125}I-NT in a total volume of 500 μl of PBS-gel. Titer is expressed as the dilution of the antiserum that gives a B/F of 1.0 (see Section IV,G).

The sensitivity permitted by an antiserum is determined by incubating it overnight (at a dilution which gives a B/F of 1.0) with varying amounts of standard (0.1–1000 fmole). Sensitivity is expressed as the amount of standard required to reduce the B/F to half its original value. The specificity of an antiserum is determined by generating competitive binding curves for standard NT and several of its partial sequences and analogs in a single experiment. Cross-reactivity with another peptide is expressed as a percent relative to NT and is defined as 100 times the dose of NT for half-displacement divided by the dose of the other peptide for half-displacement.

D. Radioiodination

Radioiodination should be carried out in a special hood equipped with an air filtration system to trap any volatile radioactive products. The procedure employing chloramine-T as oxidant is as follows: to 75 μl of phosphate buffer (0.5 M, pH 7.5) in a glass tube (10 × 75 mm) is added 5 μl NT (1.0 mg/ml in water) and 2.0 mCi Na ^{125}I (about 5.0 μl carrier-free solution in 0.1 N NaOH, New England Nuclear). The reaction is initiated by careful addition of 25 μl chloramine-T (1.0 mg/ml in 0.5 M phosphate, pH 7.4, Kodak) and the capped tube is vortexed for about 30 seconds, at which time 25 μl sodium metabisulfite (3.0 mg/ml in phosphate) is added. After thorough mixing, 0.3 ml heat-treated (60°C, 10 minutes) rat plasma (made >10 mg/ml in KI) is added and the mixture is immediately gel-filtered on a column (0.9 × 18 cm) of Sephadex G-10 using PBS-gel (0.05 M sodium phosphate, 0.15 M NaCl, pH 7.4, 0.02% sodium azide, 0.1% gelatin) as eluant. Labeled NT is excluded from this gel and elutes with the colored plasma proteins in the void volume; the excluded radioactivity, usually 75–95% of total, is pooled for further purification.

E. Purification of ^{125}I-NT

The gel-filtered ^{125}I-NT is incubated overnight at 4°C in PBS-gel with an appropriate amount of antibody–Sepharose so as to effect a selective adsorption of those iodinated derivatives of NT with the highest affinity for antibody. The gel preparation is then placed in a sintered glass funnel and washed with more than ten volumes of PBS and 1.0 M NaCl, pH 7, by vacuum suction. The tightly bound counts (usually 40–60% of total) are eluted using either 0.01 N HCl or 0.01 N NaOH into tubes containing phosphate buffer. Although it is not necessary, the preparation is usually further purified and characterized by ion-exchange chromatography on SP-Sephadex, C-25, using an elution program which adequately separates ^{125}I-NT from added NT. This is performed by diluting the pooled eluates from the affinity column to give less than 0.05 M cation concentration and adding glacial acetic acid to give a pH of less than 3. This solution is applied to a column of SP-Sephadex (10 ml) previously equilibrated with 0.05 M pyridine acetate, pH 3.1. Then the column is equilibrated with 0.05 M pyridine acetate, pH 5.5, and eluted with a linear gradient generated from 250 ml each of 0.05 M pyridine acetate pH 5.5, and 0.40 M pyridine acetate, pH 5.5. Substances elute in the following order: NT, monoiodinated derivatives of NT, and diiodinated derivatives of NT at 0.18, 0.25, and 0.3 M pyridine acetate concentrations, respectively. The purified ^{125}I-NT has a specific activity of 500–1700 μCi/μg.

Antibody–Sepharose conjugates are prepared using CNBr-activated Sepharose 4B as recommended by the manufacturer (Pharmacia Fine Chemicals). The dry Sepharose is placed in a sintered glass funnel and swollen for 15 minutes in 10^{-3} M HCl (>500 ml/gm). After suction drying, the Sepharose (1.0 gm/10–20 mg protein) is added to the antibody preparation, previously dissolved in coupling buffer (0.2 M sodium bicarbonate pH 8.3, 0.15 M NaCl) at about 5.0 mg/ml, and placed in a stoppered tube. The tube is shaken gently for one to two hours at room temperature and placed in the refrigerator overnight. The reaction is conveniently followed by monitoring the optical density of the filtered solution at 280 nm, and, if necessary, the filtered solution can be reacted with fresh Sepharose. After the reaction has gone to completion, the dry antibody–Sepharose is added to a stoppered tube containing 1.0 M ethanolamine, pH 8.3 (5 ml/gm Sepharose) which is then shaken for two hours at room temperature. The preparation is collected on a sintered glass funnel and washed cyclically with acetate buffer, pH 4, and carbonate buffer, pH 10, made with 0.5 M NaCl (500 ml/gm). This is followed with 0.01 M NaOH, 1.0 M NaCl, or 0.01 M HCl, 1.0 M NaCl (100 ml/gm), depending upon which will be used in subsequent chromatography. The dry preparation is swollen in PBS-gel and kept in the refrigerator until used. Prior to use for affinity chromatography, the ^{125}I-NT absorbing capacity of the antibody–Sepharose should be determined. This is easily done by incubating known quantities of the conjugate (10 mg) with increasing amounts of ^{125}I-NT in 1.0 ml PBS-gel overnight at 4°C and then determining the amount of radioactivity remaining in solution.

If in low titer, antibody might be purified from other plasma proteins prior to coupling to Sepharose by performing affinity chromatography on a NT–Sepharose conjugate. NT can be convalently linked to Sepharose as described above for antibody except that lower amounts of NT (0.1–1.0 mg/gm) should be used for best results. This is because the final preparations tend to leak NT, and, if used in great excess over the antibody to be purified, the leaked NT masks antibody activity in the eluates. Prior to its use for chromatography, the antibody-absorbing capacity of the NT–Sepharose should be determined; a unit of antibody might be defined as that amount which gives a B/F of 1.0 in the radioimmunoassay. Affinity chromatography of antibody can be performed by a batch or column method using antisera diluted in PBS-gel and a small excess (less than tenfold) of NT–Sepharose. We have retrieved antibody activity in good yields from NT-Sepharose using ice-cold 1.0 M NaCl (pH 12); however, since antibody stability does vary, it is advisable to perform experiments with a number of other eluates, such as 1.0 M NaCl (pH 2), 1.0 M acetic acid, and 1.0 M ammonium hydroxide.

F. Preparation of Samples

All tissues are dissected from freshly killed animals and immediately frozen on dry ice. After weighing, they are extracted by one of the following procedures. The acid–acetone method entails homogenizing the tissues in four volumes (w/v) of acetone : 1.0 N HCl (100 : 3, v/v) (solution A) in a Virtis tissue grinder. When tissue samples weigh less than 4.0 gm, acetone : 0.01 N HCl (80 : 20, v/v) (solution B) is added to make 15 ml. After homogenizing each sample, the grinder is washed with 5.0 ml of solution B which is added to the homogenate. The homogenate is then centrifuged 20 minutes at 15,000 g and the supernatant fraction is decanted and extracted three times with an equal volume of petroleum ether and rotary evaporated or boiled off. The residue is dissolved in water and lyophilized. The 2.0 N acetic acid procedure involves homogenizing the tissues in ten volumes (w/v) of 2.0 N acetic acid. After centrifugation for ten min at 15,000 g, the supernatant fluid is set aside and the precipitate is resuspended in five volumes (w/v) of 2.0 N acetic acid and recentrifuged. The combined supernatant fractions are lyophilized.

Since NT can be degraded by plasma, having a half-life of about 40 minutes at 37°C, blood samples should be chilled on ice and processed quickly. It is preferable to use heparin (10 U/ml) as anticoagulant, since EDTA can interfere in the assay. After centrifugation, plasma is isolated and a known volume is immediately extracted with acid–acetone by stirring overnight at room temperature with four volumes of solution A. The mixture is then centrifuged at 15,000 g and further processed as described above.

After lyophilization, all samples are dissolved in PBS-gel and the solutions are adjusted to pH 7 to 8 using 1.0 N NaOH and centrifuged 15 minutes at 20,000 g before being subjected to radioimmunoassay.

G. Assay Procedure and Calculations

Our assay is an equilibrium system carried out at pH 7.4 in disposable flint glass tubes (10 × 75 mm) and employing PBS-gel as diluent. The 500-μl incubation mixtures contain 100 μl ^{125}I-NT (approximately 10,000 cpm) and 100 μl standard synthetic NT or the unknown. Samples are routinely examined at three to five dilutions which span the sensitive portion of the assay, and "damage" tubes, consisting of sample in the absence of antibody, are included for each dilution. Damage is usually 2–5%, and antisera are normally used at final dilutions giving 35–50% binding (in our system, 1 : 200,000). To facilitate interassay comparisons, the standards for about 30 experiments are aliquoted into sets of assay tubes that are kept frozen at −20°C until used. The assay is set up at room temperature unless proteolytic enzymes are suspected of being present in samples (such as unextracted plasma), in which case ice water is employed. After blending on a

Vortex mixer, the mixtures are usually allowed to sit at 4°C for 18 to 24 hours, although longer incubation times (48 to 72 hours) are necessary for equilibration when lower concentrations of antisera are employed. The bound (B) and free (F) traces are separated at 4°C by the rapid addition of 1.0 ml of a 1 : 4 dilution of a stock suspension of charcoal (2.5%) and dextran T-70 (0.25%) in PBS to each tube. The tubes are immediately centrifuged for 20 minutes at 2000 rpm, and the supernatant (B) and the sedimented charcoal (F) are counted in a gamma scintillation counter.

Any of the numerous methods suggested for plotting the results is valid, provided that standard and sample are treated identically (Ekins, 1974). We choose to calculate a B/F ratio using a hand calculator and to construct a standard curve using four-cycle semilog paper. Provided that the total counts ($B + F$) delivered to the tubes varies $<1\%$, the B/F ratio may be computed by the formula, $(B_s - B_d)/F_s$, where B_s and F_s refer to counts bound and free for the sample in the presence of antibody and B_d refers to counts bound in the corresponding damage tubes. The data for the standards are graphed, plotting B/F on the linear scale and moles of added NT on the log scale. Using this standard curve, the B/F for each sample is converted to mole equivalents of NT, and the concentrations determined at the various dilutions are averaged, provided that they agree within 20%. Maximal sensitivity, as defined by 90% of the initial B/F ratio, is 2.0 fmole/tube. If nonparallelism is observed for a sample, the value obtained from the middle of the curve (half-displacement) should be taken.

Assay reproducibility is judged from the daily variation in the half-displacement point (usually 10–15%) and from the intra- and interassay coefficients of variation observed for repeated measurements on a single sample (usually about 10 and 20%, respectively).

V. CONCLUSION

Radioimmunoassay can provide one with a very sensitive, specific, and reliable means of measuring NT in biologic samples provided that proper care is taken in the design, performance, and validation of the assays. Forethought in the design of useful immunogens can be quite beneficial and may enable one to influence antibody specificity. Multiple heterogeneous and site-directed antisera can be employed to increase the selectivity of the assay for NT and to gather information about the character of NT-related substances. Radioimmunoassay will clearly be of enormous benefit to researchers as they pursue an understanding of the physiology of this interesting class of peptides, the NT family.

ACKNOWLEDGMENTS

The author is a Postdoctoral Fellow of The Arthritis Foundation. The research reported was supported in part by the following grants from the National Institute of Health: 1 R01 AM19428 and AM 16510.

REFERENCES

Assan, R., Rosselin, G., Drouet, J., Dolais, J., and Tchobroutsky, G. (1965). Glucagon antibodies. *Lancet* **2**, 590–591.

Bolton, A. E., and Hunter, W. M. (1972). A new method for labelling protein hormones with radioiodine for use in the radioimmunoassay. *J. Endocrinol.* **55**, xxx–xxxi (abstr.).

Carraway, R., and Leeman, S. E. (1973). The isolation of a new hypotensive peptide neurotensin. *J. Biol. Chem.* **248**, 6854–6861.

Carraway, R., and Leeman, S. E. (1975a). The amino acid sequence of a hypothalamic peptide, neurotensin. *J. Biol. Chem.* **250**, 1907–1911.

Carraway, R., and Leeman, S. E. (1975b). The synthesis of neurotensin; confirmation of its primary structure. *J. Biol. Chem.* **250**, 1912–1918.

Carraway, R., and Leeman, S. E. (1975c). Structural requirements for the biological activity of neurotensin, a new vasoactive peptide. *In* "Structural Chemistry and Molecular Biology of Peptides" (R. Walter and J. Meienhofer eds.), pp. 679–685. Ann Arbor Sci. Publ., Ann Arbor, Michigan.

Carraway, R., and Leeman, S. E. (1976a). Radioimmunoassay for neurotensin, a hypothalamic peptide. *J. Biol. Chem.* **251**, 7035–7044.

Carraway, R., and Leeman, S. E. (1976b). Characterization of radioimmunoassayable neurotensin in the rat. *J. Biol. Chem.* **251**, 7045–7052.

Carraway, R., Goetzl, E. J., and Leeman, S. E. (1974). Detection of a neurotensin-related antigen in human synovial fluid. VI *Pan-Am. Congr. Rheum. Dis.*

Carraway, R., Goetzl, E. J., and Leeman, S. E. (1975). Mononuclear leukocyte chemotactic activity associated with neurotensin-related antigens (NRA) in rheumatoid synovitis. *Arthritis and Rheumatism* **18**, 392.

Carraway, R., Demers, L. M., and Leeman, S. E. (1976). Hyperglycemic effect of neurotensin, a hypothalamic peptide. *Endocrinology* **99**, 1452–1462.

Chard, T., Forsling, M. L., James, M. A. R., Kitau, M. J., and Landon, J. (1970). The development of a radioimmunoassay for oxytocin: Specificity and the dissociation of immunological and biological activity. *J. Endocrinol.* **46**, 533–542.

Ekins, R. P. (1974). Radioimmunoassay and saturation analysis; basic principles and theory. *Br. Med. Bull.* **30**, 3–11.

Greenwood, F. C., Hunter, W. M., and Glover, J. S. (1963). The preparation of ^{131}I-labelled human growth hormone of high specific radioactivity. *Biochem. J.* **89**, 114–123.

Jaffe, B. M., and Walsh, J. H. (1974). Gastrin and related peptides. *In* "Methods of

Hormone Radioimmunoassay" (B. M. Jaffe and H. R. Behrman, eds.), pp. 251–273. Academic Press, New York.

Kitabgi, P., Carraway, R., and Leeman, S. E. (1976). Isolation of a tridecapeptide from bovine intestinal tissue and its partial characterization as neurotensin. *J. Biol. Chem.* **251**, 7053–7058.

Leeman, S. E., Mroz, E. A., and Carraway, R. (1977). Substance P and neurotensin. *In* "Peptides in Neurobiology" (H. Gainer, ed.), pp. 99–144.

Makino, T., Carraway, R., Leeman, S. E., and Greep, R. O. (1973). In vitro and in vivo effects of newly purified hypothalamic tridecapeptide on rat LH and FSH release. *Soc. Study Reprod.* Sixth Annual Meeting, Athens; Georgia, p. 26.

Marks, V., Morris, B. A., and Teale, J. D. (1974). Radioimmunoassay and saturation analysis; pharmacology. *Br. Med. Bull.* **30**, 80–85.

Odell, W. D., Abraham, G. A., Skowsky, W. R., Hescox, M. A., and Fisher, D. A. (1971). Production of antisera for radioimmunoassays. *In* "Principles of Competitive Protein-Binding Assays" (W. D. Odell and W. H. Daughaday, eds.), pp. 57–88. Lippincott, Philadelphia, Pennsylvania.

Orci, L., Baetens, O., Refener, C., Brown, M., Vale, W., and Guillemin, R. (1976). Evidence for immunoreactive neurotensin in dog intestinal mucosa. *Life Sci.* **19**, 559–562.

Parker, C. W. (1971). Nature of the immunological responses and antigen antibody interaction. *In* "Principles of Competitive Protein-Binding Assays" (W. D. Odell and W. H. Daughaday, eds.), pp. 25–56. Lippincott, Philadelphia, Pennsylvania.

Sundler, F., Hakanson, R., Hammer, R., Alumets, J., Carraway, R., Leeman, S. E., and Zimmerman, E. (1977a). Immunohistochemical localization of neurotensin to endocrine cells in the gut. *Cell Tissue Res.* **178**, 313–321.

Sundler, F., Alumets, J., Hakanson, R., Carraway, R., and Leeman, S. E. (1977b). Ultrastructure of the gut neurotensin cell. *Histochemistry* **53**, 25–34.

Vaitukaitis, J., Robbins, J. B., Nieschlag, E., and Ross, G. T. (1971). A method for producing specific antisera with small doses of immunogen. *J. Clin. Endocrinol. Metab.* **33**, 988–991.

PITUITARY HORMONES

9

Pituitary Gonadotropins

N. R. MOUDGAL, K. MURALIDHAR, AND
H. G. MADHWA RAJ

I. INTRODUCTION

In recent years, competitive protein binding assays in general (Odell and Daughaday, 1971), and radioimmunoassays, in particular, have been extensively employed to investigate a variety of problems in endocrine research. The radioimmunoassays for gonadotropins, by virtue of their superiority in terms of sensitivity and reproducibility, have almost completely replaced the earlier immunoassays based on

Methods of Hormone Radioimmunoassay, Second Edition
Copyright © 1979 by Academic Press, Inc.
All rights of reproduction in any form reserved. ISBN 0-12-379260-6

the complement fixation (Brody and Carlstrom, 1960) and agglutination inhibition reactions (Wide *et al.*, 1961). Needless to say, the availability of highly purified preparations of FSH and LH, the high immunogenicity of these glycoprotein hormones, the wide cross-reactivity that gonadotropin antisera exhibit (Li *et al.*, 1962; Rao and Moudgal, 1970), and the development of a relatively mild and easy method of radioiodination by Greenwood *et al.* (1963) have largely aided in the successful development of a number of radioimmunoassay systems for FSH and LH (Diczfalusy, 1969).

Although the cross-reaction of gonadotropin antisera across species barriers was recognized early (Moudgal and Li, 1961a; Madhwa Raj and Moudgal, 1971; Rao and Moudgal, 1970; Midgley *et al.*, 1972), this property was not successfully exploited to develop heterologous radioimmunoassay systems, except for the work of Niswender *et al.* (1968b). These workers used a universal antiserum against ovine LH to measure a variety of heterologous LH's. Improved milder procedures for iodination (Miyachi *et al.*, 1972; Redshaw and Lynch, 1974), simpler techniques for separation of bound from free labeled hormone (including the use of immobilized antibodies), and better description of theoretical aspects of radioimmunoassays have contributed to the large-scale acceptance of radioimmunoassays as research tools in recent years.

Most of these assays have been of the homologous type, taking five to seven days for completion. Attempts to reduce the duration of assays without appreciable loss in sensitivity or reproducibility (Kosasa *et al.*, 1976; Moudgal *et al.*, 1971), as well as attempts to apply radioimmunoassay to measure gonadotropins in urine and bound to tissue receptors, are recent events (Moudgal and Muralidhar, 1974; Moudgal *et al.*, 1971).

In this chapter, radioimmunoassay of FSH and LH as tested and routinely performed in our laboratory is described. In recent years, instrumentation has been developed in a few laboratories to increase the degree of automation, allowing simultaneous performance of a number of assays (W. M. Hunter, personal communication). The high initial expenditure and the amount of work load that required for the instrument to be kept operational may not allow such techniques to come within the reach of the average investigator. In this chapter, we describe methods which are simple and easily reproducible, and which involve minimal expenditure. We hope that the procedural details given below will enable one without prior experience in these techniques to establish the assays.

II. PROCEDURAL DETAILS OF RADIOIMMUNOASSAY

The basic materials required for conducting radioimmunoassays are radiometric facilities, pure preparations of gonadotropins for radioiodination, and antisera to these hormones. Hormones and antisera could be procured from several investigators, companies, and agencies. The National Institute of Arthritis, Metabolic and Digestive Diseases (NIAMDD), Bethesda, Maryland* provides a generous supply of these on request from investigators. However, it is advisable to prepare, wherever possible, antisera to individual gonadotropins. This would aid in better knowledge of the antibody characteristics which helps in designing newer types of heterologous radioimmunoassays.

A. Preparation of Radiolabeled Hormone

1. General Principles

Sensitive radioimmunoassays depend upon the use of radiolabeled hormone of high specific activity. This precludes use of low specific activity ^{14}C- and ^{3}H-labeled gonadotropins (Eshkol, 1969; Vaitukaitis et al., 1972). As for most other protein hormones, iodination with labeled iodine, ^{131}I or ^{125}I, has thus far been the method of choice for LH and FSH. The longer half-life of ^{125}I compared to ^{131}I (60 days versus eight days) makes the former preferable. Carrier-free radioactive iodine, essential for iodination of protein, is supplied by a number of companies. In principle, iodination involves generation of nascent radioactive iodine in a medium containing the hormone. The amount of iodine and the duration of exposure of the hormone to iodine determine the degree of iodination.

A wide variety of methods to release nascent iodine from iodide are available. These include use of oxidizing agents such as iodine monochloride (Glazer and Singer, 1964) and chloramine-T (Greenwood et al., 1963), electrolysis (Rosa et al., 1967), and the use of the enzyme lactoperoxidase (Miyachi et al., 1972). The most widely used procedure employs chloramine-T as the oxidizing agent, notwithstanding its known damaging effects on the immunologic and biologic activity of proteins. While reduction in the duration of expo-

* Inquiries may be addressed to: Hormone Distribution Officer, Office of the Director, NIAMDD, Bldg. 31, Room 9A 47, National Institutes of Health, Bethesda, Maryland.

sure partially reduces the extent of damage, hormones such as FSH and human LH have been shown to still be labile under such conditions. To remove the damaged fraction an additional chromatography on DEAE-cellulose columns has at times been found useful (Donini, 1969).

The enzymatic method (Miyachi *et al.*, 1972) yields labeled relatively undamaged LH and FSH of high specific activity. The labeled preparation has a longer shelf life compared to that prepared by the chloramine-T method (Figure 1). An improvement of the chloramine-T method has been recently described (Redshaw and Lynch, 1974). This involves generating chlorine gas and allowing the gaseous nascent chlorine to liberate iodine from $Na^{125}I$; by not allowing the protein to come into contact with chloramine-T, this minimizes damage to the peptide.

2. Iodination by Chloramine-T Method

a. Materials Required

1. Highly purified gonadotropin (LH or FSH) in 50- to 100-μg quantities. It is convenient to store gonadotropins frozen in individual vials at a concentration of 1.0–2.5 μg per 0.01 ml water. This way, every iodination requires thawing of only one vial and thereby prevents damage to highly purified hormone preparations, due to repeated freezing and thawing.
2. Chloramine-T (100–200 gm), preferably fresh stock, is stored either in bulk in a brown stoppered bottle or in a number of small vials each containing 50 mg or less.
3. Phosphate buffer, $0.5 M$, pH 7.4 (PB) (75 gm $Na_2HPO_4 \cdot 2 H_2O$, 12.5 gm $NaH_2PO_4 \cdot 2 H_2O$ made up in one liter of water).
4. Sodium metabisulfite (analytical grade) 2% solution, freshly prepared.

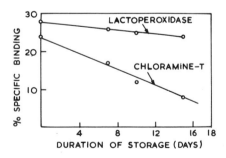

Figure 1.   Relative stability of iodinated FSH prepared by chemical and enzymatic methods.

5. Potassium iodide (analytical grade) 0.4% solution, freshly prepared.
6. $Na^{125}I$ carrier-free, 1.0–5.0 mCi in NaOH (procured from Amersham IMS-3 or IMS-300 in V vials), diluted with 100 to 200 μl 0.1 M phosphate buffer, pH 7.4, and centrifuged for ten minutes at 3000 rpm. This facilitates collection of radioactive material at the bottom of the vial and permits easier pipetting.

b. Iodination Procedure. Iodination is preferably carried out in "penicillin vials" stoppered with a rubber cap through which solutions can be conveniently injected. Gonadotropin, 2.5 μg in 5.0–10 μl water, is introduced into the vial followed by the addition of 1.0 mCi of $Na^{125}I$ in 25-μl volume. The chloramine-T, 25 μg/50 μl, is injected into the reaction vial and 30–60 seconds later, sodium metabisulfite, 250 μg/50 μl, and potassium iodide solutions, 200 μg/50 μl, are added. Each addition is followed by mixing of the solution by a swirling motion. The iodination is carried out preferably in an ice bath (0°–4°C). The separation of iodinated gonadotropin from the unreacted iodide is achieved by Sephadex gel filtration as described below.

3. Iodination by Lactoperoxidase Method

a. Materials Required

1. The enzyme lactoperoxidase is marketed by Calbiochem (Catalog No. 427466) in lots of 25 mg. The purity of the enzyme is checked by measuring the absorbance of a 200 μg/ml solution at 412 and at 280 nm. The ratio of OD_{412}/OD_{280} should be greater than 0.65. If not, it can be passed through a column of Sephadex-G200, using 0.05 M potassium phosphate, pH 7.5, as eluant. This yields a material of higher A_{412}/A_{280} ratio. For iodination, about 100 μg enzyme is weighed and dissolved in 0.5 ml 0.4 M sodium acetate buffer, pH 5.6. The enzyme powder is stored in the deep freeze.
2. Hydrogen peroxide as a 30% solution is marketed by many companies. This is stored at 4°C. Whenever required, 1.0 ml is poured into a small flask, and this is used for further dilution. It is not advisable to pipette directly from the container as heavy metal ions in the glass pipettes decompose hydrogen peroxide. Since the required concentration of hydrogen peroxide for use is low (1:50,000), it is advisable to make serial dilutions with glass-distilled water. Enzymatic iodination gives a labeled

hormone which appears quite stable over a three-week period judged from weekly binding tests (Figure 1).

3. Details of radioactive iodine and hormone are identical to the chloramine-T method described earlier. The buffer used in enzymatic iodination, however, is $0.4 M$ sodium acetate, pH 5.6.

b. Iodination Procedure. Into a small test tube (10×75 mm) containing 2.5 μg FSH or LH in 10 μl water, add in order 25 μl 0.4 M sodium acetate buffer, pH 5.6, 100–250 ng enzyme in 0.1 ml buffer, and 1.0 mCi Na ^{125}I in 20 μl. The reaction is initiated by the addition of 0.1 ml 1 : 50,000 diluted hydrogen peroxide (600 ng). Mix well, and after five minutes add another aliquot of dilute hydrogen peroxide, 600 ng/0.1 ml. Fifteen minutes after the initiation of iodination, the solution is loaded on to a Sephadex G-50 column as described below.

4. Purification by Sephadex Gel Filtration

Sephadex G-50 columns, 1.0×15 cm, are equilibrated with $0.01 M$ PBS containing 0.2% gelatin. The iodination reaction mixture from either technique is carefully layered onto the column and eluted with PBS-gelatin. One milliliter eluates are collected into individual test tubes (10×75 mm). Fifteen milliliters of eluate is sufficient to remove both the iodinated hormone and the unreacted iodide from the column. Aliquots from each tube (0.025–0.1 ml) are counted in a gamma spectrometer. Usually the iodinated protein appears in the eluate immediately after the void volume (4–6 ml). The contents of the peak tube (usually the fourth or fifth) are stored frozen in small aliquots. It is preferable to add BSA to a final concentration of 0.1% to this peak tube before aliquoting. It is advisable to repurify the labeled hormone once every two weeks by passage through a similar column.

B. Production, Purification, and Characterization of Antisera to FSH and LH

1. General Principles

Both FSH and LH are good antigens, eliciting soluble and precipitating types of antibodies, respectively, in rabbits (Rao and Moudgal, 1970; Moudgal and Li, 1961a,b). Antibodies to LH and FSH are available to qualified investigators from the NIAMDD.

Although the rabbit has been the most widely used animal, subhuman primates can also be conveniently employed for raising antibodies (Moudgal *et al.*, 1974; Prahlada *et al.*, 1974; Moudgal, 1975). A variety of immunization schedules have been employed, and they differ from one another in the total dose of hormone administered, mode of administration, and the duration of immunization. It is known that as immunization progresses, the type of antibody produced by the animal differs in many respects, especially with regard to specificity, i.e., while the specificity toward the most dominant of the antigenic determinants does not alter, less prominent determinant(s) start eliciting antibodies. Therefore, for homologous radioimmunoassays, it is preferable to employ antisera from animals that have been immunized for short periods.

When only small amounts of antigen (less than 1.0 mg) are available, the procedure outlined by Vaitukaitis *et al.* (1971) is useful.

2. Immunization of Rabbits and Monkeys

Ten to fifteen milligrams of pure hormone is sufficient. Complete Freund's adjuvant is mixed with an equal volume of saline containing 1.0 mg/ml of the hormone. Thorough shaking, to prevent phase separation, is a necessity. The first injection consists only of the hormone (500 μg) in saline. The subsequent injections are given in complete Freund's adjuvant. Intramuscular injections at weekly or 10-day intervals elicit antibody production of high titer after 10–12 injections. In the procedure of Vaitukaitis *et al.* (1971), the hormone mixed with adjuvant is injected intradermally at more than 20–30 sites. In addition to the hormone and complete Freund's adjuvant, Vaitukaitis advocates using a potent vaccine like that of *B. pertussis* to boost antibody production. Both rabbits and monkeys are amenable to such a immunization procedure. After four to five injections, a test volume (10 ml) of blood is taken from the animals (from the ear vein and femoral vein of rabbits and monkeys, respectively). The serum obtained at the test bleedings is evaluated for antibody titer by a qualitative precipitin ring test (Kabat and Mayer, 1964). A positive reaction at a dilution of 1 : 32 or 1 : 64 indicates that the animals are ready for a booster injection of the antigen in saline. Seven days after the booster injection (500 μg in 0.5 ml saline) the animals can be bled (30–40 ml) and the blood processed for serum. The animals can be continued on the immunization schedule or can be bled to death depending upon the quantity and characteristics of the antiserum one needs. The latter procedure yields a large amount of antiserum from a single batch which can be characterized and used for radioimmunoassays.

3. Immunization of Goats for Second Antibody

Goats are immunized with the γ-globulin prepared from rabbits or monkeys, depending on the animal in which the hormone antibody was prepared. The immunization schedule is the same as given above for rabbits and monkeys. The animals are bled from the jugular vein once a month (150 ml); however, injection of γ-globulin in saline is not necessary.

The volume of double antibody to be added to the individual assay tubes is computed by titrating the antiserum against normal rabbit or monkey serum as the case may be. To 0.1 ml of 1 : 100 normal rabbit or monkey serum, increasing volumes of a 1 : 1 diluted goat antiserum are added. The tubes are allowed to stand six hours at 37°C. After centrifugation, the precipitates are dissolved in 1.0 ml 0.05 N NaOH, and absorbance is measured at 280 nm in a spectrophotometer. The protein content in these pellets can be computed from a standard curve constructed using γ-globulin as standard protein. Usually the volume of double antibody added is in 20% excess of what is needed, as computed from the equivalence zone. For example, if 0.4 ml of 1 : 1 diluted goat antiserum gave maximum amount of precipitate with 0.1 ml of 1 : 100 diluted normal rabbit or monkey serum, then 0.25 ml of the undiluted goat antiserum can be added to all assay tubes.

4. Characterization of Antibodies

a. **Detection and Elimination of Antibodies to Contaminating Proteins.** Even when purified antigens are used, it is possible that the antisera raised against them contain contaminating antibodies against tissue and serum proteins. These are of both precipitating and soluble types (Rao and Moudgal, 1970). In addition, the presence of LH antibodies in FSH antisera is a major problem which has hindered the development of homologous radioimmunoassays for ovine FSH (o-FSH) (L'Hermite *et al.*, 1972). The specificity of measurement is an *a priori* condition of radioimmunoassay. When the antiserum is impure, i.e., has contaminating antibodies, choosing a purified label would partially ensure the specificity. At times sheer dilution of the antiserum would solve the problem by eliminating the low-affinity contaminating antibodies. However, if the contaminating antibodies are of equal affinity and concentration, removal by absorption is the only course. In such instances (e.g., oFSH antiserum) removal of contaminating antibodies by absorption is inevitable.

The conventional procedure to achieve this is to add to the antiserum, in small amounts, a diluted solution of the suspected antigen (normal serum or liver or kidney extract prepared in 0.01 M phosphate-buffered saline, pH 7.4). The supernatant is monitored after incubation for one day at 4°C for antibodies by the Ouchterlony technique, as described by Kabat.

The use of the suspected contaminating antigen (normal serum or tissue extract) in the form of a water-insoluble derivative, is a more precise procedure with added advantages. The water-insoluble derivative is prepared by employing any one of the techniques available for covalent coupling of proteins to polymers such as Sepharose (Cuatracasas, 1971) (see Chapter 3), or by the use of bifunctional reagents, such as ethyl chloroformate (Avrameas and Ternynck, 1967) or glutaraldehyde (Avrameas and Ternynck, 1969), or by physical absorption onto tannic acid-coated, formalinized sheep erythrocytes (Kabat and Mayer, 1964). The absorption procedure requires suspension of the immunosorbent in the antiserum for 10–12 hours at 4°C with gentle stirring and centrifugation to recover the supernatant. One or more treatments may be required depending on the capacity of the immunosorbent to remove all the contaminants. The monitoring of the contaminants in the supernatant can be done either by the Ouchterlony test or in some cases by the test of binding to radioiodinated antigen. An example of this is the removal of contaminating LH antibodies from an FSH antiserum (Table I).

The above procedure of removing contaminating antibodies has distinct advantages in that both precipitating and soluble types of antibodies can be removed, no extraneous material is introduced into the antiserum, and the immunosorbent is reusable after treatment with a dissociating agent to remove the bound protein (Muralidhar et al.,

Table I Characterization of Antisera-Labeled Hormone Binding Studies[a]

Group	Antiserum[b]	^{125}I-Labeled hormone	Specific binding (%)
I	Anti-FSH unabsorbed	FSH	58.2
II	Anti-FSH unabsorbed	LH	39.4
III	Anti-FSH absorbed	FSH	54.7
IV	Anti-FSH absorbed	LH	1.4
V	Anti-FSH	FSH	29.0
VI	Anti-FSH + 50 ng LH	FSH	28.0
VII	Anti-FSH + 1.0 ng FSH	FSH	11.0
VIII	Anti-LH	LH	43.0
IX	Anti-LH + absorbed Anti-FSH (10 μl)	LH	42.0
X	Anti-LH	FSH	89.0
XI	Anti-LH	FSH	1.8

[a] From Rao et al. (1974).

[b] In groups I, II, III, IV, X, XI, 10 μl undiluted antiserum was used. Other groups were given 100 μl 1 : 1000 diluted absorbed antiserum. See text for details of incubation.

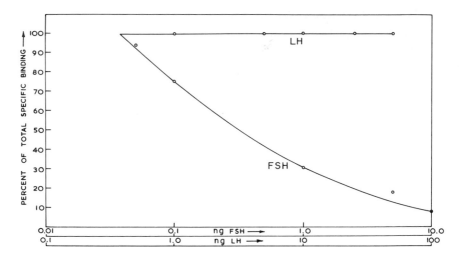

Figure 2. Homologous radioimmunoassay for ovine FSH. The FSH antiserum was freed of all contaminating antibodies by sequential treatment with a copolymer of normal sheep serum and then with LH-coated sheep erythrocytes. Note the noninterference of LH in the assay for FSH. (From Muralidhar *et al.*, 1974.)

1974). For example, using such a procedure, a homologous radioimmunoassay for ovine FSH (oFSH) can be established (Figure 2).

Prior to use in the radioimmunoassay, an antiserum must be assessed for its antibody titer. The antibody titer as evaluated by a quantitative precipitin test, is known to vary among antisera produced in different animals as well as with progressive bleedings from the same animal during the course of an immunization (Table II). For radioimmunoassay, an antiserum which shows a binding of 30–50% of the radioiodinated hormone, is chosen. Effective competition upon addition of unlabeled hormone occurs only under conditions of limited antibody. In order to determine this, the binding ability of a trace amount of the labeled hormone is tested with serial dilutions of the antiserum. Such a titration curve is shown in Figure 3.

b. Checking Binding of Labeled Hormone to Antisera. Aliquots (0.1 ml) of serial dilutions of the antiserum are incubated at 37°C for 12 hours with approximately 20,000 cpm of the labeled hormone. At the end of the incubation, 0.1 ml of 1 : 100 diluted normal rabbit serum and an amount of goat antiserum sufficient to precipitate the γ-globulin maximally are added and the incubation continued for another 10–12 hours. The tubes are then counted for total radioactivity in a gamma

Table II   Antibody Content of Various Batches of Antisera

Rabbit No.	Antigen	Bleeding No.	Antibody[b] (mg No. ml serum)
3	Ovine LH[a]	I	0.98
	Ovine LH	II	1.76
23	Ovine LH	I	2.50
	Ovine LH	IV	11.20
	Ovine LH	XII	10.64
	Ovine LH	XIV	11.20

[a] Ovine LH used was a highly purified preparation supplied by Drs. H. Papkoff and C. H. Li.

[b] Antibody content determined by the quantitative precipitin test (Kabat and Mayer, 1964). Milligram antibody equals total protein precipitated at equivalence minus antigen protein added at equivalence.

spectrometer, followed by centrifugation at 3000 rpm, preferably in the cold. The supernatant is aspirated and the pellet counted for radioactivity.

c. Species Specificity. Another aspect of the same problem is establishing cross-reactivity of an antiserum to a hormone of one species (e.g., ovine LH antiserum) with the same hormone of other species (e.g., rat, monkey, hamster LH). This would, in fact, allow development of heterologous systems, e.g., the assay of murine LH using

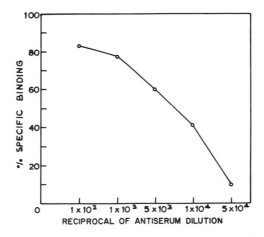

Figure 3. Binding of ^{125}I-labeled ovine LH to LH antiserum at different dilutions to assess the optimum dilution for radioimmunoassay. A dilution of 1×10^4 (1 : 10,000) is suitable for radioimmunoassay.

ovine LH antiserum. This is of particular significance, since production of antisera to gonadotropins of murine or simian origin is
not practicable for all laboratories, for want of supply of purified
antigen.

Gonadotropins (LH, FSH, and hCG) are composed of two subunits,
a hormone-specific β subunit, which has, in addition, 70% of the antigenic determinants (Papkoff *et al.*, 1971; Moudgal *et al.*, 1974;
Midgley *et al.*, 1972), and an α subunit, which is more or less similar
among the glycoprotein hormones of the same species. The cross-
reactivity of ovine LH antiserum with LH of other animals has been
attributed to a variable degree of commonality of the β subunits
(Madhwaraj and Moudgal, 1971; Moudgal *et al.*, 1974). Thus, it is
logical to expect a higher degree of inhibition by rat and hamster
pituitary extracts of the binding of ^{125}I-oLH, if antiserum to the β
subunit of ovine LH is used than when antiserum to LH is employed.
Conversely, when labeled β subunit is employed, heterologous pituitary extracts inhibit the binding of the label to antiserum to oLH but
not when ^{125}I-oLH is used. In essence, exploitation of restricted competition by choosing appropriate labels and antisera (at times at
selected dilutions) would lead to development of specific heterologous radioimmunoassays. Table III lists some of these interesting combinations to assay rat and monkey LH.

C. Methods for Separation of Bound from Free Labeled Hormone

1. Available Techniques

Separation of unreacted free labeled hormone from the antibody-
bound label in radioimmunoassays can be achieved by many methods
which utilize the difference in physicochemical properties between
the antibody and the test hormone. These include differential solubility in organic solvents (Catt, 1969; Thomas and Ferin, 1968),
molecular size (Haber *et al.*, 1965), and electrophoretic mobility
(Yalow and Berson, 1959). For routine checking of binding, use of
organic solvents with or without salts is extremely useful and rapid.
However, when serum samples are to be assayed, the results do not
appear to be satisfactory. This could possibly be due to coprecipitation
of the free label along with the antigen–antibody complex in the presence of excess protein.

Table III Representative Systems for Radioimmunoassay of Gonadotropins[c]

Hormone measured	Source	Standards	^{125}I-Labeled hormone used	Rabbit antiserum used	Separation method	Reference
LH	Human	Human LH	Human LH	Anti-hCG	DA[a]	Aono et al. (1967; Odell et al. (1966, 1969); Midgley and Jaffe (1966)
		2nd IRP hMG and hCG	hCG	Anti-hCG	DA	Midgley (1966)
		2nd IRP hMG and hCG	hCG	Anti-hCG	PA[b]	Donini et al. (1968)
	Cattle	Bovine LH	Bovine LH	Anti-bovine LH	DA	Niswender et al. (1968b)
		Bovine LH	Ovine LH	Anti-ovine LH	DA	Niswender et al. (1968b)
	Pig	Porcine LH	LER-7563	Anti-porcine LH	DA	Niswender et al. (1968b)
	Sheep	Ovine LH	Ovine LH	Anti-ovine LH	DA	Niswender et al. (1969)
		Ovine LH	Ovine LH-β	Anti-ovine LH	DA	K. Muralidhar and N. R. Moudgal (unpublished observations)
	Rabbit	Rabbit LH	Ovine LH	Anti-ovine LH	DA	Scaramuzzi et al. (1972)
	Rat	Rat LH	Rat LH	Anti-rat LH	DA	Monroe et al. (1968)
		Rat LH	Ovine LH	Anti-ovine LH	DA	Niswender et al. (1968a)
		Ovine LH	Ovine LH-β	Anti-ovine LH	PA	Muralidhar et al. (1974)
		Ovine LH	Ovine LH	Anti-ovine LH-β	DA	K. Ramasharma, K. Muralidhar, and N. R. Moudgal (unpublished observations)
	Mouse	Mouse LH	Rat LH	Anti-rat LH (NIAMDD)	DA	Beamer et al. (1972)
	Monkey	Simian LH	Simian LH	Guinea pig anti-simian LH	DA	Monroe et al. (1970)
		Simian LH	Simian LH	Anti-simian LH	DA	Monroe et al. (1970)
		Simian LH	Ovine LH	Anti-ovine LH	DA	Kirton et al. (1970)
		Human LH	Ovine LH	Anti-ovine LH	DA	Niswender et al. (1971)

(Continued)

Table III *(Continued)*

Hormone measured	Source	Standards	^{125}I-Labeled hormone used	Rabbit antiserum used	Separation method	Reference
		Human LH	Human LH	Anti-hCG-β	DA	N. R. Moudgal (unpublished observations)
		Ovine LH	Ovine LH	Anti-ovine LH-β	DA	K. Ramasharma, K. Muralidhar, and N. R. Moudgal (unpublished observations)
FSH	Human	Variety of preparations	LER-710-2	Anti-LER-735-2	DA	Midgley (1967); Ostergard et al. (1970)
		Ryan-5765-B	Ryan-5765-B	Guinea pig anti-human FSH	DA	Faiman and Ryan (1967)
		Human FSH	Human FSH	Anti-human FSH	Bentonite	Butt and Lynch (1968)
		Variety of preparations	LER-828-2	Anti-LER-735-2	DA	Aono and Taymor (1968)
		Variety of preparations	Human FSH	Anti-human FSH	Chromato-electrophoresis	Saxena et al. (1969)
	Sheep	Ovine FSH	Human FSH	Anti-ovine FSH	DA	L'Hermite et al. (1972)
		Ovine FSH	Ovine FSH	Anti-ovine FSH	DA	Muralidhar et al. (1974)

Rat	Rat FSH	Rat FSH	Anti-rat FSH	DA	NIAMDD
	Rat FSH	Rat FSH	Anti-ovine FSH	DA	C. S. Sheela Rani and N. R. Moudgal (unpublished observations)
Monkey	Human FSH	Human FSH	Anti-ovine FSH	DA	C. S. Sheela Rani and N. R. Moudgal (unpublished observations), Yamaji et al. (1973)
Placental gonadotropin Human (hCG)	hCG	hCG	Anti-hCG	DA	Midgley (1966)
	2nd IRP-hCG	hCG	Anti-hCG	DA	Franchimont (1970)
Mare (PMSG)	Ovine LH	Ovine LH	Anti-PMSG	DA	N. R. Moudgal and K. Ramasharma (unpublished observations)

[a] Double antibody.

[b] Polymerized antibody.

[c] In recent years, subunit specific antisera have been produced against hCG-β and LH-β. However, while with the hCG-β antiserum, one can measure hCG without much interference of hLH (Vaitukaitis et al., 1971), the antiserum to LH-β subunit cannot measure β subunit alone in the presence of whole LH as the cross-reaction between the two is very high. However, suitable absorption procedures (e.g., absorption of LH-β antiserum with LH) should yield a population of antibodies recognizing only the β subunit. Such antiserum will be able to measure circulating free β subunit.

187

2. Use of Isopropyl Alcohol to Separate ^{125}I-hLH–Antibody Complex from Free ^{125}I-hLH

Aliquots (0.1 ml) of suitably diluted hCG antiserum are incubated with 25,000 cpm of ^{125}I-hLH at 37°C for 12 hours. At the end of incubation, 0.1 ml human γ-globulin solution (10 mg/ml) is added, followed by mixing and addition of isopropyl alcohol to a final concentration of 55%. The final concentration of isopropyl alcohol is previously calibrated to ensure complete precipitation of the antigen–antibody complex but no precipitation of the free label. After standing at room temperature (25°C) for one hour, the tubes are counted for total radioactivity, centrifuged, the supernatants aspirated, and the tubes counted again for antibody-bound radioactivity.

Solid phase radioimmunoassay systems employing the antibody in the form of either a coated Protopol Dl/l disks (Catt et al., 1967), or polystyrene tubes (Catt and Tregéar, 1967) have been described. However, these have not yet found wide acceptance. Another method is that of Donini et al. (1968), in which the antibody used is in the form of a copolymer and involves a filtration step on cellulose acetate disks to separate antibody-bound label from free labeled hormone. This could be made simpler by introducing a simple centrifugation step, small amounts of hydroxyapatite being added to aid in procuring a good pellet.

The use of a double antibody (antibody to the γ-globulin of the animal in which the hormone antibody was prepared) to precipitate the soluble hormone–antibody complex formed during the first incubation is a widely used technique (Utiger et al., 1962). Goats immunized with rabbit γ-globulin, for example, yield antisera of suitable titer. Each batch of antiserum must be checked for titer by a quantitative precipitation test. On the other hand, anti-γ-globulin sera can be procured from several manufacturers (see Section II,B).

D. Assay Conditions

The radioimmunoassay procedure using double antibody that is widely employed is conducted at 4°C and lasts for five to seven days. Our experience, however, has shown that the total assay can be completed within 40 hours if conducted at 37°C (Table IV) without loss of sensitivity and precision (Figure 4 and Table V). The major change in the protocol of the assay when conducted at 37°C is a drastic reduction in the duration of incubation with the second antibody (Table VI), from five days to 12 hours.

Table IV A Comparison of the Conditions of Radioimmunoassay at
37° and 4°C

Conditions	37°C	4°C
Incubation of antibody with cold		
hormone or unknown (hours)	12	24
Incubation with labeled hormone (hours)	12	24
Incubation with double antibody (hours)	12	96
Total	36	144

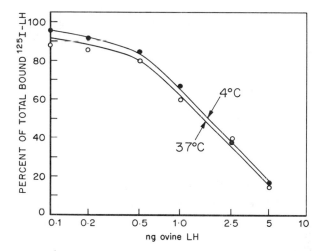

Figure 4. Comparison of standard curves for ovine LH obtained by conducting the
radioimmunoassay at 37° and 4°C. Incubation was carried out for 36 hours in the former
case and for 120 hours in the latter.

Table V Characteristics of the Elevated Temperature
Radioimmunoassay[a]

Precision at each point (ng LH)	Specific binding (% ± S.D.)
0	100 ± 5
0.1	90 ± 5
0.5	80 ± 7
1.0	65 ± 3
5.0	30 ± 1.5
10.0	5 ± 1

[a] Sensitivity, 0.5 ng; range, 0.1–10 ng; intraassay variation, 5%;
interassay variation, 10–15%.

Table VI Effect of Duration of Incubation at 37°C on the Amount of Anti-Rabbit γ Globulin Precipitated by Different Amounts of 1 : 10 Diluted Rabbit Serum[a]

Antigen NRS (1 : 10) (μl)	Antibody precipitated at different time intervals (μl) (average of two independent determinations)[b]			
	12 hours	24 hours	48 hours	96 hours[c]
25	435.0	442.5	450.0	471.0
50	870.0	870.0	710.0	690.0
100	1155.0	1140.0	1260.0	1065.0

[a] After N. R. Moudgal and S. Wyman, unpublished results.

[b] Except as otherwise stated, incubation was carried out at 37°C in a water bath. Undiluted goat anti-rabbit γ-globulin (50 μl) was added to each tube and contents made up to 1.0 ml with PBS. At the end of the indubation, the precipitate was separated by centrifugation, washed twice with 1.0 ml cold PBS, and protein in the precipitate measured by the Lowry method.

[c] Incubation carried out at 4°C for 96 hours.

Other methods of hastening the duration of the assay include use of solid-phase systems, in which the antibody is used in the form of a water-insoluble immunosorbent, making it possible for the assay to be completed within 24 hours (Isozima *et al.*, 1970). However, except in clinical laboratories where routine assays in large numbers have to be performed, solid-phase radioimmunoassay has not found wide acceptance by research investigators. A slight modification of double antibody techniques that appears promising is the double antibody solid-phase technique, in which the double antibody used is in the form of a water-insoluble derivative (Koninckx *et al.*, 1976). Either cellulose-coupled double antibody (Koninckx *et al.*, 1976) or a copolymer of the double antibody (N. R. Moudgal, K. Muralidhar, and K. Ramasharma, unpublished observations) could be used. However, conditions of actual incubation should be standardized for each of the types.

Assay Protocol

One-tenth milliliter of suitably diluted antisera is incubated at 37°C with samples and standards (0.1 to 10 ng) in phosphate buffer in duplicate in a total volume of 0.5 ml per assay tube. At the end of 12 hours, 0.1 ml of the labeled hormone containing about 20,000 cpm is added to all the tubes and incubation continued for another 12 hours at 37°C. Control tubes in duplicate are set up with an equivalent quantity of normal rabbit serum. The samples should have separate nonspecific controls (incubation mixture complete in all respects excepting antisera). The separation of antibody bound label from free label is achieved by the addition of 100–200 μl of goat antibody to rabbit γ-globulin, along with 50 μl of 1:100 diluted normal rabbit serum; incubation is continued for a further period of 10–12 hours at 37°C. The tubes are then processed for radioactive counting as described under Section II,B. It should be noted that when monkey antisera is used for radioimmunoassay, a goat antiserum to monkey γ-globulin should be used. A standard curve is constructed using known amounts of unlabeled hormone (FSH or LH) for inhibiting the binding of labeled FSH or LH to the appropriate antibody. The data can be expressed in a number of ways, as described below.

E. Calculation of Data

The data from the radioimmunoassay can be expressed in one of the following ways listed below.

1. B/F ratio versus dose of unlabeled hormone, where B is labeled hormone bound to antibody expressed as counts per minute per tube, and F is free hormone expressed as counts per minute per tube. This representation is valid only if the radiolabeled hormone is 100% immunoreactive. If this were not so, it would give low B/F ratios leading to erroneous conclusions about the binding capacity of the diluted antiserum and also would result in a less steep curve. This is especially true when the labeled hormone is stored for a long time.

2. Bound counts are expressed as a percentage of label added versus dose of unlabeled hormone. The standard curve does not have a constant slope, and this makes comparisons between assays difficult. In order to make comparisons possible and to obviate the distortion of results produced by the presence of nonimmunoreactive hormone in the label, the antibody-bound counts in all the tubes are expressed as the percentage of counts bound in the absence of competing hormone. The standard curve can be partially linearized by plotting the results against log dose.

3. With increased use of radioimmunoassays of hormones, computer analysis for a fully automated data processing system is becoming popular. The first such program was published by Rodbard and Lewald (1970). This method performs logit and log transformations on the response and dose, respectively, to obtain an almost linear dose–response curve. This is followed by least squares regression analysis.

In this analysis the relationship between logit Y, i.e., $\log[Y/(1 - Y)]$, and $\log X$ is assumed to be linear, where

$$Y = \frac{\text{net cpm of labeled hormone bound to antibody at any dose of standard}}{\text{net cpm of labeled hormone bound at zero dose}}$$

Although the linearity has been found to be valid for radioimmunoassays of hLH and hFSH, departure from linearity has been observed in some assays, especially in the low dose region.

III. APPLICATION TO MEASUREMENT OF TISSUE RECEPTOR-BOUND LH

A. General Principles

Studies on monitoring tissue receptor-bound hormone have largely been carried out using labeled hormone. The technique of radioimmunoassay, although not lacking in sensitivity, has not been fully exploited to measure gonadotropins bound specifically to tissue receptors. The reason for this has been the inability of the widely used assay at 4°C to measure tissue-bound LH. We have, however, observed that it is possible to measure receptor-bound LH by performing the radioimmunoassay at 37°C (Moudgal *et al.*, 1971; Muralidhar and Moudgal, 1976). The basis for this test is that the interaction of the hormone with either antibody or receptor is a reversible fast reaction and the equilibrium dissociation constants for both types of interactions are approximately the same, $10^{-10} M$. Therefore, it is the relative concentration of either receptor or antibody that would drive the hor-

Table VII   Results of Measurement of Tissue-Bound LH by Radioimmunoassay Performed at Two Different Temperatures

Temperature of assay (°C)	Dilution of antiserum	Sensitivity of the assay (ng)	Amount of tissue needed for the assay (mg)	ng LH bounding/mg tissue[a] control (−LH)	experimental (+LH)
4	1 : 10,000	0.5	[b]	0.01	0.01
4	1 : 1,000	200	100–200	—	—
37	1 : 10,000	0.5	2–4	0.05	0.18

[a] Rat ovarian tissue was incubated at 37°C for one hour in a Dubnoff shaker without or with ovine LH. The tissue was then processed for radioimmunoassay as described under Section III.

[b] Does not measure.

mone toward one or the other. An excess of antibody to LH can arrest LH-stimulated actions, such as cyclic AMP production and steroidogenesis (Moyle *et al.*, 1971). Even at 4°C, an excess of antiserum to LH can remove LH from the receptor (Muralidhar and Moudgal, 1976). However, a radioimmunoassay to measure tissue receptor-bound LH should also be sensitive, and this is impracticable with excess antibody required at 4°C. However, this can be achieved by exposing the tissue receptor–LH complex at 37°C to a concentration of antibody normally employed in radioimmunoassay. Thus, by conducting the radioimmunoassay throughout at 37°C, it is possible to measure physiologic levels of LH bound to receptor (Table VII).

B. Technique of Measuring Tissue-Bound LH by Radioimmunoassay

Minces of ovaries from rats under any physiologic state (pregnant, normal cycling, pseudopregnant, etc.) either exposed to LH *in vivo* or incubated with known amounts of LH at 37°C in a Dubnoff shaker for one hour, are homogenized in a loose fitting all-glass hand tissue grinder. The homogenate in the case of *in vitro* incubation is washed repeatedly with 0.05 *M* phosphate-EDTA buffered saline, pH 7.4. After three or four washes, the tissue is suspended in the same buffer at a concentration of 10–20 mg/ml. Aliquots of this suspension are pipetted out into the assay tubes. The assay procedure is the same as described earlier for the serum samples (see Section II,D).

IV. NORMAL VALUES FOR HUMAN LH AND FSH

Normal values for human FSH and LH are listed in Table VIII (Cargille *et al.*, 1969; Lee *et al.*, 1970).

Table VIII   Normal Levels of FSH and LH

	FSH (mIU/ml)	LH (mIU/ml)
Children under age 14	5.0	5.0–10
Adult men	10–15	10
Adult women		
Midcycle peak	20–30	80
Remaining cycle	10	10

V. CONCLUSIONS

The methods outlined above are by no means problem-free. We have described simple and reproducible procedures taken from our own experience. However, it is not uncommon for problems to arise, especially when strict quality control over the reagents (hormones, antisera) is not exercised. Further, this discussion attempts only to present the methods used with little consideration for the difficulties investigators would probably encounter. The methods given at each of the steps could be improved upon, and can be modified to suit the material available locally. For this very reason, we did not present an exhaustive account of historical aspects or theoretical aspects of radioimmunoassay, which can be found in standard references (Diczfalusy, 1969; Odell and Daughaday, 1971).

A brief comment about the radioimmunoassays in comparison to radioreceptor assays would not be inappropriate. In many cases, the values obtained by radioimmunoassay and radioreceptor assays have been highly correlatable. However, this does not hold true in all cases. This statement becomes more relevant in the light of recent reports that free subunits of the gonadotropins may be circulating in the plasma or are present in pituitaries (Franchimont *et al.*, 1972). Obviously, such subunits could not be measured in the conventional radioreceptor assays. Using the elevated temperature radioimmunoassay of our experience, however, it is possible to measure the β-subunit of LH bound to ovarian tissue. Therefore, radioimmunoassay, in addition to being useful in detecting subunits either in pituitaries or in plasma, can also be employed to measure that bound to tissue receptors.

REFERENCES

Aono, T., and Taymor, M. L. (1968). Radioimmunoassay for follicle stimulating hormone (FSH) with ^{125}I-labelled FSH. *Am. J. Obstet. Gynecol.* **100**, 110–117.
Aono, T., Goldstein, D. P., Taymor, M. L., and Dolch, K. (1967). A radioimmunoassay method for human pituitary luteinizing hormone (LH) and human chorionic gonadotropin (HCG) using ^{125}I LH. *Am. J. Obstet. Gynecol.* **98**, 996–1001.
Avrameas, S., and Ternynck, T. (1967). Biologically active water insoluble protein polymers. 1. Their use for isolation of antigens and antibodies. *J. Biol. Chem.* **242**, 1651–1659.
Avrameas, S., and Ternynck, T. (1969). The cross-linking of proteins with glutaraldehyde and its use for the preparation of immunoadsorbents. *Immunochemistry* **6**, 53–66.

Beamer, W. G., Murr, S. M., and Geschwind, I. I. (1972). Radioimmunoassay of mouse luteinizing and follicle stimulating hormones. *Endocrinology* **90**, 823–827.

Brody, S., and Carlstrom, G. (1960). Estimation of human chorionic gonadotropins in biological fluids by complement fixation. *Lancet* **2**, 99.

Butt, W. R., and Lynch, S. S. (1968). Radioimmunoassay of gonadotropins with special reference to follicle stimulating hormone. *Clin. Chim. Acta* **22**, 79–84.

Cargille, C. M., Ross, G. T., and Yoshimi, T. (1969). Daily variations in plasma follicle stimulating hormone, luteinizing hormone and progesterone in the normal menstrual cycle. *J. Clin. Endocrinol. Metab.* **29**, 12–19.

Catt, K. J. (1969). Radioimmunoassay with antibody-coated discs and tubes. *Proc. Symp. Immunoassay Gonadotropins, Karolinska Symp. Res. Methods Reprod. Endocrinol., 1st, 1969* pp. 222–246.

Catt, K. J., and Tregéar, G. W. (1967). A solid phase radioimmunoassay in antibody coated tubes. *Science* **158**, 1570–1572.

Catt, K. J., Niall, H. D., and Tregéar, G. W. (1967). A solid phase disc radioimmunoassay for human growth hormone. *J. Lab. Clin. Med.* **70**, 820–830.

Cuatrecasas, P. (1971). *In* "Methods in Enzymology" (W. B. Jakoby, ed.), Vol. 22, p. 345. Academic Press, New York.

Diczfalusy, E. (1969). *Proc. Symp. Immunoassay Gonadotropins, Karolinska Symp. Res. Methods Reprod. Endocrinol., 1st 1969.*

Donini, P. (1969). Radioimmunoassay employing polymerized antisera. *Immunoassay Gonadotropins, Karolinska Symp. Res. Methods Reprod. Endocrinol., 1st, 1969.*

Donini, S., D'Alessio, I., and Donini, P. (1968). Radioimmunoassay of human chorionic gonadotropin (HCG) and human luteinizing hormone (LH) using insoluble antibodies. *In* "Gonadotropins" (E. Rosemberg, ed.), pp. 263–272. Geron X, Inc., Los Altos, California.

Eshkol, A. (1969). Labelling of antigens by various isotopes. *Proc. Symp. Immunoassay Gonadotropins, Karolinska Symp. Res. Methods Reprod. Endocrinol., 1st, 1969* pp. 145–162.

Faiman, C., and Ryan, R. J. (1967). Radioimmunoassay for human follicle stimulating hormone. *J. Clin. Endocrinol. Metab.* **27**, 444–447.

Franchimont, P. (1970). The gonadotropins. *In* "Assay of Protein and Polypeptide Hormones" (C. J. Van Cauwenberg and P. Franchimont, eds.), pp. 91–123. Pergamon, Oxford.

Glazer, A. N., and Singer, F. (1964). The iodination of chymotrypsinogen. *Biochem. J.* **90**, 92–98.

Greenwood, F. C., Hunter, W. M., and Glover, J. S. (1963). The preparation of ^{131}I labelled human growth hormone of high specific radioactivity. *Biochem. J.* **89**, 114–123.

Haber, E., Page, L. B., and Richards, F. F. (1965). Radioimmunoassay employing gel filtration. *Anal. Biochem.* **12**, 163–172.

Isozima, S., Naka, O., Koyama, K., and Adachi, N. (1970). Rapid radioimmunoassay of human luteinizing hormone using polymerised anti-human chorionic gonadotropin as immunoabsorbent. *J. Clin. Endocrinol. Metab.* **31**, 693–699.

Kabat, E. A., and Mayer, M. M. (1964). "Experimental Immunochemistry." Thomas, Springfield, Illinois.

Kirton, K. T., Niswender, G. D., Midgley, A. R., Jr., Jaffe, R. B., and Forbes, A. D. (1970). Serum luteinizing hormone and progesterone concentration during the menstrual cycle of the Rhesus monkey. *J. Clin. Endocrinol. Metab.* **30**, 105–110.

Koninckx, P., Bouillon, R., and De Moor P. (1976). Second antibody chemically linked to cellulose for the separation of bound and free hormone: An improvement over soluble second antibody in gonadotropin radioimmunoassay. *Acta Endocrinol. (Copenhagen)* **81**, 436.

Kosasa, T. S., Thompson, I. E., Byer, W. B., and Taymor, M. L. (1976). A comparison between gonadotropin radioimmunoassays with the use of 48 hour and six day incubation methods. *Am. J. Obstet. Gynecol.* **124**, 116.

Lee, P. A., Midgley, A. R., Jr., and Jaffe, R. B. (1970). Regulation of human gonadotropins. IV. Serum follicle stimulating and luteinizing hormone determinations in children. *J. Clin. Endocrinol. Metab.* **31**, 248–253.

L'Hermite, M., Niswender, G. D., Reichert, L. E., Jr., and Midgley, A. R., Jr. (1972). Serum follicle stimulating hormone in sheep as measured by radioimmunoassay. *Biol. Reprod.* **6**, 325–332.

Li, C. H., Mougdal, N. R., Trenkle, A., Bourdel, G., and Sadri, K. K. (1962). Some aspects of the immunochemical methods for characterization of protein hormones. *Ciba Found. Colloq. Endocrinol. [Proc.]* **14**, 20–44.

Madhwa Raj, H. G., and Moudgal, N. R. (1971). A comparative immunochemical study of LH derived from ovine, murine, equine and human species. *Indian J. Biochem.* **8**, 314.

Midgley, A. R. (1966). Radioimmunoassay: A method for human chorionic gonadotropin and human luteinizing hormone. *Endocrinology* **79**, 10–18.

Midgley, A. R., Jr. (1967). Radioimmunoassay of human follicle stimulating hormone. *J. Clin. Endocrinol. Metab.* **27**, 295–299.

Midgley, A. R., Jr., and Jaffe, R. (1966). Human luteinizing hormone during the menstrual cycle—determination by radioimmunoassay. *J. Clin. Endocrinol. Metab.* **26**, 1375–1381.

Midgley, A. R., Jr., Niswender, G. D., Gay, V. L. and Reichert, L. E., Jr. (1972). Use of antibodies for characterization of gonadotropins and steroids. *Rec. Prog. Horm. Res.* **27**, 235.

Miyachi, Y., Vaituikaitis, J. L., Nieschlag, E., and Lipsett, M. B. (1972). Enzymatic radioiodination of gonadotropins. *J. Clin. Endocrinol. Metab.* **34**, 23–28.

Monroe, S. E., Parlow, A. F., and Midgley, A. R., Jr. (1968). Radioimmunoassay of rat luteinizing hormone. *Endocrinology* **83**, 1004–1012.

Monroe, S. E., Peckham, W. D., Neill, J. D., and Knobil, E. (1970). A radioimmunoassay for rhesus monkey luteinizing hormone. *Endocrinology* **86**, 1012–1019.

Moudgal, N. R. (1975). Passive immunization with antigonadotropin antisera as a method of menstrual regulation in the primate. *In* "Immunization with Hormones in Reproduction Research" (E. Nieschlag, ed), p. 233. North-Holland Publ., Amsterdam.

Moudgal, N. R., and Li, C. H. (1961a). An immunochemical study of sheep pituitary interstitial cell stimulating hormone. *Arch. Biochem. Biophys.* **95**, 93–98.

Moudgal, N. R., and Li, C. H. (1961b). An immunochemical study of human pituitary interstitial cell stimulating hormone. *Nature (London)* **191**, 192–193.

Moudgal, N. R., and Muralidhar, K. (1974). Some aspects of LH action on Rat ovary. *In* "Gonadotropins and Gonadal Function" (N. R. Moudgal, ed.), p. 430. Academic Press, New York.

Moudgal, N. R., Moyle, W. R., and Greep, R. O. (1971). Specific binding of luteinizing hormone to Leydig tumour cells. *J. Biol. Chem.* **246**, 4983–4986.

Moudgal, N. R., Jagannadhan Rao, A., Maneckjee, R. Muralidhar, K., Venkataramiah Mukku, and Sheela Rani, C. S. (1974). Gonadotropins and their antibodies. *Recent Prog. Horm. Res.* **30**, 47.

Moyle, W. R., Moudgal, N. R., and Greep, R. O. (1971). Cessation of steroidogenesis in Leydig cell tumors after removal of luteinizing hormone and adenosine cyclic 3', 5'-monophosphate. *J. Biol. Chem.* **246**, 4978.

Muralidhar, K., and Moudgal, N. R. (1976). Studies on rat ovarian receptors for lutropin (luteinizing hormone). Applicability of radioimmunoassay to measure lutropin bound to receptors. *Biochem. J.* **160**, 603–606.

Muralidhar, K., Samy, T. S. A., and Moudgal, N. R. (1974). Immunosorbents of gonadotropins and their antibodies. *In* "Gonadotropins and Gounadal Functions" (N. R. Moudgal, ed.), p. 169. Academic Press, New York.

Nandini, S. G., Lipner, H. J., and Moudgal, N. R. (1976). A model for studying inhibin. *Endocrinology*, **98**, 1460.

NIAMDD. Rat pituitary hormone distribution programme: Radioimmunoassay of rat follicle stimulating hormone. N.I.A.M.D.D., Bethesda, Maryland.

Niswender, G. D., Midgley, A. R., Jr., Monroe, S. E., and Reichert, L. E., Jr. (1968a). Radioimmunoassay of rat luteinizing hormone with anti-ovine LH serum and ovine LH [131]I. *Proc. Soc. Exp. Biol. Med.* **128**, 807–811.

Niswender, G. D., Midley, A. H., Jr., and Reichert, L. E., Jr. (1968b). Radioimmunological studies with murine, bovine, ovine, porcine luteinizing hormones. *In* "Gonadotropins" (E. Rosemberg, ed.), pp. 299–306. Geron-X, Inc., Los Altos, California.

Niswender, G. D., Reichert, L. E., Jr., Midgley, A. R., Jr., and Nalbandov, A. V. (1969). Radioimmunoassay for bovine and ovine luteinizing hormone. *Endocrinology* **84**, 1166–1173.

Niswender, G. D., Monroe, S. E., Peckham, W. D., Midgley, A. R., Jr., Knobil, E., and Reichert, L. E., Jr. (1971). Radioimmunoassay for rhesus monkey luteinizing hormone (LH) with anti-ovine LH serum and ovine LH I[131]. *Endocrinology* **88**, 1327–1331.

Odell, W. D., and Daughaday, W. H., eds. (1971). "Principles of Competitive Protein-Binding Assays." Lippincott, Philadelphia, Pennsylvania.

Odell, W. D., Ross, G. T., and Rayford, P. L. (1966). Radioimmunoassay of human luteinizing hormone. *Metab., Clin. Exp.* **15**, 287–289.

Odell, W. D., Ross, G. T., and Rayford, P. L. (1969). Radioimmunoassay of luteinizing hormone in human plasma or serum: Physiological studies. *J. Clin. Invest.* **46**, 248–255.

Ostergard, D., Parlow, A. F., and Townsend, D. (1970). Acute effect of castration on serum FSH and LH in the adult woman. *J. Clin. Endocrinol. Metab.* **31**, 43–47.

Papkoff, H., Solis-Wallckermann, J., Martin, M., and Li, C.H. (1971). Immunochemical properties of ovine interstitial cell stimulating hormone (ICSH) subunit. *Arch. Biochem. Biophys.* **143**, 226.

Prahlada, S., Jagannadha Rao, A., and Moudgal, N. R. (1974). Can hormone antibodies be used as a tool in fertility control? *J. Reprod. Fertil., Suppl.* **21**, 105.

Rao, A. J., and Moudgal, N. R. (1970). An immunochemical study of ovine pituitary follicle stimulating hormone (FSH). *Arch. Biochem. Biophys.* **138**, 189.

Rao, A. J., Moudgal, N. R., Madhwar Raj, H. G., Lipner, R. G., and Greep, R. O. (1974). The role of FSH and LH in the initiation of ovulation in rats and hamsters: A study of using rabbit antisera to ovine FSH and LH. *J. Reprod. Fertil.* **37**, 323.

Redshaw, M. R., and Lynch, S. S. (1974). An improved method for the preparation of iodinated antigens for radioimmunoassay. *J. Endocrinol.* **60**, 527.

Rodbard, D., and Lewald, J. E. (1970). Computer analysis of radioligand assay and radioimmunoassay data. *Steroid Assay Protein Binding, Karolinska Symp., Res. Methods Reprod. Endocrinol., 1st, 1969* pp. 79–103.

Rosa, U., Pennisi, E., Bianchi, R., Federighi, G., and Douato, L. (1967). Chemical and biological effects of iodination on human albumin. *Biochim. Biophys. Acta* **133**, 486–498.

Saxena, B. B., Leyendecker, G., Chen, W., Gandy, H. M., and Peterson, R. E. (1969). Radioimmunoassay of follicle stimulating hormone (FSH) and luteinizing hormone (LH) by chromatoelectrophoresis. *Proc. Symp. Immunoassay Gonadotropins, Karolinska Symp. Res. Methods Reprod. Endocrinol., 1st, 1969* pp. 185–206.

Scaramuzzi, R. J., Blake, C. A., Papkoff, H., Hilliard, J., and Sawyer, C. H. (1972). Radioimmunoassay of rabbit luteinizing hormone serum levels during various reproductive states. *Endocrinology* **90**, 1285–1291.

Segal, S. J., Niu, L., and Hakin, S. (1960). Immunochemical analysis of sheep pituitary FSH. *Acta Endocrinol. (Copenhagen)* **35**, Suppl. 51, 1093–1094.

Thomas, K., and Ferin, J. (1968). A new rapid radioimmunoassay for HCG (LH, ICSH) in plasma using dioxane. *J. Clin. Endocrinol. Metab.* **28**, 1667–1670.

Utiger, R., Parker, M. L., and Daughaday, W. H. (1962). Studies on human growth hormone: A radioimmunoassay for human growth hormone. *J. Clin. Invest.* **41**, 254–261.

Vaitukaitis, J. L., Robbins, J. B., Nieschlag, E., and Ross, G. T. (1971). A method for producing specific antisera with small doses of immunogen. *J. Clin. Endocrinol. Metab.* **33**, 988–991.

Vaitukaitis, J. L., Sherins, R., Ross, G. T., Hickman, J., and Ashwell, G. (1972). A method for the preparation of radioactive FSH with preservation of radioactive activities. *Endocrinology* **89**, 1356–1360.

Wide, L., Roos, P., and Gemzell, C. A. (1961). Immunological determination of human pituitary luteinizing hormone. *Acta Endocrinol. (Copenhagen)* **37**, 445–449.

Yalow, R. S., and Berson, S. A. (1959). Assay of plasma insulin in human subjects by immunological methods. *Nature (London)* **184**, 1648–1649.

Yamaji, T., Peckham, W. D., Atkinson, L. E., Diersehke, D. J., and Knobil, E. (1973). Radioimmunoassay of monkey follicle stimulating hormone. *Endocrinology* **92**, 1652–1366.

10

Prolactin

LAURENCE S. JACOBS

I. INTRODUCTION

Although prolactin (PRL) has long been recognized as a separate adenohypophyseal hormone in a variety of animal species, it has been afforded similar recognition in humans and nonhuman primates only within the last decade. This delay has been attributed to the preponderance of growth hormone (GH) over PRL in the primate pituitary, coupled with the mammotropic activity of primate GH. The human anterior pituitary gland contains 20 to 100 times more GH than PRL. The standard pigeon crop sac assay for PRL responds to GH in both the original systemic (Riddle *et al.*, 1933) and the later local (Nicoll, 1967) versions. Thus, it is hardly surprising that early attempts to

199

Methods of Hormone Radioimmunoassay, Second Edition
Copyright © 1979 by Academic Press, Inc.
All rights of reproduction in any form reserved. ISBN 0-12-379260-6

purify primate pituitary prolactins succeeded only in producing fractions which were enriched in GH. Difficulties were compounded by the then unrecognized similar general physicochemical properties of the two molecules. Although it is now clearly recognized that the crop sac assay methods are not nearly sensitive enough to detect normal concentrations of PRL in the human circulation, a number of investigators in the past have embarked on clinical studies, armed with unproved extraction methods, the crop sac assay, and considerable faith. Reviews of this valiant work have been written (Apostolakis, 1968; Kiss, 1971); it is now primarily of historical interest. A notably successful exception was the demonstration of elevated bioassayable PRL activity in serum extracts from patients with nonpuerperal galactorrhea (Canfield and Bates, 1965). In contrast to this difficult experience with serum and urine measurement attempts, the assay has been employed for many years with apparent success for pituitary PRL measurements in a wide variety of animal species. In addition, it was used successfully to demonstrate PRL activity in extracts of a human pituitary tumor when coupled with careful quantitative antibody neutralization studies for abolition of GH effects (Peake *et al.*, 1969). Up to now, the assignment of biologic potencies to highly purified animal PRL preparations has been largely accomplished by the use of the pigeon crop sac assay. A study demonstrating nonspecific responses of the assay system to relatively crude pituitary extracts (Raud and Odell, 1971) now suggests that biologic PRL assays might be better carried out by one of the more recently developed bioassay procedures which use mammalian breast tissue.

I. BIOASSAYS

Progress in the elucidation of the physiology and biochemistry of biologically active compounds is greatly facilitated by the availability both of large quantities of the compound in question and of a sensitive and specific assay method. Although primate pituitary PRL secretion rates are high relative to those of other adenohypophyseal hormones, relatively little is stored, especially in comparison to GH. Thus, neither prerequisite for progress was really at hand; then, roughly simultaneously, immunologic evidence for a separate primate prolactin was provided, and several bioassay methods of unusual sensitivity were developed. Thus, new impetus and new investigative tools simultaneously became available, roughly about 1970.

Several variations on the same bioassay theme have been reported.

The assays are based on short-term tissue culture of breast explants in complex media containing serum and supplemented with hormones (insulin, glucocorticoids); after appropriate preliminary incubation, graded doses of PRL are added, and the tissue response is measured. Histologic demonstration of milk in sections of cultured mouse (Kleinberg and Frantz, 1971) or rabbit (Forsyth and Myres, 1971) mammary explants has been used, with sensitivities of approximately 15 and 50 ng/ml of serum, respectively. The more easily quantifiable radiochemical assays of prolactin-induced lactoseamine synthetase activity (Loewenstein *et al.*, 1971) or phosphoprotein synthesis (Turkington, 1971) have also been successfully employed with mouse mammary explants. Sensitivity with these endpoints is similar to that attainable with the histologic method, precision is somewhat better, and elaborate precautions to assure objectivity of measurement are not needed. Although much more sensitive than the older crop sac methods, all these methods fall just short of detecting PRL in the sera of normal individuals. Furthermore, they respond to the intrinsic mammotropic activity of primate GH. This activity is a biologic property which is not shared by other growth hormones such as that of the cow or sheep. These assays also respond to human placental lactogen (hPL), the other peptide member of the mammosomatotropic family of hormones. Whereas primate GH may not be quite as potent in these systems as PRL, and probably exerts its effects over a smaller dosage range of peptide, hPL is essentially equipotent with pituitary PRL in inducing lactoseamine synthetase, stimulating phosphoprotein synthesis, and promoting milk formation. Thus, these bioassays cannot be used to study PRL secretion in acromegalic subjects or during pregnancy without careful quantitative application of antibody neutralization procedures. Finally, the number of specimens that can be processed is somewhat limited, even when radiochemical rather than histologic endpoints are used.

III. RADIOIMMUNOASSAYS

A. Heterologous

Several varieties of heterologous radioimmunoassays for human prolactin have been reported. Some were developed in the early 1970's, at a time when substantial quantities of purified hPRL for immunization and iodination were simply not available. Others may have been deployed due to difficulties in the iodination of hPRL. At about the same time that the mammary gland bioassays were being developed, Friesen and his colleagues carried out a series of important experiments (Friesen *et al.*, 1970, 1971, 1972; Friesen and Guyda, 1971; Guyda and Friesen, 1971; Hwang *et al.*, 1971a) demonstrating the presence of a primate and human pituitary protein immunologically related to ovine PRL. This protein was distinct from GH, was rapidly synthesized *in vitro*, and was secreted into the medium more rapidly than growth hormone. Its intrapituitary pool size was smaller than that of GH. In the experiments with normal human pituitaries and human pituitary tumors, the *in vitro* synthetic and secretory rates for this protein correlated well with the clinical status of the patients from whom the tissue was obtained; production rates were highest by tissue obtained from tumors of patients with galactorrhea. These studies led to the development of a radioimmunoassay for human PRL which was based on the reaction between anti-ovine PRL antiserum and iodinated rhesus monkey PRL (Hwang *et al.*, 1971b). At about the same time that the elegant landmark studies in Friesen's laboratory were being performed, it was reported independently that immunologic cross-reactivity could also be exploited for fluorescent microscopic identification of PRL cells, using antiserum to ovine PRL to visualize lactotroph cells in the rhesus monkey adenohypophysis (Herbert and Hayashida, 1970). Building from these leads, we (Jacobs *et al.*, 1971, 1972) and others (L'Hermite *et al.*, 1972; Midgley and Jaffe, 1973) developed radioimmunoassays for human PRL (hPRL) without the benefit of any purified human PRL. We tested animal antisera raised against ovine (oPRL) and porcine prolactins (pPRL) for cross-reactivity with human serums which we knew to be rich in hPRL on the basis of bioassay studies (Loewenstein *et al.*, 1971). Although we could demonstrate no significant displacement by hPRL when anti-ovine antiserum was reacted with labeled ovine PRL nor when anti-porcine antiserum was reacted with labeled porcine PRL, quite satisfactory displacement was observed when anti-ovine antiserum was reacted with labeled porcine PRL (Jacobs *et al.*, 1972). Similarly, competitive dose-related displacement of bound labeled ovine PRL from binding sites on anti-porcine PRL antiserum was also seen. However, the latter system was not further tested because of low binding and inadequate sensitivity. In further studies, we found that rabbit antisera to oPRL and pPRL did not tend to cross-react with the other peptide or have sufficient affinity for hPRL to allow any detectable binding. In contrast, 100% of guinea pig antisera to oPRL cross-reacted substantially with pPRL; all of these antisera were capable of binding hPRL, and no other human pituitary or placental hormone tested appeared to cross-react (Jacobs, 1974). Only a minority of these antisera (3/13) demonstrated sufficient affinity for hPRL to be useful in the measurement of circulating concentrations, however.

From this experience, it seems reasonable to conclude that guinea pig antisera to prolactins are very likely to be directed, in part, to determinants which are shared with prolactins of species other than that of the immunizing antigen. Conversely, rabbit antisera are unlikely to be directed to such determinants. This experience accords with that of other investigators (Aubert *et al.*, 1974). If one supposes, with Midgley (1973), that determinants which are shared between or among species may have evolved intact because they are more likely to be biologically important, one would predict that guinea pig antisera to prolactins might be more likely than rabbit antisera to neutralize biologic prolactin activity. Alternatively, one might speculate that failure of most rabbits to respond to these interspecific determinants could be related to similarity of these determinants to amino acid sequences in native rabbit proteins. Given the empiric nature of practical immunology, it would be hazardous to attempt to generalize too much from these data. Nonetheless, it seems fair to conclude that antisera which can bind labeled peptide hormones of a species different from the immunogen used to raise them may be binding to sites which are shared with the same peptide hormone from several animal species; hence, such antisera would be prime candidates for the development of heterologous radioimmunoassays. Whether or not such sites are at or near sites required for biologic activity is not known and would require extensive immunochemical study to prove or disprove. However, circumstantial data in favor of the bioactive site hypothesis could be obtained by demonstrating binding of the antisera in question to the same peptide hormone obtained from a large variety of species representing a substantial fraction of recent evolutionary history.

A rabbit antiserum which is an exception to these generalizations was employed for hPRL assay by L'Hermite and his collaborators (1972; Midgley and Jaffe, 1973). This antiserum to oPRL was found to be useful for assay of hPRL when employed either with oPRL or bovine PRL tracer; essentially identical results were obtained with both tracers. This assay is not heterologous in the sense defined by Midgley (Midgley *et al.*, 1971), since the species of the immunizing antigen and the tracer are the same.

Heterologous assays other than the one developed in our own laboratory which have been clinically useful include those described by Aubert *et al.* (1974), Akbar *et al.* (1975), and Boyns *et al.* (1973). The first of these used a rabbit antiserum to oPRL in conjunction with iodinated hPRL, whereas the latter two employed rabbit antiserum to hPRL and iodinated oPRL. Given the empirical nature of these matters, investigators wishing to develop new assays based on heterologous or other types of cross-reactivity systems would probably do well to try all reasonable combinations of available antisera and ligands. Assay standardizations in circumstances where purified peptide is not available may be achieved either with a crude extract of the tissue of origin or with a serum rich in the constituent of interest.

B. Homologous

The extensive studies of the synthesis, secretion, and immuno-chemistry of hPRL carried out in Friesen's laboratory during 1970 and 1971, which led to the establishment of the first satisfactory radioimmunoassay for hPRL (Hwang *et al.*, 1971b), also facilitated the purification of hPRL, affinity chromatography being the critical step. As more hPRL of high purity was accumulated, immunization and labeling using the human hormone was carried out, and a conventional homologous assay was set up. The radioimmunoassays in turn facilitated hPRL purification by classic protein chemical strategies (Hwang *et al.*, 1972). Lewis' laboratory, employing a different approach, based on the differential solubility and electrophoretic mobilities of hPRL and hGH under specified conditions, also reported purification of hPRL at about the same time (Lewis *et al.*, 1971, 1972). This laboratory then independently reported the development of an homologous radioimmunoassay for hPRL (Sinha *et al.*, 1973). Both Friesen and Lewis were prompt and generous in responding to numerous requests for assay reagents from investigators worldwide, and both donated purified peptide and antiserum for distribution by the National Pituitary Agency/NIAMDD Hormone Distribution Program. The identification code used for these materials is "F" for the various batches of peptide and antiserum from Friesen, and "VLS" for those from Vanderlaan, Lewis, and Sinha. As a result, nearly all investigators currently engaged in research involving the measurement of human prolactin by radioimmunoassay use reagents donated by these laboratories. The purified hPRL has been isolated from either frozen or acetone-preserved pituitaries, yields being better from the former source, and antisera have been generated against purified hPRL or against preparations of HGH which, in retrospect, were contaminated with hPRL (Noel *et al.*, 1972; Aubert *et al.*, 1974). All of the distributed antisera have been from rabbits.

Usually, the precision of homologous assays has been somewhat higher than that of heterologous assays, primarily because the slopes of most homologous assay displacement curves have been steeper. So long as the degree of imprecision is slight, the more gradual slope has the advantage of encompassing a wider range of values without the need for sample dilution at the high end of the spectrum. The preferred assay system of Aubert *et al.* (1974) represents an exception to this generalization; in that system, heterologous reagents yielded the most sensitive assay with the steepest slope. This report contains the most extensive published data on comparative results of homologous and heterologous radioimmunoassay systems, when applied to the same samples. The agreement was excellent and, for those reagents, would be expected to be similar in the hands of other investigators as well. In an early collaborative study, a large series of samples was assayed by Friesen's laboratory and ours concomitantly (Kastin *et al.*, 1973); although the observed differences in hPRL concentrations were not large, and the interpretation of the data was identical for both sets of results, there was a systematic overall discrepancy of about 50%, higher values being reported with our mixed heterologous assay. Since different standards were employed, one cannot say whether this difference in values was due to the different standardization of the assays or due to some other difference between them. Unfortunately, the range of values encompassed by this study was small, and few published data exist comparing homologous and heterologous assay system results in the same specimens over a wider range of values. Although it is no longer a question of practical import, the possibility certainly remains open that at least some heterologous systems may not yield similar quantitative results to those given by homologous systems.

C. Radioreceptor Assay

The use of crude rabbit mammary membranes as a source of receptor binding sites for prolactin in a prolactin radioreceptor assay was described by Shiu *et al.* (1973). This assay system detects other lactogenic hormones in addition to prolactins, i.e., primate but not other mammalian growth hormones and the placental lactogens of several species (Friesen *et al.*, 1973). The lactogenic similarity between hGH and prolactins is such that iodinated hGH may be used as the tracer in prolactin radioreceptor assay, whether mammary glands or liver is the source of the binding agent. Since prolactin is considerably more vulnerable to iodination damage than is hGH, this is frequently done.

Although bioactive peptides able to bind receptor can unquestionably be produced with chloramine-T-based iodination procedures, ordinarily this requires a low-dose or low-temperature procedure (Catt *et al.,* 1971; Lefkowitz *et al.,* 1970; Leidenberger and Reichert, 1972; Lesniak *et al.,* 1973), and many investigators performing receptor assays have preferred to iodinate with lactoperoxidase (Thorell and Johansson, 1971; Herington *et al.,* 1974).

The mammary prolactin receptor has been characterized, solubilized, and partially purified, and its biologic relevance has been established by demonstration that anti-receptor antiserum blocks the biologic actions of prolactin *in vitro* (Shiu and Friesen, 1974a,b, 1976). Physiologic modulation of hormone action probably occurs via changes in receptor number (Dijane *et al.,* 1977), as well as in receptor affinity (Perry and Jacobs, 1978).

Little information is available regarding prolactin radioreceptor activity in human serum, but what there is shows an excellent correlation with radioimmunoassay (Friesen *et al.,* 1973) over a fairly wide range of values. This agreement is also compatible with the generally good agreement between radioimmunoassay and bioassay determinations of PRL in the same samples (Frantz *et al.,* 1972).

The ability of the receptor assay to respond to lactogenic hormones of many species, including those in which endogenous growth hormone is not lactogenic, makes it an attractive tool for exploration of the physiology of placental lactogens in pregnant animals.

IV. RADIOIMMUNOASSAY METHOD

A. Immunogen and Immunization

At present, the ready availability of both purified hPRL and anti-hPRL antiserum from the Hormone Distribution Program of the NPA/NIAMDD obviate the necessity for each investigator to generate his own antiserum for radioimmunoassay purposes. However, for applications involving needs for large quantities of antiserum, such as immunoprecipitation or neutralization studies, production of antiserum might be a necessity.

Human PRL, like oPRL, bPRL, pPRL, and rat and mouse prolactins, and like the growth hormones of these same species, is somewhat hydrophobic. At high concentrations, it is incompletely solubilized near neutral pH. Thus, it is recommended that hormone be dissolved initially in a small volume of alkaline solution prior to adjustment of concentration with saline, a simple buffer, or water. Either 0.01 N NaOH or 0.05 M NaHCO$_3$ at pH 9.5 is satisfactory for this purpose. Prolonged exposure to the NaOH without dilution is to be avoided. Once diluted to a concentration of 1.0 mg/ml, the hormone solution is prepared for immunization by thorough emulsification with an equal volume of complete Freund's adjuvant. If the supply of peptide is adequate, initial immunizing doses of 0.5–1.0 mg per animal are given, followed by booster injections of 50–200 μg at two- to four-week intervals. Each immunizing and booster dose should be divided into several subcutaneous sites. Boosters should be given in the same area or limb as the initial dose, so as to maximize chances of restimulating the same lymph nodes. It should be noted that commercial laboratories now offer either the determination of hPRL by radioimmunoassay as a routine service, or sell kits which can be so used by the purchaser. Those laboratories which have purified their own peptide and raised their own antisera might have bulk quantities of either reagent available for purchase.

B. Iodination

For unknown reasons, human prolactin is extremely susceptible to iodination damage. Since successful routine iodinations have been carried out initially on batches of peptide that have subsequently been extremely difficult to iodinate successfully following general distribution, it is possible that some aspect of the handling, solubilization, lyophilization, or shipment may be, at least in part, responsible for the problems which have been apparent. Either extensive damage to the peptide has occurred, resulting in the formation of high molecular weight labeled species of little use for immunoassay, or more subtle changes in monomeric peptide (Rogol and Rosen, 1974) may be present. In the latter circumstance, detectable alteration in gel filtration elution position is not likely to occur, and thus, by the usual repurification procedure we have employed prior to assay use, such a tracer will not be distinguished from a high quality preparation. When this is the case, reasonably good initial binding (B/T) may occur, but the tracer may be poorly displaceable, resulting in overestimation of the true concentration of hormone in the unknown sample. In systems employing chemical precipitation methods, damaged unbound tracer may precipitate along with antibody-bound tracer; in adsorption-based separation systems, such as charcoal, damaged unbound tracer may be excluded from the adsorption surface, again behaving like antibody-bound species. Since the latter effects would tend to produce artifactually low results, the apparent values observed in assays with substantially damaged tracer may in fact be either high or low relative to the true value. Extensively damaged tracer may bind to antiserum so poorly that it is readily apparent that the assay in question is inadequate and requires repetition. Since the vast majority of serious assay difficulties in systems which use iodinated peptides are due to problems with the tracer, the usual best procedure to follow when faced with an unacceptable assay is to reiodinate hormone and set up a fresh assay, unless specific information suggests a different sort of assay difficulty (wrong antiserum, forgot to add second antibody, pipette malfunction, tracer added to some tubes twice, counter not working properly, etc.). Prolactin iodinated by lactoperoxidase does in fact perform more satisfactorily in both receptor assays and in radioimmunoassays than does prolactin iodinated by chloramine-T. Nonetheless, gel filtration patterns of both products are similar. That is, after initial removal of unreacted iodide and collection of the iodinated protein peak from a small column at the time of iodination (see Table I), repeat filtration on 1.5 × 30 cm columns of G-75 or G-100 Sephadex virtually always reveals three separate peaks of radioactivity. The first peak appears at the void volume of the column, the second at the position of monomeric hormone, and the third at the position of iodide or small iodopeptides. The greater the elapsed time between iodination and repurification, the larger the first and third peaks, and the smaller the monomer peak. Figure 1, which in fact represents pPRL tracer iodinated with chloramine-T, might as well be oPRL, hGH, or hPRL, whether iodinated by chloramine-T or by lactoperoxidase. Because we have frequently wished to compare radioimmunoassay and radioreceptor assay results using the same tracer (Herington et al., 1974), we have for the past several years used lactoperoxidase for iodinations to the virtual exclusion of chloramine-T. On occasion, we have also used the reagent described by Bolton and Hunter (1973); we have not observed any consistent advantage over the far less expensive lactoperoxidase procedure. Our usual lactoperoxidase iodination protocol is outlined in Table I. In our hands, the reaction has gone well both at pH 7.6 in phosphate and at pH 5.6 in acetate. The yield of this reaction for hPRL has usually been between 20 and 40% incorporation of available radioactivity into the protein. Since iodination damage increases at high levels of substitution of peptides, we have generally tried to produce labeled hormones containing an average of about 0.5 to 1.0 atoms of iodine per molecule of protein. In this way, we have tried to minimize the population of doubly and triply iodinated molecules, since they are especially sub-

Table I   Lactoperoxidase Iodination Protocol

Step	Comment
1. Into a 6 × 50 mm disposable glass tube is pipetted 25 μl 0.3 M sodium phosphate, pH 7.6, or 25 μl 0.3 M sodium acetate, pH 5.6	High ionic strength to provide sufficient buffer reserve to bring down the pH of the iodide, which is supplied in dilute NaOH
2. 2–10 μg peptide in 2–10 μl buffer is added	Buffer is usually 0.05 M sodium phosphate at pH 7.6
3. Na^{125}I is added. Usually 5–10 μl provides 500–1000 μCi	Amount added is intended to provide a product containing an average of 0.5–0.8 I atoms/molecule, taking into account the reaction yield (see Table II)
4. Hydrogen peroxide is added, usually 2–5 μl 1/15,000–1/30,000 dilution of 30% H_2O_2	10 ng/μl
5. Lactoperoxidase is added, usually 5–10 μg in 5–10 μl buffer	Calbiochem Grade B has been generally satisfactory
6. Reaction proceeds 30–60 sec, with mixing	Finger flicking of tube
7. 100 μl normal human serum is added	Macromolecular adsorption of damaged tracer
8. Reaction mixture and reaction vessel washings are placed on a 1.0 × 20 cm column of Sephadex G-25 or G-50 coarse, and fractions of about 0.5 ml are collected	Removal of unreacted iodide. Column is presaturated with protein (BSA) to minimize tracer adsorption
9. Counting of reaction vessel, transfer pipette, and fractions is carried out, and the tubes at the top and down slope of the protein peak are taken for assay use	The assumption is made that counts which stick to glassware are peptide, not iodide. Specific activity is calculated as
10. Tracer is divided into 6–10 aliquots, and stored at either 4°C or −20°C. When needed for assay use, an aliquot is first repurified on Sephadex G-75 or G-100 to separate monomer tracer from aggregated material and free iodide or small iodopeptides (Figure 1)	$$\frac{\text{Total }\mu\text{Ci added} \times \dfrac{\text{cpm peak + cpm reaction vessel + cpm transfer pipette}}{\text{total effluent cpm + cpm reaction vessel + cpm transfer pipette}}}{\mu\text{g peptide iodinated}}$$

ject to damage and to subsequent aggregation, decay catastrophe, and deiodination. As can be seen in Table II, the specific activity (microcuries per microgram) of hPRL obtained with ^{125}I, an activity which is consistent with the specified degree of substitution, is in the range of 50 to 100 μCi/μg. At 30% yield, this would mean that if one were iodinating 2.0 μg of prolactin, one would probably wish to start with about 300–600 μCi of Na^{125}I. A fuller description of iodination prac-

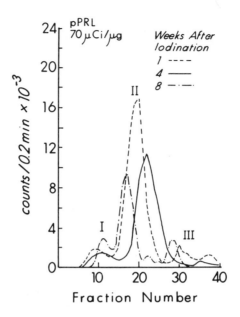

Figure 1. Repurification patterns of iodinated porcine PRL on a column of Sephadex G-100. The desalted freshly iodinated protein was aliquoted, frozen, and, at the times indicated, thawed once and gel filtered. The proportion of the total radioactivity eluted which can be accounted for by monomeric hormone (peak II) decreases progressively with time; aggregated material (peak I) and free iodide and/or small iodopeptides (peak III) increase progressively. This pattern is very similar to observations made on ovine, rat, human, and bovine prolactins and human, ovine, rat, porcine, murine, and bovine growth hormones following iodination. It seems to make little difference whether the initial iodination is done with low dose or stoichiometric chloramine-T, lactoperoxidase, or the Bolton–Hunter reagent. High dose, or conventional, chloramine-T usually results in faster aggregation and deiodination.

tices and the stability of iodinated proteins may be found in Jacobs (1978).

C. Characterization of Antisera

When an assay is being set up in a laboratory for the first time, antiserum characterization should be carried out even if the antiserum has been previously characterized in another laboratory. At the very least, determination of binding titer and assessment of affinity should probably be done. In addition, studies of hormonal cross-reactivity should be carried out if this is a key issue. These studies are required for many reasons, not the least of which is that the tracer being used is certainly a different reagent than that which was used for the initial characterization of antiserum.

Table II Specific Activity of Iodinated Hormones[a]

Hormone	Number of I atoms per molecule												
	0.1	0.2	0.3	0.4	0.5	0.6	0.7	0.8	0.9	1.0	1.2	1.4	1.6
Glucagon	66.6	133	200	267	333	400	467	533	600	667	800	933	1067
Insulin	39.1	78.2	117	156	196	235	274	313	352	391	469	547	626
PTH	24.5	49	73	98	122	147	171	196	220	245	294	343	392
GH,PRL,hPL	10.6	21.1	31.7	42.2	52.8	63.3	73.9	84.5	95	106	127	148	169
TSH	8.3	16.6	24.9	33.3	41.6	49.9	58.2	66.5	74.8	83.1	99.8	116.4	133
LH	6.7	13.3	20	26.7	33.3	40	46.7	53.3	60	66.7	80	93.3	106.7
hCG	5.8	11.7	17.5	23.3	29.2	35	40.9	46.7	52.5	58.4	70.1	81.7	93.4

[a] These calculations assume 100% isotopic abundance of ^{125}I, and are based on established molecular weights of the hormone and the fact that 1.0 mCi of ^{125}I contains 2.76×10^{14} atoms. For purposes of these calculations, the small difference in molecular weight between growth hormone and prolactin is ignored. Values are given as $\mu Ci/\mu g$.

A series of tubes should be set up which contain a constant quantity of tracer and varying dilutions of antiserum, covering a range of several logs if no prior knowledge of binding behavior exists; otherwise, a narrower range can be employed to focus with greater precision on binding in the region of greatest assay interest. In general, this proportion will fall between 30 and 60% binding of the total tracer present in the incubation mixture. Within this range, variations in antiserum dilution ordinarily have no significant effect on assay performance. Rather, the factors governing this decision will include the available quantities of antiserum, the specific activity and immunochemical integrity of the labeled hormone, and considerations of pipetting convenience. If this range is much exceeded on the high side, one begins to risk decreasing assay sensitivity because of an excessive number of available binding sites; on the low side, one begins to run into problems imposed by increased error associated with low counting rates or the necessity to use a larger gravimetric amount of tracer or a tracer of higher specific activity in order to obtain convenient counting rates. Ultimately, assay sensitivity is impaired on this side as well.

The affinity of an antiserum may be estimated by setting up a standard curve; operationally, the affinity determines the attainable sensitivity of the assay. If careful and formal definition of binding parameters is desired, then equilibrium incubation conditions should be used. It should be kept in mind that both the apparent titer of the antiserum and the observed affinity of the assay system may vary from time to time, depending on the quality of the tracer preparation used.

Antisera raised against hGH do not cross-react with hPRL and vice versa, unless the immunogens are significantly cross-contaminated with one another. However, because of this possibility, among others, no hPRL assay system should be considered validated methodologically unless it can be shown to be unresponsive to hGH. In addition, hPL should not cross-react.

D. Incubation Conditions

Most competitive binding assays proceed satisfactorily at pH values between about 7.0 and 8.6. The hPRL assay in our laboratory has usually been set up at pH 7.4–7.6, in phosphate buffer. We have preferred to use the relatively physiologic total ionic strength of 150 mM. Either 0.25% BSA or 0.25% gelatin is incorporated into the buffer to saturate glassware and plastic sites for nonspecific adsorption of proteins. EDTA at 25 mM final concentration in the buffer solution is also incorporated since chelation of divalent cations may improve performance in double antibody separation systems, due to inactivation of complement. Finally, since we use room temperature for PRL assay, we include in the buffer 0.1% sodium azide as a bacteriostatic agent.

Incubation may be carried out at room temperature for two to three days, or in the cold for four to five days, followed by overnight incubation in the cold after addition of precipitating antibody. Results are comparable for both incubation times. For maximal sensitivity, tracer addition may be delayed for one or two days prior to separation. The gain in sensitivity is approximately twofold. The assay protocol is summarized in Table III.

E. Separation Methods

In order to conduct a radioimmunoassay, one must be able to discriminate bound tracer from free; usually, this requires physical separation. A working separation method must be established, then, before antiserum can be evaluated and assays performed. Neither chemical precipitation (ammonium sulfate, etc.) nor adsorption (charcoal) methods are satisfactory for PRL assay. Large quantities of unbound labeled PRL are precipitated by concentrations of ammonium sulfate required for maximal precipitation of that bound to antibody; further, the method has an intrinsically high degree of misclassification of free hormone as bound because of trapping of incubation fluid in the rather -bulky precipitate. With ligands of molecular weight greater than about 10,000, charcoal separation techniques have often been found to be misleading; they require very careful attention to minor details in order to produce reliable results; the concentration of serum proteins, the amount of charcoal, and the coating of the charcoal (if any) may all have large influences on the performance of the method (Binoux and Odell, 1973). Both gel filtration and chromatoelectrophoresis have practical drawbacks which limit their applicability; both are tedious and time consuming and require special and expensive glassware and/or power supply and tanks.

The methods of choice for separation in PRL assay systems are double antibody and solid phase. The latter can be employed with a variety of supports ranging from cellulose through agarose and dextran to polystyrene and porous glass. Double-antibody separation has been the preferred method in our laboratory. We see the advantages as the following. (1) No chemical or physical manipulation is inflicted on unbound tracer, so that other investigations may be applied to the supernatant remaining after centrifugation. (2) A batch of second anti-

Table III hPRL Assay Protocol

Tube	Buffer (μl)	Carrier rabbit serum 1/200 (μl)	Anti-serum[a] 1:16,000 to 1:40,000 (μl)	Standard[b] (μl)	Un-known (μl)	Tracer 10,000–25,000 cpm, 200 pg (μl)	Hypox human serum (μl)	Comments
1–3	200	100	—	—	—	100	100	Blank
4–6	200	—	100	—	—	100	100	B_0
7–9, etc., to	200	—	100	100	—	100	—	Doses range from 0.15 ng to 20 ng per tube in triplicate
28–30								
31–32	200	—	100	—	100	100	—	Long-term quality control serum pools; duplicates
33–34	200	—	100	—	100	100	—	
35–36	200	—	100	—	100	100	—	Specimens repeated from last assay; duplicates
37–38	200	—	100	—	100	100	—	
39–40	200	—	100	—	100	100	—	Unknowns in duplicate
41–42	200	—	100	—	100	100	—	
43–44, etc.	200	—	100	—	100	100	—	

[a] The equivalent of 100 μl of 1/200 normal rabbit serum is incorporated into the solution containing specific antibody.

[b] Standards contain the equivalent of 100 μl human serum free of prolactin.

body which has been titered in one assay system may then be used in other systems in which the hormone antibody is from the same animal (e.g., rabbit). (3) The physical characteristics of the precipitate are such that only a minimum of unbound tracer is physically occluded within it. After completion of the immune precipitation reaction, 3.0 ml of cold distilled water is added to each assay tube prior to refrigerated centrifugation at 2500 rpm for 30 minutes. The supernatant is then aspirated either by hand or with a suction manifold.

Supernatants are routinely discarded, with only the precipitates being counted. It is worth noting that maximal cost efficiency in use of commercially purchased second antibodies may be achieved by dilution of the carrier serum so that the second antibody may also be diluted substantially. As an example, protocols which call for a final concentration of carrier serum in the range of 2.0% often require the use of 50 to 100 μl of undiluted precipitating antiserum; in contrast, final concentrations of carrier serum in the range of 0.02 to 0.05% allow the use of the same antiserum at dilutions usually in excess of 1 : 10, and often 1 : 20 or greater (100 μl per tube). A further advantage of such dilution is that peak precipitation is maintained over a much wider range of concentrations than when the reagents are more concentrated. Thus, the system tolerates slight variations in pipetting and diluting accuracy extremely well. The resultant precipitates are very small and must be handled with care after centrifugation to avoid inadvertent aspiration, but this is learned readily by technicians.

V. HORMONAL HETEROGENEITY

As is the case with many other hormones, hPRL exists in the circulation in at least two different forms and probably three (Suh and Frantz, 1974). Immunoreactivity has been detected in gel filtration column eluates not only at the position expected for monomeric hPRL but also, at the void volume, and at a position consistent with either dimeric or trimeric PRL. As with other pituitary hormones, the implications of these findings are not at all clear. The good general agreement between immunoassay and receptor assay quantitation of hPRL makes it unlikely that receptor activity is unevenly distributed among the species of molecules. Nonetheless, this possibility has yet to be tested directly. Since both "big" GH and "big" placental lactogen may be dimers held together by interchain disulfide bonds (Benveniste *et al.*, 1975; Schneider *et al.*, 1975) and these molecules are closely related to PRL, it may be that the high molecular weight form of PRL is also a disulfide dimer. Circumstantial support for this view may be taken from the demonstration of disulfide-bonded oligomers of PRL within pituitary secretory granules (Jacobs and Lee, 1975). Certain pituitary tumors appear to secrete PRL predominantly in the "big" form. Many unanswered questions remain: What is the role of "big" prolactin, if any? Is its half-life longer or shorter than that of monomeric hormone? Is it fully biologically active? Does its concentration in serum bear any systematic relationship to that of monomer? Is its main site of metabolic clearance different from that for monomeric hormone?

VI. CLINICAL RESULTS

Interesting and provocative findings have been turning up with some regularity since the development of prolactin radioimmunoassays. The difference in basal concentrations between men and women, or children and adults (Foley *et al.*, 1972), was too small to suggest an overriding role for the hormone in mammogenesis; a permissive function, wherein PRL is necessary but not alone sufficient, seems likely (Jacobs, 1977). PRL levels were found to be very high in pregnancy (Hwang *et al.*, 1971b; Jacobs *et al.*, 1972) and in neonates (Hwang *et al.*, 1971b), suggesting a role for estrogen in stimulating PRL secretion, and indicating failure of high concentrations of placental lactogen to exert any appreciable negative feedback effect on pituitary prolactin production. Extremely high concentrations of PRL were found in amniotic fluid (Friesen *et al.*, 1973); its source and role there remain speculative at present. Surprisingly, thyrotropin-releasing hormone was found to be as potent a stimulus for PRL secretion as for TSH secretion (Jacobs *et al.*, 1971, 1973), and functional thyroid status was found to be roughly inversely correlated with PRL secretion rate (Snyder *et al.*, 1973; Foley *et al.*, 1972). The ability of TRH to stimulate PRL secretion is shown in Figure 2.

PRL is frequently normal or even elevated in patients who appear by all other criteria to have hypopituitarism. The remarkable capacity of lactotroph cells to synthesize and secrete PRL, and the fact that secretion is normally restrained by hypothalamic influences both contribute to the rarity of prolactin deficiency in disease of the pituitary and hypothalamus. Representative basal concentrations of PRL in groups of patients with various hypothalamic and pituitary disorders are shown in Figure 3. The high frequency of prolactin hypersecretion in patients with pituitary adenomas is shown in Figure 3; accumulated data in several centers indicate that as many as 60–65% of all patients

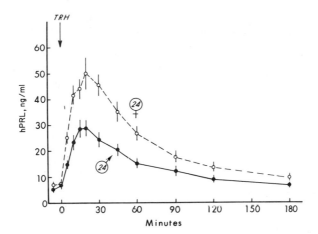

Figure 2. The hPRL response to intravenous TRH in normal adult men and women. The response is prompt and marked, and women secrete approximately twice as much acutely as men, despite the fact that the basal values are quite comparable. The dosage of TRH was 400 μg.

with pituitary adenomas hypersecrete PRL. Only a minority of these experience either gynecomastia or galactorrhea, interestingly. Prolactin measurement is, therefore, necessary for the accurate diagnosis of most prolactin-secreting pituitary adenomas; it is the most useful chemical marker in the diagnosis and treatment of such tumors.

A wide variety of neuroleptic agents, including phenothiazines, has been shown to be capable of stimulating PRL secretion, probably via hypothalamic effects. The mechanism of action appears to be depletion of, or interference with the action of, dopamine. Conversely, elevation of intrahypothalamic dopamine, either via intravenous infusion of dopamine or oral administration of L-dopa, with or without inhibition of peripheral decarboxylation, leads to suppression of PRL secretion. It is still not clear whether dopamine is the neurotransmitter which controls the secretion of hypothalamic prolactin-inhibiting factor, or whether dopamine is the prolactin-inhibiting factor itself.

Estrogens stimulate PRL secretion; the magnitude of the effect is dependent on both the dose of estrogen and the duration of the exposure. A minority of women exhibit elevated basal PRL concentrations while ingesting oral contraceptives; however, for most women, this is not enough estrogen to stimulate PRL secretion. The reproductive system effects of hyperprolactinemia have received much attention recently. It appears that hyperprolactinemia per se may be associated with both an impaired positive hypothalamic gonadotropin feedback

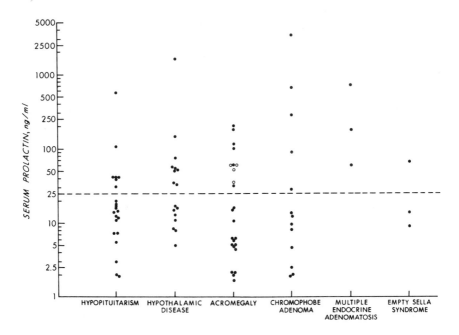

Figure 3. Fasting serum PRL concentrations in patients with a variety of pituitary and hypothalamic disorders. Most of the patients with hypopituitarism had idiopathic disease. Two patients with tumors and three postoperative patients are included. The group with hypothalamic disease includes five patients with tumors (one pinealoma, one meningioma, one optic glioma, two metastatic bronchogenic carcinomas, one metastatic tumor of unknown primary site), two with histiocytosis, and one with a basal skull fracture; the remaining five had no detectable structural lesion. The patients with acromegaly all had active disease. The four subjects indicated by the open circles were women in whom galactorrhea was part of the clinical picture. None of the patients included in the "chromophobe adenoma" group had gynecomastia, galactorrhea, or other pituitary hormone hypersecretion. The dashed line represents the upper limit of normal for fasting PRL concentration. (Reproduced from Jacobs and Daughaday, 1976, with permission of the publisher.)

response to estrogens and an imparied ovarian response to endogenous and exogenous gonadotropin. Thus, a substantial proportion of the amenorrhea seen in association with hyperprolactinemia is due to functional disarray of the hypothalamic–pituitary–gonadal axis, and not ablation of gonadotrope cells, even when a pituitary adenoma is evident. This is conclusively demonstrated when medical suppression of PRL concentrations to normal is accomplished with 2α-bromoergocryptine, a potent and long-lasting dopamine agonist. This agent frequently results in resumption of menses, ovulation, and restoration of fertility. In men, the counterpart of the amenorrhea–

galactorrhea syndrome is impotence and infertility due to functional hypogonadism. Although the normal role of prolactin in men is not known, binding sites for prolactin can be demonstrated in the prostate and seminal vesicles, and it has been proposed that PRL may have a tropic effect on these accessory sex structures. Why and how too much prolactin has an adverse effect on their functioning and the functioning of the gonads remain matters for future investigation.

REFERENCES

Akbar, A. M., Kannan, C. R., and Burke, G. (1975). The clinical utility of a heterologous radioimmunoassay for human prolactin. *Clin. Chim. Acta* **61**, 391–398.

Apostolakis, M. (1968). Prolactin. *Vitam. Horm. (N.Y.)* **26**, 197–235.

Aubert, M. L., Grumbach, M. M., and Kaplan, S. L. (1974). Heterologous radioimmunoassay for plasma human prolactin (hPRL); values in normal subjects, puberty, pregnancy, and in pituitary disorders. *Acta Endocrinol. (Copenhagen)* **77**, 460–476.

Benveniste, R., Stachura, M. E., Szabo, M., and Frohman, L. A. (1975). Big growth hormone (GH): Conversion to small GH without peptide bond cleavage. *J. Clin. Endocrinol. Metab.* **41**, 422–425.

Binoux, M. A., and Odell, W. D. (1973). Use of dextran coated charcoal to separate antibody-bound from free hormone: A critique. *J. Clin. Endocrinol. Metab.* **36**, 303–310.

Bolton, A. E., and Hunter, W. M. (1973). The labelling of proteins to high specific radioactivities by conjugation to a ^{125}I-containing acylating agent. *Biochem. J.* **133**, 529–539.

Boyns, A. R., Cole, E. N., Griffiths, K., Roberts, M. M., Buchan, R., Wilson, R. G., and Forrest, A. P. M. (1973). Plasma prolactin in breast cancer. *Eur. J. Cancer* **9**, 99–102.

Canfield, C. J., and Bates, R. W. (1965). Nonpuerperal galactorrhea. *N. Engl. J. Med.* **273**, 897–902.

Catt, K. J., Dufau, M. L., and Tsuruhara, T. (1971). Studies on a radioligand-receptor assay system for luteinizing hormone and chorionic gonadotropin. *J. Clin. Endocrinol. Metab.* **32**, 860–863.

Dijane, J., Durand, P., and Kelly, P. A. (1977). Evolution of prolactin receptors in rabbit mammary gland during pregnancy and lactation. *Endocrinology* **100**, 1348–1356.

Foley, T. P., Jr., Jacobs, L. S., Hoffman, W., Daughaday, W. H., and Blizzard, R. M. (1972). Human prolactin and thyrotropin concentrations in the serums of normal and hypopituitary children before and after the administration of synthetic thyrotropin-releasing hormone. *J. Clin. Invest.* **51**, 2143–2150.

Forsyth, I. A., and Myres, R. P. (1971). Human prolactin. Evidence obtained by the bioassay of human plasma. *J. Endocrinol.* **51**, 157–168.

Frantz, A. G., Kleinberg, D. L., and Noel, G. L. (1972). Studies on prolactin in man. *Recent Prog. Horm. Res.* **28**, 527–590.

Friesen, H. G., and Guyda, H. (1971). Biosynthesis of monkey growth hormone and prolactin *in vitro*. *Endocrinology* **88**, 1353–1362.

Friesen, H. G., Guyda, H., and Hardy, J. (1970). Biosynthesis of human growth hormone and prolactin. *J. Clin. Endocrinol. Metab.* **31**, 611–624.

Friesen, H. G., Guyda, H., and Hwang, P. (1971). Prolactin synthesis in primates. *Nature (London)* **232**, 19–20.

Friesen, H. G., Webster, B. R., Hwang, P., Guyda, H., Munro, R. E., and Read, L. (1972). Prolactin synthesis and secretion in a patient with the Forbes-Albright syndrome. *J. Clin. Endocrinol. Metab.* **34**, 192–199.

Friesen, H. G., Tolis, G., Shiu, R. P. C., and Hwang, P. (1973). Studies on human prolactin: Chemistry, radioreceptor assay, and clinical significance. *In* "Human Prolactin" (J. Pasteels and C. Robyn, eds.), Int. Congr. Ser. No. 308, pp. 11–23. Excerpta Med. Found., Amsterdam.

Guyda, H., and Friesen, H. G. (1971). The separation of monkey prolactin from monkey growth hormone by affinity chromatography. *Biochem. Biophys. Res. Commun.* **42**, 1068–1075.

Herbert, D. C., and Hayashida, T. (1970). Prolactin localization in the primate pituitary by immunofluorescence. *Science* **169**, 378–379.

Herington, A. C., Jacobs, L. S., and Daughaday, W. H. (1974). Radioreceptor and radioimmunoassay quantitation of human growth hormone in acromegalic serum: Overestimation by immunoassay and systematic differences between antisera. *J. Clin. Endocrinol. Metab.* **39**, 257–262.

Hwang, P., Friesen, H., Hardy, J., and Wilansky, D. (1971a). Biosynthesis of human growth hormone and prolactin by normal pituitary glands and pituitary adenomas. *J. Clin. Endocrinol. Metab.* **33**, 1–7.

Hwang, P., Guyda, H., and Friesen, H. (1971b). A radioimmunoassay for human prolactin. *Proc. Natl. Acad. Sci. U.S.A.* **68**, 1902–1906.

Hwang, P., Guyda, H., and Friesen, H. G. (1972). Purification of human prolactin. *J. Biol. Chem.* **247**, 1955–1972.

Jacobs, L. S. (1974). Prolactin. *In* "Methods of Hormone Radioimmunoassay" (B. M. Jaffe and H. R. Behrman, eds.), pp. 87–102. Academic Press, New York.

Jacobs, L. S. (1977). The role of prolactin in mammogenesis and lactogenesis. *In* "Comparative Endocrinology of Prolactin" (H. D. Dellman and J. A. Johnson, eds.), pp. 173–191. Plenum, New York.

Jacobs, L. S. (1978). Principles and Practice of Competitive-Binding. *In* "Gradwohl's Textbook of Laboratory Medicine" (L. Jarett and A. Sonnenwirth, eds.) 8th ed. C. V. Mosby, St. Louis, Missouri. In press.

Jacobs, L., and Daughaday, W. H. (1976). Pathophysiology and control of human prolactin secretion in patients with pituitary and hypothalamic disease. *In* "Human Prolactin" (J. L. Pasteels and C. Robyn, eds.), Int. Congr. Ser. No. 308, pp. 189–203. Exerpta Med. Found., Amsterdam.

Jacobs, L. S., and Lee, Y.-C. (1975). Polymeric growth hormone and prolactin in secretory granules: Sulfhydryl bonding masks immunoreactive sites. *Proc. 5th Annu. Meet., Am. Endocr. Soc.* Abstract No. 67. p. 84.

Jacobs, L. S., Snyder, P. J., Wilber, J. F., Utiger, R. D., and Daughaday, W. H. (1971). Increased serum prolactin after administration of synthetic thyrotropin-releasing hormone (TRH) in man. *J. Clin. Endocrinol. Metab.* **33**, 996–999.

Jacobs, L. S., Mariz, I. K., and Daughaday, W. H. (1972). A mixed heterologous radioimmunoassay for human prolactin. *J. Clin. Endocrinol. Metab.* **34**, 484–490.

Jacobs, L. S., Synder, P. J., Utiger, R. D., and Daughaday, W. H. (1973). Prolactin response to thyrotropin releasing hormone in normal subjects. *J. Clin. Endocrinol. Metab.* **36**, 1069–1073.

Kastin, A. J., Gonzalez-Barcena, D., Friesen, H., Jacobs, L. S., Schalch, D. S., Arimura, A., Daughaday, W. H., and Schally, A. V. (1973). Unaltered plasma prolactin levels in men after administration of synthetic LH-releasing hormone. *J. Clin. Endocrinol. Metab.* **36**, 375–377.

Kiss, C. S. (1971). Clinical aspects of prolactin research. *Polypeptide Horm., Proc. Congr. Hung. Soc. Endocrinol. Metab., 4th, 1969* Part V, pp. 263–267.

Kleinberg, D. L., and Frantz, A. G. (1971). Human prolactin; measurement in plasma by *in vitro* bioassay. *J. Clin. Invest.* **50**, 1557–1568.

Lefkowitz, R. J., Roth, J., Pricer, W., and Pastan, I. (1970). ACTH receptors in the adrenal; specific binding of ACTH ^{125}I and its relation to adenyl cyclase. *Proc. Natl. Acad. Sci. U.S.A.* **65**, 745–752.

Leidenberger, F., and Reichert, L. E., Jr. (1972). Studies on the uptake of human chorionic gonadotropin and its subunits by rat testicular homogenates and interstitial tissue. *Endocrinology* **91**, 135–143.

Lesniak, M. A., Roth, J., Gorden, P., and Gavin, J. R. (1973). Human growth hormone radioreceptor assay using cultured human lymphocytes. *Nature (London), New Biol.* **241**, 20–22.

Lewis, U. J., Singh, R. N. P., and Seavey, B. K. (1971). Human prolactin: Isolation and some properties. *Biochem. Biophys. Res. Commun.* **44**, 1169–1176.

Lewis, U. J., Singh, R. N. P., and Seavey, B. K. (1972). Problems in the purification of human prolactin. *Prolactin Carcinog., Tenovus Workshop, 4th, 1972*, pp. 4–12.

L'Hermite, M., Delvoye, P., Nokin, J., Vekemans, M., and Robyn, C. (1972). Human prolactin secretion as studied by radioimmunoassay: Some aspects of its regulation. *Prolactin Carcinog., Proc. Tenovus Workshop, 4th, 1972* pp. 81–97.

Loewenstein, J. E., Mariz, I. K., Peake, G. T., and Daughaday, W. H. (1971). Prolactin bioassay by induction of N-acetyllactosamine synthetase in mouse mammary gland explants. *J. Clin. Endocrinol. Metab.* **33**, 217–224.

Midgley, A. R., Jr. (1973). Heterologous and homologous radioimmunoassays: Species specificity considerations. *In* "Principles of Competitive Protein-Binding Assays" (W. D. Odell and W. H. Daughaday, eds.), pp. 419–426. Lippincott, Philadelphia, Pennsylvania.

Midgley, A. R., Jr., and Jaffe, R. B. (1973). Circulating human prolactin: A radioimmunologic analysis. *Endocrinol., Proc. Int. Congr., 4th, 1972* Int. Congr. Ser. No. 273, pp. 629–635.

Midgley, A. R., Jr., Niswender, G. D., Gay, V. L., and Reichert, L. E., Jr. (1971). Use of antibodies for characterization of gonadotropins and steroids. *Recent Prog. Horm. Res.* **27**, 235–301.

Nicoll, C. S. (1967). Bioassay of prolactin. Analysis of the pigeon crop sac response to local prolactin injection by an objective and quantitative method. *Endocrinology* **80**, 641–655.

Noel, G. L., Suh, H. K., Stone, G., and Frantz, A. G. (1972). Human prolactin and growth hormone release during surgery and other conditions of stress. *J. Clin. Endocrinol. Metab.* **35**, 840–851.

Peake, G. T., McKeel, D. W., Jarett, L., and Daughaday, W. H. (1969). Ultrastructural, histologic, and hormonal characterizations of a prolactin-rich human pituitary tumor. *J. Clin. Endocrinol. Metab.* **29**, 1383–1393.

Perry, H. M., III, and Jacobs, L. S. (1978). Rabbit mammary prolactin receptors: Demonstration of a late puerperal increase in affinity. *J. Biol. Chem.* **253**, 1560–1564.

Raud, H. R., and Odell, W. D. (1971). Studies of the measurement of bovine and porcine prolactin by radioimmunoassay and by systemic pigeon crop-sac bioassay. *Endocrinology* **88**, 991–1002.

Riddle, O., Bates, R. W., and Dykshorn, S. W. (1933). The preparation, identification, and assay of prolactin—a hormone of the anterior pituitary. *Am. J. Physiol.* **105**, 191–216.

Rogol, A. D., and Rosen, S. W. (1974). Alteration of human and bovine prolactins by chloramine T radioiodination: Comparison with lactoperoxidase-iodinated prolactins. *J. Clin. Endocrinol. Metab.* **39**, 379–382.

Schneider, A. B., Kowalski, K., and Sherwood, L. M. (1975). Big human placental lactogen: Disulfide-linked peptide chains. *Biochem. Biophys. Res. Commun.* **64**, 717–724.

Shiu, R. P. C., and Friesen, H. G. (1974a). Properties of a prolactin receptor from the rabbit mammary gland. *Biochem. J.* **140**, 301–311.

Shiu, R. P. C., and Friesen, H. G. (1974b). Solubilization and purification of a prolactin receptor from the rabbit mammary gland. *J. Biol. Chem.* **249**, 7902–7911.

Shiu, R. P. C., and Friesen, H. G. (1976). Blockade of prolactin action by an antiserum to its receptors. *Science* **192**, 259–261.

Shiu, R. P. C., Kelly, P. A., and Friesen, H. G. (1973). Radioreceptor assay for prolactin and other lactogenic hormones. *Science* **180**, 968–971.

Sinha, Y. N., Selby, F. W., Lewis, V. J., and Vanderlaan, W. P. (1973). A homologous radioimmunoassay for human prolactin. *J. Clin. Endocrinol. Metab.* **36**, 509–516.

Snyder, P. J., Jacobs, L. S., Utiger, R. D., and Daughaday, W. H. (1973). Thyroid hormone inhibition of the prolactin response to thyrotropin-releasing hormone. *J. Clin. Invest.* **52**, 2324–2329.

Suh, H. K., and Frantz, A. G. (1974). Size heterogeneity of human prolactin in plasma and pituitary extracts. *J. Clin. Endocrinol. Metab.* **39**, 928–935.

Thorell, J. I., and Johansson, B. G. (1971). Enzymatic iodination of polypeptides with ^{125}I to high specific activity. *Biochim.* Biophys. Acta **251**, 363–369.

Turkington, R. W. (1971). Measurement of prolactin activity in human serum by the induction of specific milk proteins in mammary gland *in vitro. J. Clin. Endocrinol. Metab.* **33**, 210–216.

11

Growth Hormone

GLENN T. PEAKE, JOSEPHINE MORRIS, AND
MAIRE T. BUCKMAN

I. INTRODUCTION

Methods to determine accurately circulating growth hormone concentrations in man have been available since 1963 (Glick *et al.*, 1963;

223

Methods of Hormone Radioimmunoassay, Second Edition
Copyright © 1979 by Academic Press, Inc.
All rights of reproduction in any form reserved. ISBN 0-12-379260-6

Schalch and Parker, 1964). Bioassay techniques were never sufficiently sensitive to measure growth hormone in plasma and were not entirely specific for the growth hormone molecule. Thus, radioimmunoassay has replaced the bioassay techniques for routine measurement of growth hormone. However, the bioassay is still used to quantitate the purified materials used for assay standards and is the only accepted method to determine the biologic potency of the hormone (Wilhelmi, 1973).

Successful performance of the human growth hormone (hGH) radioimmunoassay is dependent upon the quality of the protein reagents used in the assay. Great care in handling the reagents is necessary to preserve the high quality required for reproducible assays. Especially critical is the care of the radioiodinated hGH. Our procedures for the preparation and care of each reagent are listed where appropriate in the following description of the assay. The assay described here is the one we employ for routine measurements on samples obtained either from our clinical chemistry laboratory or from research studies carried out on patients.

II. PREPARATION OF BUFFERS AND COLUMNS FOR hGH ASSAY

A. Preparation of Buffers

1. Phosphosaline (0.15 M NaCl–0.01 M Phosphate)

5.14 gm $NaH_2PO_4 \cdot H_2O$
26.6 gm NaCl

Add 2.0 M NaOH dropwise to bring pH to 7.6. Add 0.1% Merthiolate as preservative. Final volume 3.0 liters. This buffer is stored at 4°C and used without further dilution.

2. 1% BSA–Phosphosaline

Dilute the commercially available 30% solution of bovine serum albumin (BSA) thirtyfold with the above phosphosaline buffer.

3. Phosphate Buffer (0.5 M)

6.9 gm $NaH_2PO_4 \cdot H_2O$ in 100 ml
7.1 gm Na_2HPO_4 in 100 ml

Add approximately one part of the monobasic to nine parts of the dibasic buffer. The volume of each buffer is adjusted until the final pH is 7.6. This buffer is stored in 10- to 20-ml aliquots at $-20°C$. For the buffer to be redissolved, it is warmed in running tap water.

4. Phosphate Buffer (0.05 M)

The 0.5 M buffer is diluted tenfold with distilled water.

5. Barbital Buffer (0.1 M Barbital)

49.44 gm sodium barbital
5.54 gm barbituric acid
0.48 gm sodium azide

Final pH should be 8.6, and final volume, 2.4 liters. This buffer is stored at 4°C and is diluted with an equal volume of distilled water prior to use.

B. Preparation of Sephadex Columns

1. Sephadex Column for Iodination

Sephadex G-50 (coarse or beaded) is placed in 0.05 M barbital buffer and is swollen at room temperature for at least one day. The Sephadex can be stored at 4°C for several days prior to use. A very small plug of glass wool is forced into a glass column with dimensions of about 0.9×30 cm. The Sephadex is then packed into the column to a height of about 20 cm. A small amount of bovine albumin (two to three drops of 30% BSA) is passed through the column to allow efficient elution of the very small amount of iodinated protein that will subsequently be passed through it. After thorough washing of the excess albumin from the column with barbital buffer, it is ready for use to separate iodinated hormone from unreacted iodine following the iodination procedure. A new column is prepared for each iodination and following its use the Sephadex is disposed of in radioactive waste.

2. Sephadex Column for Repurification of Labeled Hormone

Sephadex G-100 (coarse or beaded) is placed in 0.05 M barbital buffer and allowed to swell for three days. This Sephadex is packed into a column with the dimensions of 1.5×60 cm to a height of about 50 cm. Barbital buffer is used for elution. Eluates from this column are collected by automatic fraction collection so that about 1.5- to 2.0-ml volumes are obtained in each tube. Since the rate of elution varies from day to day, timed collections will undergo minor adjustments to maintain the volume constant. A small amount of bovine albumin (two to three drops of 30% BSA) is passed through the column prior to its first use. This column is reusable and is discarded only when the flow rate becomes very slow (greater than eight minutes to collect 1.0 ml) or when bacterial or fungal organisms grow in the column buffers. Most columns last about one month, but some have lasted as long as six months.

III. TECHNIQUE OF RADIOIMMUNOASSAY

A. Procurement and Preparation of Protein Reagents for hGH Radioimmunoassay

1. Source of the Hormone

Several commercial sources can now supply reagent grade hGH of sufficient purity to be reliably used in the assay. The authors have used the reagent grade hGH distributed by Calbiochem and have found it suitable for the assay. High-grade reagents are also available from a variety of commercial sources in the form of kits containing all or part of the reagents for the assay. Our experience has been limited to the materials distributed by Calbiochem and Abbott Laboratories, and in both instances these reagents were found to be reliable. Although the authors have no experience with other commercially available reagents, these materials have been successfully employed by numerous clinical laboratories for the hGH radioimmunoassay. In some instances, the reagents in the kits do not contain the radiolabeled hormone. This material can also be purchased from commercial sources. The authors have satisfactorily employed the labeled hormone distributed by either Abbott Laboratories or New England Nuclear.

The assay described in this chapter used human growth hormone which was originally obtained in a highly purified form from Dr. Alfred Wilhelmi. The hormone had a biologic potency of 2.0 IU/mg compared to purified bovine growth hormone, which was arbitrarily assigned a potency of 1.0 IU/mg in the hypophysectomized rat weight gain assay. The purified hGH had no significant contamination with other pituitary peptides or other proteins. Similar hGH is presently available from the NIAMDD through their Hormone Distribution Program, but is primarily intended for individuals who plan to utilize the materials for research purposes.

The purified hGH received from Dr. Wilhelmi was in powdered form and has been stored in a vacuum desiccator at $-85°C$. The hGH stored in this manner has been stable without significant loss of immunopotency over an eight-year period. When the peptide is to be used, it is removed from the desiccator, and an appropriate amount is weighed and dissolved in 0.01 N NaOH. One milligram of hGH can be readily dissolved in 200 μl NaOH. The hormone is never stored in NaOH but is immediately diluted to the desired concentration in the appropriate buffer.

2. Antibody Production to hGH

An appropriate amount of hGH (2.0–3.0 mg) is dissolved in 200 μl 0.01 N NaOH. The peptide should immediately dissolve, resulting in a clear or very slightly opalescent solution. The growth hormone is then diluted with protein-free phosphosaline buffer to a final concentration of 1.0 mg/ml. This solution of hGH is mixed vigorously with equal volumes of complete Freund's adjuvant enriched with 5.0 mg/ml *Mycobacterium butyricum*. When the solution has reached the consistency of whipped cream, 0.5 to 1.0 mg hGH is injected into two or three subcutaneous sites of a young female guinea pig. Injections are repeated at two- to three-week intervals for four injections. Three weeks following the last subcutaneous injection, 1.0 mg of hGH dissolved in the phosphosaline buffer is injected intraperitoneally. Seven days after the fluid injection of hGH, the antiserum is harvested from the guinea pig by cardiac puncture. The animals can be rebooted with 0.5 to 1.0 mg antigen subcutaneously at monthly intervals for four or five months without substantial loss in potency of the antiserum. We usually start the antigen injections with four to six animals. Perhaps two or three guinea pigs will produce antiserum of sufficiently high titer to use in the assay. If the animals do not make high titer antiserum following the first fluid boost of hGH, they are killed and the serum is discarded. Only those animals yielding a reasonably high titer antiserum are kept for future boosting and bleeding. Antibodies of higher titer have been obtained by giving four to six immunizations spaced at longer, e.g., four- to five-week, intervals. However, with this immunization schedule a substantial increase in time is required to obtain an antibody suitable for radioimmunoassay purposes. The anti-hGH serum harvested from the guinea pigs is the first antibody used in the assay. Following each bleeding, the blood is allowed to clot at room temperature for two to three hours, the serum removed,

Table I   Determination of the Immunopotency of One
Guinea Pig Anti-hGH Serum (First Antibody) in
the hGH Assay[a]

First antibody dilution	^{125}I-hGH precipitated (%)
1 : 1,000	92
1 : 5,000	85
1 : 10,000	80
1 : 20,000	63
1 : 40,000	45
1 : 80,000	40
1 : 100,000	20

[a] The first antibody was tested at the indicated
dilutions in an assay in which all other parameters
had previously been determined. Each tube contained
0.3 ml 1% BSA phosphosaline buffer, 0.1 ml of the
first antibody dilution, 0.1 ml of the labeled hGH,
and 0.1 ml of a 1 : 200 dilution of normal guinea pig
serum. After a three-day incubation at 4°C, 0.1 ml
second antibody was added. The first antibody was
subsequently tested for its displacement characteristics at a 1 : 40,000 dilution and found to be useful
in the hGH assay at this dilution.

properly identified, and frozen in about 0.5-ml aliquots for storage at
−20°C.

Each antiserum is tested for its immunopotency. Dilutions of the
antiserum from about 1 : 1000 to about 1 : 1,000,000 are prepared by
addition of 1% BSA phosphosaline buffer. The assay is set up as described below using no hGH standards or unknowns, but only labeled
hGH and different dilutions of the antisera. This usually includes
100-μl aliquots of several dilutions of the first antibody (Table I). Each
dilution of antiserum is made with a constant amount of guinea pig
carrier serum previously determined to provide maximal precipitation
of a known dilution of antiserum by the second antibody. The label
and the first antibody are allowed to react for three days before separation of antibody-bound hGH is performed, either by addition of second
antibody or chromatoelectrophoresis. Antisera which will allow for a
sensitive assay usually will precipitate 50% of the labeled hGH at a
final dilution greater than 1 : 50,000 (i.e., 100 μl of a 1 : 10,000 dilution
or greater added per tube). Although this is not invariably the case,
very few antisera at lower titer have proved sensitive in our hands.
The antiserum we presently use precipitated about 45% of the labeled
hGH when 100 μl of a 1 : 70,000 dilution was added to each assay tube.

The separation of antibody-bound and free or unreacted iodinated hGH can be achieved using several techniques. These methods have been reviewed (Daughaday and Jacobs, 1971; Odell, *et al.*, 1975). The authors prefer the second antibody technique and have generally used chromatoelectrophoresis when a second antibody is not available. Chromatoelectrophoresis is performed on 10 × 12 inch strips of Whatman DE-81 paper. Aliquots (50–100 μl) of the assay incubation mixture are mixed with 50-200 μl of dialyzed sheep serum and placed 2.0 inches from one end of the strip. Chromatoelectrophoresis is carried out at 4°C for two to three hours in 0.1 M barbital, pH 8.6, using 5.0 mA per strip. Antibody-bound labeled hGH travels cathodally.

3. Preparation of Radioimmunoassay Standard

The growth hormone is diluted with 1% BSA phosphosaline buffer to a final concentration of 100 ng/ml and stored at −20°C in 0.5-ml aliquots. One aliquot of this concentrated standard is thawed about once weekly and serially diluted with 1% BSA phosphosaline buffer to obtain standard solutions of 5.0, 2.5, 1.25, 0.625, 0.313, 0.156, and 0.078 ng/50 μl. These standards can be stored for up to two weeks at 4°C, but are seldom used for more than one week in our laboratory and are never refrozen. The standards are added directly to the assay tubes, as will be described later. Fresh hGH is weighed out at approximately six-month intervals. This material does not survive well when stored as a frozen solution.

4. Growth Hormone for Iodination

Growth hormone is weighed, dissolved in about 200 μl 0.01 N NaOH, and diluted with distilled water to a final concentration of 1.0 mg/ml. Twenty-microliter aliquots of this material are then distributed into 2.0-ml glass ampoules, sealed, and stored at −85°C until used for radioiodination.

B. Radioiodination Procedure for hGH

One ampoule containing 20 μg hGH in 20 μl is thawed and placed on ice. Iodine-125 is usually obtained from the New England Nuclear or from Amersham-Searle Corporation. High specific activity exceeding 200 mCi/ml is necessary. The radioactive iodine must be carrier-free and is supplied in a convenient conical vial. We purchase 10.0 mCi contained in a volume of about 50 μl or less. The radioactive iodine can be diluted with distilled water. To the ampoule containing hGH, 100 μl 0.5 M phosphate buffer, pH 7.6 is added. The presence of

Cl⁻ is avoided in our iodination procedure. About 1.0 mCi of the radioactive iodine is added to the ampoule. To start the iodination reaction, 35 μg of a freshly prepared solution of chloramine-T in 25 μl 0.05 M phosphate buffer, pH 7.6, is added. The iodine, hormone, and oxidant are gently agitated for 15 seconds. To stop the reaction, 125 μg of a freshly prepared solution of sodium metabisulfate in 100 μl 0.05 M phosphate buffer, pH 7.6, is added. The entire contents of the ampoule are then placed on the Sephadex G-50 column. The labeled hormone is eluted from the column with barbital buffer (0.05 M). About ten drops of this effluent per test tube are collected. The radioactive hormone is usually found in the tenth to the sixteenth tube, and elutes in a peak of three to four tubes (Figure 1). The hottest two- or three-peak tubes are pooled and diluted with 1% BSA phosphosaline buffer and divided into 10 to 20 aliquots of about 0.5 to 1.0 ml so that each contains about 10^7 cpm. The labeled hormone is then stored at $-20°C$ until used for the assay. The labeled hormone will be usable in most cases for about two months. Occasionally, the label will be unstable and last for only one or two weeks.

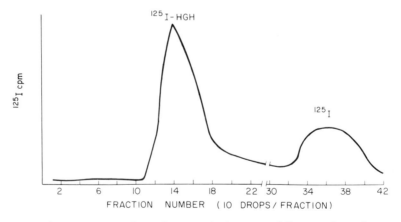

Figure 1. Elution pattern of ^{125}I from Sephadex G-50 following the iodination of human growth hormone (see text). The radioactivity is usually counted in a somewhat arbitrary fashion using the count density reading on a Geiger–Mueller-type gamma detector. In this example, the labeled hGH eluted in fraction numbers 13, 14, 15, and 16. The unreacted ^{125}I eluted from the column in tubes 32 through 40. This material is discarded in the radioactive waste. The specific activity of the labeled growth hormone can be calculated by determining the percentage of total counts of ^{125}I eluted in the first radio-active peak. In this example about 60% of the radioactive iodine was found in the first peak. If 1.0 mCi of ^{125}I was reacted with 20 μg hGH, then 0.6 mCi ^{125}I per 20 μg hGH or 30 mCi/mg was formed during the reaction. Much higher specific activities are readily obtainable, but specific activities exceeding 100 mCi/mg should not be attempted, since they frequently lead to unstable labels.

Although we frequently iodinate our own hormone, the iodinated growth hormone supplied by Abbott Laboratories, North Chicago, Illinois, has been reliably used in our assay. We find that the material they supply will be useful for one month or less from the time they iodinate the hormone, and thus, when we purchase iodinated hGH from them we never use it for more than one month. We purchase 0.1 mCi hGH, dilute it with about 5.0 ml 1% BSA phosphosaline buffer, and store it in ten equal aliquots at −20°C.

Prior to use in each assay, one aliquot of about 0.01 mCi iodinated hGH is further purified by chromatography on the Sephadex G-100 column. Fractions of 1.5 to 2.0 ml are collected by an automatic frac-

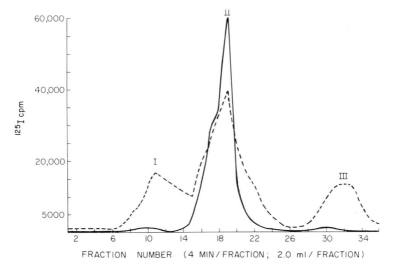

Figure 2.   Elution of labeled hGH from Sephadex G-100 on the day the assay is set up. One aliquot of the iodinated hGH was thawed and passed through the column on the day following iodination. When 10-μl aliquots of the eluate were counted, the pattern described by the solid line was obtained. Nearly all of the iodinated hGH was found in peak II, which is the best immunoreactive material and is used in the assay. About one month later, another aliquot of iodinated hGH was thawed and passed through the same column. When 10-μl aliquots of the eluate were counted, the pattern described by the dashed line was obtained. There was a substantial increase in peaks I and III at the expense of peak II. Use of the labeled hGH from peak II in an assay gave unreliable results, and the assay was discarded. Elution patterns intermediate between the solid and dashed lines produced labeled hGH in peak II, which was found to give reliable estimates of plasma hGH. Peak I represents aggregated labeled growth hormone with less immunoreactivity in the assay. Maximal precipitation of peak I with excess first antibody was only 50%. Peak II represents the best immunoreactive labeled hGH. Maximal precipitation of peak II with excess first antibody was 92%. Peak III represents smaller nonimmunoreactive substances which do not precipitate with the first antibody.

tion collector. The best immunoreactive label (peak II) is obtained in about 35 to 40 ml (Figure 2). Our experience indicates that the iodinated growth hormone can be successfully used in the assay following repurification until peak I (aggregated molecules) exceeds about 15% of the area encompassed by peak II. Occasionally the labeled hormone will rapidly degrade, forming substantial amounts of aggregated molecules within one to three days following iodination. Such a labeled hormone is not sufficiently stable during the three- or four-day incubation period to allow its use in the assay and should be discarded. Thus, if on repurification, peak I exceeds 15% of the area under peak II, we discard the label and prepare a new label.

C. Technique for Setting Up the hGH Radioimmunoassay

On the day the assay is set up, we thaw one aliquot of iodinated hGH and place it on the Sephadex G-100 column, collecting appropriately timed (one to eight minutes) fractions.

Disposable 10 × 50 mm test tubes are utilized. The number of unknowns to be assayed will determine the number of tubes in each assay. We find that 150 to 200 tubes is a convenient quantity for one person to process at one time. Many more tubes can be processed, but for convenience we rarely exceed 200 tubes in the usual assay. When the tubes have been numbered and placed in racks, the 1% BSA phosphosaline buffer is added to all tubes by a continuous pipetting apparatus.

The assay is designed in the following fashion. Tubes 1–3 will contain all of the reagents except the first antibody. The counts obtained in these tubes will be used for background subtraction from the remainder of the tubes in the assay. Tubes 4–6 will contain no standard growth hormone and no growth hormone-free control serum. These tubes will determine the precipitability of the labeled hGH in the absence of serum. Tubes 7–9 will contain no standard growth hormone, but will contain the growth hormone-free serum in order to give an estimate of the label precipitability in the presence of serum. These tubes are the "0" standards for the assay. To equalize the final volume in each of the preceding tubes, appropriate additional amounts of assay buffer are added.

Standard amounts of growth hormone are added in triplicate to tubes beginning with tube 10. We use the following standard concentrations in our routine hGH assays: 5.0, 2.5, 1.25, 0.625, 0.313, 0.156, and 0.078 ng. Each standard is added with a separate 50-μl micropipette. At this point, 30 assay tubes have been set up. To each of the standard tubes 7–30, 50 μl of serum from a hypophysectomized human patient, whose serum contains less than 0.5 ng/ml hGH, is added.

The addition of 50 μl of unknown serum begins with tube 31 and continues until duplicate aliquots of all unknown sera have been included in the assay. A separate micropipette is used for each unknown, or the pipette is washed with distilled water between different samples. All other additions to the test tubes are made with some type of continuous delivery apparatus.

The next step is to add the guinea pig anti-hGH serum (first antibody). The stored first antibody solution is appropriately diluted. An appropriate dilution of whole guinea pig serum carrier is included with the first antibody. The use of different second antibodies will alter the amount of carrier serum required in the assay to produce maximum first antibody precipitation. At present, the assay employs a first antibody dilution of 1 : 70,000 and a 1 : 600 dilution of guinea pig carrier serum. These reagents are prepared together and are added in 100-μl aliquots to each tube with the exception of tubes 1–3.

At this point, the labeled hormone should have eluted from the Sephadex column. Aliquots (5.0 or 10 μl) of the eluted fractions are counted in a well-type gamma counter to determine the peak II tubes that will be used in the assay (Figure 2). We usually select one or two tubes at the apex of the peak. These are diluted with 1% BSA phosphosaline buffer so that 100 μl contains between 10,000 and 20,000 cpm. We use one continuous pipetting apparatus for adding label that is never used for any other purpose. The label is added to every tube in 100-μl aliquots. This is usually done on the same day that the assay is set up. However, a more sensitive assay can be obtained by addition of the labeled hormone on the following day. Each assay tube should now contain 0.600 ml.

The assay tubes are shaken gently, left at room temperature for about two hours, and then placed in a refrigerator at 4°C for at least three days. After the three-day incubation, the tubes are removed from the refrigerator and the appropriate dilution of the goat anti-guinea pig serum is added (second antibody). The second antibody is diluted appropriately in 1% BSA phosphosaline buffer to obtain approximately 50% precipitation of antibody-bound labeled hGH (tubes 4–6). Aliquots of 100 μl of the second antibody are added to every tube. The tubes are gently agitated, left at room temperature for about two hours, and then placed at 4°C for at least eight hours. During the two hours at room temperature the tubes are placed in the gamma counter to obtain total counts for the assay. If desired, all tubes can be counted, but to reduce the demand on use of the gamma counter we usually get total counts only on the first 25–50 tubes of the assay.

Following incubation with second antibody the tubes are centrifuged at 2000 g for 30 minutes at 4°C in a refrigerated IEC-PR6 centrifuge. The supernatants are aspirated by vacuum suction, with care taken not to disturb the precipitates packed in the bottom of the tubes. About 50 μl of residual fluid will be left in each tube. About 2.0 ml cold phosphosaline buffer is added to each tube, and they are centrifuged as described above. The supernatants are aspirated and the precipitates are counted in the gamma counter. We have found that washing the precipitate increases reproducibility of the duplicates.

D. Calculation of Results and Reporting of Data

Numerous methods of calculating and reporting the values obtained from the human growth hormone immunoassay are available. Large-

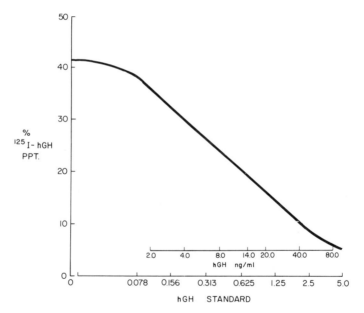

Figure 3. A typical standard curve obtained in one hGH immunoassay. Standard concentrations of hGH were prepared by serial dilution of the 5.0 ng per 50 μl standard. Increasing amounts of standard hGH produced decreasing amounts of precipitated ^{125}I-hGH. Growth hormone concentration in the unknown can be determined directly from the known amount of precipitated ^{125}I-hGH in the tube containing the unknown serum. If 50 μl aliquots of unknown are used, the scale above the abscissa gives the direct reading for nanograms hGH per milliliter plasma.

volume data production is probably best handled by logit transformation to allow computer calculation and reporting of the data (Midgley *et al.*, 1969). The following method has been useful for computing the results obtained in the usual hGH assay with less than 200 tubes. The counts obtained in tubes 1–3 are considered background and are subtracted from counts obtained for all other tubes in the assay. Many counters have a device to automatically subtract such background counts. A standard curve is constructed from the values obtained in tubes 7–30 (Figure 3). We use three-cycle semilog paper, plotting the standard hGH concentrations on the abscissa and the percent of iodinated hGH precipitated on the ordinate. The percent of ^{125}I-hGH precipitated is computed by dividing the average of the total counts obtained (denominator) into the precipitated counts obtained in each tube (numerator) and multiplying by 100.

Since we determine the hGH content on 50 μl of unknown sample, the amount of growth hormone per milliliter can be determined directly from the plotted standard curve by multiplying the numbers on the abscissa by 20. The percent of labeled hGH precipitated in the unknown tubes is computed, and the concentration of hGH is determined directly from the standard curve. Duplicate values vary less than 10%. The mean of the duplicate values is reported as nanograms hGH per milliliter serum.

E. Quality Control Measures Employed in the Assay

Even though the steps to obtain a reproducible assay are followed closely, an occasional assay will give obviously erroneous values. When the assay does not work at all, the problem usually lies in an error in dilution of antiserum, carrier serum, poorly mixed standards, omitting a reagent, or other problems in technique. These failures are troublesome but do not generally result in reporting of false values. The more important assay failures are those in which the assay appears acceptable, but falsely low or falsely elevated values for the unknowns are obtained. Knowledge of the source of the samples and the expected results helps to detect these last-mentioned assay problems. Several internal checks of the assay have been necessary to prevent the reporting of values obtained from these bad assays. When the label is not stable or the area under peak I exceeds about 15% of the area under peak II on Sephadex chromatography, the assay is likely to be invalid. If the triplicate determinations of the standards at more than one concentration are spread apart by more than 20% from the mean at that point, the assay validity must be questioned. Additionally, we employ three controls that are run in triplicate in every assay to check reproducibility. Serum which contains less than 0.5 ng per ml hGH was harvested from a hypophysectomized patient and enriched with standard concentrations of hGH so that 50-μl aliquots contained 5.0, 0.625, and 0.156 ng hGH. If the values for these samples in a particular assay vary by more than 20% from the mean values found in the previous assays, reproducibility is judged as poor and the values are not reported. In our last ten assays, the values obtained for these three samples have not varied by more than 8% from the mean for the ten assays. A further check on the stability of the labeled hGH is provided by comparing tubes 4–6, which omit serum, to tubes 7–9. The precipitability of labeled hGH should not be depressed more than 4–5% in the presence of the growth hormone-free serum. If there is greater than a 5% difference, the label is considered to be unstable. Since nearly all of this type of assay failure is attributable to the labeled hGH, the assay is repeated with freshly prepared label.

IV. CROSS-REACTIVITY WITH OTHER HORMONES

A. Growth Hormones from Other Species

The human growth hormone radioimmunoassay is highly specific. Addition of growth hormones prepared from various nonprimate species failed to displace the binding of the labeled human growth hormone to the anti-hGH serum used in the clinical assay (Figure 4). However, growth hormone from primates significantly cross-reacts with the human growth hormone assay, and this assay may be used for estimations of plasma growth hormone in monkeys. If growth hormone determinations in other species are desired, specific assays can be developed for most species generally used for experimentation. Thus, assays for bovine, ovine, porcine, rat, canine, and cat growth hormone have been developed. Varying degrees of cross-reactivity between the growth hormone assays developed for each of these species have been discovered depending on the particular antiserum available; thus, assays for one species may be suitable for measurements in another species. An example of this is the rat growth hormone immunoassay, which will detect porcine and ovine growth hormone (Birge *et al.*, 1967). In fact, early measurements of rat growth hormone utilized porcine growth hormone tracer, and some assays have employed antiserum to porcine growth hormone (Parker *et al.*, 1965; Frohman and Bernardis, 1968).

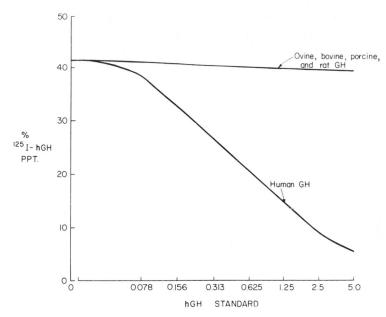

Figure 4. Cross-reaction of various animal growth hormones with the hGH immunoassay used in the authors' laboratory. When growth hormones from ovine, bovine, procine, and rat species were added up to 5.0 ng/tube, no significant effect on the hGH assay was found. Increasing the concentration of each of these growth hormones from heterologous species to 1000 ng/tube also failed to significantly displace the labeled hGH from the antibody used in this assay. This effect is a reflection of the specificity of the antiserum used and may be different for other antisera. The vertical axis is the amount of iodinated hGH recovered in the precipitate. The horizontal axis is the amount of each hormone added in nanograms to each assay tube.

B. Other Human Hormones

The steroids, cortisol, estrogen, progesterone, and testosterone, do not significantly affect the hGH immunoassay. These steroids, however, may influence secretion of the hormone in the patient. Neither thyroxine nor triiodothyronine will influence the assay, but changes in the endogenous concentration of these hormones in a patient may alter his response to tests which change growth hormone secretion. Other anterior pituitary hormones, including corticotropin, gonadotropins, thyrotropin, and prolactin, do not affect the assay. However, changes in the secretion of these hormones resulting from pathophysiologic alterations in pituitary function may alter secretion of hGH in a patient. Human placental lactogen does not cross-react with the antiserum used in the assay described here. However, many hGH antisera prepared with partially purified hGH will exhibit substantial cross-reactivity with human placental lactogen. The degree of cross-reaction will often result in falsely elevated levels of hGH during pregnancy due to the very large increases in human placental lactogen that occur during the latter stages of pregnancy.

C. "Big" Growth Hormone

The monomolecular form of hGH consists of 190 amino acids and has a molecular weight of 21,500 (Li, 1973). This monomer exhibits full biologic activity and comprises the major component (90%) of the material in highly purified reference preparations for hGH. Macromolecular forms of hGH have been found in extracts of pituitary and in plasma (Goodman *et al.*, 1972; Wright *et al.*, 1974; Gorden *et al.*, 1974; Benveniste *et al.*, 1975). Although the identity of these larger immunoreactive materials has not been fully established, most investigators feel that the major circulating component may be a dimer with a molecular weight twice that of monomeric hGH. Since "big" GH was identified by its immunologic cross-reactivity with monomeric or "little" GH, it is obvious that the big GH will be detected in the hGH radioimmunoassay. Whether it has an equivalent immunopotency to little GH is not known. However, estimates of the proportion of big GH in normal sera indicate that it may account for 14 to 40% of total circulating immunoreactive hGH. Some patients with acromegaly appear to have a diminished proportion (6–14%) of the circulating big GH (Gorden *et al.*, 1974). Estimates of the biologic potency of big GH by radioreceptor assays indicate it is only one-fourth to one-fifth as active as monomeric GH (Wright *et al.*, 1974; Gorden *et al.*, 1974; Herington *et al.*, 1974). Thus, big GH may be a relatively impotent substance biologically, but it represents a substantial proportion of circulating immunoreactive GH. Although the proportional amounts of big GH may be decreased in acromegaly, its absolute concentration may be higher than that found in normal subjects. Since the precise nature of big GH has not been defined, its role in growth hormone physiology and pathophysiology is not known.

V. MEASUREMENTS OF HORMONE IN BLOOD

A. Normal Levels

The greatest utility of hGH immunoassay is found in application to measurements of the concentration of the hormone in blood. Random measurements without regard to time of day, meals, sleep–wake cycle, hormonal status, prior activity, or sex of the subject are not diagnostically useful. All of these factors influence the levels of hGH that will be obtained. If blood is withdrawn from the patient at 8:00 to 9:00 AM in the postabsorptive state, prior to ambulation, with avoidance of undue stress, the plasma hGH concentration will rarely exceed 10 ng/ml. If blood is withdrawn from the subject following ambulation, such as traveling from home to the laboratory or doctor's office, the plasma concentration of the hormone will be variably increased (Frantz and Rabkin, 1965). Ambulatory male subjects rarely have values that exceed 25 ng/ml, but ambulatory female subjects often have values up to 50 ng/ml, and occasionally as high as 80 ng/ml. Since basal or random values are so variably influenced, stimulation and suppression tests for hGH secretion have been developed to study secretory capacity and suppressibility.

B. Suppression Tests

These maneuvers have their greatest utility in the diagnosis of acromegaly. Either oral or intravenous administration of glucose can be used. A standard oral glucose tolerance test is suitable in most instances and is the standard method used by the authors to suppress plasma hGH. Generally accepted values for normal suppression are considered to be a fall to less than 5.0 ng/ml at any point during a three-hour glucose tolerance test (Daughaday, 1968). However, patients who appear acromegalic by clinical criteria have been reported to have values from 4.0 to 10 ng/ml (Mims and Bethune, 1974). Although these subjects are rare, they have provoked doubts about the previously accepted criteria for adequate suppression following oral glucose in normal subjects. The subjects with clinical signs of acromegaly who had "normal" plasma hGH values failed to suppress following glucose administration and also failed to respond normally to provocative stimuli for hGH secretion. Thus, the diagnosis was established by defining an abnormality in the dynamics of hGH secretion. Review of the results obtained in normal subjects in the authors' laboratory has indicated that most normal individuals will suppress plasma hGH concentration to less than 2.0 ng/ml at some point during the three-hour interval following the ingestion of oral glucose. Thus, individuals who have less than 2.0 ng/ml at any time interval after oral glucose ingestion should be considered normal. If the patient has a substantial fall in plasma GH from baseline levels to less than 5.0 ng/ml, acromegaly is unlikely. Values ranging from 4.0 to 10 ng/ml that do not change following oral glucose, in a patient with features suggestive of hypersomatotropism, are indicative but not diagnostic of autonomous hGH secretion.

In an occasional patient, plasma hGH will fail to fall after oral glucose, and this will be associated with a lack of a substantial rise in the plasma glucose. In the authors' experience, the plasma glucose should exceed 100 mg% at some point during the oral glucose tolerance test to be certain that an adequate rise in glucose occurred. Although most normal subjects will have adequate suppression of the plasma hGH despite a poor increase in the plasma glucose following oral glucose administration, a rare subject will not have an adequate fall in the plasma hGH level to eliminate definitively the possibility of acromegaly. In these instances, intravenous glucose tolerance tests are performed. Twenty to fifty grams (or 0.5 gm/kg) of 50% glucose is given intravenously over a five- to ten-minute period of time and blood is withdrawn for glucose and hGH determination at 15-minute intervals during the subsequent 90 minutes. The same criteria for adequate suppression used for the oral glucose tolerance test are applied to the intravenous glucose test. This test proved useful in some of our treated acromegalic subjects who had elevations of plasma hGH on random determination and demonstrated poor suppression of hGH associated with an inadequate rise in plasma glucose on oral glucose tolerance testing. Some of the patients have responded to the intravenous glucose tolerance test with an adequate suppression of plasma hGH concentration.

C. Paradoxical Responses

Several types of patients have been reported to have substantial elevations in plasma growth hormone concentration following glucose administration rather than the expected decrease. This phenomenon was termed a paradoxical response by Beck et al. (1966). It was initially described in certain patients with acromegaly (Beck et al., 1966) and a patient with a hypothalamic tumor (Fishman and Peake, 1970). The paradoxical response has been reported to occur in newborn infants, women with metastatic breast cancer, uncontrolled diabetics, and patients with several other disorders (Martin, 1973). Children suffering from severe protein–calorie malnutrition also respond to glucose administration with unusual changes in plasma growth hormone (Pimstone et al., 1972). Some of these starved children will have paradoxical responses, but more often they fail to have a significant decrement in plasma growth hormone concentration following glucose ingestion. This defect is repaired by protein repletion over several weeks' time.

D. Stimulation Tests

These tests find their greatest usefulness in assessing hGH secretion in patients with suspected hGH deficiency, but they are also useful in establishing autonomy of hGH secretion in patients with hyper-somatotropism. Since a large number of stimuli provoke hGH secretion in normal subjects, a wide range of stimulation tests are available. For convenience, these can be divided into screening and diagnostic tests. The screening tests are those which can be performed in an outpatient setting without close physician supervision, but which are not generally accepted as diagnostic tools to define abnormalities in hGH secretion. Vigorous exercise such as jogging for 20 to 30 minutes or running up twelve flights of stairs will provoke a rise in hGH exceeding 10 ng/ml in most normal subjects within about 20 to 30 minutes after the termination of the exercise. However, about 20 to 25% of normal children evaluated for short stature by the authors failed to respond to this exercise stimulus. Since too many normal children were subsequently subjected to the more complex diagnostic studies, this test has been abandoned. Administration of the drug L-dopa regularly promotes an increase in plasma hGH in normal children (Weldon et al., 1973). This test is performed as described by Weldon et al. (1973) and has proved to be more reliable than other screening techniques used by the author.

The tests which are widely accepted as being of diagnostic value in establishing hyposomatotropism are the insulin hypoglycemia test and the arginine infusion test (Parker et al., 1967). Since a substantial number of normal individuals fail to respond to one or the other stimulus, a lack of rise in plasma growth hormone to both stimuli is generally required to establish a diagnosis of growth hormone deficiency. The tests can be performed sequentially on the same day (Penny et al., 1969). Both tests are closely supervised by a physician, and the insulin hypoglycemia test is usually performed in the hospital. The response of plasma growth hormone to arginine infusion, performed by the method described by Parker et al. (1967), in 39 normal prepuberal children studied by the authors is presented in Figure 5. Twenty of these same children also were subjected to the insulin hypoglycemia test, and comparable elevations in growth hormone occurred. The range of maximal growth hormone concentration following both stimuli was 8.0 to 80 ng/ml in these normal children. If a child

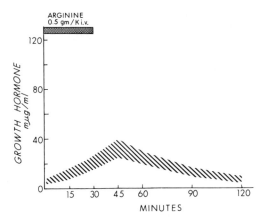

Figure 5. The rise in plasma growth hormone seen after intravenous infusion of arginine in 39 normal healthy children. Twenty of the children were male and 19 were female. No significant difference in the response was noted between the two sexes in these prepubertal children, and the data from the entire group were pooled for presentation here. The shaded band represents the mean ± one standard deviation from the mean for the entire group.

fails to show a rise in plasma growth hormone to greater than 10 ng/ml following each of these stimuli, he is considered to have hyposomatotropism. Blunted growth hormone responses to arginine infusion are also seen in adult males and in obese individuals. The response in adult males can be augmented by prior administration of estrogens (Merimee *et al.*, 1966), and some investigators routinely pretreat all subjects, other than adult females, with estrogens prior to performing the arginine provocative test. The authors have not found this to be necessary or desirable in children being evaluated for hyposomatotropism as a possible cause of short stature.

Thyrotropin-releasing hormones has been shown to increase growth hormone secretion in many patients with acromegaly. This response is confirmatory for the diagnosis of acromegaly (Samaan *et al.*, 1974).

VI. MEASUREMENTS OF THE HORMONE IN TISSUE AND URINE

Human growth hormone can be efficiently extracted from human pituitary tissue by homogenization in 0.5 ml phosphate-buffered saline (0.1 M phosphate, 0.15 M NaCl, pH 7.6) (Peake *et al.*, 1969). After centrifugation at 1000 g for 30 minutes, the supernatant containing the extracted hormone can be diluted to an appropriate concentration in the same buffer containing albumin and assayed directly. Growth hormones from other species may require somewhat different extraction methods to maximize recovery of the hormone from the tissue. Thus, in the case of rat growth hormone, $0.01\,N$ NaOH was found to be more efficient in extracting this particular hormone from pituitary tissue than other buffers (Birge *et al.*, 1967).

Several investigators have attempted to measure growth hormone excreted in the urine. A relatively recent article reviews the wide variation in estimations of growth hormone excretion obtained in different laboratories (Bala *et al.*, 1972). Since the major route of disposal of hGH is not by urinary excretion, changes in urinary excretion do not directly reflect changes in plasma content or secretory rates of the hormone. The immunoreactive material measured in urine may be a fragment of the intact circulating hormone, which would explain the varying amounts found in urine by different investigators using different antibodies to hGH.

ACKNOWLEDGMENTS

The experimental work described in this article was supported by NIH Grant No. HD 05794 and RR 00997. Dr. Maire T. Buckman is a Research and Education Associate of the Veterans Administration.

REFERENCES

Bala, R. M., Ferguson, K. A., and Beck, J. C. (1972). Growth hormone like activity in plasma and urine. *Growth Growth Horm., Proc. Int. Symp., 2nd, 1971* Excerpta Med. Found., Int. Congr. Ser. No. 244, pp. 483–498.

Beck, P., Parker, M. L., and Daughaday, W. H. (1966). Paradoxical hypersecretion of growth hormone in response to glucose. *J. Clin. Endocrinol. Metab.* **26**, 463–469.

Benveniste, R., Stachura, M. E., Szabo, M., and Frohman, L. A. (1975). Big growth hormone (GH): Conversion to small GH without peptide bond cleavage. *J. Clin. Endocrinol. Metab.* **41**, 422–425.

Birge, C. A., Peake, G. T., Mariz, I. K., and Daughaday, W. H. (1967). Radioimmunoassayable growth hormone in the rat pituitary: Effects of age, sex and hormonal state. *Endocrinology* **81**, 195–204.

Daughaday, W. H. (1968). The diagnosis of hypersomatotropism in man. *Med. Clin. North Am.* **52**, 371–380.

Daughaday, W. H., and Jacobs, L. S. (1971). Methods of separating antibody-bound from free antigen. *In* "Principles of Competitive Protein-Binding Assays" (W. D. Odell and W. H. Daughaday, eds.), pp. 303–316. Lippincott, Philadelphia, Pennsylvania.

Fishman, M. A., and Peake, G. T. (1970). Paradoxical growth in a patient with the diencephalic syndrome. *Pediatrics* **45**, 972–982.

Frantz, A. G., and Rabkin, M. T. (1965). Effects of estrogen and sex differences on secretion of human growth hormone. *J. Clin. Endocrinol. Metab.* **25**, 1470–1480.

Frohman, L. A., and Bernardis, L. L. (1968). Growth hormone and insulin levels in weanling rats with ventromedial hypothalamic lesions. *Endocrinology* **82**, 1125–1132.

Glick, S. M., Roth, J., Yalow, R. S., and Berson, S. A. (1963). Immunoassay of human growth hormone in plasma. *Nature (London)* **199**, 784–787.

Goodman, A. D., Tannenbaum, R., and Rabinowitz, D. (1972). Existence of two forms of immunoreactive growth hormone in plasma. *J. Clin. Endocrinol. Metab.* **35**, 868–878.

Gorden, P., Lesnick, M. A., Hendricks, C. M., McGuffin, W., and Gavin, J. R., III (1974). hGH · Characterization of plasma and pituitary components and application of a new radioreceptor assay. *Isr. J. Med. Sci.* **10**, 1239–1246.

Herington, A. C., Jacobs, L. S., and Daughaday, W. H. (1974). Radioreceptor and radioimmunoassay quantitation of human growth hormone in acromegalic serum: Overestimation of immunoassay and systematic differences between antisera. *J. Clin. Endocrinol. Metab.* **39**, 257–262.

Li, C. H. (1973). Growth hormone—characterization. *In* "Methods in Investigative and Diagnostic Endocrinology" (S. A. Berson and R. S. Yalow, eds.), pp. 257–261. North-Holland Pub., Amsterdam.

Martin, J. B. (1973). Neural regulation of growth hormone secretion. *N. Engl. J. Med.* **288**, 1384–1393.

Merimee, T. J., Burgess, J. A., and Rabinowitz D. (1966). Sex determined variation in serum insulin and growth hormone response to amino acid stimulation. *J. Clin. Endocrinol. Metab.* **26**, 791–793.

Midgley, A. R., Niswender, G. D., and Rebar, R. W. (1969). Principles for the assessment of the reliability of radioimmunoassay methods. *Acta Endocrinol. (Copenhagen), Suppl.* **142**, 163–184.

Mims, R. B., and Bethune, J. E. (1974). Acromegaly with normal fasting growth hormone concentrations but abnormal growth hormone regulation. *Ann. Intern. Med.* **81**, 781–784.

Odell, W., Silver, D. C., and Grover, P. K. (1975). Competitive protein binding assays. Methods of separation of bound from free. *Steroid Immunoassay, Proc. Tenovus Workshop, 5th, 1974* pp. 207–222.

Parker, M. L., Jarett, L., Schalch, D. S., and Kipnis, D. M. (1965). Rat growth hormone: Immunofluorescent and radioimmunologic studies. *Endocrinology* **76**, 928–932.

Parker, M. L., Hammond, J. M., and Daughaday, W. H. (1967). The arginine provocative test: An aid in the diagnosis of hyposomatotropism. *J. Clin. Endocrinol. Metab.* **27**, 1129–1136.

Peake, G. T., McKeel, D. W., Jarett, L., and Daughaday, W. H. (1969). Ultrastructural, histologic, and hormonal characterization of a prolactin-rich human pituitary tumor. *J. Clin. Endocrinol. Metab.* **29**, 1383–1393.

Penny, R., Blizzard, R. M., and Davis, W. T. (1969). Sequential arginine and insulin tolerance tests on the same day. *J. Clin. Endocrinol. Metab.* **29**, 1499–1450.

Pimstone, B. L., Becker, D. J., and Hansen, J. D. L. (1972). Human growth hormone in protein-calorie malnutrition. *Growth Growth Horm., Proc. Int. Symp., 2nd, 1971* Excerpta Med. Found., Int. Congr. Ser. No. 244, pp. 389–401.

Samaan, N. A., Leavens, M. E., and Jesse, R. H., Jr. (1974). Serum growth hormone and prolactin response to thyrotropin-releasing hormone in patients with acromegaly before and after surgery. *J. Clin. Endocrinol. Metab.* **38**, 957–963.

Schalch, D. S., and Parker, M. L. (1964). A sensitive double antibody immunoassay for human growth hormone in plasma. *Nature (London)* **203**, 1141–1142.

Weldon, V. V., Gupta, S. K., Haymond, M. W., Pagliara, A. S., Jacobs, L. S., and Daughaday, W. H. (1973). The use of L-dopa in the diagnosis of hyposomatotropism in children. *J. Clin. Endocrinol. Metab.* **36**, 42–46.

Wilhelmi, A. E. (1973). Growth hormone measurement-bioassay. *In* "Methods in Investigative and Diagnostic Endocrinology" (S. A. Berson and R. S. Yalow, eds.), pp. 296–302. North-Holland Pub., Amsterdam.

Wright, D. R., Goodman, A. D., and Trimble, A. D. (1974). Studies on "big" growth hormone from human plasma and pituitary. *J. Clin. Invest.* **54**, 1064–1073.

12

Adrenocorticotropic Hormone (ACTH)

DAVID N. ORTH

I. INTRODUCTION[*]

A. Biologic and Other Assays

The development of assays for adrenocorticotropic hormone (ACTH) in biologic fluids and tissues has permitted studies which have greatly expanded our knowledge about factors involved in ACTH synthesis, secretion, metabolism, and action. For years, the

[*] The nomenclature in this chapter conforms to the system of terminology for preparations of adrenocorticotropic hormone proposed by C. H. Li (1959).

245

Methods of Hormone Radioimmunoassay, Second Edition
Copyright © 1979 by Academic Press, Inc.
All rights of reproduction in any form reserved. ISBN 0-12-379260-6

burden of these studies fell upon bioassays based upon either of two major effects of ACTH on adrenal cortical cells, namely, the stimulation of steriodogenesis or the depletion of ascorbic acid observed either in the adrenal *in situ* or in portions of adrenal glands or isolated adrenal cells incubated *in vitro*. A brief bibliography is included for those who are interested (M. A. Sayers *et al.*, 1948; Guillemin *et al.*, 1958; Lipscomb and Nelson, 1962; Vernikos-Danellis *et al.*, 1966; Kloppenborg *et al.*, 1968; G. Sayers *et al.*, 1971; Chayen *et al.*, 1972; Lowry *et al.*, 1973; Nicholson and Van Loon, 1973). The radioreceptor assay technique has been applied to measurement of ACTH, using normal or neoplastic adrenocortical cells as the source of receptor (Taunton *et al.*, 1969; Lefkowitz *et al.*, 1970a,b; Wolfsen *et al.*, 1972). However, this technique has not been widely adopted, perhaps because of technical difficulties encountered by some of those who have attempted to set it up in their laboratories. In this assay, solubilized adrenal cell membrane ACTH receptor is used, rather than ACTH antibody, to bind labeled tracer. For maximum sensitivity, purified monoiodinated ^{125}I-ACTH is required, which is prepared by a shallow ammonium acetate gradient elution (0.01 M, pH 4.8, to 0.6 M, pH 5.2) from a carboxymethyl cellulose column (Lefkowitz *et al.*, 1970a). The sensitivity of the assay is reported as 1.0 pg/assay tube, or 10 pg/ml unextracted plasma (Wolfsen *et al.*, 1972). This is comparable to the radioimmunoassay and is sufficient for most physiologic studies.

An even more sensitive bioassay is the redox assay first reported by Chayen *et al.* (1971). This assay exploits the fact that ACTH depletes reducing groups in the guinea pig adrenal cortex maintained in organ culture. Using a scanning microdensitometer (No. GN2, Barr and Stroud or No. M85, Vickers Instruments) to quantitate the staining of the zona reticularis with a Prussian blue (ferriferrocyanide) reaction medium, a dose–response curve from 0.0025 to 2.5 pg/ml culture medium is obtained (Chayen *et al.*, 1972; Daly *et al.*, 1972). This assay has now been compared and validated with both ACTH bioassay and radioimmunoassay (Rees *et al.*, 1973). The scanning microdensitometer is a very expensive instrument, however, and a skilled full time technician can assay only a few samples each week. Thus, this assay procedure must be reserved for circumstances requiring extreme sensitivity.

B. Bioactivity–Immunoreactivity Relationships

The ACTH radioimmunoassay technique, while difficult, appears to have been more widely applicable than those assays just described.

Since the first potentially useful radioimmunoassay for plasma ACTH was reported by Yalow *et al.* (1964), a number of ACTH radioimmunoassay systems have been described which differ from one another in technical details. The variety of antisera employed, however, raises an issue of major consequence for ACTH and most other hormone radioimmunoassays—the relationship of biologic activity to immunologic reactivity.

The biologic actions of most hormones involve interaction with a receptor moiety within the target cell or on its surface. Hormone specificity for the cell is determined by receptor structural complementarity, since binding must occur in order to initiate the sequence of reactions which ultimately result in the biologic action of the hormone. Specificity of the hormone–antibody reaction is dependent upon mutual fit of the hormone and the immunoglobulin recognition site. However, there is no *a priori* reason why the cell receptor and the immunoglobulin should make identical demands upon the hormone molecule in terms of structural configuration required for optimal binding. This predictable dissociation of bioactivity and immunoreactivity was first described for ACTH (Besser *et al.*, 1971), rather than some other hormone, because ACTH bioassays are sensitive and relatively simple (Lipscomb and Nelson, 1962; Nicholson and Van Loon, 1973) and because biologic structure–function relationships have been defined for ACTH perhaps more extensively than for any other hormone (Ney *et al.*, 1965; Hoffman *et al.*, 1970; Seelig and Sayers, 1973).

Human ACTH consists of a chain of 39 amino acid residues (Riniker *et al.*, 1972), as it does in all species thus far studied (Table I). The complete steroidogenic potency of ACTH is possessed by its N-terminal 18-amino acid sequence. The C-terminal nonsteroidogenic part of the molecule, which is variable at residues 31 and 33, has no known biologic function. The steroidogenic potency of ACTH is rapidly lost as the chain length is decreased to less than 18 residues. The weak intrinsic melanocyte-stimulating potency of ACTH, on the other hand, increases as the chain length approaches 13 residues. In fact, α-MSH, the most potent MSH known, is N-α-acetyl-$\alpha^{1-13\text{NH}_2}$-ACTH[1] (Table I). A common 7-amino acid sequence is also shared with the lipotrophins (Chapter 13), which are now known (Bloomfield *et al.*, 1974; Tanaka *et al.*, 1976, 1978) to constitute the immunoreactive β-MSH measured by our laboratory (Abe *et al.*, 1967b, 1969) and those of others (Donald and Toth, 1973; Thody and Plummer, 1973; Donnadieu and Sevaux, 1973). Acetylation (Ney *et al.*, 1965) or oxidation of the 1-position serine with periodate (Dixon, 1956) results in almost

Table I The Chemical Structures of the Known ACTH's[a]

```
H-Ser-Tyr-Ser-Met-Glu-His-Phe-Arg-Trp-Gly-Lys-Pro-Val-Gly-Lys-Lys-Arg-Arg-Pro-Val-Lys-Val-Tyr-Pro-
  1   2   3   4   5   6   7   8   9  10  11  12  13  14  15  16  17  18  19  20  21  22  23  24
```

Beef	-Asn-	Gly-	Ala-	Glu-	Asp-	Glu-	Ser-	Ala-	Gln-	Ala-	Phe-	Pro-	Leu-	Glu-	Phe-OH
	25	26	27	28	29	30	31	32	33	34	35	36	37	38	39
Sheep	-Asn-	Gly-	Ala-	Glu-	Asp-	Glu-	Ser-	Ala-	Gln-	Ala-	Phe-	Pro-	Leu-	Glu-	Phe-OH
	25	26	27	28	29	30	31	32	33	34	35	36	37	38	39
Pig	-Asn-	Gly-	Ala-	Glu-	Asp-	Glu-	Leu-	Ala-	Glu-	Ala-	Phe-	Pro-	Leu-	Glu-	Phe-OH
	25	26	27	28	29	30	31	32	33	34	35	36	37	38	39
Man	-Asn-	Gly-	Ala-	Glu-	Asp-	Glu-	Ser-	Ala-	Glu-	Ala-	Phe-	Pro-	Leu-	Glu-	Phe-OH
	25	26	27	28	29	30	31	32	33	34	35	36	37	38	39

[a] The following are references for the original, or most recently revised, sequences for the known ACTH's: beef and sheep (Jöhl et al., 1974), pig (Gräf et al., 1971), and man (Riniker et al., 1972). All are essentially equipotent (Li, 1962; Ney et al., 1965).

complete loss of ACTH activity. The 4-position methionine is susceptible to oxidation by ambient oxygen or peroxide (Dedman *et al.*,
1961), with loss of essentially all of ACTH bioactivity (Li, 1962). Thus,
the first 18 amino acids of natural ACTH cannot be much altered without significant loss of biologic potency.

What of immunoreactivity? The antigenic portion of ACTH has
been reported to be the variable sequence C-terminal portion of the
molecule. However, antibodies can be directed to a number of sites,
even in this small molecule (Orth *et al.*, 1968). The specificities of four
such antisera are described in this chapter. The heterogeneity of antibody specificities makes one wonder, in fact, if any two are exactly
alike and must be considered when comparing results from different
radioimmunoassays.

Suppose that three antisera are directed toward three different
8-amino acid sequences of the ACTH molecule (Figure 1), antibody 1
to sequence 1–8, antibody 2 to sequence 13–20, and antibody 3 to
sequence 32–39. Now suppose that there are three degradative enzymes in our biologic system, human circulating blood; enzyme A

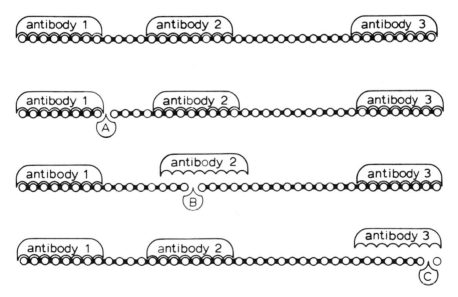

Figure 1. Diagrammatic representation of the 39-amino acid chain of ACTH and its
interactions with three antibodies. Antibody 1 reacts with the 1–8 sequence, antibody
2 with the 13–20 sequence, and antibody 3 with the 32–39 sequence of amino acid
residues. The effects on antibody binding of the action of three enzymes are indicated.
Enzyme A cleaves the 8–9 bond, enzyme B the 15–16 bond, and enzyme C the 38–39
bond. See text for discussion of potential biologic–immunologic dissociations.

cleaves ACTH at the 8–9 bond, enzyme B at the 15–16 Lys–Lys bond, and enzyme C removes the C-terminal phenylalanine. Biologic activity would be lost when enzyme A cleaved the molecule, yet reactivity would be unaffected in all three radioimmunoassays. Bioactivity and reactivity with antibody 2 would be lost by cleavage with enzyme B, but immunoassays using antibodies 1 or 3 would be unaffected. Finally, enzyme C would have no effect on bioactivity or on immunoreactivity with antibodies 1 and 2, but would destroy antibody 3 immunoreactivity. Therefore, depending on what degradative enzymes are present in the system, their relative rate constants, and the specificity of the ACTH antiserum, an ACTH radioimmunoassay might represent exactly, overestimate, or underestimate the bioactive ACTH in the specimen.

It is not necessary that the ACTH molecule be cleaved into fragments for these considerations to obtain. Alterations in the chemical nature of ACTH might have similar effects. Oxidation of the 4-methionine residue, for example, might affect the reaction with antibody 1; it certainly causes a marked reduction in bioactivity (Dedman *et al.*, 1961). Similarly, amidation of the 38-glutamic acid residue might decrease affinity for antibody 3; it would have no effect on biologic potency. In fact, recent studies in which the metabolic fate of labeled ACTH in rats was characterized in terms of both bioactivity (Nicholson and Van Loon, 1973) and radioimmunoreactivity (with the antibody whose specificity is described below and characterized in Figure 5) demonstrated that the ACTH metabolite remaining in plasma had a molecular size indistinguishable from 1–39-ACTH, despite the fact that it rapidly lost bioactivity and more slowly lost immunoreactivity (Nicholson *et al.*, 1976b). Thus, microchemical biotransformations may account for the rapid inactivation of ACTH and other polypeptide hormones in the circulation and, at least in part, for the observed dissociations of bioactivity and immunoreactivity.

Another potential source of bioactivity–immunoreactivity dissociation arises not from the metabolism of ACTH, but how it is synthesized (Orth and Nicholson, 1977b). It is now accepted that most peptide hormones are synthesized from larger precursors and that biosynthetic intermediates, as well as metabolites, may circulate in the blood (Tager and Steiner, 1974; Yalow, 1974). Since Yalow and Berson (1971, 1973) first suggested that human ACTH is synthesized from a precursor "big" ACTH, others have confirmed and extended their observations. From work in the mouse pituitary tumor cell line, AtT-20, it appears there are at least three distinct ACTH precursor forms, ranging in size from about 8000 to 31,000 daltons (Orth *et al.*, 1973b;

Eipper and Mains, 1975). Cell-free synthesis of bovine ACTH suggests that an even bigger precursor form (MW 35,000) may exist (Nakanishi *et al.*, 1976). These precursor forms appear to be glycopeptides, both in mouse (Eipper *et al.*, 1976) and man (Orth and Nicholson, 1977a). Since their bioactivity may be as little as 4% that of 1–39-ACTH (Gewirtz *et al.*, 1974) radioimmunoassay of specimens containing these precursors may greatly overestimate the amount of ACTH bioactivity present.

From these considerations certain principles can be formulated. (1) Antiserum specificity should be defined as completely as possible. (2) The antiserum should be directed at the biologically active portion of the molecule because the probability of biologic–immunologic parallelism should be greatest. (3) Biologic and immunologic comparison should be made on aliquots of the same specimens to validate the assay. (4) Since one is measuring immunoreactivity in lieu of bioactivity, the terms immunoreactive ACTH (IR-ACTH) or radioimmunoassayable ACTH (RIA-ACTH) should be used so frequently that neither the investigator nor his audience forgets it.

II. METHODS OF RADIOIMMUNOASSAY

A. Source of Hormone

The hormone used for radioiodination and standard must be as pure as possible. Although it might seem the ACTH standard should be homologous with the species being assayed, this is not always necessary. If the antibodies are directed toward a portion of the 1–24 sequence, any peptide which includes the 1–24 sequence (α^{1-24}-ACTH or any species of natural or synthetic 1–39-ACTH) should be a satisfactory standard. Appropriate allowance for the lower molecular weight of α^{1-24}-ACTH standard is made in calculating concentrations of 1–39-ACTH in the samples.

The ACTH preparations currently available include synthetic α^{1-24}-ACTH, Cortrosyn (Organon, Inc., West Orange, New Jersey). The mannitol stabilizer in Cortrosyn does not affect the radioimmunoassay or its usefulness for iodination, but Dr. Henry A. Strade of Organon has provided us with mannitol-free Cortrosyn in the past. Porcine ACTH, highly purified by chromatographic procedures, is also commercially available from Schwartz/Mann (Orangeburg, New York) and Calbiochem (Los Angeles, California) among others. Since it differs only in position 31 from human ACTH (Riniker *et al.*, 1972), it is an acceptable substitute for human ACTH in most cases.

It is esthetically satisfying and perfectly rational to use natural human ACTH as reference standard in a human ACTH radioimmunoassay, but the supply of human ACTH of sufficient purity is very limited. Dr. C. H. Li (Hormone Research Laboratories, University of California, Berkeley, California) has provided human ACTH to investigators. Dr. A. B. Lerner (Department of Dermatology, Yale University, New Haven, Connecticut) has donated his excellent ACTH preparation (Preparation 8B; Lerner *et al.*, 1968) to the National Pituitary Agency, but this material is now in extremely short supply.

Three synthetic 1–39-human ACTH preparations have been prepared. The first, synthesized by Gideon-Richter, Ltd., Budapest, Hungary (Bajusz *et al.*, 1967), was distributed by Dr. J. Mülder (Ferring AB, Mälmo, Sweden). This material was synthesized before the revised sequence of human ACTH was published (Riniker *et al.*, 1972), has only 55% of expected potency by intravenous bioassay (Lipscomb and Nelson, 1962) in our laboratory, and is unstable on storage in solution at −70°C, losing potency and generating nonparallel curves in the radioimmunoassay. The second preparation was synthesized recently by Ciba-Geigy, Ltd., Basel, Switzerland (Sieber *et al.*, 1972). It has the revised sequence of amino acids and is fully bioactive (Schenkel-Hulliger *et al.*, 1974; Nicholson *et al.*, 1976a). This material has been prepared in 50-μg quantities in sealed ampoules under conditions similar to those used for the highly successful Third International Standard for Corticotropin (Bangham *et al.*, 1962) by our laboratory (Nicholson *et al.*, 1976a) for the National Pituitary Agency. This material is suitable both for iodination and for use as standard and is available to qualified investigators from the National Pituitary Agency or the Hormone Distribution Officer, NIAMDD.* The third preparation was synthesized by Dr. C. H. Li; we have had no experience with it.

Brief mention should be made about standards for other species. If one has reason to use a C-terminal radioimmunoassay, it may be necessary to use homologous ACTH to raise antibodies, for iodination, and as a standard. If an estimate of biologic activity is sought, however, a 1–24 antiserum is desirable and has the further advantage that it can be used for any known vertebrate species. We have measured RIA-ACTH in pituitary extracts of fish, amphibian, bird, and a variety

---

* National Pituitary Agency, Suite 503, 210 W. Fayette St., Baltimore, Maryland 21201. Hormone Distribution Officer, NIAMDD, National Institutes of Health, Bethesda, Maryland 20014.

of mammals (mouse, rat, guinea pig, rabbit, cat, sheep, horse, beef, pig, and man) (Shapiro et al., 1972; Orth et al., 1968; also unpublished data) with three antisera and human ACTH tracer and standard. Parallel dose–response curves were generated and the RIA-ACTH values agreed well with bioactive ACTH. We have also measured immunoreactive plasma ACTH in rat, sheep, horse, and man. Others have described radioimmunoassays for plasma ACTH in the rat (Rees et al., 1971) and sheep (Alexander et al., 1973).

B. Production of Antibodies

1. Choice of Animal for Immunization

Over 200 guinea pigs were immunized to obtain our first useful antiserum. One bleeding (3.0 ml serum) of one animal produced antibodies sufficiently sensitive for plasma ACTH radioimmunoassay. Fortunately, the antibody titer was sufficiently high that we were able to use it in our standard ACTH radioimmunoassay for more than seven years. One can obtain antibodies with almost any ACTH preparation if one immunizes enough animals. The many reports of the "best" ACTH preparation to use, such as commercial porcine ACTH (Demura et al., 1966), zinc-porcine ACTH (Orth et al., 1968), Duracton (Berson and Yalow, 1968), or partially purified human ACTH (Landon and Greenwood, 1968; Matsukura et al., 1971) bear witness to this. It has been suggested that incomplete Freund's adjuvant should be used for booster injections, that injections should be made with charcoal-absorbed ACTH directly into the spleen or lymph nodes, and that guinea pigs generate higher affinity antibodies than rabbits. It is probable that these factors have no major influence on antibody production; the development of useful antisera may have been more serendipity than science.

However, recent experience suggests a much greater chance of success. We have raised high affinity antibodies consistently in both rabbits and sheep and no longer immunize guinea pigs because of the small amounts of antiserum obtainable and the risk of death following cardiac puncture, even by a skilled technician. Rabbits are easily bled from the marginal ear vein. The outer surface of the ear is shaved in advance. The inside of the ear is wiped with xylol, to cause vasodilatation, taking care not to get it on the outer surface. The tip of a No. 11 scalpel blade is inserted just below the marginal ear vein, then pulled up, partially transecting it. The blood is allowed to drip directly into a centrifuge tube. Alternatively, the rabbit can be bled from the central artery of the ear, which can be palpated, but not easily seen, immediately adjacent to the central vein: A heparinized, 19-gauge thin-wall needle is inserted into the artery and the blood is allowed to drip rapidly into the centrifuge tube. In either case, bleeding is readily stopped by applying pressure for a few minutes. Sheep are bled from the external jugular vein with a needle and syringe or a heparinized blood collection bag without difficulty.

2. The Antigen

Animals are immunized with α^{1-24}-ACTH conjugated to heterologous serum albumin. Others have used thyroglobulin or other protein carriers for the hapten. It is important to couple the polypeptide hapten to as many of the available exposed protein reactive carboxyl and/or amino groups as possible. Thus, a large molar excess of hapten is used in the reaction. We have used both the carbodiimide reaction (McGuire *et al.*, 1965) and the glutaraldehyde reaction (Reichlin *et al.*, 1968) to bind 1–24-ACTH, 25–39-ACTH, and other haptens to albumin. Our exact procedures for α^{1-24}-ACTH follow; they can be used for 1–39-ACTH or any other ACTH analog or fragment.

a. Carbodiimide (W. E. Nicholson and D. N. Orth, unpublished data)

i. Reagents

α^{1-24}-ACTH (Cortrosyn, Organon, Inc., West Orange, New Jersey).

Bovine serum albumin (No. A4378, Sigma Chemical Co., St. Louis, Missouri) or rabbit serum albumin (No. A3635, Sigma Chemical Co.).

ECDI;   1-ethyl-3-(3-dimethylaminopropyl)carbodiimide-HCl (Story Chemical Co., Muskegon, Michigan).

ii. Procedure. The albumin is purified by gel filtration on a 5×90 cm Sephadex G-100 resin (Pharmacia Fine Chemicals, Piscataway, New Jersey), equilibrated and developed with 0.1 M ammonium acetate buffer, pH 7.4. The albumin peak is lyophilized, redissolved in distilled water, and is again lyophilized to remove all traces of ammonium acetate. The chromatographically pure bovine serum albumin (BSA) is dissolved in distilled water, and the pH is adjusted to 7.2 with 0.1 N NaOH (36 mg BSA plus 1.1 ml H_2O and 0.1 ml NaOH). The ECDI coupling reagent is dissolved in distilled water (225 mg ECDI per 0.5 ml H_2O). The 1–24-ACTH is dissolved in 0.0001 N HCl (8.5 mg α^{1-24}-ACTH per 0.6 ml HCl).

The coupling procedure is performed at room temperature in

12 × 75 mm polypropylene tubes (No. 2053, Falcon Plastics, Oxnard, California). Two tubes, each containing 0.5 ml BSA and 0.2 ml ECDI solution (15 mg BSA and 90 mg ECDI), are prepared. To the first is added α^{1-24}-ACTH in acid solution, and to the second, which serves as a control to assess the yield, is added 0.0001 N HCl alone. Volumes of 0.1 ml ACTH solution or acid alone are added at five-minute intervals, and the tubes are agitated on a mixer (Ames Co., Division of Miles Laboratories, Inc., Elkhart, Indiana) between each addition. After the fifth addition, the tubes are agitated continuously for 30 minutes. The unused BSA and ACTH solutions are later used in estimating yield. The reaction mixture remains clear throughout and has a pH of 6.8–7.0 at the completion of the conjugation procedure.

Removal of excess coupling reagent and estimation of yield are accomplished by gel filtration on Sephadex G-50 fine resin. The control mixture, to which no ACTH was added, is diluted with an equal volume of distilled water and applied to a 1.6 × 32 cm Sephadex column which has been equilibrated with 154 mM NaCl at 4°C. The mixture is eluted with 154 mM NaCl by descending flow at 40 cm of hydrostatic pressure and a flow rate of 13 ml per hour; 2.0-ml fractions are collected. After three hours, the flow is interrupted briefly while the contents of the reaction tube containing ACTH are similarly applied to the column. Elution is then continued for another five hours or more.

Estimation of yield is based on the assumption that tryptophan ultraviolet fluorescence (283 nm excitation; 350 nm emission) of the BSA will increase in proportion to the amount of α^{1-24}-ACTH coupled, since the hormone contains one tryptophan residue. The fluorescence of fractions from the control reaction (0.1-ml aliquots of fractions 13–18 are diluted with 1.4 ml 154 mM NaCl) is measured using an Aminco-Bowman spectrophotofluorometer (Figure 2, lower curve). Native fluorescence of BSA is directly proportional to concentration over a range of 0–200 μg per ml. Consequently, the original BSA solution is diluted to 50 and 200 μg per ml with 154 mM NaCl. When the fluorescence in the fractions is related to that of the original BSA solution, it is found that 70.0% (10.5 mg; 0.162 μmole) is recovered in fractions 13–18. The fluorescence of the fractions from the ACTH reaction is similarly recorded (Figure 2, upper curve), with 0.1-ml aliquots of fractions 13–30 diluted with 1.4 ml 154 mM NaCl. When the difference in the fluorescence of the two curves is related to that of the original ACTH solution (diluted to 25 and 100 μg per ml with 154 mM NaCl), one finds that 84.7% of the 2.48 μmole added to the reaction vessel is recovered. The first peak in the upper curve (fractions 13–18, Figure 2) represents the ACTH–BSA conjugate and contains 4.00 mg

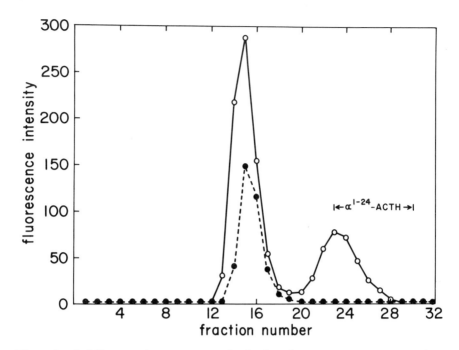

Figure 2. Gel filtration elution patterns of carbodiimide conjugation reaction products. (●---●) elution pattern of a mixture that contained 0.23 μmole bovine serum albumin (BSA) alone. (○---○) contained 0.23 μmole BSA and 2.48 μmole synthetic α^{1-24}-ACTH. The first peak is in the void volume of the column and represents BSA polymers (●---●) and α^{1-24}-ACTH–BSA conjugates (○---○), 8.6 moles α^{1-24}-ACTH per mole BSA. The second peak represents α^{1-24}-ACTH polymers. The elution volume of α^{1-24}-ACTH monomer is indicated. Sephadex G-50 fine resin, 1.6 × 32 cm column, 154 mM NaCl eluant, 13 ml/hr flow rate at 4°C, 2.0-ml fractions. Tryptophan fluorescence intensity (excitation 283 nm, emission 350 mm) is represented on an arbitrary scale.

(1.40 μmole) of ACTH. Thus, the estimated yield of conjugation is 8.6 moles of α^{1-24}-ACTH per mole of BSA.

The second peak represents polymerized α^{1-24}-ACTH, since experiments in which α^{1-24}-ACTH is coupled in the absence of BSA yield a major peak in this area. The elution volume of α^{1-24}-ACTH monomer is indicated in Figure 2. The region represented by tubes 19–30 accounts for 28.2% (2.0 mg; 0.70 μmole) of the ACTH added to the reaction vessel. Attempts to diminish further the percent of unreacted polymerized hapten results in a decreased yield of the conjugate. The α^{1-24}-ACTH–BSA conjugate (pooled fractions 13–18) is stored at 4°C until used for immunization.

Performing the procedure under the conditions described by

McGuire *et al.* (1965) results almost exclusively in the formation of polymers of the polypeptide hormone hapten. The BSA in these reactions is also almost completely polymerized, as can be shown by gel filtration on Sephadex G-100. Since these polymers dialyze poorly, if at all, simple amino acid analysis of the contents of the dialysis bag might be interpreted as demonstrating conjugation of the hapten to BSA (Goodfriend *et al.*, 1964). In fact, it represents the combined amino acid composition of the largely polymerized albumin and the polymerized polypeptides. It is not at all clear, of course, that polymerized polypeptides are inferior to conjugated ones in terms of immunogenicity, since useful antisera have been produced by conjugates produced in this manner.

b. **Glutaraldehyde** (C. D. Mount and D. N. Orth, unpublished data)

i. *Reagents*

α^{1-24}-ACTH (Cortrosyn) or other ACTH preparation.

Bovine serum albumin or rabbit serum albumin (Sigma).

Glutaraldehyde (No. G5882, Sigma Chemical Co., St. Louis, Missouri).

ii. *Procedure.* The albumin is purified, as mentioned above, by gel exclusion chromatography on a 5×90 cm Sephadex G-100 (Pharmacia) column in $0.1\,M$ ammonium acetate buffer, pH 7.4. The albumin peak is lyophilized, redissolved in distilled water, and again lyophilized to remove traces of ammonium acetate. The glutaraldehyde, unless highly purified and fresh, contains impurities, probably including glutaric acid and polymers (Gillet and Gull, 1972). This can easily be detected, since the pH of pure glutaraldehyde is 7.0–7.1; when contaminated with glutaric acid, the pH falls to much lower values. Immediately prior to use, the glutaraldehyde is purified as described by these authors [extraction of 25% glutaraldehyde two to three times with 10% (w/v) activated charcoal by shaking at 4°C for 60 minutes followed by filtration] and is stored at $-20°$C.

In a 12×75 mm polypropylene tube (No. 2053, Falcon Plastics, Oxnard, California), 0.15 μmole (10 mg) albumin is dissolved in 1.0 ml 0.1 M phosphate buffer, pH 7.0. In a similar tube, 4.2 μmole (11.4 mg) α^{1-24}-ACTH are dissolved in 0.3 ml of the same buffer containing a tracer quantity (10,000 cpm, 5–15 pg) of ^{125}I-labeled α^{1-24}-ACTH. To the albumin solution is added, dropwise and with constant stirring, 0.1 ml 21 μM glutaraldehyde in water. Ten minutes later, 0.25 ml of the ACTH solution is added with constant stirring. After ten minutes, another 0.1 ml glutaraldehyde solution is added dropwise with constant stirring; this is repeated a last time after another ten minutes. After 20–30 minutes of constant stirring, the entire reaction mixture is loaded on a 1.6×30 cm column of Sephadex G-50 fine resin, developed and eluted with $0.154\,M$ NaCl at a rate of 10 ml/hour; 20-minute fractions are collected. Percentage conjugation is calculated by comparing OD_{280} and ^{125}I cpm in the conjugate and unreacted α^{1-24}-ACTH peaks. Typically, 15–25% of hapten is coupled to BSA. Thus, the estimated ratio is 3.5–6.0 moles of α^{1-24}-ACTH per mole of BSA. Polymerized α^{1-24}-ACTH is also produced under these conditions. The use of higher concentrations of glutaraldehyde produces a heavy precipitate. The dialyzed conjugate is stored at 4°C in aliquots. This is enough material to immunize several animals.

3. Immunization

Saline containing an appropriate quantity of the dissolved antigen is sterilized by passage through a 0.22-μm Millipore filter and mixed with an equal volume of sterile adjuvant. We have used complete Freund's adjuvant (Difco), modified Perrin's adjuvant (Calbiochem), and complete Freund's adjuvant fortified with $M.$ $tuberculosis$ protein (Difco) (Vaitukaitis et al., 1971); all of these appear to be satisfactory. The antigen solution must be completely emulsified in the adjuvant, a time-consuming process requiring repeated aspiration and expulsion of the mixture through a 20-gauge needle attached to a sterile syringe or forcing the mixture from one sterile syringe to another through a female–female Luer-Lok connector. Other methods can be used (sonication, stirring with a Teflon pestle against the wall of a tube, or hand stirring, for example), but sterility can hardly be maintained, and the antigen cannot be filter-sterilized once it is emulsified. Infection is a considerable problem; it seems worthwhile to minimize it. Satisfactory emulsification has been achieved when a drop of the mixture will remain intact and spherical when dropped onto water.

The animal is injected with 50–200 μg of the hapten (total protein-plus-hapten injected depends upon the efficiency of the coupling procedure) intradermally between the shoulders in twenty or more sites, 0.05–0.1 ml per site. Injections into the weight-bearing hindfoot pads of rabbits cause great discomfort, usually become infected, and should be avoided. We usually inject 0.5 ml of $H.$ $pertussis$ vaccine at the same time in multiple intradermal sites in a different lymphatic drainage area as a nonspecific stimulus to the immune system (Vaitukaitis et al., 1971). Two to three weeks later, blood is obtained to test for titer and sensitivity. In general, animals that have no detectable antibodies are not immunized further. If a satisfactory titer and sensitivity are found, the animal can be bled repeatedly every four to eight weeks as long as the titer persists. If the titer is unsatisfactory, a booster dose of 5.0–20 μg of hapten in complete adjuvant is given in multiple intradermal sites in the same area the original dose was given. Blood is obtained 7–14 days later to assess titer. If satisfactory, the animal is bled within two to three weeks of the booster injection (30–40 ml per rabbit, 180–240 ml per sheep). Five consecutive animals (three rabbits, two sheep) have yielded highly sensitive ACTH antisera with working titers of 1 : 80,000 to 1 : 200,000. The animals can be boosted with 5.0–20 μg of hapten whenever the titer falls to unsatisfactory levels and bled every four to eight weeks as long as useful titers persist.

The rationale for the administration of low-dose antigen administration is to provide a threshold dose of antigen, but only enough to elicit blastogenic transformation of those few B cells that have very high affinity immunoglobulin receptors displayed on their surface (Edelman, 1973) and are thus able to capture the antigen. Subsequent boosters are designed only to restimulate the daughter cells of this clone, not to elicit lower affinity antibody production by other B cell clones.

4. Preparation of Antisera

The antiserum is actually plasma obtained by centrifuging lightly-heparinized blood at 1000 g, aspirating the plasma, and recentrifuging it at 6000 g for ten minutes to remove additional formed blood elements. Merthiolate (0.1 mg/ml) is added and the plasma is stored in aliquots at $-70°$C. Repeated freezing and thawing are deleterious to some antisera; we avoid it.

In order to simplify and standardize the process of setting up assays, appropriate volumes of antiserum diluted 1 : 100 in 0.05 M phosphate buffer (pH 7.6) containing 0.01% Merthiolate are accurately pipetted into several dozen 12 × 75 mm polypropylene tubes (No. 2053, Falcon Plastics, Oxnard, California) and stored at $-70°$C. A tube is thawed only once, immediately prior to each assay, and the antiserum aliquot is diluted with the same volume of buffer to achieve the desired final antibody dilution.

Even with these precautions, antisera may deteriorate with prolonged storage. We found that one antiserum, stored undiluted in multiple aliquots with 0.01% merthiolate at $-70°$C for four years without thawing, lost almost 80% of its titer and retained only one-fifth of its original sensitivity. Lyophilized antisera may be more stable during prolonged storage; we are currently testing this possibility.

C. Characterization of Antibody

Three properties of antisera must be defined: titer, sensitivity, and specificity. We usually find it necessary to incubate three to six days at 4°C for maximal sensitivity and precision. Therefore, we incubate tenfold serial dilutions of the antiserum (1 : 1000 to 1 : 1,000,000) for six days with trace quantities of ^{125}I-labeled hormone. The effective working titer binds 30–35% of tracer.

Titer alone cannot reliably predict radioimmunoassay sensitivity, of course, since it reflects both binding affinity and molar concentration of antibodies. Since one must be capable of measuring 5.0 pg/ml or less ACTH to assay normal plasma, sensitivity is assessed by adding graded quantities (1.0, 10, and 100 pg/ml) of unlabeled standard human ACTH to the incubation mixtures. Actually, we determine both titer and sensitivity of an antiserum simultaneously by setting up one incubation that includes several dilutions of antiserum and three graded doses of unlabeled standard at each dilution. While slight interpolation may be necessary to achieve optimal binding, one has a complete empirical definition of the system in one week.

Specificity must next be considered. Only one limited aspect of antiserum specificity need be considered, although others must be evaluated in antisera to be used for immunohistologic staining or affinity chromatography, for example. Thus, only the specificity of the antibodies in the antiserum that bind labeled tracer are relevant for the purposes of radioimmunoassay. If partially purified ACTH is used for immunization, antibodies to contaminating polypeptides may be produced. However, if they do not bind labeled ACTH, they are of no importance to the sensitivity or specificity of the radioimmunoassay *if* the radioiodinated ACTH tracer does not contain these contaminants. This is the reason that purity of the labeled hormone is so essential.

Characterization of ACTH antisera should include (1) definition of the portion of the ACTH molecule to which antibodies are directed and (2) cross-reactivity with α-MSH and, particularly, with γ-LPH and β-LPH, since these two human hormones possess a common heptapeptide sequence with ACTH (Chapter 13) and are secreted in parallel with it (Tanaka *et al.*, 1977).

Specificity studies obviously depend on availability of ACTH analogs for testing. A whole series of such synthetic analogs has been produced by the chemists of Ciba-Geigy, Ltd. A partial list of these includes: α-MSH (N-acetyl-$\alpha^{1-13\mathrm{NH}_2}$-ACTH), β_b-MSH, β_h-MSH, β_h-MSH-Met^{11} sulfoxide, α^{1-10}-ACTH, $\alpha^{7-13\mathrm{NH}_2}$-ACTH, $\alpha^{1-16\mathrm{NH}_2}$-ACTH, α^{1-23}-ACTH, N-acetyl-α^{1-24}-ACTH, α^{1-24}-ACTH, α^{11-24}-ACTH, α_p^{17-39}-ACTH,

$\alpha_\mathrm{p}{}^{25-39}$-ACTH, $\alpha_\mathrm{h}{}^{25-39}$-ACTH, $\alpha_\mathrm{p}{}^{1-39}$-ACTH, and $\alpha_\mathrm{h}{}^{1-39}$-ACTH. Hofmann and his co-workers at the University of Pittsburgh have also synthesized a number of analogs, including $\alpha^{1-13\mathrm{NH}_2}$-ACTH, α^{4-10}-ACTH, $\alpha^{6-13\mathrm{NH}_2}$-ACTH, α^{1-16}-ACTH, $\alpha^{1-20\mathrm{NH}_2}$-ACTH, and α^{1-19}-ACTH. Li's group at the Hormone Research Laboratories have synthesized, among others, α^{1-17}-ACTH, $\alpha^{1-17\mathrm{NH}_2}$-ACTH, $\alpha^{1-18\mathrm{NH}_2}$-ACTH, $\alpha^{1-19\mathrm{NH}_2}$-ACTH, $\alpha_\mathrm{b}{}^{1-26}$-ACTH, and $\alpha_\mathrm{h}{}^{1-39}$-ACTH. The laboratories of Sandoz and Ciba-Geigy have also produced synthetic ACTH analogs with substitutions in the 1-Ser, 4-Met, and 17,18-Arg–Arg positions. A number of these analogs are available. Thus, a rather detailed study of specificity is possible.

Competitive binding curves generated by a variety of ACTH analogs in four ACTH radioimmunoassay systems are shown in Figures 3–6. Highly purified human ACTH [Lerner-Upton-Lande 8B; 100 IU/mg, assuming 1.5 intravenous IU per ampoule of Third Inter-

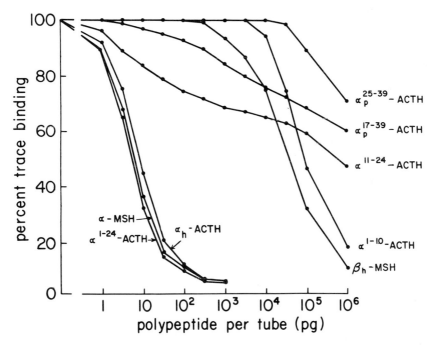

Figure 3. Specificity of the extreme N-terminal antibody (Fred 699). The percent of trace binding (the amount of labeled ACTH bound in the absence added unlabeled polypeptide) is plotted on the ordinate; the picograms of unlabeled polypeptide added per tube is plotted on the abscissa on a logarithmic scale. The competitive binding curves generated by the addition of graded amounts of a variety of unlabeled ACTH and MSH analogs are shown. The antibody reacts fully with any polypeptide containing the 1–13 sequence of amino acids of ACTH.

national Standard for Corticotropin (Bangham *et al.*, 1962)] or synthetic α_n^{1-39}-ACTH (Ciba-Geigy, Ltd.; Nicholson *et al.*, 1976a) were used as the ^{125}I-labeled tracer. The first antiserum (Fred 699) (Figure 3) was the gift of Drs. L. H. Rees, D. M. Cook, and J. W. Kendall (University of Oregon, Portland, Oregon), who injected a rabbit with α^{1-24}-ACTH (Organon) conjugated to rabbit serum albumin by the carbodiimide reaction. It is directed at the extreme N-terminal portion of the ACTH molecule and reacts with all polypeptides possessing the 1–13 sequence; the 1–10 sequence is not sufficient for full reactivity. Acetylation of the position 1 Ser residue, as in α-MSH, does not reduce immunoreactivity. Thus, this rather sensitive antibody appears to be directed at the N-terminal 11–13 amino acid segment of ACTH; it cannot distinguish between ACTH and α-MSH, but cross-reactivity with β-MSH (γ-LPH and β-LPH) is of no practical importance.

The antiserum (G-90) shown in Figure 4 that was raised in a guinea pig with commercial zinc-porcine ACTH (Organon) requires an extended N-terminal sequence for full reactivity. Analogs containing the intact 1–23 sequence are fully immunoreactive, yet none of the available subunits completely displaces labeled α-ACTH from the

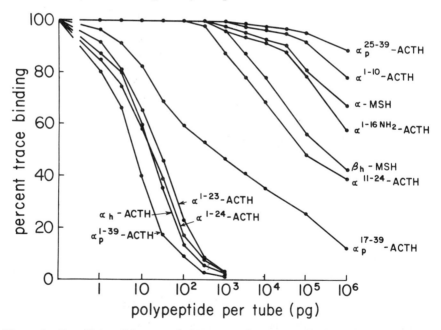

Figure 4. Specificity of the extended N-terminal ACTH antibody (G-90). The data are plotted in a manner identical to Figure 3. This antibody reacts fully with any polypeptide containing the 1–23 sequence of ACTH.

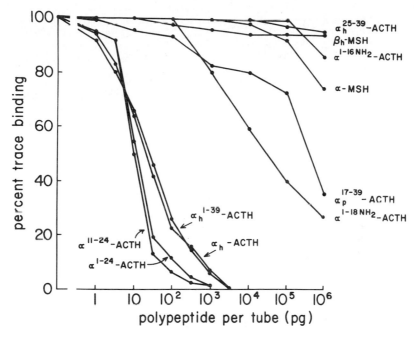

Figure 5. Specificity of the central ACTH antibody (S1B2). The data are plotted in a manner identical to Figure 3. This antibody reacts fully with any polypeptide containing the 11–24 sequence of ACTH and binds more tightly those possessing a free carboxyl-terminal 24-position prolyl residue.

antibodies. Analogs with 1-position Ser and 4-position Met substitutions are fully reactive, suggesting that the 1–4 sequence is not critical. However, the limitations of this approach are exposed by the reactivity of $\alpha_p{}^{17-39}$-ACTH; although its curve is nonparallel, indicating immunochemical nonidentity, it nevertheless causes much greater displacement than α^{11-24}-ACTH, which contains the entire sequence that $\alpha_p{}^{17-39}$-ACTH shares with α^{1-24}-ACTH. Thus, additional factors, such as total chain length and secondary structure, may be involved in binding affinity.

The third antiserum (S1B2, Figure 5) was raised in a sheep by injections of α^{1-24}-ACTH conjugated to bovine serum albumin by the carbodiimide reaction and contains antibodies directed toward the central 11–24 sequence. Interestingly, a free 24-position prolyl carboxyl terminus appears to result in a greater binding affinity, since both α^{1-24}-ACTH and α^{11-24}-ACTH have steeper competitive binding curves than $\alpha_h{}^{1-39}$-ACTH. For routine radioimmunoassay purposes, however, this is of no importance.

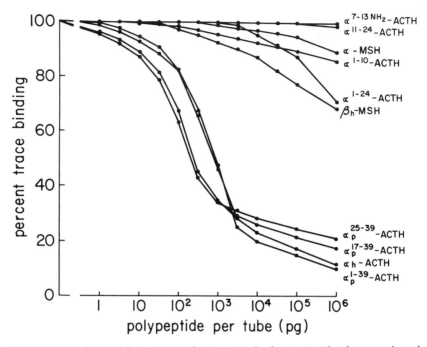

Figure 6. Specificity of the C-terminal ACTH antibody (R-12). The data are plotted in a manner identical to Figure 3. This antibody reacts fully with any polypeptide containing the 25–39 sequence of human or porcine ACTH, which differ only in position 31 (Table I).

The fourth antiserum (R-12, Figure 6) was raised in a rabbit by injections of partially purified human ACTH (Dr. Maurice Raben, 22 IU/mg) and contains antibodies to the C-terminal 25–39 sequence. A second population of antibodies, directed toward the 1–24 sequence, is manifested by the incomplete displacement of labeled ACTH with C-terminal fragments. Complete displacement can be achieved by further addition of small quantities of α^{1-24}-ACTH. Cross-reactions with α-MSH and β-MSH (γ-LPH and β-LPH) present no practical problem.

For clinical purposes, an antibody similar in specificity to those in Figures 4 or 6 that does not cross-react significantly with α-MSH or the LPH's (represented by the shared sequence in β-MSH) should be most satisfactory. An antiserum with these characteristics has been produced by Dr. Charles D. West of Salt Lake City by injecting a rabbit with Duracton (ACTH absorbed to carboxymethyl cellulose; Nordic Pharmaceuticals, Ltd., Laval, Quebec, Canada). The antibody reacts with the 11–24 sequence of ACTH and has only about 0.4% cross-reactivity with α-MSH and β-MSH (γ-LPH and β-LPH). Dr. West has given large quantities of this material to the National Pituitary Agency. Aliquots have been lyophilized for the Agency by Dr. Alfred E. Wilhelmi and are available to qualified investigators from the National Pituitary Agency or the Hormone Distribution Officer, NIAMDD.*

D. Radioiodination of ACTH

The procedure is a modification of the method of Hunter and Greenwood (1962) and is carried out in a shielded radioactive hood at 20°–23°C. Although there is less iodination damage at 4°C, the reaction takes about eight times longer. All reagents are freshly prepared just before iodination.

1. Reagents

Highly purified human ACTH (Lerner-Upton-Lande 8B) or synthetic α^{1-39}-ACTH (Ciba-Geigy, Ltd.; Nicholson *et al.*, 1976a), both provided by the National Pituitary Agency.

$Na^{125}I$ (Iso-Serve Division, Cambridge Nuclear Corp., Cambridge, Massachusetts, or Amersham-Searle, Arlington Heights, Illinois)

Chloramine-T (No. 1022, Eastman Organic Chemicals, Rochester, New York)

Sodium metabisulfite (No. 3552, J. T. Baker Chemical Co., Phillipsburg, New Jersey)

Bovine serum albumin (No. A4378, Sigma Chemical Co.)

Potassium iodide (No. 3164, J. T. Baker Chemical Co.)

Sodium phosphate dibasic, heptahydrate (No. 74243, Merck and Co., Inc., Rahway, New Jersey).

Potassium phosphate monobasic, anhydrous (No. 73351, Merck and Co., Inc., Rahway, New Jersey)

2. Procedure

Aliquots (2 μl) of 0.005 N HCl containing 2.0 μg ACTH are pipetted into 3-ml conical centrifuge tubes (No. 41000, borosilicate, Kontes Glass Corp., Vineland, New Jersey), are stored at $-70°C$, and thawed once just prior to iodination. The following are added successively, each with a calibrated disposable micropipette (Clay-Adams) and mixed by bubbling gently through the pipette after each addition: 20 μl of 0.5 M

* National Pituitary Agency, Suite 503, 210 W. Fayette St., Baltimore, Maryland 21201. Hormone Distribution Officer, NIAMDD, National Institutes of Health, Bethesda, Maryland 20014.

Sörenson's phosphate buffer, pH 7.5, 2.0 mCi (2.0–3.0 μl) Na^{125}I, 10 μl chloramine-T, 2.5 mg per ml 0.05 M Sörenson's phosphate buffer, pH 7.5, 20 μl sodium metabisulfite, 2.5 mg per ml 0.05 M phosphate buffer, pH 7.5, and 10 μl 10% aqueous KI. The reaction mixture is bubbled for only a few seconds after addition of each reagent and for 30 seconds after the addition of chloramine-T.

The whole iodination mixture is transferred immediately to a 0.9 × 55 cm column of Sephadex G-50 fine gel (Pharmacia), equilibrated and developed with 0.154 M NaCl in 0.005 M HCl, pH 2.5, at room temperature. The column is eluted by gravity flow, 55 cm hydrostatic pressure; 0.5-ml fractions are collected in 12 × 75 mm polypropylene tubes (No. 2053, Falcon Plastics) to which two drops (50 μl) BSA, 25 mg/ml in distilled water, have been added. The ^{125}I cpm in 5-μl aliquots of the fractions are counted in a gamma scintillation spectrometer (No. MS-588, Micromedic Systems, Inc., Philadelphia, Pennsylvania). The central portion of the monomeric, ^{125}I-labeled 1–39-ACTH peak ($V_e/V_0 = 1.95$) is pooled and appropriate aliquots [(3 to 4) × (the total number of ^{125}I cpm required for a typical radioimmunoassay)] are frozen at −70°C. The column is purged with 1.0 ml BSA, 25 mg/ml in water, and can be reused for many months.

Immediately prior to each assay, the ^{125}I-labeled ACTH is repurified on the same column, which is presaturated with another 1.0 ml BSA solution just before applying the labeled hormone. An elution profile is obtained as described above, and the monomeric ^{125}I-ACTH fractions are pooled, diluted appropriately with standard diluent, and used directly in the radioimmunoassay. Specific activity is estimated from the elution profile of the iodination mixture:

$$\text{Specific activity} = (^{125}\text{I}_{\text{total}} \times {}^{125}\text{I}_{\text{ACTH}})/\mu\text{g ACTH}$$

where $^{125}\text{I}_{\text{total}}$ equals μCi ^{125}I added to the reaction tube, $^{125}\text{I}_{\text{ACTH}}$ equals percent total radioactivity in the column eluate in the monomeric ACTH peak, and μg ACTH equals μg ACTH added to the reaction tube. Specific activities of 100–275 μCi/μg are usually satisfactory; 85–90% of labeled hormone will be bound by excess antibody. When specific activities of greater than 400 μCi/μg were obtained, immunoreactivity was decreased.

E. Preparation of Samples for Assay

We shall consider three types of samples for assay: (1) standards, analogs, and other relatively pure preparations, such as fractions from gel filtration columns; (2) plasma extracts; and (3) tissue extracts. In the first edition of this volume, the use of unextracted plasma was described (Orth, 1974). Since that time, however, we have found that plasma samples not infrequently produce major artifacts in the ACTH radioimmunoassay. They can either interfere with binding, resulting in a factitiously high RIA-ACTH value, or cause incubation damage, which may result in either a falsely high or low value, depending upon the separation method. This has been observed with three different antisera and with both polyethylene glycol (Desbuquois and Aurbach, 1971) and QUSO-plasma (Orth *et al.*, 1976) separation. These artifacts will not be detected unless unknowns are assayed at multiple dilutions.

1. Standards, Analogs, and Column Fractions

Standards and other pure or relatively pure compounds are made up in stock solutions in 0.001 N HCl if their concentrations are 500 μg/ml or greater. If less, they are diluted in acidified human albumin solution (Abe *et al.*, 1967a). This is prepared by dissolving 1.0 gm human serum albumin (No. 1702, Schwarz/Mann; defatted, recrystallized, and dialyzed) per liter of water and adjusting the pH to 3.0 with 20% HCl. The biologic and immunologic activities of ACTH are stable at pH less than 3.5, and ACTH, when absorbed to glassware, can be recovered with acid. At very low concentrations, however, acidification alone will not prevent significant absorption; albumin is added as a carrier for this reason. These and other types of samples are stored, in aliquots to be thawed only once, at −70°C.

2. Extracted Plasma

Plasma is prepared by first obtaining a sample of blood atraumatically in a lightly heparinized plastic syringe. It has been reported that high concentrations of heparin may interfere with antigen–antibody binding. We find that if the final concentration in the incubation is less than 3.6 U/ml, no decrease in binding is observed. We have also used sodium EDTA as anticoagulant; however, concentrations greater than 1.0 mM may also interfere with binding (D. N. Orth, unpublished data). If Vacutainer EDTA or heparin tubes are used, they must be completely filled with blood to avoid too high EDTA or heparin concentrations. The syringe is immediately placed in an ice bucket. The blood is gently expelled into a plastic tube and is centrifuged for 15 minutes at 1000 to 1500 g at 4°C. The supernate is then carefully aspirated, transferred to another plastic tube, and recentrifuged at 6000 g at 4°C for another ten minutes. This second centrifugation is very important in reducing incubation damage; it removes additional formed elements which, if frozen and then thawed for assay, apparently are ruptured and release enzymes that damage labeled and unlabeled ACTH (Besser *et al.*, 1971). The 6000 *g* plasma is decanted from the tube, taking care not to disturb the pellet, and aliquots are stored at −70°C.

Recently, it has been reported that ACTH immunoreactivity can be preserved in heparinized plasma, obtained by centrifugation of blood at 2500 *g*, by the addition of 0.01 *M* N-ethyl maleimide (NEM) (Hogan *et al.*, 1976). This agent, which alkylates cysteine sulfhydryl groups in the catalytic site of some proteolytic enzymes, completely inhibited the loss of endogenous RIA-ACTH in nonhemolyzed plasma at room temperature for as long as 72 hours, and from hemolyzed plasma under the same conditions for up to 48 hours. These authors use the extreme N-terminal antibody characterized here (Figure 3); it needs to be tested with other antisera with other specificities. However, NEM may prove to be of considerable value in preserving the ACTH in plasma and in preventing incubation damage.

In the previous edition (Orth, 1974), the use of the cationic exchange resin Amberlite CG-50 (Rohm and Haas, Philadelphia, Pennsylvania) for extracting ACTH from plasma was described. This is still a valid method, and is described below for extraction from tissue, but we now routinely use a modification of the much more rapid silicic acid extraction procedure (Donald, 1967; Orth and Woodham, 1969; Orth *et al.*, 1976).

a. **Materials**

Silicic acid (No. 2847, 100 mesh, Lot No. TBM-A, Mallinckrodt Chemical Works, St. Louis, Missouri)

Repipet (No. 3005-A-U, Labindustries, Berkeley, California) Acetone, spectrophotometric grade (No. 2348, Mallinckrodt Chemical Works)

Sodium phosphate dibasic, heptahydrate (No. 74243, Merck and Co., Inc., Rahway, New Jersey)

Potassium phosphate monobasic, anhydrous (No. 73351, Merck and Co., Inc., Rahway, New Jersey)

Merthiolate (Thiomersol powder, N. F., Eli Lilly and Co., Indianapolis, Indiana)

Biopette (No. 0010-29, Schwarz/Mann, Orangeburg, New York)

Aliquot mixer (Model No. 4651, Ames Co., Elkhart, Indiana)

b. **Procedure.** With a volumetric pipette, 2.0 ml of plasma sample is transferred to a 12 × 75 mm polypropylene tube (No. 2053, Falcon

Plastics). A Biopette is used to transfer 1.0 ml of a suspension of 200 mg silicic acid per ml 0.05 M phosphate buffer, pH 7.5, containing 0.077 M NaCl and 0.1 mg/ml Merthiolate from a beaker in which the suspension is constantly stirred with a magnetic stirring bar. The tubes are capped and mixed for 30 minutes at room temperature on the aliquot mixer. The tubes are then centrifuged at 3000 g for five minutes, and the supernates are decanted and the tubes blotted. The silicic acid pellets are washed twice with 2.5 ml distilled water, recentrifuged, and the supernates are decanted and discarded. A 2.5-ml volume of glacial acetic acid–acetone–water (1 : 20 : 80 by volume) is added with a 5.0 ml Repipet (Labindustries) and mixed for 30 minutes at room temperature on the aliquot mixer. The tubes are centrifuged at 3000 g for five minutes, and the supernates are decanted into another 12 × 75 mm polypropylene tube which is capped with a pierced polypropylene cap. Twenty-four tubes are placed in a 600-ml lyophilization flask (Virtis Co., Gardiner, New York), enough water to cover the lower half of the tubes is introduced, and the whole flask is frozen in methanol–dry ice or in a −80°C freezer. Approximately 1.0 ml distilled water is then introduced into each tube through the pierced caps with a Teflon delivery tip attached to a Repipet and frozen. Alternatively, the acetone can be blown off with dry nitrogen gas before freezing, which obviates the need for a water layer. The contents are lyophilized (Model No. 10-145-MR-BA, Virtis Co.), and the lyophilized samples are stored at −70°C until assayed.

For each assay, plasma specimens containing known concentrations of added synthetic α^{1-39}-ACTH are similarly extracted. These are used to construct the standard curve and to correct for losses of ACTH in the extraction procedure. Standard diluent solutions containing the same concentrations of added standard ACTH are assayed to quantitate the percent recovery for each extraction. In addition, specimens from two plasma pools containing high and low levels of endogenous hormone are extracted and included as internal standards.

Other methods based on adsorption to silicates and elution with acetic acid–acetone (Rees et al., 1971; Ratcliffe and Edwards, 1971) or methanol–ammonia (Landon and Greenwood, 1968) have been described.

3. Extracted Tissues

Tissue ACTH obviously must be extracted for radioimmunoassay. The tissues must either be extracted immediately or frozen directly, since ACTH cannot be extracted from formalin-fixed tissue.

a. Materials

Tissue homogenizer (Polytron, No. 2701, Brinkmann Instruments, Westburg, New York; or Tissumizer, No. SDT 182, Tekmar Co., Cincinnati, Ohio)

Rotating flash evaporator (Buchler Instruments Division, Fort Lee, New Jersey)

Borosilicate glass columns (No. K-420280, 10.5 mm I.D., 200 ml, Kontes Glass Co., Vineland, New Jersey)

Amberlite CG-50 resin (Rohm and Haas, Philadelphia, Pennsylvania)

Acetone, spectrophotometric grade (No. 2438, Mallinckrodt Chemical Works, St. Louis, Missouri)

b. Procedure. The fresh or unthawed frozen tissue is homogenized in ice-cold buffer or water, 9.0 ml/gm of wet tissue. We have recently evaluated the relative extraction efficiency of $0.1\,M$ ammonium acetate buffer, pH 7.0, and glacial acetic acid for ACTH. The results on a single fresh frozen human pituitary are tabulated below.

Extraction medium	Heated to 90°C	RIA-ACTH (μg/gm)	BIO-ACTH[a] (μg/gm)
Acetate buffer	No	364	278
Acetate buffer	Yes	282	389
Glacial acetic acid	No	860	966
Glacial acetic acid	Yes	1,010	642

[a] 1.0 μg = 100 mU of ACTH, assuming that the Third International Standard for Corticotropin has 1.5 intravenous I.U. per ampoule (Bangham *et al.*, 1962).

Although acetic acid is more efficient, it also extracts relatively more protein and is a more difficult procedure. We usually extract with water or buffer; the acetic acid extraction method is detailed, for those who are interested, in the first edition of this volume (Orth, 1974).

Three or four successive 30-second homogenizations in water or buffer at 4°C are sufficient. The homogenates are then rapidly heated at 90°C and maintained at 90°C for 10 minutes to inactivate proteolytic enzymes in the extract. The tubes are centrifuged at 50,000 g at 4°C for 20 minutes, and aliquots of the supernates are stored at −70°C.

In the case of pituitary extracts, in which ACTH concentration may be expected to be very high, further purification is unnecessary. In the case of nonpituitary tissue, ACTH concentrations are far lower (Abe *et al.*, 1967a,b; Orth *et al.*, 1968, 1973a; Ratcliffe *et al.*, 1972) and further purification is usually required. For this purpose, we use ion-exchange chromatography. The CG-50 cationic exchange resin is processed according to the method of Hirs *et al.* (1953), after which it is washed successively with 50% acetic acid, 2.0 N HCl, and 5% acetic acid (Island *et al.*, 1965). This can be done as a large-batch procedure; the resin can be stored in 5% acetic acid at 4°C for many months. The water extract of tissue is stirred with four volumes of acetone–12 N HCl (40:1) for 15 minutes at 4°C (Bornstein and Trewhella, 1950). The tube is centrifuged at 2000 g at 4°C for ten minutes, and the supernate is aspirated. The volume of the supernate is reduced to approximately the original water extract volume by washing twice for three minutes with ice-cold diethyl ether, six and four times the original extract volume, respectively, to remove the acetone (Yalow *et al.*, 1964). The acetone–ether phase is diluted 25-fold with cold 1% acetic acid, and the pH is adjusted to 3 with 5.0 N NaOH. The CG-50 resin, 3.0 cm³ packed resin per gram of wet tissue, is packed by gravity flow so that the height:diameter ratio of the column is greater than 5. The diameter of the column is selected on the basis of the amount of resin to be used. For less than 1.7 gm of tissue, the 10.5-mm inner diameter column is packed to 5.25 cm; the increased resin-to-tissue ratio does not affect recovery. The diluted tissue extract is passed through the column at 5.0 ml/cm² cross-sectional area per minute, but not exceeding 10 ml/minute, at 4°C. Flow rate is regulated with the Teflon stopcock and assisted with slight positive nitrogen pressure, if necessary. Salts and proteins are washed from the column with 5% acetic acid (3.0 ml/cm³ of resin), and the ACTH is eluted with the same volume of 50% acetic acid at 1.5 ml/cm² cross-sectional area per minute, but no faster than 10 ml/minute, at 25°C. The eluate is evaporated to dryness in a rotating flash evaporator at 40°C, and the residual acetic acid is dispelled with a stream of nitrogen. The extract is reconstituted in a small volume of 0.001 N HCl, the pH is adjusted to 3 with 0.1 N HCl, and insoluble material is removed by centrifugation at 2000 g at 4°C for ten minutes. Aliquots are stored at −70°C. Extracts equivalent to 10 gm of original tissue per milliliter can be prepared; recovery is approximately 80%.

In every case, aliquots of standards, plasmas, or plasma and tissue extracts are frozen and thawed to 4°C only once, immediately prior to assay. Repeated freeze-thawing of ACTH results in progressive, significant loss in bioactivity and immunoreactivity. The amount of extract that one wishes to add to the radioimmunoassay depends upon the concentration of ACTH in it; the amount one is able to add depends upon how much damage it causes. The incubation mixture pH of 7.4 must be maintained, of course.

F. Assay Procedure

The procedures described here are for routine ACTH assays. When special procedures, such as characterization of antisera, are being performed, certain details may be modified for convenience, but the principles are the same.

1. Materials and Equipment

> Sodium phosphate dibasic, heptahydrate (No. 74243, Merck and Co., Inc., Rahway, New Jersey)
>
> Potassium phosphate monobasic, anhydrous (No. 73351, Merck and Co., Inc., Rahway, New Jersey)
>
> Lysozyme, egg white (No. L-6876, Sigma Chemical Co., St. Louis, Missouri)
>
> Trasylol (No. 4324, 10^5 Kallikrein Inhibitory Units/10 ml ampoule, FBA Pharmaceuticals, 425 Park Avenue, New York, New York)
>
> Merthiolate (Thiomersol powder, N. F., Eli Lilly and Co., Indianapolis, Indiana)
>
> Micropipette, 100 μl (No. 8100, Oxford Laboratories, Inc., Foster City, California)
>
> Repipet (No. 3005-A-U, Ladindustries, Berkeley, California)
>
> Polypropylene 12 × 75 mm test tubes (No. 2053, Falcon Plastics, Oxnard, California)
>
> High-speed automatic dilutors (Model 25004, Micromedic Systems, Inc., Philadelphia, Pennsylvania, with 200-μl sampling and diluting pumps)
>
> Centrifuge, refrigerated high speed (RC-2B, with HS-4 swinging bucket rotor and four carriers for 24 12 × 75 mm tubes; or RC-3, with HG-4L swinging bucket rotor and eight stacking carriers for 35 12 × 75 mm tubes; Ivan Sorvall, Inc., Norwalk, Connecticut)
>
> Gamma scintillation spectrometer (MS-588, Micromedic Systems, Inc., Philadelphia, Pennsylvania)

2. Solutions

Stock aqueous solutions of 0.1 M sodium phosphate (26.81 gm $Na_2HPO_4 \cdot 7H_2O$ per liter), 0.1 M potassium phosphate (13.61 gm KH_2PO_4 per liter), and 0.9% NaCl (w/v), each containing 0.01% (w/v) Merthiolate; 10% (w/v) lysozyme in 0.05 M phosphate buffer pH 7.4; and 10% (w/v) aqueous Merthiolate are kept at 4°C. All other solutions are freshly prepared for each assay. Samples, standards, diluent plasma, antibody, and labeled hormone are stored at −70°C.

The 0.05 M phosphate buffer, pH 7.4, is prepared by adding 45 ml 0.1 M sodium phosphate and 5.0 ml 0.1 M potassium phosphate solution to 50 ml 0.9% NaCl solution. The standard diluent solution is prepared by adding to 96 ml of this buffer 1.0 ml of 6000 g dexamethasone-suppressed plasma, 2.0 ml (20,000 K.I.U.) of Trasylol, and 1.0 ml 10% lysozyme solution. The plasma acts as a carrier for antibody; Trasylol, a protease inhibitor, decreases incubation damage (higher concentrations inhibit antigen–antibody binding); lysozyme acts as a carrier for polypeptide hormones present in low concentrations. Lysozyme is used rather than 0.25% human serum albumin, as previously reported (Abe *et al.*, 1967a,b; Orth *et al.*, 1968), because foaming and degassing in the tubing and syringes of the automatic dilutor are greatly reduced. Second antibody is appropriately diluted in the standard diluent.

3. Repurification of Labeled Hormone

An aliquot of iodinated ACTH or MSH is repurified immediately prior to use by gel exclusion chromatography on a column of Sephadex G-50 fine resin, as described earlier.

4. Dilutions of Standard and Unknowns

The standard curve is prepared in triplicate at seven or more dilutions. For ACTH, the standard curve is 0.5, 1.58, 5.0, 15.8, 50, 158, 500, 1580, and 5000 pg/ml.

Unknowns are routinely assayed in duplicate at three 3.16-fold dilutions. Standard and samples are diluted with standard diluent.

Until it is found that the use of N-ethyl maleimide or some other agent completely inhibits damage at room temperature, it is very important to keep all solutions at 4°C in order to minimize damage. This is accomplished either by setting up the whole assay in a cold room or by keeping all tubes and flasks in the ice baths; technicians generally prefer the latter! Solutions from flasks kept at 4°C in ice buckets are cycled through the Micromedic dilutor syringes and tubing, which have been cooled to 4°C prior to assembly, for 15 to 20 minutes before use. Racks of tubes are kept in an ice bath while dilutions and additions are performed.

Lyophilized extracts are reconstituted with 0.5 ml diluent at 4°C immediately prior to assay. Two 100-μl aliquots of extract are pipetted into 12 × 75 mm polypropylene tubes (Falcon) with a micropipette. The remaining sample is used for dilutions. The Micromedic 200-μl sampling syringe is set to withdraw 46.25 μl (23.13%), and the diluting syringe, connected to the 4°C standard diluent, is set to deliver 100 μl

(50.0%). Although the Micromedic is exceptionally precise, the actual sampling and diluting pump settings must be calibrated, using radioactive tracer solution, to assure accurate dilutions. The 3.16-fold dilution is achieved by diluting 46.25 μl of the sample to 146.25 μl. A 46.25-μl volume is then withdrawn, leaving 100 μl of the 3.16-fold dilution, and the 46.25 μl is further diluted to 146.25 μl, a tenfold dilution. On the third cycle, 46.25 μl of the tenfold dilution is withdrawn and discarded, leaving 100 μl of the tenfold dilution. This process is repeated twice for each sample. The same procedure is followed for the standard curve, but with more serial dilutions and with triplicates of each dilution. The scheme for samples is tabulated below.

Cycle	Sample withdrawn (μl)	Diluent delivered (μl)	Total volume (μl)	Dilution
1	46.25	—	—	Undiluted
		100	146.25	1 : 3.16
2	46.25	—	100	1 : 3.16[a]
		100	146.25	1 : 10
3	46.25	—	100	1 : 10[a]
		100	146.25	Discard

[a] Tubes used in the assay (100-μl samples undiluted plasma are pipetted directly).

5. Incubation Mixture

A chilled 200-μl Micromedic diluting pump is connected by Teflon tubing to a flask in an ice bucket containing antiserum, and the dilutor is cycled for 15 minutes or so to equilibrate the system. Then, with the pump set at 50%, 100 μl of appropriately diluted antibody is added to each assay tube. Included in the incubation are three tubes for total counts per minute of tracer added and a damage control tube for each undiluted extract which contains no antibody.

The incubation mixtures are mixed by shaking them thoroughly, covered with plastic (supermarket food bags are convenient), and incubated for three days at 4°C.

After this preincubation, 100 μl standard diluent containing ^{125}I-labeled ACTH (about 2000 cpm) is similarly added, the incubations are again mixed by shaking, covered with plastic, and incubated for two more days at 4°C. The two-stage assay technique offers significant improvement in sensitivity for every radioimmunoassay to which we have applied it.

6. Separation of Antibody-Bound from Free Hormone

The ideal separation technique should afford 100% discrimination of bound from free labeled hormone. For several years, we used chromatoelectrophoresis (Yalow and Berson, 1964), which is very reliable, but very time-consuming. Furthermore, the amount of incubation mixture that can easily be applied to the moistened strip is limited to about 0.6 ml. However, other techniques, including charcoal, dextran-coated charcoal, plasma-coated charcoal, and talc, resulted in loss of precision. Only a very slight lack of optimal amounts of them failed to adsorb all the free hormone, and only a very slight excess of them adsorbed antibody-bound hormone as well. The time of exposure to the adsorbent was also critical, since free hormone was adsorbed, antibody was undamaged, and the equilibrium of Ag + Ab = Ag · Ab was disturbed, encouraging dissociation of the bound hormone from antibody. We used the polyethylene glycol (Carbowax 6000, Union Carbide, New York, New York) method (Desbuquois and Aurbach, 1971) for two years, but found that it was not reliable for detecting incubation damage and, therefore, sometimes gave erroneous results. We then used the QUSO-plasma (QUSO G-32, microfine precipitated silica, Philadelphia Quartz Co., Philadelphia, Pennsylvania) method (Berson and Yalow, 1968; Orth *et al.*, 1976) for several months. Although this method is still successfully applied to the LPH (lipotropin) radioimmunoassay (Chapter 13), we use the double-antibody method (Skom and Talmage, 1958) for all others.

The second antibody, in our case rabbit anti-sheep γ-globulin (Cappel Laboratories, Inc., Cochranville, Pennsylvania), is added at an appropriate dilution in 100 μl ice-cold standard diluent with a 200-μl Micromedic pump set at 50.0%, 48 hours after the ^{125}I-labeled ACTH tracer is added. After an additional 24 hours incubation at 4°C, 1.5 ml of ice-cold standard diluent is added with a Repipet and the tubes are centrifuged at 5000 g for 15 minutes at 4°C. The supernates are decanted, the tops of the tubes are blotted and cork-stoppered to reduce possible radioactive contamination, and the precipitates are counted in a gamma scintillation spectrometer with a tape printout.

The dilution of second antibody required for optimal precipitation is determined by adding graded quantities of second antibody to tubes which contain ^{125}I-labeled ACTH and a known concentration of ACTH antiserum and which have been incubated at 4°C long enough for the antigen–antibody reaction to reach equilibrium. In some radioimmunoassay systems, it is necessary to add carrier serum homologous with the first antiserum; in our case, adding carrier serum does not improve either total precipitation or reproducibility. We found that 3.0 μl of second antibody completely precipitates 0.008 μl of first antibody, although no pellet is visible to the unaided eye. Increasing the final volume to 1.9 ml with standard diluent prior to centrifugation reduces nonspecific counts in the pellet and/or on the walls of the tube and obviates the need for washing the pellet; in fact, reproducibility is better if the pellets are not washed. The pellets adhere well to the round bottoms of the polypropylene tubes; reproducibility is actually somewhat better when the supernates are decanted, rather than carefully aspirated. Thus, the second antibody system, which has the great advantage of *specific* precipitation of antibody-bound counts, can also be inexpensive, simple, and highly reproducible.

It should be noted that damage control tubes in the second antibody separation technique must have excess antibody added 24 hours prior to separation, since incubation-damaged ^{125}I-ACTH is not distinguished from free ^{125}I-ACTH in this separation system and can be detected only as a loss of immunoreactivity in the presence of excess antibody. Alternatively, damage control tubes containing labeled ACTH in diluent alone (assay damage) or sample-plus-diluent (sample damage) in the absence of antibody can be separated with QUSO-plasma in the same manner as in the MSH/LPH assay (Chapter 13), since this technique does distinguish between free and incubation-damaged labeled hormone (Tanaka and Orth, 1978). Results are calculated on a Wang Series 2200 computer with a teletype interface; mean estimates of ACTH concentration and confidence limits are calculated.

G. Characteristics of the Assay

The specificities of the antisera have been discussed. So many factors affect antigen–antibody binding that we assay every specimen at three dilutions to ensure that it generates a competition curve parallel to standard. Of course, one can always calculate a value from a single dilution; it just may not represent hormone concentration. The ACTH assays have sensitivities of 1.0–5.0 pg/ml of sample.

Duplication can be determined by assaying aliquots of a single specimen in one assay. The results of this procedure have been reported (Orth *et al.*, 1973a). In six duplicate determinations of four plasma pools containing approximately 120, 360, 800, and 2000 pg/ml of ACTH, the percent standard errors in the three systems were 3–8% in the extreme N-terminal assay, 3–12% in the extended N-terminal assay, and 11–20% in the C-terminal ACTH assay, using the Micromedic dilutor. Replication can be estimated by assaying aliquots of a series of samples in assays on different days. Assaying 32 plasma samples with ACTH levels ranging from 50 to 5000 pg/ml in the three ACTH assays on several different days, correlation coefficients of +0.98, +0.97, and +0.80 were obtained (Orth *et al.*, 1973a).

The normal value for plasma ACTH in man, with the antiserum shown in Fig. 4, is less than 120 pg/ml at 6:00 A.M. (mean equals approximately 55 pg/ml) and less than 75 pg/ml at 6:00 P.M. (mean equals approximately 35 pg/ml). Since the release of ACTH is extremely sensitive to stress, care must be taken to avoid stressing the subject before obtaining the blood specimen, spuriously elevating the plasma concentrations.

III. PROBLEMS

The difficulties with radioimmunoassays for ACTH have been (1) raising high affinity antibodies, which now seems possible with intradermal injections of conjugated antigen; (2) the very low plasma concentrations of ACTH, levels which can now be measured with efficient separation techniques that allow a greater ratio of plasma to labeled tracer and with extraction techniques for ACTH; and (3) the biologic and immunologic lability of ACTH *in vivo* and *in vitro*.

Dissociation of bioactivity and immunoreactivity should be minimized by using antibodies directed at the active portion of the molecule. The *in vitro* loss of activity can be minimized by avoiding prolonged storage of exogenous or endogenous ACTH in solution, plasma, tissue, or nonlyophilized extracts; by maintaining the pH at 3 and using carrier albumin at low hormone concentrations; by using 6000 g plasma; by boiling extracts immediately to inactivate some proteolytic enzymes; and by using Trasylol or N-ethyl maleimide to inhibit the proteases that survive.

Another problem is the measurement of big ACTH. Present antibodies are raised to some part of the "little" 1–39-ACTH sequence. Some of them may not react fully with "big" ACTH, however, since the sequences toward which they are directed may be partly or completely obscured by folding of the big ACTH molecule, a phenomenon suggested by the weak biologic activity of big ACTH (Yalow, 1974). Conversely, if the antibody reacts equally with big and 1–39-ACTH, then it cannot distinguish between them, and other procedures, such as gel filtration, are required to do so. Furthermore, some extraction procedures may not extract big ACTH with the same efficiency as 1–39-ACTH; this appears to be true both for CG-50 cationic-exchange chromatography and silicic acid absorption, and may also be true for other silicates, such as QUSO and porous glass.

Therefore, reliable measurement of big ACTH may require other extraction procedures, such as affinity chromatography, to separate big ACTH from other high molecular weight components of plasma and tissue and/or the development of specific assays for sequences unique to big ACTH that are applicable to unextracted plasma and relatively crude tissue homogenates.

IV. OTHER RADIOIMMUNOASSAYS

A number of ACTH radioimmunoassays have been described, most of which are listed in the bibliography. It does not seem appropriate to comment on techniques which differ from those described here but which have not been thoroughly evaluated in this laboratory. There is one variation that seems to warrant mention, however, since it appears simple to perform. It is an alternative iodination method, which avoids the use of the Sephadex column and is described in detail by Rees *et al.* (1971). After adding the sodium metabisulfite, the whole reaction vial is simply dropped into a centrifuge tube containing 20 ml 0.05 M phosphate buffer (pH 7.6) with 0.25% human serum albumin and 0.5% 2-mercaptoethanol. Ten milliliters of this mixture is transferred to a plastic tube containing 10-mg QUSO glass (G32, Philadelphia Quartz Co., Philadelphia, Pennsylvania). The tube is capped and rotated at 20 rpm on a vertical turntable for 30 minutes. The tube is centrifuged at 2000 g for ten minutes, and the supernatant is aspirated and discarded. The QUSO is washed with 2.0 ml water; the tube is centrifuged; and the supernate is aspirated and discarded. The undamaged adsorbed ACTH is eluted from the QUSO by rotating for 30 minutes with 2.0 ml 60 : 40 : 1 water–acetone–glacial acetic solution. The supernate is carefully aspirated after centrifugation, assessed for purity, and stored, appropriately diluted in the mercaptoethanol–albumin–phosphate buffer solution. Leached silica glass (No. 7930, Corning Glass Works, Corning, New York) can be used instead of QUSO, 35–50 mg per tube. The degree of purification of labeled ACTH achieved by this method is reported to be comparable to that using the Sephadex column, although we have found that gel exclusion chromatography is considerably superior.

V. RECENT DEVELOPMENTS

In addition to the entry of a number of commercial reference laboratories into the ACTH field, laboratories whose reliability is not well established, at least one ACTH radioimmunoassay kit has been marketed. Available from Amersham-Searle (Arlington Heights, Illinois), the kit is an extracted plasma assay based on principles similar to those described by Rees *et al.* (1971). In those instances when we have measured ACTH levels on the same plasma samples which others had assayed with this kit, the results were in relatively good agreement. The availability of this commercial kit and of the ampouled ACTH and ACTH antiserum from the National Pituitary Agency for investigative purposes should permit many more laboratories to set up a reliable ACTH radioimmunoassay.

ACKNOWLEDGMENTS

The author wishes to acknowledge the invaluable assistance of Donald P. Island, who iodinated ACTH for our laboratories in the past and also prepared some of the conjugated antigens; the constant support and expertise of Wendell E. Nicholson, who extracts ACTH from a variety of biologic tissues and fluids, is the bioassayer of ACTH, has produced some of the recent conjugates of ACTH, and currently iodinates and purifies ACTH; and the excellent technical assistance of Ms. Farideh Siami, Ms. Barbara Sherrell, Ms. Jean P. Woodham, Mr. Ken R. Parks, and Mr. Charles D. Mount.

These studies would not have been possible without the generous collaboration of a number of investigators, particularly Dr. Aaron B. Lerner of Yale University, those of Ciba-Geigy, Ltd., Basel, Switzerland, Dr. Henry A. Strade of Organon, Inc., West Orange, New Jersey, and the National Pituitary Agency, University of Maryland and National Institute of Arthritis and Metabolic Digestive Diseases, National Institutes of Health, Bethesda, Maryland.

This work was supported in part by National Cancer Institute Research Grant 2-R01-CA11685 and National Institutes of Health Grant 5-M01-RR00095.

REFERENCES

Abe, K., Island, D. P., Liddle, G. W., Fleischer, N., and Nicholson, W. E. (1967a). Radioimmunologic evidence for α-MSH (melanocyte stimulating hormone) in human pituitary and tumor tissues. *J. Clin. Endocrinol. Metab.* **27**, 46–52.

Abe, K. Nicholson, W. E., Liddle, G. W., Island, D. P., and Orth, D. N. (1967b). Radioimmunoassay of β-MSH in human plasma and tissues. *J. Clin. Invest.* **46**, 1609–1616.

Abe, K. Nicholson, W. E., Liddle, G. W., Orth, D. N., and Island, D. P. (1969). Normal and abnormal regulation of β-MSH in man. *J. Clin. Invest.* **48**, 1580–1585.

Alexander, D. P., Britton, H. G., Forsling, M. L., Nixon, D. A., and Ratcliffe, J. G. (1973).

Adrenocorticotrophin and vasopressin in foetal sheep and the response to stress. *In* "Endocrinology of Pregnancy and Parturition—Experimental Studies in the Sheep" (C. G. Pierrepoint, ed.), pp. 112–125. Alpha Omega Alpha Publ., Cardiff, Wales.

Bajusz, S., Medzihradsky, K., Paulay, Z., and Lang, Zs. (1967). Total synthesis of human corticotropin (α_hACTH). *Acta Chim. Acad. Sci. Hung.* **52**, 335–341.

Bangham, D. R., Musset, M. V., and Stack-Dunne, M. P. (1962). The third international standard for corticotrophin. *Bull. W.H.O.* **27**, 395–408.

Berson, S. A., and Yalow, R. S. (1968). Radioimmunoassay of ACTH in plasma. *J. Clin. Invest.* **47**, 2725–2751.

Besser, G. M., Orth, D. N., Nicholson, W. E., Bynny, R. L., Abe, K., and Woodham, J. P. (1971). Dissociation of disappearance of bioactive and radioimmunoreactive ACTH from plasma in man. *J. Clin. Endocrinol. Metab.* **32**, 595–603.

Bloomfield, G. A., Scott, A. P., Lowry, P. J., Gilkes, J. J. H., and Rees, L. H. (1974), A reappraisal of human β MSH. *Nature (London)* **252**, 492–493.

Bornstein, J., and Trewhella, P. (1950). Adrenocorticotropic activity of blood-plasma extracts. *Lancet* **2**, 678–680.

Chayen, J., Loveridge, N., and Daly, J. R. (1971). The measurable effect of low concentrations (pg/ml) of ACTH on reducing groups of adrenal cortex maintained in organ culture. *Clin. Sci.* **41**, 2P.

Chayen, J., Loveridge, N., and Daly, J. R. (1972). A sensitive bioassay for adrenocorticotrophic hormone in human plasma. *Clin. Endocrinol.* **1**, 219–233.

Daly, J. R., Loveridge, N., Bitensky, L., and Chayen, J. (1972). Early experience with a highly sensitive assay for ACTH. *Ann. Clin. Biochem.* **9**, 81–84.

Dedman, M. L., Farmer, T. H., and Morris, C. J. O. R. (1961). Studies on pituitary adrenocorticotrophin. *Biochem. J.* **78**, 348–352.

Demura, H., West, C. D., Nugent, C. A., Nakagawa, K., and Tyler, F. H. (1966). A sensitive radioimmunoassay for plasma ACTH levels. *J. Clin. Endocrinol. Metab.* **26**, 1297–1302.

Desbuquois, B., and Aurbach, G. D. (1971). Use of polyethylene glycol to separate free and antibody-bound peptide hormones in radioimmunoassays. *J. Clin. Endocrinol. Metab.* **33**, 732–738.

Dixon, H. B. F. (1956). The action of periodate on ACTH. *Biochem. J.* **62**, 25P.

Donald, R. A. (1967). A rapid method of extracting ACTH from plasma. *J. Endocrinol.* **39**, 451–452.

Donald, R. A., and Toth, A. (1973). A comparison of the β-melanocyte-stimulating hormone and corticotropin response to hypoglycemia. *J. Clin. Endocrinol. Metab.* **36**, 925–930.

Donnadieu, M., and Sevaux, D. (1973). Radioimmunoassay of melanocyte-stimulating hormone (β-MSH) in human plasma. *Biomedicine Express* **19**, 272–274.

Edelman, G. M. (1973). Antibody structure and molecular immunology. *Science* **180**, 830–840.

Eipper, B. A., and Mains, R. E. (1975). High molecular weight forms of adrenocorticotropic hormone in the mouse pituitary and in a mouse pituitary tumor cell line. *Biochemistry* **14**, 3836–3844.

Eipper, B. A., Mains, R. E., and Guenzi, D. (1976). High molecular weight forms of adrenocorticotropic hormone are glycoproteins. *J. Biol. Chem.* **251**, 4121–4126.

Gewirtz, G., Schneider, B., Krieger, D. T., and Yalow, R. S. (1974). Big ACTH: Conversion to biologically active ACTH by trypsin. *J. Clin. Endocrinol. Metab.* **38**, 227–230.

Gillett, R., and Gull, K. (1972). Glutaraldehyde—its purity and stability. *Histochemie* **30**, 162–167.

Goodfriend, T. L., Levine, L., and Fasman, G. D. (1964). Antibodies to bradykinin and angiotensin: A use of carbodiimides in immunology. *Science* **144**, 1344–1346.

Gráf, L., Bajusz, S., Patthy, A., Barát, E., and Cseh, G. (1971). Revised amide location for porcine and human adrenocorticotropic hormone. *Acta Biochim. Biophys. Acad. Sci. Hung.* **6**, 415–418.

Guillemin, R., Clayton, G. W., Smith, J. D., and Lipscomb, H. S. (1958). Measurement of free corticosteroids in rat plasma: Physiological validation of a method. *Endocrinology* **63**, 349–358.

Hirs, C. H. W., Moore, S., and Stein, W. H. (1953). A chromatographic investigation of pancreatic ribonuclease. *J. Biol. Chem.* **200**, 493–506.

Hofmann, K., Andreatta, R., Bohn, H., and Moroder, L. (1970). Studies on polypeptides. XLV. Structure-function studies in the β-corticotropin series. *J. Med. Chem.* **13**, 339–345.

Hogan, P., Rees, L. H., Lowry, P. J., Ratter, S., and Snitcher, E. J. (1976). Studies on the stability of human ACTH in biological fluids. *J. Endocrinol.* **71**, 63P-64P.

Hunter, W. M., and Greenwood, F. C. (1962). Preparation of iodine-131 labelled human growth hormone of high specific activity. *Nature (London)* **194**, 495–496.

Island, D. P., Shimizu, N., Nicholson, W. E., Abe, K., Ogata, E., and Liddle, G. W. (1965). A method for separating small quantities of MSH and ACTH with good recovery of each. *J. Clin. Endocrinol. Metab.* **25**, 975–983.

Jöhl, A., Riniker, B., and Schenkel-Hulliger, L. (1974). Identity of the structure of ovine and bovine ACTH: correction of revised structure of the ovine hormone. *FEBS Lett.* **45**, 172.

Kloppenborg, P. W. C., Island, D. P., Liddle, G. W., Michelakis, A. M., and Nicholson, W. E. (1968). A method of preparing adrenal cell suspensions and its applicability to the *in vitro* study of adrenal metabolism. *Endocrinology* **82**, 1053–1058.

Landon, J., and Greenwood, F. C. (1968). Homologous radioimmunoassay for plasma-levels of corticotrophin in man. *Lancet* **1**, 273–276.

Lefkowitz, R. J., Roth, J., Pricer, W., and Pastan, I. (1970a). ACTH receptors in the adrenal: Specific binding of ACTH-^{125}I and its relation to adenyl cyclase. *Proc. Natl. Acad. Sci. U.S.A.* **65**, 745–752.

Lefkowtiz, R. J., Roth, J., and Pastan, I. (1970b). Radioreceptor assay of adrenocorticotropic hormone: New approach to assay of polypeptide hormones in plasma. *Science* **170**, 633–635.

Lerner, A. B., Upton, G. V., and Lande, S. (1968). Purification of porcine and human ACTH. *In* "Pharmacology of Hormonal Polypeptides and Proteins" (N. Back, L. Martini, and R. Paoletti, eds.), pp. 203–212. Plenum, New York.

Li, C. H. (1959). Proposed system of terminology for preparations of adrenocorticotropic hormone. *Science* **129**, 969–970.

Li, C. H. (1962). Synthesis and biological properties of ACTH peptides. *Recent Prog. Horm. Res.* **18**, 1–40.

Lipscomb, H. S., and Nelson, D. H. (1962). A sensitive biologic assay for ACTH. *Endocrinology* **71**, 13–23.

Lowry, P. J. McMartin, C., and Peters, J. (1973). Properties of a simplified bioassay for adrenocorticotrophic activity using the steroidogenic response of isolated adrenal cells. *J. Endocrinol.* **59**, 43–55.

McGuire, J., McGill, R., Leeman, S., and Goodfriend, T. (1965). The experimental generation of antibodies to α-MSH and ACTH. *J. Clin Invest.* **44**, 1672–1678.

Matsukura, S., West, C. D., Ichikawa, Y., Jubiz, W., Harada, G., and Tyler, F. H. (1971). A new phenomenon of usefulness in the radioimmunoassay of plasma adrenocorticotropic hormone. *J. Lab. Clin. Med.* **77**, 490–500.

Nakanishi, S., Taii, S., Hirata, Y., Matsukura, S., Imura, H., and Numa, S. (1976). A large product of cell-free translation of messenger RNA coding for corticotropin. *Proc. Natl. Acad. Sci. U.S.A.* **73**, 4319–4323.

Ney, R. L., Ogata, E., Shimizu, N., Nicholson, W. E., and Liddle, G. W. Structure-function relationships of ACTH and MSH analogues. (1965). *Proc. Int. Congr. Endocrinol., 2nd, 1964* Excerpta Med. Found., Int. Congr. Ser. No. 83, pp. 1184–1191.

Nicholson, W. E., and Van Loon, G. R. (1973). Some practical innovations in the biological assay of adrenocorticotropic hormone. *J. Lab. Clin. Med.* **81**, 803–808.

Nicholson, W. E., Parks, K. R., Tanaka, K., Mount, C. D., and Orth, D. N. (1976a). Method of preparation of ampoules containing microgram quantities of polypeptide hormone for distribution and use as laboratory standards: Synthetic human ACTH and β-MSH. *J. Clin Endocrinol. Metab.* **42**:1153–1157.

Nicholson, W. E., Liddle, R. A., and Puett, D. (1976b). Corticotropin: Plasma clearance, catabolism, and biotransformations. *Endocrinology* **98**, Suppl., 59.

Orth, D. N. (1974). Adrenocorticotropic hormone and melanocyte stimulating hormone (ACTH and MSH). *In* "Methods of Hormone Radioimmunoassay" (B. M. Jaffe and H. R. Behrman, eds.), pp. 125–159. Academic Press, New York.

Orth, D. N., and Nicholson, W. E. (1977a). High molecular weight forms of human ACTH are glycoproteins. *J. Clin. Endocrinol. Metab.* **44**, 214–217.

Orth, D. N., and Nicholson, W. E. (1977b). Different molecular forms of ACTH. *Ann. N.Y. Acad. Sci.* **297**, 27–48.

Orth, D. N., and Woodham, J. P. (1969). A simple method for extraction of pituitary polypeptides from plasma. *Program 51st Annu. Meet., Am. Endocr. Soc.* p. 178.

Orth, D. N., Island, D. P., Nicholson, W. E., Abe, K., and Woodham, J. P. (1968). ACTH radioimmunoassay: Interpretation, comparison with bioassay, and clinical application. *In* "Radioisotopes in Medicine: *In Vitro* Studies" (R. L. Hayes, F. A. Goswitz, and B. E. P. Murphy, eds.), pp. 251–272. US At. Energy Comm., Div. Tech. Inf., Oak Ridge, Tennessee.

Orth, D. N., Nicholson, W. E., Mitchell, W. M., Island, D. P., and Liddle, G. W. (1973a). Biologic and immunologic characterization and physical separation of ACTH and ACTH fragments in the ectopic ACTH syndrome. *J. Clin. Invest.* **52**, 1756–1769.

Orth, D. N., Nicholson, W. E., Mitchell, W. M., Island, D. P., Shapiro, M., and Byyny, R. L. (1973b). ACTH and MSH production by a single cloned mouse pituitary tumor cell line. *Endocrinology* **92**, 385–393.

Orth, D. N., Tanaka, K., and Nicholson, W. E. (1976). The melanotropins. *In* "Hormones in Human Blood: Detection and Assay" (H. N. Antonaides, ed.), pp. 423–448. Harvard Univ. Press, Cambridge, Massachusetts.

Ratcliffe, J. G., and Edwards, C. R. W. (1971). The extraction of adrenocorticotrophin and arginine-vasopressin from human plasma by porous glass. *In* "Radioimmunoassay Methods" (K. E. Kirkham and W. M. Hunter, eds.), pp. 502–512. Williams & Wilkins, Baltimore, Maryland.

Ratcliffe, J. G., Knight, R. A., Besser, G. M., Landon, J., and Stansfeld, A. G. (1972). Tumour and plasma ACTH concentrations in patients with and without ectopic ACTH syndrome. *Clin. Endocrinol.* **1**, 27–44.

Rees, L. H., Cook, D. M., Kendall, J. W., Allen, C. F., Kramer, R. M., Ratcliffe, J. G., and

Knight, R. A. (1971). A radioimmunoassay for rat plasma ACTH. *Endocrinology* **89**, 254–261.

Rees, L. H., Ratcliffe, J. G., Besser, G. M., Kramer, R., Landon, J., and Chayen, J. (1973). Comparison of the redox assay for ACTH with previous assays. *Nature (London), New Biol.* **241**, 84–85.

Reichlin, M., Schnure, J. J., and Vance, V. K. (1968). Induction of antibodies to porcine ACTH in rabbits with nonsteroidogenic polymers of BSA and ACTH. *Proc. Soc. Exp. Biol. Med.* **128**, 347–350.

Riniker, B., Sieber, P., Rittel, W., and Zuber, H. (1972). Revised amino-acid sequences for porcine and human adrenocorticotrophic hormone. *Nature (London), New Biol.* **235**, 114–115.

Sayers, G., Swallow, R. L., and Giordano, N. D. (1971). An improved technique for the preparation of isolated rat adrenal cells: A sensitive, accurate and specific method for the assay of ACTH. *Endocrinology* **88**, 1063–1068.

Sayers, M. A., Sayers, G., and Woodbury, L. A. (1948). The assay of adrenocorticotrophic hormone by the adrenal ascorbic acid-depletion method. *Endocrinology* **42**, 379–393.

Schenkel-Hulliger, L., Maier, R., Barthe, P. L., Desaulles, P. A., Jarret, A., Riniker, B., Rittel, W., and Sieber, P. (1974). Biological activity of synthetic human corticotrophin with revised amino acid sequence. *Acta Endocrinol. (Copenhagen)* **75**, 24–32.

Seelig, S., and Sayers, G. (1973). Isolated adrenal cortex cells: ACTH agonists, partial agonists, antagonists; cyclic AMP and corticosterone production. *Arch. Biochem. Biophys.* **154**, 230–239.

Shapiro, M., Nicholson, W. E., Orth, D. N., Mitchell, W. M., Island, D. P., and Liddle, G. W. (1972). Preliminary characterization of the pituitary melanocyte stimulating hormones of several vertebrate species. *Endocrinology* **90**, 249–256.

Sieber, P., Rittel, W., and Riniker, B. (1972). Synthesis of human corticotropin (β_h-ACTH) with a revised amino acid sequence. *Helv. Chim. Acta* **55**, 1243–1248.

Tager, H. S., and Steiner, D. F. (1974). Peptide hormones. *Annu. Rev. Biochem.* **43**, 509–538.

Tanaka, K., and Orth, D. N. (1978). The detection of "purified" incubation damage by several radioimmunoassay separation methods. *J. Lab. Clin. Med.* (in press).

Tanaka, K., Mount, C. D., Nicholson, W. E., and Orth, D. N. (1976). "Big" bioactive and immunoreactive "β-MSH's" in human plasma and tumor tissues. *Clin. Res.* **24**, 10A.

Tanaka, K., Nicholson, W. E., and Orth, D. N. (1978). The nature of immunoreactive LPHs in human plasma and tissue extracts. *J. Clin. Invest.* (In press.)

Taunton, O. D., Roth, J., and Pastan, I. (1969). Studies on the adrenocorticotropic hormone-activated adenyl cyclase of a functional adrenal tumor. *J. Biol. Chem.* **244**, 247–253.

Thody, A. J., and Plummer, N. A. (1973). A radioimmunoassay for β-melanocyte-stimulating hormone in human plasma. *J. Endocrinol.* **58**, 263–273.

Vaitukaitis, J., Robbins, J. B., Nieschlag, E., and Ross, G. T. (1971). A method for producing specific antisera with small doses of immunogen. *J. Clin. Endocrinol. Metab.* **33**, 988–991.

Vernikos-Danellis, J., Anderson, E., and Trigg, L. (1966). Changes in adrenal corticosterone concentration in rats: Method of bio-assay for ACTH. *Endocrinology* **79**, 624–630.

Wolfsen, A. R., McIntyre, H. B., and Odell, W. B. (1972). Adrenocorticotropin measurement by competitive binding receptor assay. *J. Clin. Endocrinol. Metab.* **34**, 684–689.

Yalow, R. S. (1974). Heterogeneity of peptide hormones. *Recent Prog. Horm. Res.* **30**, 597–627.

Yalow, R. S., and Berson, S. A. (1964). Immunoassay of plasma insulin. *Methods Biochem. Anal.* **12**, 69–96.

Yalow, R. S., and Berson, S. A. (1971). Size heterogeneity of immunoreactive human ACTH in plasma and in extracts of pituitary glands and ACTH-producing thymoma. *Biochem. Biophys. Res. Commun.* **44**, 439–445.

Yalow, R. S., and Berson, S. A. (1973). Characteristics of "big ACTH" in human plasma and pituitary extracts. *J. Clin. Endocrinol. Metab.* **36**, 415–423.

Yalow, R. S., Glick, S. M., Roth, J., and Berson, S. A. (1964). Radioimmunoassay of human plasma ACTH. *J. Clin. Endocrinol. Metab.* **24**, 1219–1225.

13

Melanocyte-Stimulating Hormones (MSH's) and Lipotropic Hormones (LPH's)

DAVID N. ORTH, KOSHI TANAKA,
AND WENDELL E. NICHOLSON

I. INTRODUCTION*

These hormones are considered separately from adrenocorticotropic hormone (ACTH), which is treated in Chapter 12, in order to discuss certain biologic, immunologic, and methodologic features that are more or less unique to them.

* The nomenclature in this chapter conforms to the system of terminology for preparations of adrenocorticotropic hormone proposed by C. H. Li (1959a).

Methods of Hormone Radioimmunoassay, Second Edition
Copyright © 1979 by Academic Press, Inc.
All rights of reproduction in any form reserved. IS BN 0-12-379260-6

A. Structure–Function Relationships

Together with ACTH, the melanocyte-stimulating hormones (MSH's) and the lipotropic hormones (LPH's) constitute a family of polypeptides that are related both structurally and functionally. Each of these hormones contains a heptapeptide Met-Glu-His-Phe-Arg-Trp-Gly core that is required for the biologic function shared by all of them, namely, their melanocyte-stimulating activity (Li *et al.*, 1961), their corticosteroidogenic activity (Schwyzer *et al.*, 1971), and their lipolytic activity (Draper *et al.*, 1973).

The melanocyte-stimulating, or pigmentary, activity of these hormones has been studied almost exclusively in two nonmammalian species, the frog (usually *Rana pipiens*) and the so-called American chameleon (*Anolis carolinensis*). However, the dispersion of melanin granules which the MSH's stimulate in the melanocytes of these animals, causing the increase in pigmentation, is quite different from the mechanism by which they cause increased pigmentation in mammals. Thus, although it has been assumed that their relative biologic potencies are similar in man, this has never been directly proved. For those interested in MSH bioassay, a brief bibliography is provided (Smith, 1916; Hogben and Winton, 1924; Hogben and Gordon, 1930; Kleinholtz, 1938; Thing, 1952; Shizume *et al.*, 1954; Horowitz, 1958; Teague and Patton, 1960; Burgers, 1961; Kastin and Ross, 1964; Björklund *et al.*, 1972; Abe and Nicholson, 1975; Orth *et al.*, 1976).

The MSH's include: α-MSH (N-α-acetyl-α^{1-13NH_2}-ACTH), a tridecapeptide that is the most potent melanocyte-stimulating hormone known (Table I); the β-MSH's, which consist of 18 amino acid residues (22 in man, but *vide infra*) and are about 10–40% as potent as α-MSH; the ACTH's, which are 39 residues in length and are only about 1% as potent as α-MSH; the γ-LPH's, which contain 58 amino acids with the complete sequence of the respective β-MSH in positions 41–58 (37–58 in man, but *vide infra*) and which also have only about 1% the melanotropic activity of α-MSH; and the β-LPH's, which are 91 residues in length, contain the complete sequence of the respective γ-LPH in positions 1–58, and are also only about 1% as active as α-MSH in the frog skin darkening bioassay. None of them is reported to have more than 0.1% of the corticosteroidogenic activity of ACTH, although, as in the case of melanocyte-stimulating activity, none of these hormones has been tested directly with human adrenocortical cells. All of them are relatively weak lipolytic agents in animals other than the rabbit (Rudman *et al.*, 1963).

B. Biosynthetic Relationships

These hormones can be divided into those that occur only in animals whose pituitaries have a distinct intermediate lobe, such as mouse, rat, rabbit, pig, sheep, and beef, and those that occur both in these animals and in those which do not have a discrete intermediate lobe, such as man and other primates.

1. α-MSH

The first and most potent, α-MSH, apparently occurs only in the intermediate lobe. Thus, the vast majority of the biologic melanocyte-stimulating activity in the pituitaries of these species is found in this lobe (Shapiro *et al.*, 1972). Scott *et al.* (1973, 1974a,b) have proposed that ACTH actually functions as a precursor or prohormone for α-MSH. They have provided evidence that ACTH is synthesized in the intermediate lobe and have suggested that it undergoes proteolytic cleavage to form "corticotropin-like intermediate lobe peptide" (CLIP), which consists of the 18–39 sequence of ACTH (Scott *et al.*, 1974b), and a complementary N-terminal fragment that subsequently undergoes carboxypeptidase reduction in length, amidation, and acetylation to form α-MSH. This would account for the intense immunostaining of the intermediate lobe with C-terminal ACTH antisera (Phifer and Spicer, 1970) but not with N-terminal ACTH antisera (Dubois, 1972). As might be expected, α-MSH cannot be detected in human plasma, and immunoreactive α-MSH accounts for no more than 1–3% of the biologic MSH activity of human pituitary extracts (Abe *et al.*, 1967a); this is presumably the result of cross-reaction with the relatively larger concentrations of ACTH and LPH present in these extracts. Chromatographic analysis of human pituitary extracts reveals no material the size of α-MSH with MSH bioactivity or α-MSH immunoreactivity. Thus, α-MSH probably does not normally exist in the human pituitary except, perhaps, during fetal life (Silman *et al.*, 1976). In addition to the usual α-MSH tridecapeptide, two smaller analogs that share the heptapeptide core have been isolated in the dogfish shark, *Squalus acanthius* (Lowry and Chadwick, 1970).

2. β-MSH

The next of these hormones, β-MSH, also appears to be synthesized only in the intermediate lobe of the pituitary gland. Thus, β-MSH has been isolated from pig, sheep, horse, beef, and monkey pituitaries, and the amino acid sequence of the hormone has been determined for each of them (Geschwind *et al.*, 1957a,b; Dixon and Li, 1961; Lee *et al.*,

Table I The Chemical Structures and Biologic Potencies of the MSH- and LPH-Related Peptides

Peptide	Amino acid

α-MSH
  Beef, sheep,
  horse, pig,
  monkey
	Acetyl- Ser- Tyr- Ser-
	1 2 3

β-MSH Beef, sheep	H- Asp- Ser- Gly- Pro- Tyr- Lys- 1 2 3 4 5 6
Horse	H- Asp- Glu- Gly- Pro- Tyr- Lys- 1 2 3 4 5 6
Pig, sheep	H- Asp- Glu- Gly- Pro- Tyr- Lys- 1 2 3 4 5 6
Monkey	H- Asp- Glu- Gly- Pro- Tyr- Arg- 1 2 3 4 5 6
Man	H- Ala- Glu- Lys- Lys- Asp- Glu- Gly- Pro- Tyr- Arg- 1 2 3 4 5 6 7 8 9 10

[a] All of the α-MSH's thus far isolated have the same amino acid sequence and similar biologic potencies: beef, 1.0×10^{10} U/gm (Li, 1959b); sheep, 3.0×10^{9} U/gm (Lee *et al.*, 1963); horse, 1.0×10^{10} U/gm (Dixon and Li, 1961); pig, 1.5×10^{10} U/gm (Harris and Lerner, 1957; Li, 1959b); and monkey, 1.0×10^{10} U/gm (Lee *et al.*, 1961). The sequence shown is that of synthetic α-MSH (Schwyzer *et al.*, 1963a).

sequence	Melanocyte-stimulating potency *in citro* (Units/gm)

| Met- Glu- His- Phe- Arg- Trp-Gly | - Lys- Pro- Val-NH$_2$ [a] | 1.5×10^{10} [b] |
| 4   5   6   7   8   9   10 | 11   12   13 | |

| Met- Glu- His- Phe- Arg- Trp-Gly | - Ser- Pro- Pro- Lys- Asp-OH [c] | 9.7×10^{9} [b] |
| 7   8   9   10   11   12   13 | 14   15   16   17   18 | |

| Met- Glu- His- Phe- Arg- Trp-Gly | - Ser- Pro- Arg- Lys- Asp-OH [d] | 1.2×10^{9} [d] |
| 7   8   9   10   11   12   13 | 14   15   16   17   18 | |

| Met- Glu- His- Phe- Arg- Trp-Gly | - Ser- Pro- Pro- Lys- Asp-OH [e] | 3.8×10^{9} [f] |
| 7   8   9   10   11   12   13 | 14   15   16   17   18 | |

| Met- Glu- His- Phe- Arg- Trp-Gly | - Ser- Pro- Pro- Lys- Asp-OH [g] | 3.8×10^{9} [g] |
| 7   8   9   10   11   12   13 | 14   15   16   17   18 | |

| Met- Glu- His- Phe- Arg- Trp-Gly | - Ser- Pro- Pro- Lys- Asp-OH [h] | 3.3×10^{9} [f] |
| 11   12   13   14   15   16   17 | 18   19   20   21   22 | |

The following are the references for the original, or most recently revised, sequences and biologic potencies of the known melanocyte-stimulating hormones:

[b] Ney *et al*. (1965).
[c] Geschwind *et al*. (1965).
[d] Dixon and Li (1961).
[e] Geschwind *et al*. (1957a).
[f] Pickering and Li (1963).
[g] Lee *et al*. (1961).
[h] Harris (1959).
[i] Pankov (1972).
[j] Lohmar and Li (1967).
[k] Gráf and Li (1973).

[l] Lohmar and Li (1968).
[m] Gráf *et al*. (1971).
[n] Gilardeau and Chrétien (1970).
[o] Li and Chung (1976a).
[p] Chrétien and Li (1967).
[q] Gráf *et al*. (1970).
[r] Li and Chung (1976b).
[x] Ling *et al*. (1976).
[t] Guillemin *et al*. (1976).
[u] Hughes *et al*. (1975).

(Continued)

Table I (*Continued*)

Peptide	Amino acid

β-LPH
Beef

H-	xxx-	xxx-	xxx-	xxx	.....	xxx-	xxx-	xxx-	xxx-	xxx-	xxx-	xxx-	xxx-	xxx-	xxx-	xxx-	xxx-
	1	2	3	4		35	36	37	38	39	40	41	42	43	44	45	46

xxx-	xxx-	xxx-	xxx-	xxx-	xxx-	xxx-	xxx-	xxx	xxx-	xxx-	xxx-	xxx-	xxx-	Val-	Thr-	Leu-	Phe
61	62	63	64	65	66	67	68	69	70	71	72	73	74	75	76	77	78

Sheep

H-	Glu-	Leu-	Thr-	Gly	.....	Gln-	Ala-	Ala-	Glu-	Lys-	Lys-	Asp-	Ser-	Gly-	Pro-	Tyr-	Lys
	1	2	3	4		35	36	37	38	39	40	41	42	43	44	45	46

Tyr-	Gly-	Gly-	Phe-	Met	Thr-	Ser-	Glu-	Lys-	Ser-	Glu-	Thr-	Pro-	Leu-	Val-	Thr-	Leu-	Phe
61	62	63	64	65	66	67	68	69	70	71	72	73	74	75	76	77	78

Pig

H-	Glu-	Leu-	Ala-	Gly	.....	Gln-	Ala-	Ala-	Glu-	Lys-	Lys-	Asp-	Glu-	Gly-	Pro-	Tyr-	Lys
	1	2	3	4		35	36	37	38	39	40	41	42	43	44	45	46

Tyr-	Gly-	Gly-	Phe-	Met	Thr-	Ser-	Glu-	Lys-	Ser-	Gln-	Thr-	Pro-	Leu-	Val-	Thr-	Leu-	Phe
61	62	63	64	65	66	67	68	69	70	71	72	73	74	75	76	77	78

Man

H-	Glu-	Leu-	Thr-	Gly	.....	Val-	Ala-	Ala-	Glu-	Lys-	Lys-	Asp-	Glu-	Gly-	Pro-	Tyr-	Arg
	1	2	3	4		35	36	37	38	39	40	41	42	43	44	45	46

Tyr-	Gly-	Gly-	Phe-	Met	Thr-	Ser-	Glu-	Lys-	Ser-	Glu-	Thr-	Pro-	Leu-	Val-	Thr-	Leu-	Phe
61	62	63	64	65	66	67	68	69	70	71	72	73	74	75	76	77	78

γ-LPH
Sheep

H-	Glu-	Leu-	xxx-	xxx	.....	xxx-	xxx-	xxx-	xxx-	xxx-	xxx-	Asp-	Ser-	Gly-	Pro-	Tyr-	Lys-
	1	2	3	4		35	36	37	38	39	40	41	42	43	44	45	46

Pig

H-	Glu-	Leu-	Ala-	Gly	.....	Glu-	Ala-	Ala-	Glu-	Lys-	Lys-	Asp-	Glu-	Gly-	Pro-	Tyr-	Lys-
	1	2	3	4		35	36	37	38	39	40	41	42	43	44	45	46

β-Endorphin
Camel

H-	Tyr-	Gly-	Gly-	Phe-	Met	Thr-	Ser-	Glu-	Lys-	Ser-	Gln-	Thr-	Pro-	Leu-	Val-	Thr-	Leu-	Phe
	1	2	3	4	5	6	7	8	9	10	11	12	13	14	15	16	17	18

γ-Endorphin
Pig

H-	Tyr-	Gly-	Gly-	Phe-	Met	Thr-	Ser-	Glu-	Lys-	Ser-	Gln-	Thr-	Pro-	Leu-	Val-	Thr-	Leu-OH[x]
	1	2	3	4	5	6	7	8	9	10	11	12	13	14	15	16	17

α-Endorphin
Pig

H-	Tyr-	Gly-	Gly-	Phe-	Met	Thr-	Ser-	Glu-	Lys-	Ser-	Glu-	Thr-	Pro-	Leu-	Val-	Thr-OH[t]
	1	2	3	4	5	6	7	8	9	10	11	12	13	14	15	16

α-Met⁵-Enkephalin
Pig

H-	Tyr-	Gly-	Gly-	Phe-	Met -OH[u]
	1	2	3	4	5

sequence	Melanocyte-stimulating potency *in vitro* (Units/gm)

<table>
<tr><td>

xxx- xxx- xxx- xxx- xxx- xxx-xxx - xxx- xxx- xxx- xxx- xxx- xxx-xxx-
47   48   49   50   51   52   53   54 55 56 57 58 59 60

..... Lys- Lys- Gly- Gln-OH[i]
    88   89   90   91

</td><td>2.0×10^{7j}</td></tr>
</table>

Met- Glu- His- Phe- Arg- Trp-Gly - Ser- Pro- Pro- Lys- Asp- Lys-Arg-
47   48   49   50   51   52   53   54 55 56 57 58 59 60

..... Lys- Lys- Gly- Gln-OH[k]
    88   89   90   91

2.0×10^{7l}

Met- Glu- His- Phe- Arg- Trp-Gly - Ser- Pro- Pro- Lys- Asp- Lys- Arg-
47   48   49   50   51   52   53   54 55 56 57 58 59 60

..... Lys- Lys- Gly- Gln-OH[m]
    88   89   90   91

1.5×10^{7n}

Met- Glu- His- Phe- Arg- Trp-Gly - Ser- Pro- Pro- Lys- Asp- Lys- Arg-
47   48   49   50   51   52   53   54 55 56 57 58 59 60

..... Lys- Lys- Gly- Glu-OH[o]
    88   89   90   91

—

Met- Glu- His- Phe- Arg- Trp-Gly - Ser- Pro- Pro- Lys- Asp-OH[p]
47   48   49   50   51   52   53   54 55 56 57 58

1.6×10^{7p}

Met- Glu- His- Phe- Arg- Trp-Gly - Ser- Pro- Pro- Lys- Asp-OH[q]
47   48   49   50   51   52   53   54 55 56 57 58

—

..... Lys- Lys- Gly- Gln-OH[r]
    28   29   30   31

—

—

—

—

1961). In each case, the peptide is 18 amino acid residues in length and has from 10 to 40% the biologic activity of α-MSH. It was long believed that β-MSH was also synthesized by the anterior pituitary of man. Human β-MSH was obtained by prolonged weak acetic acid extraction of acetone-dried human pituitaries as a by-product of the preparation of growth hormone (Dixon, 1960) and was subsequently sequenced (Harris, 1959) and synthesized (Rittel, 1968). In contrast to the β-MSH's of other species, human β-MSH had a tetrapeptide amino-terminal extension, making its overall length 22 amino acid residues. It was later noted that the additional tetrapeptide was identical to the sequence preceding the β-MSH sequence in the β-lipotropins from sheep (Li et al., 1965; Pankov, 1972) and pig (Gráf et al., 1971; Gráf and Li, 1973) pituitaries. However, it was not until the chromatographic behavior of immunoreactive human "β-MSH" on molecular sieve resin columns was examined in pituitary glands (Scott and Lowry, 1974) and circulating plasma (Bloomfield et al., 1974) that it was suggested that human β-MSH did not, in fact, exist and that it was an artifact of the original extraction procedure. This observation has now been confirmed by our laboratory (Tanaka et al., 1976a,b; 1978a). It appears that the 58-amino acid analog, γ-LPH, is the smallest β-MSH-related peptide found in normal human tissue and plasma, although a molecule about the size of β-MSH on gel filtration may be associated with ectopic tumor production of ACTH and lipotropins (Tanaka et al., 1978a; Hirata et al., 1976). The regular observation of a material the size of β-MSH by some investigators (Hirata et al., 1976) but not by others (Scott and Lowry, 1974; Bloomfield et al., 1974; Tanaka et al., 1976a,b, 1978a) may relate to how the tissues are handled prior to freezing or during extraction and chromatography.

What, then, was the material measured by radioimmunoassays for "β-MSH" (Abe et al., 1967b, 1969; Donald and Toth, 1973; Thody and Plummer, 1973; Donnadieu and Sevaux, 1973; Hirata et al., 1975)? It was, in the case of some, apparently primarily γ-LPH [Donald and Toth's (1973) antiserum (NZ) characterized by Gilkes et al. (1975)] and, in others, both β-LPH and γ-LPH [the antiserum of Abe et al. (1967b, 1969) characterized by L. H. Rees and G. A. Bloomfield (personal communication), and that of Tanaka et al., (1978a)]. In the other cases, one or the other or both presumably were measured, although the degree of reactivity with human β- and γ-LPH has not actually been reported for these antisera.

The studies of Phifer et al. (1970, 1974), employing antisera raised to synthetic bovine β-MSH (Schwyzer et al., 1963b) and the

C-terminal 25–39 sequence of porcine ACTH (Ciba-Geigy), demonstrated that ACTH and immunoreactive β-MSH, which we now believe to represent β- and γ-LPH, are synthesized in the same human adenohypophysal cells. In animals that possess an intermediate lobe, immunostaining experiments with an antiserum that was raised to ovine β-LPH and does not react with the β-MSH sequence (Desranleau *et al.*, 1972) indicate that β-LPH is synthesized in the same intermediate lobe cells that contain immunoreactive ACTH (Pelletier *et al.*, 1977). Thus, these intermediate lobe melanotrophs presumably produce α-MSH and CLIP from an ACTH precursor and use β-LPH as a precursor for the production of β-MSH, an amino terminal molecule of undetermined biologic significance, and a 59–91 carboxyl-terminal fragment that contains the sequences of methionine–enkephalin (Hughes *et al.*, 1975) and the endorphins (Guillemin *et al.*, 1976; Li and Chung, 1976b; Ling *et al.*, 1976). The enkephalins and endorphins are endogenous opiate-like peptides which compete with labeled naloxone (a morphine analog) for receptors on cells of the central nervous system and gastrointestinal tract and are the subject of intensive biochemical, physiologic, and pharmacologic investigations at present.

3. ACTH

ACTH, which is considered in detail in Chapter 12, is a relatively weak melanocyte-stimulating hormone. It is presumably synthesized from high molecular weight precursors (Orth *et al.*, 1973; Coslovsky *et al.*, 1975; Eipper and Mains, 1975; Mains and Eipper, 1975; Orth and Nicholson, 1977a), the first and largest of which has a molecular mass of about 31,000 daltons and is a glycopeptide (Eipper *et al.*, 1976; Nakanishi *et al.*, 1976; Orth and Nicholson, 1977b). In the intermediate lobe, ACTH itself appears to be a precursor for the production of α-MSH and CLIP, as mentioned earlier.

4. β-LPH and γ-LPH

As discussed above, both β- and γ-LPH appear to be synthesized in the adenohypophysis, where they are the final products of the biosynthetic pathway, and in the pars intermedia, where they are merely precursors for the synthesis of β-MSH and quite possibly the enkephalin–endorphin series of opiate polypeptides. In man, it is not yet clear which of the two LPH's predominates in the circulation; γ-LPH may predominate under some conditions (Jeffcoate *et al.*, 1977; Tanaka *et al.*, 1978), while β-LPH may predominate in others

(Bloomfield *et al.*, 1974; Bachelot *et al.*, 1977). However, the identity of the circulating LPH's has not yet been accurately defined in many physiologic or pathologic conditions.

5. Possible Common Prohormone

Evidence currently being obtained with AtT-20/D16v mouse pituitary adenocarcinoma cells (B. A. Eipper and R. E. Mains, personal communication) and with messenger RNA obtained from these cells translated in a cell-free system (Roberts *et al.*, 1977) indicates that ACTH, α-MSH, β-MSH, CLIP, β-LPH, γ-LPH, and the endorphins may, at least in this cell line, derive from a common precursor molecule with a molecular mass of about 31,000 daltons. The amino-terminus consists of a large fragment of as yet undetermined sequence and function, the central portion contains the ACTH (and, therefore, α-MSH and CLIP) sequence, and the extreme carboxy-terminus is the β-LPH (and, thus, γ-LPH, β-MSH and the enkephalin–endorphin) sequence. The different way in which this prohormone is processed in the anterior pituitary and intermediate lobe melanocorticotrophic cells presumably depends upon the presence of specific enzymes in these cells.

C. Immunologic Considerations

As in the case of ACTH (Chapter 12), there are a variety of potential problems in relating MSH/LPH immunologic reactivity to biologic activity and chemical identity. One of these has already been discussed in detail, the misinterpretation of the identity and, therefore, the biologic potency of immunoreactive "human β-MSH." Thus, although the data of Abe *et al.* (1967b, 1969) and others were correct, the assumption that the data reflected β-MSH concentration was not. If β-LPH and γ-LPH are weak melanocyte-stimulating hormones in man, as currently available data would suggest, then the conclusion that β-MSH is "the principal pigmentary hormone in man" (Abe *et al.*, 1969) requires reevaluation, and ACTH may well deserve that title.

The question of enzymatic degradation, already considered in Chapter 12, also obtains for the MSH/LPH peptides. Let us consider the specificities of a series of antibodies and what they might measure in biologic specimens. The known sequences of the MSH/LPH peptides are presented in Table I. Figure 1 is a diagrammatic representation of this series of hormones and of 11 antisera to various sequences of amino acid residues. Antibody 1, raised to β- or γ-LPH, is directed to some portion of the 1–40 sequence. It reacts indistinguishably with

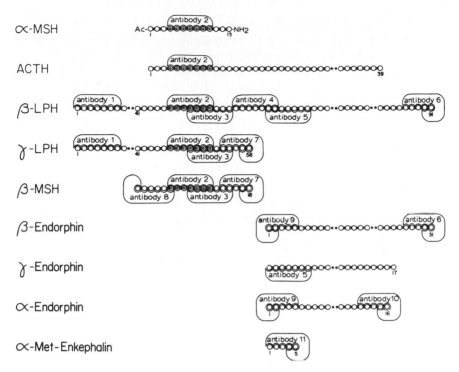

Figure 1. Diagrammatic representation of the primary structures of the MSH- and LPH-related hormonal peptides and their interactions with 11 representative antibodies. The heptapeptide Met-Glu-His-Phe-Arg-Trp-Gly sequence common to the melanocyte-stimulating members of this series is represented by (O) and reacts with antibody 2. See text for discussion of other antibodies.

β-LPH and γ-LPII, but does not react with the 41–58 sequence representing β-MSH. Such an antiserum has been raised to ovine β-LPH (Desranleau *et al.*, 1972) and, more recently, to human β-LPH (Jeffcoate *et al.*, 1977). Antibody 2 might have been raised to a number of antigens, since it reacts with heptapeptide core common to all of the ACTH/MSH/LPH hormones and might be expected not to distinguish one from another. Antibody 3 might have been raised to β-MSH, β-LPH, or γ-LPH and is directed toward a sequence near the carboxy-terminus of β-MSH and γ-LPH; it reacts with β-MSH, β-LPH, and γ-LPH. The antisera of Abe *et al.* (1967b, 1969), Bloomfield *et al.* (1974), and Tanaka *et al.* (1976a,b, 1978a) have this characteristic. Antibody 4 reacts with sequence containing the 59–60 Lys–Arg dipeptide connecting the 1–58 (γ-LPH) fragment to the 61–91 (β-endorphin) fragment of β-LPH and, thus, might react fully only with β-LPH. Antibody 5 is directed toward the 61–67 sequence and would not, therefore, distinguish between β-LPH and the endorphins, although it might have less affinity for methionine–enkephalin. Antibody 6 reacts with the carboxy-terminal 85–91 sequence, requires the terminal glutamyl residue, and measures β-LPH and β-endorphin indistinguishably. Such an antiserum has been developed (R. Guillemin, personal communication). Antibody 7 requires the carboxy-terminal asparaginyl residue and reacts on an equimolar basis with β-MSH and γ-LPH; it does not react with β-LPH. It could be produced by immunizing with either β-MSH or γ-LPH. The "NZ" antiserum of Donald and Toth (1973) appears to be such an antiserum, according to the results of Gilkes et al. (1975). The next antibody, antibody 8, might have been raised to β-MSH and requires the amino-terminal prolyl residue; it would react only with β-MSH. Antibody 9 requires the free amino-terminal tyrosyl residue of the enkephalin/endorphin peptides and would react with all of them, but not with β-LPH. Antibody 10 might be raised to α-endorphin and requires the carboxy-terminal threonyl residue; it reacts only with α-endorphin. Such an antiserum has been developed (R. Guillemin, personal communication). Finally, antibody 11 might be raised to methionine–enkephalin conjugated to a carrier protein. It would react only with methionine–enkephalin.

Thus, it can be seen that in designing immunogens, characterizing antisera, and interpreting results obtained with these antisera, both the structural interrelationships and the metabolic fates of these molecules must be considered.

II. METHODS OF RADIOIMMUNOASSAY

A. Source of Hormone

1. α-MSH

There are both purified and synthetic α-MSH preparations available. Dr. A. B. Lerner (Department of Dermatology, Yale University, New Haven, Connecticut) has produced highly purified α-MSH (Lerner and Lee, 1962) of porcine origin. We have not used this preparation in radioimmunoassay, but it is fully bioactive (Ney et al., 1965). We have used synthetic α-MSH (Schwyzer et al., 1963a) generously provided by Ciba-Geigy, Basel, Switzerland, for iodination and as reference standard. Others have synthesized α-MSH (Guttmann and Boissonnas, 1959; Hofmann et al., 1970; Blake et al., 1970), but we have had no experience with these preparations. With the availability of solid-phase synthesis (Merrifield, 1969), α-MSH has also become available from commercial sources, such as Beckman, Palo Alto, California.

2. β-MSH

Human β-MSH has been synthesized by Ciba-Geigy, Ltd. We have prepared sealed ampoules of this synthetic peptide under contract for the National Pituitary Agency to distribute to qualified investigators (Nicholson *et al.,* 1976). Each ampoule contains 50 μg synthetic peptide, which is suitable for use either for radioiodination or for reference standard. Human β-MSH has also been synthesized by Dr. H. Yajima of Kyoto University, Kyoto, Japan; we have not had personal experience with this preparation. Ciba-Geigy, Ltd., has also provided us with synthetic β_b-MSH (Schwyzer *et al.,* 1963b). The experience of Shapiro *et al.* (1972) would suggest that homologous standards may be required in at least some β-MSH radioimmunoassays; rat and mouse MSH's were distinctly nonparallel in their β_h-MSH assay, and even β_b-MSH and β_p-MSH had shallower competition curves than did β_h-MSH. It is obviously not possible to calculate the concentration of MSH in a specimen that generates a nonparallel curve, although, if the slopes are not too dissimilar, one can obtain an approximation using the point of 50% displacement of labeled tracer.

Commercial preparations of porcine ACTH contain significant quantities of contaminating porcine β-MSH, which differs in only one residue from the 41–58 sequence of human β-LPH. Several excellent antisera have been generated with these commercial preparations.

2. β-LPH and γ-LPH

As yet, there are no readily available sources of purified β-LPH and γ-LPH, and neither has yet been synthesized. Dr. C. H. Li (Hormone Research Laboratories, University of California, Berkeley, California) provided us with sufficient quantities of highly purified human β-LPH (Li and Chung, 1976a) for a number of studies, and Dr. P. J. Lowry (Chemical Pathology Research Laboratories, St. Bartholomew's Hospital, London, England) has provided us with highly purified human β-LPH and γ-LPH preparations (Scott and Lowry, 1974). Ovine β-LPH has been purified by Dr. C. H. Li (Li *et al.,* 1965) and by Dr. M. Chrétien (Institut de Recherches Cliniques, Montreal, Canada) and has been made available to various investigators. Because of the great current interest in the related enkephalin and endorphin peptides, it is probable that other investigators will undertake the purification of these hormones, although synthesis seems unlikely at this time because of their relatively large size. In the meantime, commercial ACTH preparations may again prove a valuable resource, as they may be contaminated with porcine LPH's as well as with β-MSH. A radioimmunoassay has been developed, using such an immunogen, which reacts with human β-LPH and γ-LPH, but not with the 37–58 ("β-MSH") sequence of these molecules (X. Bertagna and F. Girard, personal communication).

B. Production of Antibodies

1. Choice of Animal to Immunize

At present, there are no commercial or other sources of antisera to β-MSH, β-LPH, or γ-LPH, so one must produce his own. The choice of animal does not appear to be of any great importance. Useful antisera have been produced in guinea pigs (Abe et al., 1967b; Tanaka et al., 1976a,b) and rabbits (Donald and Toth, 1973; Thody and Plummer, 1973; Donnadieu and Sevaux, 1973; Ances and Pomerantz, 1974; Gilkes et al., 1975; Tanaka et al., 1978a).

2. The Antigen

The choice of antigen is restricted by availability. Synthetic human β-MSH is in too short supply for general use as an immunogen, and insufficient amounts of β-LPH and γ-LPH have been purified to make them widely available. However, as noted above, synthetic α-MSH is commercially available, and commercial ACTH preparations may contain both β-MSH and the LPH's. Antisera to α-MSH were obtained using synthetic α-MSH conjugated to rabbit serum albumin by the carbodiimide reaction (McGuire et al., 1965). Both rabbits injected produced very satisfactory antisera, one of which was highly specific and quite sensitive (Abe et al., 1967a). The other was even more sensitive, but reacted significantly with ACTH. Workers in several laboratories have obtained very useful antisera to β-MSH by immunizing guinea pigs or rabbits with commercially available ACTH, and we have obtained antisera by immunizing rabbits with synthetic human β-MSH conjugated to bovine serum albumin by either the carbodiimide or glutaraldehyde reactions, described in detail in Chapter 12.

If purified or synthetic peptides or fragments become more widely available, the considerations represented in Figure 1 dictate that care be exercised in the peptides used and the manner in which they are conjugated to protein carriers. For example, if one wished to produce an antibody with the specificity of antibody 8 (Figure 1), one might conjugate β-MSH by its amino-terminus, leaving the carboxy-terminus free for interaction with the B lymphocyte recognition site.

3. Immunization

The principles and procedures are precisely the same as those for ACTH, and are described in detail in Chapter 12.

C. Characterization of Antibody

As in the case of ACTH, antisera must be defined in terms of titer, sensitivity, and specificity. These properties are examined in precisely the same way as described for ACTH in Chapter 12.

Among the synthetic analogs produced by the chemists of Ciba-Geigy, Ltd., are α-MSH, α^{1-10}-ACTH, α^{7-13NH_2}-ACTH, β_b-MSH, β_h-MSH and β_h-MSH-Met[11]-sulfoxide. Dr. K. Hofmann and his co-

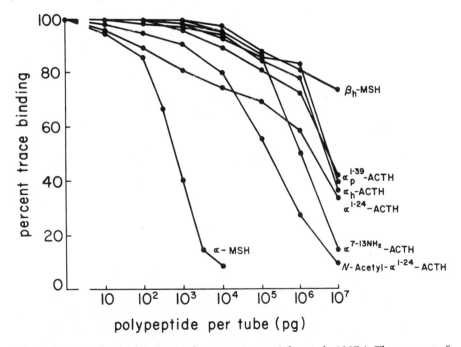

Figure 2. Specificity of α-MSH radioimmunoassay (Abe et al., 1967a). The percent of trace binding ($B/B_0 \times 100$) is plotted against picograms of unlabeled MSH and ACTH analogs added per tube. Peptides other than α-MSH react only weakly with this antiserum (R-31-1).

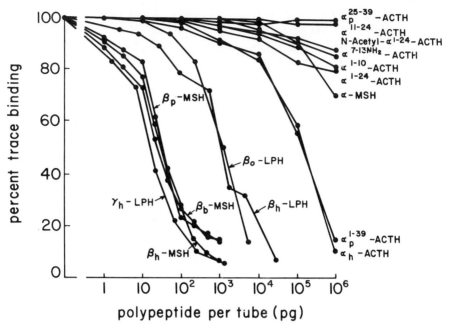

Figure 3. Specificity of β_h-MSH radioimmunoassay using antiserum G-82 (Abe *et al.*, 1967b, 1969). The data are plotted similarly to those in Figure 2. Human, bovine, and porcine β-MSH's generate similar competitive binding curves using ^{125}I-β_h-MSH tracer. Human and ovine β-LPH and γ_h-LPH also generate parallel curves. On a molar basis, β_h-LPH and γ_h-LPH appeared to be about 67 and 300% as effective as synthetic β_h-MSH (Ciba-Geigy, Ltd.) in displacing tracer from the antibodies, respectively. Other peptides react only weakly with this antiserum. The data on β_h-LPH and γ_h-LPH were provided by Drs. G. A. Bloomfield and L. H. Rees (personal communication). Ovine β-LPH was the gift of Dr. M. Chrétien.

workers at the University of Pittsburgh have synthesized a variety of analogs, including α^{1-13NH_2}-ACTH, α^{4-10}-ACTH, and α^{6-13NH_2}-ACTH. In addition, Dr. H. Yajima and his associates at Kyoto University have synthesized α-MSH, β_h-MSH, and a number of related peptides.

The competitive binding curve of an α-MSH antiserum (R-31-1) is shown in Figure 2. It can be seen that only α-MSH itself reacts well with the antibodies; there is no significant cross-reaction with human ACTH or "β-MSH" (and, thus, with β-LPH or γ-LPH) or even with N-acetyl-α^{1-24}-ACTH (which has the same amino-terminal configuration as α-MSH) or α^{7-13NH_2}-ACTH (which has the same carboxy-terminal configuration as α-MSH) (Abe *et al.*, 1967a).

Figures 3–5 show the specificities of the β-MSH antiserum (G-82) used by Abe *et al.* (1967b, 1969) and those (G-106, R-3) used by

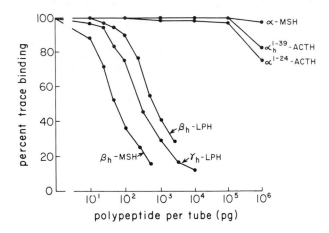

Figure 4. Specificity of β_h-MSH radioimmunoassay using antiserum G-106 (Tanaka *et al.*, 1976a,b). The data are plotted like those in Figure 2. On a molar basis, β_h-LPH and γ_h-LPH (provided by C. H. Li and P. J. Lowry, respectively) appeared to be about 58 and 82% as effective as synthetic β_h-MSH (Ciba-Geigy, Ltd.) in competing with ^{125}I-β_h-MSH for antibody binding sites. The data on α-MSH, α^{1-24}-ACTH, and α_h-ACTH were provided by Dr. K. Abe (personal communication).

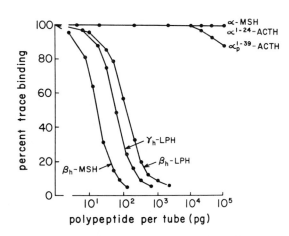

Figure 5. Specificity of β_h-MSH radioimmunoassay using antiserum R-3 (Tanaka *et al.*, 1976a,b). The data are plotted as in Figure 2. On a molar basis, β_h-LPH and γ_h-LPH (provided by Drs. C. H. Li and P. J. Lowry, respectively) appeared to be about 34 and 56% as effective as synthetic β_h-MSH (Ciba-Geigy, Ltd.) in competing with ^{125}I-labeled β_h-MSH for antibody binding sites.

Tanaka *et al.* (1976a,b, 1978a,b). Although the immunizing antigen was porcine β-MSH contaminating commercial ACTH for G-82 and G-106 (Orth, 1974) and synthetic human β-MSH conjugated to bovine serum albumin for R-3, the radioimmunoassays are sensitive and react significantly only with the various species of β-MSH, each of which differs in only one amino acid residue from the β-MSH peptide used for immunization and the LPH's that contain the respective β-MSH sequences.

D. Radioiodination of MSH

The preparation of radioiodinated α-MSH, β-MSH, β-LPH, and γ-LPH has been accomplished by minor modifications (Abe *et al.*, 1967a; Orth *et al.*, 1976; Tanaka *et al.*, 1978a) of the method of Hunter and Greenwood (1962). The procedure is essentially identical to that described for ACTH in Chapter 12, except that the peptide is contained in 5.0 μl 0.005 M HCl and only 1.0 mCi of ^{125}I is added to the iodination mixture.

The labeled peptide is separated from other iodination reagents and products by adding 3.0 ml 6000 g plasma from a dexamethasone-suppressed donor and 50 mg QUSO G-32 (microfine precipitated silica, Philadelphia Quartz Company, Philadelphia, Pennsylvania) to the iodination tube. The mixture is transferred to a 12×75 mm polypropylene tube (No. 2053, Falcon Plastics, Oxnard, California), mixed on a Vortex mixer for four to five seconds, and centrifuged; the supernatant fluid is removed. The QUSO pellet is washed two times with 3.0 ml distilled water and the labeled peptide is eluted from the QUSO with 4.0 ml acetic acid–acetone–water (1 : 20 : 80, v/v), mixing with a Vortex mixer until the pellet is completely resuspended. The supernate is decanted after centrifugation, and 0.1- to 0.2-ml aliquots are stored frozen at $-56°$C in polypropylene test tubes.

Aliquots of the QUSO-purified labeled peptide (10,000 to 30,000 cpm) are analyzed to determine the degree of purity and iodination damage by gel filtration through Sephadex G-25 or G-50 fine resin (Pharmacia Fine Chemicals, Piscataway, New Jersey) for β-MSH and the LPH's, respectively. Similar aliquots are also incubated overnight at 4°C in the presence of excess antibody in order to assess the degree of immunoreactivity of the labeled hormone. The specific activity averages about 250 μCi/μg and binding by excess antibody averages about 80 to 85%. In contrast to the experience of Gilkes *et al.* (1975), we find that this purification procedure is very satisfactory and that labeled hormone is stable at $-56°$C for up to three months. However, as in the case of ACTH, the labeled tracer is repurified immediately prior to use in each radioimmunoassay.

E. Preparation of Samples for Assay

Plasma is prepared by first obtaining a sample of blood atraumatically in a lightly heparanized syringe or by completely filling a Vacutainer EDTA or heparin collection tube. Although EDTA concentrations less than 7.6 mM do not inhibit the binding of β-MSH by antibodies, heparin concentrations of as little as 10 U/ml are inhibitory (Figure 6), as we and others have also found for ACTH (Chapter 12; Galskov, 1972). The samples are chilled and the plasma is separated in the same way as for ACTH (Chapter 12). The MSH/LPH peptides are extracted from plasma in exactly the same way as described for ACTH radioimmunoassay in Chapter 12, except that 200 mg silicic acid (No. 2847, 100 mesh, Lot No. TBM-A, Mallinckrodt Chemical Works, St.

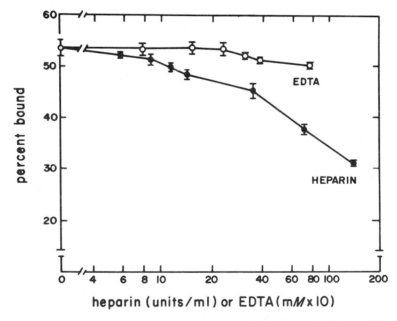

Figure 6. Effects of heparin and EDTA on antibody binding of ^{125}I-β_h-MSH. Trace concentrations of ^{125}I-labeled β_h-MSH (2-6 pg) and an antibody concentration sufficient to bind 50% of labeled tracer were incubated with graded concentrations of sodium heparin and disodium EDTA at 4°C for three days. In this and subsequent figures, the points represent the means of several values and the brackets represent the standard errors of the means (S.E.M.).

Louis, Missouri) is used for the extraction procedure (Orth *et al.*, 1976). As shown in Figure 7, the plasma concentration and sample volume have relatively little effect on the efficiency of extraction of labeled human β-MSH. Similar results have been obtained with β-LPH and γ-LPH (Tanaka *et al.*, 1978a). Both the adsorption and elution of peptide are essentially complete within 20 minutes (Figures 8 and 9), making the procedure a rapid one. Although more peptide is extracted as the concentration of silicic acid is increased (Donald, 1967), elution efficiency is also reduced and the net efficiency of the procedure hardly changes from 100 to 200 mg of silicic acid per extraction tube. (Figure 10). Thus, without varying the procedure, it is possible to extract a variety of plasma volumes depending, for example, upon the anticipated hormone concentration or the volume of sample available.

The extracts are frozen, lyophilized, stored, and reconstituted in 1.5 ml of standard diluent in the same way as those intended for ACTH radioimmunoassay (Chapter 12).

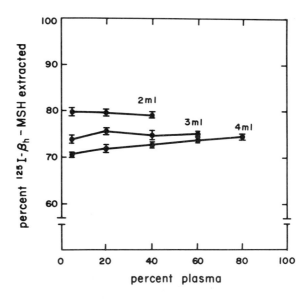

Figure 7.   Effects of sample volume and plasma concentration on silicic acid extraction of ^{125}I-labeled β_h-MSH. Three different volumes of buffer containing 5–80% plasma and ^{125}I-β_h-MSH were each extracted with 200 mg silicic acid by mixing for 30 minutes at room temperature. The labeled β_h-MSH was eluted with 2.5 ml acetic acid–acetone–water (1 : 20 : 80, v/v).

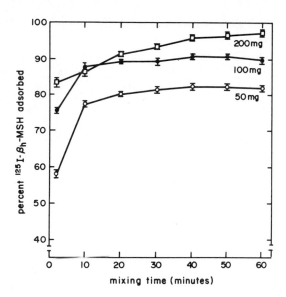

Figure 8. Effect of time on adsorption of ^{125}I-β_h-MSH to various amounts of silicic acid. A 2.0-ml volume of plasma to which ^{125}I-labeled β_h-MSH was added was mixed with silicic acid at room temperature on an aliquot mixer for the times indicated. The silicic acid was then washed twice with 2.5 ml distilled water and the percent of labeled β_h-MSH adsorbed was determined.

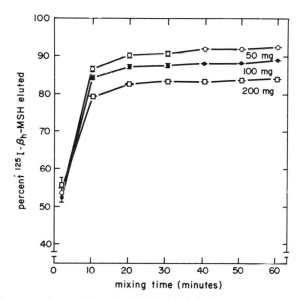

Figure 9. Effect of time on elution of ^{125}I-labeled β_h-MSH adsorbed to various amounts of silicic acid. Silicic acid to which labeled β_h-MSH was adsorbed was mixed with 2.5 ml acetic acid–acetone–water (1:20:80, v/v) on an aliquot mixer at room temperature for the times indicated, and the percent elution of adsorbed β_h-MSH was determined.

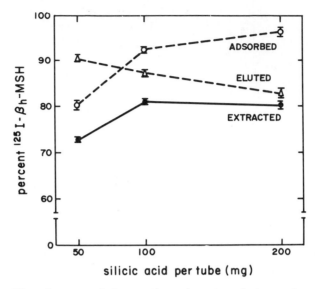

Figure 10.   Effect of amount of silicic acid on adsorption, elution, and net extraction of ^{125}I-β_h-MSH from plasma. Two milliliters of human plasma to which labeled β_h-MSH had been added was mixed with 50, 100, or 200 mg of silicic acid in 1.0 ml phosphate buffer for 30 minutes at room temperature. The silicic acid was centrifuged, washed twice with 2.5 ml distilled water, and mixed with 2.5 ml acetic acid–acetone–water for 30 minutes at room temperature. Percent adsorption, elution, and extraction (percent adsorption × percent elution) were determined.

F. Assay Procedure

The procedure is identical to that described for ACTH, with the exception of the separation of antibody-bound from free hormone.

The ideal separation should afford 100% discrimination of bound from free labeled hormone, should be simple, convenient, rapid, and inexpensive and should provide an accurate assessment of the amount of damage to the labeled hormone resulting from the incubation. The MSH's and LPH's all appear quite susceptible to damage, even when the whole procedure is carried out at 4°C. Damage is most marked when unextracted plasma is added to the incubation tubes, although recentrifugation at 6000 g prior to freezing appears to reduce this (Besser *et al.*, 1971). However, even plasma extracts can cause damage, and the degree of damage varies from one extract to another.

Of all the separation methods we have evaluated, QUSO (QUSO G-32, microprecipitated silica, Philadelphia Quartz Co., Philadelphia, Pennsylvania) appears to be as satisfactory as any for the MSH's and

LPH's and meets all of the criteria for an ideal separation method except for 100% discriminatory capacity and total assessment of damage. Efficient separation requires the presence of at least 30% unextracted plasma (Orth *et al.*, 1976). Bovine serum albumin (Cohn fraction V) and bovine globulin (Cohn fraction II) are not satisfactory substitutes. The final volume (incubation mixture plus QUSO–plasma–buffer) is also important, since the percent adsorption of ^{125}I-labeled hormone is greater in a small volume, but so is the percent of antibody-bound labeled hormone nonspecifically trapped with the pellet. To the 0.3 ml incubation mixture we add 2.2 ml 0.05 M phosphate buffer, pH 7.5, containing 45.5% outdated human blood bank plasma and 22.7 mg/ml QUSO at 4°C. This QUSO–plasma–buffer must be stirred constantly and vigorously with a magnetic stirring bar in order to prevent settling. It is dispensed with a 5.0-ml Repipet (Lab Industries). The tubes are mixed immediately for two to three seconds on a Vortex mixer and are centrifuged at 4000 g for five minutes at 4°C. The supernates are decanted, the tubes are drained, blotted, and capped, and the QUSO pellets, which contain free ^{125}I-labeled hormone, are counted in a gamma scintillation spectrometer.

G. Characteristics of the Assays

The specificities of the antisera have been discussed. Each sample is assayed at three or more dilutions to ensure that it generates a competitive binding curve parallel to that of the standard. The β-MSH assay has a sensitivity of about 5.0 pg/ml of extracted plasma, and the α-MSH assay about 50 pg/ml. The interassay and the intraassay coefficients of variation are about 11 and 7%, respectively. Since excessive concentrations of heparin or EDTA, high molarity, extremes of pH, and high protein concentrations can all inhibit antigen–antibody binding, these variables must be monitored and kept constant, insofar as possible, in every tube in an assay.

The normal values for human plasma immunoreactive β-MSH (i.e., LPH) are similar to those of immunoreactive ACTH, suggesting that, under most conditions, equimolar quantities of each are released by the pituitary corticomelanotrophic cell. Normal subjects have maximal plasma immunoreactive β-LPH levels of 58 ± 5.7 pg/ml early in the morning and minimal levels of 15 ± 2.1 pg/ml late in the evening (Tanaka *et al.*, 1978b). Because the release of the LPH's, like that of ACTH, is extremely sensitive to stress, care must be taken to avoid stressing the subject before obtaining the blood specimen, which may spuriously elevate the plasma concentration of these hormones.

III. PROBLEMS

The difficulties have been (1) raising high-affinity antibodies, a problem which now appears to have been overcome by intradermal injection of small amounts of conjugated antigens, (2) lack of materials for immunization, a problem which has not yet been solved, (3) lack of material for use as tracer and standard, a problem which has been corrected for human "β-MSH" radioimmunoassay, at least, and (4) interpretation of results and correlation with biologic activity. It is now clear that in man the "β-MSH" is the size of γ-LPH or greater. There is a need for homologous bioassays for the MSH's to confirm that the *in vitro* frog skin bioassay accurately reflects the relative potencies of the melanocyte-stimulating hormones in man.

ACKNOWLEDGMENTS

The authors wish to acknowledge the primary role played by Dr. Kaoru Abe in the development of the α-MSH and original β-MSH radioimmunoassays, the assistance of Ms. Barbara Sherrell in compiling the references, and that of Ms. Linda D'Errico in transcribing the manuscript.

These studies have involved the generous collaboration of a number of investigators, particularly Dr. Aaron B. Lerner of Yale University, New Haven, Connecticut; Drs. Glenys A. Bloomfield, Philip J. Lowry, and Lesley H. Rees of St. Bartholomew's Hospital, London, England; Dr. Choh Hao Li of the Hormone Research Laboratories, University of California, Berkeley, California; and those of Ciba-Geigy, Ltd., Basel, Switzerland, and the National Pituitary Agency, National Institute of Arthritis, Metabolism and Digestive Diseases, National Institutes of Health, Bethesda, Maryland, and University of Maryland, Baltimore, Maryland.

This work was supported in part by National Cancer Institute Research Grant 2-R01-CA11685 and National Institutes of Health grant 5-M01-RR00095.

REFERENCES

Abe, K., and Nicholson, W. E. (1975). Bioassay of pigmentary hormones. *In* "Methods in Enzymology" (B. W. O'Malley and J. G. Hardman, eds.), Vol. 37, pp. 121–130. Academic Press, New York.

Abe, K., Island, D. P., Liddle, G. W., Fleischer, N., and Nicholson, W. E. (1967a). Radioimmunologic evidence for α-MSH (melanocyte stimulating hormone) in human pituitary and tumor tissues. *J. Clin. Endocrinol. Metab.* **27**, 46–52.

Abe, K., Nicholson, W. E., Liddle, G. W., Island, D. P., and Orth, D. N. (1967b).

Radioimmunoassay of β-MSH in human plasma and tissues. *J. Clin. Invest.* **46,** 1609–1616.

Abe, K., Nicholson, W. E., Liddle, G. W., Orth, D. N., and Island, D. P. (1969). Normal and abnormal regulation of β-MSH in man. *J. Clin. Invest.* **48,** 1580–1585.

Ances, I. G., and Pomerantz, S. H. (1974). Serum concentration of β-melanocyte-stimulating hormone in human pregnancy. *Am. J. Obstet. Gynecol.* **119,** 1062–1068.

Bachelot, I., Wolfsen, A. R., and Odell, W. D. (1977). Pituitary and plasma lipotropins: Demonstration of the artifactual nature of β-MSH. *J. Clin. Endocrinol. Metab.* **44,** 939–946.

Besser, G. M., Orth, D. N., Nicholson, W. E., Byyny, R. L., Abe, K., and Woodham, J. P. (1971). Dissociation of disappearance of bioactive and radioimmunoreactive ACTH from plasma in man. *J. Clin. Endocrinol. Metab.* **32,** 595–603.

Björklund, A., Meurling, P., Nilsson, G., and Nobin, A. (1972). Standardization and evaluation of a sensitive and convenient assay for melanocyte-stimulating hormone using anolis skin in vitro. *J. Endocrinol.* **53,** 161–169.

Blake, J. J., Crooks, R. W., and Li, C. H. (1970). Solid-phase synthesis of (5-glutamine)-α-melanotropin. *Biochemistry* **9,** 2071–2074.

Bloomfield, G. A., Scott, A. P., Lowry, P. J., Gilkes, J. J. H., and Rees, L. H. (1974). A reappraisal of human β MSH. *Nature (London)* **252,** 492–493.

Burgers, A. C. J. (1961). Occurrence of three electrophoretic components with melanocyte-stimulating activity in extracts of single pituitary glands from ungulates. *Endocrinology* **68,** 698–703.

Chrétien, M., and Li, C. H. (1967). Isolation, purification, and characterization of γ-lipotropic hormone from sheep pituitary glands. *Can. J. Biochem.* **45,** 1163–1174.

Coslovsky, R., Schneider, B., and Yalow, R. S. (1975). Characterization of mouse ACTH in plasma and in extracts of pituitary and of adrenotropic pituitary tumor. *Endocrinology* **97,** 1308–1315.

Desranleau, R., Gilardeau, C., and Chrétien, M. (1972). Radioimmunoassay of ovine beta-lipotropic hormone. *Endocrinology* **91,** 1004–1010.

Dixon, H. B. F. (1960). Chromatographic isolation of pig and human melanocyte-stimulating hormones. *Biochim. Biophys. Acta* **37,** 38–42.

Dixon, J. S., and Li, C. H. (1961). The isolation and structure of β-melanocyte-stimulating hormone from horse pituitary glands. *Gen. Comp. Endocrinol.* **1,** 161–169.

Donald, R. A. (1967). A rapid method of extracting ACTH from plasma. *J. Endocrinol.* **39,** 451–452.

Donald, R. A., and Toth, A. (1973). A comparison of the β-melanocyte-stimulating hormone and corticotropin response to hypoglycemia. *J. Clin. Endocrinol. Metab.* **36,** 925–930.

Donnadieu, M., and Sevaux, D. (1973). Radioimmunoassay of melanocyte stimulating hormone (β-MSH) in human plasma. *Biomedicine* **19,** 272–274.

Draper, M. W., Merrifield, R. B., and Rizack, M. A. (1973). Lipolytic activity of Met-Arg-His-Phe-Arg-Trp-Gly, a synthetic analog of the ACTH (4-10) core sequence. *J. Med. Chem.* **16,** 1326–1330.

Dubois, M. P. (1972). Localisation cytologique par immunofluorescence des sécretions corticotropes, α- et β-mélanotropes au niveau de l'adénohypophyse des bovins, ovins et porcins. *Z. Zellforsch. Mikrosk. Anat.* **125,** 200–209.

Eipper, B. A., and Mains, R. E. (1975). High molecular weight forms of adrenocorticotrophic hormone in the mouse pituitary and in a mouse pituitary tumor cell line. *Biochemistry* **14**, 3836–3844.

Eipper, B. A., Mains, R. E., and Guenzi, D. (1976). High molecular weight forms of adrenocorticotropic hormone are glycoproteins. *J. Biol. Chem.* **251**, 4121–4126.

Galskov, A. (1972). Radioimmunochemical corticotropin determination. *Acta Endocrinol. (Copenhagen)* **162**, Suppl., pp 117–121.

Geschwind, I. I., Li, C. H., and Barnafi, L. (1957a). The structure of the β-melanocyte-stimulating hormone. *J. Am. Chem. Soc.* **79**, 620–625.

Geschwind, I. I., Li, C. H., and Barnafi, L. (1957b). The isolation and structure of a melanocyte-stimulating hormone from bovine pituitary glands. *J. Am. Chem. Soc.* **79**, 1003–1004.

Gilardeau, C., and Chrétien, M. (1970). Isolation and characterization of β-lipolytic hormone from porcine pituitary gland. *Can. J. Biochem.* **48**, 1017–1021.

Gilkes, J. J. H., Bloomfield, G. A., Scott, A. P., Lowry, P. J., Ratcliffe, J. G., Landon, J., and Rees, L. H. (1975). Development and validation of a radioimmunoassay for peptides related to β-melanocyte-stimulating hormone in human plasma: The lipotropins. *J. Clin. Endocrinol. Metab.* **40**, 450–457.

Gráf, L., and Li, C. H. (1973). Action of plasmin on ovine beta-lipotropin: Revision of the carboxyl terminal sequence. *Biochem. Biophys. Res. Commun.* **53**, 1304–1309.

Gráf, L., Barát, E., Cseh, G., and Sajgó, M. (1970). Amino acid sequence of porcine γ-lipotropic hormone. *Acta Biochim. Biophys. Acad. Sci. Hung.* **5**, 305–307.

Gráf, L., Barát, E., Cseh, G., and Sajgó, M. (1971). Amino acid sequence of porcine β-lipotropic hormone. *Biochim. Biophys. Acta* **229**, 276–278.

Guillemin, R., Ling, N., and Burgus, R. (1976). Endorphines, peptides d'origine hypothalamique et neurohypophysaire à activité morphinomimétique. Isolement et structure moléculaire de l'alpha-endorphine. *C. R. Hebd. Seances Acad. Sci., Ser. D* **282**, 783–785.

Gutmann, S., and Boissonnas, R. A. (1959). Synthèse de l'α-melantropine (α-MSH) de porc. *Helv. Chim. Acta* **42**, 1257–1264.

Harris, J. I. (1959). Structure of a melanocyte-stimulating hormone from the human pituitary gland. *Nature (London)* **184**, 167–186.

Harris, J. I., and Lerner, A. B. (1957). Amino-acid sequence of the α-melanocyte-stimulating hormone. *Nature (London)*, **179**, 1346–1347.

Hirata, Y., Yamamoto, H., Matsukura, S., and Imura, H. (1975). *In vitro* release and biosynthesis of tumor ACTH in ectopic ACTH producing tumors. *J. Clin. Endocrinol. Metab.* **41**, 106–114.

Hirata, Y., Matsukura, S., Imura, H., Nakamura, M., and Tanaka, A. (1976). Size heterogeneity of β-MSH in ectopic ACTH-producing tumors: Presence of β-LPH-like peptides. *J. Clin. Endocrinol. Metab.* **42**, 33–40.

Hofmann, K., Andreatta, R., Bohn, H., and Moroder, L. (1970). Studies on polypeptides. XLV. Structure-function studies in the β-corticotropin series. *J. Med. Chem.* **13**, 339–345.

Hogben, L., and Gordon, C. (1930). Studies on the pituitary. VII. The separate identity of the pressor and melanophore principles. *J. Exp. Biol.* **7**, 286–292.

Hogben, L. T., and Winton, F. R. (1924). The pigmentary effector system. III. Colour response in the hypophysectomised frog. *Proc. R. Soc. London* **95**, 15–31.

Horowitz, S. B. (1958). The energy requirements of melanin granule aggregation and dispersion in the melanophores of *Anolis carolinensis*. *J. Cell. Comp. Physiol.* **51**, 341–357.

Hughes, J., Smith, T. W., Kosterlitz, H. W., Fothergill, L. A., Morgan, B. A., and Morris,

H. R. (1975). Identification of two related pentapeptides from the brain with potent opiate agonist activity. *Nature (London)* **258**, 577–580.

Hunter, W. M., and Greenwood, F. C. (1962). Preparation of iodine-131 labelled human growth hormone of high specific activity. *Nature (London)* **194**, 495–496.

Jeffcoate, W. J., Gilkes, J. J. H., Rees, L. H., Lowry, P. J., and Besser, G. M. (1977). The use of radioimmunoassays for human β-lipotropin. *Endocrinology* **100**, Suppl., 215.

Kastin, A. J., and Ross, G. T. (1964). Modified *in vivo* assay for MSH. *Experientia* **20**, 461–462.

Kleinholz, L. H. (1938). Studies in reptilian colour changes. II. The pituitary and adrenal glands in the regulation of the melanophores of *Anolis carolinensis J. Exp. Biol.* **15**, 474–491.

Lee, T. H., Lerner, A. B., and Buettner-Janusch, V. (1961). The isolation and structure of α- and β-melanocyte-stimulating hormones from monkey pituitary glands. *J. Biol. Chem.* **236**, 1390–1394.

Lee, T. H., Lerner, A. B., and Buettner-Janusch, V. (1963). Melanocyte-stimulating hormones from sheep pituitary glands. *Biochim. Biophys. Acta* **71**, 706–709.

Lerner, A. B., and Lee, T. H. (1962). The melanocyte-stimulating hormones. *Vitam. Horm. (N.Y.)* **20**, 337–346.

Li, C. H. (1959a). Proposed system of terminology for preparations of adrenocorticotropic hormone. *Science* **129**, 969–970.

Li, C. H. (1959b). The relation of chemical structure to the biologic activity of pituitary hormones. *Lab. Invest.* **8**, 574–587.

Li, C. H., and Chung, D. (1976a). Primary structure of human β-lipotrophin. *Nature (London)*, **260**, 622–624.

Li, C. H., and Chung, D. (1976b). Isolation and structure of an untriakontapeptide with opiate activity from camel pituitary glands. *Proc. Natl. Acad. Sci. U.S.A.* **73**, 1145–1148.

Li, C. H., Schnabel, E., Chung, D., and Lo, T. (1961). Synthesis of L-methionyl-L-glutamyl-L-histidyl-L-phenylalanyl-L-arginyl-L-tryptophyl-glycine and its melanocyte-stimulating and corticotropin-releasing activity. *Nature (London)* **189**, 143.

Li, C. H., Barnafi, L., Chrétien, M., and Chung, D. (1965). Isolation and amino-acid sequence of β-LPH from sheep pituitary glands. *Nature (London)* **208**, 1093–1094.

Ling, N., Burgus, R., and Guillemin, R. (1976). Isolation, primary structure, and synthesis of α-endorphin and γ-endorphin, two peptides of hypothalamic–hypophysial origin with morphinomimetic activity. *Proc. Natl. Acad. Sci. U.S.A.* **73**, 3942–3946.

Lohmar, P., and Li, C. H. (1967). Isolation of bovine β-lipotropic hormone. *Biochim. Biophys. Acta* **147**, 381–383.

Lohmar, P., and Li, C. H. (1968). Biological properties of ovine β-lipotropic hormone. *Endocrinology* **82**, 898–904.

Lowry, P. J., and Chadwick, A. (1970). Interrelations of some pituitary hormones. *Nature (London)* **226**, 219–222.

McGuire, J., McGill, R., Leeman, S., and Goodfriend, T. (1965). The experimental generation of antibodies to α-MSH and ACTH. *J. Clin Invest.* **44**, 1672–1678.

Mains, R. E., and Eipper, B. A. (1975). Molecular weights of adrenocorticotropic hormone in extracts of anterior and intermediate-posterior lobes of mouse pituitary. *Proc. Natl. Acad. Sci. U.S.A.* **72**, 3565–3569.

Merrifield, R. B. (1969). Solid-phase peptide synthesis. *Adv. Enzymol.* **32**, 221–296.

Nakanishi, S., Taii, S., Hirata, Y., Matsukura, S., Imura, H., and Numa, S. (1976). A large product of cell-free translation of messenger RNA coding for corticotropin. *Proc. Natl. Acad. Sci. U.S.A.* **73,** 4319–4323.

Ney, R. L., Ogata, E., Shimizu, N., Nicholson, W. E., and Liddle, G. W. (1965). Structure–function relationships of ACTH and MSH analogues. *Proc. Int. Congr. Endocrinol., 2nd, 1964* Excerpta Med. Found. Int. Congr. Ser. No. 83, pp. 1184–1191.

Nicholson, W. E., Parks, K. R., Tanaka, K., Mount, C. D., and Orth, D. N. (1976). Method for preparation of ampoules containing microgram quantities of polypeptide hormones for distribution and use as laboratory standards: synthetic human ACTH and β-MSH. *J. Clin. Endocrinol. Metab.* **42,** 1153–1157.

Orth, D. N. (1974). Adrenocorticotropic hormone and melanocyte stimulating hormone (ACTH and MSH). *In* "Methods of Hormone Radioimmunoassay" (B. M. Jaffe and H. R. Behrman, eds.), 1st ed., pp. 125–159. Academic Press, New York.

Orth, D. N., and Nicholson, W. E. (1977a). Different molecular forms of ACTH. *Ann. N.Y. Acad. Sci.* **297,** 27–48.

Orth, D. N., and Nicholson, W. E. (1977b). High molecular weight forms of human ACTH are glycoproteins. *J. Clin. Endocrinol. Metab.* **44,** 214–217.

Orth, D. N., Nicholson, W. E., Mitchell, W. M., Island, D. P., and Liddle, G. W. (1973). Biologic and immunologic characterization and physical separation of ACTH and ACTH fragments in the ectopic ACTH syndrome. *J. Clin. Invest.* **52,** 1756–1769.

Orth, D. N., Tanaka, K., and Nicholson, W. E. (1976). The melanotropins. *In* "Hormones in Human Blood: Detection and Assay" (H. N. Antoniades, ed.), pp. 423–448. Harvard Univ. Press, Cambridge, Massachusetts.

Pankov, Y. A. (1972). C-terminal sequence of amino acid residues in bovine β-lipotropic hormone molecule. *Biokhimiya* **37,** 1095–1096.

Pelletier, G., Leclerc, R., Labrie, F., Cote, J., Chrétien, M., and Lis, M. (1977). Immunohistochemical localization of β-lipotropic hormone in the pituitary gland. *Endocrinology* **100,** 770–776.

Phifer, R. F., and Spicer, S. S. (1970). Immunohistologic and immunopathologic demonstration of adrenocorticotropic hormone in pars intermedia of the adenohypophysis. *Lab. Invest.* **23,** 543–550.

Phifer, R. F., Spicer, S. S., and Orth, D. N. (1970). Specific demonstration of the human hypophyseal cells which produce adrenocorticotropic hormone. *J. Clin. Endocrinol. Metab.* **31,** 347–361.

Phifer, R. F., Orth, D. N., and Spicer, S. S. (1974). Specific demonstration of the human hypophyseal adrenocortico-melanotropic (ACTH/MSH) cell. *J. Clin. Endocrinol. Metab.* **39,** 684–692.

Pickering, B. T., and Li, C. H. (1963). On the properties of human β-melanocyte-stimulating hormone. *Biochim. Biophys. Acta* **74,** 156–157.

Rittel, W. (1968). Techniques for the synthesis of ACTH and MSH peptides and analogues. *Adv. Exp. Med. Biol.* **2,** 35–47.

Roberts, J. L., Phillips, M. A., and Herbert, E. (1977). Messenger RNA directed synthesis of a high molecular weight form of ACTH. *Endocrinology* **100,** Suppl., 57.

Rudman, D., Brown, S. J., and Malkin, M. F. (1963). Adipokinetic actions of adrenocorticotrophin, thyroid-stimulating hormone, vasopressin, α- and β-melanocyte stimulating hormones, fraction H, epinephrine and norepinephrine in rabbit, guinea pig, hamster, rat, pig, and dog. *Endocrinology* **72,** 527–542.

Schwyzer, R., Costopangiotis, A., and Sieber, P. (1963a). Zwei Synthesen des αMSH mit Hilfe leicht entfernbarer Schutzgruppen. *Helv. Chim. Acta* **46,** 870–889.

Schwyzer, R., Isselin, B., Kappeler, H., Riniker, B., Rittel, W., and Zuber, H. (1963b).

Die Synthese des β-MSH mit der Aminosaurensequenz des bovinen Hormons. *Helv. Chim. Acta* **46**, 1975–1996.

Schwyzer, R., Schiller, P., Seelig, S., and Sayers, G. (1971). Isolated adrenal cells: Log dose response curves for steroidogenesis induced by $ACTH_{1-24}$, $ACTH_{1-10}$, $ACTH_{4-10}$ and $ACTH_{5-10}$. *FEBS Lett.* **19**, 229–231.

Scott, A. P., and Lowry, P. J. (1974). Adrenocorticotrophic and melanocyte-stimulating peptides in the human pituitary. *Biochem. J.* **139**, 593–602.

Scott, A. P., Ratcliffe, J. G., Rees, L. H., Landon, J., Bennet, H. P. J., Lowry, P. J., and McMartin, C. (1973). Pituitary peptide. *Nature (London), New Biol.* **244**, 65–67.

Scott, A. P., Lowry, P. J., Ratcliffe, J. G., Rees, L. H., and Landon, J. (1974a). Corticotrophin-like peptides in the rat pituitary. *J. Endocrinol.* **61**, 355–367.

Scott, A. P., Lowry, P. J., Bennett, H. P. J., McMartin, C., and Ratcliffe, J. G. (1974b). Purification and characterization of porcine corticotrophin-like intermediate lobe peptide. *J. Endocrinol.* **61**, 369–380.

Shapiro, M., Nicholson, W. E., Orth, D. N., Mitchell, W. M., Island, D. P., and Liddle, G. W. (1972). Preliminary characterization of the pituitary melanocyte stimulating hormones of several vertebrate species. *Endocrinology* **90**, 249–256.

Shizume, K., Lerner, A. B., and Fitzpatrick, T. P. (1954). *In vitro* bioassay for the melanocyte stimulating hormone. *Endocrinology* **54**, 553–560.

Silman, R. E., Chard, T., Lowry, P. J., Smith, I., and Young, I. M. (1976). Human foetal pituitary peptides and parturition. *Nature (London)* **260**, 716–718.

Smith, P. E. (1916). The effect of hypophysectomy in the early embryo upon the growth and development of the frog. *Anat. Rec.* **11**, 57–64.

Tanaka, K., Mount, C. D., Nicholson, W. E., and Orth, D. N. (1976a). "Big" bioactive and immunoreactive "β-MSH's" in human plasma and tumor tissue. *Clin. Res.* **24**, 10A.

Tanaka, K., Mount, C. D., and Orth, D. N. (1976b). High molecular weight forms of bioactive and immunoreactive "β-MSH" in human plasma, pituitary and tumor tissue. *Endocrinology* **98**, Suppl., 121.

Tanaka, K., Nicholson, W. E., and Orth, D. N. (1978a). The nature of immunoreactive LPHs in human plasma and tissue extracts. *J. Clin. Invest.* (In press).

Tanaka, K., Nicholson, W. E., and Orth, D. N. (1978b). Diurnal rhythm and disappearance half-time of endogenous plasma immunoreactive β-MSH (LPH) and ACTH in man. *J. Clin. Endocrinol. Metab.* **46**, 883–890.

Teague, R. S., and Patton, J. R. (1960). Analysis of the spectrophotometric reflectance response of frogs to melanophore hormone. *J. Cell. Comp. Physiol.* **56**, 15–24.

Thing, E. (1952). Melanophore reaction and adrenocorticotrophic hormone. I. Comparison of methods based upon photoelectric measurements and microscopic observations of the melanophores. *Acta Endocrinol. (Copenhagen)* **10**, 295–319.

Thody, A. J., and Plummer, N. A. (1973). A radioimmunoassay for β-melanocyte-stimulating hormone in human plasma. *J. Endocrinol.* **58**, 263–273.

14

Thyrotropin

ROBERT D. UTIGER

I. INTRODUCTION

Thyrotropin (TSH) is largely responsible for the maintenance of normal thyroid hormone synthesis and secretion. In addition to its ability to bind to thyroid cell membranes and stimulate thyroidal iodide metabolism and thyroid hormone synthesis and release, TSH stimulates many other metabolic processes in the thyroid gland such as cyclic AMP generation, glucose oxidation, oxygen consumption, and phospholipid and protein synthesis. Many of these actions of TSH have been used as endpoints for the biologic assay of TSH. However, available TSH bioassay methods, even newer cell membrane binding assays, do not have sufficient sensitivity for the measurement of TSH in plasma, except in situations wherein plasma TSH concentrations are elevated. The one exception to this rule, the very sensitive TSH cytobiochemical assay, is technically difficult and requires special

315

Methods of Hormone Radioimmunoassay, Second Edition
Copyright © 1979 by Academic Press, Inc.
All rights of reproduction in any form reserved. ISBN 0-12-379260-6

equipment (Bitensky *et al.*, 1974). Assay specificity is also a problem, since other hormones, such as human chorionic gonadotropin (HCG) and thyroid-stimulating immunoglobulins (the long-acting thyroid stimulator and related substances), also produce positive bioassay responses.

When highly purified human TSH first became available (Condliffe, 1962), the development of TSH radioimmunoassays became feasible. It soon became clear that human TSH differed immunochemically from that of other species (Utiger *et al.*, 1963), even though there is no species specificity of the biologic activity of TSH. Thus, satisfactory human TSH radioimmunoassay systems have all employed human TSH and anti-human TSH serum. TSH is one of the three carbohydrate-containing protein hormones of the anterior pituitary, the others being luteinizing hormone (LH) and follicle-stimulating hormone (FSH). These three hormones (TSH, LH, and FSH), as well as chorionic gonadotropin (HCG), have considerable chemical and thus immunologic similarities. This has posed certain problems in the radioimmunoassay of TSH, as will be described below. The immunoglobulin thyroid-stimulating hormones, of which LATS is the prototype, have no immunochemical similarity to TSH and thus are not detected by the TSH radioimmunoassay.

II. METHOD OF RADIOIMMUNOASSAY

A. Source of Hormone

Initially, highly purified human TSH prepared by Condliffe (1962) was used both for labeling with radioactive iodide and as standard in the radioimmunoassay. More recently, purified TSH has been available from the National Pituitary Agency and is now also commercially available. This material, usually prepared as a 0.5 to 1.0 mg/ml solution in $0.05 M$ phosphate buffer, pH 7.5, is used for labeling. It should be pointed out that most purified TSH preparations contain 1.0–2.0% LH biologic activity by weight. As standard for the radioimmunoassay, a partially purified human TSH preparation, Human Thyrotropin Research Standard A (HTRS-A), prepared and distributed under the auspices of the World Health Organization and available from the National Institute for Medical Research, Great Britain, is used. This material is available in ampoules containing 50 mU. The contents of an ampoule of this material are readily soluble in 20 ml 0.25% bovine serum albumin (BSA), $0.01 M$ phosphate, $0.15 M$ NaCl, pH 7.5. This solution thus contains 2.5 mU/ml. It is quite stable when stored in small aliquots in the frozen state.

B. Antibody Production

Initially, anti-human TSH sera were prepared by immunization of rabbits with highly purified TSH emulsified in complete Freund's adjuvant, in a dose of 100–300 μg/injection (Utiger *et al.*, 1963). Serum obtained four weeks after the second or third monthly injection proved to have a high titer, 50% binding of 0.05–0.1 ng ^{125}I-TSH usually occurring at a final dilution of $> 1 : 100,000$. The affinity of these anti-TSH sera is such that 0.1 ng purified TSH or 0.3 μM of the HTRS-A standard can be detected. The anti-TSH serum now in use in this laboratory is that available from the National Pituitary Agency, prepared by a similar method and having similar characteristics. It is available in ampoules containing a 1 : 100 dilution of the antiserum.

C. Characterization of Antibody

As indicated previously, the TSH preparations available for use as immunogen have all had detectable LH biologic activity and may contain FSII as well. Therefore, the anti-TSH serum obtained contains anti-LH and anti-FSH antibody as well as anti-TSH antibody. This has been demonstrated by the finding that highly purified LH and FSH preparations inhibit the binding of labeled TSH to the anti-TSH serum (Odell *et al.*, 1968; Jacquet *et al.*, 1971). The LH and FSH dose–response relationship is usually parallel to that of TSH, although larger quantities of the gonadotropins are required. HCG has also been found to inhibit binding of labeled TSH to anti-TSH serum, although in this case the dose–response inhibition pattern is very different from that of TSH (Utiger, 1965). All of these hormones (TSH, LH, FSH, and HCG) have two polypeptide subunits, and there is evidence that one of these subunits (the α subunit) is similar or identical in structure in the four hormones (Cornell and Pierce, 1973). On the other hand, the other subunit (β) of these hormones differs substantially, and it is the β subunit which confers the biologic specificity of the hormone. The reactivity of the several gonadotropins with anti-TSH sera may reflect in part the presence of antibody to the non-TSH specific α subunit of the TSH molecule as well as gonadotropin contamination of the TSH immunogen. Reactivity of anti-TSH serum with gonadotropins can be reduced by absorption of anti-TSH serum with HCG. Reactivity with both α and β subunits of TSH can still be demonstrated when HCG-absorbed anti-TSH is used, but the quantities required are large and may reflect the presence of small amounts of intact TSH in the subunit preparations (Binoux *et al.*, 1974). Absorption is easily accomplished by incubating the anti-TSH serum with HCG in a ratio of 3000–5000 I.U. HCG for each ml of 1 : 100 diluted anti-TSH serum for 48 hours at 5°C. The absorbed anti-TSH serum is then frozen and aliquots are used as needed. When anti-TSH serum is absorbed in this manner, HCG no longer inhibits the binding of labeled TSH to antiserum. While absorption with HCG is probably mandatory only when the TSH concentration of serum from pregnant women is to be determined, it is in practice easier to use HCG-absorbed anti-TSH serum in all assays.

Other human pituitary hormones and other thyroid-stimulating hormones, such as serum or serum concentrates rich in thyroid-stimulating immunoglobulins, have no reactivity with the anti-TSH serum (Odell *et al.*, 1967; Utiger, 1968; Raud and Odell, 1969). Similarly, little reactivity with bovine, rat, and mouse pituitary tumor TSH has been observed (Utiger *et al.*, 1963).

D. Preparation of ^{125}I-TSH

TSH is labeled with ^{125}I by the method of Greenwood *et al.* (1963), using 2.0 μg purified TSH (20 μl), 1.0 mCi ^{125}I, and 35 μg chloramine-T (40 μl). The reaction is carried out in 0.5 M phosphate at pH 7.5 and is allowed to proceed for 30 seconds. Sodium metabisulfite (24 μg) is then added. The ^{125}I-TSH is recovered from the reaction mixture by fractionation on a 1.0 × 15 cm column of Sephadex G-50 prepared and eluted with 0.01 M PO$_4$, 0.15 M NaCl, pH 7.5. The first four milliliters to emerge from the column are discarded. The next four milliliters are collected and diluted with 10–12 ml 5% BSA, 0.01 M PO$_4$, and 0.15 M NaCl, pH 7.5, and frozen in small aliquots. Using this procedure, ^{125}I-TSH with calculated specific activities of 50–100 μCi/μg is obtained, and up to 90% of the product is immunoreactive when incubated with an excess of anti-TSH serum.

For use in the radioimmunoassay, the ^{125}I-TSH is purified by gel filtration on Sephadex G-100 (2.0 × 40 cm) at the time it is to be added to the assay. The column is eluted with 0.01 M PO$_4$, 0.15 M NaCl, pH 7.5, and thirty to forty 2-ml fractions are collected and their radioactivities are determined. Radioactivity eluted in the void volume (V_0) of the column (20–25 ml) represents ^{125}I-TSH aggregates and is poorly immunoreactive (Figure 1). ^{125}I-TSH of high immunoreactivity is eluted between 50 and 60 ml. Subsequent fractions contain degraded ^{125}I-TSH or ^{125}I and are also poorly immunoreactive. As time elapses after

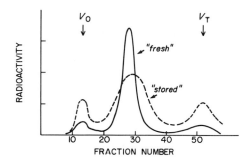

Figure 1. Chromatography of ^{125}I-TSH. The solid line shows the pattern of elution of radioactivity of freshly iodinated TSH and the dashed line that of iodinated TSH stored at $-5°C$ for 60 days.

initial preparation of ^{125}I-TSH, the proportion of radioactivity remains high. A recent study by Pekary and co-workers (1975) has carefully defined the optimal conditions for storage of ^{125}I-TSH in order to minimize radiation damage and ^{125}I dissociation, as assessed by Sephadex G-75 gel filtration. They found that storage of ^{125}I-TSH in 0.25% BSA at $-60°C$ was best. It is evident that careful storage and Sephadex G-75 or G-100 purification enable use of a ^{125}I-TSH preparation for several months.

E. Preparation of Samples for Assay

Comparative studies have shown that measurement of TSH in either serum or plasma gives similar results in the TSH radio-immunoassay (Adams *et al.*, 1972). Furthermore, serum or blood kept at room temperature for 72 hours contained no less TSH than serum frozen two to three hours after collection. TSH is not lost in serum stored at $-5°C$ for up to five years.

F. Assay Procedure

The specific TSH radioimmunoassay procedure now in use in this laboratory is described here. This protocol is designed for use with an automatic pipetting station (Micromedic Systems, Inc.), but is equally suited for manual preparation. The assay is carried out in 12×75 mm disposable glass tubes, and all reactions are carried out at $5°C$. The assay buffer is 0.25% BSA, $0.01\,M$ PO$_4$, $0.15\,M$ NaCl, pH 7.5.

1. Day 1

a. Two hundred microliters (in quadruplicate) of the standard TSH (HTRS-A) is serially diluted with BSA–PO$_4$–NaCl so that each tube contains 20, 10, 5.0, 2.5, 1.25, 0.62, 0.31, and 0.155 μU TSH and 200 μl of serum from a patient with severe hyperthyroidism or a normal subject who had received large doses of exogenous thyroid hormone. Serum or plasma samples are assayed in volumes of 200 and 100 μl unless high serum TSH concentrations are anticipated, in which case smaller volumes are used. Serum containing no TSH, as described above, is added so that the total volume of serum in each tube is 200 μl. For quality control, aliquots of a serum pool prepared to contain a normal or slightly elevated TSH concentration are assayed in two doses in quadruplicate.

b. One hundred microliters of anti-human TSH serum (NPA) absorbed with HCG as described above and diluted 1 : 20,000 with BSA–PO$_4$–NaCl containing 0.05 M EDTA, pH 7.5, is added. This is sufficient to precipitate 40–50% of the added ^{125}I-TSH. The antibody solution also contains commercial rabbit IgG immunoglobulin in a concentration of 25 μg/ml. This is added to ensure optimal precipitation of antibody-bound ^{125}I-TSH, since the amount of IgG in the anti-TSH serum alone in each tube is not sufficient for the formation of an immune precipitate when the second antibody is added.

2. Day 2

Following purification of the ^{125}I-TSH by Sephadex G-100 gel filtration as described previously, the appropriate fractions are pooled and diluted so that the solution has about 60,000 to 80,000 cpm/ml. One hundred microliters of this solution is added to each assay tube. The addition of the ^{125}I-TSH one day after initiation of the assay has been found to increase assay sensitivity by a factor of two.

3. Day 4

One hundred microliters of goat anti-rabbit IgG serum is added to each tube. This antiserum may be prepared by immunization of goats with 40 mg rabbit IgG emulsified in complete Freund's adjuvant. Potent anti-rabbit IgG sera are also available commercially. Each batch of goat anti-rabbit IgG is fractionated by ammonium sulfate precipitation, followed by extensive dialysis of the dissolved precipitate against 0.01 M PO$_4$, 0.15 M NaCl, pH 7.5. Each batch of second antibody must be tested to ensure that a quantity which maximally precipitates antibody-bound ^{125}I-TSH radioactivity is used.

4. Day 5

To each tube is added 1.5 ml of 0.01 M PO_4, 0.15 M NaCl, pH 7.5, and the tubes are centrifuged at 3000 rpm for 45 minutes at 5°C. The supernatant is aspirated, and the precipitate radioactivity is determined. The addition of buffer before centrifugation has been found to obviate the need for washing of the precipitates and thus reduces the manual work necessary for completion of the assay. For calculation of results, the precipitate radioactivity is plotted as a function of the logarithm of the TSH content of the tubes containing the standard TSH. The result-ing plot usually has a sigmoidal shape; only the linear part of the plot is employed for calculation of the TSH content of unknown samples. The resulting value then is converted to μU/ml.

G. Verification of the Assay

The effect of purified TSH, partially purified TSH (HTRS-A), and TSH in serum on the binding of ^{125}I-TSH to anti-TSH serum is shown in Figure 2. The finding of similar slopes of inhibition of binding of ^{125}I-TSH to anti-TSH by the three TSH-containing solutions suggests

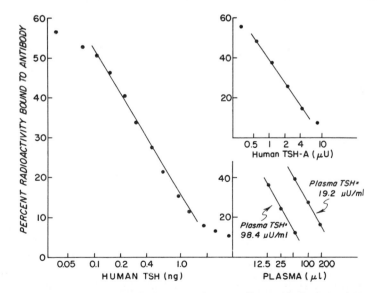

Figure 2. Effects of highly purified TSH (left), partially purified TSH, WHO Human Thyrotropin Research Standard (upper right), and plasma in the TSH radioimmunoas-say. The plasma samples were obtained from a patient with hypothyroidism before and after three weeks of therapy with L-thyroxine, 0.1 mg/day. Reprinted with permission from Utiger (1968).

the TSH in them is immunochemically similar and constitutes one measure of verification of the assay. Slight chromatographic differences between pituitary and serum TSH have been reported by Dimond and Rosen (1974). The β subunit of TSH and the glycoprotein hormone α subunit have been found in serum (Kourides et al., 1975; Edmonds et al., 1975), but their concentrations are low and, as noted previously, their reactivities in the TSH radioimmunoassay are minimal.

The problem of reactivity of anti-TSH serum with various gonadotropins, its minimization by absorption of the anti-TSH serum with HCG, and the lack of reactivity of other pituitary hormones and other thyroid stimulators has been previously discussed. Validation of the assay also comes from two other types of observations. The first is that both radioimmunoassay and bioassay of serum or serum concentrate TSH levels, in assays in which the same standard (HTRS-A) was used, yielded comparable results (Raud and Odell, 1969; Adams et al., 1972). Second, serum TSH concentrations have been found to change appropriately in a variety of pathologic states or after various physiologic manipulations, i.e., elevated serum TSH levels which return to normal during thyroid hormone therapy in patients with primary hypothyroidism and undetectable levels in patients with hyperthyroidism. Pregnant women, whose serum contains large quantities of HCG, have serum TSH concentrations similar to those of normal nonpregnant subjects.

The assay as described above has a sensitivity of 0.2 to 0.3 μU, permitting the detection of 1 to 1.5 μU TSH per milliliter of serum. Recovery of TSH added to serum varies from 90 to 104%. When purified human TSH is used as immunoassay standard, the serum values range from <0.4 to 2.0 ng/ml (about 1.0×10^{-11} M), but since even this material is not pure, the true weight of TSH per milliliter of serum is probably lower. Precision, as defined by the coefficient of variation, averages 5.6% for serum TSH levels determined in the same assay, and 10.2% for samples determined in different assays. In normal subjects, serum TSH concentrations range from <1.0 to 8.0 μU/ml (mean, 3.2 μU/ml), measurable TSH being detected in serum from approximately 90% of normal individuals. On the basis of results of TSH assays of serum concentrates, in which serum levels were found to be approximately one-third of those found by direct assay of serum, it appears that direct assay of serum using this method overestimates its TSH content (Adams et al., 1972). This is further supported by the findings of Patel and co-workers (1971) and Pekary et al. (1975), who, utilizing more sensitive assays, reported that serum TSH concentrations in normal subjects averaged 1.0 and 1.5 μU/ml, respectively.

In one extraction technique (Adams and Kennedy, 1968; Adams *et al.*, 1969), one volume of serum is mixed with an equal volume of 1.75 M $CaCl_2$ and two volumes of acetone for two to three hours. After centrifugation, the precipitate is washed three times each with two volumes of acetone–5% NaCl, 1 : 1. The supernatant and washings are pooled and made up to 75% acetone. After standing for two to three hours, the precipitate is collected by centrifugation, washed once with 85% acetone, dialyzed against two changes of distilled water (20 volumes, two to three hours each), and lyophilized. The TSH-containing extracts (concentrated ten- to fortyfold) can be reconstituted in buffer. This technique is cumbersome and far from, ideal.

III. OTHER IMMUNOASSAYS

TSH radioimmunoassays using the reagents available from the National Institutes of Health and the World Health Organization (HTRS-A) have been developed and are in use in many laboratories. Other workers have prepared their own reagents, although HTRS-A is universally used as the assay standard at the present time. Most of the reported assays are similar in detail to that described here, although a number of minor modifications in the assay procedure have been introduced. These include variations in the reaction time of the assay, variations in the buffer used and in the method used for separation of free and antibody-bound labeled TSH, such as chromatoelectrophoresis (Utiger, 1965), and use of the solid phase technique (Glatstein *et al.*, 1971). Other variations employed include the use of different methods, such as gel filtration on Sephadex G-200 (Jaquet *et al.*, 1971), adsorption to QUSO (Hall *et al.*, 1971), and polyvinylchloride electrophoresis (Gordin and Saarinen, 1972), for the purification of ^{125}I-TSH for use in the assay. Perhaps a more significant question concerns the need for absorption of anti-TSH serum with HCG. As indicated previously, it is the experience in this laboratory that the anti-TSH serum must be absorbed with HCG or else spuriously high serum TSH concentrations, especially in pregnant women and postmenopausal females, will be obtained. Other workers, apparently using the same anti-TSH serum, find no difference in TSH values using unabsorbed serum, except in pregnant women (Mayberry *et al.*, 1971; Gordin and Saarinen, 1972). The explanation for these differences is not apparent. Thus, even though a number of minor assay modifications have been described, all of the methods described have a roughly similar sensitivity threshold, and most yield serum TSH concentrations in the same order of magnitude [mean values reported ranging from 1.0 μU/ml (Patel *et al.*, 1971) to 13.2 μU/ml

(LeMarchand-Beraud, 1970)]. This is undoubtedly because most workers use the same TSH for iodination, the same anti-TSH serum, and the HTRS-A as immunoassay standard. The variations found in results reported are probably due to differences in labeling techniques, differences in how the labeled TSH is purified or whether it is repurified, and whether or not HCG absorbed anti-TSH serum is used.

REFERENCES

Adams, D. D., and Kennedy, T. H. (1968). Measurement of the thyroid-stimulating hormone content of serum from hypothyroid and euthyroid people. *J. Clin. Endocrinol. Metab.* **28**, 325–331.
Adams, D. D., Kennedy, T. H., and Purves, H. D. (1969). Comparison of the thyroid-stimulating hormone content of serum from thyrotoxic and euthyroid people. *J. Clin. Endocrinol. Metab.* **29**, 900–903.
Adams, D. D., Kennedy, T. H., and Utiger, R. D. (1972). Comparison of bioassay and immunoassay measurements of serum thyrotropin (TSH) and study of TSH levels by immunoassay of serum concentrates. *J. Clin. Endocrinol. Metab.* **24**, 1074–1079.
Binoux, M., Pierce, J. G., and Odell, W. D. (1974). Radioimmunological characterization of human thyrotropin and its subunits: Applications for the measurement of human TSH. *J. Clin. Endocrinol. Metab.* **38**, 674–682.
Bitensky, L., Alaghband-Zadeh, J., and Chayen, J. (1974). Studies on thyroid stimulating hormone and the long-acting thyroid stimulating hormone. *Clin. Endocrinol.* **3**, 363–374.
Condliffe, P. (1963). Purification of human thyrotropin. *Endocrinology* **72**, 893–896.
Cornell, J. S., and Pierce, J. (1973). Subunits of human pituitary thyroid-stimulating hormone: Isolation, properties and composition. *J. Biol. Chem.* **248**, 4327–4334.
Dimond, R., and Rosen, S. W. (1974). Chromotographic differences between circulating and pituitary thyrotropin. *J. Clin. Endocrinol. Metab.* **39**, 316–325.
Edmonds, M., Molitch, M., Pierce, J., and Odell, W. D. (1975). Secretion of alpha and beta subunits of TSH by the anterior pituitary. *Clin. Endocrinol.* **4**, 525–530.
Glatstein, E., McHardy-Young, S., Brast, N., Eltringham, J. R., and Kriss, J. P. (1971). Alterations in serum thyrotropin (TSH) and thyroid function following radiotherapy in patients with malignant lymphoma. *J. Clin. Endocrinol. Metab.* **32**, 833–841.
Gordin, A., and Saarinen, P. (1972). Methodological study of the radioimmunoassay of human thyrotropin. *Acta Endocrinol. (Copenhagen)* **71**, 24–36.
Greenwood, F. C., Hunter, W. L., and Glover, J. J. (1963). The preparation of ^{131}I-labeled growth hormone of high specific activity. *Biochem. J.* **89**, 114–123.
Hall, R., Amos, J., and Ormston, B. J. (1971). Radioimmunoassay of human serum thyrotropin. *Br. Med. J.* **1**, 582–585.
Jaquet, P., Ketelslegers, J. M., Jakubowski, H., Hellman, G., and Franchimont, P. (1971). Dosage radio-immunologique de l'hormone thyreotrope humaine (H-TSH). I. Etude de la Communaté antigénique entre TSH humaine, bovine, porcine et les autres hormone glycoprotéiques (H. FSH, H. LH, HCG). *Ann. Endocrinol.* **32**, 423–495.
Kourides, I. A., Weintraub, B. D., Ridgway, E. C., and Maloof, F. (1975). Pituitary

secretion of free alpha and beta subunit of human thyrotropin in patients with thyroid disorders. *J. Clin. Endocrinol. Metab.* **40**, 872–885.

LeMarchand-Beraud, T. (1970). Comparison between antibodies to bovine and human thyrotropin (TSH) for radioimmunoassay in plasma: Cross-reaction studies with clinical results. *Acta Endocrinol. (Copenhagen)* **64**, 610–629.

Mayberry, W. E., Gharib, H., Bilstad, J. M., and Sizemore, G. W. (1971). Radioimmunoassay for human thyrotropin. *Ann. Intern. Med.* **74**, 471–480.

Odell, W. D., Wilber, J. F., and Utiger, R. D. (1967). Studies of thyrotropin physiology by means of radioimmunoassay. *Recent Prog. Horm. Res.* **23**, 47–78.

Odell, W. D., Vanslager, L., and Bates, R. W. (1968). Radioimmunoassay of human thyrotropin. *AEC Symp. Ser.* **13**, 185–202.

Patel, Y. C., Burger, H. G., and Hudson, B. (1971). Radioimmunoassay of serum thyrotropin: Sensitivity and specificity. *J. Clin. Endocrinol. Metab.* **33**, 768–774.

Pekary, A. E., Hershman, J. M., and Parlow, A. F. (1975). A sensitive and precise radioimmunoassay for human thyroid-stimulating hormone. *J. Clin. Endocrinol. Metab.* **41**, 676–684.

Raud, H. R., and Odell, W. D. (1969). The radioimmunoassay of human thyrotropin. *Br. J. Hosp. Med.* **2**, 1366–1372.

Utiger, R. D. (1965). Immunoassay of human plasma TSH. *Curr. Top. Thyroid Res., Proc. Int. Thyroid Conf., 5th, 1965* pp. 513–526.

Utiger, R. D. (1968). Thyrotropin in blood. *Clin. Endocrinol.* **2**, 25–39.

Utiger, R. D., Odell, W. D., and Condliffe, P. G. (1963). Immunological studies of purified human and bovine thyrotropin. *Endocrinology* **73**, 359–363.

15

Oxytocin

AVIR KAGAN AND SEYMOUR M. GLICK

INTRODUCTION AND HISTORY

Since the previous edition of this chapter (Kagan and Glick, 1974), the radioimmunoassay for oxytocin has not been widely applied. This fulfills the prediction of Chard (1973), who felt that technical problems and sensitivity limitations would slow its widespread use. The radioimmunoassay has not yet resolved the controversy (Kumaresan *et al.*, 1975) over the origin of oxytocin during delivery and the role played by oxytocin during labor.

Thus, it appears reasonable to assume that bioassay techniques, in-

Methods of Hormone Radioimmunoassay, Second Edition
Copyright © 1979 by Academic Press, Inc.
All rights of reproduction in any form reserved. ISBN 0-12-379260-6

cluding measurements of rat breast intraductal pressure (Bisset *et al.*, 1967) and extrusion of milk from lactating breast tissue (van Dongen and Hays, 1966), will remain useful for some time.

II. METHODS OF RADIOIMMUNOASSAY

A. Immunization

Without an antiserum of high affinity and reasonable titer, no radioimmunoassay can be developed. Sensitivity depends upon the antibody affinity, which ultimately determines the steepness of the standard curve slope (Yalow and Berson, 1964). Although it is possible to maximize the effectiveness of a particular radioimmunoassay (Chard *et al.*, 1970b), the affinity of the individual antiserum is the basic limiting factor affecting assay sensitivity. Gilliland and Prout (1965) first demonstrated that unconjugated oxytocin in Freund's adjuvant could induce an immunologic response. The first sensitive radioimmunoassay (Wheeler *et al.*, 1966) for oxytocin was developed in our laboratory only after we were able to produce antibodies of sufficient titer and affinity. Despite the importance of the antiserum, we do not emphasize the need for a specific rigorous schedule of immunization, primarily because we have no confidence in one particular schedule over another. The fortuitous availability of a particularly susceptible animal seems more important than the immunization schedule. Since only a small proportion of animals responded favorably to the injection of unconjugated oxytocin, we now use oxytocin conjugated to albumin with glutaraldehyde, as described for ACTH (Vance *et al.*, 1969). Adsorption to carbon microparticles has also been reported to be successful (Chard *et al.*, 1970a).

Oxytocin (450 U/mg) in pure powdered form can be obtained from the Parke, Davis & Company. The oxytocin is dissolved in acid water, pH 3 (distilled H_2O acidified with HCl), at 1.0 mg/ml. If stored below $-20°C$, this solution can be used for at least one year for both immunization and iodination. All further dilutions for standards are made with oxytocin buffer (diluent) to be described later.

The glutaraldehyde coupling procedure is simple: 20 mg bovine serum albumin (Pentex or Sigma) is mixed with 2.0 mg oxytocin and dissolved in 2 ml 0.1 M phosphate buffer, pH 7.5. One milliliter of glutaraldehyde (0.02 M) is added dropwise with constant stirring. In order to determine the degree of conjugation, an aliquot of the reaction mixture is subjected to Sephadex G-25 gel filtration. Virtually complete coupling of the oxytocin is documented by the detection of all the trace label oxytocin and the oxytocin immunoreactivity in the albumin fraction.

Ten milliliters of a 40–50 U/ml (0.1 mg/ml) dilution of coupled oxytocin is mixed and added to 10 ml complete Freund's adjuvant (Difco). The mixture is homogenized in a Virtis homogenizer at maximum speed until emulsification is complete as evidenced by an opaque, glistening, creamy-white appearance with the consistency of soft ice cream. The utensils must be scrupulously clean to prevent immunization with other antigens. Two milliliters of the resulting mixture (40–50 U or 0.1 mg) is injected into each animal (New Zealand white rabbits, weighing 3–5 kg) as follows: 0.5 ml into each front foot pad and 1.0 ml subcutaneously in the back. In 14 days, the injection is repeated using 0.5 ml into each rear foot pad and 1.0 ml subcutaneously. Thereafter, all injections are made at two-week intervals subcutaneously, since each foot pad can tolerate only one dose. Ten to fourteen days after a third injection, 5.0–10 ml of blood is drawn from the ear vein.

B. Antibody Selection

The rabbit plasma is subsequently tested by dilution with a tracer amount of labeled oxytocin (except where noted, in this chapter, oxytocin ^{131}I and ^{125}I can be used interchangeably). If 50% of the tracer is not bound at a dilution of 1 : 10, the animal is useless and should be discarded. After a second series of immunizations, one should continue immunizing only those animals with titers above 1 : 200. After a third series, all chosen animals will usually show titers of 1 : 1000 or greater. At this point, standard curve titrations should be performed with each antiserum and further immunizations and testing should be limited to animals whose antisera show steep falls in B/F upon addition of small amounts of unlabeled oxytocin. Although reasonable titers are desirable so that many assays can be performed with antiserum selected, the choice of antisera depends primarily on the steepness or fall of the slope of B/F. Adsorption of contaminating antibodies against bovine albumin can be accomplished by the addition of 25 mg bovine serum albumin to each 1.0 ml antiserum and removal of any resultant precipitate.

C. Iodination

Iodination is accomplished by a modification of the Hunter and Greenwood method (Greenwood *et al.*, 1963). We have eliminated the metabisulfite step, since metabisulfite alters the migration of iodinated oxytocin on chromatoelectrophoresis (see below) and on thin-layer ascending chromatography (butanol–acetic acid) (Glick *et al.*, 1968). This modification may not be necessary in other systems (Chard, 1973). A typical iodination is carried out as shown below.

1. Reagents

Buffer, 0.25 M phosphate, pH 7.4
Oxytocin, 5.0 μg (5.0 μl of a 1.0 mg/ml solution)
Chloramine-T, 10 mg in 2.8 ml buffer
Human serum albumin, 0.3 gm/ml
Na^{131}I or Na^{125}I (Union Carbide, Sterling Forest, New York—high specific activity, carrier-free)

The volume of radioactive iodine used depends on concentration and desired specific activity. If, for example, the ^{131}I was provided at a concentration of 1000 mCi/ml and a specific activity of 400 mCi/mg was desired, since the efficiency of iodination is usually 90%, 2.0 μl (2.0 mCi) of the Na^{131}I solution would be used in the reaction. Iodine-125 should be added at lower specific activities (50–100 mCi/mg), since its elemental iodine content per millicurie is about eight times that of ^{131}I, and the use of higher specific activities may result in undesirable iodination damage.

2. Procedure

Buffer (20 μl) is pipetted into a test tube. Using a syringe micro-pipette (Hamilton), graduated 1.0–10 μl, the appropriate amount of ^{131}I or ^{125}I is added to the buffer liquid. Any excess liquid on the tip of the needle is carefully touched to the inside of the test tube just above the buffer. Five microliters of oxytocin solution (5.0 μg), 20 μl chloramine-T, and 50 μl of albumin are added in rapid sequence, mixing these reagents by gently bubbling during pipetting. The last pipette (albumin) has enough labeled oxytocin on its tip so that by dipping it into 2.0 ml of diluent (see below) an aliquot of the iodination mixture large enough for analysis is deposited in the diluent. In order to determine the amount of damage, this mixture is now subjected to chromatoelectrophoresis (10–20 μl of label, 40 μl bromphenol blue-dyed normal human plasma, Whatman 3MC or Toyo 514 paper strips 1$\frac{3}{8}$ inches wide, 4°C, 0.05 M phosphate, pH 7.4, 600 mv). The remaining product is either purified immediately or preserved in the frozen state.

3. Estimation of Iodination Results

By means of chromatoelectrophoresis (see above for details), three peaks can be ascertained: free hormone (slightly beyond the origin), damaged hormone (with the blue protein front), and free iodide (beyond the dyed plasma). The estimation of iodination damage is calculated as follows:

$$\text{Percentage damage} = \frac{100 \times \text{damaged counts}}{\text{free hormone counts} + \text{damaged counts}}$$

The estimation of degree of iodination is shown below:

$$\text{Percentage iodination} = \frac{100 \times (\text{damaged counts} + \text{free hormone counts})}{\text{Total counts (including free iodide)}}$$

D. Oxytocin Buffer (Diluent)

Five milliliters of human serum albumin (0.3 mg/ml) and 5.0 ml normal rabbit plasma (Pel Freeze) are added to each liter of 0.05 M phosphate buffer, pH 7.5. To this solution are added 48 mg of cystine, 372 mg of EDTA, and 5.0 mg phenanthroline (dissolved in 50 μl 95% ethyl alcohol). The albumin prevents loss of peptide on glassware. The rabbit plasma provides globulin for a reasonable precipitate during the second antibody reaction and also prevents loss of peptide on glass. The cystine, EDTA, and phenanthroline retard damage to oxytocin. Merthiolate (1 : 10,000) is added to prevent bacterial growth.

E. Purification of Labeled Oxytocin

About 100 μl of the iodination mixture is mixed with 100 μl normal human plasma (dyed blue with bromphenol blue dye) and layered on the top of a 2 × 18 cm column of Sephadex G-25 Fine (Pharmacia). The Sephadex is equilibrated and eluted with the oxytocin diluent, collecting 1.0–2.0-ml fractions. A significant portion of the radioactivity leaves the column in the first 10–20 ml of effluent with blue-dyed protein. This fraction represents damaged and aggregated oxytocin attached to protein. The next 20–60 ml of effluent usually contains the useful labeled oxytocin peak. Some unreacted ^{131}I is present in this peak and can be removed (Glick et al., 1969) by mixing the peak fraction tubes with a pinch of Amberlite-400 resin (Mallinckrodt). After the resin settles to the bottom of the fraction tube, the oxytocin fraction can be separated by aspiration. On Sephadex G-25, the oxytocin peak is not a homogeneous one (Glick et al., 1969), since the labeled oxytocin is retarded by the gel, giving increasing specific activity in the latter fractions of the oxytocin peak. This phenomenon was described first for vasopressin by Roth *et al.* (1966). We have found that trial incubation of the iodinated hormone fractions with antibody prior to beginning an assay is useful in determining which fraction is most suitable.

To tubes containing the same concentration of antibody (enough to give a B/F with tracer oxytocin of 1 to 3), the same quantity of radioactivity of each purified iodinated fraction is added and incubated for several hours at room temperature. The bound and free hormone is then separated in the usual manner (see Section II,G). Room temperature is used to speed up the initial reaction so that this entire trial should take about 24 to 36 hours. Since the same quantity of radioactivity is used, those fractions having the highest B/F (usually the downward slope of the peak) are selected for use in the radioimmunoassay. Fractions that yield lower B/F ratios either contain significant amounts of unlabeled oxytocin or contain labeled molecules with impaired immunoreactivity. Fractions chosen with the highest B/F in this screening test are usually more than 90% bindable by excess antibody.

F. Assay Incubation

Table I shows a sample protocol that can be used for the oxytocin radioimmunoassay using our antibody. The smallest tracer giving reasonable counting rates on the available equipment should be used (less than 50 pg or approximately 1500 cpm). A concentration of antiserum yielding an initial B/F of 1.0 is ideal. Our current antiserum is used at a final dilution of 1 : 50,000. Either unlabeled standard oxytocin, 0.5–400 pg, or the unknown samples are added, and the final volume is adjusted to 1.0 ml. The incubation is carried out at 4°C for four to six days.

G. Separation of Bound from Free Oxytocin

At the end of the assay incubation period, 0.05–0.15 ml of sheep anti-rabbit globulin serum is added, and the resultant precipitate is separated after 12 to 18 hours of further incubation of 4°C. When calculating the assay results, the precipitate contains the antibody-bound counts (B) whereas the supernatant contains unbound label or free (F).

This second antiserum can be readily produced in sheep by the intramuscular injection of 50 mg of rabbit globulin (Pentex) in Freund's adjuvant every two weeks. Ten to fourteen days after the third injection, 600 ml of blood can be removed from the sheep. Continued reimmunization and bleeding provide the necessary supply. The optimal quantity of second antibody to be used can be determined by adding varying quantities to tracer tubes and using that amount which precipitates the most iodinated oxytocin counts. It must be emphasized that each batch of second antibody must be completely evaluated before use in the radioimmunoassay.

Second antibody added to the precipitate control tube (Table I) yields a precipitate free of first antibody. The percentage of oxytocin ^{131}I counts precipitated in this tube represents nonspecific precipitation, and this percentage should be subtracted from all precipitated counts in the assay, as follows: true bound counts in assay tube equals total precipitate counts in assay tube minus (percentage of counts in precipitate control tube × total counts in assay tube). When using the double antibody method, damage control tubes are prepared as suggested by Quabbe (1969) and Roth et al. (1968). The "damage control" tube for each sample is set up with identical composition as the assay tubes (diluent, antibody, labeled hormone, and plasma). Twelve hours

Table I   Standard Protocol

Oxytocin weight[a] (pg)	Oxytocin units[a] (μU)	Labeled hormone solution (μl)	Unlabeled oxytocin 25 μU/ml (μl)	Unlabeled oxytocin 250 μU/ml (μl)	Diluent (μl)	Antisera (μl)
0.5[b]	0.25	100	10	0	790	100
1.0	0.5	100	20	0	780	100
2.0	1.0	100	40	0	760	100
4.0	2.0	100	80	0	720	100
10	5.0	100	200	0	600	100
20	10	100	400	0	400	100
20	20	100	0	80	720	100
100	50	100	0	200	600	100
200	100	100	0	400	400	100
400	200	100	0	800	0	100
Tracer[c] 0 pg added	0	100	0	0	800	100
Precipitate control	0	100	0	0	900	0
Sample[d]	—	100	0[e]	0	700	100

[a] Rounded out for simplification at 500 U/mg.
[b] All tubes in duplicate.
[c] In quadruplicate (two tubes to act as damage control).
[d] In duplicate, but one extra tube per patient for damage control.
[e] 100 μl plasma or extract solution added.

before the second antibody is added to the assay tubes, an excess of first antibody (anti-oxytocin) is added to the damage control tube. It is advisable to use enough antibody to ensure maximum binding of labeled oxytocin tracer, i.e., we have used 10–20 μl undiluted antisera, a quantity which would ordinarily give a B/F of greater than 1.0 at 1 : 4000 dilutions. This large excess of antibody molecules ensures rapid binding of all the tracer oxytocin that is bindable. Obviously, we use one of our antisera with poorer affinity, since all that is necessary is that it bind oxytocin not that it has a steep slope in a standard curve. Second antibody is added to these damage control tubes at the same time it is added to the assay. The addition of excess first antibody in the damage control tubes may change the amount of second antibody that must be added to the control tubes in order to achieve maximum precipitation. Similar damage control tubes are prepared for the tracer tubes in the standard curve (Table I) and used for calculation of standard curve B/F. The damage control tubes estimate the maximum bindability of the tracer which is impaired in part by changes induced by iodination and in part by changes occurring with incubation. Incubation damage is greater in test tubes containing plasma. In both standard curve and sample tubes, nonbindable iodinated oxytocin remains in the supernatant so that the free (F) counts must be corrected by the following formula:

$$F \text{ correction factor} = 100\% - (\% \text{ maximally precipitable counts in the control tube})$$

$$\text{True } F = \text{ total } F \text{ counts} - (F \text{ correction factor} \times \text{ total sample tube counts})$$

Ammonium sulfate precipitation (Chard *et al.*, 1970a) or polyethylene glycol (Kumaresan *et al.*, 1974) may be useful but is not preferred with our antiserum. The use of polyethylene glycol is described elsewhere in this volume in the chapter on vasopressin (Chapter 16).

III. SENSITIVITY, CROSS-REACTIVITY, AND VALIDATION

Our antiserum can detect less than 1.0 pg (0.5 μU oxytocin per milliliter). The antiserum reported by Chard *et al.* (1970a,b) has a sensitivity of 10 to 20 pg (5–10 μU/ml).

The structure of oxytocin is

Cys-Tyr-Ile-Gln-Asn-Cys-Pro-Leu-Gly-NH$_2$

Our antiserum cross-reacts to less than 1% with lysine vasopressin and arginine vasopressin and to varying degrees with related but noncirculating analogs: 1-D-amino oxytocin, 110%; 4-Val-oxytocin, 80%; 1-D-amino-4-Val-oxytocin, 90%; 5-Val-oxytocin, 1-D-amino-5-Val-oxytocin, 8-Ala-oxytocin, and 1-D-amino-8-Ala-oxypressin, all less than 1%, (Glick *et al.*, 1969). In addition, our antiserum blocks oxytocin activity in two *in vitro* bioassays, the lactating rat mammary gland strip (van Dongen and Hays, 1966) and the uterine strip assay (performed by Dr. W. Sawyer, Columbia University).

IV. OXYTOCIN IN PLASMA

A. Extraction of Oxytocin

Radioimmunoassay of oxytocin, while quite sensitive and specific, still requires extraction of plasma (Chard, 1973; Kagan and Glick, 1974) in order to detect the low levels of oxytocin found in human plasma. Depending upon the specific antibody, extraction procedures may lead to erroneous results (Chard, 1973). We have not solved the occasional artifact that our acetone extraction causes, i.e., artifactual lowering of the B/F ratio resulting in falsely elevated levels of oxytocin (Kagan and Glick, 1974). Thus, while Fuller's earth absorption and acetone precipitation can yield recoveries of up to 90%, plasma studies are still plagued with problems. Indeed, we feel that this is the reason for the slow application of the oxytocin radioimmunoassay alluded to earlier in this chapter.

Using this system, Kumaresan *et al.* (1974) have assayed unextracted plasma at a dilution of 1 : 5. While this eliminates artifacts secondary to extraction, the endogenous oxytocin and the assay itself are then more easily susceptible to the damaging effects of pregnancy plasma. Kumaresan feels that the presence of phenanthroline can inhibit the effects of oxytocinase.

At the present time, we recommend the use of the following extraction procedure: To 1.0 ml of plasma, 2.0 ml of acetone is added. After mixing and centrifugation, the acetone supernatant is aspirated from the precipitated proteins. Lipids are removed from the acetone by thorough mixing with 3.0 ml of petroleum ether. The liquid ether phase layers on the top of the liquid acetone phase and is removed by careful aspiration. The remaining acetone phase containing the extracted oxytocin is then dried. The dried oxytocin can be reconstituted directly in diluent for assay purposes, or the assay reagents can be added directly to the extraction tubes. This procedure gives recoveries of 80 to 90%.

B. Collection of Blood

Since plasma contains oxytocinase during pregnancy, phenanthroline (0.005 mg/ml of blood) is added immediately after venipuncture of pregnant subjects. Fifteen milligrams of phenanthroline is dissolved in 100 μl of 95% ethyl alcohol and mixed into 1.116 gm of EDTA dissolved in 30 ml distilled water, and 100 μl of the resultant stock solution is then added to each 10 ml of freshly drawn blood. In both pregnant and nonpregnant states, the plasma should be quickly separated and stored at $-20°C$. Phenanthroline in this concentration does not affect the radioimmunoassay of oxytocin, does inhibit oxytocinase degradation, and is not responsible for the extraction problems mentioned above. A method of blood collection recommended by Chard (1973) is acidification of the separated plasma. Collection of blood should be performed under chilled conditions and refrigerated centrifugation.

C. Effect of Degradation

We have shown that the biologic and immunologic activity of oxytocin can be dissociated (Kumaresan et al., 1969). Oxytocin, reduced by thioglycollate to biologic inactivity, retains almost complete immunoreactivity. Something in the plasma of pregnant women affected biologic activity more than immunologic activity, and placental extracts destroyed both biologic and immunologic activity.

D. Levels of Oxytocin in Plasma

Oxytocin levels in normal males and nonpregnant women reported by Chard and associates (1970c) and by Kumaresan et al. (1974) and measured in our laboratory are quite low (1.5 to 2.0 pg/ml). In most samples collected during human pregnancy and labor, the Chard group reported equally low maternal plasma levels. In contrast, Kumaresan found levels up to 300 pg/ml during pregnancy and labor. Since these latter data were derived using a technique that is significantly affected by oxytocinase, they have been controversial. Since both groups noted high fetal levels of oxytocin, further controversy exists concerning both the origin of oxytocin in either mother or fetus, and the possible role that oxytocin plays in labor. It should be pointed out that in the guinea pig (utilizing extraction with glass beads and the assay of Chard), oxytocin levels have been evaluated by Burton *et al.* (1974). Maternal levels were low before the expulsive phase of labor occurred. During this phase, they were significantly elevated, with a mean level of 503 pg/ml (range of 96–2900). The sequence of the rise in oxytocin levels in the guinea pig litters suggested that the mother was the active producer of oxytocin. In the mare (Allen *et al.*, 1973), qualitatively similar but less dramatic results have been found. While these last two reports lend support to Kumaresan's data, the values found in unextracted plasma should be confirmed in an inde-

Table II Comparison of Two Oxytocin Radioimmunoassays

Step	Chard *et al.* (1970a, b, c)	Glick *et al.* (1969)	Comment
Iodination	At high specific activity; uses metabisulfite step	Lower specific activity; no metabisulfite	High specific activity and metabisulfite probably alter oxytocin molecule
Purification	Dowex resin	Sephadex	Increase in specific activity offered by Sephadex not needed if iodination carried out at high specific activity
Separation	NH$_4$ acetate	Double antibody	NH$_4$ acetate faster; double antibody precipitate firmer; double antibody expensive and must be continually reproduced
Immunization	Oxytocin adsorbed to carbon microparticles	Oxytocin coupled to albumin	Albumin coupling has produced more sensitive antisera
Extraction	Fuller's earth, and glass beads	Acetone; controversial Kumaresan unextracted plasma modification	Fuller's earth extraction apparently free of interfering factors. Glass beads simpler. Acetone extraction yields higher recovery
Sensitivity	10 pg/ml (5.0 μU/ml)	1.0 pg/ml (0.5 μU/ml)	Depends on antiserum

pendent laboratory utilizing the same techniques. Distinct elevations of oxytocin in response to suckling and milking continue to be confirmed by radioimmunoassay (Forsling *et al.*, 1974).

V. DISCUSSION

From the previous section, it is obvious that neither of the two major assays described in the literature is completely satisfactory as yet. Table II compares the two assays. Until the sensitivity and extraction problems are resolved, the role of maternal oxytocin during labor will probably remain unsettled. Since that is the case, as yet there is no defined clinical use for this assay during pregnancy.

ACKNOWLEDGMENTS

This manuscript was prepared with the help of Noemi Artau Kagan, R.N., and Pearl Sasso. We once again thank Dr. Perianna Kumaresan, who supplied useful information. Partial support from the N.I.H. Grant No. 5Ro1AM16175 is acknowledged.

REFERENCES

Allen, W. E., Chard, T., and Forsling, M. D. (1973). Peripheral plasma levels of oxytocin and vasopressin in the mare during parturition. *J. Endocrinol.* **57**, 175–176.

Bisset, G. W., Clark, B. J., Haldar, J., Harris, M. C., Lewis, G. P., and Rocha e Silva, M. (1967). The assay of milk ejecting activity in the lactating rat. *Br. J. Pharm. Pharmacol.* **31**, 537–549.

Burton, A. M., Illingworth, D. V., Challis, J. R. G., and McNeilly, A. S. (1974). Placental transfer of oxytocin in the guinea pig and its release during parturition. *J. Endocrinol.* **60**, 499–506.

Chard, T. (1973). The radioimmunoassay of oxytocin and vasopressin. *J. Endocrinol.* **58**, 143–160.

Chard, T., Kitau, M. J., and Landon, J. (1970a). The development of a radioimmunoassay for oxytocin: Radioiodination, antibody production, and separation techniques. *J. Endocrinol.* **46**, 269–278.

Chard, T., Forsling, M. D., James, M. A. R., Kitau, M. J., and Landon, J. (1970b). The development of a radioimmunoassay for oxytocin: Specificity and the dissociation of immunological and biological activity. *J. Endocrinol.* **46**, 533–542.

Chard, T., Boyd, N. R. H., Forsling, M. L., McNeill, A. S., and Landon, J. (1970c). The development of a radioimmunoassay for oxytocin: The extraction of oxytocin from plasma and its measurement during parturition in human and goat blood. *J. Endocrinol.* **48**, 223–234.

Forsling, M. L., Reinhardt, V., and Himmler, V. (1974). Neurohypophysial hormones and prolactin release. *J. Endocrinol.* **63**, 579–580.

Gilliland, P. F., and Prout, T. E. (1965). Immunological studies of octapeptides II. Production and detection of antibodies to oxytocin. *Metab.* **14**, 918–923.

Glick, S. M., Wheeler, M., Kagan, A., and Kumaresan, P. (1968). Radioimmunoassay of oxytocin. *In* "Pharmacology of Hormonal Polypeptides and Proteins" (N. Back, L. Martini, and R. Paoletti, eds.), pp. 93–100. Plenum, New York.

Glick, S. M., Kumaresan, P., Kagan, A., and Wheeler, M. (1969). Radioimmunoassay of oxytocin. *Protein Polypeptide Proc. Int. Symp., 1968.* Excerpta Med. Found., Int. Congr. Ser. No. 161, pp. 81–83.

Greenwood, F. C., Hunter, W. M., and Glover, J. S. (1963). The preparation of 131I labeled human growth hormone of high specific radioactivity. *Biochem. J.* **89**, 114–123.

Kagan, A., and Glick, S. M. (1974). Oxytocin. *In* "Methods of Hormone Radioimmunoassay" (B. M. Jaffe and H. R. Behrman, eds.), 1st ed., pp. 173–185. Academic Press, New York.

Kumaresan, P., Kagan, A., and Glick, S. M. (1969). Oxytocin: Effects of degradation on radioimmunologic and biologic activity. *Science* **166**, 1160–1161.

Kumaresan, P., Anandarangam, P. B., Dianzon, W., and Vasicka, A. (1974). Plasma oxytocin levels during human pregnancy and labor determined by radioimmunoassay. *Am. J. Obstet. Gynecol.* **119**, 215–223.

Kumaresan, P., Han, G. S., Anandarangam, P. B., and Vasicka, A. (1975). Oxytocin in maternal and fetal blood. *Obstet. Gynecol.* **46**, 272–274.

Quabbe, H. J. (1969). Sources of error in the immunoprecipitation system of radioimmunoassays. *Protein Polypeptide Horm., Proc. Int. Symp., 1968.* Excerpta Med. Found., Int. Congr. Ser. No. 161, pp. 21–25.

Roth, J., Klein, L. A., and Peterson, M. J. (1966). Vasopressin antibodies and a sensitive radioimmunoassay. *J. Clin. Invest.* **45**, 1064.

Roth, J., Gorden, P., and Pastan, I. (1968). "Big insulin": A new component of plasma insulin detected by immunoassay. *Proc. Natl. Acad. Sci. U.S.A.* **61**, 138–145.

Vance, V. L., Schure, J. J., and Reichlin, M. (1969). Induction of antibodies to porcine ACTH in rabbits with nonsteroidogenic polymers of BSA and ACTH. *Protein Polypeptide Horm., Proc. Int. Symp., 1968.* Excerpta Med. Found., Int. Congr. Ser. No. 161, pp. 380–384.

van Dongen, C. G., and Hays, R. L. (1966). A sensitive in vitro assay for oxytocin. *Endocrinology* **78**, 1–6.

Wheeler, M., Kagan, A., and Glick, S. M. (1966). Radioimmunoassay of oxytocin *Clin. Res.* **14**, 479.

Yalow, R. S., and Berson, S. A. (1964). Immunoassay of plasma insulin. *Methods Biochem. Anal.* **12**, 69–96.

16

Vasopressin

SEYMOUR M. GLICK AND AVIR KAGAN

I. INTRODUCTION AND HISTORY

The value of the vasopressin radioimmunoassay has been adequately proved (Husain *et al.*, 1973; Robertson *et al.*, 1973; Robertson and Athar, 1976). A major reason for this success has been the production of antisera with great affinity for vasopressin (Oyama *et al.*, 1971). Antibodies to vasopressin were first developed by Roth *et al.* (1966), and a radioimmunoassay was soon developed (Robertson *et al.*, 1970; Permutt *et al.*, 1966). Unfortunately, these assays had difficulties with large quantities of nonvasopressin cross-reacting materials. Our own laboratory initially attempted to avoid the cross-reacting plasma artifacts by assaying urine (Oyama *et al.*, 1971). Subsequently we noted that the antiserum we had developed could be used for the assay of

341

Methods of Hormone Radioimmunoassay, Second Edition
Copyright © 1979 by Academic Press, Inc.
All rights of reproduction in any form reserved. ISBN 0-12-379260-6

plasma (Husain *et al.*, 1973; Robertson *et al.*, 1973) with little difficulty.

II. METHODS OF RADIOIMMUNOASSAY

A. Immunization and Antibody Selection

Synthetic arginine vasopressin (Spectrum Medical Industries, Los Angeles, California, 250 U/mg) is dissolved in dilute acetic acid (0.25 ml glacial acetic in 100 ml distilled H_2O) at a concentration of 1.0 mg/ml. In this state, it can be stored at $-20°C$ for two or more years and used for iodination, immunization, and incubation as standard in radioimmunoassay curves. Storage in concentrations less than 1.0 μg/ml for more than four months is discouraged (Robertson *et al.*, 1973). We used the same method of glutaraldehyde coupling to bovine serum albumin as was used for oxytocin (see Chapter 15). This immunization technique, immunization schedule, and selection of the best antiserum were identical to the methods described for oxytocin. The dose of arginine vasopressin (AVP) at each injection was 0.1 mg per animal.

B. Iodination

The Hunter and Greenwood method (Greenwood *et al.*, 1963) (without metabisulfite) is used to label vasopressin to specific activities of approximately 100 mCi/mg ^{131}I and 50 mCi/mg ^{125}I. The efficiency of iodination is 80–90%, so 0.25 to 0.5 mCi is used to iodinate 5.0 μg. Variations of the more gentle lactoperoxidase iodination method give much poorer iodination efficiency (1–25%) without lower levels of iodination damage (A. Kagan and S. Greenstein, unpublished data). Our iodination procedure is identical to that described in this volume, Chapter 15. It should be pointed out that not all authors (Chard, 1973) agree with the need for eliminating the metabisulfite step. The degree of damage is estimated by chromatoelectrophoresis ($1\frac{3}{8}$-inch strips of Toyo 514 paper at 4°C; 0.067 M phosphate, pH 7; 10–20 μl of reaction mixture, 40 μl bromphenol blue-dyed normal human plasma; 600 mV); iodinated vasopressin remains at the origin, damaged label migrates with the blue marker, and free iodine moves beyond the dye marker. Even when stored at $-20°C$, the labeled vasopressin should not be used after four weeks.

C. Purification of Radioiodinated Vasopressin

A 25 × 1.45 cm column of Sephadex G-25 Fine (Pharmacia) is equilibrated and eluted with 0.25% acetic acid containing 1.25 mg/ml human serum albumin (Pentex). Of the iodination mixture, 100 μl is mixed with 100 μl bromphenol blue-dyed normal human plasma and layered onto the top of the column. The first peak of radioactivity emerges along with the blue protein and represents damaged and aggregated radioactive vasopressin bound to plasma protein. The small iodine peak emerges next. Vasopressin [125]I (except where noted, ^{125}I and ^{131}I are interchangeable in this article) is retarded by the Sephadex gel and emerges last. This retardation, first described for vasopressin by Roth et al. (1966) and also reported by this laboratory for oxytocin (Glick et al., 1969), can be exploited to increase the specific activity of the labeled hormone fraction which is chosen (see Chapter 15, this volume). A retarded fraction (on the downward slope of the vasopressin peak) is used for further purification. When initial iodination at very high specific activity is attempted, a fourth elution peak (second vasopressin peak) becomes prominent. It is not useful for the assay (Husain et al., 1973).

We have found that repurification on an identical Sephadex G-25 and 0.25% acetic acid column is useful. A 3-ml fraction taken from the retarded portion of the vasopressin peak (after the initial acetic acid–Sephadex fractionation) is mixed with 100 μl of blue-dyed normal human plasma and gently layered onto the top of the second Sephadex G-25–acetic acid column. Fractions taken from the retarded portion of the vasopressin ^{125}I peak in this fractionation are of great purity, high specific activity (estimated at close to 2000 mCi/mg), and 90–99% bindable to antibody. Before setting up an assay, it is often useful to evaluate which fraction has the highest specific activity and maintains the best binding properties. This evaluation is accomplished by means of testing with antisera as outlined previously in this volume, Chapter 15.

D. Assay Incubation

Table I shows a sample protocol that can be used for the vasopressin radioimmunoassay with our antibody. The smallest tracer giving reasonable counting rates on the available equipment should be used and usually is 1.0–2.0 pg (2000 cpm). Standards range from 0.05 to 20 pg. The slope of the fall in B/F with our antiserum is extremely steep (Oyama et al., 1971; Husain et al., 1973; Robertson et al., 1973), and we have

Table I Standard Protocol

Vasopressin concentration (pg/ml)	Labeled vasopressin (μl)	1.0 pg/ml unlabeled vasopressin (μl)	10 pg/ml unlabeled vasopressin (μl)	100 pg/ml unlabeled vasopressin (μl)	Diluent (μl)	Antibody (μl)
0.05[a]	100	50	0	0	750	100
0.1	100	100	0	0	700	100
0.2	100	200	0	0	600	100
0.3	100	300	0	0	500	100
0.5	100	500	0	0	300	100
0.75	100	0	75	0	725	100
1.0	100	0	100	0	700	100
1.5	100	0	150	0	650	100
2.0	100	0	200	0	600	100
3.0	100	0	300	0	500	100
5.0	100	0	500	0	300	100
7.5	100	0	0	75	725	100
10.0	100	0	0	100	700	100
20.0	100	0	0	200	600	100
Trace[b] 0 pg	100	0	0	0	800	100
Precipitate Control[c]	100	0	0	0	900	0
Sample[d]	100	0[e]	0	0	700	100

[a] All tubes in duplicate.
[b] In quadruplicate (two tubes to act as damage control).
[c] To check nonspecific trapping of counts during precipitation with polyethylene glycol.
[d] In duplicate, but one extra tube per patient plasma used for damage control.
[e] 100 μl of plasma or extract solution added.

found that a concentration of antiserum yielding an initial B/F of 2 to 4 gives us best results. Our current antiserum is used at a final titer of 1:200,000. The incubation is carried out for six days at 4°C in a final volume of 1.0 ml.

E. Vasopressin Assay Diluent

Disodium EDTA (Mallinckrodt) (372 mg), 48 mg L-cystine (Mann), 5.0 ml control rabbit plasma (Pel Freeze), and 5.0 ml 30% human serum albumin (Pentex) are made up to 1.0 liter with 0.05 phosphate buffer, pH 7.5. The proteins minimize loss of peptides on glassware and aid in the formation of a precipitate during separation of the bound from free hormone. Cystine and EDTA delay damage to iodinated vasopressin.

F. Separation of Bound from Free Hormone

Our first assays utilized chromatoelectrophoresis at 4°C on Toyo 514 (Nuclear Associates, Carle Place, New York) paper (Oyama et al., 1971). The assay tube contents (200 μl) were mixed with 40 μl bromophenol blue-dyed normal human plasma and pipetted onto strips 1⅜ inches wide. We have always felt that, where possible, a radioimmunoassay using chromatoelectrophoresis is advantageous because of its ability to effect precise separation and quantitation of damaged AVP and free iodine. Chromatoelectrophoresis in a refrigerated room is, however, physically exhausting and time-consuming to perform. We still use it whenever an assay is small. For a large number of samples, we use polyethylene glycol separation, developed by Dr. G. Robertson (1973) and patterned after the work of Desbuquois and Aurbach (1971).

Sufficient protein to form a good precipitate is provided by adding 100 μl of a 2% solution of powdered bovine globulin to all assay, standard curve, and control tubes. The bovine globulin solution is made by dissolving 2.0 gm powdered bovine globulin (fraction II—Pentex Research Labs.) in 100 ml 0.05 M phosphate buffer, pH 7.4. A polyethylene glycol solution is made by dissolving 250 mg powdered polyethylene glycol (Union Carbide) in 1.0 liter of distilled water. This solution must always be kept at 4°C. Of this 25% solution, 2.0 ml is then added to each assay tube, after which the reaction tubes are vortexed for at least ten seconds. The entire separation to this point must be performed either in the cold room at 4°C or in an ice-water bath. After shaking the assay tubes, the rest of the procedures can be performed at room temperature. The tubes are centrifuged at 2000 rpm for 20 minutes, resulting in a visible precipitate coating the bottom of the tube. The supernatant contains the free hormone (F) and the precipitate contains the bound hormone (B); bound hormone is separated from free hormone by decanting the supernatant. Damage control tubes which contain identical ingredients with either sample assay tubes (trace, diluent, plasma, antibody) or trace tubes in the standard curve (trace, diluent, antibody) are separated in the same manner. Of a 1 : 1000 dilution of anti-vasopressin antiserum, 50 μl is added to the damage control tubes 18 hours before separation. This excess antiserum will rapidly bind all the unbound radioactive vasopressin and thereby permit a calculation of the maximal binding of the trace to the antibody. In some laboratories, it is felt that the use of extracted plasma eliminates the need for a damage control with plasma (Robertson *et al.*, 1973) with a trace control tube still essential. Nonspecific trapping of labeled vasopressin is corrected by using precipitate control tubes. The reader is referred to this volume, Chapter 15, for further discussion of the method for calculating bound and free hormone using the two control tubes. The techniques are the same except for the manner of separation. The percentage of nonspecific precipitate counts in the vasopressin assay is usually 2%; 10–14% damage is expected using the damage control tubes.

III. SENSITIVITY, CROSS-REACTIVITY, AND VALIDATION

The specificity of the antiserum for vasopressin has been well established, and it is useful in evaluating plasma and urine during physiologic changes (Oyama *et al.*, 1971; Robertson *et al.*, 1973; Husain *et al.*, 1973). Our antibody cannot distinguish between synthetic arginine vasopressin, natural arginine vasopressin, and lysine vasopressin. Mesotocin, isotocin, and vasotocin (Table II) cross-react weakly (less than 1 : 200, 1 : 10,000, and 1 : 10,000, respectively); oxytocin cross-reacts more than 200-fold less strongly than arginine vasopressin.

Table II **Structure of Vasopressin Analogs**

	1	2	3	4	5	6	7	8	9
Arginine vasopressin	Cys-	Tyr-	Phe-	Gln-	Asn-	Cys-	Pro-	Arg-	Gly-NH$_2$
Lysine vasopressin	Cys-	Tyr-	Phe-	Gln-	Asn-	Cys-	Pro-	Lys-	Gly-NH$_2$
Mesotocin	Cys-	Tyr-	Phe-	Gln-	Asn-	Cys-	Pro-	Ile-	Gly-NH$_2$
Isotocin	Cys-	Tyr-	Ile-	Ser-	Asn-	Cys-	Pro-	Ile-	Gly-NH$_2$
Vasotocin	Cys-	Tyr-	Ile-	Gln-	Asn-	Cys-	Pro-	Arg-	Gly-NH$_2$
Oxytocin	Cys-	Tyr-	Ile-	Gln-	Asn-	Cys-	Pro-	Leu-	Gly-NH$_2$

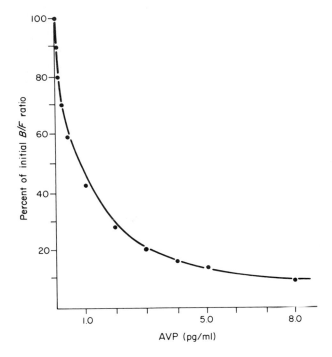

Figure 1. Vasopressin standard curve. (Reproduced from Husain *et al.*, 1973, with permission of the publisher.)

Our antiserum detects less than 0.5 pg arginine vasopressin per milliliter of extracted plasma (Figure 1) with a high degree of reproducibility (intraassay coefficient of variability, 16.7%; interassay coefficient of variability, 17.2%).

IV. VASOPRESSIN IN PLASMA

A. Extraction of Vasopressin

The presence of large amounts of cross-reacting materials in plasma has been described by Robertson *et al.* (1970). These macromolecular substances are not significant factors in assaying unextracted urine with our antiserum (Oyama *et al.*, 1971). As shown in Table III, various plasma extraction procedures have been utilized by several laboratories (reviewed by Chard, 1973; Glick and Kagan, 1974). Although our antiserum was less susceptible to the interfering factors noted with

Table III Comparison of Radioimmunoassays of Vasopressin

Immunization	Separation	Extraction	Sensitivity	Reference
Glutaraldehyde coupling to albumin	Polyethylene glycol (also chromato-electrophoresis)	Acetone and petroleum ether	0.1 pg or less	Oyama et al. (1971), Husain et al. (1973), Robertson et al. (1973)
Carbodiimide coupling to albumin (lysine vasopressin)	Charcoal	Trichloroacetic acid, Amberlite CG-50 adsorption and dilution	Appears to be a few pg	Shade and Share (1975)
Coupling to thyroglobulin	NH$_4$SO$_4$	Florisil–glass beads	1–5 pg	M. L. Forsling (personal communication)
Absorption to carbon particles; toluene diisocyanate coupling to ovine albumin	NH$_4$SO$_4$ (also double antibody)	Adsorption to glass beads	8.0 pg	Edwards et al. (1972)
Glutaraldehyde coupling to albumin	Charcoal–dextran	Fuller's earth, methanol, NH$_3$–ethanol	About 7.0–10 pg/ml	Johnston (1972)
Carbodiimide coupling to albumin	Double antibody	Florisil	10 pg/ml (pure AVP in standard curve)	Beardwell (1971)
Coupling to thyroglobulin	Not stated	Bentonite	1.0 pg/ml after 4.0 ml plasma extracted	Skowsky and Fisher (1972)

other antisera, extraction was still necessary for reliable results in plasma. Robertson first reported success with the present antibody and our method for extraction of oxytocin as described in this volume, Chapter 15. This extraction procedure yields a recovery of 65–75% (Husain *et al.*, 1973; Robertson *et al.*, 1973).

One milliliter of plasma is mixed with 2.0 ml acetone (spectral quality, Matheson-Coleman-Bell Co.). After centrifugation, the resultant precipitate, which contains plasma proteins, is then separated from the vasopressin-containing supernatant by decanting. Petroleum ether (4.0 ml) is then mixed with the acetone phase in order to extract plasma lipids. The ether phase is removed by aspiration. The remaining acetone solution is then air-dried and reconstituted in 1.0 ml vasopressin diluent. [In Robertson's hands (Robertson *et al.*, 1973), the acetone solution is not completely air-dried.] Aliquots (100 μl) of the mixture are used for assay, or, alternatively, the reconstituted solution is frozen and stored for subsequent assay. Standing at room temperature for one hour and freezing and thawing do not have significant effects upon the recovery of vasopressin from plasma. Heparinization of collecting tubes has no apparent effect on plasma vasopressin values. The extraction procedure should be performed as soon as possible after collection of the blood, since significant losses can occur after 24 hours even at 20°C (Robertson *et al.*, 1973). Both thioglycollate and pregnancy plasma have an effect (although incomplete) upon vasopressin immunoreactivity (Husain *et al.*, 1973).

B. Values in Blood and Urine

Water-loaded man excretes 0.35 mU/hour (120 U/mg) of vasopressin into urine, and dehydrated normals excrete 1.2–6.5 mU/hour (Oyama *et al.*, 1971). Mean plasma levels are 1.5 pg/ml or less in healthy recumbent men; the mean level after dehydration is 3.7 pg/ml, and it is 0.45 pg/ml after water loading (Husain *et al.*, 1973). Extremely high plasma values (up to 200 pg/ml) are found after nicotine (cigarettes) stimulation (Husain *et al.*, 1973). These marked elevations can be suppressed with alcohol (Husain *et al.*, 1975). The vasopressin radioimmunoassay has allowed precise evaluation of the relationship of vasopressin secretion, blood volume, and osmotic control (Dunn *et al.*, 1973; Robertson and Athar, 1976; Shade and Share, 1975). It has also demonstrated the presence of small amounts of vasopressin in some cases of diabetes insipidis (Robertson *et al.*, 1973). Suppression by norepinephrine (Shimamoto and Miyahara, 1976) and stimulation by surgery (Glick and Haas, 1977) have also been demonstrated.

V. COMPARISON WITH OTHER ASSAYS

Table III compares our assay with several others. It is presented to show variations of vasopressin assays. There are numerous other examples (reviewed by Glick and Kagan, 1974; Chard, 1973).

Because of our success with both vasopressin and oxytocin we would suggest the glutaraldehyde–albumin coupling technique for immunization. The use of the polyethylene glycol separation of bound and free hormone may require modification in different laboratories, but it is simpler than chromatoelectrophoresis and is much cheaper than the double antibody technique. Our oxytocin extraction method works very well for vasopressin and does not present the problems we have encountered with oxytocin. This extraction method has been aided by the great sensitivity of our antiserum. Less sensitive antisera may require the extraction of larger volumes of plasma and greater amounts of reagents which could, therefore, lead to the problems encountered with oxytocin. Other extraction methods may be superior when other antisera are used.

ACKNOWLEDGMENTS

This paper was prepared with the help of Noemi Artau Kagan, R.N., Joseph Ernst, and Pearl Sasso. It was supported by N.I.H. Grant No. 5R01AM16175.

REFERENCES

Beardwell, C. G. (1971). Radioimmunoassay of arginine vasopressin in human plasma. *J. Clin. Endocrinol. Metab.* **33,** 739–744.

Chard, T. (1973). The radioimmunoassay of oxytocin and vasopressin. *J. Endocrinol.* **58,** 143–160.

Desbuquois, B., and Aurbach, G. D. (1971). Use of polyethylene glycol to separate free and antibody-bound peptide hormones in radioimmunoassays. *J. Clin. Endocrinol. Metab.* **33,** 737–738.

Dunn, F. L., Brennan, T. J., Nelson, A. E., and Robertson, G. L. (1973). The role of blood osmolality and volume in regulating vasopressin secretion in the rat. *J. Clin. Invest.* **52,** 3212–3219.

Edwards, C. R. W., Chard, T., Kitau, M. J., Forsling, M., and Landau, J. (1972). The development of a radioimmunoassay for arginine vasopressin: Production of antisera and labeled hormone; separation techniques; specificity and sensitivity of the assay in aqueous solution. *J. Endocrinol.* **52,** 279–288.

Glick, S. M., and Hass, M. (1977). Plasma vasopressin alterations with surgery. *Endocrinol., Proc. Int. Congr. Endocrinol. 5th, 1976,* Abstracts, p. 196.

Glick, S. M., and Kagan, A. (1974). Vasopressin. *In* "Methods of Hormone Radioimmunoassay" (B. M. Jaffe and H. R. Behrman, eds.), 1st ed., pp. 187–195. Academic Press, New York.

Glick, S. M., Kumaresan, P., Kagan, A., and Wheeler, M. (1969). Radioimmunoassay of oxytocin. *Protein Polypeptide Horm., Proc. Int. Symp., 1968.* Excerpta Med. Found., Int. Congr. Ser. No. 161, pp. 81–83.

Greenwood, F. C., Hunter, W. M., and Glover, J. S. (1963). The preparation of 131I labeled human growth hormone of high specific radioactivity. *Biochem. J.* **89**, 114–123.

Husain, M. K., Fernando, N., Shapiro, M., Kagan, A., and Glick, S. M. (1973). Radioimmunoassay of arginine vasopressin in human plasma. *J. Clin. Endocrinol. Metab.* **37**, 616–625.

Husain, M. K., Frantz, A. G., Ciarochi, F., and Robinson, A. G. (1975). Nicotine stimulated release of neurophysin and vasopressin in humans. *J. Clin. Endocrinol. Metab.* **41**, 1113–1117.

Johnston, C. I. (1972). Radioimmunoassay for plasma antidiuretic hormone, *J. Endocrinol.* **52**, 69–78.

Oyama, S. N., Kagan, A., and Glick, S. M. (1971). Radioimmunoassay of vasopressin: Application to unextracted human urine. *J. Clin. Endocrinol. Metab.* **33**, 739–744.

Permutt, M. A., Parker, C. W., and Utiger, R. D. (1966). Immunochemical studies with lysine vasopressin. *Endocrinology* **78**, 809–818.

Robertson, G. L., and Athar, S. (1976). The interaction of blood osmolality and blood volume in regulating plasma vasopressin in man. *J. Clin. Endocrinol. Metab.* **42**, 613–620.

Robertson, G. L., Klein, L. A., Roth, J., and Gorden, P. (1970). Immunoassay of plasma vasopressin in man. *Proc. Natl. Acad. Sci. U.S.A.* **66**, 1298–305.

Robertson, G. L., Mahr, E. A., Athar, S., and Sinha, T. (1973). Development and clinical application of a new method for the radioimmunoassay of arginine vasopressin in human plasma. *J. Clin. Invest.* **52**, 2340–2352.

Roth, J., Glick, S. M., Klein, L. A., and Peterson, M. J. (1966). Specific antibody to vasopressin in man. *J. Clin. Endocrinol. Metab.* **26**, 671–675.

Shade, R. E., and Share, L. (1975). Volume control of plasma antidiuretic hormone concentration following acute blood volume expansion in the anesthetized dog. *Endocrinology* **97**, 1048–1057.

Shimanoto, K., and Miyahara, M. (1976). Effect of noreprinephrine infusion on plasma vasopressin levels in normal human subjects. *J. Clin. Endocrinol. Metab.* **43**, 201–204.

Skowsky, W. R., and Fisher, D. A. (1972). Vasopressin (VP) kinetics in man and the rhesus monkey fetus using radioimmunoassay measurements. *J. Clin. Invest.* **51**, 91a.

THYROID AND PARATHYROID HORMONES

17

Human Calcitonin: Application of Affinity Chromatography

ARMEN H. TASHJIAN, JR., AND EDWARD F. VOELKEL

I. INTRODUCTION

All known calcitonins (CT) consist of a 32-amino acid polypeptide chain which contains a 1–7 disulfide bridge at the NH_2-terminus and prolinamide as the C-terminal amino acid residue. Human, porcine, bovine, ovine, eel, and salmon CT's differ in many specific residues within the chain, and these differences in structure are reflected in

355

Methods of Hormone Radioimmunoassay, Second Edition
Copyright © 1979 by Academic Press, Inc.
All rights of reproduction in any form reserved. ISBN 0-12-379260-6

profound differences in immunologic activity (Tashjian and Levine, 1969; Tashjian et al., 1970a,b). Because of these differences, homologous immunoassay methods are usually required to measure the concentrations of CT present in biologic fluids. In this chapter, we shall discuss assay procedures that apply exclusively to human CT. Readers interested in specific immunoassay methods for CT of other species should refer to Deftos et al. (1968, 1972), Tashjian (1969), Tashjian et al. (1972), Roos and Deftos (1976), and Cooper et al. (1976).

II. METHOD OF RADIOIMMUNOASSAY

A. Source of Peptide

Synthetic CT M (monomer), synthesized by Ciba-Geigy, Basel, Switzerland, or N. V. Organon, Oss, The Netherlands, is used for labeling with radioiodine. As standard in the radioimmunoassay, either synthetic CT (Ciba) or MRC human synthetic calcitonin, tumor sequence 70/234 (National Institute for Medical Research, London) is used.

B. Preparation of Antiserum

Antibodies to human CT have been prepared in guinea pigs and rabbits; both natural material extracted from medullary thyroid carcinoma tissue (Clark et al., 1969; Tashjian et al., 1970b; Deftos, 1971) and the synthetic peptide (Dietrich and Rittel, 1970; Deftos, 1971) have been used as immunogens. We have found it satisfactory to extract fresh medullary carcinoma tissue by homogenization in cold 0.1 N HCl (10–20 ml/gm fresh weight) in a Waring blender for 30 to 60 seconds. After standing for 15 minutes at 2°–4°C, the insoluble material is separated by centrifugation (8000 g, 15–20 minutes, 4°C). An aliquot of the supernatant solution containing 5.0–20 MRC units of human calcitonin can be mixed with an equal volume of complete Freund's adjuvant and used for immunization, or the crude extract can be further fractionated and purified before use as an immunogen. Conjugation of calcitonin to carriers is not necessary. No single approach appears to stand out as particularly reliable. In one technique, animals were successfully immunized with 0.25–1.0 mg CT dissolved in 0.001 N HCl and emulsified with an equal volume of Freund's adjuvant (final volume, 0.8 ml). Immunizations were repeated at three-week intervals, and animals were bled ten days later. As with most moderately small peptide immunogens, a number of animals are immunized, and the various sera obtained are screened for binding and displacement of label by conventional techniques (Yalow and Berson, 1970; Ekins *et al.*, 1970) in order to identify an antiserum useful for assay purposes.

C. Preparation and Purification of Labeled Calcitonin

Synthetic human CT is radioiodinated by minor modifications of the chloramine-T method of Hunter and Greenwood (1962). Two millicuries of ^{131}I or ^{125}I are used for 4.0 μg of CT in 0.5 M phosphate, pH 7.4. Twenty micrograms of chloramine-T in 0.05 M phosphate, pH 7.4, is added, the mixture is agitated for 10 seconds, and 100 μg of $Na_2S_2O_5$ (in 0.05 M phosphate, pH 7.4) is added (final volume, 0.17 ml), followed immediately by 1.5 ml of 5% egg albumin–0.05 M 2-mercaptoethanol in 0.1 M Tris, pH 7.5. Approximately one-half (800 μl) of the reaction mixture is transferred to a tube containing 3.0 mg of QUSO G-32, microfine granules of precipitated silica (Philadelphia Quartz Co.). After brief mixing, the suspension is separated by centrifugation. The supernatant solution is aspirated, and the precipitate is washed once or twice with 2.0 ml of a solution of 0.05 M mercaptoethanol. Following centrifugation and removal of the wash solution, labeled CT is eluted from the QUSO with 1.0 ml of a solution containing 20% acetone, 1% acetic acid, and 0.05 M mercaptoethanol, and an aliquot is taken for determination of radioactivity. The entire iodination procedure is performed at room temperature and is essentially the same technique as has been described in detail porcine CT (Tashjian, 1969). Using this procedure, labeled CT of specific radioactivities of 150 to 450 μCi/μg is regularly obtained. The majority of experiments in this laboratory have been carried out with ^{131}I-CT. We have not made detailed comparisons between [131]I- and ^{125}I-labeled CT.

Freshly prepared ^{131}I-CT shows very little damage when examined by chromatoelectrophoresis (Tashjian, 1969); 97–99% of the radioactivity remains at the origin as a sharp symmetrical peak. In nearly all experiments reported from this laboratory, freshly prepared ^{131}I-CT or ^{125}I-CT is added to assay incubation tubes within one to three hours of labeling. This rapid addition of labeled CT results in lower incubation damage (see below) than if the labeled peptide is prepared one or two days in advance of use. Deftos (1971) has suggested that additional fractionation of ^{125}I-CT on columns of Biogel P-10 gives a labeled preparation with less damage and higher affinity for antibody than the original QUSO eluate.

D. Samples

Either serum or plasma can be used in the immunoassay, and no systematic differences between the two have been noted. Because clots occasionally form during incubation with plasma samples, serum is preferable. It is stored at $-70°C$ until assay.

Urine, also stored at $-70°C$, can be assayed directly at $25-\mu l$ aliquots (final dilution of $1:20$) or less without nonspecific effects on the assay, or urine concentrates (Voelkel and Tashjian, 1971) may be used (Tashjian *et al.*, 1972).

Acid extracts of tissues (see above) (Tashjian and Voelkel, 1967) can be diluted $1:5$ in assay diluent (see below) and tested at $100-\mu l$ aliquots (final dilution $1:25$) or less without nonspecific effects.

E. Incubation Procedure

The diluent is $0.10\ M$ Tris buffer, pH 7.5, containing 10% human serum from an athyreotic patient or from a normal subject with unmeasurable CT in the sample (<0.10 ng/ml), and 500 KI units of kallikrein-trypsin inhibitor (Trasylol, FBA Pharmaceuticals, Inc.) per milliliter. Fresh diluent is made up for each assay. The Tris buffer, stored at 4°C, should not be more than one month old.

Incubation mixtures are prepared in acid-washed, flint glass tubes in a total volume of 500 μl to contain the same concentration of ^{131}I-CT ($2–20$ pg/0.1 ml) and antiserum (0.1 ml), but variable concentrations of standard unlabeled CT ($5–2500$ pg/tube) or unknown sample (up to 100 μl). Antiserum is used at a final dilution (currently $1:80,000$) which gives 40–60% binding of the labeled peptide at the end of the incubation period. Sensitivity is improved in a nonequilibrium system in which the unlabeled standard and unknown are preincubated at 4°C with antiserum for three to five days and then for an additional three to five days with labeled CT ($5000–10,000$ cpm). No-antibody controls are included for each unknown sample when the final dilution is $1:20$ or less. Samples are usually tested at multiple dilutions (at least two and often three to five separate dilutions per sample).

At $1:10$ dilution of serum, incubation damage is in the range of 7 to 12%; at $1:5$ dilution, it usually does not exceed 10–15%. Incubation damage appears to rise as serum samples age at $-20°C$. It is, therefore, preferable to assay samples as soon as possible after drawing and to store them at $-70°C$. CT in human serum stored at $-70°C$ is quite stable, loss of immunologic activity being less than 10–15% in three to six months. Samples having incubation damage of greater than 20%

are retested at higher dilution, if possible, or the values obtained are rejected as being of uncertain significance.

F. Separation of Bound and Free Labeled Calcitonin

Free labeled CT can be separated from antibody-bound material by chromatoelectrophoresis (Tashjian, 1969), dextran–charcoal (Clark *et al.*, 1969; Dietrich and Rittel, 1970; Tashjian *et al.*, 1970b; Deftos, 1971), and dioxane (Deftos, 1971). Presumably other liquid phase separation methods would also be suitable.

In this laboratory, chromatoelectrophoresis is the standard method against which other techniques are judged. However, because of the relative slowness of this method for large numbers of samples (more than 200 per assay), the dextran–charcoal procedure is used as follows. A stock dextran–charcoal suspension is made by stirring equal volumes of a 5% charcoal suspension (Norit "A" N. F. X., Amend Drug and Chemical Co., Inc.) in 0.13 M borate buffer, pH 8.0, with a 0.5% dextran solution (Dextran 250, Pharmacia Fine Chemicals, Inc.) in borate buffer for two hours. From this stable stock suspension a diluted working suspension is prepared immediately before use. The well-mixed stock suspension is diluted 1 : 25 in 0.10 M Tris buffer, pH 7.5, to give the working suspension. The working suspension is stirred continuously as aliquots are removed.

When the assay is ready for separation, the incubation tubes are moved from the cold (4°C) to room temperature for about 30 minutes. Thereafter, 1.0 ml of the working dextran–charcoal suspension is added to each tube which is immediately agitated on a Vortex mixer and then allowed to stand for 30 minutes. The suspensions are then centrifuged at 2000–3000 rpm for 30 minutes at room temperature. The supernatant solution containing the antibody-bound ^{131}I-CT is carefully decanted into another test tube. Both the charcoal pellet and supernatant solution are counted in an automatic gamma spectrometer system for a time sufficient to provide a counting accuracy of 1 to 2%.

III. INTERPRETATION OF RADIOIMMUNOASSAY DATA

A. Sensitivity

The working sensitivity (Yalow and Berson, 1970) of any immunoassay depends heavily on the particular antiserum used and on the variability of the zero point of the standard curve, for only when this variability is significantly exceeded ($p < 0.05$) can a given amount of antigen be said to be detected by the assay. For the CT assay currently in use in our laboratory, the range of two standard deviations of the percentage labeled CT bound for the zero point is ± 2.8 to $\pm 3.7\%$ when ten blank samples are included in the assay. In practice we usually determine two to four blank points in each assay and require that any unknown sample produce at least 5–7% inhibition from the zero point ($p < 0.05$) before a CT value for that sample is read from the standard curve. This procedure gives a working sensitivity for the assay of 0.05 to 0.10 ng/ml for serum or plasma with 100 μl as the largest sample size used, and an absolute sensitivity of about 5.0 pg of CT per assay tube. Unknown samples are regularly tested at multiple dilutions and a mean CT concentration is calculated from these dilutions. Most serum samples containing measurable CT show a linear decrease with dilution (Tashjian *et al.*, 1970b).

B. Specificity

Deftos and co-workers (1971) have emphasized that certain serum or plasma samples can produce nonspecific (presumably not due to CT) inhibition of the percentage labeled CT bound to antibody. We have observed this effect as well. It is not clear whether it is an effect on the antigen–antibody reaction, the phase separation method, or both. That such nonspecific effects are not due merely to serum or protein concentrations is shown by the data in Table I. Because the nonspecific effects are unpredictable and vary from serum to serum, values for CT concentration in serum in the range of less than 0.10 to 1.0 ng/ml are subject to uncertainty. For concentrations above 1.0 ng/ml, the serum can be diluted 1 : 10 to 1 : 50 in the assay tube, and nonspecific effects are not seen. For reasons discussed below (Section V), we believe that affinity chromatography offers advantages over charcoal adsorption in order to prove that estimates of low levels of CT in serum (<1.0 ng/ml) are real.

The homologous immunoassay for human CT has high specificity for the human peptide. At concentrations up to 10^4 times those of human CT, porcine and salmon CT's show essentially no cross-reaction in the human CT assay. Likewise, 10^2 to 10^3 times (based on biologic activity) more eel or avian (chicken or pigeon) CT does not cross-react. On the other hand, certain antisera against human CT cross-react substantially with rat CT (Burford *et al.*, 1975; Roos and Deftos, 1976; Bell and Queener, 1976).

Table I Effects of Serum Concentration on the Binding of Labeled CT to Specific Antibody[a]

Serum concentration (%)	No. of samples	Zero point[b] (% labeled CT bound)
10	5	41.7 ± 0.58
15	5	40.6 ± 0.58
30	5	41.5 ± 0.58

[a] The same amount of ^{131}I-CT was incubated with the same dilution of anti-CT for three days in the presence of 10, 15, or 30% normal human serum in the buffer (500 μl total volume per tube). There was no unlabeled CT in any tube. All samples were then separated by the dextran–charcoal method and the percentage labeled CT bound to antibody was determined. The same result was obtained if incubations were all carried out in 10% serum buffer and then additional serum was added to 15 or 30% to two groups of tubes immediately before phase separation.

[b] Mean values ± SE. No significant differences were detected.

C. Reproducibility

Serum samples containing low (<0.1 ng/ml) and high (up to 60 ng/ml) concentrations of CT have been assayed in two or more assays separated in time by three to six weeks. The samples were stored at −70°C between studies. The results of replicate assays were in good agreement, interassay variation usually being <25% (Tashjian, 1973). Intraassay variation, calculated from multiple dilutions of the same sample (Tashjian *et al.*, 1970b), or from separate determinations at the same dilution, is likewise generally <25%.

D. Comparison of Biologic and Immunologic Assay Methods

We have assayed for CT biologically (Cooper *et al.*, 1967) in serum samples from patients with medullary carcinoma of the thyroid gland, a disease in which high levels of CT are found in the circulation. The same samples were assayed by the radioimmunoassay method described in this chapter. The results showed excellent agreement between the two assay methods when the concentrations of CT were between 10 and 50 MRC mU/ml. For values above 50 mU/ml (1 MRC mU = 3.33 ng), the results obtained by bioassay tended to be higher by 20–65% (Tashjian, 1973). These results gave no evidence, at least at high blood levels, that immunologically active but biologically inert CT peptides circulate in peripheral human plasma.

On the other hand, as knowledge of the heterogeneity of CT in human plasma has accumulated (Singer and Habener, 1974; Sizemore and Heath, 1975; Deftos *et al.*, 1975; Snider *et al.*, 1977), it has become important to evaluate the biologic activity of each of the various immunoreactive forms of CT in plasma (Tashjian, 1977). Preliminary results with a highly sensitive *in vitro* bone culture assay method for CT indicate that not all of the immunoreactive peaks are biologically active (Wright *et al.*, 1977a; Tashjian, 1977).

We have found large discrepancies between the amounts of CT in urine or urine concentrates measured by both bioassay and immunoassay methods. It is clearly established that biologically active CT-like material can be measured in urine (Voelkel and Tashjian, 1971), but it is also clear that this material has much higher serologic than biologic activity (Tashjian *et al.*, 1972).

IV. CONCENTRATIONS OF CALCITONIN IN HUMAN SERUM AND URINE

The average concentration of CT in basal (fasting) normal human serum is <0.50 ng/ml in most (see Deftos *et al.*, 1971; Tashjian *et al.*, 1974; Hillyard *et al.*, 1977) but not all (Samaan *et al.*, 1973; Silva *et al.*, 1974; Heynen and Franchimont, 1974) laboratories performing such assays. In the majority of normal subjects, the concentration appears to be <0.10 ng/ml (Deftos *et al.*, 1971; Melvin *et al.*, 1972; Tashjian *et al.*, 1974; Parthemore and Deftos, 1975; Hillyard *et al.*, 1977). Because of the low levels present and the problems of nonspecific inhibition of the radioimmunoassay at high concentrations of certain sera, it still appears that the absolute range of normal values remains to be defined in a large number of human subjects. It is to be hoped that either greatly improved assay sensitivity or concentration of CT from normal serum by affinity chromatography (see below), immunoprecipitation and immunoextraction (Parthemore and Deftos, 1975), or adsorption techniques (Hillyard *et al.*, 1977) will aid in the resolution of these uncertainties.

In patients with medullary carcinoma of the thyroid gland, concentrations of CT in serum are regularly detectable, and if the disease is clinically evident, the values are usually greater than 1.0 ng/ml, often 10–1000 ng/ml (Tashjian *et al.*, 1970b; Deftos *et al.*, 1971; Melvin *et al.*, 1972). In early or clinically covert disease, the levels may be <0.1–1.0 ng/ml, but often they can be stimulated by calcium infusion to values of greater than 1.0 ng/ml, a technique which can enable the very early diagnosis of the tumor with a high degree of reliability (Melvin *et al.*, 1971, 1972; Bloch *et al.*, 1972; Tashjian *et al.*, 1974). CT concentrations in serum before and during a provocative calcium infusion test correlate well with the extent of the medullary carcinoma and offer a means for quantitatively monitoring the effects of therapy. In addition to the standard four-hour calcium infusion test (15 mg calcium/kg body weight) (Tashjian *et al.*, 1970b), both short-term calcium infusions (Parthemore *et al.*, 1974; Rude and Singer, 1977) and rapid pentagastrin injections (0.5 μg/kg body weight over 5–10 seconds intravenously) (Hennessy *et al.*, 1974; Rude and Singer, 1977) are being used as provocative agents to stimulate the secretion of CT in patients at risk for medullary thyroid carcinoma. The one-minute calcium injection and pentagastrin injection procedures show promise as methods which may replace the four-hour calcium infusion because of the relative ease of administration and brevity of tests. However, to date, insufficient data have been collected to indicate that they are diagnostically superior (have a lower false negative yield) to the four-hour calcium infusion (Wright *et al.*, 1977b).

The occurrence of elevated CT concentrations in plasma in conditions other than medullary thyroid carcinoma have been documented. Patients with hyperparathyroidism and varying degrees of chronic hypercalcemia have been reported to have either undetectable or minimally elevated CT levels (Heynen and Franchimont, 1974; Silva *et al.*, 1974; Tashjian *et al.*, 1972). Little information is available on calcitonin concentrations in patients with hypercalcemia of other etiologies, but the results are similar to those obtained in hyperparathyroid patients. Subjects with chronic hypocalcemia of several causes have been reported to have unmeasurable basal levels (Deftos *et al.*, 1972, 1973). However, these patients released unusually large amounts of CT in response to even minor elevations of serum calcium, presumably because the amounts of CT in thyroid gland stores increased during hypocalcemia.

Increased CT concentrations in plasma have also been reported in patients with carcinoid tumors (Milhaud *et al.*, 1970), Zollinger–Ellison syndrome (Sizemore *et al.*, 1973), pernicious anemia (Heynen and Franchimont, 1974), a child with pycnodysostosis (Baker *et al.*, 1973), and in maternal and fetal serum at term (Tashjian *et al.*, 1972, 1974; Samaan *et al.*, 1975). Elevated concentrations have also been regularly observed in both acute and chronic renal failure (Heynen and Franchimont, 1974; Ardaillou *et al.*, 1975). Little is known about the pathophysiology and clinical significance of these findings. Lastly, hypercalcitoninemia has been reported in association with malignancies of non-C cell origin (Tashjian *et al.*, 1975; Coombes *et al.*, 1976a,b; Silva *et al.*, 1975). In such cases, it is usually not difficult to differentiate between medullary thyroid carcinoma and other malignancies on the basis of the absolute levels of CT in plasma, the genetic history, and the clinical findings.

In unconcentrated normal human urine, immunoreactive CT concentrations are less than 1.0 ng/ml; however, the values may be very high (up to 3.0 μg/ml) in patients with medullary carcinoma. Concentrates of normal urine do, however, contain both immunoreactive and biologically active CT-like material (Tashjian *et al.*, 1972), a finding that is consistent with the proposition that biologically active CT circulates normally at low levels in man.

V. AFFINITY CHROMATOGRAPHY

A. A Specific Method for the Removal of Calcitonin from Samples before Immunoassay

The problem of nonspecific inhibition of the labeled hormone–antibody interaction has been discussed earlier in this chapter with special reference to unknown samples which contain low concentrations (<1.0 ng/ml) of CT. One approach to the solution of this problem has been suggested by Deftos *et al.* (1971). They treated serum with charcoal in order to remove CT from the sample. The serum was then assayed before and after adsorption. Their results showed that the bulk of the immunoreactive CT was removed from CT-rich plasma by such treatment. This method certainly has utility; however, it is well established that charcoal treatment removes many components from plasma. Therefore, loss of immunologic reactivity after charcoal treatment does not constitute strong evidence that the material in plasma, which inhibited the labeled CT–anti-CT reaction before but not after treatment with charcoal, was indeed CT. In order to strengthen the approach to the selective removal of CT from unknown samples, we have used the more specific technique of affinity chromatography (Cuatrecasas and Anfinsen, 1971a; Wright *et al.*, 1977).

1. Preparation and Testing of Anti-calcitonin Affinity Columns

The antiserum was prepared in a rabbit against human tumor calcitonin using procedures similar to those described for the guinea pig by Tashjian *et al.* (1970b). Anti-CT for coupling to agarose (Sepharose) was partially purified from one to four milliliters of antiserum by precipitation with 40% saturated ammonium sulfate at 4°C. This was repeated twice and the final precipitate was dissolved in 0.05 M sodium phosphate, pH 7.4, and dialyzed against the same buffer. The CT binding capacity of the final solution and that of intermediate fractions and the starting antiserum are given in Table II.

Antibodies and other proteins (20–40 mg) were coupled at pH 7.8 to 10–20 ml wet Sepharose 4B (Pharmacia) which had been activated by treatment with cyanogen bromide (Cuatrecasas and Anfinsen, 1971b). After coupling, the Sepharose was washed extensively with 0.5 M sodium bicarbonate and then with 6 M guanidine-HCl (pH 3.0). The washes were tested for CT binding activity (Table III). In exactly parallel experiments, normal rabbit serum was fractionated by ammonium sulfate precipitation, and the globulin fraction was coupled to Sepharose.

Small columns of substituted Sepharose (anti-CT or normal rabbit globulins) were prepared in disposable Pasteur pipettes (bed volumes of 0.5 to 2.0 ml). The columns were equilibrated with 0.15 M NaCl–0.01 M sodium phosphate, pH 7.4. All chromatography was performed at room temperature.

The operation of the anti-CT affinity chromatography system was tested in several ways. Labeled CT, parathyroid hormone (PTH), and prolactin (PRL) were added to human serum and chromatographed on anti-CT columns. CT, but not PTH or PRL, was efficiently removed from serum (Table IV). Labeled calcitonin did not bind to columns of Sepharose coupled with normal rabbit globulins (Table IV). The

Table II   Binding of Labeled CT by Ammonium Sulfate Fractions of Rabbit Anti-human Calcitonin

Fraction	Final dilution	Percentage ^{131}I-CT bound[a]
Original antiserum	1 : 25,000	21
	1 : 5000	60
First, second, and third $(NH_4)_2SO_4$ supernatant solutions	1 : 1000	0
	1 : 200	11–14
Final $(NH_4)_2SO_4$ globulin fraction in solution after dialysis	1 : 25,000	16
	1 : 5000	49
	1 : 1000	75

[a] Incubated for 18 hr at 4°C with 10,000 cpm/ml of ^{131}I-CT. Phase separation was by dextran–charcoal adsorption of the free labeled CT. Each value is the mean of duplicate samples.

Table III   Lack of Binding of Labeled CT by Sodium Bicarbonate and Guanidine–HCl Eluates of Rabbit Anti-CT Coupled to Sepharose 4B

Fraction	Absorbancy at 277 nm (undiluted)	Volume (ml)	Dilution tested for binding	Percentage ^{131}I-CT bound[a]
Original antiserum	—	—	1:25,000	21
			1:5000	60
NaHCO$_3$ eluates				
1st	0.042	30	1:200	2.0
2nd	0.026	30	1:200	0
4th	0.000	30	1:200	0
6th	0.000	30	1:200	0
7th	0.000	30	1:200	0
12th	0.000	200[b]	1:200	0
Guanidine eluates				
1st	0.024	10	1:200	0
2nd	0.003	10	1:200	0
4th	0.000	10	1:200	0
6th	0.000	10	1:200	0

[a] Incubated for 18 hr at 4°C with 10,000 cpm/ml of ^{131}I-CT. Phase separation was by dextran–charcoal adsorption of the free labeled CT. Each point was determined in duplicate.

[b] The volumes of elution were increased after sample number 7. The volume collected in the 12th fraction was 200 ml, and the cumulative volume of eluate was 4000 ml.

Table IV   Chromatography on Affinity Columns of Normal Human Serum Containing Labeled Human CT, Bovine Parathyroid Hormone, and Rat Prolactin[a]

Labeled hormone added to serum	Percentage labeled hormone absorbed[b]	Percentage absorbed labeled hormone eluted with	
		Guanidine[b]	Acetic acid[b]
Columns of Sepharose–anti-CT			
Calcitonin	88 ± 1.2	91 ± 1.1	64 ± 5.6
PTH	6.0	2.0	—
Prolactin	7.0	<1.0	—
Columns of Sepharose–normal rabbit globulins			
Calcitonin	3.0	—	—

[a] Iodine (^{131}I or ^{125}I) labeled hormones (25,000–40,000 cpm) were added individually to 0.5–1.0 ml of normal human serum which contained <0.10 ng/ml of immunoreactive CT. The sera containing the labeled hormones were then chromatographed without dilution on columns of either anti-CT or normal rabbit globulins.

[b] Mean values ± SE for eight separate columns or the average of duplicate columns (single figures).

Table V   Inhibition by Pure Synthetic Human CT of the Binding of Labeled CT
to Anti-CT Affinity Columns[a]

Human CT added (μg)	Percentage ^{131}I-CT bound to column	Percentage inhibition of binding
0	89	—
0.005	40	55
0.50	25	72
50.0	2.0	98

[a] ^{131}I-CT (25,000–35,000 cpm) was added to each 0.5 ml of normal human serum that contained <0.10 ng/ml of immunoreactive CT. To 0.5-ml aliquots of this mixture either zero or known amounts of unlabeled synthetic human CT were added and the samples (0.5 ml) were chromatographed on small columns of anti-CT. The data shown are the results of two separate but similar experiments.

labeled CT could be eluted in excellent yield from anti-CT columns with 6.0 M guanidine or less effectively with 1.0 M acetic acid (Table IV) and was fully immunoreactive. The binding of labeled CT to anti-CT columns was inhibited by mixing, prior to chromatography, synthetic calcitonin together with human serum containing a known amount of labeled CT (Table V).

2. Application of Anti-calcitionin Affinity Columns to Removal of Calcitionin from Human Serum

The ability of anti-CT columns to remove CT from human serum was tested in two ways. First, sera from patients with histologically proved medullary carcinoma of the thyroid gland were assayed immunologically in order to determine the concentrations of CT before chromatography. When the levels were sufficiently high, the results of immunoassay were confirmed by biologic assay of the same samples. Sera with widely varying, but clearly measurable, CT were then chromatographed on columns of anti-CT, and the effluent fractions were assayed quantitatively for CT by immunoassay. The data, summarized in Table VI, show that endogenous calcitonin in the serum of patients with medullary carcinoma is largely removed by a single passage through a column of anti-CT. In control experiments, when CT-rich sera were passed through normal rabbit serum globulin–Sepharose columns, essentially no CT was removed (recovery of CT was 90–100%).

In a second type of experiment, normal human serum which contained less than 0.10 ng/ml of endogenous CT (determined by immunoassay) was enriched with CT by adding a known quantity of synthetic CT to the serum. Such sera were immunoassayed before and

Table VI Removal of CT from Human Sera by a Single Passage through Affinity Columns of Anti-CT

Sample	CT in sample applied to column (ng)	CT recovered in effluent from column (ng)	Percentage CT removed by column
Medullary carcinoma sera			
Expt. No. 1[a]			
M. W.	10	1.5	85
M. J.	26	3.4	87
M. J.	4.5	0.54	88
M. J.	4.6	0.50	89
M. J.	7.7	2.0	74
M. S.	3.5	1.2	66
K. C.	10	2.5	75
			81 ± 2.3[c]
Expt. No. 2[b]			
M. C.	6.1	0.79	87
C. T.	1.1	0.22	80
R. T.	0.8	0.10	88
R. T.	4.2	0.72	83
M. G.	5.3	0.66	88
G. W.	3.2	0.38	88
G. W.	30	3.3	89
R. P.	3.0	0.37	88
R. P.	31	2.4	92
S. K.	2.1	0	100
S. K.	20	2.2	89
S. K.	39	2.4	94
A. C.	10	1.6	84
A. C.	48	4.4	91
E. J.	52	6.5	88
H. F.	4.0	0.91	77
H. F.	20	3.1	84
H. F.	40	5.1	87
H. F.	80	13	84
			87 ± 1.4[c]
Normal human serum[d]			
Not incubated	10	0.20	98
Incubated 37°C, one hr	10	0.10	99

[a] Experiments performed with batch TEV-485 of Sepharose–anti-CT, which had a binding efficiency for ^{131}I-CT of 80 ± 4.0%.

[b] Experiments performed with batch TEV-508 of Sepharose–anti-CT, which had a binding efficiency for ^{131}I-CT of 88 ± 1.2%.

[c] Mean values ±SE.

[d] Synthetic calcitonin M (10 ng/0.5 ml) was added to normal serum containing <0.10 ng/ml of endogenous CT.

after chromatography on anti-CT columns. Essentially all of the added CT was removed by chromatography (Table VI). In these experiments the samples were analyzed before and after incubation at 37°C for one hour in order to rule out any association of CT with serum macromolecules at 37°C which might prevent or inhibit binding to anti-CT coupled to Sepharose.

We have used this affinity chromatography technique to show that the immunoreactive material in the serum of a child with pycnodysostosis is CT (Baker *et al.*, 1973). Similar studies have been performed on plasma from patients with C-cell hyperplasia.

B. Use of Affinity Chromatography to Concentrate Calcitonin

Weintraub (1970) has shown the utility of affinity chromatography to concentrate very small amounts of antigen (hCS) from serum and the application of this procedure to radioimmunoassay. Parthemore and Deftos (1975) have used immunorecipitation and immunoextraction to measure CT in normal human plasma. Because we have demonstrated that CT can be removed from serum by affinity chromatography and can be eluted from the affinity column in an immunoreactive form, we anticipate that this technique will prove useful in seeking solutions to several unresolved problems such as: (1) What are the basal circulating concentrations of CT in normal human sera? (2) Does CT play any significant role in normal human physiology or development? (3) What subtle abnormalities of CT secretion exist that have not been detected by direct radioimmunoassay of unconcentrated plasma? (4) What is the nature of the material in urine that behaves like CT by bioassay, while having an unusually high ratio of serologic to biologic activity? (5) What is the biologic significance, if any, of the immunoheterogeneity of CT in plasma?

ACKNOWLEDGMENTS

The development of the radioimmunoassay for CT and of the affinity chromatography procedure was supported in part by a research grant from the National Institute of Arthritis, Metabolism and Digestive Diseases (AM 10206), and aspects of the clinical studies were aided by the American Cancer Society (CI-65).

REFERENCES

Ardaillou, R., Beaufils, M., Nivez, M.-P., Isaac, R., Mayaud, C., and Sraer, J.-D. (1975). Increased plasma calcitonin in early acute renal failure. *Clin. Sci. Mol. Med.* **49**, 301–304.

Baker, R. K., Wallach, S., and Tashjian, A. H., Jr. (1973). Plasma calcitonin in pycnodysostosis: Intermittently high basal levels and exaggerated responses to calcium and glucagon infusions. *J. Clin. Endocrinol. Metab.* **37**, 46–55.

Bell, N. H., and Queener, S. F. (1976). A radioimmunoassay for serum calcitonin in the rat. *Proc. Soc. Exp. Biol. Med.* **152**, 516–519.

Bloch, M. A., Jackson, C. E., and Tashjian, A. H., Jr. (1972). Medullary thyroid carcinoma detected by serum calcitonin assay. *Arch. Surg.* (*Chicago*) **104**, 579–585.

Burford, H. J., Ontjes, D. A., Cooper, C. W., Parlow, A. F., and Hirsch, P. F. (1975). Purification, characterization and radioimmunoassay of thyrocalcitonin from rat thyroid glands. *Endocrinology* **96**, 340–348.

Clark, M. B., Byfield, P. G. H., Boyd, G. W., and Foster, G. V. (1969). A radioimmunoassay for human calcitonin. *Lancet* **2**, 74–77.

Coombes, R. C., Ellison, M. L., Easty, G. C., Hillyard, C. J., James, R., Galante, L., Girgis, S., Heywood, L., MacIntyre, I. and Neville, A. M. (1976a). The ectopic secretion of calcitonin by lung and breast carcinomas. *Clin. Endocrinol.* **5**, Suppl., 387s–396s.

Coombes, R. C., Ward, M. K., Greenberg, P. B., Hillyard, C. J., Tulloch, B. R., Morrison, R., and Joplin, G. F. (1976b). Calcium metabolism in cancer. *Cancer* **38**, 2111–2120.

Cooper, C. W., Hirsch, P. F., Toverud, S. U., and Munson, P. L. (1967). An improved method for the biological assay of thyrocalcitonin. *Endocrinology* **81**, 610–616.

Cooper, C. W., Obie, J. F., and Hsu, W. H. (1976). Improvement and initial *in vivo* application of the radioimmunoassay of rat thyrocalcitonin. *Proc. Soc. Exp. Biol. Med.* **151**, 183–188.

Cuatrecasas, P., and Anfinsen, C. B. (1971a). Affinity chromatography. *Annu. Rev. Biochem.* **40**, 259–278.

Cuatrecasas, P., and Anfinsen, C. B. (1971b). Affinity chromatography. *In* "Methods in Enzymology" (W. B. Jakoby, ed.), Vol. 22, pp. 345–378. Academic Press, New York.

Deftos, L. J. (1971). Immunoassay for human calcitonin. I. Method. *Metab., Clin. Exp.* **20**, 1122–1128.

Deftos, L. J., Lee, M. R., and Potts, J. T., Jr. (1968). A radioimmunoassay for thyrocalcitonin. *Proc. Natl. Acad. Sci. U.S.A.* **60**, 293–299.

Deftos, L. J., Bury, A. E., Habener, J. F., Singer, F. R., and Potts, J. T., Jr. (1971). Immunoassay for human calcitonin. II. Clinical studies. *Metab., Clin. Exp.* **20**, 1129–1137.

Deftos, L. J., Murray, T. M., Powell, D., Habener, J. F., Singer, F. R., Mayer, G. P., and Potts, J. T., Jr. (1972). Radioimmunoassays for parathyroid hormones and calcitonins. *In* "Calcium, Parathyroid Hormone and the Calcitonins" (R. V. Talmage and P. L. Munson, eds.), Int. Congr. Ser. No. 243, pp. 140–151. Excerpta Med. Found., Amsterdam.

Deftos, L. J., Powell, D., Parthemore, J. G., and Potts, J. T., Jr. (1973). Secretion of calcitonin in hypocalcemic states in man. *J. Clin. Invest.* **52**, 3109–3114.

Deftos, L. J., Roos, B. A., Bronzert, D., and Parthemore, J. G. (1975). Immunochemical heterogeneity of calcitonin in plasma. *J. Clin. Endocrinol. Metab.* **40**, 409–412.

Dietrich, F. M., and Rittel, W. (1970). Antigenic site(s) of synthetic human calcitonin M. *Nature (London)* **225**, 75–76.

Ekins, R. P., Newman, G. B., and O'Riordan, J. L. H. (1970). Saturation assays. In "Statistics in Endocrinology" (J. W. McArthur and T. Colton, eds.), pp. 345–378. MIT Press, Cambridge, Massachusetts.

Hennessy, J. F., Wells, S. A., Jr., Ontjes, D. A., and Cooper, C. W. (1974). A comparison of pentagastrin injection and calcium infusion as provocative agents for the detection of medullary carcinoma of the thyroid. *J. Clin. Endocrinol. Metab.* **39**, 487–495.

Heynen, G., and Franchimont, P. (1974). Human calcitonin radioimmunoassay in normal and pathological conditions. *Eur. J. Clin. Invest.* **4**, 213–222.

Hillyard, C. J., Cooke, T. J. C., Coombes, R. C., Evans, I. M. A., and MacIntyre, I. (1977). Normal plasma calcitonin: Circadian variation and response to stimuli. *Clin. Endocrinol.* **6**, 291–298.

Hunter, W. M., and Greenwood, F. C. (1962). Preparation of iodine-131 labeled human growth hormone of high specific activity. *Nature (London)* **194**, 495–496.

Melvin, K. E. W., Miller, H. H., and Tashjian, A. H., Jr. (1971). Early diagnosis of medullary carcinoma of the thyroid gland by means of calcitonin assay. *N. Engl. J. Med.* **285**, 1115–1120.

Melvin, K. E. W., Tashjian, A. H., Jr., and Miller, H. H. (1972). Studies in familial (medullary) thyroid carcinoma. *Recent Prog. Horm. Res.* **28**, 399–460.

Milhaud, G., Calmettes, C., Raymond, J. P., Bignon, J., and Moukhtar, M. S. (1970). Carcinoïde sécrétant de la thyrocalcitonine. *C. R. Hebd. Seances Acad. Sci., Ser. D* **18**, 2195–2198.

Parthemore, J. G., Bronzert, D., Roberts, G., and Deftos, L. J. (1974). A short calcium infusion in the diagnosis of medullary thyroid carcinoma. *J. Clin. Endocrinol. Metab.* **39**, 108–111.

Parthemore, J. G., and Deftos, L. J. (1975). The regulation of calcitonin in normal human plasma as assessed by immunoprecipitation and immunoextraction. *J. Clin. Invest.* **56**, 835–841.

Roos, B. A., and Deftos, L. J. (1976). Radioimmunoassay of calcitonin in plasma, normal thyroid, and medullary thyroid carcinoma of the rat. *J. Lab. Clin. Med.* **88**, 173–182.

Rude, R. K., and Singer, F. R. (1977). Comparison of serum calcitonin levels after a 1-minute calcium injection and after pentagastrin injection in the diagnosis of medullary thyroid carcinoma. *J. Clin. Endocrinol. Metab.* **44**, 980–983.

Samaan, N. A., Hill, C. S., Jr., Beceiro, J. R., and Schultz, P. N. (1973). Immunoreactive calcitonin in medullary carcinoma of the thyroid and in maternal and cord serum. *J. Lab. Clin. Med.* **81**, 671–681.

Samaan, N. A., Anderson, G. D., and Adam-Mayne, M. E. (1975). Immunoreactive calcitonin in the mother, neonate, child and adult. *Am. J. Obstet. Gynecol.* **121**, 622–625.

Silva, O. L., Snider, R. H., and Becker, K. L. (1974). Radioimmunoassay of calcitonin in human plasma. *Clin. Chem.* **20**, 337–339.

Silva, O. L., Becker, K. L., Primack, A., Doppman, J. L., and Snider, R. H. (1975). Hypercalcitoninemia in bronchogenic cancer: Evidence for thyroid origin of the hormone. *J. Am. Med. Assoc.* **234**, 183–185.

Singer, F. R., and Habener, J. F. (1974). Multiple immunoreactive forms of calcitonin in human plasma. *Biochem. Biophys. Res. Commun.* **61**, 710–716.

Sizemore, G. W., and Heath, H., III. (1975). Immunochemical heterogeneity of calcitonin in plasma of patients with medullary thyroid carcinoma. *J. Clin. Invest.* **55**, 1111–1118.

Sizemore, G. W., Go, V. L. W., Kaplan, E. L., Sanzenbacher, L. J., Holtermuller, K. H., and Arnaud, C. D. (1973). Relations of calcitonin and gastrin in the Zollinger–Ellison syndrome and medullary carcinoma of the thyroid. *N. Engl. J. Med.* **288**, 641–644.

Snider, R. H., Silva, O. L., Moore, C. F., and Becker, K. L. (1977). Immunochemical heterogeneity of calcitonin in man: Effect on radioimmunoassay. *Clin. Chim. Acta* **76**, 1–14.

Tashjian, A. H., Jr. (1969). Immunoassay of thyrocalcitonin. I. The method and its serological specificity. *Endocrinology* **84**, 140–148.

Tashjian, A. H., Jr. (1973). Calcitonin radioimmunoassay. *In* "Methods in Investigative and Diagnostic Endocrinology" (S. A. Berson and R. S. Yalow, eds.), pp. 1010–1019. North-Holland Publ., Amsterdam.

Tashjian, A. H., Jr. (1977). Calcitonin 1976: A review of some recent advances. *Endocrinol., Proc. Int. Congr. Endocrinol., 5th, 1976,* Excerpta Med. Found., Int. Congr. Ser. No. 403, Vol. 2, pp. 256–261.

Tashjian, A. H., Jr., and Levine, L. (1969). Taxonomic specificity of growth hormones and thyrocalcitonins as measured immunologically. *Prog. Endocrinol., Proc. Int. Congr. Endocrinol., 3rd, 1968,* Excerpta Med. Found., Int. Congr. Ser. No. 184, pp. 440–452.

Tashjian, A. H., Jr., and Voelkel, E. F. (1967). Decreased thyrocalcitonin in thyroid glands from patients with hyperparathyroidism. *J. Clin. Endocrinol. Metab.* **27**, 1353–1357.

Tashjian, A. H., Jr., Bell, P. H., and Levine, L. (1970a). Immunochemistry of thyrocalcitonins: species differences and studies of the relationships between structure and immunological activity. *Calcitonin, Proc. Int. Symp., 2nd, 1969* pp. 359–375.

Tashjian, A. H., Jr., Howland, B. G., Melvin, K. E. W., and Hill, C. S., Jr. (1970b). Immunoassay of human calcitonin: clinical measurement, relation to serum calcium and studies in patients with medullary carcinoma. *N. Engl. J. Med.* **283**, 890–895.

Tashjian, A. H., Jr., Melvin, K. E. W., Voelkel, E. F., Howland, B. G., Zuckerman, J. E., and Minkin, C. (1972). Calcitonin in blood, urine and tissue: Immunological and biological studies. *In* "Calcium, Parathyroid Hormone and the Calcitonins" (R. V. Talmage and P. L. Munson, eds.), Int. Congr. Ser. No. 243, pp. 97–112. Excerpta Med. Found., Amsterdam.

Tashjian, A. H., Jr., Wolfe, H. J., and Voelkel, E. F. (1974). Human calcitonin: Immunological assay, cytological localization and studies on medullary thyroid carcinoma. *Am. J. Med.* **56**, 840–849.

Tashjian, A. H., Jr., Voelkel, E. F., Wolfe, H. J., Gagel, R., DeLellis, R. A., Franklin, R., and Jackson, C. E. (1975). Calcitonin and prostaglandins: Significance, relevance and uncertainties. *In* "Calcium-Regulating Hormones" (R. V. Talmage, M. Owen, and J. A. Parsons, eds.), Int. Congr. Ser. No. 346, pp. 135–148. Excerpta Med. Found., Amsterdam.

Voelkel, E. F., and Tashjian, A. H., Jr. (1971). Measurement of thyrocalcitonin-like activity in urine of patients with medullary carcinoma. *J. Clin. Endocrinol. Metab.* **32**, 102–109.

Weintraub, B. D. (1970). Concentration and purification of human chorionic somatomammotropin (HCS) by affinity chromatography: Application to radioimmunoassay. *Biochem. Biophys. Res. Commun.* **39**, 83–89.

Wright, D. R., Voelkel, E. F., Sides, K. M., Tice, J. E., and Tashjian, A. H., Jr. (1977a). Heterogeneous forms of human calcitonin: Direct assessment of biologic activity. *Clin. Res.* **25**, 404A.

Wright, D. R., Voelkel, E. F., and Tashjian, A. H., Jr. (1977b). Measurement of human calcitonin by affinity chromatography and radioimmunoassay. *In* "Handbook of Radioimmunoassay" (G. E. Abraham, ed.), pp. 391–423. Dekker, New York.

Yalow, R. S., and Berson, S. A. (1970). Radioimmunoassays. *In* "Statistics in Endocrinology" (J. W. McArthur and T. Colton, eds.), pp. 327–344. MIT Press, Cambridge, Massachusetts.

18

Thyroxine and Triiodothyronine

JEEREDDI A. PRASAD AND CHARLES S. HOLLANDER

I. INTRODUCTION

It has long been recognized that two thyroid hormones, thyroxine (T4) and triiodothyronine (T3), are normally present in peripheral blood. Although reverse T3 (rT3) (3,3′,5′-triiodothyronine) and 3,3′-diiodothyronine (T2) were recognized about 20 years ago in the serum and thyroglobulin of the rat (Roche *et al.*, 1955a,b, 1956a,b), they were not measured in human serum until very recently (Chopra, 1974; Nicod *et al.*, 1976; Meinhold *et al.*, 1975). Nevertheless, early estimates of thyroid hormone levels by iodine analysis (protein-bound iodine and thyroxine by column) were reasonably accurate reflections of T4 levels (Trevorrow, 1939; Riggs *et al.*, 1942; Man *et al.*, 1951; Wynn, 1960; Pileggi *et al.*, 1961), because T4 accounts for 85–90% of organic iodine-containing compounds in the circulation. The development of competitive protein-binding analysis (Murphy and

375

Methods of Hormone Radioimmunoassay, Second Edition

Pattee, 1964) and radioimmunoassay techniques for T4 (Mitsuma *et al.*, 1972a; Chopra, 1972) have permitted more specific measurements of this hormone. In contrast, the minute concentration of T3 normally present in serum made quantitation by routine chemical means a formidable task. The development of competitive protein-binding analysis (Nauman *et al.*, 1967; Sterling *et al.*, 1969) and gas–liquid chromatography (Hollander, 1968) for T3 were useful in providing pioneering studies on T3, but these methods were cumbersome and generally overestimated T3 concentration. The more recent development of radioimmunoassay techniques for measuring T3 has allowed for a greater understanding of the contribution of T3 to thyroidal economy. In addition, the availability of methods for quantitation of rT3 secretion (Chopra, 1974) and measurements of tetraiodothyroacetic acid (Burger, 1977) and T2 (Wu *et al.*, 1976) have shed new light on the metabolism of thyroxine (T4).

It is interesting to note that the application of radioimmunoassay techniques for measurement of T3, rT3, and T4 lagged behind the development of radioimmunoassays by approximately a decade. Presumably, the small size of the thyroxine molecule dissuaded investigators from considering it a suitable antigen, but as has been subsequently shown for T3, T4, rT3, T2, tetraiodothyroacetic acid (tetrac), and other small antigens as well, small size does not preclude antigenicity if appropriate methods are employed. After the demonstration by Brown *et al.* (1970) that antibodies to T3 could be raised in animals injected with a poly-L-lysine–T3 conjugate, other investigators were stimulated to develop serum T3 and T4 radioimmunoassays suitable for routine clinical and laboratory use.

II. PRINCIPLES OF T3 AND T4 RADIOIMMUNOASSAY

As with radioimmunoassays of other hormones, the methods for T3 and T4 radioimmunoassays employ variations of three basic steps: (1) preparation of specific anti-T3 or anti-T4 antibodies, (2) addition of isotopically labeled T3 or T4 to standards or serum to be tested and reaction with anti-T3 or anti-T4 antibody, and (3) separation of antibody-bound and free T3 or T4.

There are several potential pitfalls in these radioimmunoassays that require special attention. The first arises from the presence in serum of proteins with high affinity for T3 and T4 [i.e., thyroxine-binding globulin (TBG) and thyroxine-binding prealbumin (TBPA)] which compete with anti-T3 and anti-T4 antibodies for available T3 and T4.

This has been circumvented either by extraction of serum prior to assay or by the addition of a number of agents to block the binding of the thyroid hormones to serum proteins. A second possible problem which applies to the T3 radioimmunoassay is the presence in serum of far higher concentrations of T4 than T3. Since these substances differ by only one iodine atom, the potential for error, even with small degrees of cross-reactivity of anti-T3 antibody with T4, is very great. Moreover, preliminary separation of T3 and T4 may be hazardous, since it may prove incomplete and induce conversion of T4 to T3 (Taurog, 1963). Using specific antisera with minimal cross-reactivity and T3 and T4 labeled with different iodine isotopes, we have developed a rapid simultaneous radioimmunoassay for T3 and T4.

III. RAPID SIMULTANEOUS RADIOIMMUNOASSAY FOR T3 AND T4 IN UNEXTRACTED SERUM

In this section, we will describe the method we have developed for measuring T3 which can be completed in three hours and has the additional advantage of permitting the simultaneous measurement of T4 as well.

A. Preparation of Reagents

1. T3 and T4 Immunogens: Production of Anti-T3 and Anti-T4 Antibodies

T3 and T4 were obtained as the free acids (Sigma Chemical, St. Louis, Missouri) and in the presence of trace label were purified by five consecutive paper (Whatman 3MM) chromatographic separations in a t-amyl alcohol : hexane : 2.0 N ammonia system (1 : 5 : 6, v/v/v) (Sterling *et al.*, 1969) to a constant specific activity and eluted with methanol–1.0 N HAc (5 : 1) as previously described (Nihei *et al.*, 1971). After purification, T3 was coupled directly to bovine serum albumin. To accomplish this, 50 mg of chromatographically purified T3 was dissolved in 2.5 ml 0.15 N NaOH and added, with stirring, to 5.0 ml of a solution of 100 mg bovine serum albumin (BSA) (Sigma Chemical) per 5.0 ml distilled deionized water. Carbodiimide (300 mg) was then introduced with continued stirring and the pH of the reaction mixture adjusted to 9 with hydrochloric acid. The mixture was incubated at 4°C overnight and dialyzed for five days against six liters of distilled deionized water which was changed daily.

The resulting immunogens, emulsified in complete Freund's adjuvant (Difco Labs Detroit, Michigan) were injected into the toepads of rabbits at 0.75 mg/0.2 ml. This amount of immunogen was administered at the same site at four, five, eight, and nine weeks after the initial injection, and blood for antiserum was drawn one week after the last dose and every two weeks thereafter. Fifty adult 2700-gm female rabbits of the New Zealand white strain (Zartman Farms, Douglasville, Pennsylvania) were immunized with the T3–bovine serum albumin conjugate.

^{125}I-T3 (Abbott Laboratories) was chromatographically purified before use. Barbital buffer, 0.08 M, containing 1.0 gm/liter of bovine serum albumin to prevent adsorption to glassware (barbital diluent) was used for dilution of the antisera, radioactive T3 (^{125}I-T3), and, subsequently, for test samples.

Rabbit serum in dilutions of 1 : 10, 1 : 50, 1 : 100, and 1 : 500 was screened for the presence of antibody to T3 in the following manner: 3 pg ^{125}I-T3 (specific activity 70–90 μCi/μg; Abbott Laboratories, North Chicago, Illinois) was added to 0.1 ml of the diluted test antiserum. The mixture was incubated at 4°C for 24 hours. In this system, after incubation, 1.0 ml of a slurry of activated charcoal, 0.5 gm Norit A, and 0.05 gm dextran 80 in 100 ml barbital diluent prepared as previously described (Brown *et al.*, 1970; Herbert *et al.*, 1965) was added, the mixture reincubated for five minutes, centrifuged at approximately 675 g for 15 minutes, the supernatant decanted, and the bound-to-free ratio determined as described below in the section on preparation of standard curves. A B/F ratio in excess of 2 at the lower dilutions (1 : 10, 1 : 50), indicated the presence of potentially usable antibody. Antiserum to T4 can be produced and detected in analogous fashion.

2. Antiserum Solution

The antiserum solution employed in our assay was prepared by mixing antiserum to T3 and antiserum to T4 in the same vessel with barbital diluent (0.08 M sodium barbital, 0.1 gm/100 ml bovine serum albumin, pH 8.4). In our system, the anti-T3 antiserum was diluted 1 : 2000 and the anti-T4 antiserum 1 : 200.

3. T3,T4-Free Serum

Serum free of T3 and T4 (T3,T4-free serum) was prepared by incubating 100 ml of normal human serum with 20 gm activated Norit A charcoal (Sigma Chemical, St. Louis, Missouri) for 24 hours at 4°C. The resulting slurry was centrifuged three times at 20,000 g. This procedure removes over 99% of the T3 and T4 from serum, and does not affect total protein concentration, pH, or T4-binding capacity.

4. Nonradioactive Standards of T3 and T4

These were obtained from Sigma Chemical in the free acid form. T3 was dissolved in ethanol : 1.0 N HCL (2 : 1), T4 in 0.13 M NaOH in 70% ethanol solution. The standards were prepared in T3,T4-free serum.

5. ^{125}I-T3 and ^{131}I-T4

The isotopes were obtained from the Abbott Laboratories, North Chicago, Illinois. The isotope mixture used in this assay was prepared by diluting both isotopes in barbital buffer in the same vessel at a concentration of 30 pg ^{125}I-T3 (70–90 μCi/μg) and 50 pg ^{131}I-T4 (30–50 μCi/μg) per 0.1 ml diluent.

Thyroid hormones can be iodinated using chloramine-T (Burger and Ingbar, 1974). Hormone, 1.0 nmole in 0.01 ml methanol, is mixed with Na ^{125}I and titrated to pH 6.2 with 0.05 ml 0.1 M phosphate buffer. Chloramine-T, 4 μg in 10 μl phosphate buffer, is added, and after two minutes, the reaction is stopped by adding 20 μl one-tenth saturated sodium metabisulfite. Disposable 2.5-ml plastic syringes are filled with 1.5 ml Sephadex LH-20 in phosphate buffer. After application of the reaction mixture, the column is washed successively with 1.0 ml phosphate buffer, 4.0 ml water, and 1.2 ml methanol–2 N NH$_3$ (99 : 1). The purified labeled hormone is eluted with 4.0 ml methanol–ammonia, dried under a stream of nitrogen, and further purified by paper chromatography as described above.

6. 8-Anilino-1-Naphthalene Sulfonic Acid (ANS)

To accurately measure serum T3 and T4, it is necessary to prevent binding of the hormones to serum proteins. This was accomplished for both T3 and T4 by using barbital buffer to inhibit binding to thyroxine-binding prealbumin and adding ANS (Eastman Kodak) to block binding to thyroxine-binding globulin (TBG). To control for effects of ANS and/or the barbital buffer on binding, serum samples and standards were diluted identically. A concentration of 175 μg ANS per 0.2 ml was employed in assays in which serum or standards were diluted 1 : 4; 350 μg per 0.2 ml was used for serum samples or standards which were diluted 1 : 2.

B. Assay Procedure

The assay procedure was performed in quadruplicate in 10×75 mm disposable glass tubes by the sequential addition of 0.1 ml of the unknown sample or standard (which has been diluted 1 : 2 or 1 : 4 in barbital diluent), 0.1 ml of the isotope solution, 0.2 ml of the ANS solution, and 0.1 ml of the antibody solution. The assay mixture was agitated in a Vortex mixer and incubated for 90 minutes at 37°C in a gently shaking water bath. After incubation, the samples were allowed to cool for 10 minutes in a 4°C cold room where the separation was carried out by the addition of 1.0 ml of a stock solution of dextran–charcoal. The stock solution was prepared by mixing 5.0 gm activated Norit A charcoal and 0.05 gm dextran 80 (molecular weight 86,000; K and K Labs, Hollywood, California) in 100 ml barbital diluent and constantly stirring with a magnetic stirrer to prevent settling during the procedure. The reaction mixture was agitated in a Vortex mixer, incubated at 4°C for 20 minutes, and centrifuged at 100 g for 15 minutes. The supernatant containing the antibody-bound hormone was decanted off the hard charcoal pellet containing the free hormone. The two fractions were then counted in a two-channel gamma counter (Nuclear Chicago) equipped with a 300-sample automatic changer. It

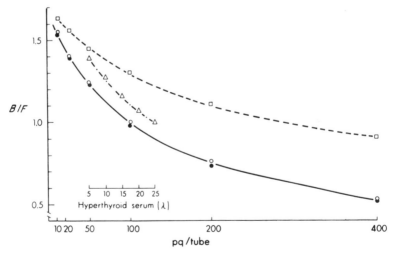

Figure 1.   The T3 standard curve has been prepared by the addition of T3 to barbital diluent (●) and to T3,T4-free serum in the presence of ANS (○) and without ANS (□). Concentrations of 0, 12.5, 25, 50, 100, 200, and 400 pg T3 per tube were prepared, representing T3 concentrations of 0, 50, 100, 200, 400, 800, and 1600 ng T3/100 ml serum. A parallel curve was obtained with dilutions of hyperthyroid serum (△). (Reproduced from Mitsuma *et al.*, 1972a, with the permission of the publishers.)

must be emphasized that the specific dilutions of antibody and re-agents and incubation times described here are clearly a function of the antibody employed and would require some modifications for use with another antibody. Figures 1 and 2 show typical standard curves for T3 and T4 prepared in buffer and also in T3,T4-free serum with and without ANS. The serum standard curves for both T3 and T4 obtained with ANS are almost identical to those obtained with buffer alone. Routinely, a concentration of 175 μg per tube successfully inhibits TBG binding of T3 and T4 in hypothyroid, normal pregnant, and hyperthyroid subjects. The antigen–antibody reaction reaches equilibrium within 60 minutes at 37°C. We chose a 90-minute incubation time, which was found to fall well within the plateau of the equilibrium curve. At 4°C, the dextran–charcoal binding of hormone reached equilibrium within 15 minutes. Twenty minutes was therefore selected for the second incubation.

Neither the anti-T3 nor the anti-T4 antisera used in our assay showed measurable cross-reaction with monoiodotyrosine, diiodotyrosine, or ANS. The anti-T3 antiserum showed less than

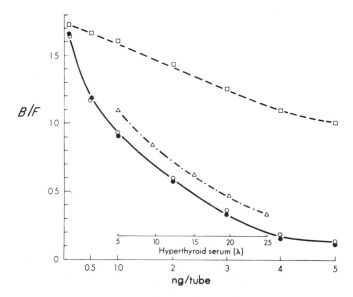

Figure 2. The T4 standard curve has been prepared by the addition of T4 to barbital diluent (●) and to T3,T4-free serum in the presence of ANS (○) and without ANS (□). Concentrations of 0, 0.1, 0.5, 1, 2, 4, and 5 ng T4 per tube were prepared representing concentrations of 0, 0.4, 2, 4, 8, 16, and 20 μg T4/100 ml serum. A parallel curve was obtained with dilutions of hyperthyroid serum (△). (Reproduced from Mitsuma *et al.*, 1972a, with the permission of the publishers.)

1 : 5000 cross-reaction with chromatographically purified T4. In view of the very minor cross-reaction between the anti-T3 antibody and T4, no significant effect on immunoassayable T3 would be anticipated from clinically observed variations in the T4 concentrations of a hypothyroid serum, which initially contained 60 ng/100 ml T3 and less than 0.2 μg/100 ml T4 after adding 0.4, 2,10,20, and 40 μg/100 ml T4 *in vitro*. A similar series of determinations was performed on a T3-free serum sample which was devoid of measurable T4 (i.e., less than 0.2 μg/100 ml of T4) to which 200 ng/100 ml of T3 had been added. In both cases, no change in the measured T3 concentration was observed with additions of T4 (Figure 3). Likewise, the anti-T4 antiserum did not cross-react with T3. Recovery experiments were performed by the addition of known amounts of T3 and T4 to T3 and T4-free serum and normal serum. The mean recovery of T3 in ten separate experiments was 103.8% (Figure 4). Twenty-five similar experiments with T4 demonstrated a recovery of 100.8 ± 1.4%.

Intraassay reproducibility, assessed by measuring the identical sample 33 times was 4.4% for T3 and 4.1% for T4. Interassay variation evaluated by determining 18 paired specimens in two successive assays was 6.8% for T3 and 7.4% for T4.

The T4 values obtained in this assay were compared with determinations on the identical specimens by competitive protein-binding analysis (Boston Medical Labs). In 40 specimens, from 14 hypothyroid patients, 11 hyperthyroid subjects, and 15 normal subjects, the agreement was excellent (coefficient of correlation, 0.98).

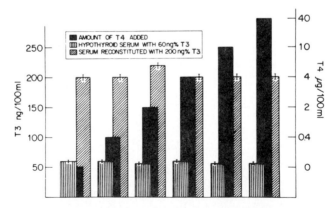

Figure 3.   Effect of added T4 on the measured T3 concentration. Note that additions of T4 throughout the physiologic range do not alter the measured serum T3 in a hypothyroid serum or in a T3-free serum sample to which 200 ng/100 ml T3 had been added (see text).

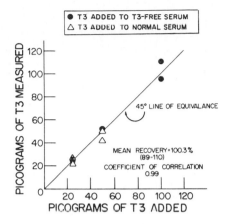

Figure 4. Recovery of T3 added to normal and T3-free serum. T3 measured is plotted on the vertical axis versus T3 added on the horizontal axis. All points hover about the 45° line of equivalence.

The principles involved in the radioimmunoassays of reverse T3 (Chopra, 1974), 3-3′ diiodothyronine (T2) (Wu *et al.*, 1976), monoiodotyrosine (MIT) (Nelson *et al.*, 1977), and tetraiodothyroacetic acid (tetrac) (Burger, 1976) are similar to the T3 and T4 radioimmunoassays and detailed descriptions of the relevant methodologies have been published (Chopra, 1974; Wu *et al.*, 1976; Nelson *et al.*, 1977; Burger, 1977).

IV. COMPARISON OF VARIOUS T3 AND T4 RADIOIMMUNOASSAY TECHNIQUES AND RESULTS

In the past four years, many investigators have developed radioimmunoassays for T3. Each of these laboratories has employed somewhat different methods to solve the technical problems of such assays. In spite of differences in methodology, it is interesting to note that results obtained by the various investigators have, in general, agreed quite well (Table I).

Anti-T3 antibodies have been produced in good titer using a variety of antigen complexes. Brown and co-workers (1970) successfully employed the carbodiimide condensation product of T3 and succinylated poly-L-lysine as immunogen. Carbodiimide condensation of T3 to bovine or human serum albumin has subsequently been used to produce suitable antigens (Mitsuma *et al.*, 1971, 1972a; Doctor *et al.*, 1972; Gharib *et al.*, 1970, 1971; Huefner and Hesch, 1973; Larsen,

Table I Comparison of Various T3 Radioimmunoassays

References	Range of T3 values (ng/100 ml)[a]			Antigen employed for raising T3 antibody	Blocker	Method of separation (second step)
	Hypothyroid	Normal	Hyperthyroid			
Alexander and Jennings (1974)	24 ± 22	96 ± 26	263 ± 58	—	None: used Sephadex G-25 columns	—
Beckers et al. (1973a, 1974)	—	141 ± 0.04 (SEM)	726 ± 72.4 (SEM)	Thyroglobulin	ANS	Second antibody
Brown et al. (1970); Williams et al. (1972)	—	87.5–176 (range)	—	T3–poly-L-lysine	—	Methyl cellulose charcoal
Burger et al. (1972, 1975)	—	153 ± 58 (SD)	—	Hemocyanin	ANS	QAE Sephadex columns
Chopra et al. (1971, 1972)	40.1 ± 7.6 (SEM)	112.8 ± 3.3 (SEM)	490.7 ± 42.3 (SEM)	Thyroglobulin	T4 (250 ng per tube)	Second antibody (goat anti-rabbit γ-globulin)
Docter et al. (1972)	—	140 ± 22 (SD)	294–700 (range)	T3–bovine serum albumin complex	Sodium salicylate	Second antibody
Gharib et al. (1970, 1971)	103 ± 43 (SD)	218 ± 55 (SD)	760 ± 289 (SD)	T3–bovine or human serum albumin complex	Merthiolate(?)	Second antibody (goat anti-rabbit γ-globulin)

Huefner and Hesch (1973)	25–80 (range)	90–150 (range)	300–3000 (range)	T3–bovine serum albumin complex	Sodium salicylate	Dextran-coated charcoal
Larsen (1972)	39 ± 21 (SD)	110 ± 25 (SD)	546 ± 44.2 (SD)	T3–bovine serum albumin complex	Sodium salicylate	Dextran-coated charcoal
Lieblich and Utiger (1972)	99 ± 24 (SD)	145 ± 25 (SD)	429 ± 14.6 (SD)	T3–bovine serum albumin complex	Dilantin	Second antibody (goat anti-rabbit γ-globulin)
Mitsuma et al. (1971, 1972a,b)	67 ± 2.2 (SEM) 52–78 (range)	134 ± 6.2 (SEM) 96–170 (range)	486 ± 77 (SEM) 320–1200 (range)	T3–bovine serum albumin complex	ANS	Dextran-coated charcoal
Nejad et al. (1972)	20–50 (range) 44 (mean)	140 ± 40 (SD)	300–1000 (range) 560 (mean)	T3–bovine fibrinogen complex	Dilantin	Dextran-coated charcoal
Sterling and Milch (1974)	47 ± 39	189 ± 30	838 ± 398	T3–bovine serum albumin complex	Heating (60°C)	Polyethylene glycol
Surks et al. (1972)	44 ± 26 (SD)	146 ± 24 (SD)	665 ± 289 (SD)	T3–bovine serum albumin complex	None: extraction by Sephadex column chromatography employed	Dextran-coated charcoal

[a] T3 values have been expressed as either the mean ± standard error of the mean (SEM), mean ± standard deviation (SD), and/or the range of observed concentrations.

1972; Lieblich and Utiger, 1972). Reichlin's group has reported on the use of a T3–fibrinogen complex (Nejad *et al.*, 1972), and two other laboratories have employed thyroglobulin to produce anti-T3 antibody (Beckers *et al.*, 1973a; Chopra *et al.*, 1971). Burger *et al.* (1975) coupled T3 to hemocyanin by diazotized benzidine and used it to produce anti-T3 antibody.

The problem of plasma-binding protein interference with the T3 assay has also been solved in several different ways. Most of the presently reported techniques for measuring T3 in unextracted serum employ a chemical blocking agent or blocker to prevent T3 binding to TBG. Both Chopra (Chopra *et al.*, 1972) and Beckers (Beckers *et al.*, 1973a, 1974) utilized ANS. Although we initially employed tetrachlorothyronine for this purpose (Mitsuma *et al.*, 1971), difficulty in obtaining this compound in pure form led us to use ANS instead. Lieblich and Utiger (1972) as well as Reichlin's group (Nejad *et al.*, 1972) have used Dilantin as blocker. Merthiolate (Gharib *et al.*, 1970, 1971), sodium salicylate (Docter *et al.*, 1972), and thyroxine (Chopra *et al.*, 1971, 1972) have also been employed by others. Sterling and Milch (1974) used 60°C incubation temperature to inactivate the thyroxine-binding globulin. They also noted that the antigen–antibody reaction is greatly accelerated at 60°C. An alternate approach to the problem of plasma protein interference has been developed by Surks *et al.* (1972) and Alexander and Jennings (1974). In their method, T3 is initially separated from plasma proteins by a preliminary extraction on Sephadex G25 and then assayed. Patel and Burger (1973) and Werner *et al.* (1974) used ethanol extraction of serum to denature the thyroxine-binding globulins prior to assay.

Separation of bound and free hormone after incubation with anti-T3 antibody has been accomplished either with second antibody (Docter *et al.*, 1972; Gharib *et al.*, 1971; Lieblich and Utiger, 1972; Beckers *et al.*, 1973a; Chopra *et al.*, 1971, 1972), dextran-coated charcoal (Mitsuma *et al.*, 1972a, 1971; Larsen, 1971; Surks *et al.*, 1972; Nejad *et al.*, 1972), methyl cellulose charcoal (Williams *et al.*, 1972), polyethylene glycol (Werner *et al.*, 1974; Desbuquois and Aurbach, 1971; Sekadde *et al.*, 1973; Sterling and Milch, 1974), dextran-coated charcoal with bovine serum albumin (Kirkegaard *et al.*, 1974), QAE Sephadex A25 columns (Burger *et al.*, 1975), or a resin. One additional methodological difference between the various T3 radioimmunoassays is the vehicle used for preparation of standard curve. Both we and Larsen (1972) have noted that T3-free serum displaces labeled T3 from anti-T3 antibody. To eliminate this artifact, we have employed T3,T4-free serum as the vehicle in which the standard curve is constructed. Larsen has utilized a similar technique. Chopra *et al.* (1971, 1972) have constructed their standard curve with serum from hypothyroid sheep, while Lieblich and Utiger (1972) have used 4% human serum albumin.

Despite these rather considerable differences in methods of assay, there appears to be general agreement that the normal T3 concentration is approximately 100–160 ng per 100 ml. The relatively small variations noted between various investigators may be simply methodological. Alternatively, they could represent true differences in thyroid hormone levels depending on demographic characteristics in the populations studied. Similarly, results of T3 levels in untreated hyperthyroid patients have ranged from 300 to 3000 ng per 100 ml, mean values from different groups varying from 430 to 760 ng per 100 ml. Larsen (1972), Chopra *et al.* (1972), Surks and co-workers (1972), and our group have obtained mean T3 levels ranging from 30 to 67 ng per 100 ml in hypothyroid patients. Lieblich and Utiger (1972) and Gharib *et al.* (1970, 1971) have observed higher mean levels, 99 and 103 ng per 100 ml, respectively. It is of interest that values obtained utilizing preliminary extraction procedures instead of a blocker are in good agreement with those obtained in unextracted serum.

Several radioimmunoassays for T4 have been developed. Chopra (1972) has described a method for measuring T4 in unextracted serum which employs anti-T4 antibody produced by immunizing rabbits with human thyroglobulin–T4 complex, ANS as a blocker, and second antibody to separate bound from free T4. Values obtained generally agree with results by competitive protein-binding methods. However, in sera from some hyperthyroid patients and from several euthyroid subjects given TSH, thyroxine levels by radioimmunoassay were higher than those by competitive protein-binding methods. Beckers *et al.* (1973b) also observed similar discrepancies between serum T4 values by radioimmunoassay and competitive protein-binding analysis in hyperthyroid patients. In his studies, mean T4 levels in hyperthyroid patients were 50% higher than with competitive protein-binding assays. But, T4 levels by radioimmunoassay in euthyroid patients, pregnant women, and hypothyroid individuals were compatible with T4 levels by competitive protein-binding techniques. Ratcliffe *et al.* (1974) also compared T4 levels using both techniques. They found that T4 levels by radioimmunoassay were slightly higher in hyperthyroid patients but generally correlated well with those obtained by CPB. Thus, they failed to confirm the large differences in T4 levels estimated by radioimmunoassay and competitive protein-binding analysis reported by Chopra (1972) and Beckers *et al.* (1973b). Variations of this magnitude between the two techniques have also not been observed in our combined T3–T4 radioimmunoassay (Mitsuma *et al.*, 1972a) and in the T4 radioimmunoassay of Larsen *et al.* (1973). The reasons for these possible discrepancies (Chopra, 1972) have not been completely clarified and may be related to the presence of T4 covalently linked to serum proteins. As in the T3 assay, several chemical blockers of TBG binding, such as salicylate (Larsen *et al.*, 1973), ANS (Chopra, 1972), and heating (Dunn and Foster, 1973), are used for radioimmunoassay of serum T4.

Recently, a radioimmunoassay for 3,3′,5′-triiodothyronine [reverse T3 (rT3)] in human serum has been developed by Chopra (1974) and Meinhold *et al.* (1975) that requires prior extraction with ethanol. Nicod *et al.* (1976) have developed a radioimmunoassay for rT3 in unextracted human serum using ANS as a blocker. The principle and method of assay of rT3 is very similar to T3 radioimmunoassay. Chopra immunized animals with rT3 conjugated to human serum albumin (HSA). In this procedure, 9 mg of rT3 (Werner-Lamber Research Institute) in 2.0 ml of N,N-dimethylformamide and 0.1 ml of $0.4\,M$ NaOH was incubated with 1.0 ng ^{125}I-rT3 (400–500 mCi/mg) (Abbott) to monitor the degree of conjugation (mean 37%), 25 mg HSA in 12.5 ml $0.01\,M$ phosphate, $0.14\,M$ NaCl, pH 7.5, and 20 mg 1-cyclohexyl-3 (2-morpholinoethyl) carbodiimide metho-p-toluene sulfonate (Aldrich Chemical, Milwaukee, Wisconsin) for 18 hours in the dark at 20°C. The dialyzed conjugate was emulsified in complete Freund's adjuvant for immunization. Both Chopra (1974) and Meinhold *et al.* (1975) used second antibody to separate bound and free ^{125}I-rT3, whereas Nicod *et al.* (1976) used small QAE Sephadex A-25 columns to separate bound from free ^{125}I-rT3. In Chopra's technique, 0.5-ml serum samples were extracted with 1.0 ml 95% ethanol. The 1000 g supernatant [and in standard tubes, an identical volume of 95% ethanol–water (2 : 1)] was added directly to the assay incubation tube. Mean serum rT3 levels in normal subjects were 405 pg/ml (Chopra, 1974), 182 ± 118 pg/ml (Meinhold *et al.*, 1975), and 450 ± 200 pg/ml (Nicod *et al.*, 1976).

For radioimmunoassay of T2, Wu *et al.* (1976) conjugated T2 (River Research, Toledo, Ohio) to HSA as described above. Three-milliliter serum samples were extracted with 6.0 ml ethanol. After centrifugation at 1000 g for 30 minutes, the supernatants were mixed with 14 ml water, lyophilized, reconstituted in 1.4 ml $0.075\,M$ barbital buffer, pH 8.6, containing 1% normal rabbit serum, and centrifuged at 1000 g for 30 minutes. Aliquots (0.5 ml) of supernatant, representing 0.83 ml of serum, were used directly in the assay. ^{125}I-T2 (300–400 mCi/mg) was obtained from Abbott Laboratories. The separation of bound from free labeled ligand was accomplished using double antibody precipitation. Normal levels of T2 averaged 7.6 ± 2.4 ng per 100 ml ($n = 44$); levels in hyperthyroid patients and newborns were significantly elevated, 20.2 ± 7.5 and 16.4 ± 3.8 ng/100 ml, respectively.

V. PHYSIOLOGICAL CONSIDERATIONS

The radioimmunoassay for T4 is more rapid and sensitive than competitive protein-binding assays, but provides essentially similar information. Since prior methods for T3 were inadequate, the advent of simple and accurate radioimmunoassay methods for quantitating scrum T3 levels has permitted more precise delineation of the important role of T3 in thyroid hormone physiology. In conventional hyperthyroidism, regardless of cause (i.e., whether the thyrotoxicity results from toxic diffuse goiter, toxic nodular goiter, or autonomously functioning adenoma), T3 levels are invariably elevated. In a series of 64 patients with the usual forms of thyrotoxicosis, we found that T3 varied from 232 to 1700 ng per 100 ml, with a mean of 495 ng per 100 ml. This contrasts with the findings in normal and hypothyroid subjects. Eighty-two normal subjects had T3 concentrations ranging from 96 to 172 ng per 100 ml with a mean of 138 ng per 100 ml (Mitsuma et al., 1971). Forty-five patients with primary hypothyroidism had a mean serum T3 level of 62 ± 9 ng per 100 ml, and four patients with hypothyroidism secondary to pituitary disease had a mean serum T3 level of 57 ng per 100 ml. In general, patients with hypothyroidism had T3 levels which were approximately one-half those found in normals. Similar results have been noted by others, although some workers have found some overlap between normal and hypothyroid patients (see Table I). The T3 levels may be depressed in many euthyroid subjects, e.g., those with chronic illnesses (Bermudez et al., 1975; Carter et al., 1974), hepatic cirrhosis (Chopra, 1976; Nomura et al., 1975), complete fasting (Portnay et al., 1974; Vagenakis et al., 1975), after operations (Burr et al., 1975), protein–calorie malnutrition (Chopra and Smith, 1975), diabetic coma (Naeije et al., 1976), anorexia nervosa (Miyai et al., 1975), dexamethasone treatment (Chopra et al., 1975a) and in the elderly (Rubenstein et al., 1973; Burger et al., 1975; Snyder and Utiger, 1972; Brunelle and Bohuon, 1972). Because of all these decrements in serum T3 levels in nonthyroidal disorders, T3 is of limited value in evaluating patients with hypothyroidism.

Since the development of radioimmunoassays for 3,3'5'-triiodothyronine (rT3) (Chopra, 1974), these variations in thyroid hormone levels in nonthyroidal disorders and T4 metabolism are better understood. T4 undergoes a number of transformations in addition to the one which produces T3. One well-documented alternate pathway involves deamination of the side chain to give rise to tetraiodothyroacetic acid (tetrac). Recent studies have confirmed that tetrac is indeed a normal product of thyroxine metabolism in man (Braverman et al., 1970). Burger (1977) noted reduced serum tetrac levels in acute illness and fasting in man. Pharmacologic blockade of T3 production with propylthiouracil increased tetrac levels. Moreover, tetrac was unmeasurable in T3-substituted hypothyroid subjects (Burger, 1977). Considerable attention has also been focused upon alternative monodeiodination pathways in which a single iodine is lost from the inner carboxyl ring instead of the phenolic ring to give rise to 3,3′,5′-triiodothyronine (rT3). Reverse T3 is a noncalorigenic and biologically inactive congener of T3 (Vagenakis et al., 1975). Peripheral conversion of T4 accounts for the large bulk of rT3 production with thyroidal secretion constituting only 2.5% of its production (Wenzel and Meinhold, 1975; Chopra 1976). Recent studies indicate that serum rT3 is increased in several conditions, e.g., starvation (Vagenakis et al., 1975), hepatic cirrhosis, chronic renal failure, acute febrile illness, protein–calorie malnutrition (Chopra et al., 1975b), after dexamethasone treatment (Chopra et al., 1975a; Burr et al., 1976; Duick et al., 1974), after surgical operations (Burr et al., 1975) and in amniotic fluid (Chopra and Crandall, 1975). The reciprocal changes in serum T3 and rT3 levels during caloric deprivation revert to normal with refeeding (Vagenakis et al., 1975). In addition, Spaulding et al. (1976) found decreased serum T3 levels during caloric restriction on the basis of a decrease in carbohydrate intake, but observed no change inserum T3 and rT3 concentrations when caloric restriction was coupled with a high-carbohydrate diet. These findings may suggest a possible role of carbohydrates in T3 production in man. It should be emphasized that despite the considerable physiologic importance of these findings, rT3 measurements in serum are not needed for clinical management.

Since first calling attention to the syndrome of T3 toxicosis, i.e., thyrotoxicosis caused by excessive secretion of T3 rather than T4 (Hollander, 1968), we have identified 40 additional patients over the course of three years (Hollander et al., 1972a). Similar patients have been described by others (Larsen, 1971; Sterling et al., 1970; Wahner and Gorman, 1971; Sakurada et al., 1969; Bellabarba, 1972). Twenty-nine of our patients appeared to have Graves' disease, eight, autonomous adenoma, and three, toxic multinodular goiter. These patients all had normal total and free T4 concentrations, normal thyroid-binding proteins, and a normal or elevated thyroidal uptake of radioiodine that could not be suppressed with exogenous thyroid hormone. All had elevated total T3 levels, ranging from 228 to 2000 ng per 100 ml, and high free T3 levels as well. The clinical picture and the response to therapy in patients with T3 toxicosis were indistinguishable from those with conventional thyrotoxicosis. More recently, we have seen this syndrome develop in children (Mitsuma *et al.*, 1972b). Moreover, we have noted several patients with a past history of conventional thyrotoxicosis who, after a euthyroid interval varying from several months to 30 years, developed a clinical recurrence of the thyrotoxic state with normal T4 but elevated T3 levels (Shenkman *et al.*, 1972b). It would appear, therefore, that some patients with recurrent hyperthyroidism may present as T3 toxicosis.

Also of interest is the observation that hyperthyroid patients may pass through a stage of T3 toxicosis before developing the usual form of thyrotoxicosis (Hollander *et al.*, 1971). Over the past years, we have had the opportunity to observe ten hyperthyroid patients during the early phase of their disease. Although all had a clearly elevated serum T3 level, they were followed without therapy because their symptoms were relatively mild. After one to ten months, four of these patients developed more overt thyrotoxicosis with classic physical and laboratory findings consistent with conventional toxic diffuse goiter including a high serum T4 level. In these four instances, high circulating T3 levels were an early premonitory finding in toxic diffuse goiter. The other six patients remained symptomatic but failed to manifest an increased T4 over 12–18 months.

As would be anticipated, the elevated T3 levels in subjects with conventional hyperthyroidism fell to normal with the induction of the euthyroid state by surgery, radioiodine, or antithyroid drugs (Mitsuma *et al.*, 1971). However, we have observed several patients with conventional hyperthyroidism who, early in the course of antithyroid drug therapy, remained clinically toxic despite a fall in their T4 levels to normal (Hollander *et al.*, 1972b). Interestingly, in these patients, T3 levels had not yet fallen to normal, and probably accounted for the toxic state. Similar observations have been made by Bellabarba (1972). Sterling *et al.* (1970) and Bellabarba *et al.* (1972) have observed the maintenance of normal clinical states in patients who have normal or elevated T3 but low serum T4 concentration after ^{131}I therapy for thyrotoxicosis. More recently, Marsden and McKerron (1973) have critically examined the diagnostic value of T3 in hyperthyroidism and have confirmed our findings. We think T3 estimation in serum is the best single thyroid function test in hyperthyroidism.

After the intramuscular administration of bovine thyrotropin, serum T3 levels rise earlier and relatively higher than serum T4. Likewise, intravenous administration of thyrotropin-releasing hormone, by causing a rise of endogenous TSH, results in a more striking elevation of serum T3 than T4 levels (Hollander *et al.*, 1972c; Shenkman *et al.*, 1972a). This latter observation may permit simultaneous assessment of pituitary and thyroid status.

VI. SCREENING FOR CONGENITAL HYPOTHYROIDISM

Congenital hypothyroidism is the most frequent known endocrine or metabolic cause of mental deficiency in the newborn. Its incidence in most series has varied from 1 in 3000 to 1 in 10,000. The most commonly cited figure is the order of 1 in 5000 to 1 in 7000.

Prevention of mental deficiency due to congenital hypothyroidism requires early detection and treatment of hypothyroidism before the age of three months (Klein *et al.*, 1972; Raiti and Newns, 1971). Unfortunately, prompt clinical diagnosis of congenital hypothyroidism is often difficult (Klein *et al.*, 1974, 1975). The recent development of more sensitive and specific measures of thyroid hormones and TSH by filter paper methods (Larsen *et al.*, 1976; Larsen and Broskin, 1975; Dussault *et al.*, 1973, 1975, 1976b; Grajwar *et al.*, 1976) has prompted a number of workers to undertake large-scale screening of infants to detect congenital hypothyroidism at birth. Published compilations of screening programs of this sort have emanated from Quebec (Dussault *et al.*, 1975, 1976a,b), Pittsburgh (Klein *et al.*, 1976), and Toronto (Walfish, 1976). The observations suggest that 10–15% of cases would be missed if screening is conducted with TSH alone (Dussault *et al.*, 1976a). For this reason, screening for congenital hypothyroidism using the filter paper T4 method, with filter paper TSH testing of suspicious samples, is advised (Fisher *et al.*, 1976) in order to minimize the number of cases missed.

Some workers have also suggested the use of rT3 measurement as a screening test for congenital hypothyroidism, although further studies are needed to properly assess its usefulness in this regard. One potential application for the rT3 assay would be for the antepartum diagnosis of congenital hypothyroidism in mothers at increased risk of bearing hypothyroid infants, i.e., pregnant women on high doses of antithyroid drugs, those who have inadvertently received therapeutic doses of radioiodine, or who have previously given birth to a cretin.

VII. SUMMARY AND CONCLUSIONS

Despite the small size of the thyroid hormones, several radioimmunoassays have been developed for measuring these compounds in serum. Because these hormones are tightly bound to serum proteins, the various methods have either employed a preliminary extraction procedure or, more commonly, a chemical substance, such as ANS, Dilantin, salicylate, or Merthiolate, to interfere with this binding. Separation of the bound and free hormone has been achieved either by use of a second antibody, dextran-coated charcoal, methyl cellulose, charcoal, or polyethylene glycol. In this chapter, a rapid simultaneous radioimmunoassay for T3 and T4 has been described and compared with other available radioimmunoassays. The development of the T3 radioimmunoassay has permitted delineation of a number of clinical situations wherein T3 has a major role, the most dramatic being T3 toxicosis. Moreover, the advent of a T3 radioimmunoassay affords, for the first time, a simple, reproducible, and accurate assay suitable for routine clinical use. Although reliable methods for assaying T4 have been available for some time, the radioimmunoassay for T4 could supplant competitive-binding analysis by virtue of its greater simplicity and sensitivity in the lower range.

More recently, radioimmunoassays have been developed for reverse T3, a noncalorigenic congener of T3, tetrac, T2, and monoiodotyrosine. Physiologic studies with these assays have led to better understanding of T4 metabolism. However, their potential role in clinical medicine remains to be clarified.

REFERENCES

Alexander, N. M., and Jennings, J. F. (1974). Radioimmunoassay of serum triiodothyronine reusable sephadex column. *Clin. Chem.* **20**, 1353–1361.

Beckers, C., Cornette, C., and Thalasso, M. (1973a). Serum triiodothyronine. Importance of its determination in thyroid disorders and in the study of hypothalamuspituitary interplay. *Proc. Eur. Thyroid Assoc., 1973.* Abstract No. 12.

Beckers, C., Cornette, C., and Thalasso, M. (1973b). Evaluation of serum thyroxine by radioimmunoassay. *J. Nucl. Med.* **14**, 317–320.

Beckers, C., Cornette, C., and Thalasso, M. (1974). Serum L-Triiodothyronine radioimmunoassay measurements in normal subjects and in thyroid patients. *Int. J. Nucl. Med. Biol.* **1**, 121–129.

Bellabarba, D. (1972). Further observations on T3 thyrotoxicosis. *Clin. Res.* **20**, 421.

Bellabarba, D., Bernard, B., and Langlois, M. (1972). Serum pattern of thyroxine (T4), a triiodothyronine (T3) and thyroid stimulating hormone (TSH) after treatment of thyrotoxicosis. *Clin. Res.* **20**, 421.

Bermudez, F., Surks, M. I., and Oppenheimer, J. H. (1975). High incidence of decreased serum triiodothyronine concentration in patients with non-thyroidal disease. *J. Clin. Endocrinol. Metab.* **41**, 27–40.

Braverman, L. E., Ingbar, S. H., and Sterling, K. (1970). Conversion of thyroxine (T4) to triiodothyronine (T3). *J. Clin. Invest.* **49**, 855–864.

Brown, B. L., Ekins, R. P., Ellis, S. M., and Reith, W. S. (1970). Specific antibodies to triiodothyronine. *Nature (London)* **226**, 359.

Brunelle, P., and Bohuon, C. (1972). Decrease of triiodothyronine in serum of senescent persons. *Clin. Chim. Acta* **42**, 201–203.

Burger, A. (1977). The pathophysiological significance of tetraiodothyroacetic acid (Tetrac). *Endocrinol., Proc. Int. Cong. Endocrinol., 5th, 1976* Excerpta Med. Found., Int. Congr. Ser. No. 400, Abstract No. 129.

Burger, A., and Ingbar, S. H. (1974). Labeling of thyroid hormones and their derivatives. *Endocrinology* **94**, 1189–1192.

Burger, A., Miller, B., Sakoloff, C., and Vallotton, M. B. (1972). Thyroxine et triiodothyronine seriques. *Schweiz. Med. Wochenschr.* **102**, 1280–1281.

Burger, A., Sakoloff, C., Staeheli, V., Vallotton, M. B., and Ingbar, S. H. (1975). RIA of 3-5-3′ triiodo-L-thyronine with and without prior extraction step. *Acta Endocrinol. (Copenhagen)* **80**, 58–69.

Burr, W. A., Griffith, R. S., Black, E. G., Hoffenberg, R., Meinhold, H., and Wenzel, K. W. (1975). Serum triiodothyronine and reverse triiodothyronine concentration after surgical operation. *Lancet* **2**, 1277–1279.

Burr, W. A., Ramsden, D. B., Griffiths, R. S., Black, E. G., Hoffenberg, R., Meinhold, H., and Wenzel, K. W. (1976). Effect of single dose of dexamethasone on serum concentration of thyroid hormones. *Lancet* **2**, 58–61.

Carter, J. N., Eastman, G. J., Corcoran, J. M., and Lazarus, L. (1974). Effect of severe chronic illness on thyroid function. *Lancet* **2**, 971–974.

Chopra, I. J. (1972). A radioimmunoassay for measurement of thyroxine in unextracted serum. *J. Clin. Endocrinol. Metab.* **35**, 938–947.

Chopra, I. J. (1974). A radioimmunoassay for measurement of 3,3′5′-triiodothyronine (reverse T3). *J. Clin. Invest.* **54**, 583–592.

Chopra, I. J. (1976). An assessment of daily production and significance of 3,3′,5′-triiodothyronine (reverse T3) in man. *J. Clin. Invest.* **58**, 32–40.

Chopra, I. J., and Crandall, B. F. (1975). Thyroid hormones and thyrotropin in amniotic fluid. *N. Engl. J. Med.* **293**, 740–743.

Chopra, I. J., and Smith, S. R. (1975). Circulating thyroid hormones and thyrotropin in adult patients with protein–calorie malnutrition. *J. Clin. Endocrinol. Metab.* **40**, 221–227.

Chopra, I. J., Solomon, D. H., and Beall, A. N. (1971). Radioimmunoassay for measurement of triiodothyronine in human serum. *J. Clin. Invest.* **50**, 2033–2041.

Chopra, I. J., Ho, R. S., and Lam, R. (1972). An improved radioimmunoassay of triiodothyronine in serum: Its application to clinical and physiological studies. *J. Lab. Clin. Med.* **80**, 729–739.

Chopra, I. J., Williams, D. E., and Orgiazzi, J. (1975a). Opposite effects of dexamethasone on serum concentrations of 3,3'5'-triiodothyronine (reverse T3) and 3,3'5-triiodothyronine (T3). *J. Clin. Endocrinol. Metab.* **41**, 911–920.

Chopra, I. J., Chopra, U., Smith, S. R., Reza, M., and Solomon, D. H. (1975b). Reciprocal changes in serum concentration of 3,3',5'-triiodothyronine (reverse T3) and 3,3'5 triiodothyronine (T3) in systemic illnesses. *J. Clin. Endocrinol. Metab.* **41**, 1043–1049.

Desbuquois, B., and Aurbach, G. D. (1971). Use of polyethylene glycol to separate free and antibody bound peptide hormones in radioimmunoassays. *J. Clin. Endocrinol. Metab.* **33**, 732–738.

Docter, R., Hennemann, A., and Bernard, H. (1972). A radioimmunoassay for measurements of triiodothyronine (T3) in serum. *Isr. J. Med. Sci.* **8**, 1870.

Duick, D. S., Warren, D. W., Nicoloff, J. T., Otis, C. L., and Croxsan, M. S. (1974). Effect of single dose dexamethasone on the concentration of serum triiodothyronine in man. *J. Clin. Endocrinol. Metab.* **39**, 1151–1154.

Dunn, R. T., and Foster, L. B. (1973). Radioimmunoassay of thyroxine in unextracted serum by a single antibody technique. *Clin. Chem.* **19**, 1063–1066.

Dussault, J. H., and Laberge, C. (1973). Thyroxine (T4) determination in dried blood by radioimmunoassay: Screening method for neonatal hypothyroidism. *Union Med. Can.* **102**, 2062–2064.

Dussault, J. H., Coulombe, P., Laberge, C., Letarte, J., Guyda, H., and Khoury, K. (1975). Preliminary report on a mass screening program for neonatal hypothyroidism. *J. Pediatr.* **86**, 670–674.

Dussault, J. H., Letarte, J., Guyda, H., and Laberge, C. (1976a). Thyroid function in neonatal hypothyroidism. *J. Pediatr.* **89**, 541–545.

Dussault, J. H., Parlow, A., and Laberge, C. (1976b). TSH measurements on blood spots on filter paper: A confirmatory screening test for neonatal hypothyroidism. *J. Pediatr.* **89**, 550–552.

Fisher, D. A., Burrow, G. N., Dussault, J. H., Hollingsworth, D. R., Larsen, P. R., Man, E. B., and Walfish, P. G. (1976). Recommendations for screening programs for congenital hypothyroidism. *J. Pediatr.* **89**, 692–694.

Gharib, H., Mayberry, W. E., and Ryan, R. J. (1970). Radioimmunoassay for triiodothyronine: A preliminary report. *J. Clin. Endocrinol. Metab.* **31**, 709–712.

Gharib, H., Ryan, R. J., Mayberry, W. E., and Hockert, T. (1971). Radioimmunoassay for triiodothyronine (T3). I. Affinity and specificity of the antibody for T3. *J. Clin. Endocrinol. Metab.* **33**, 509–516.

Grajwar, L. A., Lam, R. W., Bruce, V. A., Parlow, A. F., and Fisher, D. A. (1976). A sensitive TSH radioimmunoassay for new born thyroid screening. *Clin. Res.* **24**, 192A.

Herbert, V., Lau, K. S., Gottlieb, C. W., and Bleicher, S. J. (1965). Coated charcoal immunoassay of insulin. *J. Clin. Endocrinol. Metab.* **25**, 1375–1384.

Hollander, C. S. (1968). On the nature of circulating thyroid hormone: Clinical studies of triiodothyronine and thyroxine in serum using gas chromatographic methods. *Trans. Assoc. Am. Physicians* **81**, 76–91.

Hollander, C. S., Mitsuma, T., Shenkman, L., Blum, M., Kastin, A. J., and Anderson, D. G. (1971). Hypertriiodothyroninaemia as a premonitory manifestation of thyrotoxicosis. *Lancet* **2**, 731–733.

Hollander, C. S., Mitsuma, T., Nihei, N., Shenkman, L., Burday, S. Z., and Blum, M. (1972a). Clinical and laboratory observations in forty cases of triiodothyronine toxicosis confirmed by radioimmunoassay. *Lancet* **1**, 609–611.

Hollander, C. S., Shenkman, L., Mitsuma, T., and Asper, S. P. (1972b). Triiodothyronine toxicosis developing during anti-thyroid drug therapy for hyperthyroidism. *Johns Hopkins Med. J.* **131**, 184–188.

Hollander, C. S., Mitsuma, T., Shenkman, L., Woolf, P., and Gershengorn, M. C. (1972c). Thyrotropin releasing hormone: Evidence for thyroid response to intravenous injection in man. *Science* **175**, 209–210.

Huefner, M., and Hesch, R. D. (1973). Radioimmunoassay for triiodothyronine in human serum. *Acta Endocrinol. (Copenhagen)* **72**, 464–474.

Kirkegaard, C., Friis, T., and Siersbock-Nielsen, K. (1974). Measurements of serum triiodothyronine by radioimmunoassay. *Acta Endocrinol. (Copenhagen)* **77**, 71–81.

Klein, A. H., Meltzer, S., and Kenny, F. M. (1972). Improved prognosis in congenital hypothyroidism treated before the age of three months. *J. Pediatr.* **81**, 912–915.

Klein, A. H., Augustin, A. V., and Foley, T. P. (1974). Successful laboratory screening for congenital hypothyroidism. *Lancet* **2**, 77–79.

Klein, A. H., Augustin, A. V., Hopwood, N. J., Pericelli, A., Johnson, L., and Foley, T. P., Jr. (1975). Thyrotropin screening for congenital hypothyroidism. *Pediatr. Res.* **9**, 291.

Klein, A. H., Foley, T. P., Larsen, P. R., Augustin, A. V., and Hopwood, N. J. (1976). Neonatal thyroid function in congenital hypothyroidism. *J. Pediatr.* **89**, 545–549.

Larsen, P. R. (1971). Technical aspects of the estimation of triiodothyronine in human serum: Evidence of conversion of thyroxine to triiodothyronine during assay. *Metab., Clin. Exp.* **20**, 609–624.

Larsen, P. R. (1972). Direct immunoassay of triiodothyronine in human serum. *J. Clin. Invest.* **51**, 1939–1949.

Larsen, P. R., and Broskin, K. (1975). Thyroxine (T4) immunoassay using filter paper blood samples for screening of neonates for hypothyroidism. *Pediatr. Res.* **9**, 604–609.

Larsen, P. R., Dockalova, J., Sipula, D., and Wu, F. M. (1973). Immunoassay of thyroxine in unextracted human serum. *J. Clin. Endocrinol. Metab.* **37**, 177–182.

Larsen, P. R., Merker, A., and Parlow, A. F. (1976). Immunoassay of human TSH using dried blood samples. *J. Clin. Endocrinol. Metab.* **42**, 987–990.

Lieblich, J., and Utiger, R. D. (1972). Triiodothyronine radioimmunoassay. *J. Clin. Invest.* **51**, 157–166.

Man, E. B., Kydd, D. M., and Peters, J. P. (1951). Butanol-extractable iodine of serum. *J. Clin. Invest.* **30**, 531–538.

Marsden, P., and McKerron, C. G. (1973). Serum T3 concentration in the diagnosis of hyperthyroidism. *Clin. Endocrinol.* **4**, 183–189.

Meinhold, H., Wenzel, K. W., and Schürnbrand, P. (1975). Radioimmunoassay of 3,3′,5′-triiodothyronine (reverse T3) in human serum and its application in different thyroid states. *Z. Klin. Chem. Klin. Biochem.* **13**, 571–574.

Mitsuma, T., Nihei, N., Gershengorn, M. C., and Hollander, C. S. (1971). Serum triiodothyronine: Measurements in human serum by radioimmunoassay with collaboration by gas liquid chromatography. *J. Clin. Invest.* **50**, 2679–2688.

Mitsuma, T., Colucci, J., Shenkman, L., and Hollander, C. S. (1972a). Rapid simultaneous radioimmunoassay for triiodothyronine and thyroxine in unextracted serum. *Biochem. Biophys. Res. Commun.* **46**, 2107–2113.

Mitsuma, T., Owens, R., Shenkman, L., and Hollander, C. S. (1972b). T3 toxicosis in childhood: Hyperthyroidism due to isolated hypersecretion of triiodothyronine. *J. Pediatr.* **81**, 982–984.

Miyai, K., Yamamoto, T., Azaikizawa, M., Kaichiro, I., and Kumahara, Y. (1975). Serum thyroid hormones and thyrotropin in anorexia nervosa. *J. Clin. Endocrinol. Metab.* **40**, 334–338.

Murphy, B. E. P., and Pattee, C. J. (1964). Determination of thyroxine utilizing the property of protein binding. *J. Clin. Endocrinol. Metab.* **24**, 187–196.

Naeije, R., Clumeck, N., Somers, G., Vanhaelst, L., and Golstein, J. (1976). Letters to the Editor. *Lancet* **1**, 1070–1071.

Nauman, J. A., Nauman, A., and Werner, S. C. (1967). Total and free triiodothyronine in human serum. *J. Clin. Invest.* **46**, 1346–1355.

Nejad, I. F., Bollinger, V. A., Mitnick, M. A., and Reichlin, S. (1972). Importance of T3 (triiodothyronine) secretion in altered states of thyroid function in the rat: Cold exposure subtotal thyroidectomy and hypophysectomy. *Trans. Assoc. Am. Physicians* **85**, 295.

Nelson, J. C., Palmer, F. J., and Lewis, J. E. (1977). Radioimmunoassay of serum monoiodotyrosine (MIT). *Endocrinol., Proc. Int. Congr. Endocrinol., 5th, 1976,* Excerpta Med. Found., Int. Congr. Ser. No. 40, Abstract No. 128.

Nicod, P., Burger, A., Staeheli, V., and Vallotton, M. B. (1976). A radioimmunoassay for 3,3',5' triiodothyronine in unextracted serum: Method and clinical results. *J. Clin. Endocrinol. Metab.* **42**, 823–829.

Nihei, N., Gershengorn, M. C., Stringham, L. R., Coldy, A., Kuchmy, B., and Hollander, C. S. (1971). Measurements of triiodothyronine and thyroxine in human serum by gas–liquid chromatography. *Anal. Biochem.* **43**, 433–445.

Nomura, S., Pittman, C. S., Chambers, J. B., Jr., Buck, M. W., and Shimizu, T. (1975). Reduced peripheral conversion of thyroxine to triiodothyronine in patients with hepatic cirrhosis. *J. Clin. Invest.* **56**, 643–652.

Patel, Y. C., and Burger, H. G. (1973). A simplified radioimmunoassay for triiodothyronine. *J. Clin. Endocrinol. Metab.* **36**, 187–190.

Pileggi, V. J., Lee, N. D., Golub, O. J., and Henry, R. J. (1961). Determination of iodine compounds in serum. I. Serum thyroxine in the presence of some iodine contaminants. *J. Clin. Endocrinol. Metab.* **21**, 1272–1279.

Portnay, G. I., O'Brian, J. T., Bush, J., Vagenakis, A. G., Azizi, F., Arky, R. A., Ingbar, S. H., and Braverman, L. E. (1974). The effect of starvation on the concentration and binding of thyroxine and triiodothyronine in serum and the response to TRH. *J. Clin. Endocrinol. Metab.* **39**, 191–194.

Raiti, S., and Newns, G. H. (1971). Cretinism: Early diagnosis and its relation to mental prognosis. *Arch. Dis. Child.* **46**, 692–694.

Ratcliffe, W. A., Ratcliffe, J. G., McBridge, A. D., Hartland, W. A., and Randall, T. W. (1974). The radioimmunoassay of thyroxine in unextracted human serum. *Clin. Endocrinol.* **3**, 481–488.

Riggs, D. S., Lavietes, P. H., and Man, E. B. (1942). Investigations on the nature of blood iodine. *J. Biol. Chem.* **143**, 363–372.

Roche, J., Michel, R., Wolf, W., and Nunez, J. (1955a). Sur la présence dans thyroglobuline de la 3:3'-diiodothyronine, nouvelle hormone thyroidïenne. *C. R. Hebd. Seances Acad. Sci.* **240**, 921–923.

Roche, J., Michel, R., Nunez, J., and Wolf, W. (1955b). Sur la présence dans la plasma de la 3:3'-diiodothyronine, nouvelle hormone thyroidïenne. *C. R. Seances Soc. Biol. Ser Fil.* **149**, 884–887.

Roche, J., Michel, R., Wolf, W., and Nunez, J. (1956a). Sur deux nouveaux constituants hormanaux du corps thyroide, la 3:3'diiodothyronine et la 3:3'5' triiodothyronine. *Biochim. Biophys. Acta* **19**, 308–317.

Roche, J., Michel, R., and Nunez, J. (1956b). Sur le métabolisme de la 3:3':5' triiodothyronine dans le sang de rat. *C. R. Seances Soc. Biol. Ser Fil.* **150**, 20–24.

Rubenstein, H. A., Butler, V. P., Jr., and Werner, S. C. (1973). Progressive decrease in serum triiodothyronine concentrations with human aging. Radioimmunoassay following extraction of serum. *J. Clin. Endocrinol. Metab.* **37**, 247–253.

Sakurada, T., Saito, S., Ingaki, K., Tayama, J., and Turikai, T. (1969). Quantitative determination of total and free triiodothyronine and thyroxine. *Tohoku J. Exp. Med.* **99**, 179–188.

Sekadde, C. B., Slaunwhite, W. R., Jr., and Aceto, T., Jr. (1973). Rapid radioimmunoassay of triiodothyronine. *Clin. Chem.* **19**, 1016–1021.

Shenkman, L., Mitsuma, T., Suphavai, A., and Hollander, C. S. (1972a). T3 and TSH response to thyrotropin releasing hormone—a new test of thyroidal and pituitary reserve. *Lancet* **1**, 111–112.

Shenkman, L., Mitsuma, T., Blum, M., and Hollander, C. S. (1972b). Recurrent hyperthyroidism presenting as triiodothyronine toxicosis. *Ann. Intern. Med.* **77**, 410–413.

Snyder, P. J., and Utiger, R. D. (1972). Response to thyrotropin releasing hormone in normal man. *J. Clin. Endocrinol. Metab.* **34**, 380–385.

Spaulding, S. W., Chopra, I. J., Sherwin, R. W., and Lyall, S. S. (1976). Effect of caloric restriction and dietary composition on serum T3 and reverse T3 in man. *J. Clin. Endocrinol. Metab.* **42**, 197–200.

Sterling, K., and Milch, P. O. (1974). Thermal inactivation of thyroxine binding globulin for direct radioimmunoassay of triiodothyronine in serum. *J. Clin. Endocrinol. Metab.* **38**, 866–875.

Sterling, K., Bellabarba, D., Newman, E. S., and Brenner, M. A. (1969). Determination of triiodothyronine concentration in human serum. *J. Clin. Invest.* **48**, 1150–1158.

Sterling, K., Refetoff, S., and Selenkow, H. A. (1970). T3 thyrotoxicosis due to elevated serum triiodothyronine levels. *J. Am. Med. Assoc.* **213**, 571–575.

Surks, M. I., Schadlow, A. R., and Oppenheimer, J. H. (1972). A new radioimmunoassay for plasma L-triiodothyronine: Measurements in thyroid disease and in patients maintained on hormonal replacement. *J. Clin. Invest.* **51**, 3104–3113.

Taurog, A. (1963). Spontaneous deiodination of I^{131} labelled thyroxine and related iodophenols on filter paper. *Endocrinology* **73**, 45–56.

Trevorrow, V. (1939). Studies on the nature of the iodine in blood. *J. Biol. Chem.* **127**, 737–750.

Vagenakis, A. G., Burger, A., Portnay, G. I., Rudolph, M., O'Brien, J. T., Azizi, F., Arky, R. A., Nicod, P., Ingbar, S. H., and Braverman, L. E. (1975). Diversion of peripheral thyroxine metabolism from activating to inactivating pathways during complete fasting. *J. Clin. Endocrinol. Metab.* **41**, 191–194.

Wahner, W. H., and Gorman, C. A. (1971). Interpretation of serum triiodothyronine levels measured by sterling technique. *N. Engl. J. Med.* **284**, 225–230.

Walfish, P. G. (1976). Evaluation of three thyroid function screening tests for detection of neonatal hypothyroidism. *Lancet* **1**, 1208–1210.

Wenzel, K. W., and Meinhold, H. (1975). T3/rT3 balance and thyroxine metabolism. *Lancet* **2**, 413.

Werner, S. C., Acevedo, A., and Radichevich, I. (1974). Rapid radioimmunoassay for both T3 and T4 in the same sample of human serum. *J. Clin. Endocrinol. Metab.* **38**, 493–495.

Williams, E. S., Pharoah, P., Lawton, N. F., Ekins, R., and Ellis, S. M. (1972). Serum triiodothyronine concentration in subjects from an area of endemic goiter. *Isr. J. Med. Sci.* **8**, 1871.

Wu, Sing-Yung, Chopra, I. J., Nakamura, Y., Solomon, D. H., and Bennet, L. R. (1976). A radioimmunoassay of 3-3′ diiodothyronine (T2). *J. Clin. Endocrinol. Metab.* **43**, 682–685.

Wynn, J. (1960). Organic iodine constituents in human serum. *Arch. Biochem. Biophys.* **87**, 120–124.

19

Parathyroid Hormone

BERNARD A. ROOS AND LEONARD J. DEFTOS

I. INTRODUCTION

In 1963, Berson and his colleagues reported on the development of the first radioimmunoassay for parathyroid hormone (PTH). Subsequent to this pioneering achievement, PTH immunoassays have been developed and modified in many other laboratories (Reiss and Canterbury, 1968; Arnaud et al., 1971; O'Riordan et al., 1971; Conaway and Anast, 1974; Deftos, 1974; Fischer et al., 1974; Hawker, 1975). They have been used to measure endogenous PTH in the human, bovine, ovine, canine, and murine species (Sherwood et al., 1966; Slatopolsky et al., 1971; Deftos, 1974; Hargis et al., 1974). This wide range of clinical and experimental studies has greatly increased our knowledge of the importance of PTH in calcium and skeletal

401

Methods of Hormone Radioimmunoassay, Second Edition
Copyright © 1979 by Academic Press, Inc.
All rights of reproduction in any form reserved. ISBN 0-12-379260-6

metabolism. *In vitro* as well as *in vivo* studies have discovered the complex nature of PTH biosynthesis, secretion, and metabolism (Sherwood *et al.*, 1970; Hamilton *et al.*, 1971; Habener *et al.*, 1972). This important progress is well summarized in several review articles (Reiss and Canterbury, 1974; Fischer *et al.*, 1975; Hawker, 1975).

In this chapter we will outline methodology for the parathyroid hormone immunoassay. Although in general there is considerable similarity among the published immunoassay methods for PTH measurement, some important differences do exist, varying among different laboratories and with different procedures. These differences will be considered in relationship to the procedures we have selected to develop clinically useful immunoassays for the measurement of human parathyroid hormone.

II. METHODOLOGY

A. Preparations of Parathyroid Hormone

Most PTH radioimmunoassays have been based on the bovine species of the hormone. This species of parathyroid hormone was the first to be purified for tracer and the first to be available in sufficient quantities for immunization (Berson *et al.*, 1963). Porcine PTH has also been used in some assay systems (Arnaud *et al.*, 1971; Woodhead and O'Riordan, 1971).

Human PTH has recently been isolated, purified, and used in the development of radioimmunoassays (O'Riordan *et al.*, 1971; Fischer *et al.*, 1974; Segré and Potts, 1976). However, it is not likely that sufficient human PTH will soon be readily available for wide-scale use in assays for the hormone. The controversy regarding the exact amino sequence of the hormone needs resolution before large-scale synthesis, difficult in itself, is undertaken to provide sufficient human PTH for assay development and use (Segré and Potts, 1976). Since bovine PTH is available and is immunochemically similar to, if not indistinguishable from, human PTH, bovine PTH will probably provide the basis for most radioimmunoassays for human PTH for the foreseeable future.

Bovine PTH is extracted from bovine parathyroid glands and purified by chromatography (Potts *et al.*, 1968; Keutmann *et al.*, 1971). Hormone of varying degrees of purity is commercially available (Inolex, Park Forest, Illinois). Although partially purified hormone can be used to raise antibodies, only highly purified PTH can be used for iodination. Some commercial lots of highly purified hormone seem to be suitable for tracer (Inolex, Park Forest, Illinois). However, there can be a lack of correlation between biochemical and immunochemical purity and suitability for labeling, so that some PTH preparations that are apparently pure and have a high specific activity do not label well. Therefore, if one either produces or obtains a preparation of PTH that does label well, it should be reserved exclusively for labeling, and other preparations should be used for standards and for immunization.

B. Radioiodination

For radioiodination, the purest form of PTH is required. Some lots of commercial preparations and preparations supplied by the Medical Research Council (Zanelli, 1977) may be suitable for labeling. However, it is often necessary to further purify a preparation to obtain PTH that can be used for tracer. For example, the partially purified preparation of bovine PTH supplied by Inolex (Sephadex G-100) can be further purified by linear gradient elution from carboxymethyl cellulose. The starting buffer is $0.07\,M$ ammonium acetate in $8.0\,M$ urea, pH 4.9, conductivity of 0.6 mmho; the limiting buffer is $0.3\,M$ ammonium acetate in $8.0\,M$ urea, pH 6.85, conductivity of 16 mmho. The major component of pure PTH comes off at a conductivity of three to four mmho. The urea is removed either by rerunning the PTH on the same column in the absence of urea or by desalting on BioGel P-2 (Keutmann *et al.*, 1971).

Using this pure preparation of PTH, one may radiolabel it according to the method outlined in Figure 1. All of the steps should be carried out as quickly as possible. Most of the reagents can be added with disposable (Corning) micropipettes (steps 1–4) or Pasteur pipettes (steps 5–9). The reaction can be performed in disposable 75×10 mm flint glass test tubes. For many theoretical considerations, as well as the practical consideration of the longer half-life, ^{125}I is to be preferred over ^{131}I (Freedlander, 1969). Radioiodine should be accurately added as a small volume of approximately 10 to 20 μl. To achieve this, commercial solutions of ^{125}I can be diluted with distilled water.

The suggested ratios of hormone to iodine to reagents in Figure 1 should only serve as a rough guide. Different preparations of hormone vary in their labeling characteristics, so some experimentation with these ratios will be necessary for each preparation (Hughes, 1958). In this connection, some general comments deserve mention. The conditions should be kept sufficiently mild so that the hormone is not immunochemically altered. However, the oxidation must be vigorous

RADIOIODINATION OF PARATHYROID HORMONE

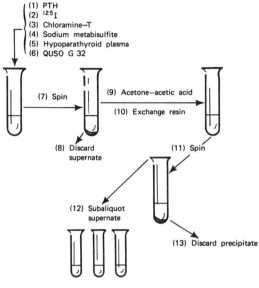

Comments:

1. 2 μg PTH in 75 μl 0.5 *M* phosphate buffer, pH 7.5
2. 1500 μC in 10–20 μl
3. 20 μl of a solution of 25 mg in 10 ml phosphate buffer
4. 50 μl of a solution of 36 mg in 10 ml phosphate buffer
5. 1 ml of 10% plasma in phosphate buffer
6. 10 mg
7. & 11. Desk–top centrifuge (e.g., International)
9. 1 ml of 20% acetone, 1% acetic acid
10. Bio–Rad Ag–1–x 10, 200–400 mesh, chloride form, 0.5 ml
12. Store at –20°C

Figure 1. Protocol for the radioiodination of parathyroid hormone. See text for additional discussion.

enough to achieve high specific activity of tracer. The greatest variation in specific activity can be achieved by altering the ratio of hormone to iodine. Altering the ratio (or time of exposure) of chloramine-T to hormone has much less pronounced effects on specific activity, but relatively more chloramine-T will increase tracer damage. (Damage is defined as that fraction of tracer which, in the absence of antibody, behaves during phase separation as though it were bound to antibody.) Consequently, no more than 15 to 30 seconds should expire between steps 3 and 4. It is of interest that porcine PTH, which contains no tyrosine, can be radioiodinated to acceptable specific activity (Woodhead and O'Riordan, 1971). The iodine is probably incorporated into the histidine of the porcine peptide.

Alternative methods of labeling have also been described. The use of lactoperoxidase affords a gentler procedure, which may alter the hormone less than the vigorous oxidation produced by chloramine-T (Robinson *et al.*, 1974). Despite this theoretical advantage, lactoperoxidase, in limited trials by the authors, does not seem to be superior to chloramine-T. Similarly, the use of a recently described method by Bolton and Hunter (1973) involving conjugation to an ^{125}I-containing acylating agent does not seem to have any advantages for the labeling of PTH. Electrolytic labeling has been used for the preparation of biologically active PTH rather than for radioimmunoassay tracer (Sammon *et al.*, 1973).

C. Purification of Tracer

At the end of the reaction, silica (QUSO, supplied by Philadelphia Quartz, Philadelphia, Pennsylvania) is added to the mixture because it has the property of adsorbing the undamaged radioiodinated PTH from the reaction mixture (step 6) (Palmieri *et al.*, 1971). The addition of plasma (PTH-deficient is preferred but not required) in step 5 serves at least two purposes. One is to prevent the PTH from sticking to the glass of the reaction tube (and subsequent storage and incubation tubes). The other purpose is to allow the protein in the plasma to compete with the damaged tracer for sites on the silica and thus to minimize the amount of damaged tracer that will adhere to the silica and be subject to subsequent elution from the silica by acetone–acetic acid (step 9).

The unreacted iodine does not readily adhere to the silica. However, any remaining free iodine can be eliminated by a distilled water wash between steps 7 and 8 and/or by the addition of the ion-exchange resin in step 10. The latter is more reliable and easier, eliminating an additional centrifugation step which would be necessary if a distilled water wash were used. The ion-exchange resin is most conveniently added by packing it into a plastic tuberculin syringe, the tip of which has been cut off, and by injecting 0.5 ml of the dry powder into the reaction mixture. Since repeated freezing and thawing increase tracer damage, the labeled hormone should be stored in multiple aliquots which can be used in their entirety (or discarded) when thawed.

Freshly labeled PTH, which is purified on silica as described above, usually contains little (<10%) damaged hormone, although there can be considerable variation in this regard among different preparations. Consequently, recently labeled hormone can be directly added to assay incubations. However, some preparations of freshly labeled hormone or labeled hormone that has been stored for several days have a significant proportion (>15–20%) of damage. In such instances it is necessary to further purify the tracer.

The further purification of labeled PTH by column chromatography can greatly improve assay performance. The result is most dramatic when tracer that has been stored for several days is purified. However, even freshly labeled tracer benefits from chromatography. Several types of gel seem to be suitable for this important purification step. We have recently adopted a duo-gel procedure to purify PTH tracer after labeling (Figure 2), since this technique gives more peaks and better separation. In this gel filtration technique, the top half of the column is BioGel P-10 and the bottom half is A-0.5m. Elution is performed using the assay buffer (see below).

D. Preparation of Antibodies

Although there are several commercial sources of anti-parathyroid hormone antibody (Immunonuclear, Stillwater, Minnesota; Inolex, Park Forest, Illinois; Wellcome Research Laboratories, Beckenham, England; Calbiochem, La Jolla, California), the serious investigator should be encouraged to raise his own antisera (Tanaka *et al.*, 1974; Mallet and Brunell, 1975). Guinea pigs, rabbits, chickens, and goats have been most widely used to raise antibodies (Berson *et al.*, 1963; Parthemore *et al.*, 1978; Reiss and Canterbury, 1968; Deftos and Potts,

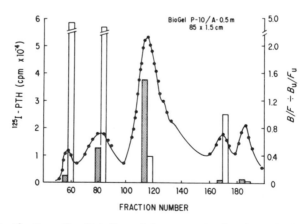

Figure 2. Purification of radioiodinated bovine PTH by duo-gel chromatography. Shaded bars represent tracer bound to antibody; open bars represent "damaged" tracer. The subscript "u" designates unfractionated tracer. Salt and void volumes are fractions 60 and 182, respectively.

1969; Arnaud *et al.*, 1971; Fischer *et al.*, 1974). There is no theoretical reason that one species should be preferable and, in fact, sensitive antibodies have been produced in each species. Various immunizing schedules have been advocated; there are no control studies which demonstrate the superiority of one over others (Vaitukaitis *et al.*, 1971; Fischer *et al.*, 1974). The most important consideration is to immunize as large a number of animals as can be accommodated by one's budget and space. It is also important to bleed the animals frequently to evaluate their antibody production. It does not appear to be fruitful to boost animals which have not produced useful antibodies after several immunizations. Partially purified preparations of PTH can be used for immunizing without conjugation to immunogenic carriers. A suggested schedule is to immunize chickens with 0.2 to 0.4 mg of hormone and rabbits with 0.4 to 0.8 mg of hormone every three to six weeks. However, much smaller amounts of hormone have been used with success (Fischer *et al.*, 1974).

The hormone should be emulsified with complete Freund's adjuvant at least for the priming dose, which can be given in footpads. Bleeding should be performed seven to 14 days after each subsequent immunization. Since titer and avidity of antisera may change independently during the course of immunization, they should be evaluated for each bleeding (see further discussion in Section II,F).

E. Assay Standards

It is theoretically preferable to use a preparation of human PTH as a standard in order to approximate a homologous assay system. Since a pure preparation of human PTH is not necessary for the standard, alternative sources for the hormone are available. These range from partially purified extracts of glandular PTH to plasma from patients with hyperparathyroidism that are instituted as standards (Reiss and Canterbury, 1968; Arnaud *et al.*, 1971). The advantage of homology between test sample and standard when human hormone is used as standard may be outweighed by the practical difficulty of obtaining a sufficient amount of human hormone to serve as standard for a significant period of time. Because of this, a well-characterized preparation of bovine PTH that is available in adequate supply may be a preferred assay standard (Zanelli, 1977).

F. Incubation Conditions

Antisera can vary in their pH of optimal binding, although optimal binding usually occurs close to neutrality (Deftos *et al.*, 1972; Fischer *et al.*, 1974). For our most useful PTH antisera, 0.05 M barbital buffer at pH 8.6 is better than phosphate, borate, or Tris buffer. For maximizing assay performance, the optimal pH of binding should be determined separately for each antibody used. Merthiolate (0.05%) or sodium azide can be used as bacteriostatic agents, and Trasylol (FBA Pharmaceuticals, New York) as a protease inhibitor, but they do not seem to have a dramatic effect in the performance of the PTH assay.

The amount and type of protein used in the buffer are critical. The type of protein can greatly influence the tracer damage and the amount of tracer that adsorbs to glass. As in other peptide hormone immunoassays, the concentration of protein can influence the estimation of antibody binding and tracer damage which is achieved by phase separation (Roos and Deftos, 1976). (This point is discussed in greater detail in Section II,G.) The concentration of protein should be sufficient to prevent labeled hormone from sticking to glass and sufficient to compete with damaged tracer for binding to charcoal (or any similarly acting phase reagent such as silica, talc, or paper), but should be low enough so that tracer damage is not seriously increased. Although there is no ideal protein solution, 10% hypoparathyroid plasma (in buffer) seems to offer a close approximation.

The protein content of the incubation mixture is, of course, greatly influenced by the addition of plasma sample. Since too great a protein concentration can increase tracer damage and can have spurious effects on tracer performance (see Section II,G for further discussion of this problem), the final concentration of protein in the incubation mix-

Table I   **Parathyroid Hormone RIA Protocol**

	Samples (μl)		Standards (μl)	
	Test	Control[b]	Test	Control[b]
Tracer[a]	100	100	100	100
Antibody[a]	100	—	100	—
Test plasma[c,d]	50	50	—	—
PTH standard[a]	—	—	100	100
Diluent	250	350	150	250
Hypoparathyroid plasma[c]	—	—	50	50

[a] Added in diluent (10% hypoparathyroid plasma, 0.05 M barbital buffer, pH 8.6).

[b] The damage control has slightly less protein than other samples since it contains no antibody; however, since antibody is so dilute, the difference is negligible.

[c] The sum of test plasma and hypoparathyroid plasma should be held constant to minimize nonspecific protein effects. For example, if 25 μl of test plasma is used, 75 μl of hypoparathyroid plasma should be used.

[d] Run in varying amounts (dilutions) to determine linearity.

ture should not exceed 20% (Roos and Deftos, 1976). It is equally important that great care be taken to equalize the protein concentration in all standards and samples. To do so, it may be necessary to add extra protein (e.g., hypoparathyroid plasma) to the standard curve and to dilutions of test sample. Furthermore, each sample should have a damage control containing exactly duplicate constituents (with the exception of antibody) as the test sample. A typical scheme for assay incubation is outlined in Table I. For some antisera, a preincubation period before tracer is added may improve assay sensitivity. In general, an incubation period after tracer addition that is approximately 75% of the preincubation period offers maximal sensitivity. The exact lengths of the preincubation period and the period after tracer addition yielding optimal assay sensitivity depend on the antiserum; optimal incubation conditions should be determined for each antiserum (Figure 3).

G. Phase Separation

The method used for phase separation (i.e., the separation of antibody-bound hormone from free tracer) can significantly affect im-

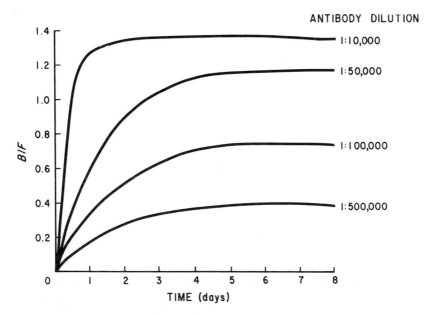

Figure 3. The effect of antibody dilution on binding of ^{125}I-bPTH (B/F) as a function of incubation time.

munoassay performance. Many procedures are currently used for phase separation in PTH assays, but dextran-coated charcoal seems to have the widest application (Reiss and Canterbury, 1968; Deftos and Potts, 1969; Arnaud *et al.*, 1971; Palmieri *et al.*, 1971; Habener *et al.*, 1973; Conaway and Anast, 1974). In our system, 2.5 gm dextran T-70 and 25 gm charcoal are mixed in 1000 ml assay buffer overnight at 4°C. Under standard conditions, the reaction tubes are allowed to equilibrate at 4°C for one hour after adding 0.8 ml of a 1 : 4 dilution (in water)

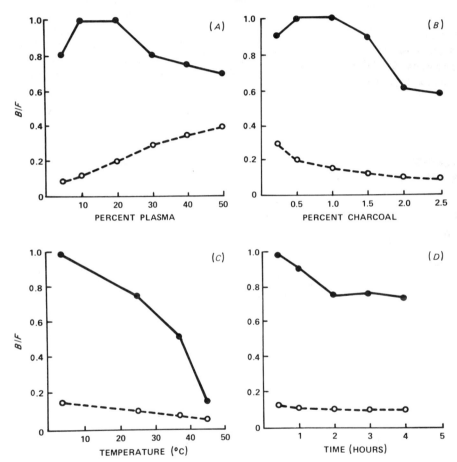

Figure 4.   Effect of several variables on parathyroid hormone immunoassay performance. Closed circles represent *B/F* of test samples; open circles represent *B/F* of "damage" controls (no added antibody; see Table I). There is an obvious effect on assay performance by each of the variables depicted: protein concentration (A); charcoal concentration (B); temperature (C); and time (D) used for phase separation. See text for further discussion.

of the stock dextran–charcoal solution. Samples are centrifuged 20 minutes at 3000 rpm, separated by decanting or aspiration, and counted. It is preferable to count both the bound and the free phases, but this may be limited by practical considerations. Many factors can influence the results of phase separation. Some of these (the effect of protein concentration, phase reagent concentration, and time and temperature of its addition) are illustrated in Figure 4. These factors can cause over- and underestimation of hormone concentration. Time may become a factor in large assays in which the tube taken down at the beginning of phase separation may have a different time of exposure to the dextran–charcoal than samples taken down at the end of the experiment. Temperature may play a role if samples are allowed to remain on the bench top for variable periods of time while awaiting decanting or aspiration of supernate. The concentration of dextran–charcoal may be variable if the suspension is not kept agitated at all times during its addition. Finally, and perhaps most important, the concentration of protein can greatly influence assay results. Vigorous attempts should be made to equalize the protein concentration in all samples, each sample should have its own control for nonspecific binding of tracer (Table I), and total protein concentration should be kept to a minimum.

Our recent experience confirms reports that the use of second antibody for separation of free and antibody-bound parathyroid hormone reduces nonspecific binding of tracer, increases radioimmunoassay sensitivity and reproducibility, and is more convenient (Conaway and Anast, 1974; Scurry, 1975). The second-antibody method is more expensive and its use requires consideration of possible interference resulting mainly from significant affinity of human γ-globulin for the second antibody) with phase separation. To minimize the competition effects of human globulin on phase separation we use relatively large amounts of carrier serum from a normal animal of the same species used for production of first (anti-parathyroid hormone) antibody and increased amounts of second antibody.

III. INTERPRETATION OF RADIOIMMUNOASSAY DATA

A. Biologic and Immunologic Behavior

Many of the problems of the PTH radioimmunoassay derive from the intrinsic characteristics of the assay procedure itself. The measurement of the hormone is based on its immunochemical rather than biologic activity, and for PTH there is a distinct dissociation between the two (Tregéar *et al.*, 1974; Fischer *et al.*, 1975). Newer methods such as radioreceptor assays, immunoradiometric assays, or cytochemical assays may be necessary to overcome this fundamental problem (Addison *et al.*, 1971; Barling *et al.*, 1975; Hesch *et al.*, 1975; McIntosh and Hesch, 1975). In addition, the secretory activity of the gland may not be accurately assessed by the measurement of hormone concentration in blood. Serial measurements and measurements during functional tests of hormone secretion can help with these limitations, but more sophisticated measurements of secretory activity, such as isotopic dilution techniques, may be ultimately necessary for accurate determinations of PTH secretory rates (Judd *et al.*, 1970).

B. Possible Artifacts in the PTH Radioimmunoassay System

In addition to these fundamental limitations of radioimmunoassays in general, the difficulty of the PTH assay is compounded by its peculiar methodologic problems, some of which have been discussed in the previous sections. For example, the importance of appropriate damage or nonspecific controls (Table I) cannot be overemphasized, and the possibility of assay artifacts constantly must be considered. In addition, because the basal concentration of hormone in normal human subjects and in some hyperparathyroid subjects is low relative to the sensitivity of most PTH immunoassays, PTH measurements must often be made from the least reliable portion of the standard curve. Accordingly, in many instances it is necessary to make complicated statistical adjustments in order to estimate hormone levels in plasma samples (Arnaud *et al.*, 1971). It has been shown for other radioimmunoassay systems that such measurements of hormone concentration can be misleading (Deftos, 1971). The implication of these observations is that extreme care must be exercised in performing assays of hormone concentrations in plasma samples, especially for samples which contain low (relative to assay sensitivity) concentrations of PTH.

All samples should be assayed in multiple dilutions to demonstrate a progressive displacement of tracer from antibody, and the assay borderline samples should be compared before and after some procedure designed to remove PTH from the sample, such as charcoal or immunologic adsorption, to verify the presence of hormone (Roos and Deftos, 1976; Roos *et al.*, 1978).

C. Immunochemical Heterogeneity

Many of the difficulties associated with the PTH assay are related to the phenomenon of immunochemical heterogeneity, a finding which was described by Berson and Yalow (1968) and which has been further studied in several other laboratories (reviewed in Fischer *et al.*, 1975). These studies have pointed out that PTH exists in multiple forms in gland and peripheral blood (Sherwood *et al.*, 1970; Hamilton *et al.*, 1971; Cohn *et al.*, 1972; Habener *et al.*, 1972; Kemper *et al.*, 1972, 1974; Silverman and Yalow, 1973; Arnaud *et al.*, 1974; Cohn *et al.*, 1974). These forms, in order of decreasing molecular size, include (1) preproparathyroid hormone, a biosynthetic precursor of proparathyroid hormone, (2) proparathyroid hormone, a biosynthetic precursor of parathyroid hormone, (3) PTH, and (4) PTH derivatives of smaller molecular size. PTH seems to be the predominant form of hormone that is secreted into the circulation. Under some circumstances, proparathyroid hormone may also be secreted, but it is unlikely that preproparathyroid hormone, which seems to have a transitory intracellular existence, is ever secreted (Kemper *et al.*, 1974; Habener *et al.*, 1976b). In addition to native hormone and its precursor molecules, fragments of PTH are also present in peripheral blood. Those fragments can be secreted by the gland or can result from glandular and/or peripheral degradation of secreted hormone and precursors (Habener *et al.*, 1971; Potts *et al.*, 1971; Segré *et al.*, 1972; Silverman and Yalow, 1973; Arnaud *et al.*, 1974). The fragments that have received most attention are an amino-terminal fragment which may be biologically active and a carboxy-terminal fragment which is biologically inactive (Canterbury *et al.*, 1973; Arnaud *et al.*, 1974; Habener, 1976). There are also isohormonal forms of PTH (Keutmann *et al.*, 1971). Therefore, multiple forms of PTH can exist in peripheral plasma, forms varying in immunochemical and biologic activity.

The heterogeneity of plasma PTH is compounded by the fact that different antisera to PTH have differing immunochemical specificity (Segré *et al.*, 1972; Fischer *et al.*, 1974). Because of this, the permutation of possible antigen–antibody reactions in different PTH assays becomes formidable. Consequently, it is not surprising that assay results can vary among laboratories that are using different assay systems (Figure 5).

These complexities in PTH measurement are the subject of active research in several laboratories. Their resolution will provide important fundamental and clinical information about the biosynthesis, secretion, and metabolism of this important hormone (Habener *et al.*,

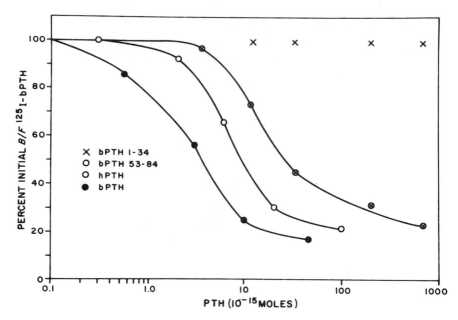

Figure 5. Specificity and sensitivity of a PTH radioimmunoassay. The carboxy-terminal fragment of bPTH (O) is reactive whereas the amino-terminal fragment (×) is not.

1976a). These complexities notwithstanding, it is still possible to develop and establish clinically useful radioimmunoassays for PTH (Arnaud *et al.*, 1971; Hawker, 1975; Parthemore *et al.*, 1978). Some of the procedures discussed earlier can help to improve the clinical value of a PTH assay. In addition, some antisera may be more valuable than others in certain clinical situations (Berson and Yalow, 1968; Habener *et al.*, 1976a). It seems that antisera with carboxy-terminal reactivity are more useful in the differential diagnosis of hypercalcemic states (in which case PTH data are frequently related to a standard serum from a patient with hyperparathyroidism and expressed as μl-Eq/ml) and that antisera with amino-terminal reactivity are more useful in acute studies of PTH secretion (reviewed in Fischer *et al.*, 1975). However, these considerations represent an oversimplification of a very complex situation (Habener, 1976). Until the fundamental issues are resolved it remains necessary to characterize fully a given assay system by clinical application in order to determine its diagnostic value. It is difficult for each investigator to prepare his own reagents, although this would be the way to assure quality control. Commercial preparations of hormone may be suitable for raising antibodies and for tracer preparation and standard, as discussed earlier. Some companies are beginning to supply labeled PTH (Immunonuclear, Stillwater, Minnesota) and the commercially available antisera mentioned earlier seem to be useful (Tanaka *et al.*, 1974; Mallet and Brunell, 1975). With the judicious use of available commercial reagents in combination with reagents otherwise available to the investigator (Zanelli, 1977), experienced clinical scientists should be able to set up a diagnostically useful radioimmunoassay for PTH. Careful patient follow-up and comparison of PTH measurements with concurrent analyses of PTH obtained in other laboratories (with PTH immunoassays of known clinical value) serve to validate PTH measurements obtained with a newly established PTH radioimmunoassay (Parthemore *et al.*, 1978).

ACKNOWLEDGMENTS

The authors are indebted to the technical skills of Tom Cantor, Cheryl Chalberg, A. L. Frelinger, Michiko Moriguchi, Cherie Redelings, Mike Tom, and Rob Van Horn, and the secretarial skills of Susan Murphy.

Supported by grants from The American Cancer Society, The National Institutes of Health, and The Veterans Administration.

REFERENCES

Addison, G. M., Hales, C. N., Woodhead, J. S., and O'Riordan, J. L. H. (1971). Immunoradiometric assay of parathyroid hormone. *J. Endocrinol.* **49**, 521–530.

Arnaud, C. D., Tsao, H. S., and Littledike, T. (1971). Radioimmunoassay of human parathyroid hormone in serum. *J. Clin. Invest.* **50**, 21–34.

Arnaud, C. D., Goldsmith, R. S., Bordier, P. J., and Sizemore, G. W. (1974). Influence of immunoheterogeneity of circulating parathyroid hormone on results of radioimmunoassays of serum in man. *Am. J. Med.* **56**, 785–793.

Barling, P. M., Hendy, G. N., Evans, M. C., and O'Riordan, J. L. H. (1975). Region-specific immunoassays for parathyroid hormone. *J. Endocrinol.* **66**, 307–318.

Berson, S. A., and Yalow, R. S. (1968). Immunochemical heterogeneity of parathyroid hormone in plasma. *J. Clin. Endocrinol. Metab.* **28**, 1037–1047.

Berson, S. A., Yalow, R. S., Aurbach, G. D., and Potts, J. T., Jr. (1963). Immunoassay of bovine and human parathyroid hormone. *Proc. Natl. Acad. Sci. U.S.A.* **49**, 613–617.

Bolton, A. E., and Hunter, W. M. (1973). The labelling of proteins to high specific radioactivities by conjugation to a ^{125}I-containing acylating agent. *Biochem. J.* **133**, 529–539.

Canterbury, J. M., Levey, G. S., and Reiss, E. (1973). Activation of renal cortical adenylate cyclase by circulating immunoreactive parathyroid hormone fragments. *J. Clin. Invest.* **52**, 524–527.

Cohn, D. V., MacGregor, R. R., Chu, L. L. H., Kimmel, J. R., and Hamilton, J. W. (1972). Calcemic fraction: A biosynthetic peptide precursor of parathyroid hormone. *Proc. Natl. Acad. Sci. U.S.A.* **69**, 1521–1525.

Cohn, D. V., MacGregor, R. R., Chu, L. L. H., Huang, D. W. Y., Anast, C. S., and Hamilton, J. W. (1974). Biosynthesis of proparathyroid hormone and parathyroid hormone. *Am. J. Med.* **56**, 767–773.

Conaway, H. H., and Anast, C. S. (1974). Double-antibody radioimmunoassay for parathyroid hormone. *J. Lab. Clin. Med.* **83**, 129–138.

Deftos, L. J. (1971). Immunoassay for human calcitonin. I. Method. *Metab., Clin. Exp.* **20**, 1122–1128.

Deftos, L. J. (1974). Parathyroid hormone. *In* "Methods of Hormone Radioimmunoassay" (B. M. Jaffe and H. R. Behrman, eds.), pp. 231–247. Academic Press, New York.

Deftos, L. J., and Potts, J. T., Jr. (1969). Radioimmunoassay for parathyroid hormone and calcitonin. *Br. J. Hosp. Med.* **11**, 1813–1827.

Deftos, L. J., Bury, A. E., Habener, J. F., Singer, F. R., and Potts, J. T., Jr. (1971). Immunoassay for human calcitonin. II. Clinical studies. *Metab., Clin. Exp.* **20**, 1129–1137.

Deftos, L. J., Habener, J. F., Mayer, G. P., Bury, A. E., and Potts, J. T., Jr. (1972). Radioimmunoassay for bovine calcitonin. *J. Lab. Clin. Med.* **79**, 480–490.

Fischer, J. A., Binswanger, U., and Dietrich, F. M. (1974). Human parathyroid hormone. Immunological characterization of antibodies against a glandular extract and the synthetic amino-terminal fragments 1-12 and 1-34 and their use in the determination of immunoreactive hormone in human sera. *J. Clin. Invest.* **54**, 1382–1394.

Fischer, J. A., Blum, J. W., Hunziker, W., and Binswanger, U. (1975). Regulation of circulating parathyroid hormone levels: Normal physiology and consequences in disorders of mineral metabolism. *Klin. Wochenschr.* **53**, 939–954.

Freedlander, A. E. (1969). Practical and theoretical advantages for the use of ^{125}I in radioimmunoassay. *Protein Polypeptide Horm., Proc. Int. Symp., 1968*, p. 351.

Habener, J. F. (1976). New concepts in the formation, regulation of release, and metabolism of parathyroid hormone. *Polypept. Horm.: Mol. Cell. Aspects, Ciba Found. Symp.* **41**, 197–224.

Habener, J. F., Powell, D., Murray, T. M., Mayer, G. P., and Potts, J. T., Jr. (1971). Parathyroid hormone: Secretion and metabolism in vivo. *Proc. Natl. Acad. Sci. U.S.A.* **68**, 2986–2991.

Habener, J. F., Kemper, B., Potts, J. T., Jr., and Rich, A. (1972). Proparathyroid hormone: Biosynthesis by human parathyroid adenomas. *Science* **178**, 630–633.

Habener, J. F., Mayer, G. P., Powell, D., Murray, T. M., Singer, F. R., and Potts, J. T., Jr. (1973). Dextran–charcoal and dioxane phase separation methods in the radioimmunoassays for parathyroid hormone and calcitonin. *Clin. Chim. Acta* **45**, 225–233.

Habener, J. F., Mayer, G. P., Dee, P. C., and Potts, J. T., Jr. (1976a). Metabolism of amino- and carboxyl-sequence immunoreactive parathyroid hormone in the bovine: Evidence for peripheral cleavage of hormone. *Metab., Clin. Exp.* **25**, 385–395.

Habener, J. F., Stevens, T. D., Tregéar, G. W., and Potts, J. T., Jr. (1976b). Radioimmunoassay of human proparathyroid hormone: Analysis of hormone content in tissue extracts and in plasma. *J. Clin. Endocrinol. Metab.* **42**, 520–530.

Hamilton, J. W., MacGregor, R. R., Chu, L. L. H., and Cohn, D. V. (1971). The isolation and partial purification of a non-parathyroid hormone calcemic fraction from bovine parathyroid glands. *Endocrinology* **89**, 1440–1447.

Hargis, G. K., Bowser, E. N., Henderson, W. J., and Williams, G. A. (1974). Radioimmunoassay of rat parathyroid hormone in serum and tissue extracts. *Endocrinology* **94**, 1644–1649.

Hawker, C. D. (1975). Parathyroid hormone: Radioimmunoassay and clinical interpretation. *Ann. Clin. Lab. Sci.* **5**, 383–398.

Hesch, R. D., McIntosh, C. H. S., and Woodhead, J. S. (1975). New aspects of radioimmunochemical measurement of human parathyroid hormone using the labelled antibody technique. *Horm. Metab. Res.* **7**, 347–352.

Hughes, W. L. (1958). The chemistry of iodination. *Ann. N.Y. Acad. Sci.* **70**, 3–18.

Judd, H. L., Scully, R. E., Atkins, L., Neer, R. M., and Kliman, B. (1970). Pure gonadal dysgenesis with progressive hirsuitism. *N. Engl. J. Med.* **282**, 881–885.

Kemper, B., Habener, J. F., Potts, J. T., Jr., and Rich, A. (1972). Proparathyroid hormone: Identification of a biosynthetic precursor to parathyroid hormone. *Proc. Natl. Acad. Sci. U.S.A.* **69**, 643–647.

Kemper, B., Habener, J. F., Mulligan, R. C., Potts, J. T., Jr., and Rich, A. (1974). Preproparathyroid hormone: A direct translation product of parathyroid messenger RNA. *Proc. Natl. Acad. Sci. U.S.A.* **71**, 3731–3735.

Keutmann, H. T., Aurbach, G. D., Dawson, B. F., Niall, H. D., Deftos, L. J., and Potts, J. T., Jr. (1971). Isolation and characterization of bovine parathyroid iso-hormones. *Biochemistry* **10**, 2779–2787.

McIntosh, C. H. S., and Hesch, R. D. (1975). Labelled antibody membrane assay for parathyroid hormone. A new approach to the measurement of receptor bound hormone. *Biochem. Biophys. Res. Commun.* **64**, 376–383.

Mallet, E., and Brunell, P. (1975). Technique de dosage radioimmunologique de la parathormone humaine. Utilisation d'un antiserum disponible et d'un etalon international. *Clin. Chim. Acta* **64**, 11–18.

O'Riordan, J. L. H., Potts, J. T., Jr., and Aurbach, G. D. (1971). Isolation of human parathyroid hormone. *Endocrinology* **89**, 234–239.

Palmieri, G. M. A., Yalow, R. S., and Berson, S. A (1971). Adsorbent techniques for the separation of antibody bound from free peptide hormones in radioimmunoassay. *Horm. Metab. Res.* **3**, 301–305.

Parthemore, J. G., Roos, B. A., Parker, D. C., Kripke, D. F., and Deftos, L. J. (1978). Assessment of acute and chronic changes in parathyroid hormone secretion by a radioimmunoassay with predominant specificity for the carboxy-terminal region of the molecule. *J. Clin. Endocrinol. Metab.* In press.

Potts, J. T., Jr., and Deftos, L. J. (1974). Parathyroid hormone, calcitonin, vitamin D, bone and bone mineral metabolism. *In* "Duncan's Diseases of Metabolism" (P. K. Bondy, ed.), 7th ed., vol. 20, pp. 1225–1430. Saunders, Philadelphia, Pennsylvania.

Potts, J. T., Jr., Keutmann, H. T., Niall, H. D., Deftos, L. J., Brewer, H. B., and Aurbach, G. D. (1968). Covalent structure of bovine parathyroid hormone in relation to biological and immunological activity. *Parathyroid Horm. Thyrocalcitonin (Calcitonin), Proc. Parathyroid Conf., 3rd, 1967*, Excerpta Med. Found. Int. Congr. Ser. No. 159, p. 44.

Potts, J. T., Jr., Murray, T. M., Peacock, M., Niall, H. D., Tregéar, G. W., Keutmann, H. T., Powell, D., and Deftos, L. J. (1971). Parathyroid hormone: Sequence, synthesis, immunoassay studies. *Am. J. Med.* **50**, 639–649.

Reiss, E., and Canterbury, J. M. (1968). A radioimmunoassay for parathyroid hormone in man. *Proc. Soc. Exp. Biol. Med.* **128**, 501–504.

Reiss, E., and Canterbury, J. M. (1974). Emerging concepts of the nature of circulating parathyroid hormones: Implications for clinical research. *Recent Prog. Horm. Res.* **30**, 391–429.

Robinson, C. J., Reit, B., and Martin, T. J. (1974). Effect of iodination by the chloramine-T and lactoperoxidase methods upon the biological activity of parathyroid hormone. *J. Endocrinol.* **63**, 27P–28P.

Roos, B. A., and Deftos, L. J. (1976). Radioimmunoassay of calcitonin in plasma, normal thyroid, and medullary thyroid carcinoma of the rat. *J. Lab. Clin. Med.* **88**, 173–182.

Roos, B. A., Cooper, C. W., Frelinger, A. L., and Deftos, L. J. (1978). Calcitonin in the rat. I. Changes in immunoreactive and biologically active plasma calcitonin. *Endocrinology.* In press.

Sammon, P. J., Brand, J. S., Neuman, W. F., and Raisz, L. G. (1973). Metabolism of labelled parathyroid hormone. I. Preparation of a biologically active ^{125}I-labelled PTH. *Endocrinology* **92**, 1596–1603.

Scurry, M. T. (1975). Serum parathyroid hormone: A double antibody radioimmunoassay. *Tex. Rep. Biol. Med.* **33**, 457–464.

Segré, G. V., and Potts, J. T., Jr. (1976). Immunological comparisons of two synthetic human parathyroid hormone-(1-34) peptides. *Endocrinology* **98**, 1294–1301.

Segré, G. V., Habener, J. F., Powell, D., Tregéar, G. W., and Potts, J. T., Jr. (1972). Parathyroid hormone in human plasma. Immunochemical characterization and biological implication. *J. Clin. Invest.* **51**, 3163–3172.

Sherwood, L. M., Potts, J. T., Jr., Care, A. D., Mayer, G. P., and Aurbach, G. D. (1966). Intravenous infusion of calcium and EDTA in the cow and goat. *Nature (London)* **209**, 52–55.

Sherwood, L. M., Rodman, J. S., and Lundberg, W. B. (1970). Evidence for a precursor to circulating parathyroid hormone. *Proc. Natl. Acad. Sci. U.S.A.* **167**, 1631–1638.

Silverman, R., and Yalow, R. S. (1973). Heterogeneity of parathyroid hormone: Clinical and physiologic implications. *J. Clin. Invest.* **52**, 1958–1971.

Slatopolsky, E., Caglar, S., Pennell, J. P., Taggart, D. D., Canterbury, J. M., Reiss, E., and Bricker, N. S. (1971). On the pathogenesis of hyperparathyroidism in chronic experimental renal insufficiency in the dog. *J. Clin. Invest.* **50**, 492–499.

Tanaka, M., Abe, K., Adachi, I., Miyakawa, S., and Kumaoka, S. (1974). Radioimmunoassay of parathyroid hormone in human plasma and tissue using commercially available antiserum and modified iodination. *Endocrinol. Jpn.* **21**, 173–178.

Tregéar, G. W., van Rietschoten, J., Greene, E., Niall, H. D., Keutmann, H. T., Parsons, J. A., O'Riordan, J. L. H., and Potts, J. T., Jr. (1974). Solid-phase synthesis of the biologically active N-terminal 1-34 peptide of human parathyroid hormone. *Hoppe Seyler's Z. Physiol. Chem.* **355**, 415–421.

Vaitukaitis, J., Robbins, J. B., Nieschlag, E., and Ross, G. T. (1971). A method for producing specific antisera with small doses of immunogens. *J. Clin. Endocrinol. Metab.* **33**, 988–991.

Woodhead, J. S., and O'Riordan, J. L. H. (1971). The immunological properties of porcine parathyroid hormone. *J. Endocrinol.* **49**, 79–85.

Zanelli, J. M. (1977). Preliminary international collaborative immunochemical studies on a possible reference preparation of human parathyroid hormone (hPTH). *Endocrinol., Proc. Int. Congr. Endocrinol., 5th, 1976*, p. 226.

RENAL HORMONES

20

Erythropoietin

JOSEPH F. GARCIA

I. INTRODUCTION

It is now generally accepted that the control of the production of red blood cells is humorally mediated by erythropoietin (Krantz and Jacobson, 1970). Erythropoietin can be extracted from the plasma and urine of a variety of animal species including man. The two main sources of this hormone have been the plasma of phenylhydrazine-anemic sheep and the urine of severely anemic humans. It has been purified to specific activities in the order of 8000–12,000 U/mg by Espada and Gutnisky (1970) and Dukes et al. (1971) using the urine from anemic humans and by Goldwasser and Kung (1971) utilizing the plasma of anemic sheep. Erythropoietin has been characterized as a glycoprotein hormone with an estimated molecular weight of 45,000, made up of approximately 70% protein and 30% carbohydrate of which 10.8% is sialic acid (Goldwasser and Kung, 1971). The most convincing evidence would support the kidney as the source for this hormone (Jacobson et al., 1957).

421

Methods of Hormone Radioimmunoassay, Second Edition
Copyright © 1979 by Academic Press, Inc.
All rights of reproduction in any form reserved. ISBN 0-12-379260-6

In assaying for erythropoietin, the initial studies consisted of hematocrit, hemoglobin concentration, or reticulocyte studies (Erslev, 1953; Borsook *et al.*, 1954). Later, the *in vivo* incorporation of radioiron into red cells became the common means of assay for this hormone. A variety of recipient animal preparations were used; two such were the hypophysectomized and fasted rats (Garcia and Van Dyke, 1959). Both of these preparations have depressed erythropoiesis and respond quantitatively to the administration of erythropoietin with increased radioiron incorporation into red blood cells. More recently, the polycythemic mouse has been almost exclusively used for the bioassay of erythropoietin (DeGowin *et al.*, 1962). Such an assay animal, with a hematocrit of approximately 70%, will show essentially no radioiron incorporation into red cells. The injection of as little as 0.05 U of erythropoietin will result in a significant increase in radioiron incorporation. While this bioassay is capable of measuring increased plasma levels of erythropoietin, it is still inadequate for the measurement of erythropoietin levels in normal subjects. In fact, generally, quite a profound anemia must be present before erythropoietin can be detected in plasma or serum by bioassay (Van Dyke *et al.*, 1961). It is also now recognized that the polycythemic mouse erythropoietin assay can respond to other materials, such as testosterone, prolactin, serotonin, cyclic AMP, and prostaglandins. A variety of *in vitro* bioassay systems for erythropoietin have been developed utilizing cultures of bone marrow, spleen, or fetal liver. Generally, such *in vitro* systems have not been useful for measuring erythropoietin concentrations in plasma or serum below 0.05 U/ml.

Since the first demonstration of the ability to produce antibody which can neutralize the biologic activity of erythropoietin (Schooley and Garcia, 1962), various investigators have been concerned with the application of immunologic techniques to the measurement of erythropoietin. Goudsmit *et al.* (1967) have developed an immunologic technique utilizing an Ouchterlony-type double diffusion system for the assay of human plasma erythropoietin. Lange *et al.* (1969) have utilized a hemagglutination inhibition system for the measurement of circulating erythropoietin levels in normal individuals. Studies utilizing the radioimmunoassay approach to the measurement of erythropoietin in human plasma or serum (Garcia, 1972, 1974; Lertora *et al.*, 1975) have been presented. Also, Cotes (1973) has developed a radioimmunoassay for sheep plasma erythropoietin. This chapter will summarize the currently available methodology for the radioimmunoassay for human erythropoietin.

II. ERYTHROPOIETIN SOURCES

The unit accepted as the standard for erythropoietin had its origin in the work of Goldwasser *et al.* (1958). One unit was defined as the amount of erythropoietin that would produce a response in the fasted male Sprague–Dawley rat assay equivalent to that produced by 5 μM of cobaltous chloride. An International Reference Preparation of Erythropoietin has been established (Cotes and Bangham, 1966; Annable *et al.*, 1972) and can be obtained from the National Institute for Biological Standards and Control, Hampstead, London, United Kingdom. Dr. Joaquin Espada, Facultad de Medicina, U.N.N.E., Corrientes, Argentina has supplied us with limited amounts of highly purified human urinary erythropoietin with specific activities in the order of 8000 U/mg protein. Human urinary erythropoietin with specific activities as high as 9000 to 12,000 U/mg protein can be obtained from the Division of Blood Diseases and Resources, National Heart and Lung Institute, Bethesda, Maryland. Sheep plasma erythropoietin can be obtained from the Connaught Laboratories, West Willowsdale, Ontario, Canada. A satisfactory preparation of human urinary erythropoietin, suitable for immunization, can be simply prepared by ultrafiltration of urine from severely anemic patients (Van Dyke *et al.*, 1957). Urine can be ultrafiltered by forcing urine through a collodion membrane under 20 lb nitrogen pressure. The membrane can be dissolved in 50% ether–ethanol, and the precipitate can be obtained by centrifugation and washed with ether and dried. The product can be dissolved in physiologic saline for characterization of biologic activity and immunization.

III. RADIOIMMUNOASSAY

A. Erythropoietin Antibody

Antibody to erythropoietin was produced in rabbits immunized with erythropoietically active human urinary extracts from severely anemic patients prepared by pressure filtration through a collodion membrane (Van Dyke *et al.*, 1957). Ten milligrams of such an extract, containing approximately 200 U of erythropoietin, was dissolved in 1.0 ml of distilled water, emulsified with 1.0 ml of complete Freund's adjuvant, and given in four subcutaneous sites at weekly intervals for

3–4 weeks. This procedure usually resulted in erythropoietin neutralizing antiserum in more than half the rabbits immunized.

Precipitin lines can be demonstrated when anti-erythropoietin antiserum is allowed to react in Ouchterlony plates with a wide variety of purified human plasma protein fractions. However, if the antiserum is absorbed with these proteins, no reduction in the erythropoietin neutralizing ability of the antiserum is observed (Schooley and Garcia, 1965). Thus, the anti-erythropoietin antiserum contains a mixture of antibodies against a variety of proteins, as well as antibody specifically directed against erythropoietin.

The anti-erythropoietin activity can be assessed by its effect in depressing the radioiron incorporation into red cells of normal mice. In this technique, erythropoietin (before and after absorption with antibody) is given subcutaneously. Fifty-six hours later, 0.5 μCi of ^{59}FeCl$_3$ is injected intravenously. The mice are sacrificed after 3 days and blood is harvested from the aorta for estimation of incorporation of labeled iron. The presence of erythropoietin antibody can also be determined by combining antiserum with a standard amount of erythropoietin in vitro at 37°C for 1 hour and overnight at 40°C and assaying in the polycythemic mouse (hypertransfused with 1.4 ml of 70% homologous erythrocytes) for any remaining erythropoietin (Schooley and Garcia, 1962).

Although the anti-erythropoietin antiserum was produced in rabbits immunized with human erythropoietin, it was shown that, in addition to human erythropoietin, increased erythropoietin levels produced in a variety of animal species, including mice, rats, rabbits, and sheep, could also be neutralized with such antisera (Garcia and Schooley, 1963). These data suggest that portions of the erythropoietin molecule in all these species may be similar.

Because of the neutralization of rabbit erythropoietin by antiserum produced in rabbits immunized with human erythropoietin, the hematological state of the rabbits being immunized was explored (Garcia, 1972). A transient anemia developed in the rabbits following immunization, and as the hematocrit fell, erythropoietin neutralizing ability was present in the serum. It appears that the presence of anti-erythropoietin in the serum reacted with the endogenous erythropoietin in the rabbit. The presence of anti-erythropoietin activity in the rabbit serum disappeared along with the anemia. This is usually observed in rabbits immunized with human urinary erythropoietin. However, one rabbit, after an initial immunization with human erythropoietin, was given an intravenous booster of sheep erythropoietin, and after the disappearance of the usual transient anemia, the serum of this rabbit retained the ability to neutralize human erythropoietin for more than 1 year. The *in vitro* incubation of serum from this rabbit with rabbit erythropoietin showed that it no longer could neutralize rabbit erythropoietin (Garcia, 1972). These data suggest that although there are similarities between human and rabbit erythropoietin giving rise to antibody which will neutralize both, there must also be molecular differences between these two erythropoietins which can give rise to antibody which will neutralize one and not the other.

More quantitative studies of our antisera produced in rabbits immunized with human urinary erythropoietin have revealed other species differences in their ability to neutralize various erythropoietins. Although many of our antisera can neutralize 25 U of human erythropoietin per milliliter, they can neutralize only about one-tenth of this amount of rat erythropoietin. Rioux and Erslev (1968) have also observed immunologic differences between sheep and mouse erythropoietins. These species differences in erythropoietins can be highly significant in attempts at radioimmunoassay. So far we have not been able to show competition with sheep and rabbit erythropoietin in our radioimmunoassay for human erythropoietin.

The antiserum used in the radioimmunoassay described here was obtained from a single bleeding of one rabbit. This rabbit had previously been immunized with a series of subcutaneous injections of relatively crude human urinary erythropoietin plus complete Freund's adjuvant, and as described above, had responded with a transient anemia coincident with erythropoietin neutralizing serum. It was later given a single booster immunization of 13 μg (approximately 100 U) of highly purified erythropoietin of human urinary origin. The rabbit was bled 9 days after this immunization and at this time the serum had a very high neutralizing ability for human erythropoietin. One milliliter of this antiserum neutralized more than 300 U of human erythropoietin. Fractionation of this antiserum on Sephadex G-200 revealed that both the erythropoietin neutralizing ability and the ability to bind labeled erythropoietin resided with the 7 S γ-globulins (Garcia, 1972). This antiserum is used in the radioimmunoassay for human erythropoietin described here at a final incubation dilution of 1 : 1,000,000.

The antiserum was not absorbed with normal human plasma because of the possibility of losing the most reactive anti-erythropoietin antibody in the presence of the small amounts of erythropoietin existing in normal plasma. Since the only reaction of consequence in a radioimmunoassay scheme is that between labeled antigen and its antibody, the presence of antibodies against other proteins should offer no interference if such proteins do not exist in the labeled form. Thus, in attempting to achieve a sensitive radioimmunoassay for erythropoietin, we concentrated on the possibility of obtaining a labeled fraction which consisted only of labeled erythropoietin molecules.

B. Labeled Erythropoietin

The human erythropoietin used for labeling was obtained from Dr. Espada. It was extracted from the urine of anemic patients and purified by a series of chromatographic steps to a specific activity of approximately 8000 U/mg (Espada and Gutnisky, 1970). This lyophilized material was dissolved in distilled water, and divided into 50-μl aliquots containing 6.5 μg, and 50 U of erythropoietin. The glass ampoules were sealed and kept frozen until the product was used for labeling. The erythropoietin was labeled with ^{125}I, using the method of Greenwood et al. (1963). Usually 2 mCi of ^{125}I (New England Nuclear, as carrier-free Na^{125}I, 400 mCi/ml, pH 8–10) and 5.0 to 6.5 μg of erythropoietin were used in each iodination. One hundred μl of phosphate buffer (0.5 M, pH 7.5) and 5 μl of Na^{125}I were added to the ampoule containing the erythropoietin, which was then stoppered with a rubber cap. The other reagents were added through the rubber cap by the use of microsyringe. They were added in the following order with mild agitation: 10 μl chloramine-T (4 mg/ml), 100 μl sodium metabisulfite (2.4 mg/ml), and 200 μl potassium iodide (10 mg/ml). These reagents were made up in phosphate buffer (0.05 M, pH 7.5). Approximately 30 seconds were allowed following the addition of the chloramine-T, whereas the other reagents were added moderately rapidly. The total contents of the ampoule were then immediately transferred to a small Sephadex G-50 column and eluted in approximately 1-ml aliquots with barbital buffer (0.07 M, pH 8.6). Usually the labeled erythropoietin was eluted in the third and fourth tube, and the remaining unreacted radioiodide peaked at approximately the eighth tube (Figure 1). This procedure resulted in preparations of labeled erythropoietin which usually had specific activities greater than 100 μCi/μg. In our early studies concerning the production of antibody to human erythropoietin, in addition to immunizing rabbits with erythropoietically active human urinary extracts, we also immunized some rabbits with a similar extract prepared from normal human urine (Schooley and Garcia, 1962). Some of the antiserum prepared against normal human urinary protein was combined with the labeled erythropoietin and submitted to gel filtration on a 1.5 × 30 cm column of Sephadex G-150. Such a fractionation resulted in two peaks of

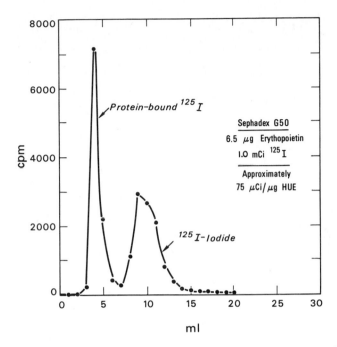

Figure 1. Separation on Sephadex G-50 of labeled erythropoietin from free iodide following the iodination procedure. (Reproduced from Garcia, 1972, with permission of the publisher.)

radioactivity (Figure 2). The first peak, occurring at the void volume, contained any erythropoietin damaged in the labeling process and any labeled protein contaminants to which antibody was present in the antiserum against the normal urinary extract. The second peak, at approximately 1.6 times the void volume, contained undamaged labeled erythropoietin molecules freed of some of its labeled contaminants. In our experience, biologically active erythropoietin occurs at approximately 1.6 times the void volume on Sephadex G-150 and at 1.8 times the void volume on Sephadex G-200 (Garcia, 1974). The second peak, containing the labeled erythropoietin, at 1.6 times the void volume was combined with an anti-erythropoietin antiserum and again placed on the Sephadex G-150 column (Figure 3). Again two peaks of radioactivity occurred. The first peak, at the void volume, consisted of labeled erythropoietin molecules bound to anti-erythropoietin γ-globulin. The second peak consisted of labeled material which was not recognized by either of the antisera used. Garcia and Schooley (1971) have shown that the biologic activity of erythropoietin in an

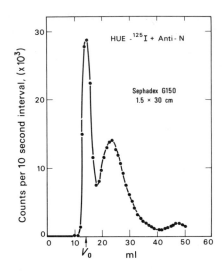

Figure 2. Gel filtration on Sephadex G-150 of previously combined urinary extract with some anti-normal urinary extract antiserum. (Reproduced from Garcia, 1972, with permission of the publisher.)

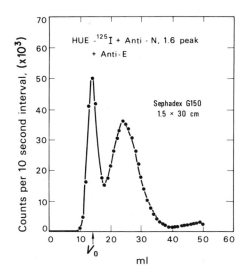

Figure 3. Gel filtration on Sephadex G-150 of previously combined material from the second radioactive peak shown in Figure 2 with some anti-erythopoietin antiserum. (Reproduced from Garcia, 1972, with permission of the publisher.)

erythropoietin–anti-erythropoietin complex can be recovered by an acidification–heating procedure similar to that used by Borsook *et al.* (1954). The labeled erythropoietin was dissociated from its antibody by acidification to pH 5.5 and heating in a boiling water bath for 5 minutes. The labeled erythropoietin resulting from such a procedure is thus freed of any damaged labeled erythropoietin, some labeled contaminants, and some labeled nonantigenic material. Gel filtration on G-200 Sephadex, of such immunologically purified labeled erythropoietin, shows a single symmetrical peak of radioactivity coinciding with both biologic and immunologic erythropoietin activity at approximately 1.8 times the void volume (Garcia, 1974). This immunologically purified labeled erythropoietin was also characterized in electrofocusing studies (Garcia, 1972). The major peak of radioactivity occurred at pH 3.5, which is in agreement with the data of Lukowsky and Painter (1972), who observed similar results for the biologic activity of sheep plasma erythropoietin.

C. Erythropoietin Radioimmunoassay

The radioimmunoassay presented here was designed for the measurement of plasma or serum concentrations of human erythropoietin. A double antibody technique was used for the final separation of the antibody-bound labeled erythropoietin. Goats immunized with rabbit γ-globulin were used as a source of the precipitating second antibody. Initially, the first International Reference Preparation of human erythropoietin was used as the standard. More recently, the second International Reference Preparation has been used, with similar results. The erythropoietin standard was dissolved in a diluent made up of 5% human serum albumin in 0.05 M phosphate buffer, pH 7.5. Halving concentrations of the erythropoietin standard from 100 down to 0.78 mU/ml were made using the same 5% human serum albumin–phosphate diluent. This was done in an attempt to keep the concentration of this protein constituent in the erythropoietin standards similar to that in normal plasma or serum.

One milliliter of the varying erythropoietin standard dilutions was pipetted into a 15-ml test tube. Other test tubes were set up with 1.0 ml of plasma or serum to be assayed. Two milliliters of the immunologically purified labeled erythropoietin containing 5000–10,000 cpm and approximately 0.1–0.2 mU of erythropoietin were added to each tube. This was followed by the addition of 2.0 ml of a 1 : 400,000 dilution of the rabbit anti-erythropoietin. The diluent for both the labeled erythropoietin and the anti-erythropoietin consisted of 0.05 M

phosphate buffer, pH of 7.5, containing 0.05% bovine serum albumin. The tubes were then capped and incubated at 4°C for a period of 4–5 days. After the incubation period 1.0 ml of a 1 : 10 dilution of normal rabbit serum was added as a source of carrier rabbit γ-globulin. This was followed by an amount of goat anti-rabbit γ-globulin serum which had previously been determined would maximally precipitate the rabbit γ-globulin in the assay tube and thus, any labeled erythropoietin which was antibody bound. After a 2-hour period at 4°C, the test tubes were centrifuged at 700 g in a refrigerated centrifuge for 30 minutes, and the supernatants were decanted. Using such an excess of rabbit γ-globulin resulted in a readily visible precipitate which held together as a pellet in the bottom of the test tube on decanting. The radioiodide in the precipitates was then counted in a Nuclear Chicago automatic well-type scintillation counter. Curves were plotted using semi-logarithmic paper with the standard erythropoietin concentration (i.e., the initial concentration in the 1.0 ml used) on the logarithmic scale and the percent of the labeled erythropoietin bound to antibody on the linear scale. This allows for a direct reading of the concentration of erythropoietin in the 1.0 ml of plasma or serum used in the assay. A curve of a typical radioimmunoassay for human erythropoietin is presented in Figure 4. With the antibody concentration and the incubation period used, the percentage of labeled erythropoietin bound is approximately 70% when no unlabeled erythropoietin is added. As shown in Figure 4, human erythropoietin in plasma or serum can be assayed when the concentration lies between 1 and 100 mU/ml. The separated 7 S γ-globulin of the anti-erythropoietin antiserum can equally be used in the radioimmunoassay and will result in a similar curve.

Removal of the sialic acid from erythropoietin by use of the enzyme neuraminidase does not appear to interfere either with the labeled erythropoietin or the unlabeled erythropoietin used for the development of the standard curve, although this treatment completely destroys the biologic activity of erythropoietin. The curve obtained with neuraminidase-treated erythropoietin was identical to that obtained with nontreated erythropoietin.

Although 100 mU of the human erythropoietin standard results in maximal competition, 1000 mU of rabbit or sheep erythropoietin do not compete with the binding of labeled human erythropoietin for the antibody. Thus the radioimmunoassay appears to be specific for human erythropoietin and, unfortunately, is not useful for animal studies.

Dilutions of human sera having high erythropoietin values result in

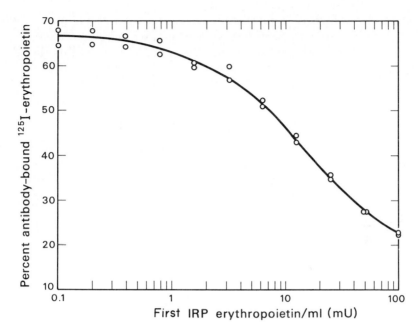

Figure 4.   A typical standard curve for the radioimmunoassay of human erythropoietin. (Reproduced from Garcia, 1974, with permission of the publisher.)

a parallel relationship with the erythropoietin standard, thus supporting the identity of the immunoreactive material in the sera with the erythropoietin standard.

IV. MEASUREMENTS OF ERYTHROPOIETIN IN BLOOD

Using the radioimmunoassay for human erythropoietin on a large series of samples of serum from normal individuals resulted in an average of 4.3 ± 0.2 mU/ml for females as compared to 4.9 ± 0.2 mU/ml for males (Garcia, 1974). This small difference was significant with a P value of <0.02. No difference was seen between heparinized plasma and serum taken at the same time. Serum samples taken in the morning from normal subjects all gave higher values than samples taken in the afternoon on the same subjects, suggesting a diurnal pattern.

Although erythropoietin bioassay systems have generally been insensitive to the concentrations in plasma or serum of normal individuals, it has been possible to measure the excretion of erythropoietin in concentrates of urine from normal individuals (Adamson *et al.*, 1966). Using such urinary concentrates, Alexanian (1966) has observed a greater excretion of erythropoietin in normal men as compared to normal women. Also, Adamson *et al.* (1966) have observed diurnal variations in the excretion pattern of erythropoietin in normal individuals.

With the radioimmunoassay for erythropoietin, it was possible to demonstrate an increase in serum erythropoietin following a moderate bleeding of a normal individual (Garcia, 1974), whereas no change in erythropoietin was demonstrable when these same serum samples were assayed in the polycythemic mouse bioassay. However, by utilizing concentrates of urine, it was possible to show a rise in the excretion of erythropoietin, as measured by increased radioiron incorporation in polycythemic mice. This increase coincided with the observed rise in serum erythropoietin as measured by the radioimmunoassay.

Thus, results obtained in normal individuals by radioimmunoassay of serum are in agreement with those obtained for urine concentrates measured by bioassay.

Using the radioimmunoassay presented here, sera from anemic patients contained higher amounts of erythropoietin than those from normal subjects (Table I). Generally, these results are not as high as results obtained by bioassay of the same samples. In one case, a severely anemic patient (Fanconi) with a high bioassayable serum erythropoietin showed a normal value for serum erythropoietin in the radioimmunoassay. Also, a great discrepancy has been observed utilizing this radioimmunoassay on the sera of severely anemic patients with renal failure, either anephrics, or patients with kidney disease undergoing hemodialysis. These patients have very high serum immunoreactive erythropoietin levels, although no erythropoietin was

Table I   Serum Levels of Erythropoietin

Source of serum	Number of patients	Mean hemo-globin conc (gm/100 ml)	Erythropoietin (mU/ml ± S.E.M.)
Normal			
Male	311	15.1	4.9 ± 0.2
Female	457	13.6	4.3 ± 0.2
Iron deficiency anemia	37	9.0	32.3 ± 5.4
Polycythemia vera	30	16.8	8.9 ± 0.9
Hemochromatosis	68	13.9	11.8 ± 0.4
Anephric patients	10	5.8	261.0 ± 41.0
End stage renal disease	19	6.4	211.0 ± 21.0

detectable in the serum of anephric patients with the polycythemic mouse assay (Garcia, 1974). The results in the anephric patients have a model in the results obtained with neuraminidase-treated erythropoietin, in that, whereas the erythropoietin immunoreactivity is retained, its biologic activity in the polycythemic mouse is completely lost. No other clinical material so far examined by erythropoietin radioimmunoassay has yielded results as high as those observed in patients with renal disease, with the exception of three of four patients diagnosed as having chronic lymphatic leukemia, who also had similarly high values.

The possible effect of enhancing or inhibiting factors may account for some of the discrepancies seen between the radioimmunoassay and bioassay for erythropoietin. In the bioassay, such factors could express themselves by modifying the biologic activity of the erythropoietin molecules, whereas the radioimmunoassay may be more correlated with the number of erythropoietin molecules present in the serum. In this respect, Wallner *et al.* (1975) concluded on the basis of an *in vitro* bioassay that there is a substance in the serum of uremic patients which suppresses heme synthesis and that this uremic toxin may be responsible for the clinically severe anemia seen in these patients. High immunoreactive serum erythropoietin levels in anemic uremic patients have also been observed by Lange *et al.* (1970) and Lertora *et al.* (1975).

V. FINAL COMMENTS

The radioimmunoassay for erythropoietin must still be considered to be in its experimental stages. Unfortunately the biochemistry of erythropoietin has not yet evolved to the point where absolutely pure hormone is available for labeling. Highly purified human erythropoietin was labeled, despite the fact that the contaminating proteins were being labeled as well as the erythropoietin molecules. Then an attempt was made to separate the labeled erythropoietin molecules from the labeled contaminants using immunologic techniques. This approach may be useful in considering the adaptation of radioimmunoassay techniques to other, as yet, impure materials.

Generally, no bioassay system for erythropoietin is sensitive enough to measure erythropoietin concentrations in plasma or serum much below 50 mU/ml. Details of a radioimmunoassay for erythropoietin have been presented in this chapter which allows for the measurement of erythropoietin concentrations of approximately 1 mU/ml in unextracted human serum. Although a reasonable correlation with bioassay of urinary concentrates has been observed when the radioimmuno-assay was used on serum or plasma of normal individuals, the results obtained with certain patient material has shown inconsistencies.

The final radioimmunoassay for erythropoietin must await the final purification of this hormone. The explanation of some of the discrepancies observed here may then become obvious.

ACKNOWLEDGMENTS

The author gratefully acknowledges with thanks the assistance of Ms. Carol Ford in the preparation of this manuscript. This work was supported by the United States Energy Research and Development Administration.

REFERENCES

Adamson, J. W., Alexanian, R., Martinez, C., and Finch, C. A. (1966). Erythropoietin excretion in normal man. *Blood* **28**, 354–364.

Alexanian, R. (1966). Urinary excretion of erythropoietin in normal men and women. *Blood* **28**, 344–353.

Annable, L., Cotes, P. M., and Mussett, M. V. (1972). The second international reference preparation of erythropoietin, human, urinary, for bioassay. *Bull. W. H. O.* **47**, 99–112.

Borsook, H., Graybiel, A., Keighley, G., and Windsor, E. (1954). Polycythemic response in normal adult rats to a nonprotein plasma extract from anemic rabbits. *Blood* **9**, 734–742.

Cotes, P. M. (1973). Erythropoietin—measurement. *In* "Methods in Investigative and Diagnostic Endocrinology" (S. A. Berson and R. W. Yalow, eds.), Part III, pp. 1110–1123. North-Holland Publ., Amsterdam.

Cotes, P. M., and Bangham, D. R. (1966). The international reference preparation of erythropoietin. *Bull. W. H. O.* **35**, 751–760.

DeGowin, R. L., Hofstra, D., and Gurney, C. W. (1962). A comparison of erythropoietin bioassays. *Proc. Soc. Exp. Biol. Med.* **110**, 48–51.

Dukes, P. P., Hammond, D., Shore, N. A., and Ortega, J. A. (1971). Differences between *in vivo* and *in vitro* activities of various erythropoietin preparations. *Isr. J. Med. Sci.* **7**, 919–925.

Erslev, A. J. (1953). Humoral regulation of red cell production. *Blood* **8**, 349–357.

Espada, J., and Gutnisky, A. (1970). Purificacion de eritropoyetina urinaria humana. *Acta Physiol. Lat. Am.* **20**, 122–129.

Garcia, J. F. (1972). The radioimmunoassay of human plasma erythropoietin. *In* "Regulation of Erythropoiesis" (A. S. Gordon, M. Condorelli, and C. Peschle, eds.), pp. 132–153. The Publishing House "Il Ponte," Milano.

Garcia, J. F. (1974). Radioimmunoassay of human erythropoietin. *In* "Radioimmunoassay and Related Procedures in Medicine," Vol. I, pp. 275–287. IAEA, Vienna.

Garcia, J. F., and Schooley, J. C. (1963). Immunological neutralization of various erythropoietins. *Proc. Soc. Exp. Biol. Med.* **112**, 712–714.

Garcia, J. F., and Schooley, J. C. (1971). Dissociation of erythropoietin from
erythropoietin–anti-erythropoietin complex. *Proc. Soc. Exp. Biol. Med.* **138**, 213–
215.

Garcia, J. F., and Van Dyke, D. C. (1959). Dose–response relationships of human urinary
erythropoietin. *J. Appl. Physiol.* **14**, 233–236.

Goldwasser, E., and Kung, C. K.-H. (1971). Purification of erythropoietin. *Proc. Natl.
Acad. Sci. U.S.A.* **68**, 697–698.

Goldwasser, E., Jacobson, L. O., Fried, W., and Plzak, L. F. (1958). Studies on erythropoiesis. V. The effect of cobalt on the production of erythropoietin. *Blood* **13**,
55–60.

Goudsmit, R., Krugers-Dagneaux, P. G. L. C., and Krijnen, H. W. (1967). Een im-
munochemische bepaling van erythropoietine. *Folia Med. Neerl.* **10**, 39–45.

Greenwood, F. C., Hunter, W. M., and Glover, J. S. (1963). The preparation of ¹³¹I-
labelled human growth hormone of high specific radioactivity. *Biochem. J.* **89**,
114–123.

Jacobson, L. O., Goldwasser, E., Fried, W., and Plzak, L. (1957). Role of the kidney in
erythropoiesis. *Nature (London)* **179**, 633–634.

Krantz, S. B., and Jacobson, L. O. (1970). "Erythropoietin and the Regulation of Erythropoiesis." Univ. of Chicago Press, Chicago, Illinois.

Lange, R. D., McDonald, T. P., and Jordan, T. (1969). Antisera to erythropoietin: Partial
characterization of two different antibodies. *J. Lab. Clin. Med.* **73**, 78–90.

Lange, R. D., McDonald, T. P., Jordan, T. A., Trobaugh, F. E., Jr., Kretchmar, A. I., and
Chernoff, A. I. (1970). The hemagglutination-inhibition assay for erythropoietin: A
progress report. *In* "Hemopoietic Cellular Proliferation" (F. Stohlman, Jr., ed.),
pp. 122–132. Grune & Stratton, New York.

Lertora, J. J., Dargon, P. A., Rege, A. B., and Fisher, J. W. (1975). Studies on a radioimmunoassay for human erythropoietin. *J. Lab. Clin. Med.* **86**, 140–151.

Lukowsky, W. S., and Painter, R. H. (1972). Studies on the role of sialic acid in the
physical and biological properties of erythropoietin. *Can. J. Biochem.* **50**, 909–917.

Rioux, E., and Erslev, A. J. (1968). Immunologic studies of a partially purified sheep
erythropoietin. *J. Immunol.* **101**, 6–11.

Schooley, J. C., and Garcia, J. F. (1962). Immunochemical studies of human urinary
erythropoietin. *Proc. Soc. Exp. Biol. Med.* **109**, 325–328.

Schooley, J. C., and Garcia, J. F. (1965). Some properties of serum obtained from rabbits
immunized with human urinary erythropoietin. *Blood* **25**, 204–217.

Van Dyke, D. C., Garcia, J. F., and Lawrence, J. H. (1957). Concentration of highly
potent erythropoietic activity from urine of anemic patients. *Proc. Soc. Exp. Biol.
Med.* **96**, 541–544.

Van Dyke, D. C., Layrisse, M., Lawrence, J. H., Garcia, J. F., and Pollycove, M. (1961).
Relation between severity of anemia and erythropoietin titer in human beings.
Blood **18**, 187–201.

Wallner, S. F., Ward, H. P., Vautrin, R., Alfrey, A. C., and Mishell, J. (1975). The anemia
of chronic renal failure: *In vitro* response of bone marrow to erythropoietin. *Proc.
Soc. Exp. Biol. Med.* **149**, 939–944.

21

Vitamin D Metabolites

JOHN G. HADDAD, JR.

I. INTRODUCTION

Vitamin D can be synthesized endogenously or can be assimilated from dietary sources (Bills, 1954). Under normal conditions, the bulk of available vitamin D is cholecalciferol (D_3), which is produced by the action of 280–310 nm light on 7-dehydrocholesterol in the skin. In situations or climates where effective solar irradiation is limited, dietary sources of D_3 and ergocalciferol (D_2) become important. Even in areas where D_2 supplementation of foods is common, however, indirect evidence establishes the skin as the dominant source of vitamin D (Haddad and Hahn, 1973). Thus, except for unusual conditions, vitamin D is an endogenous product and resembles a hormone more closely than a vitamin.

437

Methods of Hormone Radioimmunoassay, Second Edition
Copyright © 1979 by Academic Press, Inc.
All rights of reproduction in any form reserved. ISBN 0-12-379260-6

Following cutaneous synthesis or intestinal absorption, the calciferols are transported on a specific serum α-globulin and lipoproteins to the liver or adipose storage sites. Calciferol is hydroxylated at the C-25 position by a hepatic microsomal hydroxylase. The product, 25-hydroxycalciferol (25-OHD), inhibits the 25-hydroxylase, which is also under other poorly defined constraints. Provision of sufficient substrate overwhelms these regulatory influences and produces increased serum levels of 25-OHD (Haddad and Stamp, 1974).

The hepatic metabolite is transported to the kidney via the same serum α-globulin. In the kidney, 25-OHD is hydroxylated at the C-1 or C-24 position to 1,25-dihydroxycalciferol [1,25-$(OH)_2D$] or 24,25-dihydroxycalciferol [24,25-$(OH)_2D$], respectively. The renal hydroxylation steps are regulated by ionic and hormonal factors. Parathyroid hormone, decreased serum calcium, and decreased serum inorganic phosphorus all stimulate the 25-OHD 1α-hydroxylase. Conversely, increased 24,25-$(OH)_2D$ synthesis is observed with reductions in serum parathyroid hormone and increases in serum calcium or phosphorus. It is also recognized that 1,25-$(OH)_2D$ inhibits the renal 1α-hydroxylase and stimulates the 24-hydroxylase. Another metabolite, 25,26-dihydroxycalciferol [25,26-$(OH)_2D$] has been identified, but its origin and function are not yet understood.

The recognition of these modulations of 25-OHD metabolism in the kidney certainly introduced a new dimension in our understanding of mineral homeostasis (DeLuca, 1976). Parallel with this development, our ability to quantitate antiricketic sterols has also advanced in recent years. Earlier methods based on bioassay were tedious and inconvenient (Warkany and Mabon, 1940). The administration of hepatic or renal metabolites is followed by earlier biologic responses, and these metabolites are more potent than the parent vitamin. Thus, bioassay of crude extracts yielded imprecise data. Although the 1,25-$(OH)_2D$ metabolite is currently considered to be the most potent and its production is most closely regulated, direct physiologic roles for other metabolites have not been excluded from consideration (Birge and Haddad, 1975).

The development and application of competitive protein-binding radioassays for vitamin D metabolites have occurred over the past seven years. Although successful immunoassays have not been reported to date, efforts in this direction are underway in many laboratories. However, successful assays have been developed by utilizing the naturally occurring binding proteins in serum and tissue. It is my intent to review the features of the currently applied assays for 25-OHD, 1,25-$(OH)_2D$, and 24,25-$(OH)_2D$.

II. 25-OHD ASSAYS

A. Binding Proteins

Since earlier reports of the association between antiricketic sterols and serum protein fractions (Haddad and Chyu, 1971a; Rikkers and DeLuca, 1967), a considerable amount of information characterizing these binding proteins has been reported (Haddad and Walgate, 1976a; Imawari *et al.*, 1976). In mammals, an α-globulin with a sedimentation coefficient of 3.46 S (MW ~58,000) is recognized to bind 25-OHD$_3$, 25-OHD$_2$, 24,25-(OH)$_2$D$_3$, and 25,26-(OH)$_2$D$_3$ with equal affinity. In contrast, vitamins D$_2$ and D$_3$, as well as 1,25-(OH)$_2$D$_3$, are less tightly bound by this serum protein. The human and rat (Botham *et al.*, 1976) serum-binding proteins have been isolated and partially characterized. The dissociation constant for the pure human serum binding protein and 25-OHD$_3$ at 4°C is 6.8×10^{-8} M. Saturation analyses (Haddad *et al.*, 1976a) and radioimmunoassay (Haddad and Walgate, 1976b) of serum DBP (serum binding protein for vitamin D and its metabolites) content indicate that the DBP concentration is normally 7.0×10^{-6} to 9.0×10^{-6} M. In contrast, the serum content of vitamin D and its metabolites is estimated to be 1×10^{-7} to $2.0 \times 10^{-7} M$. Thus, the dominant moiety of DBP is the apoprotein under normal conditions and forms the basis for the observation that normal serum is a suitable source of binding protein for the assay.

In all nucleated mammalian tissues examined to date (Haddad *et al.*, 1973, 1976b; Haddad and Birge, 1975), a specific 25-OHD-binding protein is present in the high-speed supernatant. This protein sediments at 5 S to 6 S in the ultracentrifuge, and has a ligand-binding specificity very similar to that of the serum DBP. Binding of 25-OHD by these tissue cytosols is of slightly greater affinity than that of serum DBP. The precise nature of the tissue-binding protein is presently unclear. Tissue DBP may represent an aggregate form of serum DBP or interaction between a prosthetic group and serum DBP.

Because of its availability, serum DBP is often used, but rat kidney cytosol has also been widely utilized. Tissue is homogenized with four volumes of 0.05 M phosphate, pH 7.4, in a Teflon pestle, using 20 strikes in ice over one minute. The material is centrifuged at 105,000 g for 45 minutes and adjusted to 200 μg protein per milliliter. Both serum and tissue DBP are stable during frozen storage or in the lyophilized state, and neat dilutions work well as binding protein sources.

B. Extraction and Chromatographic Techniques

A variety of organic solvent extraction procedures can be used to effectively extract the polar vitamin D metabolites from serum. Complete extractions are effected with three extractions with four volumes of chloroform–methanol, 1 : 2, and dichloroethane–methanol, 1 : 1, is almost as effective. Another less effective solvent which has the benefit of quicker drying is anhydrous ethyl ether. Serum organic solvent mixtures are homogenized with a Teflon pestle or shaken in a motor-driven horizontal shaker, and allowed to phase. The lipid extracts are pooled and dried under a stream of nitrogen.

Since metabolites other than 25-OHD can compete in the assays utilizing serum or tissue DBP (Haddad *et al.*, 1976c; Taylor *et al.*, 1976), isolation of 25-OHD (both 25-OHD$_2$ and 25-OHD$_3$) is usually achieved by chromatography on short silicic acid columns (4.0 cm in Pasteur pipettes plugged with glass wool with n-hexane–ether mixtures (Table I) or by liquid–gel partition chromatography on 1.0×17 cm columns of Sephadex LH-20 with chloroform–n-hexane, 65 : 35, monitoring the eluates by absorbtion at 264 nm. Early eluates from either of these column procedures contain cholesterol and its esters, as well as vitamin D and its esters, and these are easily removed. 25-OHD elutes later, but before 24,25-$(OH)_2D$, 1,25-$(OH)_2D$, and 25,26-$(OH)_2D$. The 25-OHD fraction contains 25-OHD$_2$ and 25-OHD$_3$, which are equally recognized by mammalian DBP (Figure 1).

Table I   Procedures in the Saturation Analysis of 25-OHD

1. Recovery tracer 25-OH-[^{3}H]D$_3$ (~500 dpm) added to serum
2. Organic solvent extraction of serum or plasma (ether, or CHCl$_3$–CH$_3$OH, or CH$_2$Cl$_2$–CH$_3$OH), followed by drying under N$_2$ stream
3. Chromatography of lipid extract
   a. Silicic acid columns (8 ml) n-hexane–ether (2 : 1, v/v) and discard eluate; 8.0 ml of 100% ether flush saved
   b. Sephadex LH-20 columns, CHCl$_3$–n-hexane (65 : 35, v/v) as only solvent
4. Column fraction dried under N$_2$ stream and solubilized in ethanol
5. Aliquot (0.25 ml) removed for estimation of recovery from the extraction and column chromatographic procedures and counted in a toluene-based scintillation solution
6. 0.05-ml aliquots of sample or standard in ethanol, and 0.05 ml of assay tracer 25-OH-[^{3}H]D (5000 cpm) added to assay tubes. 1.0 ml of cold diluted serum or tissue cytosol in buffer is added and the tubes are briefly mixed and placed in an ice bath.
7. After one-hour incubation, 0.25 ml of the dextran-coated charcoal suspension (1.0 gm Norit A charcoal, 100 mg Dextran 20 in 250 ml 0.05 M phosphate, pH 7.5) is added. After mixing, the tubes are placed in the ice bath for 15 minutes and mixed again. After centrifugation at 2000 rpm for 15 minutes, 1.0-ml aliquots of the supernate are transferred to Hydromix cocktail (Yorktown Research) for assay of radioactivity.

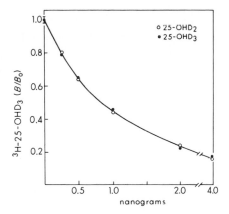

Figure 1. Competitive binding radioassay of 25-OHD utilizing a 1:5000 dilution of normal human serum as the source of binding protein. 25-OHD$_2$ and 25-OHD$_3$ are equipotent competitors for the displacement 25-OH-[^{3}H]D$_3$.

There have been reports of direct assays of 25-OHD in which the chromatographic steps are omitted (Belsey *et al.*, 1974; Garcia-Pascual *et al.*, 1976; Offerman and Dittmar, 1974). Although the lower binding affinity of DBP for vitamin D is established, other metabolites, such as 24,25-(OH)$_2$D and 25,26-(OH)$_2$D, are potential sources of overestimation by these nonchromatographic methods (Haddad *et al.*, 1976c; Taylor *et al.*, 1976). If the quantity and variation in content of these other metabolites prove to be substantial, direct 25-OHD assays would be inaccurate and possibly suitable only for detection of deficiency states. A study of the chromatographic and nonchromatographic assays has revealed that the chromatographic step is necessary for accurate results (Skinner and Wills, 1977). At present, therefore, it is reasonable to consider the valid DBP binding assays of 25-OHD in serum to be those which are preceded by the chromatographic isolation of 25-OHD.

C. Assay Procedures

An outline of the steps in the assay for 25-OHD is provided in Table I. In addition, features of several of the published methods are shown in Table II. Following extraction and chromatographic steps, the 25-OHD fraction is solubilized in ethanol, and aliquots are used for estimation of recovery and for the assay. Usually, small amounts of ethanol (10% or less) are included in the incubation tubes to enhance solubilization and binding, but suitable binding can also be demon-

Table II Serum 25-OHD Assay Methods[a]

Extraction	Chromatography	Tracer recovery(%)	Binding protein	Incubation	Separation	Normal range (ng/ml)	Reference
Ether	Silicic acid columns	64	Rat kidney cytosol or serum	One hour at 25°C	Dextran–charcoal	11–55	Haddad and Chyu (1971b)
Chloroform–methanol	Silicic acid columns	80	Rat serum	Ten days at 4°C	Heparin–MnCl$_2$	18–36	Belsey et al. (1971)
Dichloromethane methanol	Silica gel thin layer	25	Human serum	20 hours at 4°C	Florisil	10–23	Bayard et al. (1972)
Chloroform–methanol	Sephadex LH-20 columns	77	Rat serum	30 minutes at 25°C	Dextran–charcoal	8–30	Edelstein et al. (1974)
Chloroform–methanol–water	Silicic acid columns	87	Rat serum	15 hours at 4°C	Dextran–charcoal	4–33	Preece et al. (1974)
Dichloromethane methanol–water	Sephadex LH-20 columns	82	Rat or human serum	One hour at 0°C	Dextran–charcoal	5–22	Bouillon et al. (1976)

[a] Optimal 25-OHD binding by DBP occurs at neutral to alkaline pH (Haddad and Chyu, 1971a).

strated if the sterols' vehicle is dried prior to addition of the DBP solution.

The dilution of serum or cytosol and amount of assay tracer used are largely a matter of preference, depending on the sensitivity required. Approximately 5000 cpm 25-OH-[³H]D₃ at a specific activity of 10–12 Ci/mmole in 50 μl ethanol, and 1.0 ml of normal human serum at 1:5000 or rat serum at 1:3000 dilution or 1.0 ml rat kidney cytosol (200 μg protein) provide a reasonable displacement curve over 0.25 to 6.0 ng of reference 25-OHD₃. Assay incubations can be shorter than one hour at 0°–4°C since the association time is quite short. Care must be taken that the amount of and exposure to coated charcoal are uniform, since variations can result in variable binding as a result of over- or under-adsorption of free sterol. Although there are pitfalls, the coated charcoal procedure can provide reproducible results. A representative displacement curve is shown in Figure 1.

In practice, less than 25% of the chromatographic isolate is used in the incubation, since larger fractions of some sera presumably contain sufficient lipid material to interfere with the association of the ligand and protein and/or the adsorbent removal of ligand not specifically bound to DBP. Since our recovery averages greater than 60%, our usual sensitivity is in the order of 2.0 ng/ml. As needed, utilization of less DBP and assay tracer provides more sensitive displacement curves.

Because of the marked lability of the antiricketic sterols, considerable care must be taken to avoid their excessive exposure to air, light, heat, or decreased pH. All assay procedures are carried out in the absence of direct exposure to 280–310 nm light, and extracts and eluates are dried under nitrogen. If not dried, solutions of sterols are kept in a nitrogen atmosphere. We routinely purify the recovery and assay tracer 25-OH-[³H]D₃ by silicic acid or Sephadex LH-20 chromatography prior to assay. Reference sterols are weighed, solubilized in ethanol, and analyzed for their absorption of 264 nm light. Appropriate adjustment is made according to their molar extinction coefficients (E_M of 25-OHD₃ equals 18,000), and multiple aliquots are prepared and dried under nitrogen. Each reference tube is kept cold and used only once. Reference sterols in solution can deteriorate, and these precautions prevent difficulty.

Quite recently, other laboratories have reported modifications in the assay procedure for 25-OHD (Ellis and Dixon, 1977) or some of the problems associated with this competitive binding assay (Mason and Posen, 1977). An alternative assay procedure, which correlates well with the saturation analysis, is to quantitate these sterols [25-OHD and

24,25-$(OH)_2D$] by analyzing their ultraviolet light absorbance during their elution from high-pressure liquid chromatographic columns (Gilbertson and Stryd, 1977; Lambert *et al.*, 1977).

III. 1,25-$(OH)_2D$ ASSAY

A. Binding Proteins

In contrast to serum and tissue DBP's, lower affinity binding of 1,25-$(OH)_2D$, extracts from avian and rat intestinal mucosa have been shown to contain a protein which binds 1,25-$(OH)_2D_3$ with high affinity (Brumbaugh and Haussler, 1974; Frolik and DeLuca, 1976; Lawson and Wilson, 1974). A similar binding protein has been demonstrated in avian parathyroid extracts (Brumbaugh *et al.*, 1975) and in human parathyroid adenomata (Haddad *et al.*, 1976b).

Recently, competitive radioassays for 1,25-$(OH)_2D_3$ have been developed on the basis of the ability of avian intestinal mucosal extract to bind this sterol with high affinity. Attempts to detect a similar material in mammalian gut cytosol have been made without success (Haddad *et al.*, 1973). In contrast to the tissue cytosol 5 S to 6 S binding protein, the 1,25-$(OH)_2D_3$ binding protein is apparently in lower concentration and is more labile. It has not been isolated, but it, like serum DBP, sediments at 3 S to 4 S in the ultracentrifuge.

Binding protein can be purified from vitamin D-deficient white leghorn chickens. Duodena are removed and rinsed with 5.0 ml 0.05 M phosphate and 0.05 M KCl, pH 7.4. The mucosa is scraped off, minced in five volumes of buffer, and centrifuged at 2000 g for 10 minutes. The material is washed twice with five volumes of buffer, and the supernatants are discarded. The mucosal pellet is resuspended in two volumes of buffer and homogenized at 0°C. The homogenate is centrifuged at 50,000 rpm for 45 minutes; the lipid layer is aspirated; and the clear cystosol is lyophilized (Eisman *et al.*, 1976b).

Several factors contribute to the difficulty of the 1,25-$(OH)_2D_3$ assay: (a) serum content of 1,25-$(OH)_2D$ is much lower than serum 25-OHD, (b) 1,25-$(OH)_2D_3$ cochromatographs with 25,26-$(OH)_2D_3$ in the silicic acid and Sephadex LH-20 chromatographic procedures, (c) very high specific activity, 1,25-$(OH)_2$-[^{3}H]D_3 has not, until recently, been available except by *in vitro* biosynthesis from 25-O^{3}HD_3 by avian kidney, and (d) the lability of the 1,25-$(OH)_2D_3$ binding protein. In spite of these obstacles, workers have developed techniques which enable them to isolate and assay this important metabolite.

B. Extraction and Chromatographic Techniques

Following the addition of 3500 dpm $1,25(OH)_2$-$[^3H]D_3$ to serum to monitor recovery, large volumes (5.0–20 ml) of serum are extracted with chloroform–methanol, 1:2, or six volumes of dichloromethane. The chloroform layer is dried under N_2 prior to chromatography.

Initially, arduous series of chromatographic steps were employed to isolate the $1,25$-$(OH)_2D$. Silicic acid columns were used but have recently been deleted in favor of two successive 1.0×15 cm columns of Sephadex LH-20 eluting with 65% chloroform in hexane. Final purification relied on the liquid–liquid partition of these eluates on columns of Celite using on this column a stationary phase of 55% aqueous ethanol and a mobile phase of 10% ethyl acetate in hexane; $1,25$-$(OII)_2D$ emerged between 7.0 and 22 ml (Haussler *et al.*, 1976).

Superior resolution of the metabolites has been reported with high-pressure liquid chromatography on a 0.4×30 cm column of 10 μm silicic acid in 10% isopropanol in Skelly solve B at 1.8 ml/minute and 800 psi (Ikekawa and Koizumi, 1976; Jones and DeLuca, 1975). For the purpose of assays, an initial 0.7×9.0 cm Sephadex LH-20 column step in *n*-hexane–chloroform: methanol, 9:1:1, is followed by high-speed chromatography on microparticulate silicic acid columns in 10% isopropanol in hexane at 800 psi nitrogen pressure. The resolution of D metabolites is excellent in high-pressure systems, and an example is illustrated in Figure 2.

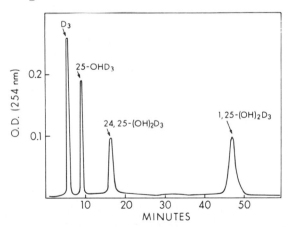

Figure 2. High-pressure liquid chromatography of vitamin D metabolites on a 0.22×50 cm column of 10 μm silica gel. 10% isopropanol in *n*-hexane under 375 psi of N_2 gas resulted in a flow rate of 0.25 ml/minute. Reference sterols, in the column solvent, were injected via a stop-flow valve, and the eluate was continuously monitored at 254 nm.

C. Assay Procedures

The two reported techniques vary in the preparation of the avian intestinal mucosal binding protein. In one instance, an intestinal cytosol–chromatin complex is utilized by preparing 100,000 g supernatant and detergent-extracted chromatin from 6.0 gm of intestinal mucosa from vitamin D-depleted chickens (Brumbaugh et al., 1974a,b; Hughes et al., 1976; Haussler et al., 1976). In the other method, only the high-speed supernatant of extracts of mucosa is used and is prepared in the presence of 0.05 M KCl (Eisman et al., 1976a,b). Optimal pH for either method is in the 7–8 range.

The cytosol–chromatin assay utilizes incubations of 200 μl of binding protein solution, 1,25-$(OH)_2$-$[^3H]D_3$, and either standards or unknowns in 20 μl ethanol at 25°C for 20 minutes, followed by the addition of 1.0 ml cold 1% Triton-X-100 in 0.01 M Tris, pH 7.5, and filtration of the suspension on glass fiber filters. Following rinsing with detergent buffer, the filters containing bound 1,25-$(OH)_2$-$[^3H]D_3$ are heated in counting vials containing 5 ml CH_3OH–$CHCl_3$ (2 : 1, v/v), the solvent is dried, and radioactivity is assayed in toluene-based scintillating fluid.

The cytosol assay utilizes 1.0-ml dilutions (1.0 mg protein per tube) of binding protein, 70 pg 1,25-$(OH)_2$-$[^3H]D$, and either standards (10–140 pg) or unknowns, and is conducted at 25°C for 1 hour. As with the cytosol–chromatin assay, radioactive and nonradioactive sterols are introduced in small amounts (50 μl) of ethanol. After one hour, tubes are placed at 0°C, and 1.0 ml of cold 40% polyethylene glycol is added. The tube contents are mixed and centrifuged at 4800 g for 30 minutes at 4°C, and the supernatants are discarded. The precipitates are solubilized and counted in a dioxane-based scintillation solution.

Variable sensitivity has been reported using 6–12 Ci/mmole tracer 1,25-$(OH)_2$-$[^3H]D_3$ synthesized from 25-OH-$[^3H]D_3$ by chicken kidney homogenates. Recently, high specific activity 1,25-$(OH)_2$-$[^3H]D_3$ has been synthesized (78 Ci/mmole) and shall permit greater sensitivity, as well as smaller serum samples to be processed. Although the source of the binding protein used is identical in these assays, the cytosol–chromatin assay recognizes 1,25-$(OH)_2D_2$ less well, but the cytosol assay is reported to not distinguish between the ergo and chole forms of this dihydroxy metabolite. The apparent contradiction demands additional study in order to resolve this issue.

At present, the 1,25-$(OH)_2D$ assays are difficult because of the necessity of at least two chromatographic procedures. Either Celite columns or high-pressure chromatographic systems are required to isolate 1,25-$(OH)_2D_3$ from other metabolites. The use of cytosol-binding protein seems to represent an improvement over the preparation of sub-

Table III   Serum 1,25-$(OH)_2D$ Assay Methods

Step	Method 1[a]	Method 2[b]
Serum extraction	20 ml of CH_3OH–$CHCl_3$ (2 : 1)	5.0 ml dichloromethane
Chromatography	a. Two columns of Sephadex LH-20, 1.0 × 15 cm [$CHCl_3$–hexane (65 : 35)] b. Celite 0.8 × 8.5 cm (aqueous ethanol and ethyl acetate–hexane)	a. Sephadex LH-20 (0.7 × 9 cm) [hexane–$CHCl_3$–CH_3OH (9 : 1 : 1)] b. High-pressure (silica 10 μm) (isopropanol–hexane)
Recovery	40–75	68
Binding protein	Avian small intestine; cytosol–chromatin suspension	Avian small intestine; cytosol preparation
Assay	25°C for 20 minutes	25°C for 60 minutes
Harvest	Glass filters with Triton-X-100 rinse	PEG 6000; count precipitate
Sensitivity	20 pg/tube	10 pg/tube
Normal level (human blood)	64 ± 12 pg/ml (Brumbaugh *et al.*, 1974b) (n = 20); 33 ± 6 pg/ml (Brumbaugh *et al.*, 1974a; Haussler *et al.*, 1976); (n = 29)	29 ± 2.0 pg/ml (Eisman *et al.*, 1976a) (N = 20)

[a] Brumbaugh *et al.* (1974a,b), Haussler *et al.* (1976), and Hughes *et al.* (1976).
[b] Eisman *et al.* (1976a,b).

cellular fraction mixtures, and the widespread availability of high specific activity 1,25-$(O^3H)_2D_3$ should attract more workers into this area of investigation. The features of these assays are depicted in Table III.

Very recently, two groups of workers have reported success in raising antisera to vitamin sterols (Clemens *et al.*, 1978; Schaefer *et al.*, 1978).

IV. 24,25-$(OH)_2D$ ASSAYS

A. Binding Proteins

In contrast to the assays previously mentioned, the assay of 24,25-$(OH)_2D_3$ has been described only recently. The important observations which made these assays possible were the recognition that rat serum diluted 1 : 3500 (Haddad *et al.*, 1976c) and rat kidney cytosol (Taylor *et al.*, 1976) were capable of binding 24,25-$(OH)_2D_3$ with high affinity. In fact, 25-OHD_3 and 24,25-$(OH)_2D_3$ are equipotent in their ability to displace 25-O^3HD_3 from these binding proteins (Figure 3). Avian sera do not bind either of these sterols as tightly as sera from

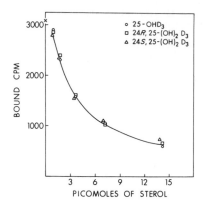

Figure 3.   Competitive binding radioassay of 24,25-(OH)₂D₃ utilizing a 1 : 3000 dilution of normal rat serum as the source of binding protein. 25-OHD₃ and 24,25-(OH)₂D₃ are equipotent competitors for the displacement of 25-OH-[³H]D₃. (Reproduced from Haddad *et al.*, 1976c, with permission of the publisher.)

mammals, and avian sera bind the ergocalciferol compounds less tightly than the cholecalciferol metabolites.

It is clear that both 25-OHD₃ and 25-OHD₂ are equally measured in mammalian DBP assays, but the recognition of 24,25-(OH)₂D₃ is presumed now to be equal to 24,25-(OH)₂D₂ recognition, since reference 24,25-(OH)₂D₂ is not currently available. In biologic fluids, it is recognized that the hydroxyl group at the C-24 position is the *R* isomer, and 24*R*,25-(OH)₂D₃ is equal to 25-OHD₃ in its ability to displace 25-OH-[³H]D₃ from mammalian DBP.

B. Extraction and Chromatography

The procedures are similar to those previously described for extraction of vitamin D metabolites from serum. Thus far, Sephadex LH-20 chromatography seems to offer the most convenient isolation technique. In one technique (Taylor *et al.*, 1976) 0.9 × 30 cm columns are eluted with CHCl₃–*n*-hexane (6 : 4, v/v), and the 24,25-(OH)₂D₃ fraction is then rechromatographed (size exclusion only) in methanol. Alternatively, 1.0 × 15 cm columns of Sephadex LH-20 slurried in CHCl₃–*n*-hexane, 65 : 35 (v/v) can be used as a single step (Haddad *et al.*, 1977). 24,25-(OH)₂D elutes between 33 and 45 ml.

Validation of the isolation performed on small Sephadex LH-20 columns has been done with longer columns and in a high-speed liquid chromatographic system (see Figure 2). 24,25-(OH)₂-[³H]D₃ is not commercially available at present and must be biosynthesized *in vitro* in order to trace its recovery during the extraction and chromatography steps. Although 24,25-$(OH)_2$-[^{3}H]D_3 can be used as the assay tracer (Taylor *et al.*, 1976), 25-OH-[^{3}H]D_3 serves as well, and is commercially available (Figure 3).

C. Assay Procedures

The methods employed for the assay of 24,25-$(OH)_2$D are very similar to those described for the 25-OHD assay. After isolation, aliquots are used in the assay (50 μl) and for estimation of recovery. Incubation conditions and adsorbent separation steps are identical to those used in the 25-OHD assay. To date, few measurements have been reported, but the levels of 24,25-$(OH)_2$D in human sera are apparently in the 1.0–5.0 ng/ml range. Of considerable interest is the presence of 24,25-$(OH)_2$D in sera from patients who have had total nephrectomy, indicating extrarenal 24-hydroxylase activity (Haddad *et al.*, 1977). The availability of agents and the relative ease of this assay ensure its future application to a variety of disorders of mineral homeostasis.

V. SUMMARY

Saturation analyses of vitamin D metabolites have been developed utilizing natural binding protein sources, relatively high specific activity radioactive sterols, and a variety of chromatographic techniques. A method for the measurement of the parent vitamin has been reported (Belsey *et al.*, 1971), but has not proved reliable (Edelstein *et al.*, 1974). Analyses based on gas–liquid chromatography and mass spectrometry have been reported (Björkhem and Holmberg, 1976; Sklan *et al.*, 1973), and such applications deserve continued scrutiny. Although only a few antisera have been developed, it is anticipated that such materials, coupled with effective isolation procedures (Figure 2), will also provide the means for quantitation of these sterols in the near future.

REFERENCES

Bayard, F., Bec, P., and Louvet, J. P. (1972). Measurement of plasma 25-hydroxycholecalciferol in man. *Eur. J. Clin. Invest.* **2**, 195–198.
Belsey, R. E., DeLuca, H. F., and Potts, J. T., Jr. (1971). Competitive binding assay for vitamin D and 25-OH-vitamin D. *J. Clin. Endocrinol. Metab.* **33**, 554–557.

Belsey, R. E., DeLuca, H. F., and Potts, J. T., Jr. (1974). A rapid assay for 25-OH-vitamin D without preparative chromatography. *J. Clin. Endocrinol. Metab.* **38**, 1046–1051.

Bills, C. E. (1954). Vitamin D group. *In* "The Vitamins" (W. Sebrell and R. Harris, eds.), 1st ed., Vol. 2, Chapter 6, pp. 132–266. Academic Press, New York.

Birge, S. J., and Haddad, J. G. (1975). 25-hydroxycholecalciferol stimulation of muscle metabolism. *J. Clin. Invest.* **56**, 1100–1107.

Björkhem, I., and Holmberg, I. (1976). A novel specific assay of 25-hydroxyvitamin D_3. *Clin. Chim. Acta* **68**, 215–221.

Botham, K. M., Ghazarian, J. G., Kream, B. E., and DeLuca, H. F. (1976). Isolation of an inhibitor of 25-hydroxyvitamin D_3-1-hydroxylase from rat serum. *Biochemistry* **15**, 2130–2135.

Bouillon, R., VanKerkhove, P., and DeMoor, P. (1976). Measurements of 25-hydroxyvitamin D_3 in serum. *Clin. Chem.* **22**, 364–370.

Brumbaugh, P. F., and Haussler, M. R. (1974). 1α,25-dihydroxycholecalciferol receptors in intestine. *J. Biol. Chem.* **249**, 1258–1262.

Brumbaugh, P. F., Haussler, D. H., Bursac, K. M., and Haussler, M. R. (1974a). Filter assay for 1α,25-dihydroxyvitamin D_3. Utilization of the hormone's target tissue chromatin receptor. *Biochemistry* **13**, 4091–4097.

Brumbaugh, P. F., Haussler, D. H., Bressler, R., and Haussler, M. R. (1974b). Radioreceptor assay for 1α,25-dihydroxyvitamin D. *Science* **183**, 1089–1091.

Brumbaugh, P. F., Hughes, M. R., and Haussler, M. R. (1975). Cytoplasmic and nuclear binding components for 1α,25-dihydroxyvitamin D in chick parathyroid glands. *Proc. Natl. Acad. Sci. U.S.A.* **72**, 4871–4875.

Clemens, T. L., Hendy, G. N., Graham, R. F., Baggiolini, E. G., Uskokovic, M. R., and O'Riordan, J. L. H. (1978). A radioimmunoassay for 1,25-dihydroxycholecalciferol. *Clin. Sci. Mol. Med.* **54**, 329–332.

DeLuca, H. F. (1976). Recent advances in our understanding of the vitamin D endocrine system. *J. Lab. Clin. Med.* **87**, 7–26.

Edelstein, S., Charman, M., Lawson, D. E. M., and Kodicek, E. (1974). Competitive protein binding assay for 25-hydroxycalciferol. *Clin. Sci. Mol. Med.* **46**, 231–240.

Eisman, J. A., Hamstra, A. J., Kream, B. E., and DeLuca, H. F. (1976a). 1,25-dihydroxyvitamin D in biological fluids: A simplified and sensitive assay. *Science* **193**, 1021–1023.

Eisman, J. A., Hamstra, A. J., Kream, B. E., and DeLuca, H. F. (1976b). A sensitive, precise and convenient method for determination of 1,25-dihydroxyvitamin D in human plasma. *Arch. Biochem. Biophys.* **176**, 235–243.

Ellis, G., and Dixon, K. (1977). Sequential-saturation-type assay for serum 25-hydroxyvitamin D. *Clin. Chem.* **23**, 855–862.

Frolik, C. A., and DeLuca, H. F. (1976). Solubilization and partial purification of a rat intestinal 1,25-dihydroxyvitamin D_3 binding protein. *Steroids* **27**, 433–440.

Garcia-Pascual, B., Peytremann, A., Courvoisier, B., and Lawson, D. E. M. (1976). A simplified competitive protein assay for 25-hydroxycalciferol. *Clin. Chim. Acta* **68**, 99–105.

Gilbertson, T. J., and Stryd, R. P. (1977). High performance liquid chromatographic assay for 25-hydroxyvitamin D_3 in serum. *Clin. Chem.* **23**, 1700–1704.

Haddad, J. G., and Birge, S. J. (1975). Widespread, specific binding of 25-hydroxycholecalciferol in rat tissue. *J. Biol. Chem.* **250**, 299–304.

Haddad, J. G., and Chyu, K. J. (1971a). 25-hydroxycholecalciferol-binding globulin in human plasma. *Biochim. Biophys. Acta* **248**, 471–481.

Haddad, J. G., and Chyu, K. J. (1971b). Competitive protein-binding radioassay for 25-hydroxycholecalciferol. *J. Clin. Endocrinol. Metab.* **33**, 992–995.

Haddad, J. G., and Hahn, T. J. (1973). Natural and synthetic sources of 25-hydroxyvitamin D in man. *Nature (London)* **244**, 515–517.

Haddad, J. G., and Stamp, T. C. B. (1974). Circulating 25-hydroxy-vitamin D in man. *Am. J. Med.* **57**, 57–62.

Haddad, J. G., and Walgate, J. (1976a). 25-hydroxyvitamin D transport in human plasma: Isolation and partial characterization of calcifidiol-binding protein. *J. Biol. Chem.* **251**, 4803–4809.

Haddad, J. G., and Walgate, J. (1976b). Radioimmunoassay of the binding protein for vitamin D and its metabolites in human serum. *J. Clin. Invest.* **58**, 1217–1222.

Haddad, J. G., Hahn, T. J., and Birge, S. J. (1973). Vitamin D metabolites: Specific binding by rat intestinal cytosol. *Biochim. Biophys. Acta* **329**, 93–97.

Haddad, J. G., Hillman, L. S., and Rojanasathit, S. (1976a). Human serum binding capacity and affinity for 25-hydroxyergocalciferol and 25-hydroxycholecalciferol. *J. Clin. Endocrinol. Metab.* **43**, 86–91.

Haddad, J. G., Walgate, J., Min, C., and Hahn, T. J. (1976b). Vitamin D metabolite binding proteins in human tissue. *Biochim. Biophys. Acta* **444**, 921–925.

Haddad, J. G., Min, C., Walgate, J., and Hahn, T. J. (1976c). Competition by 24, 25-dihydroxycholecalciferol in the competitive radioassay of 25-hydroxycalciferol. *J. Clin. Endocrinol. Metab.* **43**, 712–715.

Haddad, J. G., Mendelsohn, M., Min, C., Slatopolsky, E., and Hahn, T. J. (1977). Competitive protein binding radioassay of 24,25-dihydroxyvitamin D in sera from normal and anephric subjects. *Arch. Biochem. Biophys.* **182**, 390–395.

Haussler, M. R., Baylink, D. J., Hughes, M. R., Brumbaugh, P. F., Wergedal, J. E., Shen, F. H., Nielsen, R. L., Counts, S. J., Bursac, K. M., and McCain, T. A. (1976). The assay of 1α,25-dihydroxyvitamin D_3: Physiologic and pathologic modulation of circulating hormone levels. *Clin. Endocrinol.* **5**, 151s–165s.

Hughes, M. R., Baylink, D. J., Jones, P. G., and Haussler, M. R. (1976). Radioligand receptor assay for 25-hydroxyvitamin D_2/D_3 and 1α,25-dihydroxyvitamin D_2/D_3. *J. Clin. Invest.* **58**, 61–70.

Ikekawa, N., and Koizumi, N. (1976). Separation of vitamin D_3 metabolites and their analogues by high-pressure liquid chromatography. *J. Chromatogr.* **119**, 227–232.

Imawari, M., Kida, K., and Goodman, D. S. (1976). The transport of vitamin D and its 25-hydroxymetabolite in human plasma. Isolation and partial characterization of vitamin D and 25-hydroxyvitamin D binding protein. *J. Clin. Invest.* **58**, 514–523.

Jones, G., and DeLuca, H. F. (1975). High pressure liquid chromatography: Separation of the metabolites of vitamins D_2 and D_3 on small-particle silica columns. *J. Lipid Res.* **16**, 448–453.

Lambert, P. W., Syverson, B. J., Armand, C. D., and Spelsberg, T. C. (1977). Isolation and quantitation of endogenous vitamin D and its physiologically important metabolites in human plasma by high pressure liquid chromatography. *J. Steroid Biochem.* **8**, 929–938.

Lawson, D. E. M., and Wilson, P. W. (1974). Intranuclear localization and receptor proteins for 1,25-dihydroxycholecalciferol in chick intestine. *Biochem. J.* **144**, 573–583.

Mason, R. S., and Posen, S. (1977). Some problems associated with assay of 25-hydroxycalciferol in human serum. *Clin. Chem.* **23**, 806–810.

Offerman, G., and Dittmar, F. (1974). A direct protein-binding assay for 25-hydroxycalciferol. *Horm. Metab. Res.* **6**, 534.

Preece, M. A., O'Riordan, J. L. H., Lawson, D. E. M., and Kodicek, E. (1974). A competitive protein binding assay for 25-hydroxycholecalciferol. *Clin. Chim. Acta* **54**, 235–242.

Rikkers, H., and DeLuca, H. F. (1967). An in vivo study of the carrier proteins of ³H-vitamins D_3 and D_4 in rat serum. *Am. J. Physiol.* **213**, 380–386.

Skinner, R. K., and Wills, M. R. (1977). Serum 25-hydroxyvitamin D Assay: Evaluation of Chromatographic and Non-chromatographic Procedures. *Clin. Chim. Acta* **80**, 543–554.

Sklan, D., Budowski, P., and Katz, M. (1973). Determination of 25-hydroxycholecalciferol by combined thin layer and gas chromatography. *Anal. Biochem.* **56**, 606–609.

Taylor, C. M., Hughes, S. E., and deSilva, P. (1976). Competitive protein binding assay for 24,25-dihydroxycholecalciferol. *Biochem. Biophys. Res. Commun.* **70**, 1243–1249.

Warkany, J., and Mabon, H. E. (1940). Estimation of vitamin D in blood serum II. Level of vitamin D in human blood serums. *Am. J. Dis. Child.* **60**, 606–614.

ADDENDUM

Very recently, two groups of workers have reported success in raising antisera to vitamin D sterols [Clemens, T. L., Hendy, G. N., Graham, R. F., Baggiolini, E. G., Uskokovic, M. R., and O'Riordan, J. L. H. (1978). A radioimmunoassay for 1,25-dihydroxycholecalciferol. *Clin. Sci. Mol. Med.* **54**, 329–332; Schaefer, P. C., Lifschitz, M. D., Fadem, S. Z., and Goldsmith, R. S. (1978). Radioimmunoassay of 1α,25-dihydroxycholecalciferol in patients with renal disease. *Progr. Annu. Meeting Endocr. Soc.*, *60th*. Abstract No. 490].

HORMONES OF THE GASTROINTESTINAL TRACT

22

Gastrin and Related Peptides

BERNARD M. JAFFE AND JOHN H. WALSH

I. INTRODUCTION

Although gastrin was initially described by Edkins (1906), its molecular structure was not elucidated until 1964 (Gregory *et al.*, 1964). The molecular form described was an acidic heptadecapeptide (G-17) with an N-terminal pyroglutamate and a C-terminal amide group (Gregory, 1966). The molecule exists in two forms, one in which the Tyr in position 12 is sulfated, gastrin II (G17-II), and one in which it is not, gastrin I (G17-I). Tracy and Gregory (1964) demonstrated that the C-terminal four amino acid residues (gastrin tetrapeptide) were responsible for the full range of physiologic actions of the parent

455

Methods of Hormone Radioimmunoassay, Second Edition
Copyright © 1979 by Academic Press, Inc.
All rights of reproduction in any form reserved. ISBN 0-12-379260-6

hormone. Since biologic assay systems are not sensitive enough to measure fasting concentrations of gastrin in peripheral serum (Colin-Jones and Lennard-Jones, 1972; Barrett, 1966), the availability of semipurified and purified human and porcine gastrins rapidly stimulated the development of radioimmunoassay systems for gastrin (McGuigan 1968a; Yalow and Berson, 1970a). Recently, it has been discovered that the principal circulating form of gastrin is a larger molecule with a less negative charge (Yalow and Berson, 1970b). This molecular form has been isolated from Zollinger–Ellison tissue (Gregory and Tracy, 1972), and its biologic activity characterized (Walsh *et al.*, 1974). Larger [i.e., big, gastrin (Yalow and Berson, 1972) and component I (Rehfeld, 1972; Rehfeld *et al.*, 1974)] and smaller [i.e., minigastrin (Gregory and Tracy, 1974) and amino-terminal fragment (Dockray and Walsh, 1975)] forms of gastrin have been identified and characterized. The heterogeneity of gastrin enormously complicates the radioimmunoassay measurement of this hormone and necessitates thorough characterization of antibody specificity.

II. METHODS OF RADIOIMMUNOASSAY

A. Development of Antibodies

1. Immunogens and Immunization Schedules

Antibodies to gastrin have been elicited using both pure and semipurified gastrin as immunogens. Jeffcoate (1969) utilized partially purified porcine gastrin (mixture of gastrins I and II) coated onto positively charged latex particles. Yip and Jordan (1970) used semipurified porcine gastrin conjugated to bovine serum albumin.

Yalow and Berson (1970a) used two preparations of semipurified porcine gastrin directly as immunogens, "gastrin A," 0.5% gastrin, and "stage II gastrin," 10% gastrin (Wilson Laboratories, Chicago, Illinois). Either gastrin A (200 mg) or stage II gastrin (10 mg), utilized to immunize three guinea pigs, was dissolved in 1.0 ml of 0.1 M glycine, pH 9.5, and titrated to lower pH with 1.0 ml of 0.25 M phosphate, pH 7.4. The aqueous solutions were emulsified with 2.0 ml of Freund's adjuvant and administered subcutaneously. Immunizations were repeated at monthly intervals and animals were bled 8–12 days later. Sera with anti-gastrin antibodies with affinity suitable for use in the radioimmunoassay were frequently noted after three immunizations, and approximately 40% of the animals responded.

McGuigan (1968a) first described the use as immunogen of synthetic human gastrin I (residues 2–17, Imperial Chemical Industries) conjugated to serum albumin. We have prepared this antigen by initially dissolving 10 mg of 2–17-gastrin in 0.7 ml of N, N-dimethylformamide, and then adding bovine serum albumin, 20.1 mg in 0.7 ml of 0.05 M phosphate buffer, pH 7.4, and a tenfold excess of carbodiimide [1-ethyl-3-(3-diethylaminopropyl) carbodiimide, Ott Chemical Company], 91 mg in 0.5 ml of phosphate. The reaction mixture was stirred at room temperature for 24 hours, during which time it became slightly opalescent. The conjugate was thoroughly dialyzed against 0.15 M NaCl, 0.01 M phosphate, pH 7.4. Since each molecule of 2–17-human gastrin contains five glutamic acid residues, the degree of conjugation has been evaluated by amino acid analysis; an average of 8.5 moles of 2–17-gastrin has been conjugated to each mole of BSA. As described, the conjugation reaction is very consistent, and amino acid analysis of each conjugate is not necessary. A simpler method to follow conjugation is the inclusion of a trace amount of ^{125}I-2–17-gastrin in the initial reaction. An alternate method is to measure absorbance at 280 nm of the reaction mixture before and after dialysis. Using the molar extinction coefficient of gastrin (12,700), one can calculate the amount of gastrin dialyzed off, and the difference represents the amount conjugated (plus a small amount of nondialyzed and unconjugated gastrin).

For immunization, conjugate (5.0 mg/ml) should be emulsified with an equal volume of complete Freund's adjuvant and rabbits are immunized with 2.0 mg of antigen subcutaneously in the foot pads, 0.2 ml per foot pad. Similar immunizations except using incomplete Freund's adjuvant are repeated one and six months later; animals are bled 10–20 days after each injection. Detectable antibodies have been frequently noted after the second immunization, but anti-gastrin antibodies suitable for radioimmunoassay are more consistently obtained after the third immunization. The timing of subsequent immunizations is best judged by following the antibody titers; when titers in an animal decline, reimmunization is suggested. In a modification of this technique, much smaller amounts of antigen, i.e., 50 μg given by multiple intradermal injections, usually result in antibodies after a single immunization.

Although both of these methods result in very similar anti-gastrin antibodies, we suggest the use of conjugated human gastrin as antigen. Its big advantage is its consistency. Of 14 guinea pigs, we have immunized with crude porcine gastrin, only three have produced antibodies, whereas every rabbit immunized with human gastrin conjugated to BSA has yielded antibodies suitable for radioimmunoassay. Although there are theoretical advantages to using 2–17-gastrin rather than the whole molecule for conjugation (the former has a free amino group available for conjugation), since carbodiimide reacts with either carboxyl or amino groups and 2–17-gastrin has six of the former and only one of the latter, in fact, both compounds are equally effective. Rehfeld and associates (1972) have carefully studied the production of antibodies to gastrin and have made very similar observations.

2. Evaluation of Antisera

The optimal titer of antibody is determined by testing serial dilutions of antisera in a series of tubes containing small amounts (1.0–8.0 pg) of labeled gastrin. Tubes are incubated at 4°C for one to three days before separation of bound and free gastrin. The range to be covered can be determined empirically by making a wide range of dilutions. The dilution of the antibody used in the assay may be taken as the dilution at which 50% of label is bound to antibody ($B/F = 1.0$). We suggest preparing prediluted antibody (Millipore-filtered to reduce chances of bacterial contamination) in 0.15 M NaCl containing 2% nonimmune serum from the same species from which the antibody was derived and Merthiolate or sodium azide as a preservative. This solution can be stored for years at 4°C, and aliquots can be diluted further for use in the assay. Concentrated antibodies are stored at $-40°$ to $-70°$C for prolonged storage. Prediluted antibody is made up 50–100 times more concentrated than the final dilution used in the assay incubation.

B. Radioiodination of Gastrin

1. Iodination Techniques

Gastrin is iodinated by a modification of the technique of Hunter and Greenwood (1962). To a small glass test tube are added in sequence 50 μl of 0.25 M phosphate, pH 7.4, 25 μl of a 40 nmole/ml solution of pure human or porcine gastrin I, 10 μl of Na^{125}I, 100 mCi/ml (in NaOH), and 10 μl phosphate buffer containing chloramine-T, 2.0 mg/ml. In order to minimize damage to the peptide, the iodination is terminated within 15 seconds by the addition of 20 μl sodium metabisulfite, 5 mg/ml in phosphate buffer. This formula produces labeled gastrin with a calculated specific activity of 500 mCi/mg. Other specific activities can be obtained by adjusting the ratio of gastrin to iodide.

2. Purification of Labeled Gastrin

The reaction mixtures contain unlabeled gastrin, mono- and diiodinated gastrin, damaged labeled gastrin, free iodide, and the several small molecular components of the incubation. Isolation of usable labeled gastrin has been accomplished using starch gel electrophoresis (Yalow and Berson, 1970a; Smithies, 1959), gel filtration on Sephadex G-10 (McGuigan, 1968a), and ion-exchange chromatography (Stadil and Rehfeld, 1972a).

Starch gel is prepared according to the manufacturer's instructions and allowed to set up in the refrigerator for six to 18 hours prior to use. Each slit in the starch holds 0.04 ml. The reaction mixture is pipetted into one or two slits in the starch. Adjacent slits on either side receive 0.04 ml each of bromphenol blue in phosphate buffer to serve as migration markers. The surface is sealed with paraffin. Electrophoresis is performed at 4°C in a vertical position with the cathode at the top and the anode at the bottom. At a constant voltage, 200–250 V or 15–30 mA, the marker is allowed to migrate two-thirds the length of the gel, usually requiring four to six hours.

The starch gel is removed from the mold and placed on a sheet of Parafilm. Labeled gastrin migrates slightly more anodally than the bromphenol blue marker. Using the marker as a guide, eight to 12 serial 0.5-cm sections are cut anodally starting from the blue markers. Each section is placed in a 16×100 mm glass tube, and is counted. Those sections with the greatest amounts of radioactivity (usually Nos. 2–5) are saved for extraction. The starch fractions are frozen for several hours, after which 1.0–2.0 ml of 0.15 M NaCl is added to each tube, and extraction is performed by mechanically pressing the starch with a 13×100 mm test tube. The solution of ^{125}I-gastrin is poured off, an aliquot is saved for evaluation (Figure 1), and the remainder is frozen.

Gel filtration is performed at 4°C on a 1.0×30 cm column of Sephadex G-10. The reaction mixture is applied to the column and eluted with 0.05 or 0.1 M phosphate, pH 7.4. Fractions (one-milliliter) are collected and 0.01-ml aliquots are sampled and counted. Labeled gastrin emerges in the first peak of radioactivity with the void volume, usually starting at fraction 6. Aliquots of each fraction of the first peak of radioactivity are saved for evaluation, and the remainder is diluted in buffer containing egg albumin, 10 mg/ml, and frozen.

In the ion-exchange technique, we use a preliminary gel filtration step. The reaction mixture is diluted with 0.4 ml 0.25 M phosphate buffer, pH 7.5, and applied to a 1.0×10 cm column of Sephadex G-15. Labeled gastrin is eluted with 0.025 M ammonium bicarbonate (con-

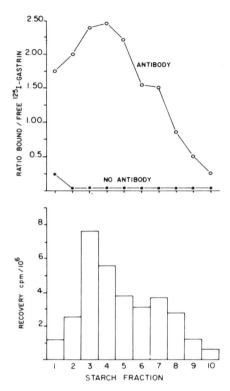

Figure 1.   Typical elution pattern obtained after starch gel electrophoresis of iodination mixture. The origin is the left and is not shown. Fractions (0.5 cm) were cut in anodal direction from leading edge of bromphenol blue marker (fraction 1). In this instance the fractions with highest concentration of radioactivity exhibited optimal binding properties. Iodination at higher specific activity leads to increased size of second peak, probably representing doubly iodinated gastrin, which binds poorly with gastrin antibody. Free iodide migrates off the starch and into the anodal reservoir.

taining 0.2% Plasmatine) in the void volume peak. Aminoethyl-cellulose (AE-41) (Whatman) is prepared according to the instructions of the manufacturer. Thirty grams of AE-41 is washed successively with 1.0 liter water and 500 ml 0.5 M NaOH followed by 1.0 liter water (four times). The pH is adjusted to pH 6.0 with 1.0 M HCl, and the residue is washed with 1.0 liter water four times and then 0.5 M ammonium bicarbonate. The material is stored at 4°C with a few drops of toluene. A 1.0 × 10 cm column is packed with AE-41 resin and equilibrated with 0.05 M ammonium bicarbonate, pH 8.0. After application of the sample, monoiodinated gastrin is eluted using a linear gradient from 0.05 to 0.4 M ammonium bicarbonate (125 ml in each mixing flask). The column is run at 8.0 ml/hour and 1.0-ml fractions are collected. The results of a typical ion-exchange chromatographic

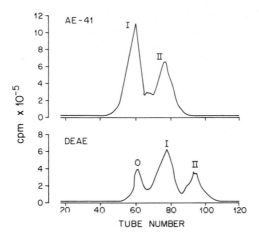

Figure 2. Separation of labeled gastrin components by two different ion-exchange systems. The iodination mixture contained 0.95 nmole natural human G-17-I, 1.0 mCi (0.57 nmole) $Na^{125}I$, 71 nmoles chloramine-T, and 526 nmoles $Na_2O_5S_2$ added sequentially in a final volume of 0.1 ml 0.25 M sodium phosphate buffer, pH 7.4. Labeled gastrin was separated from free iodide by preliminary gel filtration on a 1.0 × 10 cm Sephadex G-10 column; the yield was 36% incorporation. The two peak tubes from G-10 were pooled and rechromatographed on either Whatman AE-41 or DEAE-Sephadex anion exchange columns (top and bottom panels, respectively). The AE-41 column was equilibrated with 0.05 M NH_4HCO_3; the sample was applied at slightly lower ionic concentration. The gradient was developed by pumping 0.5 M NH_4HCO_3 into a 125-ml mixing vessel containing 0.05 M NH_4HCO_3 at 6.0 ml per hour. Pump, mixing vessel, and 1.0 × 10 cm column were arranged into a continuous system. Fractions of 1 ml were collected at 10-minute intervals and analyzed for radioactivity. The DEAE column was treated similarly, except that the starting buffer was 0.02 M NH_4HCO_3 + 0.08 M NaCl, and the gradient was made by adding 0.02 M NH_4HCO_3 + 0.98 M NaCl to a 50-ml mixing vessel. In both systems, unlabeled gastrin eluted before peak I. Autoinhibition studies revealed that peak I from each column was composed of moniodinated gastrin and peak II was composed of diiodinated gastrin. Both forms were fully immunoreactive, but the specific activity of peak II was twice that of peak I. The peak labeled "0" on the DEAE elution profile was not immunoreactive.

purification is illustrated in Figure 2. An alternative method involves the use of DEAE-Sephadex A-25 instead of AE-41. The conditions and technique are similar except that the resin is made up in 1.7 M ammonium bicarbonate and a more concentrated buffer is needed for the gradient, 0.5–20 M ammonium bicarbonate. Monoiodinated gastrin elutes at 0.3 M from AE-41 and at 1.5 M from DEAE-Sephadex. The usual efficiency of iodination is about 30–40% under these conditions.

Ion-exchange chromatography is the best technique. It is relatively rapid and yet separates mono- and diiodinated gastrins. AE-41 is produced in very small quantities and is, therefore, quite difficult to obtain. However, the adaptation of the method to DEAE-Sephadex has obviated this problem. Although starch gel electrophoresis effectively separates mono- and diiodinated gastrins, it is time-consuming and sloppy. Gel filtration is rapid and simple but does not separate gastrin with zero, one, or two iodines; it is useful in situations in which maximal sensitivity is not necessary.

3. Evaluation of Purified Labeled Gastrin

Regardless of how the gastrin was iodinated and purified, three parameters are important: nonspecific binding or damage in the separation system, maximal binding with excess antibody, and specific activity.

Nonspecific binding and maximal binding are determined by overnight incubation of 2000 to 3000 cpm of each fraction of labeled gastrin to be evaluated in duplicate sets of assay tubes. One set contains no antibody, the other contains a tenfold excess of antibody. Antibody-bound and free label are separated as described below. Nonspecific binding is the fraction of radioactivity bound in tubes which contain no antibody; we discard label which shows more than 10% nonspecific binding. Maximal binding varies with the preparation of gastrin used for iodination and the antibody used for testing. We expect a corrected B/F ratio greater than 2.0 (more than 67% bound) in the best fractions (Figure 1). The fractions found suitable for assay may be pooled and diluted appropriately so that each aliquot contains enough counts for a single assay, and frozen in individual tubes to avoid repeated freezing and thawing. A single iodination should suffice for six to eight weeks. Nonspecific binding and maximal binding should be rechecked periodically. Deterioration of either parameter indicates the need for making new label.

Specific activity is not tested routinely for each iodination but should be done several times to define the usual yield and to confirm the immunologic homogeneity of labeled and unlabeled gastrin. This is done by preparing two standard curves (see below). In one curve the counts of labeled gastrin per tube are constant, and doubling concentrations of unlabeled gastrin (preferably the same material used for labeling) are added to a series of tubes over the range appropriate for the antibody used. The other curve is constructed by adding doubling concentrations of radioactive gastrin, starting with the number of counts used in the first curve and ending with a 32- or 64-fold higher radioactivity. Inhibition curves are plotted for each. If binding kinetics are identical for labeled and unlabeled gastrin, the scale can be adjusted so that the additional counts added will produce a curve which superimposes on the curve plotted for concentration of unlabeled gastrin added. The number of counts added per milliliter which equals 1.0 pg/ml or 1.0 fmole (or 10^{-15} mole) per ml can be read directly from the curve. In a gamma counter with 80% efficiency, 600–800 cpm of good labeled gastrin is equivalent to 1.0 pg of unlabeled gastrin. Thus, an incubation mixture containing 4000 cpm per tube contains approximately 6.0 pg of labeled gastrin. A quick estimate of specific activity may be obtained with each batch of labeled gastrin by comparing the inhibition of binding produced with a fourfold excess of labeled gastrin with inhibition produced by unlabeled gastrin. Preparations of low specific activity will cause great inhibition and require the use of less radioactivity or more concentrated antibody in the assay.

C. Standards

Synthetic human gastrin is available from the Imperial Chemical Industries of Britain, but some laboratories have found differences in potency among different vials. Porcine gastrin II and synthetic human gastrin I standards are available from the Medical Research Council of England.

The Center for Ulcer Research and Education, Los Angeles, California, makes available standards of heptadecapeptide gastrins (G17-I and G17-II) as well as big gastrin (G34-I) and minigastrin (G14-I) for calibration of assays.

If possible, it is a good idea to use two or more standard gastrin preparations in each assay as a check for dilution mistakes or losses in potency of a single standard. It is also desirable to have independent confirmation of chemical and biologic potency for each standard used. Chemical potency of pure gastrin on a molar basis can be calculated by measuring absorbance at 280 nm and using the molar extinction coefficient of 12,700. Biologic activity is best determined in dogs with gastric pouches, but this is generally not necessary because gastrin preparations have good correlation between immunoreactivity and biologic activity. Some vials of synthetic human gastrin have been found to have diminished potency in both immunochemical and biologic systems when compared with the molar concentrations as determined by optical density measurements. Use of a standard with low potency will produce artificially elevated results for unknown specimens.

Gastrin is a relatively stable molecule, and frozen solutions are not likely to lose activity, especially if stored at $-40°C$ or colder. There is little tendency for absorption to glass. Gastrin will precipitate at low pH, so solutions should be slightly alkaline. Standards used in radioimmunoassay are much more dilute than those used for radioiodination. Therefore, serial tenfold dilutions of the solution used for iodination may be prepared in aliquots and used repeatedly. We maintain standards of 3.0 to 10 ng/ml (1.6–4.8 pmoles/ml) and dilute further for each assay. Periodically, a vial which is not used routinely should be tested and compared with the usual standard to eliminate the possibility of changing potency or chemical degradation.

D. Incubation Procedure

The radioimmunoassay is performed in duplicate; in addition to the assay tubes, each sample is measured with a damage control tube to which no antibody is added.

When the immunoassay is to be separated with ion-exchange resin, 0.02 M Veronal, pH 8.6, is suitable for the gastrin assay. The buffer should contain 1–2% serum albumin or normal rabbit or guinea pig serum to minimize nonspecific absorption of antibody and peptide to glass.

Sample (0.2 to 0.02 ml) is diluted to a final volume of 1.0 ml with standard diluent, giving final concentrations of 1 : 10 and 1 : 100 in the assay incubation. Standards and other samples which contain high concentrations of gastrin are prediluted before this step. Standard curves are prepared by diluting the gastrin standards to contain 1000, 100, and 10 fmole/ml. Each diluted standard is pipetted in duplicate tubes to contain 0.2, 0.1, 0.05, and 0.02 ml, producing a ten-point curve with two points of overlap. With antibodies of high affinity, 0.2-ml samples of normal serum (1 : 10 final dilution) produce inhibition which falls in the midportion of the curve.

After all standards and unknown samples have been pipetted to a final volume of 1.0 ml, labeled gastrin and antibody are added to the tubes in an additional 1.0 ml volume. Labeled gastrin is diluted in standard diluent to a concentration of approximately 2000–3000 cpm/ml. To each assay tube is added 0.8 ml diluted label plus 0.2 ml of diluted antibody (1 : 10,000–1 : 250,000 final dilution); to each control tube is added 0.8 ml of diluted label and 0.2 ml of standard diluent or similarly diluted preimmunization serum. Tubes are mixed by agitation, sealed, and kept at 4°C for incubation.

If the radioimmunoassay is to be separated with precipitating second antibody, there are some minor modifications in the incubation methodology. Although the Veronal buffer might be satisfactory, we have used phosphate-buffered saline, pH 7.4, containing egg albumin, 2.5–10 mg/ml. In order to form a satisfactory sized precipitate, 1.0–5.0 μg of carrier normal rabbit γ-globulin is added in 0.1 ml. McGuigan and Trudeau (1970) have suggested the importance of inclusion of 0.1

ml of 0.1 M EDTA in the reaction mixture. The final reaction volume (including precipitating antibody) is limited to 1.0 ml.

With many antibodies it is possible to premix label and antibody before addition to the tubes. However, with some antibodies a variable proportion of the antibody-labeled gastrin complex is not completely reversible by addition of excess unlabeled gastrin. Before this procedure is followed, it is essential to test the reversibility of the antigen–antibody reaction by adding excess gastrin to such mixtures at timed intervals.

The optimal incubation time may be determined by preparing a series of tubes which contain label and antibody but no additional unlabeled gastrin. These reaction mixtures are separated at frequent intervals (daily or more frequently). Most uniform results are obtained when the reaction has come to equilibrium, that is when additional incubation produces no further increase in binding. Optimal incubation times for gastrin radioimmunoassay range from one to three days.

E. Separation of Antibody-Bound from Free Labeled Gastrin

A number of techniques have been employed for this step including charcoal (Schrumpf and Sand, 1972; Hansky and Cain, 1969), ethanol precipitation (Jeffcoate, 1969), anion-exchange resin (Yalow and Berson, 1970a), and double antibody precipitation (McGuigan, 1968a; Ganguli and Hunter, 1972). The latter two procedures have been used most frequently and will be described in detail.

Amberlite IRP-58M (Rohm and Haas) is prepared as a suspension by mixing 10 gm resin per 100 ml 0.02 M Veronal buffer and allowed to stand with shaking for at least one hour. Each tube to be separated should contain at least 0.1 ml serum. This can be added immediately before adding resin to each tube which contains less serum. The flask containing resin suspension is stirred vigorously while 0.2 ml of resin is transferred to each reaction tube. Prolonged contact of resin and incubation mixtures can cause some separation of bound hormone from antibody. Therefore, no more than 48 tubes should be separated at a time, and the other tubes should remain in the refrigerator. As soon as the resin has been added, the tubes are agitated briefly and then centrifuged for five to ten minutes in a refrigerated centrifuge. After centrifugation, supernatant solutions are poured off into additional tubes and both the resin pellets and supernatants are counted.

Free labeled gastrin is absorbed by the resin, whereas antibody-bound trace remains in the supernatant.

Serum samples or nonheparinized plasma are suitable for resin separation, as is very lightly heparinized plasma. Excess heparin leads to increased nonspecific binding, probably by competing with gastrin for resin binding sites.

For separation by the double antibody technique (Morgan and Lazarow, 1963) an antibody to species-specific (rabbit) γ-globulin is required. Purified rabbit γ-globulin (Cohn Fraction II, Pentex Corp.) dissolved in saline is emulsified with an equal volume of complete Freund's adjuvant and injected into multiple subcutaneous sites in a goat (2 mg/kg). The goat is bled from the jugular vein three weeks later. Immunizations and bleedings are repeated as necessary. The amount of anti-rabbit γ-globulin (second or precipitating) antibody necessary to bind the rabbit globulin (anti-gastrin antibody) in the assay tubes is determined by quantitative precipitin analysis.

After the radioimmunoassay tubes have incubated 1–2 days, precipitating antibody is added and the assay is left at 4°C an additional 24 hours. After precounting, the assay tubes are centrifuged at 4°C for 15 minutes at 2000 rpm and the supernatants are aspirated. The precipitates which are counted contain goat anti-rabbit γ-globulin bound to rabbit anti-gastrin antibody bound to labeled gastrin.

The use of anion-exchange resin is more rapid, but it precludes the use of over-heparinized plasma, and the resin competes with antibody for free label requiring rapid processing. The double antibody technique is slower, requires inactivation of complement (McGuigan and Trudeau, 1970), and introduces an additional variable, but it is specific, is not generally interfered with by heparin, and, since the precipitates are rather stable, obviates the problem of rapid processing (an entire assay can be taken down at one time).

F. Calculations

Standard curves are prepared by plotting the nonspecific binding blank-corrected B/F ratios or percentage bound on the ordinate and the concentration of gastrin standard per milliliter incubation on the abcissa. Unknown values are read from the curve by finding the concentration of gastrin that produces the B/F ratio, or percentage bound obtained with the specimen. This value is multiplied by the dilution of specimen to derive the concentration of gastrin in the original specimen.

Serum values can be expressed as fmole/ml or as pg/ml. Currently, picogram per milliliter is used with pure gastrin I as the standard. More appropriate, however, is fmole/ml since, as described later, gastrin circulates in multiple forms with varying molecular weights. The conversion factor is fmole/ml $\times$ 2.1 = pg gastrin I/ml, 2.2 for G17-II, 3.8 for G34-I, and 1.8 for G14-I.

III. EVALUATION OF RADIOIMMUNOASSAY DATA

A. Sensitivity and Precision

Many antisera have now been produced which are of sufficient affinity to eliminate the problem of sensitivity from the gastrin assay. When used at optimal dilution with 1.0 pg of labeled gastrin, these antisera are capable of detecting 1.0 pg (or less) of added gastrin. Even at 1 : 10 serum dilutions, serum gastrin can be measured in virtually all subjects, since the minimum fasting gastrin even in gastrectomized patients is seldom less than 20–30 pg/ml (Stern and Walsh, 1973).

Precision, expressed as the coefficient of variation of multiple gastrin determinations in the same serum samples, varies with the part of the dose–response curve covered. It is less at the extremes of high and low gastrin concentrations. In the midportion of the curve, 30–70% inhibition of binding, precision of duplicate samples is approximately 5–10%. For optimal precision, samples containing high gastrin concentrations should be diluted so that they produce inhibition in the most precise portion of the curve.

B. Standardization and Validation

Initial standardization of the gastrin radioimmunoassay should be performed using the English Medical Research Council synthetic human and natural porcine standards as well as by comparing data and standards with other laboratories using the same technique. Validation of measurement using a biologic assay system is not feasible for routine analysis; it is possible only in serum from patients with the Zollinger–Ellison syndrome (Moore *et al.*, 1967; Wilson *et al.*, 1968) in which there are very high levels of circulating gastrin (McGuigan and Trudeau, 1968). However, it is important to validate the assay by measuring dilutions of patients' samples; parallelism between the dilutions of serum and the gastrin standards provides further evidence that the radioimmunoassay is measuring gastrin in the sample.

Table I   Structure of Gastrins and Gastrinlike Peptides

Peptide	Molecular weight	
Human G34-II	3839	(Pyro)Glu-Leu- Gly- Pro- Gln- Gly- His- Pro- Ser-Leu- Val- Ala-
Human G17-II	2178	
Human G17-I	2098	
Human G14-I	1833	
Porcine G17-I	2116	
Sheep G17-I	2023	
Dog G17-I	2058	
CCK–PZ variant	4678	Tyr- Ile-Gln- Gln- Ala- Arg- Lys- Ala- Pro- Ser- Gly- Arg- Val- Ser-Met- Ile- Lys-
CCK–PZ	3918	Lys- Ala- Pro- Ser- Gly- Arg- Val- Ser-Met- Ile- Lys-
CCK–PZ octapeptide	1094	
Caerulein	1352	
Pentagastrin	784	
Tetrapeptide	613	

C. Cross-Reactivity

1. Other Gastrointestinal Hormones

The only hormone in serum that is known to pose any significant cross-reactivity problem is cholecystokinin–pancreozymin (CCK–PZ), which possesses the same C-terminal five amino acid residues as gastrin (Mutt and Jorpes, 1967) (Table I). The degree of cross-reactivity varies considerably among antibodies. Antibodies prepared against C-terminal fragments show a high degree of cross-reactivity (McGuigan, 1968b; Jaffe et al., 1970a). Antibodies prepared against the whole gastrin molecule, conjugated or unconjugated, usually have only slight cross-reactivity, 0.1 to about 4%; in this range, CCK–PZ should not introduce any problem into the measurement of gastrin in serum. Other related peptides (Table I), not known to be present in serum, produce higher degrees of cross-reactivity. These include caerulein (Erspamer et al., 1967; McGuigan, 1969b), the C-terminal octapeptide of CCK–PZ (McGuigan, 1969b), and pentagastrin (McGuigan, 1968b).

2. Species-Specific Gastrin Molecules

The gastrin molecules of humans, pigs, sheep, cows, cats, and dogs have been isolated and characterized. They differ from one another only by one or two amino acid substitutions (Gregory, 1966) (Table I).

```
           1   2    3    4    5    6    7    8    9   10   11   12   13   14   15   16   17
Asp- Pro- Ser- Lys- Lys- Gln- Gly- Pro- Trp-Leu- Glu- Glu- Glu- Glu- Glu- Ala- Tyr- Gly- Trp-Met- Asp- Phe-NH₂
                                                                      SO₃H
          (Pyro) Glu- Gly- Pro- Trp-Leu- Glu- Glu- Glu- Glu- Glu- Ala- Tyr- Gly- Trp-Met- Asp- Phe-NH₂
                                                                      SO₃H
          (Pyro) Glu- Gly- Pro- Trp-Leu- Glu- Glu- Glu- Glu- Glu- Ala- Tyr- Gly- Trp-Met- Asp- Phe-NH₂
                           Trp-Leu- Glu- Glu- Glu- Glu- Glu- Ala- Tyr- Gly- Trp-Met- Asp- Phe-NH₂
          (Pyro) Glu- Gly- Pro- Trp-Met- Glu- Glu- Glu- Glu- Glu- Ala- Tyr- Gly- Trp-Met- Asp- Phe-NH₂
          (Pyro) Glu- Gly- Pro- Trp- Val- Glu- Glu- Glu- Glu- Ala- Ala- Tyr- Gly- Trp-Met- Asp- Phe-NH₂
          (Pyro) Glu- Gly- Pro- Trp-Met- Glu- Glu- Ala- Glu- Glu- Ala- Tyr- Gly- Trp-Met- Asp- Phe-NH₂
Asn-Leu- Gln- Ser-Leu- Asp- Pro- Ser- His- Arg- Ile- Ser- Asp- Arg- Asp- Tyr- Gly- Trp-Met- Asp- Phe-NH₂
                                                                      SO₃H
Asn-Leu- Gln- Ser-Leu- Asp- Pro- Ser- His- Arg- Ile- Ser- Asp- Arg- Asp- Tyr- Met- Gly- Trp-Met- Asp- Phe-NH₂
                                                                      SO₃H
                                              Asp- Tyr- Met- Gly- Trp-Met- Asp- Phe-NH₂
                                                        SO₃H
                              (Pyro)Glu-Gln-Asp- Tyr- Met- Gly- Trp-Met- Asp- Phe-NH₂
                                                        SO₃H
                                                 t-BOC-βAla- Trp-Met- Asp- Phe-NH₂
                                                             Trp-Met- Asp- Phe-NH₂
```

Human and porcine gastrin demonstrate similar immunochemical behavior and vary only slightly in their abilities to inhibit antibody-binding of label (Yalow and Berson, 1970a). There is also significant cross-reactivity between other species of gastrin (McGuigan, 1969a; McGuigan *et al.*, 1970). When working with nonhuman species, the ideal standards would be natural gastrins derived from the same species, but such standards (except porcine) are not generally available. Since these substituted gastrins react in parallel fashion with human (and porcine) gastrin, it is acceptable to express results as human (or porcine) equivalents. With this technique, absolute values may be artificially low, but reflect relative serum gastrin concentrations.

3. Molecular Forms of Gastrin

The various molecular forms in which gastrin circulates complicate the interpretation of radioimmunoassay data. There are two major approaches to dealing with the heterogeneity of gastrin, developing and utilizing antibodies with specificity for various determinants of the gastrin molecule, and chromatographic separation of the different forms of gastrin.

Although gastrins I and II are equally potent stimulants of gastric acid secretion, they are not immunologically identical. Thus, specific antisera appear to preferentially recognize one or the other form, and

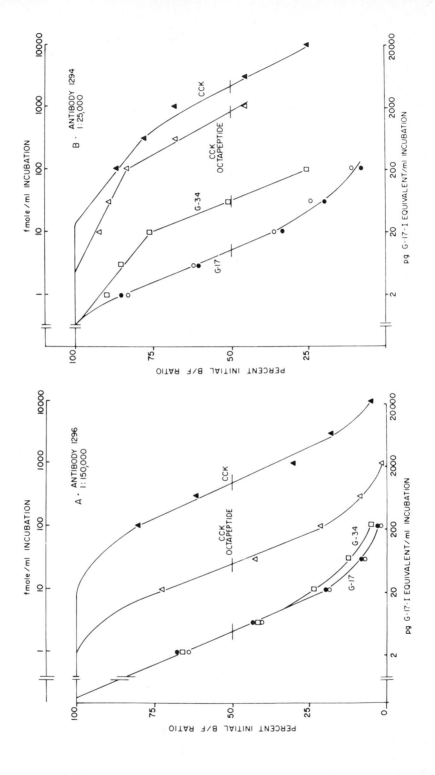

Table II   Relative Inhibitory Potency (Compared with PG 17-I)

Antibody	G17-I	G17-II	G34-I	S-7G17-I	1-13G17-I	Octa CCK
1296	1.00	0.91	1.00	0.80	<0.01	0.08
1295	1.00	1.38	<0.01	<0.01	0.88	<0.01
1294	1.00	1.08	0.18	0.07	0.31	0.01
L6	1.00	1.42	<0.01	<0.01	<0.01	<0.01
1611	1.00	1.05	0.70	0.85	<0.01	0.01

use of such antisera results in gastrin concentrations different from those obtained using antisera that recognize gastrins I and II equally well (Hansky *et al.*, 1973). In addition to the heptadecapeptide form, gastrin is present in tissues (Berson and Yalow, 1971) and serum (Yalow and Berson, 1970b) in a big form, a 33-amino acid molecule which yields the 17-amino acid form upon trypsinization (Gregory and Tracy, 1975), and which also has sulfated and nonsulfated varieties. As illustrated in Figure 3 and summarized in Table II, antibodies vary considerably in their ability to bind big as compared to heptadeca-peptide gastrin. Antibody 1296 recognizes equally all forms of gastrin with intact carboxyl-terminal fragments, and thus measures total gastrin activity. On the other hand, antibodies which react less well with the big form (1294 and, particularly, 1295) give lower values for serum specimens when a 17-amino acid gastrin standard is used, particularly since the big gastrin predominates in the circulation (Yalow and Berson, 1970b) and has a longer circulating half-life (Walsh *et al.*, 1973). Antibody 1925 is directed mainly against the amino-terminal portion of the gastrin molecule; big gastrin does not inhibit the binding of ^{125}I-G17-I, but the 1–13 fragment of G17 displaces bound labeled ligand virtually as well as the intact heptadecapeptide form. Finally, L6 (Dockray and Taylor, 1976) requires both carboxy- and amino-terminal determinants. As a specific anti-heptadecapeptide antibody, it can be used to evaluate the role of G17 in a number of physiologic situations.

Chromatographic separation of the various forms of gastrin is ac-

Figure 3.   Standard curves obtained with two different anti-gastrin rabbit sera for determination of sensitivity and specificity. A, Antibody 1296 (1 : 150,000); B, antibody 1294 (1 : 25,000). Sulfated (PG 17-II) and nonsulfated (PG 17-I) porcine little gastrin, nonsulfated human big gastrin (HG 33-I), natural porcine cholecystokinin (CCK), and the C-terminal octapeptide of CCK (octa-CCK) were evaluated. HG 33-I is equally potent on a molar basis compared with PG 17-I in antibody 1296, but is less potent in antibody 1294. Since G-34 predominates in the circulation, serum gastrin values obtained with antibody 1294 should be lower than those obtained with antibody 1296 if G-17 was utilized as standard.

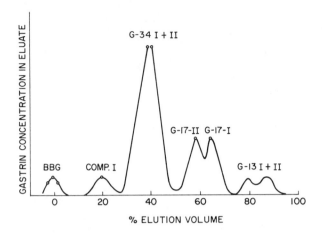

Figure 4. Schematic elution profile showing relative concentration of serum gastrin components (ordinate) after gel filtration on Sephadex G-50. Percent elution volume (abcissa) is measured from protein peak (0%) to salt peak (100%). Individual components are described in the text (Reproduced from Walsh and Grossman, 1975, with permission of the publisher.)

complished on a 1.0×95 cm column of Sephadex G-50 superfine, eluting at 4°C at 15 ml/hour using 0.02 M barbital buffer, pH 8.4. The columns are calibrated with ^{125}I-BSA, ^{125}I-G-17-I, and Na^{125}I. A schematic representation of the elution pattern is displayed in Figure 4. Serum samples can be applied directly. Tissue samples must be extracted prior to chromatography. This is easily done by boiling tissue in water (1 : 100, w/v) for five minutes, centrifuging the extracts at 4°C for five minutes at 3300 g, and chromatographing the supernatants.

D. Levels of Circulating Gastrin

Normal values must be established for each laboratory. They will vary according to the exact methodology, the type and potency of standard, and specificity of the antibody used.

In most laboratories, including our own, normal fasting values range from 20–100 pg/ml when heptadecapeptide gastrin is used as the standard (McGuigan and Trudeau, 1970; Stadil and Rehfeld, 1971; Yalow and Berson, 1970a). The mean fasting gastrin concentrations in normal and duodenal ulcer subjects do not differ significantly (Hansky *et al.*, 1971; Trudeau and McGuigan, 1970). Elevated levels of gastrin have been reported in achlorhydria associated with pernicious anemia and chronic atrophic gastritis (Ganguli *et al.*, 1971; Korman *et al.*, 1971b), chronic renal failure (Korman *et al.*, 1972), short bowel syndrome (Straus *et al.*, 1974), pheochromocytoma (Hayes *et al.*, 1972), vitiligo (Howitz and Rehfeld, 1974), gastric carcinoma (McGuigan and Trudeau, 1973), rheumatoid arthritis (Rooney *et al.*, 1973), hyperparathyroidism (Dent *et al.*, 1972), as well as in patients with the Zollinger–Ellison syndrome (McGuigan and Trudeau, 1968; Jaffe *et al.*, 1972a; Deveney *et al.*, 1977) Gastrin release has been documented following feeding (Jaffe *et al.*, 1972b, 1974; Forrester and Ganguli, 1970), calcium infusion (Reeder *et al.*, 1970), ethanol (Becker *et al.*, 1974), caffeine (Cohen *et al.*, 1974), and vagal stimulation (Jaffe *et al.*, 1970b; Stadil and Rehfeld, 1972b; Korman *et al.*, 1971a).

IV. MEASUREMENT OF GASTRIN TETRAPEPTIDE

Antibodies to the gastrin tetrapeptide (GT) have been readily elicited using GT conjugated to protein carriers (Jaffe *et al.*, 1970a; McGuigan, 1967, 1968c). GT (Cyclo Chemical Company) was conjugated to ribonuclease (RNAsc, Sigma Chemical Company) and bovine serum albumin (BSA) using two different water-soluble carbodiimides [1-ethyl-3-(3-diethylaminopropyl)carbodiimide-HCl (EDC) (Ott Chemical Company) and 1-cyclohexyl-3-morpholinyl-(4)-ethyl carbodiimide metho-*p*-toluene sulfonate, (CMC) (Aldrich Chemical Company)]. Aqueous solutions of carrier protein, 30–80 mg/ml, were adjusted to pH 6.5–7. A 30-fold molar excess of GT in a small volume of *N,N*-dimethylformamide and water was added, after which a threefold molar excess of carbodiimide was added. With constant stirring for 24 hours at room temperature, the initially clear solution developed a precipitate. The reaction mixture was extensively dialyzed against water and lyophilized. The degree of conjugation (moles of peptide per mole of carrier) was determined by (1) change in optical density at 278 nm (E_m = 5910), (2) amino acid analysis, and (3) titration with N-bromosuccinimide in 8.0 M urea titrated to pH 4 with acetic acid (Patchornik *et al.*, 1958). BSA–EDC–GT contained 12 moles of GT per mole of BSA; RNAse–CMC–GT contained four moles of GT per mole of RNAse. Rabbits were immunized with 4.0–6.0 mg of conjugate subcutaneously in complete Freund's adjuvant at zero, one, two, and six months and were bled 10–20 days later. The presence of anti-GT antibodies was confirmed using gel filtration and equilibrium dialysis with ³H-acetyl-GT. Attempts to induce antibodies to highly substituted conjugates of poly-L-lysine and poly-L-glutamic acid were unsuccessful, whereas all 26 rabbits immunized with GT–protein conjugates produced useful antibodies.

An iodinatable GT-containing marker was made by conjugating GT to a random copolymer of glutamic acid, alanine, and tyrosine, 75, 25, and five molar equivalents, respectively (Pilot Chemical Company) (Newton *et al.*, 1970). Since the two carbodiimides cross-react extensively with each other, the immunogen and labeled tracer must be prepared with different carbodiimides. Conjugated as above (Glu-Ala-Tyr)$_n$–EDC–GT had 6 moles of GT per mole of copolymer and (Glu-Ala-Tyr)$_n$–CMC–GT had 3 moles per mole. Conjugates can be radioiodinated by the method of Hunter and Greenwood (1962) to specific activities of 0.75 to 2.5 mCi/μg.

^{125}I-(Glu-Ala-Tyr)$_n$–GT functions as a labeled GT in a radioimmunoassay system. Anti-GT (0.1 ml) diluted 1 : 1000, 0.1 ml Pentex rabbit γ-globulin (10 μg/ml), 6000 cpm ^{125}I-(Glu-Ala-Tyr)$_n$–GT in 0.1 ml, and 0.1 ml containing GT standards (0.05–50 ng) all in phosphate-buffered saline, pH 7.4, containing egg albumin (2.5 mg/ml) are incubated at 4°C for 24 hours. Antibody-bound label is separated from free tracer by the double antibody technique.

This artificial system is capable of detecting less than 60 pg of GT. Depending on the specific antibody used, gastrin is 0.12 to 0.02 times as effective an inhibitor of binding as is GT.

REFERENCES

Barrett, A. M. (1966). Specific stimulation of gastric acid secretion by a pentapeptide derivative of gastrin. *J. Pharm. Pharmacol.* **18**, 633–639.
Becker, H. D., Reeder, D. D., and Thompson, J. C. (1974). Gastrin release by ethanol in man and in dogs. *Ann. Surg.* **179**, 906–909.
Berson, S. A., and Yalow, R. S. (1971). Nature of immunoreactive gastrin extracted from tissues of the gastrointestinal tract. *Gastroenterology* **60**, 215–222.
Cohen, M. M., Debas, H. T., Holubitsky, I. B., and Harrison, R. C. (1974). Caffeine and pentagastrin stimulation of human gastric secretion. *Gastroenterology* **61**, 440–444.
Colin-Jones, D. G., and Lennard-Jones, J. E. (1972). The detection and measurement of circulating gastrin-like activity by bioassay. *Gut* **13**, 88–94.
Dent, R. I., James, J. H., Wang, C., Deftos, L. J., Talamo, R. and Fischer, J. E. (1972). Hyperparathyroidism, gastric acid secretion, and gastrin. *Ann. Surg.* **176**, 360–369.
Deveney, C. W., Deveney, K. S., Jaffe, B. M., Jones, R. S., and Way, L. W. (1977). Use of calcium and secretin in the diagnosis of gastrinoma (Z–E syndrome). *Ann. Intern. Med.* **87**, 680–686.
Dockray, G. J., and Taylor, I. L. (1976). Heptadecapeptide gastrin: Measurement in blood by specific radioimmunoassay. *Gastroenterology* **71**, 971–977.

Dockray, G. J., and Walsh, J. H. (1975). Amino terminal gastrin fragment in serum of Zollinger–Ellison syndrome patients. *Gastroenterology* **68**, 222–230.

Edkins, J. S. (1906). The chemical mechanism of gastric secretion. *J. Physiol. (London)* **34**, 133–144.

Erspamer, V., Bertaccini, G., DeCarlo, G., Endean, R., and Impicciatore, M. (1967). Pharmacological actions of caerulein. *Experientia* **23**, 702–703.

Forrester, J. M., and Ganguli, P. C. (1970). The effects of meat extract (Oxo) on plasma gastrin concentration in human subjects. *J. Physiol. (London)* **211**, 33P–35P.

Ganguli, P. C., and Hunter, W. M. (1972). Radioimmunoassay of gastrin in human plasma. *J. Physiol. (London)* **220**, 499–510.

Ganguli, P. C., Cullen, D. R., and Irvine, W. J. (1971). Radioimmunoassay of plasma gastrin in pernicious anemia, achlorhydria without pernicious anemia, hypochlorhydria, and controls. *Lancet* **1**, 155–158.

Gregory, R. A. (1966). Memorial lecture: The isolation and chemistry of gastrin. *Gastroenterology* **51**, 953–959.

Gregory, R. A., and Tracy, H. J. (1972). Isolation of two "big" gastrins from Zollinger–Ellison tumor tissue. *Lancet* **2**, 797–799.

Gregory, R. A., and Tracy, H. J. (1974). Isolation of two minigastrin from Zollinger–Ellison tumor tissue. *Gut* **15**, 683–685.

Gregory, R. A., and Tracy, H. J. (1975). The chemistry of the gastrins; some recent advances. *In* "Gastrointestinal Hormones" (J. C. Thompson, ed.), pp. 13–24. Univ. of Texas Press, Austin.

Gregory, R. A., Hardy, P. M., Jones, D. S., Kenner, G. W., and Sheppard, R. C. (1964). The antral hormone gastrin. *Nature (London)* **204**, 931–933.

Hansky, J., and Cain, M. D. (1969). Radioimmunoassay of gastrin in human serum. *Lancet* **2**, 1388–1390.

Hansky, J., Korman, M. G., Cowley, D. J., and Baron, J. H. (1971). Serum gastrin in duodenal ulcer. *Gut* **12**, 959–962.

Hansky, J., Soveny, C., and Korman, M. G. (1973). What is immunoreactive gastrin? Studies with two antisera. *Gastroenterology* **64**, 740.

Hayes, J. R., Ardill, J., Kennedy, T. L., Shanks, R. G., and Buchanan, K. D. (1972). Stimulation of gastrin release by catecholamines. *Lancet* **1**, 819–821.

Howitz, J., and Rehfeld, J. F. (1974). Serum-gastrin in vitiligo. *Lancet* **1**, 831–833.

Hunter, W. M., and Greenwood, F. C. (1962). Preparation of iodine-131 labelled human growth hormone of high specific activity. *Nature (London)* **194**, 495–496.

Jaffe, B. M., Newton, W. T., and McGuigan, J. E. (1970a). The effect of carriers on the production of antibodies to the gastrin tetrapeptide. *Immunochemistry* **7**, 715–725.

Jaffe, B. M., McGuigan, J. E., and Newton, W. T. (1970b). Immunochemical measurement of the vagal release of gastrin. *Surgery* **68**, 196–201.

Jaffe, B. M., Peskin, G., and Kaplan, E. L. (1972a). Diagnosis of occult Zollinger–Ellison tumors by gastrin radioimmunoassay. *Cancer* **29**, 694–700.

Jaffe, B. M., Clendinnen, B. G., Clarke, R. J., and Williams, J. A. (1972b). Gastrin response to parietal and selective vagotomies. *Surg. Forum* **23**, 323–324.

Jaffe, B. M., Clendinnen, B. G., Clarke, R. J., and Williams, J. A. (1974). Effect of selective and proximal gastric vagotomy on serum gastrin. *Gastroenterology* **66**, 944–953.

Jeffcoate, S. L. (1969). Radioimmunoassay of gastrin: Specificity of gastrin antisera. *Scand. J. Gastroenterol.* **4**, 457–461.

Korman, M. G., Soveny, C., and Hansky, J. (1971a). Radioimmunoassay of gastrin. *Scand. J. Gastroenterol.* **6**, 71–75.

Korman, M. G., Strickland, R. G., and Hansky, J. (1971b). Serum gastrin in chronic gastritis. *Br. Med. J.* **2**, 16–18.

Korman, M. G., Laver, M. C., and Hansky, J. (1972). Hypergastrinemia in chronic renal failure. *Br. Med. J.* **1**, 209–210.

McGuigan, J. E. (1967). Antibodies to the carboxyl-terminal tetrapeptide of gastrin. *Gastroenterology* **53**, 697–705.

McGuigan, J. E. (1968a). Immunochemical studies with synthetic human gastrin. *Gastroenterology* **54**, 1005–1011.

McGuigan, J. E. (1968b). Antibodies to the C-terminal tetrapeptide of gastrin. *Gastroenterology* **54**, 1012–1017.

McGuigan, J. E. (1968c). Antibodies to the carboxyl-terminal tetrapeptide amide of gastrin in guinea pigs. *J. Lab. Clin. Med.* **71**, 964–970.

McGuigan, J. E. (1969a). Studies of the immunochemical specificity of some antibodies to human gastrin. *Gastroenterology* **56**, 429–438.

McGuigan, J. E. (1969b). Binding of caerulein by antibodies to human gastrin. *Gastroenterology* **56**, 858–861.

McGuigan, J. E., and Trudeau, W. L. (1968). Immunochemical measurement of elevated levels of gastrin in the serum of patients with pancreatic tumors of the Zollinger–Ellison variety. *N. Engl. J. Med.* **278**, 1308–1313.

McGuigan, J. E., and Trudeau, W. L. (1970). Studies with antibodies to gastrin. *Gastroenterology* **58**, 139–150.

McGuigan, J. E., and Trudeau, W. L. (1973). Serum and tissue gastrin concentrations in patients with carcinoma of the stomach. *Gastroenterology* **64**, 22–25.

McGuigan, J. E., Jaffe, B. M., and Newton, W. T. (1970). Immunochemical measurement of endogenous gastrin release. *Gastroenterology* **59**, 499–504.

Moore, F. T., Murat, J. E., Endahl, G. L., Baker, J. L., and Zollinger, R. M. (1967). Diagnosis of ulcerogenic tumor of the pancreas by bioassay. *Am. J. Surg.* **113**, 735–737.

Morgan, C. R., and Lazarow, A. (1963). Immunoassay of insulin: Two antibody system. *Diabetes* **12**, 115–126.

Mutt, V., and Jorpes, J. E. (1967). Isolation of aspartyl-phenylalanine amide from cholecystokinin–pancreozymin. *Biochem. Biophys. Res. Commun.* **26**, 392–397.

Newton, W. T., McGuigan, J. E., and Jaffe, B. M. (1970). Radioimmunoassay of peptides lacking tryosine. *J. Lab. Clin. Med.* **75**, 886–892.

Patchornik, A., Lawson, W. B., and Witkop, B. (1958). Selective cleavage of peptide bonds. II. the tryptophyl bond and the cleavage of glucagon. *J. Am. Chem. Soc.* **80**, 4747.

Reeder, D. D., Jackson, B. M., Ban, J., Clendinnen, B. G., Davidson, W. D., and Thompson, J. C. (1970). Influence of hypercalcemia on gastric secretion and serum gastrin concentrations in man. *Ann. Surg.* **172**, 540–546.

Rehfeld, J. F. (1972). Three components of gastrin in human serum. *Biochim. Biophys. Acta* **285**, 364–372.

Rehfeld, J. F., Stadil, F., and Rubin, B. (1972). Production and evaluation of antibodies for the radioimmunoassay of gastrin. *Scand. J. Clin. Lab. Invest.* **30**, 221–232.

Rehfeld, J. F., Stadil, F., and Vikelsoe, J. (1974). Immunoreactive gastrin components in human serum. *Gut* **15**, 102–111.

Rooney, P. J., Vince, J., Kennedy, A. C., Webb, J. Lee, P., Dick, W. C., Buchanan, K. D., Hayes, J. R., Ardill, J., and O'Connor, F. (1973). Hypergastrinemia in rheumatoid arthritis: Disease or iatrogenesis. *Br. Med. J.* **2**, 752–753.

Schrumpf, E., and Sand, T. (1972). Radioimmunoassay of gastrin with activated charcoal. *Scand. J. Gastroenterol.* **7**, 683–687.

Smithies, O. (1959). Zone electrophoresis in starch gels and its application to studies of serum proteins. *Adv. Protein Chem.* **14**, 65–113.

Stadil, F., and Rehfeld, J. F. (1971). Radioimmunoassay of gastrin in human serum. *Scand. J. Gastroenterol., Suppl.* **9**, 61–65.

Stadil, F. and Rehfeld, J. F. (1972a). Preparation of ^{125}I-labelled synthetic human gastrin I for radioimmunoanalysis. *Scand. J. Clin. Lab. Invest.* **30**, 361–368.

Stadil, F., and Rehfeld, J. F. (1972b). Hypoglycemic response of gastrin in man. *Scand. J. Gastroenterol.* **7**, 509–514.

Stern, D. H., and Walsh, J. H. (1973). Gastrin release in postoperative ulcer patients: evidence for release of duodenal gastrin. *Gastroenterology* **64**, 363–369.

Straus, E., Gerson, C. D., and Yalow, R. S. (1974). Hypersecretion of gastrin associated with the short bowel syndrome. *Gastroenterology* **66**, 175–180.

Tracy, H. J., and Gregory, R. A. (1964). Physiological properties of a series of synthetic peptides structurally related to gastrin. I. *Nature (London)* **204**, 935–938.

Trudeau, W. L., and McGuigan, J. E. (1970). Serum gastrin levels in patients with peptic ulcer disease. *Gastroenterology* **59**, 6–12.

Walsh, J. H., and Grossman, M. I. (1975). Gastrin. *N. Engl. J. Med.* **292**, 1324–1332 and 1377–1384.

Walsh, J. H., Debas, H. T., and Grossman, M. I. (1973). Pure natural big gastrin: biological activity and half-life in the dog. *Gastroenterology* **64**, 873.

Walsh, J. H., Debas, H. T., and Grossman, M. J. (1974). Pure human big gastrin: Immunochemical properties, disappearance half time, and acid stimulating action in dogs. *J. Clin. Invest.* **54**, 477–485.

Wilson, S. D., Mathison, J. A., Schulte, W. J., and Ellison, E. L. (1968). The role of bioassay in the diagnosis of ulcerogenic tumors. *Arch. Surg. (Chicago)* **97**, 437–443.

Yalow, R. S., and Berson, S. A. (1970a). Radioimmunoassay of gastrin. *Gastroenterology* **58**, 1–14.

Yalow, R. S., and Berson, S. A. (1970b). Size and charge distinctions between endogenous human plasma gastrin in peripheral blood and heptadecapeptide gastrin. *Gastroenterology* **58**, 609–615.

Yalow, R. S., and Berson, S. A. (1972). And now "big, big" gastrin. *Biochem. Biophys. Res. Commun.* **48**, 391–395.

Yip, B. S. S. C., and Jordan, P. H., Jr. (1970). Radioimmunoassay of gastrin using antiserum to porcine gastrin. *Proc. Soc. Exp. Biol. Med.* **134**, 380–385.

23

Secretin

GUENTHER BODEN AND ROBERT M. WILSON

I. INTRODUCTION

In 1902, Bayliss and Starling found that a substance capable of stimulating water and bicarbonate secretion from the pancreas was released from the small intestine. They named this substance secretin and postulated that it belonged to a class of substances, which they later called hormones, which were secreted into the bloodstream, exerting their effects at sites distant from their origin. Hence, the discovery of secretin can be considered the beginning of endocrinology.

Although the hormonal activity of secretin has been known for 75 years, elucidation of secretin's chemical nature and physiologic effects has been a slow and difficult process. Purification of porcine secretin was not accomplished until 1961 (Jorpes and Mutt, 1961); the elucidation of its primary amino acid sequence was reported in 1966 (Mutt and Jorpes, 1966) (Figure 1); and the synthesis of the complete 27-amino acid polypeptide was accomplished in 1966 (Bodanszky *et al.*, 1966).

479

Methods of Hormone Radioimmunoassay, Second Edition
Copyright © 1979 by Academic Press, Inc.
All rights of reproduction in any form reserved. ISBN 0-12-379260-6

His – Ser – Asp – Gly – Thr – Phe – Thr – Ser – Glu – Leu – Ser – Arg – Leu – Arg – Asp – Ser – Ala – Arg –
1   2   3   4   5   6   7   8   9   10   11   12   13   14   15   16   17   18

Leu – Gln – Arg – Leu – Leu – Gln – Gly – Leu – Val – NH$_2$
19   20   21   22   23   24   25   26   27

Figure 1. Primary amino acid sequence of secretin.

It has been established that secretin is synthesized and stored in the S cells of the small intestine (Polak *et al.*, 1971). The greatest density of these cells is found in the duodenum, with their concentration decreasing distally along the small bowel. The only established mechanism for release of secretin is intestinal acidification (Boden *et al.*, 1974; Ward and Bloom, 1974; Schaffalitzy de Muckadell *et al.*, 1977), and the only known inhibitor of its release is somatostatin (Boden *et al.*, 1975; Hanssen *et al.*, 1977). Numerous studies have determined the biologic effects of secretin, the most important of which is its ability to stimulate water and bicarbonate secretion from the pancreas. Other effects have been reviewed and include stimulation of water and bicarbonate output by the gallbladder, inhibition of gastrin release and gastrin-stimulated acid release, inhibition of smooth muscle activity in the GI tract, stimulation of insulin release from the pancreas, and lipolysis in adipose tissue (Jorpes and Mutt, 1973). Some of these effects of secretin are physiologic while others may not be.

Until recently secretin could only be measured by bioassay techniques which were relatively nonspecific and which lack the sensitivity necessary for physiologic measurements (Harper, 1967; Heatley, 1968; Jorpes and Mutt, 1966). After pure preparations of secretin were available, the development of a radioimmunoassay became possible; in 1973, Boden and Chey reported an accurate, sensitive, specific, and reproducible radioimmunoassay for secretin. The remainder of this chapter presents the details of this radioimmunoassay, as well as a summary of the present knowledge of the radioimmunologic determination of secretin.

II. METHODS OF RADIOIMMUNOASSAY

A. Preparation of Antibodies

Secretin in different states of purity has been employed to generate antibodies. Young *et al.* (1968) injected crude porcine secretin (Sigma) conjugated to rabbit serum albumin into rabbits. Buchanan *et al.* (1972) used very small amounts (25–90 μg) of either synthetic secretin

(Squibb) absorbed to microfine carbon particles or pure natural secretin (GIH) coupled to egg albumin. Boden and Chey (1973) utilized purified synthetic secretin coupled with carbodiimide to bovine serum albumin in random bred white New Zealand rabbits. Straus *et al.* (1975) injected synthetic human secretin (Schwarz-Mann) coupled to guinea pig albumin into rabbits. Fahrenkrug *et al.* (1976) immunized rabbits with either unconjugated synthetic porcine secretin or with that secretin preparation coupled to bovine serum albumin. The antiserum presently used in this laboratory was prepared by Kolts and McGuigan (1977), who immunized random-bred New Zealand white rabbits with highly purified porcine secretin conjugated to bovine serum albumin. The conjugate was prepared by incubating 525 μg purified natural porcine secretin, 2.0 mg bovine serum albumin, and 50.0 mg 1-ethyl-3-(3-diethylaminopropyl)carbodiimide in 2.0 ml 0.05 M potassium phosphate buffer, pH 7.4. The reactants were stirred for 24 hours at 2°C, and the resultant suspensions were exhaustively dialyzed against phosphate-buffered saline (0.01 M phosphate, pH 7.4, 0.15 M NaCl) at 4°C. The conjugate was emulsified using an equal volume of complete Freund's antigen. The antigen was administered to eight rabbits by foot pad injection (27 μg of secretin/foot pad) at two-month intervals. Antisera were harvested by ear vein bleeding for the first time, two weeks after the third immunization and then two weeks after each subsequent immunization. The presence of antiserum was detected by reacting dilutions of immune serum with radiolabeled secretin. The antiserum which gave the greatest sensitivity is presently used in a final dilution of a $1:1 \times 10^6$.

B. Antibody Characterization

All secretin antisera produced in different laboratories have been described to be specific for secretin. There has been no cross-reactivity with insulin, human gastrin I, 90% pure CCK, glucagon, or GIP. Porcine and avian vasoactive intestinal peptide (VIP) preparations have shown minimal cross-reactivity with secretin antibodies (immunologic potencies: 1:1000 and 1:600, respectively) (Kolts and McGuigan, 1977). The weak cross-reactivity of VIP may represent contamination with trace amounts of secretin or may indicate true cross-reactivity. This uncertainty cannot be resolved until a pure preparation of synthetic VIP again becomes available. However, even a true cross-reactivity of 1:600 would not be of practical importance except in circumstances in which high levels of VIP are encountered, such as in tumors secreting VIP (Said and Faloona, 1975).

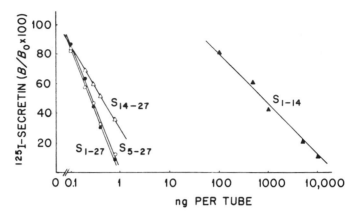

Figure 2. Immunoreactivity of synthetic secretin and three synthetic secretin fragments with the antiserum. Shown are the means of triplicate determinations and the calculated lines of regression. B, precipitated radioactivity in presence of unlabeled secretin. B_0, precipitated radioactivity in absence of unlabeled secretin. (Reproduced from Boden and Chey, 1973, with permission of the publishers.)

The antiserum described by Boden and Chey (1973) has also been evaluated with respect to its binding affinities for several synthetic secretin fragments. Figure 2 shows that the antiserum reacted equally with the complete secretin molecule (S 1–27) and the carboxyterminal tricosapeptide (S 5–27). Its affinity to the carboxyterminal tetradecapeptide (S 14–27) was approximately 50% that of the complete secretin molecule. In comparison, an amino-terminal tetradecapeptide (S 1–14) exhibited only minimal cross-reaction. These observations indicated that the binding sites of this antiserum react predominantly with the carboxy-terminal end of the secretin molecule. Similarly, the Kolts antibody also recognizes the C-terminal portion of the secretin molecule (G. Boden, unpublished data).

C. Preparation of Radioactive Secretin

1. Radioiodination

The radioiodination of secretin, which contains no tyrosine residues, was considered very difficult by many investigators (Berson and Yalow, 1972). There is, however, good evidence that histidine can be iodinated in peptides that are free of tyrosine (Bassiri and Utiger, 1972; Li, 1944; Ramachandran, 1956; Savoie *et al.*, 1973). Indeed,

Pauly (1910) demonstrated that iodine can form sulfite-resistant combinations with the carbon atoms of the imidazole ring of histidine. Young *et al.* (1968) were the first to report successful iodination of pure synthetic secretin, using the conventional chloramine-T method of Hunter and Greenwood (1962). Desbuquois (1974) has demonstrated that when Na^{125}I is incorporated into synthetic secretin, all of the radioactivity can be recovered as iodohistidines. Na^{125}I can be incorporated into secretin using either the chloramine-T method of Hunter and Greenwood or an enzymatic method utilizing lactoperoxidase (Holohan *et al.*, 1973). Additionally, secretin can be radiolabeled by using tyrosine analogs of secretin such as 1-Tyr- or 6-Tyr-secretin. The following section will present the details of these methods and results of their use in our laboratory.

Table I lists sources of secretin that can be iodinated. The pure

Table I   Sources of Secretin

Material	Activity	Source
A. Suitable for iodination		
Synthetic secretin	3.1 CU/μg	Squibb Institute for Medical Research, New Brunswick, New Jersey
Natural porcine secretin	3.5 CU/μg	Professor V. Mutt, GIH Research Laboratory, Karolinska Institutet, Stockholm, Sweden
Synthetic porcine secretin	3.5 CU/μg	Synthesized by H. C. Beyerman, Delft, Netherlands. Available through M. I. Grossman, M.D., Los Angeles, California
6-Tyrosine secretin		Schwarz/Mann, Orangeburg, New York
B. Suitable for use as standard		
Pure natural secretin in cysteine hydrochloride	75 CU/ampule	GIH Research Laboratory, Karolinska Institutet, Stockholm, Sweden
Synthetic secretin in cysteine-HCl (E. R. Squibb & Sons)	3 CU/μg	Available through Dr. G. Kitzes, Bethesda, Maryland. Gastrointestinal Resource of the Digestive Disease Program of the NIAMDD

Table II   Iodination of Secretin with Chloramine-T or Lactoperoxidase

Chloramine-T method	Lactoperoxidase method
1.0 mCi Na^{125}I (0.002 ml)[a]	1.0 mCi Na^{125}I (0.002)[a]
Secretin or 6-Tyr-secretin 1.0 μg/μl in 0.1 N HCl (0.003 ml)	Secretin in 1.0 μg/μl of 0.1 N HCl (0.003 ml)
0.5 M phosphate buffer, pH 7.5 (0.025 ml)	0.5 M phosphate buffer, pH 6.0 (0.100 ml)
Add Chloramine-T (0.6 mg/ml in 0.05 M phosphate buffer) (0.020 ml)	Add lactoperoxidase (50 μg/ml in 0.5 M phosphate buffer) (0.010 ml)
Shake gently for one minute	Add H$_2$O$_2$ (0.86 mM) (0.010 ml)
Add Na metabisulfite (2.4 mg/ml in 0.05 M phosphate buffer) (0.080 ml)	Incubate 15 minutes at 20°C
Add normal human serum (0.100 ml)	Add Na metabisulfite (2.4 mg/ml in 0.5 M phosphate buffer) (0.080 ml)
	Add normal human serum (0.100 ml)

[a] Volume varies slightly with specific activity of Na^{125}I.

synthetic secretin from the Squibb Institute has been used exclusively in this laboratory for iodination. This material is, however, no longer available. The natural secretin from Professor Mutt is equal in all respects to the synthetic secretin from Squibb (Boden *et al.*, 1973).

In the chloramine-T iodination method (Table II), the reagents are mixed in a small conical test tube. After the chloramine-T is added, the reaction is allowed to proceed for one minute and is then stopped by the addition of sodium metabisulfite. Immediately thereafter human serum is added to bind damaged secretin. The lactoperoxidase method is a modification of that described by Holohan *et al.* (1973). Best results were obtained when 5.0 μg of enzyme was used and the incubation was carried out for 15 minutes at room temperature. Results of the three methods of iodination after purification are compared in Table III. Although the specific activity and yield are higher with the lactoperoxidase method, this method has not resulted in any clear-cut advantage with respect to assay sensitivity. The use of 6-Tyr-

Table III   Comparison of Results Obtained with Different Iodination Techniques

Method	Yield[a] (%)	Specific activity (μCi/μg)	% Intact ^{125}I-secretin
Chloramine-T: secretin	44.0	143	12.7
Chloramine-T: 6-tyrosine-secretin	86.6	290	52.3
Lactoperoxidase: secretin	62.5	208	43.6

[a] Percent incorporation of radioactivity into peptide.

secretin also results in a higher yield and specific activity, but its use in the assay has not resulted in greater assay sensitivity. In our hands, and in the experience of others, the use of 6-Tyr-secretin, in fact, yielded inferior results, probably because of the relative impurity of the 6-Tyr-secretin used.

2. Purification

Although Hanssen and Torjesen (1977) and Shaffalitzky de Muck-adell and Fahrenkrug (1976) have purified labeled secretin using gel filtration on Sephadex G-25 columns, in our procedure, the purification of radiolabeled secretin is carried out in two steps using talc tablets and cellulose (Table IV) (Rosselin et al., 1966). This procedure is used regardless of the iodination method. One hundred microliters of the original iodination mixture are added to a talc tablet which has been crushed in a plastic test tube. Intact ^{125}I-secretin is absorbed by the talc; after the talc has been washed with serum and water to remove unreacted Na^{125}I and damaged ^{125}I-secretin, the intact ^{125}I-secretin is eluted from the talc with acetic acid–acetone (0.1 ml glacial acetic acid, 5.9 ml water, 4.0 ml acetone). The eluate is then transferred in a Pasteur pipette to a small column (10 × 7.0 cm) packed with Whatman-CF-1 cellulose powder. (The eluate is gently blown into but not through the cellulose powder.) The column is washed twice with 2.0 ml of 0.05 M phosphate buffer containing 0.5% bovine serum albumin. Labeled intact secretin is eluted from the column with 0.1 N HCl. The eluate is collected in three 1.0-ml fractions; the first is discarded,

Table IV   Two-Step Purification of Radiolabeled Secretin

Talc step
1. Add 100 μl original iodination to crushed talc tablet
2. Add 1.5 ml serum, vortex, centrifuge, discard supernatant
3. Add 1.5 ml distilled H$_2$O, vortex, centrifuge, discard supernatant
4. Add 2.0 ml acetic acid–acetone, vortex, centrifuge, save supernatant
    ↓
Cellulose step
1. Transfer supernatant to column
2. Wash column twice with 0.5 M PO$_4$ buffer containing bovine serum albumin
3. Add 2.0 ml 0.1 N HCl, discard first 1.0 ml collect remainder
4. Add 1.0 ml 0.1 N HCl, collect entire amount

while the second and third are collected and kept separate for assessment of purity.

The purity of radiolabeled secretin can be assessed in several ways. The method used routinely in this laboratory is hydrodynamic flow paper chromatography using Whatman 3 MM or 3 MC paper in $0.075 M$ Veronal buffer, pH 8.6, at room temperature. Fifty microliters of the reaction solution, mixed with 10 μl bromphenol blue (0.8 mg/ml) in 5% bovine serum albumin, is added to $12 \times 1\frac{1}{2}$ inch paper strips. The paper strips are vertically suspended from glass rods into the buffer solution. Intact secretin remains at the origin whereas the damaged ^{125}I-secretin and Na^{125}I move upward with the bromphenol blue marker. To calculate the final purity of the radiolabeled secretin, the paper strips are cut in the middle and both halves are counted separately for radioactivity.

Another method for assessing purity is hydrodynamic flow chromatoelectrophoresis (Yalow and Berson, 1960). Fifty microliters of reaction solution, mixed with 10 μl bromphenol blue containing 5% bovine serum albumin, is added to 14×4 cm strips of Whatman 3 MM paper. Veronal buffer, $0.075 M$, pH 8.6, is added to the chambers of a LKB electrophoresis apparatus. The paper strips, which have been moistened in the buffer, are gently stretched horizontally across the apparatus with each end of the paper strip extending an equal distance into the buffer. The electrophoresis is run for one hour at room temperature with a current of 0.5 mA/cm of paper width. Intact ^{125}I-secretin remains at the origin, while unreacted Na^{125}I and damaged secretin move at different rates toward the anode. At the end of 1 hour the strips are removed and dried. After drying, the strips are cut into 24 0.5-cm strips beginning at a point 2.0 cm behind the origin. Each strip is then counted for radioactivity.

Figure 3 demonstrates the increased purity with each purification step as assessed by chromatoelectrophoresis. Since this procedure separates unreacted Na^{125}I and damaged ^{125}I-secretin, it permits calculation of specific activity and incorporation of radioactivity into intact secretin.

The two outlined procedures are based on the observation that undamaged ^{125}I-secretin binds to cellulose, whereas damaged ^{125}I-secretin and Na^{125}I move freely along the paper strip. A third method more specifically assesses the capacity of the labeled secretin to bind with an excess of anti-secretin antibody. The use of this method is limited by the supply of antibody. The purity of ^{125}I-secretin as assessed by excess antibody binding was usually between 90 and 95%.

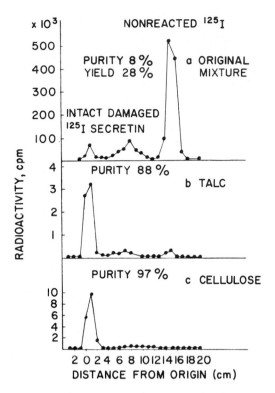

Figure 3. Chromatoelectrophoretograms of an original iodination mixture (a) before purification, (b) after purification by talc, and (c) after purification by a cellulose column.

3. Stability

The purified labeled hormone was found to be stable for at least four days when kept in 0.1 N HCl at 4°C (Boden and Chey, 1973). Holohan *et al.* (1973) have reported that ^{125}I-labeled secretin retained its immunoreactivity for three months if stored in acidified ethanol at −20°C. We found that secretin, as other polypeptides, has a strong tendency to adsorb to glass. As much as 25% of the radiolabeled secretin remained adsorbed to the test tube after a solution of ^{125}I-secretin in phosphate buffer was incubated at 4°C for 30 minutes, decanted, and the test tube rinsed with distilled water. Adsorption was reduced to 10% by incubation in 0.1 N HCl and to 5% when bovine serum albumin (0.5%, w/v) or serum (10%, v/v) was added to the buffer. Several factors have been identified which have a negative effect on the quality of the labeled hormone and on the sensitivity of the radioimmunoassay. These were (1) the use for the iodination of radioactive iodine older than two weeks, (2) the use for the iodination of secretin which had been in solution for more than two to three months, and (3) use for the assay of ^{125}I-secretin which was iodinated more than two to three weeks prior to purification.

D. Preparation of Sample for the Radioimmunoassay

We observed that the immunoreactivity of secretin was lost at a rather rapid rate during incubation in normal human serum at 37°C (Figure 4). The loss can be significantly reduced by incubation at 4°C. These findings confirm the early observations of Greengard *et al.* (1941), who demonstrated that secretin was inactivated by incubation in whole blood, serum, or plasma. Therefore, to keep the loss of endogenous secretin immunoreactivity to a minimum, blood should be collected in iced tubes and subsequent steps carried out at 4°C. Plasma or serum may be used in the assay. When serum is used, the blood is allowed to clot and is centrifuged at 4°C. Fibrin clots when present should be removed and the serum recentrifuged. The use of plasma avoids the problem of fibrin clots. In this case, the blood is collected into iced tubes containing an anticoagulant and the plasma is separated by centrifugation at 4°C. When plasma is used, dextran-coated charcoal should be used for separation of bound from free

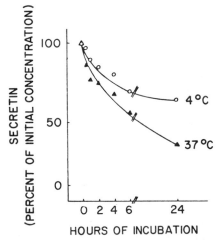

Figure 4. Decrease of serum immunoreactive secretin (IRS) concentration during incubation at 4° and 37°C. Pure porcine secretin was added to three freshly prepared human sera before incubation. IRS was determined in aliquots taken at intervals during the incubation.

^{125}I-secretin, whereas with serum, either the charcoal separation or the double antibody technique may be used. Plasma and serum are stored at $-15°C$ until assayed. No loss of immunoactivity has been observed in several samples kept frozen for over one year.

E. Assay Procedure and Separation Techniques

Table V shows the preparation of standard and test solutions. Standard solutions are prepared to contain 2.0, 5.0, 10, 25, 50, 75, 100, and 200 pg in 1.25 ml of buffer. Microgram amounts (20–50 μg) of GIII secretin (obtained from the GIH Research Laboratory, Karolinska Institutet, Stockholm, Sweden) are weighed on a Cahn electrobalance, dissolved in 0.1 N HCl, and diluted with 0.075 M borate buffer, pH 8.0, containing 0.1% crystalline bovine serum albumin, 0.1% gelatin, Merthiolate (1 : 10,000 w/v), and 2% secretin-free normal rabbit serum

Table V   Reactants and Volumes of the Radioimmunoassay for Secretin

	Standard (ml)	Sample (ml)
Buffer[a]	1.0	1.00
Plasma or serum sample		0.25
Trasylol (1000 KIU)	0.10	0.10
Anti-secretin serum	0.10	0.10
Incubation for three days at 4°C		
Addition of ^{125}I-secretin	0.05	0.05
Incubation for two days at 4°C		
Separation of bound from free ^{125}I-secretin by technique A or B (see below).		

Separation techniques	Volumes (ml)
A. Double antibody separation procedure	
1. Addition of sheep anti-rabbit γ-globulin serum	0.10
(1 : 20) and normal guinea pig serum (1 : 200)	
2. Incubation for 12 hours at 4°C	0.10
3. Centrifugation, decantation, counting	
B. Charcoal separation	
1. Serum (human) is added to standards	0.25
2. Charcoal–dextran mixture is added to all tubes	0.4
3. 1% gelatin in borate buffer, pH 8.0, is added to all tubes	0.1
4. All tubes are then	
a. mixed on a Vortex mixer	
b. incubated at 4°C for 30 minutes	
c. centrifuged at 4°C for 15 minutes, decanted, and counted	

[a] Buffer: 0.075 M borate buffer, pH 8.0, containing 0.1% crystalline bovine serum albumin, 0.1% gelatin, Merthiolate (1 : 10,000, w/v), and 2% secretin-free normal rabbit serum.

(NRS). Secretin-free serum is prepared by passing aged serum through 1×40 cm carboxymethylcellulose columns several times at 37°C. The gelatin, NRS, and albumin are added to prevent absorption of hormone to the test tube, while the Merthiolate is added to prevent bacterial growth.

Test solutions are prepared by adding 0.25 ml of the test samples to 1.0 ml of the borate buffer containing bovine serum albumin, gelatin, Merthiolate, and 2% NRS. All standard and test solutions are prepared in triplicate.

To each tube is added 0.1 ml of rabbit anti-secretin serum (diluted in borate buffer containing bovine serum albumin and Merthiolate, to give a final concentration of $1 : 10^6$) and 0.1 ml Trasylol (1000 KIU). Trasylol (Aprotinin, FBA Pharmaceutical, New York), a kallikrein inhibitor, was shown to reduce to an acceptable minimum the degradation of ^{125}I-secretin by serum (Boden and Chey, 1973). After incubation for three days at 4°C, 0.05 ml of freshly purified ^{125}I-secretin (5–10 pg) is added and the incubation is continued for two more days at 4°C. The three-day preincubation without tracer followed by a two-day incubation with tracer has been found to give optimal sensitivity.

The final step in the assay procedure is the separation of free labeled secretin from antibody-bound ^{125}I-secretin. Previously, this was accomplished in our laboratory by adding a second antibody to rabbit γ-globulin to precipitate the antibody–secretin complex. It was found, however, that postprandial human and canine sera contained factors that interfered with the precipitation of bound ^{125}I-secretin by the second antibody and thus led to spuriously high secretin values. In dogs, the postprandial rise in serum lipids accounted for most of this interference. The problem, however, can be circumvented by use of the dextran-coated charcoal technique (Herbert et al., 1965). The charcoal–dextran mixture is prepared by mixing equal volumes of 1.0% Norit-A charcoal (Fisher Scientific Co.) and 0.5% Dextran-80 in 0.075 M borate buffer (pH 8.0). The mixture is kept in an ice bath and is stirred on a magnetic mixer for at least 15 minutes prior to use. After 0.25 ml of plasma has been added to all tubes not containing plasma, to equalize the protein concentration, 0.4 ml of the charcoal–dextran mixture and 0.1 ml of 1% gelatin in borate buffer, pH 8.0, are added to all tubes. The tubes are then shaken briefly on a Vortex mixer, incubated for 20 minutes at 4°C, and then centrifuged for 10 minutes at 3000 rpm at 4°C. The supernatants are decanted into a separate test tube, and both supernatants and precipitate are counted for radioactivity.

With the use of the charcoal separation technique, the mean fasting

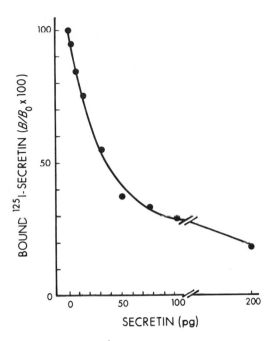

Figure 5. Typical standard curve. B, precipitated radioactivity in presence of un-labeled secretin. B_0, precipitated radioactivity in absence of unlabeled secretin.

level of normal human serum was 37 ± 8 pg/ml. Figure 5 shows a typical standard curve obtained using the described technique.

F. Plasma Problems

It was recently found that some human and all rat sera so far tested contained factors which interfered with binding in the radioim-munoassay and led to spuriously high immunoreactive secretin val-ues. Thus far, we have not identified these factors. The problem, how-ever, can be circumvented. The serum is precipitated with methanol $(1:9, \text{v/v})$, and the supernate is utilized for the radioimmunoassay. We have recently begun to assay all human sera in three different dilutions. Whenever dilution resulted in differing immunoreactive secretin values, the sample was extracted with methanol and the supernate was reassayed. Following this procedure, measured immunoreactive se-cretin values of all sera decreased linearly with dilution.

Hanssen and Torjesen (1977) have similarly utilized methanol ex-traction of plasma. In their technique, 1.8 ml of methanol is added to

1.0 ml of plasma and the mixture is centrifuged. The supernatant is evaporated *in vacuo* and dissolved in 0.5 ml of assay buffer. Schaffalitzky de Muckadell and Fahrenkrug (1977) have extracted plasma with two volumes of absolute ethanol; after centrifugation, the supernatant is evaporated and reconstituted in the original volume of assay buffer.

III. EVALUATION AND VALIDATION OF THE METHOD

The reproducibility of this assay has been previously reported (Boden and Chey, 1973). The intraassay variation was 9%, and the interassay variation was 17%. The sensitivity of this assay utilizing the Kolts antiserum at a $1:1 \times 10^6$ final dilution is presently 2.0 pg/tube or 8.0 pg/ml of plasma. When known amounts of secretin were added to sera, mean recoveries were 86 and 87% after addition of 125 and 250 pg, respectively (Boden and Chey, 1973). An important criterion for specificity is that measured immunoreactive secretin levels decrease linearly with dilution. This was demonstrated for secretin values of several human sera which contained high endogenous hormone levels (Boden and Chey, 1973). Finally, evidence for the physiologic validity of the radioimmunologic measurement of secretin has been provided by the demonstration of severalfold increase in circulating IRS in dogs and man following intraduodenal HCl infusion, presently the only well-established stimulus for the release of secretin (Boden *et al.*, 1974).

ACKNOWLEDGMENTS

Supported by United States Public Health Service Grants AM Ca 19397-01 and 5 M01 RR 349-10, National Institutes of Health, General Clinical Research Centers Branch.

REFERENCES

Bassiri, R. M., and Utiger, R. D. (1972). The preparation and specificity of antibody to thyrotropin releasing hormone. *Endocrinology* 90, 722–727.
Berson, S. A., and Yalow, R. S. (1972). Radioimmunoassay in gastroenterology. *Gastroenterology* 62, 1061–1084.
Bodanszky, M., Ondetti, M. A., Levine, S. D., Marajan, V. L., von Saltza, J. T., Williams, N. J., and Sabo, E. T. (1966). Synthesis of a heptacosapeptide amide with the hormonal activity of secretin. *Chem. Ind. (London)* 42, 1757–1758.

Boden, G., and Chey, W. Y. (1973). Preparation and specificity of antiserum to synthetic secretin and its use in a radioimmunoassay (RIA). *Endocrinology* **92**, 1617–1624.

Boden, G., Dinoso, V., and Owen, O. E. (1973). Immunological comparison of natural and synthetic secretins. *Horm. Metab. Res.* **5**, 237–240.

Boden, G., Essa, N., Owen, O. E., and Reichle, F. A. (1974). Effects of intraduodenal administration of HCl and glucose on circulating immunoreactive secretin and insulin concentrations. *J. Clin. Invest.* **53**, 1185–1193.

Boden, G., Sivitz, M. C., Owen, O. E., Essa-Koumar, N., and Landor, J. H. (1975). Somatostatin suppresses secretin and pancreatic exocrine secretion. *Science* **190**, 163–165.

Buchanan, K. D., Teale, J. D., and Harper, G. (1972). Antibodies to unconjugated synthetic and natural secretins. *Horm. Metab. Res.* **4**, 507.

Desbuquois, B. (1974). The interaction of vasoactive intestinal polypeptide and secretin with liver cell membranes. *Eur. J. Biochem.* **46**, 439–450.

Fahrenkrug, J., Schaffalitzky de Muckadell, O. B., and Rehfeld, J. (1976). Production and evaluation of antibodies for radioimmunoassay of secretin. *Scand. J. Clin. Lab. Invest.* **36**, 281–287.

Greengard, H., Stein, I. F., and Ivy, A. C. (1941). Secretinase in blood serum. *Am. J. Physiol.* **133**, 121–127.

Hanssen, L. E., and Torjesen, P. (1977). Radioimmunoassay of secretin in human plasma. *Scand. J. Gastroenterol.* **12**, 481–488.

Hanssen, L. E., Hanssen, K. F., and Myren, J. (1977). Inhibition of secretin release and pancreatic bicarbonate secretion by somatostatin infusion in man. *Scand. J. Gastroenterol.* **12**, 391–394.

Harper, A. A. (1967). Hormonal control of pancreatic secretion. *Handb. Physiol., Sect. 6: Aliment. Canal* **2**, 972–974.

Heatley, N. G. (1968). The assay of secretin in the rat. *J. Endocrinol.* **42**, 535–547.

Herbert, V., Lau, K., Gottlieb, C. W., and Bleicher, S. J. (1965). Coated charcoal immunoassay of insulin. *J. Clin. Endocrinol. Metab.* **25**, 1375.

Holohan, K. W., Murphy, R. F., Flanagan, R. W. J., Buchanan, K. D., and Elmore, D. T. (1973). Enzymatic iodination of the histidyl residue of secretin: A radioimmunoassay of the hormone. *Biochim. Biophys. Acta* **322**, 178–180.

Hunter, W. M., and Greenwood, F. A. (1962). Preparation of iodine-131 labeled human growth hormone of high specific activity. *Nature (London)* **194**, 495–496.

Jorpes, J. E., and Mutt, V. (1961). On the biological activity and the amino acid composition of secretion. *Acta Chem. Scand.* **15**, 1790–1791.

Jorpes, J. E., and Mutt, V. (1966). On the biological assay of secretin. The reference standard. *Acta Physiol. Scand.* **66**, 316–325.

Jorpes, J. E., and Mutt, V. (1973). "Biological Actions of Gastrointestinal Hormones." *Handb. Exp. Pharmakol.* **34**, 54–133.

Kolts, B. E., and McGuigan, J. E. (1977). Radioimmunoassay measurement of secretin half-life in man. *Gastroenterology* **72**, 55–60.

Li, C. H. (1944). Kinetics of reactions between iodine and histidine. *J. Am. Chem. Soc.* **66**, 225–30.

Mutt, V., and Jorpes, J. E. (1966). Secretin: Isolation and determination of structure. *Proc. Int. Symp. Chem. Nat. Prod.*, Section 2C-3.

Pauly, H. (1910). Uber Jodierte Abkommlinge des Imidazols und des Histidins. *Ber. Dsch. Chem. Ges.* **43**, 2243–2261.

Polak, J., Bloom, S. R., Goulling, I., and Pearse, A. G. G. (1971). Immunofluorescent localization of secretin in the canine duodenum. *Gut* **12**, 605–610.

Ramachandran, L. K. (1956). Protein–iodine interaction. *Chem. Rev.* **56**, 199–218.

Rosselin, G., Assan, R., Yalow, R. S., and Berson, S. D. (1966). Separation of antibody bound and unbound peptide hormones labeled with iodine-131 by talc powder and precipitated silica. *Nature (London)* **212**, 355–358.

Said, S. I., and Faloona, G. R. (1975). Elevated plasma and tissue levels of vasoactive intestinal polypeptide in the watery-diarrhea syndrome due to pancreatic, bronchogenic and other tumors. *N. Engl. J. Med.* **293**, 155–160.

Savoie, J. C., Massin, J. P., and Savoie, F. (1973). Studies on mono and diiodohistidine. *J. Clin. Invest.* **52**, 116–125.

Schaffalitzky de Muckadell, O. B., and Fahrenkrug, J. (1976). Preparation of ^{125}I-labelled synthetic porcine secretin for radioimmunoassay. *Scand. J. Clin. Lab. Invest.* **36**, 661–668.

Schaffalitzky de Muckadell, O. B., and Fahrenkrug, J. (1977). Radioimmunoassay of secretin in plasma. *Scand. J. Clin. Lab. Invest.* **37**, 155–160.

Schaffalitzky de Muckadell, O. B., Fahrenkrug, J., and Holst, J. J. (1977). Plasma secretin concentration and pancreatic exocrine secretion after intravenous secretin or intraduodenal HCl in anesthetized pigs. *Scand. J. Gastroenterol.* **12**, 267–272.

Straus, E., Urbach, H.-J., and Yalow, R. S. (1975). Comparative reactivities of ^{125}I-secretin and ^{125}I-6-tyrosyl secretin with guinea pig and rabbit anti-secretin sera. *Biochem. Biophys. Res. Commun.* **64**, 1036–1040.

Ward, A. S., and Bloom, S. R. (1974). The role of secretin in the inhibition of gastric secretion by intraduodenal acid. *Gut* **15**, 889–897.

Yalow, R. S., and Berson, S. A. (1960). Immunoassay of endogenous plasma insulin in man. *J. Clin. Invest.* **39**, 1157–1175.

Young, J. D., Lazarus, L., Chisholm, D. J., and Atkinson, F. F. V. (1968). Radioimmunoassay of secretin in human sera. *J. Nucl. Med.* **9**, 641–642.

24

Cholecystokinin–Pancreozymin

RICHARD F. HARVEY

I. INTRODUCTION

Cholecystokinin (CCK) was first described half a century ago (Ivy and Oldberg, 1928), and its effect on pancreatic enzyme secretion (pancreozymin) was documented by Harper and his colleagues only a few years later (Harper and Vass, 1941; Harper and Raper, 1943). The slow process of purification of cholecystokinin by Jorpes and Mutt, working in the Karolinska Institutet, Stockholm, has led to most of the recent advances in our understanding of this hormone. Jorpes and Mutt (1966) demonstrated that cholecystokinin and pancreozymin are one and the same substance. The molecule was soon shown to be a 33-amino acid polypeptide, whose biologic activity resides in the C-terminal sequence, where there is a close structural similarity to

495

Methods of Hormone Radioimmunoassay, Second Edition
Copyright © 1979 by Academic Press, Inc.

the corresponding sequence of the gastrin molecule (Mutt and Jorpes, 1968; Jorpes and Mutt, 1973). The availability of increasingly pure cholecystokinin, prepared by Professor Viktor Mutt, has enabled large numbers of physiologic studies to be carried out, and more recently has made it possible to develop radioimmunoassay systems for the measurement of physiologic amounts of cholecystokinin in the body. The methods used have, in general, been the same as those used in the case of gastrin, but some of the problems encountered have proved to be more difficult to overcome.

II. METHODS

A. Production of Antisera

1. Antigens

A variety of different materials are capable of stimulating production of antisera which can bind radioactively labeled cholecystokinin. Apart from preparations of cholecystokinin itself, of varying degrees of purity, synthetic C-terminal fragments of the molecule and a variety of analogs showing some chemical similarity to cholecystokinin have also been shown to be capable of eliciting production of cholecystokinin-binding antibodies. The antigens employed to date and the approximate results obtained with them are summarized in Table I.

Cholecystokinin is widely believed to be a poor immunogen. This is one hypothesis put forth to explain the relative lack of success in radioimmunoassay methods for measurement of this hormone. While it is possible that this may be true, examination of the results summarized in Table I suggests that success in raising antisera may in part be influenced by the purity of the antigen employed. When pure antigens coupled to protein are used, virtually 100% of animals will produce antisera, and if an antibody of suitable affinity and cross-reactivity is produced, these are usually of sufficiently high titer to supply one laboratory for many years. On the other hand, with the various impure cholecystokinin preparations, the success rate is generally only 10–20%, and the antibody titers achieved are usually much lower.

At present, highly purified cholecystokinin is not available in sufficient quantity to be routinely used as an immunogen, and, with the exception of Go *et al.* (1974), most workers have used preparations containing less than 20% cholecystokinin by weight. In our own

Table I   Antibody Production

Antigen	Approximate success rate (%)	Antibody titer	Quality of antibody	References
Very impure CCK (<0.1%)	5	1 : 400	High affinity and specificity	Harvey et al. (1974a)
Impure (5–20%) CCK	10–20	1 : 100– 1 : 1,000	Generally high affinity and specificity	Young et al. (1969a); Reeder et al. (1973); Englert (1973); Harvey et al. (1974a); Rayford et al.) (1975); Thompson et al. (1975)
Impure (50% or more) CCK	10–20	1 : 600– 1 : 10,000	Moderate affinity, good specificity (one antibody porcine-specific)	Go et al. (1971, 1974)
Octapeptide[a]	100	1 : 50,000– 1 : 300,000	Often high affinity usually strong cross-reaction with gastrins	Unpublished data
Dodecapeptide[a]	100	1 : 5,000– 1 : 50,000	Often high affinity usually strong cross-reaction with gastrins	Unpublished data
Tetrapeptide or pentagastrin[a]	100	1 : 500– 1 : 10,000	Often high affinity usually strong cross-reaction with gastrins	McGuigan (1968); Jaffe et al. (1970); Young et al. (1969b); Unpublished data
Gastrin (HG 17-I)[a]	100[b]	Up to 1×10^6	—[b]	Lanciault et al. (1976)

[a] Conjugated to protein prior to injection. This has not always been the case when the whole molecule of cholecystokinin has been used as antigen.

[b] Although gastrin-binding antibodies can be raised in virtually 100% of immunized animals, with suitable technique (Jaffe and Walsh, 1974; Fabri and McGuigan, 1976), only a small proportion (probably <10%) will show sufficient cross-reaction with CCK to allow measurement of plasma cholecystokinin levels: a 1 : 1 cross-reaction on a molar basis is probably the best that can be achieved.

studies (Harvey *et al.*, 1974a), the antibody response to injections of a very impure cholecystokinin preparation (Pancreozymin, The Boots Company, Ltd.) was very poor; only five of 43 animals produced detectable antibodies, only two of which were suitable for use in a radioimmunoassay, and the antibody titers were invariably very low. For these reasons, this cholecystokinin preparation is not recommended for antibody production. Most antisera in published studies have been raised in response to 10–20% pure cholecystokinin (G.I.H. Research Laboratory, Karolinska Institute), but the total numbers published are still very small, since most workers have stopped immunizing new animals when one responded. Thus, Young *et al.* (1969a) produced a usable antiserum in one of five animals, Go *et al.* (1974) in one of six, our group (Harvey *et al.*, 1974a) in one of eight, and Thompson's group (Reeder *et al.*, 1973) in one of eleven. This success rate of approximately 10–20% may well be either an overestimate, because successful workers will naturally be more inclined to publish their results than those who are not so lucky, or an underestimate, because some workers may succeed in producing antisera but fail to recognize the fact because of difficulties with the labeled hormone. Since the success rate is unlikely to be much more than 10–20% when using this cholecystokinin preparation, provision should be made for immunization of at least ten animals in any planned program of antibody production to give a better than even chance of success.

2. Animals

At present, there seems no reason to suppose that one species of animal is more likely to produce antisera than another. While relatively exotic species occasionally have been used to raise antisera, for example, white leghorn chickens (Young *et al.*, 1969b), most workers have successfully employed rabbits, guinea pigs, or sheep (see Table I). In our hands, guinea pigs appeared to be less satisfactory, but this may well have been due to the fact that a very impure antigen was used (Harvey *et al.*, 1974a).

3. Immunization Methods

The best dose route of administration of the antigen and frequency of immunization have not been properly evaluated in the case of cholecystokinin antibodies. However, it seems very probable that, as with gastrin (Fabri and McGuigan, 1976), only small doses of cholecystokinin or its analogs are required to induce antibody formation (i.e., 10–100 μg hapten per animal per injection). Injections into the foot pad are believed by many workers to be generally more likely to induce antibody formation, but in our experience this has not been necessary.

Antibodies to pure analogs of cholecystokinin, such as the C-terminal octapeptide (Squibb Institute), can be produced reliably in the following way. Cholecystokinin octapeptide (5.0 mg) is first coupled to human or bovine serum albumin (5.0 mg) by dissolving each in 3.0 ml 0.05 M phosphate buffer, and adding to the mixture 10–20 mg 1-ethyl-3-(3-diethylaminopropyl) carbodiimide, stirring continuously at room temperature in the dark for 24 hours. The mixture is then dialyzed against deionized water for a further 24 hours, lyophilized, and weighed. It is doubtful whether it is either possible or useful to determine accurately the recovery of octapeptide after the conjugation procedure; in our hands, it has been fairly constant, varying between 60 and 75%. The conjugate is divided into three aliquots, each of which will provide enough for a single immunizing injection of about 200 μg hapten for each of five rabbits. For immunization, the aliquot is taken up into 1.0 ml of normal saline and emulsified with an equal volume of complete Freund's adjuvant, and 200 μl of the emulsion is injected into multiple intradermal sites over the back of each of the five rabbits. The amounts of antigen and the volumes can be varied, depending on the number of animals to be immunized. Using this technique, we have obtained antibodies in 100% of animals after a single immunization, the titer continuing to increase over at least a two month period (Figure 1). As will be apparent from Table I, this pattern of response is probably similar for all of the smaller cholecystokinin fragments and analogs, which are relatively easily available in pure form and injected after conjugation to a protein. Antibody production using these fragments should thus present little difficulty.

It is much more difficult to produce antisera using the whole cholecystokinin molecule as the immunogen than it is when using C-terminal fragments. Multiple injections have almost invariably been required, usually being given at one- to three-monthly intervals, and it may be well over a year from the first injection before antibodies are detected (Young *et al.*, 1969a; Reeder *et al.*, 1973; Harvey *et al.*, 1974a). The reason for using cholecystokinin itself as antigen, as opposed to C-terminal fragments of the molecule, is that although the antisera are much more difficult to produce and are of lower titer, they have been less likely to cross-react with gastrin. A policy decision must, therefore, be made at the outset by workers wishing to raise antisera to cholecystokinin. They may decide either to immunize a relatively small number of animals with an octapeptide–protein conjugate (which should in a short time produce high titer antisera in

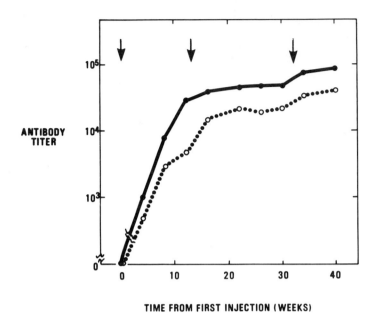

TIME FROM FIRST INJECTION (WEEKS)

Figure 1. Changes in antibody titer in two rabbits, in response to immunizing injections of a CCK octapeptide–human serum albumin conjugate, made as described in the text. Titers adequate for radioimmunoassay are usually obtained after a single injection, but the levels continue to rise for at least three months. Antibody titer is defined here as the reciprocal of the antiserum dilution at which 50% of labeled hormone is bound (B/F ratio = 1.0). The arrows indicate the times at which three immunizing injections were given.

virtually all of the animals, with some cross-reactivity with the various gastrins), or, alternatively, if they require more specific antisera, they must make a much greater investment of time, animals, and antigen with the risk that even this may not produce a suitable antiserum. Schlegel and Raptis (1976) have suggested that N,N'-carbonyl-diimidazole might be a more suitable agent than carbodiimide for coupling labile peptides, such as CCK, to proteins prior to immunization, since it is less likely to denature the peptide. If this suggestion is correct, it may prove possible in the future to avoid some of these problems.

4. Testing for Antiserum Production

Regardless of the immunization policy adopted, the animals must be bled at intervals and the antisera tested. Initially, serial dilutions of antisera are incubated with small amounts of radioactively labeled

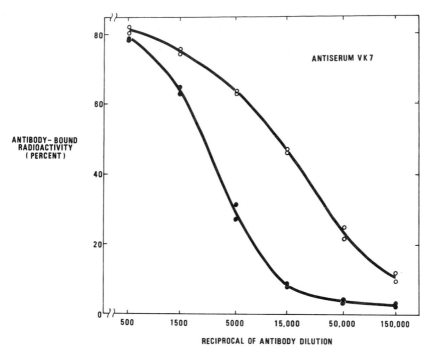

Figure 2. Antibody dilution curve for an antiserum (VK7) obtained after injection of a CCK octapeptide–human serum albumin conjugate, as shown in Fig. 1, incubated in the absence (O——O) or in the presence (●——●) of excess nonradioactive hormone (10 ng per incubation tube). The addition of nonradioactive hormone to the dilution curve is not essential in the case of a high-titer antiserum, as shown here, but may be very important in the case of antisera to cholecystokinin which are of low titer but high affinity.

cholecystokinin for 24–48 hours at 4°C before separation of free from antibody-bound labeled hormone. It is particularly important in the case of cholecystokinin to add excess nonradioactive hormone (e.g., 10 ng per incubation tube) to a dilution curve run at the same time to ensure that a low-titer, high-affinity antiserum is not missed (Figure 2). While one normally would not consider routinely using an antiserum to gastrin that bound less than 20% of labeled gastrin at an antibody dilution of only 1 : 1000, in the case of cholecystokinin antisera, this would be more the rule than the exception, judging by the recent experience of various workers (Young *et al.*, 1969a; Englert, 1973; Harvey *et al.*, 1973; Reeder *et al.*, 1973; Go *et al.*, 1974; Schlegel and Raptis, 1976). All antisera that show binding of labeled hormone, and displacement of labeled hormone by nonradioactive cholecystokinin, should be evaluated further by more detailed studies of affinity, specificity, and suitability for use in an assay system. The undiluted antisera may be stored frozen or may be lyophilized in aliquots of suitable size.

B. Radioiodination of Cholecystokinin

1. Iodination Methods

Production of radioactively labeled cholecystokinin which is sufficiently immunoreactive and stable for use in a radioimmunoassay has proved to be unexpectedly difficult, considering the relative lack of problems with labeling gastrin. Cholecystokinin can be iodinated by various methods, but the techniques used most often have been based on the chloramine-T method (Hunter and Greenwood, 1962), as in the method used in our laboratory, as follows. Forty microliters of Sorensen's phosphate buffer, 0.05 M, pH 7.4, containing 500 ng of highly purified CCK, is placed in a 5.0 × 30 mm glass tube. Radioactive iodine (500 μCi of either ^{125}I or ^{131}I may be used), and 20 μg chloramine-T in 10 μl phosphate buffer, are then added in quick succession, with mixing. After 10–15 seconds, 50 μg sodium metabisulfite in 10 μl phosphate buffer is added, and the reaction mixture is diluted with excess potassium iodide (2.0 M KI in 0.2 ml phosphate). Although several chromatographic columns, including Sephadex G-10 (Young et al., 1969a), Sephadex G-25 (Reeder et al., 1973; Englert, 1973), Bio-Gel P2 (Go et al., 1971), and BioGel P10 (Go et al., 1974) have been used, we have generally then purified the labeled hormone using Sephadex G-15 column chromatography (Figure 3). Sephadex G-15 is better than G-10 at separating a third peak of radioactivity, intermediate between the first peak, immediately after the void volume and the iodide peak. This third peak is often seen, especially after prolonged exposure to chloramine-T; we have regarded it (without any definite evidence) as an iodinated fragment of cholecystokinin, possibly the C-terminal octapeptide (Figure 4). When octapeptide is labeled, most of the peptide-linked radioactivity elutes in the same position as this fraction, a pattern which perhaps would support this hypothesis (Figure 4).

A major problem which we faced initially was to decide whether failure to detect antibodies during immunization might be due to difficulties with the labeled hormone, or a failure to induce antibody formation. This is now less of a problem, since antisera of proved ability to bind labeled cholecystokinin can be exchanged between workers to test their labeled hormone preparations and assay systems.

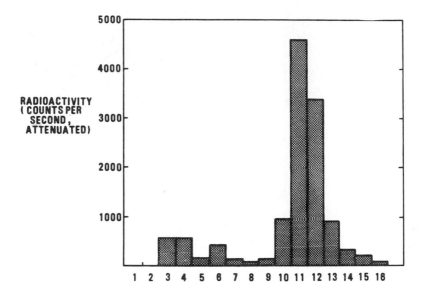

FRACTION NUMBER

Figure 3.   Passage of the iodination mixture through a column of Sephadex G-15 separates the radioactivity into two or three distinct peaks. The first peak corresponds to radioiodinated CCK-33, and elutes immediately after the void volume. The third and largest peak is radioactive iodide. The intermediate peak is not definitely identified, but may be a radioiodinated CCK fragment, possibly the octapeptide, since labeled octapeptide generally elutes in this position (see Figure 4).

In the early stages of our studies with cholecystokinin assays, an alternative method of assessing labeled hormone preparations was used, which depended on the hypothesis that undamaged labeled hormone should bind specifically to receptors in its target tissues. Different fractions of the reaction mixture, eluted from Sephadex G-15 columns, were injected into guinea pigs, which were killed 15 minutes later, and the distribution of radioactivity in different organs measured (Table II). Although too much significance should not be attached to such a crude experiment, the results suggested that the first radioactive fraction to emerge from Sephadex G-15 columns contains radioactive material which is concentrated in target organs for cholecystokinin; this is presumably undamaged labeled hormone. With most antisera, this later proved to be the fraction which bound most strongly and showed greatest displacement by nonradioactive hormone in the radioimmunoassay system. This biologic test system may, therefore, be useful as a preliminary test of labeled cholecystokinin fractions,

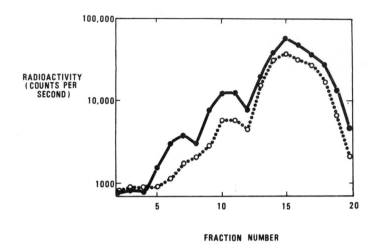

RADIOACTIVITY
(COUNTS PER
SECOND)

FRACTION NUMBER

Figure 4. Pattern of radioactivity in fractions eluted from a Sephadex G15 column after Chloramine-T iodination of CCK-33 or CCK-8. (Note that the scale is logarithmic.) Labeled octapeptide is better separated from iodide on a G-10 column; on G-15 columns it elutes in an intermediate position between labeled cholecystokinin and iodide, in the same fractions as the second peak of radioactivity after labeling of CCK-33.

although the correspondence between immunoreactivity of the labeled hormone with its ability to bind to tissue receptors need not always be as close as seen with our antiserum MS6/72 (for example, if the antiserum employed is directed at a part of the cholecystokinin molecule other than the C-terminus). Other possible methods of iodination include the lactoperoxidase method or the use of Bolton–Hunter reagent [N-succinimidyl-3-(4-hydroxy[3,5-^{125}I] iodophenyl)-

Table II   Distribution of Radioactivity in Different Organs[a]

Fraction	Pancreas	Gall-bladder	Jejunum	Colon	Kidney	Thyroid
3	126.2	72.7	72.7	45.8	98.3	13.9
6	57.4	65.9	48.9	21.8	107.5	25.2
12	32.4	41.6	82.0	71.7	90.2	147.8

[a] Distribution of radioactivity [cpm per milligram of tissue (wet weight) (as a percentage of the radioactivity in the blood at the same time)] for each of three representative eluate fractions. This table shows the results of a single experiment using the eluates shown in Fig. 3 (two guinea pigs used per fraction). Fraction 3 gave highest concentrations of radioactivity in the pancreas and gallbladder, lowest in the thyroid: conversely fraction 12 gave highest concentrations in thyroid, lowest in pancreas and gallbladder. Fraction 6 gave intermediate results. Fraction 3 was thus "CCK-like" in distribution, and fraction 12 "iodine-like."

propionate]. There is no published experience on the use of these two techniques for radioiodination of cholecystokinin. Both methods successfully incorporate radioactive iodine, but the stability of the labeled hormone preparations produced by these means is apparently no better than after chloramine-T iodination, at least in our hands (see below).

2. Stability of Labeled Hormone

When the first radioactive fraction eluted from the Sephadex G-15 column is rechromatographed after storage on another Sephadex G-15 column, various patterns have been seen. After a "bad" iodination, the labeled hormone has been extremely unstable, so that much of the radioactive iodine dissociates and appears as a large peak in the iodide position (Figure 5). Up to 20% of the radioactive iodine may be seen in this second peak within one hour of iodination. Much less rapid rates of deterioration would still preclude use of such labeled hormone in radioimmunoassay systems, and this seems to be a particular problem with labeled cholecystokinin (Berson and Yalow, 1972; Go *et al.,*

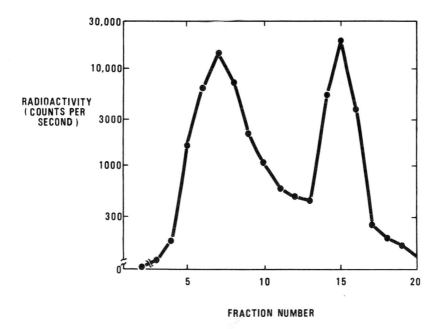

FRACTION NUMBER

Figure 5. Pattern of radioactivity in eluates from a Sephadex G-15 column to which Chloramine-T radioiodinated CCK was applied after storage for 24 hours. A large proportion of the total radioactivity apparently consists of free iodide (second peak) which has spontaneously become detached from the peptide.

1971). The same amount of deiodination has been seen as often after two days' storage of labeled CCK-PZ as after two months' storage of labeled gastrin under the same conditions. With chloramine-T iodinations, there seem to be two different patterns of loss of immunoreactivity, as judged by Sephadex G-15 chromatography patterns. The iodine can simply become dissociated (Figure 5), or there may be apparent fragmentation of the labeled hormone with the appearance of a third peak of radioactivity (Figure 6), which we have presumed to be a fragment of the cholecystokinin molecule, possibly the same one which is often seen after the initial iodination (Figure 4). The extent to which deterioration of labeled cholecystokinin preparations occurs has been quite unpredictable, and in our hands has varied considerably using the same iodination technique. This unpredictable variability in the success of iodination is a well-known phenomenon with the chloramine-T method, whatever hormone is being labeled, but it seems to be more marked in the case of CCK-PZ than other hormones. Various maneuvers have been used to try to reduce spontaneous damage of labeled hormone preparations, including dilution of the labeled peptide in protein-containing buffers and the use of enzyme inhibitors such as Trasylol. Both of these techniques have inhibited spontaneous damage to labeled cholecystokinin (Figure 7). It is interesting that the

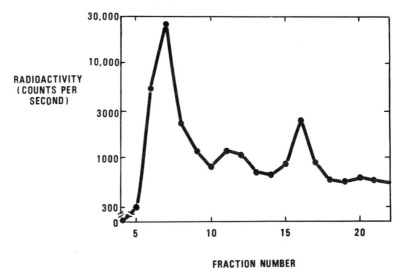

Figure 6. Repurification of labeled cholecystokinin on Sephadex G-15 at 68 hours after a less damaging iodination than in the case of Figure 5, showing the appearance of a third peak of radioactivity between the labeled cholecystokinin peak and the iodine peak.

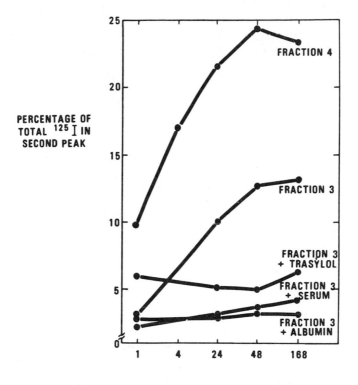

PERCENTAGE OF TOTAL ^{125} I IN SECOND PEAK

FRACTION 4

FRACTION 3

FRACTION 3 + TRASYLOL

FRACTION 3 + SERUM

FRACTION 3 + ALBUMIN

TIME AFTER IODINATION (HOURS)

Figure 7. Patterns of loss of radioactive iodine from labeled CCK under different conditions of storage. The most stable radioiodinated hormone generally elutes first from the column after the initial iodination (Fraction 3, see Figure 3). Later fractions tend to show a varying degree of instability (Fraction 4, see Figure 3), as shown by more rapid loss of iodide. The rate of deiodination is greatest in the first day or two after iodination. Enzyme inhibitors and proteins both appear to protect the labeled hormone from such spontaneous damage, although this effect is variable and unpredictable.

rate of deterioration (as judged by the rate of appearance of free iodide) has been greatest in the period soon after iodination (Figure 7), since this may mean that the labeled hormone contains different populations, some being inherently unstable, but others being much less liable to spontaneous damage. If this were the case, then the labeled hormone might paradoxically perform better in an assay after a period of storage followed by repurification than if used immediately. This seems to be so in the case of iodination with the Bolton–Hunter reagent, as well as when chloramine-T or lactoperoxidase are used. Thus, when labeled cholecystokinin has been repurified soon after iodina-

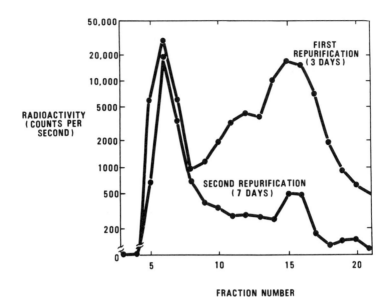

Figure 8. Effect of time on stability of cholecystokinin labeled with iodinated *p*-hydroxyphenylpropionic acid *N*-hydroxysuccinimide ester (Bolton and Hunter, 1973). Labeled hormone was repurified by column chromatography on Sephadex G-15 at three days. At this time a large proportion of the radioactivity had become dissociated, no longer appearing immediately after the void volume. The nature of the later radioactive peaks is uncertain. A further repurification four days later of the first peak obtained at three days showed a much slower rate of loss of radioactivity from the first peak (presumed to be labeled cholecystokinin) during the second period of storage.

tion, damage was shown to be proceeding at a much greater rate than was apparent one week later (Figure 8). It is recommended that workers suspecting that their labeled cholecystokinin preparation is unstable evaluate the time course of spontaneous damage in this way to see whether maneuvers such as prolonged storage followed by repurification may be helpful.

3. Choice of Hormone for Labeling

With any peptide radioimmunoassay, the hormone used for radioiodination should be the purest available. For practical purposes, it is a waste of time to try to set up cholecystokinin assays using 20% pure hormone for radioiodination, particularly now that highly purified CCK preparations are easier to obtain than previously. The effect of using impure hormone for radioiodination was clearly shown by Thompson and his colleagues (Rayford *et al.*, 1975) (Figure 9).

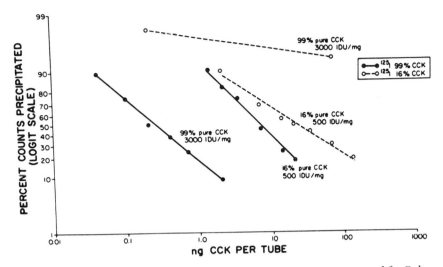

Figure 9. Influence of impurities in the cholecystokinin preparation used for Bolton–Hunter radioiodination on the inhibition curve. Sensitivity is greatest when 99% pure CCK is used for labeling. It is interesting that when 16% pure CCK was used as tracer, highly purified CCK was less immunoreactive than 16% CCK. This suggests that the antiserum used in these studies contained antibodies to other constituents present in 16% pure CCK, and that these other constituents were both radioiodinated and bound by antibody. (Reproduced from Rayford *et al.*, 1975, with permission of the publisher.)

Several biologically active forms of cholecystokinin are available in a relatively pure state, including CCK-variant (CCK-39) and cholecystokinin (CCK-33), both natural porcine forms purified by Professor Viktor Mutt and his colleagues at the Karolinska Institute, and available in limited quantities through the Gastrointestinal Hormone Resource. Synthetic C-terminal fragments are also available in relatively pure form, notably the octapeptide (CCK-8) from the Squibb Institute for Medical Research, New Brunswick, New Jersey. All three forms can be radioiodinated. Since at least two and possibly all three forms exist naturally (Mutt and Jorpes, 1968; Debas and Grossman, 1973; Harvey *et al.*, 1974b; Oliver and Harvey, 1977; Rehfeld, 1978), it is likely that region-specific radioimmunoassays for each form may have to be developed in time so that proper studies of levels of individual cholecystokinin components can be carried out. To some extent, the choice of the labeled preparation will depend on the antiserum with which it is to be used. Thus, C-terminal-reacting antisera should detect all three forms, but N-terminal-reacting antisera may only bind labeled CCK-33 or CCK-39. These problems are discussed more fully later.

C. Incubation and Separation Procedures

1. Conditions of Incubation

It is probably of no great value to give detailed accounts of the incubation and separation procedures involved in an individual radioimmunoassay, since the optimal assay conditions depend to such a great extent on various properties of the antiserum employed. Since it is not possible to influence these properties during the immunization procedure, each individual antiserum needs to be tested in various ways to assess the relative suitability of the different incubation and separation techniques. A large number of factors influence the antigen–antibody reaction, and the effect of each must be tested with individual antisera (Harvey, 1976). Most radioimmunoassays work best at a neutral or slightly alkaline pH (7.0–8.6) in various buffers, particularly phosphate, phosphosaline, Herbert, Tris, or Veronal, usually at molar concentrations varying between 0.1 and 0.01 M. Phosphate-based buffers have generally been used in the various cholecystokinin assays (Young et al., 1969a; Go et al., 1971; Englert, 1973; Reeder et al., 1973; Harvey et al., 1974a), and proteins of some sort (e.g., bovine albumin, egg albumin, rabbit or human serum) have generally been added to minimize adsorption to the assay tubes and to give some protection against spontaneous "damage" to the labeled hormone.

The optimal duration of incubation depends on the rate at which cholecystokinin is bound by the antiserum, but may also be influenced by other factors. Since the labeled preparations are so often unstable, prolonged incubation (e.g., 48–72 hours) is likely to be associated with more damage than with shorter incubation periods (24 hours or less). It may, therefore, be necessary to reach a compromise between achieving the greatest amount of antibody binding and the least amount of damage (as shown generally by increased nonspecific binding and/or flattening of the standard curve with loss of sensitivity). Generally speaking, the incubation is best carried out at 4°C, since this helps to minimize interassay variation.

The exact order and timing of addition of the various components of the incubation mixture may be of considerable importance with some antisera. If the dissociation rate of the cholecystokinin–antibody complex is very slow, the nonradioactive standards and unknown samples should be added to the antibody before the addition of labeled hormone, or the standard curve slope will be very flat, since the incubation period may not be long enough for complete equilibrium to be reached. This situation can easily be tested for by varying the relative times of addition of labeled and unlabeled cholecystokinin. Similarly, the effect of varying the pH, temperature, and ionic composition of the buffer should be tested, together with the effect of additives such as Trasylol or EDTA. Our assay has been performed in a total of 0.3 ml 0.05 M Sorensen's phosphate buffer. We have incubated 0.1 ml ^{131}I-CCK-PZ, antiserum, and either standard CCK-PZ (1.0–10 pg) or serum samples (heated to 100°C for five to ten minutes and the supernatant diluted 1 : 20) for 24–48 hours at 4°C.

2. Separation Methods

A number of different methods have been used for this step, including adsorption with ion-exchange resin [5.0 mg Amberlite CG-400, type II, 200 mesh in 1.0 ml 0.05 M phosphate (Young *et al.*, 1969a; Harvey *et al.*, 1974a)] or dextran-coated charcoal [1.0 ml 0.05 M phosphate containing 5.0 mg Norit OL charcoal and 0.25 mg dextran T70 (Harvey *et al.*, 1974a)], or precipitation of antibody-bound hormone with polyethylene glycol (Go *et al.*, 1974) or ammonium sulfate. To date, the method most commonly used has been a double antibody separation (Englert, 1973; Go *et al.*, 1971; Harvey *et al.*, 1973, 1974a; Reeder *et al.*, 1973), and this has appeared to be the most satisfactory method in our hands. All of the various methods are standard, and have been used in many radioimmunoassays. The choice of method will depend on the nature of the cholecystokinin antibody, the association and dissociation rates of the labeled hormone–antibody complex, and the susceptibility of the reaction to nonspecific interference. Thus, with one antiserum (HO/2/75) to guanosine 3',5'-cyclic monophosphate (cGMP) (Harvey, 1976), we found a dissociation rate so rapid that adsorption methods of separation were unsuitable because of rapid "stripping" of labeled hormone from its complex with the antibody. Since the isotopically labeled cGMP used required liquid scintillation counting, a precipitating technique of separation was rather inconvenient, so Millipore filtration was used for this purpose (Albano *et al.*, 1976). Similarly, one of our cholecystokinin antisera (MS6/72) was rather susceptible to nonspecific interference during the separation procedure, interference which could only be eliminated by the use of a preprecipitated double antibody technique (Harvey *et al.*, 1973). Details of the various methods for separating free from antibody-bound labeled cholecystokinin can be found in the general references at the end of this chapter, and have also been reviewed quite recently (Ratcliffe, 1974).

D. Calculation of Results

Standard dose–response curves (standard curves) are drawn by plotting the percentage of labeled cholecystokinin bound to antibody [or else the bound to free ratio (B/F)] against the amounts of standard hormone added to the various incubation tubes. Unknown samples are incubated under conditions which are as nearly identical as possible to those of the standards (although the limitations of this theoretical goal should be recognized), and their content of cholecystokinin is taken as equivalent to that amount of standard which produces the identical inhibition of antibody binding of labeled hormone. Appropriate calculations are then made to allow for the volume and degree of dilution of the unknown sample. The various pitfalls inherent in these assumptions should be recognized (Harvey, 1976).

E. Standards

No preparation of cholecystokinin of proved stability, purity, and potency is currently available for use as a radioimmunoassay standard, although it is hoped that this situation may change in the near future (World Health Organization Expert Committee on Biological Standardization, 1975). The various pure hormone preparations have been described briefly (Section II,B,3), and one would expect that any of these would prove to be usable as internal standard after it is divided into aliquots and stored frozen or lyophilized until use. It is worrisome, however, that some workers have found considerable variation in the amount of immunoreactivity apparently present in different batches of highly purified hormone (Go et al., 1974), although we have not found this in our studies. Impure preparations of CCK-PZ show gross discrepancies in their content of both biologically and immunologically measured hormone, Boots Pancreozymin being much more potent than expected when compared with Karolinska Institute CCK-PZ (Oliver and Harvey, 1977). It is clear that only the provision of a fully evaluated standard preparation can resolve doubts about the quality of standards used in different laboratories. Since cholecystokinin, like gastrin, is heterogeneous, a series of standards analogous to the CURE gastrin standards (available from J. H. Walsh and M. I. Grossman, Veterans Administration Center, Los Angeles, California) will probably be required eventually. In the meanwhile, all workers reporting results of CCK radioimmunoassays should be encouraged to quote the source and batch number of the standard they used, to facilitate comparison between laboratories.

III. EVALUATION OF THE RADIOIMMUNOASSAY

A. Initial Validation

The demonstration that an antibody has been obtained which can bind isotopically labeled cholecystokinin, and that such binding is inhibited by nonradioactive hormone in a dose-dependent manner, is only the first step in the development of a suitable radioimmunoassay. Undoubtedly, many of the odd results obtained with radioimmunoassays in early stages of development are due to neglect of the various validating procedures which must be undertaken after this stage (Harvey, 1976). A large amount of data is required before an assay can be regarded as properly characterized, and various recommendations as to what is necessary have been made (*Journal of Endocrinology*, 1974; World Health Organization, 1975). In the present state of knowledge of cholecystokinin, it is not always possible to satisfy such criteria fully, but a number of tests can easily be carried out, and the results should be reported when any new assay system is described.

1. Recovery Tests

The assay should be able to measure accurately various amounts of hormone added to unknown samples. This is seldom a problem when assays are carried out in buffer solutions alone, but plasma, serum, and tissue extracts may all contain substances which interfere in the assay in some way (e.g., by inhibiting antibody binding of the labeled hormone). An extension of this test is to inject or infuse the hormone into a subject and use the assay to measure the blood levels achieved. These levels should not differ greatly from those expected. These have been performed with our radioimmunoassay techniques. Recovery has varied from 93.8 to 110%.

2. Parallelism

Serial dilutions of cholecystokinin-containing biologic samples (e.g., jejunal mucosal extracts, postprandial plasmas, or sera) should produce inhibition curves parallel with that obtained with standard amounts of hormone (standard curve). Logit/log transformation of the data is usually required for statistical handling of the data, although, with experience, reading of the curves by eye is probably sufficient for preliminary screening. Parallelism should be demonstrable over at least two orders of magnitude.

3. Biologic Situations

Some of the cholecystokinin assays described are barely capable of detecting significant elevations in plasma levels after a mixed meal. While this might be taken as evidence that cholecystokinin is not significantly released after food, it is more probable that something is wrong with such assays. An assay which cannot detect appropriate changes in cholecystokinin levels when the biologic action of the hormone is apparent should be regarded with some suspicion.

B. Sensitivity

The potential sensitivity of a radioimmunoassay depends on the affinity of the antigen–antibody reaction. This is an inherent property of the antibody and cannot be altered. A low-affinity antibody will never be capable of achieving a high degree of sensitivity in an assay, whatever manipulations may be carried out. High-affinity antisera

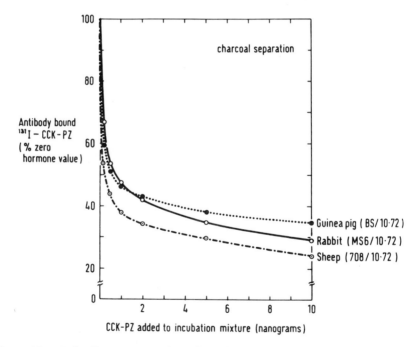

Figure 10. High-affinity antisera from three different species, showing the very steep initial slope of the standard curve. Each of these antisera could detect approximately 5.0 pg/ml of cholecystokinin in the unknown sample. (From Harvey *et al.*, 1974a, with permission of the publisher.)

have a high value for the equilibrium constant (K value); for peptide hormones, this is usually greater than 10^8 liters/mole. The K value can be calculated from a Scatchard plot, which will also show the degree of homogeneity of the antiserum. It is not necessary to calculate the K value in order to get an idea of the assay sensitivity, since this can be tested directly by finding the smallest amount of added cholecystokinin to produce a significant inhibition of antibody binding of the labeled hormone. With high-affinity antisera, a very steep initial slope of the standard curve is seen, and such antisera have been produced in various species of immunized animals (Figure 10). The degree of sensitivity required of a cholecystokinin antiserum will depend on the purpose for which it is to be used. For plasma or serum samples, a high degree of sensitivity is required, as normal levels averaged 60.4 pg/ml. Thus, even with our most sensitive assay, fasting serum cholecystokinin levels were undetectable (<5.0 pg/ml) in about one in four normal subjects. For studies with tissue extracts, a much lower degree of sensitivity would be perfectly acceptable. Assay sensitivity can be increased to a limited extent by dilution of the ingredients and by use of smaller amounts of antibody and labeled hormone.

C. Specificity

1. Species Specificity

Since all the varieties of cholecystokinin at present available are porcine in origin, all radioimmunoassays measure porcine hormone. Go *et al.* (1971) had the misfortune to develop a radioimmunoassay for porcine cholecystokinin which did not react with the human hormone; the antiserum employed presumably was directed against a part of the molecule where the two cholecystokinins are structurally different. Such problems are probably less likely with antisera reacting with the C-terminal (biologically active) end of the cholecystokinin molecule; since the porcine hormone is biologically active in man, the porcine and human hormones are probably structurally similar at the C-terminus. Failure to detect elevation in plasma cholecystokinin levels after food in man (as previously discussed) might be due to the use of antisera which react poorly with human CCK. It should be possible to assess this further, as Go and his colleagues (1971) did, by showing that a food-related rise in plasma levels can be detected in the pig but not in man, and that hormone can be measured in jejunal mucosa of the pig but not of man, and by demonstrating that the antiserum is not

C-terminal reacting (e.g., cannot measure C-terminal octapeptide of cholecystokinin).

2. *Biologic Activity*

One of the greatest limitations of hormone radioimmunoassays is that it is not possible to be certain that measured immunoreactivity corresponds with biologic activity. This has been a major problem since radioimmunoassays were first introduced (Bangham and Cotes, 1974; Odell and Ross, 1971; Yalow and Berson, 1960, 1971). In the case of cholecystokinin, several potential bioassay methods are available which may be sensitive enough to measure physiologic levels of the hormone in blood. We have used the superfused rabbit gallbladder method (Berry and Flower, 1971; Johnson and McDermott, 1973; Johnson *et al.*, 1975; Rey *et al.*, 1977) as a bioassay method to attempt to check our radioimmunoassay findings. Figure 11 shows an early study in which the two methods were compared to check our finding of raised fasting cholecystokinin levels in patients with pancreatic exocrine deficiency. The bioassay has a high blank effect, as most such assays do, so the comparison is not absolute. Nevertheless, these data seemed to confirm that the elevated levels of "CCK-like immunoreactivity" in such patients consist of biologically active hormone. Other biologic methods could probably be adapted for this purpose, in particular, measurement of ^{45}Ca efflux from primed isolated

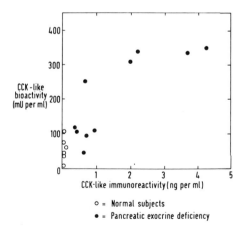

Figure 11. Comparison of CCK-like bioactivity with CCK-like immunoreactivity in fasting serum samples from six control subjects and ten patients with pancreatic disease. Despite the high blank on the bioassay, the difference in CCK-like bioactivity between the groups is significant ($p < 0.01$).

pancreatic acinar cells (Gardner *et al.*, 1975) or else a cytochemical microbioassay method (Chayen *et al.*, 1974), both of which are capable of a high degree of sensitivity. Until the cholecystokinin radioimmunoassay methods have become considerably more refined than they are at present, there will be a continuing need for some sort of sensitive *in vitro* bioassay method to check the radioimmunoassay findings.

3. Molecular Forms of Cholecystokinin

At least two types of cholecystokinin can be extracted from the intestinal mucosa of the pig (Mutt and Jorpes, 1968). These have now been chemically characterized (Table III). Cholecystokinin itself is a 33 amino acid peptide (CCK-33), and the other type, named CCK-variant, differs by the addition of a further 6-amino acid sequence on the N-terminal end, giving a total length of the peptide chain of 39 amino acids (CCK-39). In boiled extracts, separated by passage down a 50–100 cm column of Sephadex G-50, immunoreactivity using a C-terminal-reacting antiserum is separated into three distinct peaks (Figure 12). Two of these peaks correspond in position to cholecystokinin and CCK-variant; the third has not yet been identified with certainly, but is presumably a small C-terminal fragment, possibly the octapeptide (Harvey *et al.*, 1974b). Recently, both the carboxyl-terminal octapeptide and intact immunoreactive CCK-PZ have been identified in the brain of several species (Dockray, 1976; Muller *et al.*, 1977). It is possible that other molecular forms of cholecystokinin are also present in the body, and this would make interpretation of radioimmunoassay results very difficult. The different forms of cholecystokinin may be expected to show patterns of biologic activity similar to those seen with gastrin; the smaller forms are biologically more active on a weight basis, but will probably turn out to have a shorter half-life in blood and a shorter duration of action. It is possible to convert larger to smaller forms *in vitro* (Figure 13), but it is not known whether such conversion takes place *in vivo*. The presence of molecular forms of cholecystokinin that will probably differ in their immunoreactivity with different antisera, and also in their biologic activities, means that in time specific assays for each form may be required. This would probably only be possible by using several region-specific antisera, and different preparations of labeled hormone and hormone fragments. CCK-33, CCK-39, and CCK-8 are all available, and a start in this direction can be made by testing the immunoreactivity of each of these cholecystokinins in any new CCK-PZ radioimmunoassay.

Table III Structures of the Cholecystokinin–Gastrin Family[a]

Cholecystokinin variant (CCK-39)	Tyr-Ile-Glu-Ala-Arg-Lys-Ala-Pro-Ser-Gly-Arg-Val-Ser-Met-Ile-Lys-Asn-Leu-Gln-Ser-Leu-Asp-Pro-Ser-His-Arg-Ile-Ser-Asp-Arg-Asp-Tyr(SO₃H)-Met-Gly-Trp-Met-Asp-Phe-NH₂
Cholecystokin (CCK-33)	Lys-Ala-Pro-Ser-Gly-Arg-Val-Ser-Met-Ile-Lys-Asn-Leu-Gln-Ser-Leu-Asp-Pro-Ser-His-Arg-Ile-Ser-Asp-Arg-Asp-Tyr(SO₃H)-Met-Gly-Trp-Met-Asp-Phe-NH₂
Caerulein	Glp-Gln-Asp-Tyr(SO₃H)-Thr-Gly-Trp-Met-Asp-Phe-NH₂
Octapeptide (CCK-8)	Asp-Tyr(SO₃H)-Met-Gly-Trp-Met-Asp-Phe-NH₂
Tetrapeptide (?"tiny gastrin")	Trp-Met-Asp-Phe-NH₂
Minigastrin (G-14 II)	Trp-Leu-Glu-Glu-Glu-Ala-Try(SO₃H)-Gly-Trp-Met-Asp-Phe-NH₂
Little gastrin (G-17 II)	Glp-Gly-Pro-Trp-Leu-Glu-Glu-Glu-Glu-Glu-Ala-Tyr(SO₃H)-Gly-Trp-Met-Asp-Phe-NH₂
Big gastrin (G-34 II)	Glp-Leu-Gly-Pro-Gln-Gly-His-Pro-Ser-Leu-Val-Ala-Asp-Pro-Ser-Lys-Lys-Gln-Gly-Pro-Trp-Leu-Glu-Glu-Glu-Glu-Glu-Ala-Tyr(SO₃H)-Gly-Trp-Met-Asp-Phe-NH₂

[a] The structures given are for porcine hormone in the case of CCK, and human in the case of gastrin. Gastrins exist in two forms, I and II. In form I the C-terminal tyrosine has no SO₃H attached. The N-terminal amino acid of caerulein, G-17, and G-34 is pyroglutamyl (Glp).

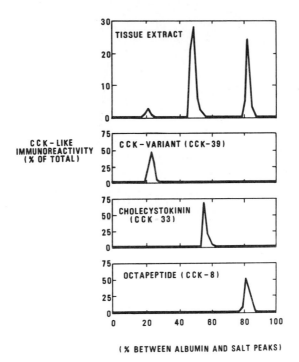

Figure 12. Patterns of CCK-like immunoreactivity obtained when different cholecystokinin preparations were eluted through a Sephadex G-50 column. Upper panel: extract obtained by boiling jejunal mucosa. Immunoreactivity separates into three distinct peaks. These peaks correspond in position to pure preparations of cholecystokinin and CCK-variant (courtesy of Professor Viktor Mutt) and of C-terminal octapeptide (courtesy of Dr. Miguel Ondetti), as shown in the lower panels. CCK-like immunoreactivity in each case was measured by a C-terminal-reacting antiserum. Absolute amounts of each fraction present in the tissue extract cannot be given, since suitable standards are not available, and in any case, the extraction procedure used may well have altered the relative proportions of the different peptides.

4. Cross-Reactivity with the Gastrins

Of the known hormones present in man, only the gastrin family [because of structural similarities of the C-terminal sequence (see Table III)] are likely to show immunologic cross-reactivity with cholecystokinin and thereby interfere in the cholecystokinin radioimmunoassay. This is a common problem with C-terminal-reacting antisera (see Table I), so the effect of different gastrins should always be tested for (for example, by using the CURE standards for HG 17-I, HG 17-II, HG 14-I, and HG 34-I). A small degree of cross-reactivity (e.g., 1 : 1000) can probably be tolerated, but

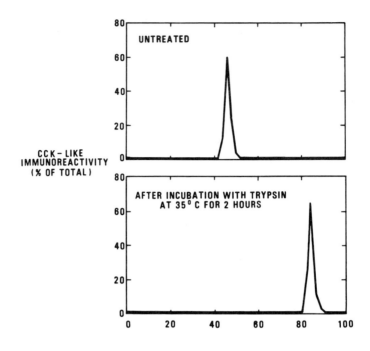

VOLUME ELUTED (% BETWEEN ALBUMIN AND SALT PEAKS)

Figure 13.   Alteration of elution pattern of cholecystokinin by incubation with trypsin. The peak which appears lower panel elutes in a similar position to octapeptide and the third peak in the tissue extract (Figure 12), and is probably octapeptide or a mixture of octapeptide and C-terminal dodecapeptide.

if a more specific antiserum is not available, greater degrees of cross-reactivity by gastrins in the cholecystokinin assay should be corrected for by measuring the gastrin content of the unknown samples and sub-tracting the appropriate amount from the measured cholecystokinin level. This is neither particularly satisfactory nor accurate, since it is improbable that the different molecular forms of gastrin would react similarly in the two assays. Thus, for example, minigastrin (G-14) might react more strongly than little gastrin (G-17) in the cholecysto-kinin assay, but less strongly than G-17 in the gastrin assay; in these circumstances, accurate correction might be very difficult, unless the exact amounts of all the different gastrins in the sample were known, information which is not obtainable with currently available methods.

5. Measurement of Cholecystokinin with a Gastrin Assay

In certain circumstances, immunologic cross-reaction of gastrin with cholecystokinin might be regarded as a useful property for an antiserum to possess. Some gastrin antisera and gastrin assays which show sufficient cross-reactivity can be used to measure cholecystokinin levels (Figure 14), but appropriate corrections must be carefully made to allow for the gastrin content of the samples (Dockray, 1976).

D. Precision

Intraassay and interassay variation should be measured. It should be recognized that even the best radioimmunoassays in the most experi-

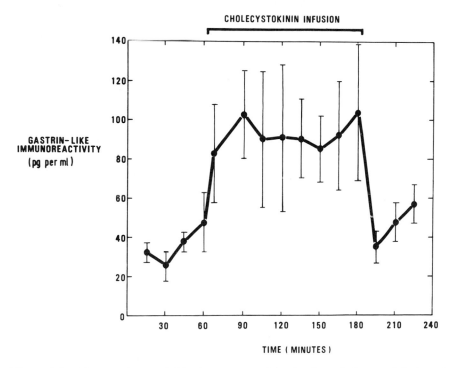

Figure 14. Changes in gastrinlike immunoreactivity in dogs during an infusion of cholecystokinin. The authors were unable to explain these findings and suggest that either the cholecystokinin preparation they used contained gastrin, or else endogenous gastrin was released by an unidentified substance present in it. However, the antiserum used in this study to measure gastrin showed strong cross-reaction with cholecystokinin (about 1 : 4 on a molar basis), and it can be calculated that, when using such an antiserum, a rise in gastrinlike immunoreactivity of the order observed could be produced by cross-reaction alone. (Data from Lanciault *et al.*, 1976.)

enced hands show a degree of inter- and intraassay laboratory variations which can be surprisingly marked (Cotes *et al.*, 1969; Harvey, 1976).

IV. RESULTS OBTAINED WITH CHOLECYSTOKININ RADIOIMMUNOASSAYS

Cholecystokinin-pancreozymin radioimmunoassays are still at such an early stage of development that most have only been reported as preliminary communications (Young *et al.*, 1969a; Harvey *et al.*, 1973), or in abstract form (Englert, 1973; Go *et al.*, 1974; Del Mazo *et al.*, 1976), and only five groups have described their studies in any detail (Go *et al.*, Go and Reilly, 1975; Reeder *et al.*, 1973; Thompson *et al.*, 1975; Rayford *et al.*, 1975; Harvey *et al.*, 1974a, Schlegel *et al.*, 1977a; Rehfeld, 1978).

Endogenous release of immunoreactive CCK-PZ has been demonstrated in response to a variety of stimuli, including normal mixed meals, carbohydrate or amino acid solutions, magnesium sulfate, and oral or intraduodenal fat (Harvey *et al.*, 1973; Reeder *et al.*, 1973; Grayburn *et al.*, 1975; Low-Beer *et al.*, 1975; Spence *et al.*, 1976; Schlegel *et al.*, 1977a, 1977b; Harvey *et al.*, 1978).

Because of the presence in the body of multiple molecular forms of CCK-PZ that differ in their biologic activities and immunoreactivities, an exact measurement of CCK-PZ levels is still not possible. Nevertheless, a number of physiologic and clinical studies have been performed. The distribution of CCK-PZ in the mucosa of the small intestine has been confirmed, the levels being greatest in the duodenum and upper jejunum, and decreasing steadily down to the terminal ileum (Harvey, 1975). Little or no CCK-PZ is found elsewhere in the body, with the exception of the nervous system, where a CCK-PZ-like peptide has been reported in the brain (Dockray, 1976; Muller *et al.*, 1977; Rehfeld, 1978). Radioimmunoassay studies have suggested that, in both tissues and plasma CCK-PZ exists in several different molecular forms, and the octapeptide of CCK-PZ may be a major contributor to the total biologic activity of the hormone (Harvey *et al.*, 1974b; Rehfeld, 1978).

Infusion studies suggest (subject to inaccuracies of measurement resulting from molecular heterogeneity) that, in man, CCK-PZ has an *in vivo* half-life of about 2.5 minutes (Rayford *et al.*, 1975; Harvey *et al.*, 1978), the kidney being a major organ for its removal from the blood. In man, after a normal mixed meal, the endogenous secretion rate of CCK-PZ has been estimated to be equivalent to 1.0–2.0 Ivy dog units of GIH Research Laboratories CCK-PZ per kg hour (Harvey *et al.*, 1978). Secretion of CCK-PZ is completely inhibited by somatostatin infusion (Schlegel *et al.*, 1977b).

Since CCK-PZ is a hormone having a number of important actions on the gastrointestinal tract, notably on the gallbladder, biliary tract, pancreas, stomach, and intestine (Jorpes and Mutt, 1973; Harvey, 1975a,b; Go, 1978), it can be predicted that disturbances in its secretion or actions may be important in various clinical disorders of these organs. A small but growing number of studies, using radioimmunoassays to measure serum cholecystokinin levels, indicate that this may well be the case in patients with pancreatic insufficiency (Harvey *et al.*, 1973, 1977; Schlegel *et al.*, 1977c; Ederle *et al.*, 1977), coeliac disease (Low-Beer *et al.*, 1975), the Zollinger–Ellison syndrome (Thompson *et al.*, 1975, Rayford *et al.*, 1975), and other gastrointestinal disorders (Harvey, 1978). Despite the many problems involved, the further development and application of radioimmunoassays for CCK-PZ should be exciting and productive endeavors for future research.

ACKNOWLEDGMENTS

The studies reported here would have been impossible without the help of many friends and colleagues in Bristol and elsewhere. Jane Oliver, Lyn Dowsett, Jean-Francois Rey, Andrea Ederle, Janet Albano, and Caroline Owens did much of the work, and I am most grateful to them. Martin Hartog, Jon Grayburn, Tom Low-Beer, Paul Salmon, and Professor Alan Read gave encouragement and advice throughout, together with much practical help in the collection of plasma samples. In such a complex field, progress is difficult enough at the best of times, and would be impossible without the collaboration of workers in other centers. I am particularly grateful for helpful advice and gifts of gastrointestinal hormones or CCK antisera from Professor Viktor Mutt, V. J. Birkinshaw, John Bourne, Guy Clendinnen, Graham Dockray, Provash Ganguli, Professor A. A. Harper, Bernard Jaffe, Alan Johnson, Chris Marshall, J. S. Morley, Neil Mortensen, Miguel Ondetti, Ian Ramus, Jens Rehfeld, Werner Schlegel, and John Walsh. I am grateful to Dr. J. C. Thompson for permission to reproduce Figure 9. Our own studies are supported by the Medical Research Council.

REFERENCES

Albano, J. D. M., Bhoola, K. D., and Harvey, R. F. (1976). Intracellular messenger role of cyclic GMP in the exocrine pancreas. *Nature (London)* **262**, 404–406.

Bangham, D. R., and Cotes, P. M. (1974). Standardisation and standards. *Br. Med. Bull.* **30**, 12–17.

Berry, H., and Flower, R. J. (1971). The assay of endogenous cholecystokinin and factors influencing its release in the dog and cat. *Gastroenterology* **60**, 409–420.

Berson, S. A., and Yalow, R. S. (1972). Radioimmunoassay in gastroenterology. *Gastroenterology* **62**, 1061–1084.

Bolton, A. E., and Hunter, W. M. (1973). The labelling of proteins to high specific radioactivities by conjugation to a ^{125}I-containing acylating agent. *Biochem. J.* **133**, 529–539.

Chayen, J., Bitensky, L., and Daly, J. R. (1974). Cytochemical bioassay of hormones. *Life Sci.* **15**, 191–201.

Cotes, P. M., Musset, M. V., Berryman, I., Ekins, R., Glover, S., Hales, N., Hunter, W. M., Lowy, C., Neville, R. W. J., Samols, E., and Woodward, P. M. (1969). Collaborative study of estimates by radioimmunoassay of insulin concentration in plasma samples examined in groups of five or six laboratories. *J. Endocrinol.* **45**, 557–569.

Debas, H. T., and Grossman, M. I. (1973). Pure cholecystokinin: Pancreatic protein and bicarbonate response. *Digestion* **9**, 469–481.

Del Mazo, J. (1976). Radioimmunoassay of cholecystokinin-pancreozymin. *Gastroenterology* **68**, 957 (abstr.).

Dockray, G. J. (1976). Immunochemical evidence of cholesystokinin-like peptides in brain. *Nature (London)* **264**, 568–570.

Ederle, A., Vantini, I., Harvey, R. F., Piubello, W., Oliver, J., Benini, L., Cavallini, G. and Read, A. E. (1977). Fasting serum cholecystokinin levels in chronic relapsing pancreatitis. *Irish J. Med. Sci.* **146**, 30.

Englert, E. (1973). Radioimmunoassay (RIA) of cholecystokinin. *Clin. Res.* **21**, 207 (abstr.).

Fabri, P. J., and McGuigan, J. E. (1976). Optimisation of antibody production for radioimmunoassay of gastrin. *Gastroenterology* **68**, 883.

Gardner, J. D., Conlon, T. P., Klaeveman, H. L., Adams, T. D., and Ondetti, M. (1975). Action of cholecystokinin and cholinergic agents on Calcium transport in isolated pancreatic acinar cells. *J. Clin. Invest.* **56**, 366–375.

Go, V. L. W. (1978). The physiology of cholecystokinin. *In* "Gut Hormones" (S. R. Bloom, ed.), pp. 203–207. Churchill Livingstone, Edinburgh.

Go, V. L. W., and Reilly, W. M. (1975). Problems encountered in the development of the cholecystokinin radioimmunoassay. *In* "Gastrointestinal Hormones" (J. C. Thompson, ed.), pp. 295–299. Univ. of Texas Press, Austin.

Go, V. L. W., Ryan, R. J., and Summerskill, W. H. J. (1971). Radioimmunoassay of porcine cholecystokinin–pancreozymin. *J. Lab. Clin. Med.* **77**, 684–689.

Go, V. L. W., Cataland, S., and Reilly, W. (1974). Radioimmunoassay (RIA) of cholecystokinin–pancreozymin (CCK-PZ) in human serum. *Gastroenterology* **63**, 700 (abstr.).

Grayburn, J. A., Harvey, R. F., Dowsett, L., Hartog, M., and Jennings, R. D. (1975). Relationships between changes in serum cholecystokinin–pancreozymin and serum insulin after different stimuli. *Diabetologia* **11**, 35–38.

Harper, A. A., and Raper, H. S. (1943). Pancreozymin, a stimulant of the secretion of pancreatic enzymes in extracts of the small intestine. *J. Physiol. (London)* **102**, 115–125.

Harper, A. A., and Vass, C. C. N. (1941). The control of the external secretion of the pancreas in cats. *J. Physiol. (London)* **99**, 415–435.

Harvey, R. F. (1975a). The secretion and actions of cholecystokinin. *In* "Modern Trends in Gastroenterology" (A. E. Read, ed.), pp. 175–202. Butterworth, London.

Harvey, R. F. (1975b). Hormonal control of gastrointestinal motility. *Am. J. Dig. Dis.* **20**, 523–539.

Harvey, R. F. (1976). Radioimmunoassay. *In* "Topics in Gastroenterology" (S. C. Truelove and J. A. Ritchie, eds.), pp. 231–261. Blackwell, Oxford.

Harvey, R. F. (1978). Pathology of cholecystokinin in man. *In* "Gut Hormones" (S. R. Bloom, ed.), pp. 219–223. Churchill Livingstone, Edinburgh.

Harvey, R. F., Dowsett, L., Hartog, M., and Read, A. E. (1973). A radioimmunoassay for cholecystokinin–pancreozymin. *Lancet* **2**, 826–828.

Harvey, R. F., Dowsett, L., Hartog, M., and Read, A. E. (1974a). Radioimmunoassay of cholecystokinin–pancreozymin. *Gut* **15**, 690–699.

Harvey, R. F., Dowsett, L., and Read, A. E. (1974b). Studies on the nature of cholecystokinin–pancreozymin in small-intestinal mucosal extracts. *Gut* **15**, 838–839.

Harvey, R. F., Rey, J. F., Howard, J. M., Read, A. E., Ederle, A., Vantini, I., Groarke, J. F., FitzGerald, O. (1977). Bioassay and radioimmunoassay of serum cholecystokinin in patients with pancreatic disease. *Rendiconti di Gastroenterologia* **9**, 15–16.

Harvey, R. F., Ederle, A., Vantini, I., Scuro, L. A., Oliver, J. M., and Read, A. E. (1978). Half-life, clearance, and endogenous secretion rates of cholecystokinin–pancreozymin in man. *Rendiconti di Gastroenterologia* **10**, 121–126.

Hunter, W. M., and Greenwood, F. C. (1962). Preparation of iodine-[131]-labelled human growth hormone of high specific activity. *Nature (London)* **194**, 495–6.

Ivy, A. C., and Oldberg, E. (1928). A hormone mechanism for gall-bladder contraction and evacuation. *Am. J. Physiol.* **86**, 599–613.

Jaffe, B. M., and Walsh, J. H. (1974). Gastrin and related peptides. *In* "Methods of Hormone Radioimmunoassay" (B. M. Jaffe and H. R. Behrman, eds.), pp. 251–273. Academic Press, New York.

Jaffe, B. M., Newton, W. T., and McGuigan, J. E. (1970). The effect of carriers on the production of antibodies to the gastrin tetrapeptide. *Immunochemistry* **7**, 715–725.

Johnson, A. G., and McDermott, S. (1973). Sensitive bioassay of cholecystokinin in human serum. *Lancet* **2**, 589–591.

Johnson, A. G., Marshall, C. E., Dowsett, L., and Harvey, R. F. (1975). Correlation between bioassay and radioimmunoassay of serum cholecystokinin. *Gut* **16**, 398–399.

Jorpes, E., and Mutt, V. (1966). Cholecystokinin and pancreozymin, one single hormone? *Acta Physiol. Scand.* **66**, 196–202.

Jorpes, J. E., and Mutt, V. (1973). Secretin and cholecystokinin (CCK). *Handb. Exp. Pharmakol.* **34**, 1–179.

Journal of Endocrinology. (1974). The validation of assays and the statistical treatment of results. *J. Endocrinol.* **63**, 1–4.

Lanciault, G., Ertan, A., Adair, L. S., and Brooks, F. P. (1976). Effect of cholecystokinin–pancreozymin on circulating gastrin levels in man and dog. *Am. J. Dig. Dis.* **21**, 39–43.

Low-Beer, T. S., Harvey, R. F., Read, A. E., and Davies, E. R. (1975). Abnormalities of serum cholecystokinin and gallbladder emptying in coeliac disease. *New Engl. J. Med.* **292**, 961–963.

McGuigan, J. E., (1968). Antibodies to the C-terminal tetrapeptide of gastrin. *Gastroenterology* **54**, 1012–1017.

Muller, J. E., Straus, E., and Yalow, R. S. (1977). Cholecystokinin and its COOH-terminal octapeptide in the pig brain. *Proc. Natl. Acad. Sci. U.S.A.* **74**, 3035–3037.

Mutt, V., and Jorpes, J. E. (1968). Structure of porcine cholecystokinin–pancreozymin. Cleavage with thrombin and with trypsin. *Eur. J. Biochem.* **6**, 156–162.

Odell, W. D., and Ross, G. T. (1971). Correlation of bioassay and immunoassay potencies for FSH, LH, TSH and HCG. *In* "Principles of Competitive Protein-Binding Assays" (W. D. Odell and W. H. Daughaday, eds.), pp. 401–413. Lippincott, Philadelphia, Pennsylvania.

Oliver, J. M., and Harvey, R. F. (1977). Hormonal content of commercial preparations of cholexytokinin–pancreozymin. *Gut* **18**, A982.

Ratcliffe, J. G. (1974). Separation techniques in saturation analysis. *Br. Med. Bull.* **30**, 32–37.

Rayford, P. L., Fender, H. R., Ramus, N. I., Reeder, D. D., and Thompson, J. C. (1975). Release and half-life of CCK in man. *In* "Gastrointestinal Hormones (J. C. Thompson, ed.), pp. 301–318. Univ. of Texas Press, Austin.

Reeder, D. D., Becker, H. D., Smith, N. J., Rayford, P. L., and Thompson, J. C. (1973). Measurement of endogenous release of cholecystokinin by radioimmunoassay. *Ann. Surg.* **177**, 304–310.

Rehfeld, J. F. (1978). Multiple molecular forms of cholecystokinin. *In* "Gut Hormones (S. R. Bloom, ed.), pp. 213–218. Churchill Livingstone, Edinburgh.

Rey, J.-F., Howard, J., and Harvey, R. F. (1977). Studies with a bioassay for serum cholecystokinin. *Digestion* **16**, 217.

Schlegel, W., and Raptis, S. (1976). On a reliable method for generating antibodies against pancreozymin, secretin and gastrin. *Clin. Chim. Acta* **73**, 439–444.

Schlegel, W., Raptis, S., Grube, D., and Pfeiffer, E. F. (1977a). Estimation of cholecystokinin–pancreozymin (CCK) in human plasma and tissue by a specific radioimmunoassay and the immunohistochemical identification of pancreozymin-producing cells in the duodenum of humans. *Clin. Chim. Acta* **80**, 305–316.

Schlegel, W., Raptis, S., Harvey, R. F., Oliver, J. M., and Pfeiffer, E. F. (1977b). Inhibition of cholecystokinin–pancreozymin release by somatostatin. *Lancet* **2**, 166–168.

Schlegel, W., Raptis, S., Dollinger, H. C., and Pfeiffer, E. F. (1977c). Inhibition of secretin, pancreozymin and gastrin release and their biological activities by somatostatin. *In* "Hormonal Receptors in Digestive Tract Physiology" (Bonfils, S., Fromageot, P., and Rosselin, G., eds.), pp. 361–377. North-Holland, Amsterdam.

Spence, R. W., Celestin, L. R., and Harvey, R. F. (1976). Effect of metiamide on basal and stimulated serum cholecystokinin levels in duodenal ulcer patients. *Gut* **17**, 920–923.

Thompson, J. C., Fender, H. R., Ramus, N. I., Villar, H. V., and Rayford, P. L. (1975). Cholecystokinin metabolism in man and dogs. *Ann. Surg.* **182**, 496–504.

World Health Organisation Expert Committee on Biological Standardisation. (1975). Twenty sixth report. *W.H.O., Tech. Rep. Ser.* **565**.

Yalow, R. S., and Berson, S. A. (1960). Immunoassay of endogenous plasma insulin in man. *J. Clin. Invest.* **39**, 1157–1175.

Yalow, R. S., and Berson, S. A. (1971). Problems of validation of radioimmunoassays. *In* "Principles of Competitive Protein-Binding Assays" (W. D. Odell and W. H. Daughaday, eds.), pp. 374–400. Lippincott, Philadelphia, Pennsylvania.

Young, J. D., Lazarus, L., Chisholm, D. J., and Atkinson, F. F. V. (1969a). Radioimmunoassay of pancreozymin cholecystokinin in human serum. *J. Nucl. Med.* **10**, 743–745.

Young, J. D., Byrnes, D. J., Chisholm, D. J., and Griffiths, F. B. (1969b). Radioimmunoassay of gastrin in human serum using antiserum against pentagastrin. *J. Nucl. Med.* **10**, 746–748.

25

Serotonin

BERNARD M. JAFFE

I. INTRODUCTION

Serotonin was identified as 5-hydroxytryptamine in 1954. Since that time, this amine has been implicated in a large number of biologic effects on the cardiovascular, endocrine, neurologic, alimentary, coagulation, and pulmonary systems. Despite these suggestions, until recently, physiologic experiments have been hampered by the lack of suitable techniques for measuring serotonin. Spectrophotofluorometry (Udenfriend et al., 1958) is neither sensitive nor specific (i.e., it measures other 5-hydroxyindoles) enough, and it is slow and cumbersome, requiring butanol extraction of deproteinized samples and addition of ninhydrin (Snyder et al., 1965). Although they are more sensitive, enzymatic-isotopic methods (Saavedra et al., 1973) are rather demand-

Methods of Hormone Radioimmunoassay, Second Edition
Copyright © 1979 by Academic Press, Inc.
All rights of reproduction in any form reserved. ISBN 0-12-379260-6

ing and are not suitable for measurement of large numbers of samples. Application of the serotonin radioimmunoassay has permitted large-scale measurement of this amine in a number of experimental and physiologic situations and has enormously simplified the diagnosis of hyperserotoninemic disorders, especially the carcinoid syndrome. The techniques for serotonin radioimmunoassay developed in our laboratory (Kellum and Jaffe, 1976a) will be described in detail in this chapter.

II. METHODS OF RADIOIMMUNOASSAY

A. Preparation of Immunogen

The technique utilized is that of Peskar and Spector (1973), in which serotonin is diazotized to a conjugate of bovine serum albumin (BSA) and aminophenylalanine. The reactions are summarized in Figure 1.

Fifty milligrams each of DL-p-aminophenylalanine, BSA, and 1-ethyl-3-(3-dimethylaminopropyl)carbodiimide (all from Sigma Chemical Company, St. Louis) are incubated in 5.0 ml water for 24 hours at room temperature. The reaction mixture is dialyzed at 4°C against at least 12 liters of water over three to four days. The pH of the solution is adjusted to 1.5 with 0.7 ml 1.0 N HCl. Diazotization is performed by adding 100 mg NaNO$_2$ and 50 mg ammonium sulfamate

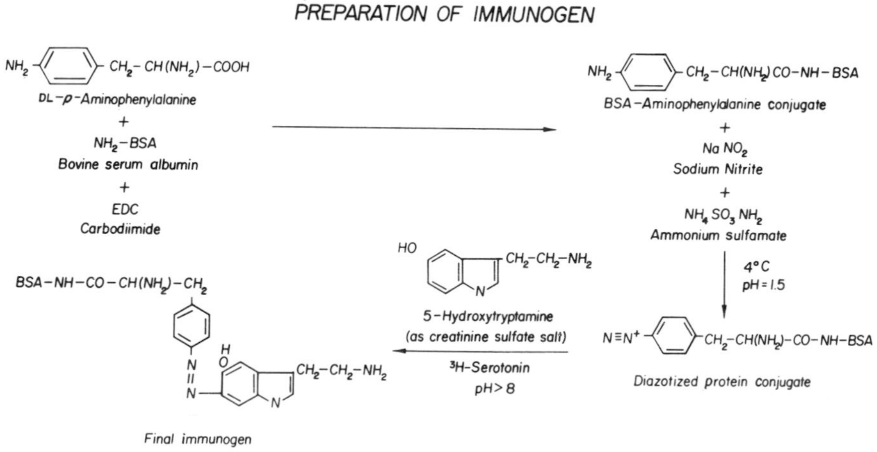

PREPARATION OF IMMUNOGEN

Figure 1.   Schematic representation of the conjugation technique.

dropwise in 1.0 ml water. After thorough mixing, the diazotized protein solution is added dropwise to 10 ml 0.1 M borate buffer, pH 9, containing 100 mg serotonin (either as the oxalate or creatinine sulfate salts (Sigma Chemical Company) and tracer amounts (7.6 pmoles) of ^{3}H-serotonin binoxylate, 5000 mCi/mmole (New England Nuclear, Boston) to evaluate the degree of conjugation of serotonin. The reaction mixture rapidly develops a deep red color. The pH of the reaction mixture must be maintained above 8 by addition of borate buffer. The reaction is allowed to proceed for 24 hours in the dark at 4°C, after which time the conjugate is exhaustively dialyzed against cold distilled water and lyophilized. In several immunogen preparations, 11.3% of the ^{3}H-serotonin was conjugated to the protein carrier, resulting in an average serotonin : BSA molar ratio of 39 : 1.

B. Immunization and Antibody Characterization

1. Immunization

Standard immunization techniques have been quite satisfactory. Eight female New Zealand white rabbits have each been immunized with 1.0 mg antigen dissolved in 0.5 ml 0.05 M phosphate buffer, pH 7.4, and emulsified with 0.5 ml complete Freund's adjuvant. The immunogen was injected subcutaneously into the foot pads. At three, eight, and 16 weeks, rabbits were boosted with 0.5 mg of conjugate in incomplete Freund's adjuvant.

At zero, two, four, nine, and 17 weeks, the rabbits were bled from the central artery of the ear into siliconized and heparinized centrifuge tubes. In order to prevent interference by platelet-bound endogenous serotonin, platelet-poor plasma (PPP) was utilized as the antibody source and was stored in aliquots at −20°C. Platelet-poor plasma is prepared by successive centrifugations at 1200 g for ten minutes and 2250 g for 45 minutes.

2. Antibody Titer

Every animal immunized produced anti-serotonin antibodies. In four of eight rabbits, antibody activity was detectable by four weeks after the initiation of immunization (after two immunizations). With successive immunizations, antibody titers increased. By 17 weeks, 1 : 50 dilutions of plasma samples from all the rabbits were capable of binding significant amounts of ^{3}H-serotonin. The antibody utilized in subsequent studies specifically binds >30% of ^{3}H-serotonin at a dilution of 1 : 1250; at a comparable dilution, the preimmune plasma from

Table I   Cross-Reactivity of Serotonin Analogs

Analog	pmoles required for 50% inhibition of bound ^{3}H-serotonin
5-Hydroxytryptamine (serotonin)	11.4
5-Methoxytryptamine	42.1
Tryptamine	2309
5-Hydroxytryptophan	>5000
5-Hydroxyindole	>5000
L-Tryptophan	>5000
L-Tryosine	>5000
5-Hydroxyindoleacetic acid	>5000

the same rabbit binds an average of 4.1%. The binding of ^{3}H-serotonin is totally inhibited by the addition of excess serotonin; in the presence of 250 ng serotonin, antibody binds less than 5% of ^{3}H-serotonin.

3. Antibody Specificity

Specificity of the anti-serotonin antibody was evaluated by addition to the assay tubes (see below) of equimolar amounts (0.5, 5.0, 50, 500, 2500, and 5000 pmoles) of a large number of serotonin analogs. The results of this study are listed in Table I. Only 5-methoxytryptamine and tryptamine cross-reacted significantly. However, since these compounds normally circulate at concentrations of 5.0–20 ng/ml and 20–50 ng/ml, respectively (Gross and Fransen, 1965), they do not interfere with the radioimmunoassay measurement of physiologic levels of serotonin.

C. Preparation of Samples and Standards

1. Whole Blood

Serotonin is measured after extraction of the amine into a protein-free supernatant (PFS). Blood must be collected using siliconized syringes, transferred immediately into heparinized and siliconized tubes, and kept at 4°C. Within 30 minutes, serotonin is extracted using the technique of Udenfrend et al. (1958). Five milliliters of water is added to 1.0 ml whole blood to lyse the platelets and cellular elements. In order to precipitate plasma proteins, 1.0 ml 10% $ZnSO_4$ and 0.5 ml 1.0 N NaOH are added with thorough mixing after each addition. The mixture is centrifuged at 1200 g for 30 minutes at 4°C and the supernatant (pH 6.9) is aspirated. Serotonin is stable in the protein-free supernatant for at least six months at $-20°C$.

In experiments designed to quantitate serotonin recovery from whole blood, both radioactive (0.7 pmoles ^{3}H-serotonin in 0.1 ml) and cold (200 to 2000 pg in 0.1 ml) serotonin was added to control whole blood samples. Protein-free supernatants were prepared as described above. Duplicate 0.1-ml aliquots of ^{3}H-serotonin-containing PFS were solubilized in 0.5 ml Nuclear Chicago Solubilizer and counted in a toluene-based scintillation solution. In 15 replicate analyses, recovery averaged 34.4 ± 2.0%. Recovery of unlabeled exogenous serotonin, assessed by measuring serotonin concentrations by radioimmunoassay, averaged 36.3% and did not vary with the quantity of unlabeled serotonin added. Since recovery is only 35%, immunoreactive serotonin concentrations are corrected for recovery by adding ^{3}H-serotonin to blood samples prior to processing.

2. Platelet-Rich Plasma

Virtually all circulating serotonin is bound to platelets. Thus, accurate serotonin analyses can be performed in platelet-rich plasma (PRP).

Platelet counts are performed on aliquots of whole blood samples, after which time platelet-rich plasma is prepared by centrifugation at 1400 g for three minutes. Platelet counts are performed on 0.1-ml aliquots of PRP, after which PFS is prepared as described above. Serotonin concentrations are expressed as nanograms per 10^9 platelets.

Experiments performed on 15 normal subjects supported the feasibility of this technique (Kellum and Jaffe, 1976a). Platelet-rich plasma and whole blood contained 337 ± 40 ng per 10^9 platelets and 341 ± 37 ng per 10^9 platelets, respectively. Regression analysis of the plot of the individual serotonin concentrations (nanograms per 10^9 platelets) in PRP versus those in whole blood yielded a straight line with a slope of 0.851 and a correlation coefficient of 0.822.

The data described above suggested that virtually all immunoreactive serotonin is bound to platelets. Further support for this observation includes: (1) platelet-poor plasma contained only 7.2 ± 2.0% of whole blood serotonin; thus, 93.8% of the serotonin circulating in peripheral venous blood was associated with platelets, (2) in portal venous blood, 92% of endogenously released serotonin is bound to platelets (Jaffe et al., 1977), and (3) antibodies to serotonin compete with platelet receptors for free molecules of serotonin (O'Brien et al., 1975).

3. Tissue

Tissue samples (approximately 300 mg) are homogenized with 2.0 ml $0.1 N$ HCl per gram wet weight. The pH of the extracts is adjusted to 10 using anhydrous sodium carbonate. Five milliliters of butanol- and salt-saturated $0.5 M$ borate buffer, pH 10, containing 0.2 pmole ³H-serotonin is added and the extracts are mixed. The volume of the extract is made up to 15 ml, after which 15 ml of n-butanol and 5.0 gm NaCl are added and the extracts are shaken vigorously for 10 minutes. After centrifugation at 2500 rpm for 10 minutes, 10 ml of the supernatant is added to 20 ml heptane and 1.5 ml serotonin-free PFS (see below). The organic phase is discarded and the aqueous solution is utilized directly for radioimmunoanalysis. In 15 experiments, recovery of ³H-serotonin averaged $78.8 \pm 3.2\%$ (Kellum and Jaffe, 1976b).

4. Serotonin Standards

Radioimmunoassay standards (0, 0.05, 0.1, 1.0, 10, 50, and 100 ng) are made up by appropriately diluting dissolved serotonin into serotonin-free PFS. Protein-free supernatants are made from 100 ml outdated bank blood. This PFS is incubated for six hours at 4°C with an equal volume of dextran-coated charcoal (500 mg activated Norit A and 50 mg dextran T-70 diluted in 200 ml $0.05 M$ phosphate, $0.15 M$ NaCl, pH 7.5). The suspension is centrifuged for ten minutes at $1200 g$, and the resultant supernatant is filtered twice using Whatman CF-1 paper. The resultant solution contains no immunoreactive serotonin, which is appropriate, since treatment of PFS with dextran–charcoal removed $98.9 \pm 0.5\%$ of added ³H-serotonin.

D. Assay Procedure and Separation Techniques

Assays are carried out in duplicate in 12×75 mm glass tubes. The additions include 0.1 ml each of a $1:200$ dilution of antibody-containing plasma (or preimmune plasma for blank tubes), EDTA at a final concentration of 1.0 mM, and 0.2 ml of ³H-serotonin containing 0.2 pmole (10,000 cpm) diluted in $0.05 M$ phosphate, $0.15 M$ NaCl, pH 7.5, containing 0.1% egg albumin. Standards and unknowns are added in 0.1 ml of serotonin-free PFS. After incubation at 4°C for 24 hours, 0.4 ml ice-cold saturated ammonium sulfate is added dropwise with constant vortexing. After an additional 60 minutes at 4°C, the tubes are centrifuged at $1200 g$ for 60 minutes. In our initial studies, precipitates were washed with 1.0 ml cold 40% saturated ammonium sulfate, but since this step did not increase the reproducibility of the assay, it is no longer performed in our laboratory. After aspiration of the supernatants by vacuum, the precipitates are dissolved in 0.5 ml NCS (Nuclear Chicago Solubilizer), transferred to 10 ml of scintillation solution [22.8 gm PPO and 0.194 gm POPOP (Fischer) per gallon of scintillation-grade toluene] and counted. For calculation of data, the amount of radioactivity added to each assay tube is determined in at least duplicate by counting 0.05-ml aliquots of the ^{3}H-serotonin solution in serotonin-free PFS after dissolution in 0.5 ml NCS. Serotonin concentrations in unknown PFS samples are calculated from the standard curve (Figure 2) and corrected for recovery.

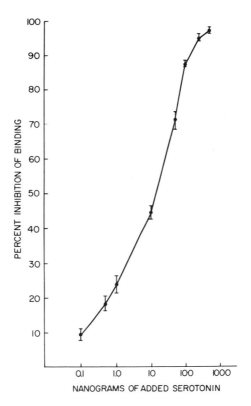

Figure 2. Calibration curve produced by averaging data from 12 successive experiments. (Reproduced from Kellum and Jaffe, 1976a, with permission of the publisher.)

III. VALIDATION AND CHARACTERIZATION OF THE ASSAY

A. Sensitivity and Precision

Since serotonin circulates in relatively high concentrations (see below) sensitivity is not a serious limiting factor. The radioimmunoassay is sensitive to 100 pg (0.78 pmole) of serotonin; in 12 experiments, 100 pg of serotonin caused $9.5 \pm 0.9\%$ inhibition of binding, significantly different from 0 ($p < 0.01$). In our laboratory, 0.1–1.0 ml of whole blood is diluted 1 : 40 to 1.80 during the preparation of samples for radioimmunoanalysis.

Based on replicate analyses of 80 samples, the intraassay coefficient of variation averaged $9.4 \pm 1.1\%$; based on 13 determinations, the interassay coefficient of variation averaged $9.4 \pm 1.7\%$. Since serotonin immunoreactivity is somewhat unstable and deteriorates with repeated freezing and thawing, duplicate analyses must be performed on frozen aliquots of PFS.

B. Comparison with Spectrophotofluorometry

In our laboratory, spectrophotofluorometric analysis of serotonin is performed using the technique of Snyder et al. (1965). PFS from 2.0-ml blood samples are titrated to pH 10 using about 2.0 ml of 1.0 N NaOH. Fifteen milliliters of n-butanol, 0.5 ml 0.5 M borate buffer, pH 10, and 1.5 gm NaCl are added and the mixtures shaken vigorously for ten minutes. The organic phases are aspirated by Pasteur pipette and washed for three minutes with 2.0 ml salt-saturated 0.5 M borate, pH 10. Fifteen milliliters of n-heptane and 1.4 ml 0.05 M phosphate buffer, pH 7.0, are added to 10-ml aliquots of the washed supernatants and shaken for two minutes. After discarding the organic phases, 1.2-ml aliquots of the aqueous phases are incubated at 75°C for 30 minutes with 0.1 ml 0.1 M ninhydrin. After allowing 60 minutes for the mixtures to cool to room temperature, the solutions are transferred to quartz cuvettes. Fluorescence is measured in an Aminco Bowman specrophotofluorometer at 20°C with activation at 385 nm and fluorescence at 490 nm. Serotonin standards added to PFS are carried through the procedure to permit quantitation of the unknowns. Recovery for the extraction procedure, as measured by recovery of added 0.1 pmole ^{3}H-serotonin, far exceeds 90% and need not be corrected for.

In our initial experiments, three normal blood samples were measured simultaneously by radioimmunoassay and spectrophotofluorometry. The data agreed within 12.5%.

O'Brien and Spector (1975) compared human, rat, guinea pig, and rabbit platelet concentrations of serotonin determined by both techniques. The data agreed within 9%.

C. Endogenous and Exogenous Serotonin

In order to validate the assay, we compared the ability of endogenous and exogenous serotonin to displace antibody-bound ^{3}H-serotonin. PFS samples containing high endogenous concentrations of serotonin were derived from blood from a normal rabbit and from a patient with metastatic ileal carcinoid tumor (serotonin level 2143 ng/ml). Dilutions in serotonin-free PFS (0, 1 : 1, 1 : 4, 1 : 10, and 1 : 50) were superimposable on a calibration curve produced by adding exogenous serotonin to a serotonin-free PFS diluent (Figure 3). These data imply that endogenous and exogenous serotonin behave identically in the radioimmunoassay system.

Infusions of serotonin significantly elevate circulating immunoreactive serotonin levels. In thirteen experiments performed on three dogs, at a dose of 6.0 μg/kg/minute, serotonin levels increased from basal values of 243 ± 31 to 372 ± 153 ng/ml at ten minutes and 467 ± 109 ng/ml at 30 minutes (Jaffe et al., 1977). These levels agree quite well with values calculated based on the circulating blood volume.

D. Normal Levels

In 55 normal human subjects, the mean whole blood concentration of serotonin was 168 ± 13 ng/ml. In the fasting state, serotonin levels ranged from 39 to 361 ng/ml. Based on 95% confidence limits, normal serotonin levels are between 45 and 345 ng/ml. These data are in good agreement with levels reported by Udenfriend et al. (1958) using spectrophotofluorometry and Zucher and Borrelli (1955) utilizing a perfused rabbit ear bioassay.

Normal human platelet concentrations of immunoreactive serotonin average 341 ± 34 ng per 10^9 platelets. These data are in good agreement with those of Crawford et al. (1967) using spectrophotofluorometry and Humphrey and Jacques (1954) utilizing rat colon bioassay.

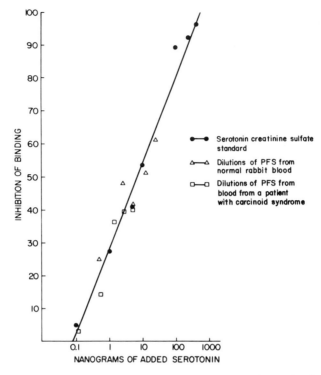

Figure 3. Comparison of dilutions (0, 1:1, 1:4, 1:10, and 1:50) of endogenous serotonin in PFS from normal rabbit blood and from a patient with a carcinoid tumor with a calibration curve prepared by adding exogenous serotinin to a serotinin-free PFS diluent. (Reproduced from Kellum and Jaffe, 1976a, with permission of the publisher.)

In the canine gastrointestinal tract, the duodenum contains the highest concentration of serotonin (15.4 ng/gm). Corresponding data for the stomach, jejunum, and terminal ileum are 3.4, 6.8, and 9.7 ng/gm.

E. Physiologic Observations and Inactivation

In normal human subjects, serotonin is released into the peripheral circulation following a mixed meal. In 17 normal volunteers, a meal (consisting of one egg, two strips of bacon, one piece of buttered toast, 120 ml orange juice, and 240 ml milk) increased serotonin levels from the mean basal value of 198 ± 37 ng/ml to 362 ± 67 ng/ml and 402 ± 116 ng/ml at 30 and 60 minutes, respectively ($p < 0.02$). By two hours circulating serotonin levels returned to the basal range (Figure 4).

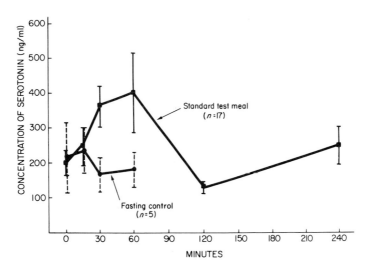

Figure 4. Response of 17 normal humans to a standard meal. Time 0 is immediately before eating (fasting) and other time points refer to the length of time postcibal. Fasting control data in five patients are included. (Reproduced from Kellum and Jaffe, 1976a, with permission of the publisher.)

In order to explore the mechanism and site of release of serotonin, canine experiments were conducted to evaluate the role of intraduodenal administration of acid (50 ml of $0.1 N$ HCl) and hypertonic glucose (50%). Figure 5 displays the results of eight experiments in which serotonin levels were measured in the portal, hepatic, and peripheral veins following duodenal administration. Basal levels in these three veins were nearly identical, 77 ± 34, 81 ± 26, and 82 ± 23 ng/ml, respectively. Saline irrigation of the duodenum did not release serotonin, whereas acid provoked an immediate increase in portal venous serotonin levels. Although the response in the inferior vena cava was delayed (peak at ten minutes), the peak level (342 ± 131 ng/ml) was significantly elevated. In four additional studies, hypertonic glucose alone was found to be a relatively weak stimulant of serotonin release, whereas 50% glucose at pH 2 resulted in a marked (threefold) increase in peripheral venous serotonin levels.

A number of investigators including Feldstein and Williamson (1968) and Thomas and Vane (1967) have suggested that the liver plays a major role in the inactivation of serotonin. Canine experiments were performed to evaluate the usefulness of the radioimmunoassay in assessing the metabolism of serotonin. Intraportal administration of exogenous serotonin resulted in elevations in peripheral venous

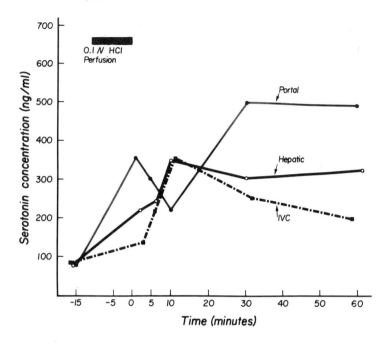

Figure 5. The serotonin response to duodenal acidification in the portal vein, hepatic vein, and inferior vena cava (IVC).

serotonin levels that were not significantly different from those that resulted after intracaval infusion under the same conditions. These data demonstrated that significant amounts of serotonin escaped hepatic inactivation. However, in contrast to endogenously released serotonin, after intraportal administration of serotonin (via a mesenteric tributary), only 59% of the immunoreactive serotonin within the portal vein was bound to platelets.

IV. SUMMARY

The radioimmunoassay for serotonin is sensitive and specific enough to facilitate physiologic studies of the role of this compound. The immunoassay system also has important clinical applications. We have found immunoreactive serotonin levels to be far superior to other diagnostic modalities in the diagnosis of hyperserotoninemia in the carcinoid syndrome. Furthermore, our preliminary studies have suggested that peak serotonin levels following intraduodenal or intrajejunal administration of 50% glucose can be useful in the diagnosis of the postgastrectomy dumping syndrome. In future studies, modifications of the procedure should permit the development of radioimmunoassay systems for analogs and metabolites of serotonin; those latter assays may well be useful in evaluating the specific compounds synthesized and released by carcinoid tumors of fore-, mid-, and hindgut origin.

REFERENCES

Crawford, N., Sutton, M., and Horsfield, G. I. (1967). Platelets in the carcinoid syndrome: A chemical and ultrastructural investigation. *Br. J. Haematol.* **13,** 181–188.

Feldstein, A., and Williamson, O. (1968). 5-hydroxytryptamine metabolism in rat brain and liver homogenates. *Br. J. Pharmacol.* **34,** 38–46.

Gross, H., and Fransen, F. (1965). Tryptamine, *N,N*-dimethyltryptamine, *N,N*-dimethyl-5-hydroxytryptamine and 5-methoxytryptamine in human blood and urine. *Nature (London)* **206,** 1052.

Humphrey, J. H., and Jacques, R. (1954). The histamine and serotonin content of the platelets and polymorphonuclear leukocytes of various species. *J. Physiol. (London)* **124,** 305–310.

Jaffe, B. M., Kopen, D. F., and Lazan, D. W. (1977). Endogenous serotonin in the control of gastric acid secretion. *Surgery* **82,** 156–163.

Kellum, J. M., Jr., and Jaffe, B. M. (1976a). Validation and application of a radioimmunoassay for serotonin. *Gastroenterology* **70,** 516–522.

Kellum, J. M., Jr., and Jaffe, B. M. (1976b). Release of immunoreactive serotonin following acid perfusion of the duodenum. *Ann. Surg.* **184,** 633–636.

O'Brien, R. A., and Spector, S. (1975). Determination of platelet serotonin by radioimmunoassay and comparison with the spectrophotofluorometric method. *Anal. Biochem.* **67,** 336–338.

O'Brien, R. A., Boublik, M., and Spector, S. (1975). Immunopharmacological studies using 5-hydroxytryptamine antibody. *J. Pharmacol. Exp. Ther.* **194,** 145–153.

Peskar, B., and Spector, S. (1973). Serotonin: Radioimmunoassay. *Science* **179,** 1340–1341.

Saavedra, J. M., Brownstein, M., and Axelrod, J. (1973). A specific and sensitive enzymatic-isotopic microassay for serotonin in tissues. *J. Pharmacol. Exp. Ther.* **186,** 508–515.

Snyder, S. H., Axelrod, J., and Zweig, M. (1965). A sensitive and specific fluorescence assay for tissue serotonin. *Biochem. Pharmacol.* **14,** 831–835.

Thomas, D. P., and Vane, J. R. (1967). 5-hydroxytryptamine in the circulation of the dog. *Nature (London)* **216,** 335–337.

Udenfriend, S., Weissbach, H., and Brodie, B. B. (1958). Assay of serotonin and related metabolites, enzymes, and drugs. *Methods Biochem. Anal.* **6,** 95–130.

Zucker, M. B., and Borelli, J. (1955). Quantity assay and release of serotonin in human platelets. *J. Applied Physiol.* **7,** 425–431.

26

Gastric Inhibitory Polypeptide

JOHN C. BROWN AND JILL R. DRYBURGH

I. INTRODUCTION

Physiologic evidence for the existence of a substance with enterogastrone activity present in GIH cholecystokinin–pancreozymin preparations was described by Brown and Pederson (1969), and partial purification of the material was achieved in the same year (Brown *et al.*, 1969). The polypeptide nature of this material has been ascertained (Brown *et al.*, 1970), and the amino acid composition and sequence were reported (Brown, 1971; Brown and Dryburgh, 1971):

Tyr-Ala-Glu-Gly-Thr-Phe-Ile-Ser-Asp-Tyr-Ser-Ile-Ala-Met-Asp-Lys-Ile-Arg-
Gln-Gln-Asp-Phe-Val-Asn-Trp-Leu-Leu-Ala-Gln-Gln-Lys-Gly-Lys-Lys-Ser-Asp-
Trp-Lys-His-Asn-Ile-Thr-Gln

            GIP

Methods of Hormone Radioimmunoassay, Second Edition
Copyright © 1979 by Academic Press, Inc.
All rights of reproduction in any form reserved. ISBN 0-12-379260-6

The polypeptide has subsequently been referred to as gastric inhibitory polypeptide (GIP). Two major biologic activities have been demonstrated for GIP, namely, the inhibition of canine gastric secretion (Pederson and Brown, 1972) and the stimulation of insulin release in man (Dupré *et al.*, 1973) and dog (Pederson *et al.*, 1975a,b). A radioimmunoassay for GIP has been described (Kuzio *et al.*, 1974) and applied successfully to the study of the physiology of the peptide.

II. METHOD OF RADIOIMMUNOASSAY

A. Source of Hormone

Natural porcine GIP isolated by the published methods is currently prepared as a collaborative venture between V. Mutt of the Karolinska Institutet and J. Brown, University of British Columbia. It is available from the Department of Physiology, University of British Columbia. A standard preparation, suitable for immunoassay standards, will be available from the National Institute for Biological Standards and Control (Medical Research Council, United Kingdom). In the following sections, GIP purified to EG stage III (Brown *et al.*, 1970) or EG stage IV, an extra purification step including gel filtration on Sephadex G-50 (fine), has been employed. This material is approximately 95% pure.

B. Production and Characterization of Antisera

1. Production of Antisera

GIP has been a poor antigen, and to date it has proved impossible to raise antibodies to unconjugated polypeptide, either in rabbits or guinea pigs. Antibodies have been raised in both New Zealand white rabbits and guinea pigs using porcine GIP conjugated to bovine serum albumin (BSA) by use of carbodiimide condensation (Goodfriend *et al.*, 1964). Fifty micrograms of GIP calculated from the composition of the conjugate were used for each immunization. GIP–BSA conjugate was emulsified with an equal volume of complete Freund's adjuvant, and immunization was achieved using at least five sites for intradermal injections. In rabbits, injections were made in the suprascapular region, and in the lower abdomen or upper thigh region for guinea pigs. Animals were bled 10–13 days following immunization, and reimmunization in complete adjuvant took place 30 days following the initial event. Animals showing no antibody titer 10–13 days following the second immunization were removed from the series. A third immunization with conjugate was made, but following that nonconjugated peptide was used.

2. Characterization of Antisera

Antisera demonstrating useful titers, i.e., in excess of $1 : 10 \times 10^3$, were checked for cross-reactivity with other hormones, especially those of the secretin family. Antiserum GP 08 was shown not to cross-react with secretin, glucagon, CCK–PZ, gastrin, motilin (Kuzio *et al.*, 1974), insulin, and VIP, when concentrations of up to 10 nanograms per 500 μl were introduced into the assay system.

Further characterization of antisera was obtained using fragments of GIP molecule produced by cleavage at the methionine residue with cyanogen bromide (Brown, 1971). These fragments referred to as N-terminal GIP (1–14) and C-terminal GIP (15–43) were purified and separated from uncleaved polypeptide using carboxymethyl cellulose (CM 11) and 0.01 M NH$_4$HCO$_3$ buffer. Studies with these fragments revealed that the antigenic site or sites were located in the C-terminal fragment of the molecule (GIP (15–43)). No displacement of ^{125}I-GIP from antibody could be achieved by the N-terminal fragment GIP (1–14).

C. Preparation, Purification, and Storage of ^{125}I-GIP

GIP was labeled with ^{125}I by the method of Greenwood *et al.* (1963). A typical iodination, with volumes of reactants, was carried out as described. Five micrograms of GIP, purified to stage III, was dissolved in 100 μl 0.4 M PO$_4$ buffer, pH 7.5. To this was added 1.0 mCi of carrier-free ^{125}I usually with a specific activity of 100 mCi/ml. Mixing was achieved by gently expelling air from a 1.0-ml tuberculin syringe attached to the appropriate size of micropipette. Chloramine-T at a concentration of 40 μg per 10 μl was added. The solution was mixed, and the reaction was allowed to continue for 15 seconds before the addition of 252 μg sodium metabisulfite in 20 μl 0.4 M PO$_4$ buffer, pH 7.5.

The reaction mixture was transferred to a column of Sephadex G-25 fine (0.9 × 27.5 cm) that had been equilibrated with 0.2 M acetic acid containing 2% Trasylol (10,000 KIU/ml) and 0.5% bovine serum albumin (Fraction V, Sigma). Fractions of 300 μl were collected until 15 ml had eluted from the column. Aliquots of 10 μl were counted for 0.1 minute and a radiochromatogram was plotted. A charcoal binding assay (as described below) across the ^{125}I-GIP peak was performed immediately on samples diluted to 5×10^3 cpm per 100 μl aliquots to determine the extent of damaged labeled hormone. Fractions showing the highest concentration of radioactivity which was bound to charcoal were pooled, diluted with equal amounts of eluant buffer and acid–alcohol (100 ml of 99% ethanol and 1.5 ml concentrated HCl) to 1.5×10^6 cpm per 100 μl, and stored at $-20°$C until required for use. The labeled GIP, of average specific activity 90 mCi/mg, was stable for one month at $-20°$C.

The damage assay and binding studies revealed that the best fractions for radioimmunoassay were found eluting on the descending limb of the radiochromatogram immediately following the peak. The fractions on the ascending limb and at the peak invariably demonstrated greatest damage and poorest binding to antibody. Characteristically, there can also be seen a shoulder toward the end of the descending limb. This shoulder increased with lengthening exposure time to chloramine-T. Exposure of GIP to chloramine-T and followed by separation using polyacrylamide electrophoresis showed an increasing degradation of the GIP molecule with time. It is suggested that this shoulder is composed of ^{125}I-tyrosine-containing peptides of the GIP molecule that are not immunoreactive. The above cleavage sites have not as yet been confirmed.

D. Assay Procedure

1. Incubation Conditions

a. **Diluent Buffer.** The composition of the diluent buffer used to dilute the label, antibody, standards, and samples and to finalize the volume to 1.0 ml was as follows: 0.04 M phosphate buffer, pH 6.5, stored, as stock solution at 0.4 M at 4°C; 5% plasma (charcoal-extracted outdated blood bank plasma); and 7500 KIU Trasylol per 100 ml buffer.

b. **Duration and Temperature of Incubations.** Assays were performed in a cold tray, at 4°C, and all solutions were refrigerated prior to use. Incubations were of the equilibrium type at 4°C for 48 or 72 hours. No difference was observed during this period of time.

c. **Glassware.** All glassware used in the assay was pretreated with a siliconizing agent, dimethyldichlorosilane, 1% in benzene (Bio-Rad laboratories). Siliconizing was accomplished by placing a beaker containing 10 ml of the agent into a desiccator, with glassware, and evacuating using a vacuum pump.

2. Preparation of Reactants

a. **Standards.** Porcine GIP was used. Several hundred micrograms were weighed using a Cahn microbalance and dissolved in 0.2 M acetic acid with 2% Trasylol and 0.5% bovine serum albumin so that a final concentration of 1.0 μg per 100 μl was achieved. Aliquots of 100 μl were transferred to siliconized glass tubes and lyophilized. The lyophilized aliquots were stored at $-20°$C until required. One aliquot was dissolved in 0.04 M phosphate, pH 6.5, with 0.5% BSA and 750 μl Trasylol, 10,000 KIU/ml (per 100 ml), to a final concentration of 8.0 ng/ml. Peptide for preparation of standards was stored in 1.5-ml microtest tubes [polypropylene test tubes (Eppendorf) supplied by Brinkman Instruments] at $-20°$C until required. In the assay, standards at concentrations of 6.25 to 400 pg per 100 μl were used. These were prepared by serial dilution from 8.0 ng/ml stock.

b. **Antibody.** Several antibodies with varying affinity constants have now been raised in both guinea pigs and rabbits. However, GP 08 (originally referred to as GP 76) has been used in all studies published to date and was the material supplied to other groups. After bleeding by cardiac puncture (guinea pigs) or ear vein (rabbits), 200-μl aliquots were placed into glass tubes and the solution was lyophilized. The stock antiserum was stored in the dry state at $-20°$C. One 200-μl aliquot was reconstituted with 200 μl of distilled water, followed by 1.8 ml of diluent buffer. Aliquots, depending upon the titer of the antiserum, were dispensed into siliconized glass tubes and stored at $-20°$C until needed. The initial dilution of the antiserum was achieved using the diluent buffer. In our assay, we have utilized antibodies at 1 : 35,000 final dilution.

c. **[125]I-GIP.** An aliquot of the prepared ^{125}I-GIP, containing approximately 1.5×10^6 cpm was diluted with diluent buffer to achieve 5×10^3 cpm per 100 μl. The volume of buffer to be added was calculated immediately after the label was prepared and was adhered to in subsequent assays until the useful life of the ^{125}I-GIP had expired. Label was considered to have expired when nonspecific binding in an assay situation showed in excess of 15%.

d. **Control Sera.** Artificial control sera were used in checking for inter- and intraassay variability. GIP is dissolved in 0.04 M PO$_4$ with

2% Trasylol and 5% charcoal-extracted aged plasma (immunoreactive GIP-free) to a concentration of 200 pg per 100 μl. It is stored at $-20°$C in Eppendorf microtest tubes (Brinkmann Instruments) and used at the beginning and end of assays.

e. Samples. Both serum and plasma samples were assayed for immunoreactive GIP and no differences were observed. Serum was preferred because of the occasional clot formation when plasma was incubated. Tissue extracts, as described in Chapter 30, have also been assayed, and if nonspecific binding tubes were included for each extract, little difference was noted if acidic, neutral, or basic preparations were used. Samples for immunoreactive GIP determinations in tissues invariably had to be diluted and the diluent buffer used.

3. Separation Technique

Separation of free ^{125}I-GIP from peptide bound to antibody was achieved by dextran-coated charcoal. One hundred milliliters of phosphate buffer 0.04 M, pH 6.5, containing 2500 KIU Trasylol was cooled in an ice bath. Dextran T-70 (0.25 gm), was suspended in this solution by gently stirring. Charcoal, 1.25 gm carbon decolorizing (Neutral, Norite) was then added and stirring was continued for one hour. Two hundred microliters of the charcoal suspension was added as rapidly as possible to each tube at 4°C. The tubes were vortexed and immediately centrifuged at 2800 rpm for 20 minutes at 4°C. The tubes were decanted and the charcoal pellet was covered with 60°C wax and counted.

III. EVALUATION OF RADIOIMMUNOASSAY DATA

A. Sensitivity and Precision

The sensitivity of the assay system with antiserum GP 08 allowed reproducible detection of immunoreactive GIP at a concentration of 250 pg/ml (Figure 1). Accuracy deteriorates between 125 and 250 pg/ml, and also with the age of the ^{125}I-GIP. At 250 pg/ml, displacement was between 10 and 15%, from the zero binding which was held at 30% following subtraction of nonspecific binding effects.

B. Standardization

Inter- and intraassay variabilities have been compared routinely in assays, using artificially prepared controls. A pooled serum for these

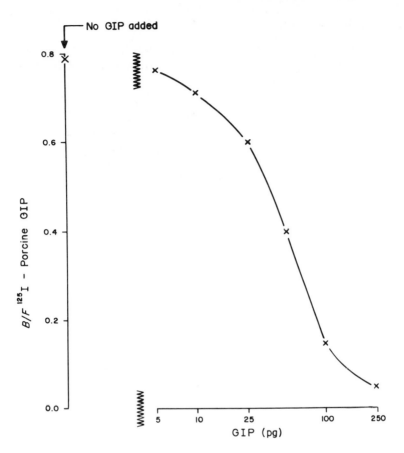

Figure 1.   Standard curve for immunoassay using antiserum GP 76 at a final dilution of 1:20,000. (From Kuzio *et al.*, 1974, with permission of the publisher.)

controls was discontinued when the heterogeneity of circulating im-munoreactive GIP was observed (Brown *et al.*, 1975). The composi-tion of the control has been described earlier, and the preparation which was used was GIP, with a molecular weight of approximately 5100. Immunoreactive GIP values from controls in 50 arbitrarily cho-sen assays in which the control was measured at the beginning and the end of the assay give the following results: 254 ± 43 pg/100 μl (mean ± 1 S.D.) for the first control and 258.3 ± 49.7 pg/100 μl for the second control. Assays were considered suspect if the controls were greater than, or varied within, the assay by ±1 S.D. from these mean values.

C. Specificity of Antisera

As shown in Figure 2, no other gastrointestinal hormone cross-reacted significantly in the assay. Immunoreactive GIP has been shown to exist in serum in at least three forms (Brown *et al.*, 1975) and in at least two forms in tissue extracts from the duodena of hogs (Dryburgh and Brown, 1976). Serum samples, when subjected to Sephadex G-50 chromatography (1.0×100 cm column; eluant either $0.2\,M$ acetic acid or $0.04\,M$ phosphate, pH 7.5), showed a large molecular component eluting with V_0. This component was not present when serum samples were pretreated with $6.0\,M$ urea and is probably an artifact. The two immunoreactive forms detectable in

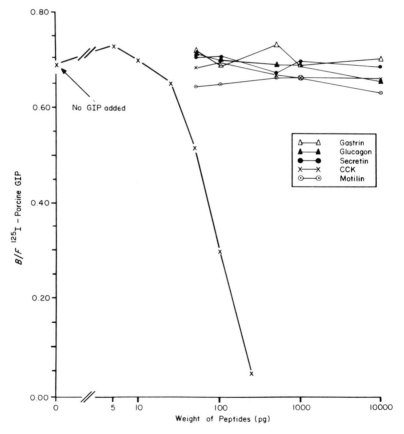

Figure 2. Comparative immunoreactivities of porcine GIP, synthetic gastrin (15-Leu), synthetic glucagon, pure natural porcine secretin, porcine CCK–PZ, and natural porcine motilin. (From Kuzio *et al.*, 1974, with permission of the publisher.)

both serum and tissues had molecular weights of approximatively 5000 and 7500; these represent authentic GIP and a less basic molecular form. Preliminary studies with antiserum GP 08 have shown that both molecular forms were indistinguishable in routine assay conditions. Sera obtained at varying times from subjects following ingestion of glucose, fat, or a mixed meal, and assayed for immunoreactive GIP at several dilutions could be superimposed upon a standard curve, even though these samples showed differing ratios of immunoreactive GIP 5000 : 7500. Human, baboon, and dog sera apparently cross-react identically with antisera GP 08.

D. Normal Circulating Levels

Kuzio *et al.* (1974) reported that the mean total immunoreactive GIP level in 48 normal human subjects was 237 ± 98 pg/ml (mean $\pm$ S.D.), following a 12-hour fast. The normal range was considered to be from nondetectable (less than 10% of the samples) to 400 pg/ml. Ingestion of a large mixed breakfast produced an increase in circulating immunoreactive GIP levels to 1200 pg/ml within 45 min of ingestion of food and remained significantly elevated for a period of time in excess of 270 minutes (Figure 3). Oral glucose was shown to be a se-

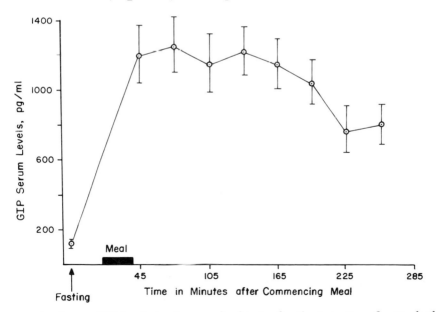

Figure 3. Serum GIP levels in six normal subjects after the ingestion of a standard meal (mean $\pm$ S.E.M.). (From Kuzio *et al.*, 1974, with permission of the publisher.)

cretagogue for GIP release (Cataland *et al.*, 1974). In this study, mean fasting immunoreactive GIP levels were reported as 319 ± 83 pg/ml (mean ± S.D.), which increased to 589 ± 244 pg/ml 15 minutes after ingestion of 75 gm of glucose, with a peak of 747 ± 271 pg/ml at approximately 45 minutes. Ingestion of 100 gm of triglyceride suspension (Lipomul) has also been shown to be a potent stimulus for immunoreactive GIP release (Brown, 1974). Serum immunoreactive GIP levels rose to approximately 750 pg/ml at 120–150 minutes, remaining significantly elevated above fasting levels in excess of 210 minutes. Cleater and Gourlay (1975) have observed a small increase in serum immunoreactive GIP following ingestion of 75 gm of galatose, and Thomas *et al.* (1976) reported a rapid increase in serum immunoreactive GIP following amino acid perfusion of the duodenum. The effect was transitory, declining from a peak of 523 pg at 15 minutes to basal within approximately two hours.

E. Clinical Observations

GIP has been described as having both an "enterogastrone-like" and an "incretin-like" action. Most of the clinical observations made to date have been concerned with problems related to impaired carbohydrate metabolism. Creutzfeldt *et al.* (1977) studied immunoreactive GIP levels in normal subjects and patients admitted to hospital for a weight-reducing procedure. The obese patients were subdivided into two groups, based upon an oral glucose tolerance test: those with a pathological test (pOGTT) and those with a normal test (nOGTT). Fasting immunoreactive GIP levels were higher in the pOGTT group than in the nOGTT group and the normals. Administration of a test meal showed that the integrated immunoreactive GIP release was greatest in the pOGTT obese group 298.2 ± 34.8 ng per three hours, measured in 1.0-ml samples at 15-minute intervals, as compared to the nOGTT obese group (200.6 ± 21.4 ng) and the control group (74.1 ± 108 ng). After complete starvation, immunoreactive GIP levels diminished in parallel fashion with insulin levels. Similar changes in immunoreactive GIP and immunoreactive insulin (IRI) were observed when obese individuals were placed on a low caloric diet (800 ml) for five days. Creutzfeldt *et al.* (1976) have studied six patients with partial duodenopancreatectomy, six patients with coeliac disease, and 15 controls before and after a test meal. Fasting and postprandial immunoreactive GIP levels increase significantly after duodenopancreatectomy. Basal levels in the controls were 194.4 ± 16.5 pg/ml and the integrated response to the test meal, 106.16 ± 9.39

ng/ml in five hours. In the patients with duodenopancreatectomy, basal levels were 894 ± 127 pg/ml, and following a test meal, a total immunoreactive GIP release of 455.0 ± 90.2 ng/ml in five hours was observed. The patients with coeliac disease had fasting immunoreactive GIP levels of 254 ± 19.8 pg/ml and following the test meal the integrated output was 17.4 ± 2.7 ng/ml in five hours. Botha *et al.* (1976) and Ebert *et al.* (1976) studied immunoreactive GIP levels in patients with chronic pancreatitis following ingestion of 50 gm of glucose in 150 ml water and compared this response with control subjects. There were significantly higher immunoreactive GIP levels in the pancreatitis group than in the controls. In the pancreatitis group, a peak immunoreactive GIP response of 1.8 ng/ml was observed at 30 minutes, as compared to a response of 700 pg/ml at the 30-minute period in the control subjects. Brown *et al.* (1975) demonstrated an exaggerated release of immunoreactive GIP in a group of patients who had non-insulin-dependent diabetes. These patients were being treated by diet alone at the time of the study. A 50-gm load of glucose was administered orally, and peak immunoreactive GIP levels were observed at 30 minutes. The peak response was double that seen in a control group of individuals.

REFERENCES

Botha, J. L., Vinik, A. I., and Brown, J. C. (1976). Gastric inhibitory polypeptide (GIP) in chronic pancreatitis. *J. Clin. Endocrinol. Metab.* **42,** 791–797.

Brown, J. C. (1971). A gastric inhibitory polypeptide. I. The amino acid composition and the tryptic peptides. *Can. J. Biochem.* **49,** 255–261.

Brown, J. C. (1974). Gastric inhibitory polypeptide (GIP). *Endocrinol., Proc. Int. Congr., 4th, 1972,* pp. 276–284.

Brown, J. C., and Dryburgh, J. R. (1971). A gastric inhibitory polypeptide. II. The complete amino acid sequence. *Can. J. Biochem.* **49,** 867–872.

Brown, J. C., Dryburgh, J. R., Ross, S. A., and Dupré, J. (1975). Identification and actions of gastric inhibitory polypeptide PTO. *Rec. Progr. Horm. Res.* **31,** 487–532.

Brown, J. C., and Pederson, R. A. (1969). A multiparameter study on the action of preparations containing cholecystokininpancreozymin. *Scand. J. Gastroenterol.* **5,** 537–541.

Brown, J. C., Pederson, R. A., Jorpes, E., and Mutt, V. (1969). Preparation of highly active enterogastrone. *Can. J. Physiol. Pharmacol.* **47,** 113–114.

Brown, J. C., Mutt, V., and Pederson, R. A. (1970). Further purification of a polypeptide demonstrating enterogastrone activity. *J. Physiol. (London)* **209,** 57–64.

Cataland, S., Crockett, S. E., Brown, J. C., and Mazzaferri, E. L. (1974). Gastric inhibitory polypeptide (GIP). Stimulation by oral glucose in man. *J. Clin. Endocrinol. Metab.* **39,** 223–228.

552   John C. Brown and Jill R. Dryburgh

Cleater, I. G. M., and Gourlay, R. H. (1975). Release of immunoreactive gastric inhibitory polypeptide (IR-GIP) by oral ingestion of substances. *Am. J. Surg.* **130**, 128–135.

Creutzfeldt, W., Ebert, R., Arnold, R., Frerichs, and Brown, J. C. (1976). Gastric inhibitory polypeptide, gastrin and insulin: Response to test meal in coeliac disease and after duodenopancreatectomy. *Diabetologia* **12**, 279–286.

Creutzfeldt, W., Ebert, R., Willms, B., Frerichs, H., and Brown, J. C. (1977). Gastric inhibitory polypeptide (GIP) and insulin in obesity: Increased response to stimulation and defective feedback control of serum levels. *Diabetalogia* **14**, 15–24. (submitted on).

Dryburgh, J. R., and Brown, J. C. (1976). Immunoreactive forms of gastric inhibitory polypeptide in serum and tissue. *Can. Physiol.* **7**, 28.

Dupré, J., Ross, S. A., Watson, D., and Brown, J. C. (1973). Stimulation of insulin secretion by gastric inhibitory polypeptide in man. *J. Clin. Endocrinol. Metab.* **37**, 826–828.

Ebert, R., Creutzfeldt, W., Brown, J. C., Frerichs, H., and Arnold, R. (1976). Response of gastric inhibitory polypeptide (GIP) to test meal in chronic pancreatitis—relation to exocrine and endocrine insufficiency. *Diabetalogia* **12**, 609–912.

Goodfriend, T. L., Levine, L., and Fasman, G. D. (1964). Antibodies to bradykinin and angiotensin: A use of carbodiimides in immunology. *Science* **144**, 1344–1346.

Greenwood, F. C., Hunter, W. M., and Glover, J. S. (1963). The preparation of ^{131}I labelled human growth hormone of high specific radioactivity. *Biochem. J.* **89**, 114–123.

Kuzio, M., Dryburgh, J. R., Malloy, K. M., and Brown, J. C. (1974). Radioimmunoassay for gastric inhibitory polypeptide. *Gastroenterology* **66**, 357–364.

Pederson, R. A., and Brown, J. C. (1972). Inhibition of histamine-, pentagastrin-, and insulin-stimulated canine gastric secretion by pure "gastric inhibitory polypeptide." *Gastroenterology* **62**, 393–400.

Pederson, R. A., Schubert, H. E., and Brown, J. C. (1975a). The insulinotropic action of gastric inhibitory polypeptide. *Can. J. Physiol. Pharmacol.* **53**, 217–223.

Pederson, R. A., Schubert, H. E., and Brown, J. C. (1975b). Gastric inhibitory polypeptide. Its physiological release and insulinotropic action in the dog. *Diabetes* **24**, 1050–1056.

Thomas, F. B., Mazzaferri, E. L., Crockett, S. E., Makhjian, H. S., Gruemer, H. D., and Cataland, S. (1976). Stimulation of secretion of gastric inhibitory polypeptide and insulin by intraduodenal amino acid perfusion. *Gastroenterology* **70**, 523–527.

27

Vasoactive Intestinal Peptide

S. R. BLOOM

I. INTRODUCTION

Vasoactive intestinal peptide (VIP) is a basic 28-amino acid molecule with considerable sequence homologies with gastric inhibitory peptide (GIP), secretin, and glucagon (Figure 1) (Bodanszky *et al.*, 1973). It was isolated in 1970 by Said and Mutt using as reference its property of vasodilation in the canine femoral artery. It has subsequently been found to have many other actions, however. Like glucagon, it causes hepatic glycogenolysis; like secretin, it stimulates watery bicarbonate juice production (Said and Mutt, 1972); and like GIP, it inhibits gastric acid (Villar *et al.*, 1976) and also stimulates insulin production (Bloom and Iversen, 1976). Furthermore, VIP is a

Methods of Hormone Radioimmunoassay, Second Edition
Copyright © 1979 by Academic Press, Inc.
All rights of reproduction in any form reserved. ISBN 0-12-379260-6

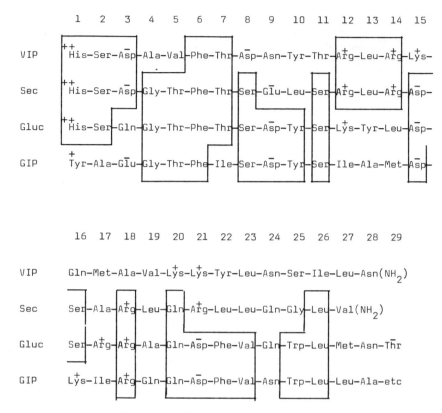

Figure 1.   Amino acid sequence of porcine VIP, secretin, glucagon, and GIP (up to residue 28).

potent stimulus of small intestinal juice production (Barbezat and Grossman, 1971) and causes a dramatic rise in mucosal cyclic AMP concentrations (Schwartz *et al.*, 1974). Although originally isolated from the gut, it has been found to be widely distributed in the body and is present in high concentrations in the central nervous system (Bryant *et al.*, 1976). Immunocytochemistry has shown that it occurs not only in endocrine cells in the mucosa but also in fine nerve fibers (Larsson *et al.*, 1976). It is present in particularly high concentration in the synaptosome fraction of tissue isolates (Giachetti *et al.*, 1976). Since no other member of the secretin–glucagon group is present in the nervous system (Bryant *et al.*, 1976), the potential dual role of VIP active in both brain and periphery suggests that it may be the evolutionary precursor hormone of the group.

The physiology of VIP is not known, but as it probably acts partly as a neurotransmitter and partly as a local hormone (paracrine system), it is likely that elevated blood levels rarely occur under physiologic circumstances. Certainly, no group working in the field has yet detected a physiologic stimulus which causes a biologically significant rise in plasma VIP. This may, however, be a reflection of the present assay sensitivity, since it is possible that even very small increments of plasma VIP are of importance. Thus, at the present time, radioimmunoassay of VIP is very useful as a research tool. Even a crude and insensitive assay can yield valuable information on the changes of tissue VIP content. There is one circumstance, however, in which measurement of plasma VIP is also of considerable clinical utility. Although rare, VIP-producing tumors of the pancreas (Bloom *et al.*, 1973) are both potentially fatal and yet often easy to cure when diagnosed. Pancreatic VIPomas are about as common as the other three pancreatic endocrine tumors, glucagonomas, gastrinomas, and insulinomas. They present as intermittent watery diarrhea, usually of several months' or years' duration. On further clinical investigation, no other abnormality can be detected. The diarrhea is often of such severity (1–5 liters per day) that hypokalemia develops, which, together with the dehydration, may rapidly prove fatal. Once the diagnosis is made, the patient can be completely cured by surgery, since at least half the tumors are benign (Verner and Morrison, 1974). The main problem in the past has been the reluctance of clinicians to operate on a patient whose only symptom is diarrhea and who has no other obvious abnormality (Kraft *et al.*, 1970). This has led to many untimely deaths due both to the complications of severe diarrhea and also to the spread of the tumor itself. Now that a radioimmunoassay for VIP is available, the diagnosis of a functioning VIPomas is made extremely easily by the measurement of a single fasting blood sample (Bloom and Polak, 1975). VIP levels in excess of 65 pmole/liter are associated with clinical symptoms of diarrhea, and the patients with the VIPoma syndrome usually have levels very greatly in excess of this. Other diarrheal diseases, for example, medullary carcinoma of the thyroid, are associated with low VIP levels, a phenomenon which makes the differential diagnosis extremely straightforward. The dual need for VIP radioimmunoassay, e.g., clinical and research, has led to considerable attention being paid to improvement of reliability, specificity, and sensitivity.

II. METHOD OF RADIOIMMUNOASSAY

A. Source of Hormone

VIP occurs in some abundance in many tissues of the body and, being highly charged, is quite easy to extract (see below). At the present time, however, the only source of natural VIP is the Gastrointestinal Hormone Research Unit, Karolinska Institutet, Stockholm, under the direction of Professor V. Mutt. He has made a certain amount of hormone available to the National Institute of Arthritis, Metabolism and Digestive Diseases (NIAMDD), from where it can be obtained upon application to the Gastrointestinal Hormone Resource. Porcine VIP has also been prepared synthetically by Professor Bodanszky in the United States and by Professors Yanaihara and Yajima in Japan. The amounts available are small.

VIP was initially purified from a methanol extract of small intestine (Said and Mutt, 1970). The next purification step was ion-exchange chromatography on carboxymethyl cellulose. The active fraction was retained on the column when the buffer was 0.0125 M phosphate, but was eluted with 0.2 M HCl. A further carboxymethyl cellulose purification was then utilized, the buffer being 0.1 M ammonium bicarbonate. The material was thereafter subjected to 200-tube transfer countercurrent distribution, using a system of 1-butanol and 0.1 M ammonium bicarbonate, and the final purification step was gel filtration on Sephadex G-25, using 0.2 M acetic acid as the elutant.

B. Antibody Production

VIP antibodies have been successfully raised in rabbits using VIP–bovine serum albumin conjugates. The antigenicity is approximately equal to that of glucagon, and, with optimal techniques, about 20% of the rabbits respond with reasonable titers of antibodies. A high coupling yield can be obtained by use of fresh 1-ethyl-3-(3-dimethyl aminopropyl)carbodiimide, which condenses the VIP via amino or carboxyl groups to the carrier albumin, leaving a water-soluble acyl urea. 1.0 mg VIP is incubated with 10 mg albumin and 100 mg carbodiimide in 1.0 ml distilled water at pH 7 for 18 hours at 4°C. The resulting solution, which contains VIP coupled to albumin in a molar ratio of between 1 : 1 and 2 : 1, is then administered directly to the animals so that each rabbit receives 300 μg VIP. The degree of conjugation is determined using trace amounts of ^{125}I-VIP. The VIP conjugate is diluted in distilled water to make 300 μg/ml and then emulsified with an equal volume of complete Freund's adjuvant, taking care that oil is in the continuous phase. The emulsion is administered in four subcutaneous sites (0.5 ml per site). Injections are given every three months, and useful antisera are usually available after a primary and two boosters. The author has immunized about 200 rabbits and 100 guinea pigs. Only two of the rabbits have produced antisera of the highest affinity necessary for the measurement of fasting plasma levels. An additional twenty rabbits, however, produced antisera which would have been adequate either to diagnose the hyper-VIPemia of the VIPoma syndrome or to measure the VIP content of tissue extracts.

C. Iodination

Since VIP possesses two tyrosines (see Figure 1), its iodination theoretically presents little problem. Two amino acids, namely, tryptophan and methionine, are known to be particularly susceptible to oxidation damage. Although VIP does not contain tryptophan, a methionine residue exists at position 17. Thus, oxidative iodination is likely to produce a highly charged methionine sulfoxide group. This problem is obviated by using the trace iodination technique. This method, which is coming into much wider use for small peptides, relies on iodination of only a small fraction of the peptide and separation of the iodinated peptide by high-resolution chromatography, usually ion exchange. The schedule for VIP iodination is given in Table I. It can be seen that the specific activity of the crude product will not exceed 100 μCi/μg (0.3 mCi/mole), whereas the theoretical value for pure monoiodinated VIP approaches 700 μCi/μg (2.2 mCi/mole). The

Table I   VIP Iodination Protocol

6.0 nmole Porcine VIP (20 μg)
100 μl   Acetate buffer (50 mmole/liter, pH 5.0)
1.0 nmole [125]I (approx. 2.0 mCi Amersham IMS 30)

plus

1.8 nmole H_2O_2 (20 μl 0.86 mmole/liter)
22 pmole   Lactoperoxidase (Sigma milk-derived) (20 μl 25 μg/ml)

Mix; react 15 minutes, 18°C

500 μl   Acetate buffer, as above
       Elute from 1.5 × 30 cm CM Sephadex C25 column at 4°C over 36 hours
       using 160 mmole/liter phosphate buffer pH 8.5 (containing 0.4 mmole/liter
       human serum albumin and 0.4 MKIU/liter aprotinin).

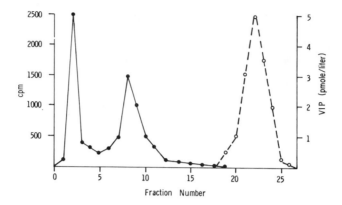

Figure 2. Elution pattern from CM Sephadex C-25 ion-exchange column (1.5 × 30 cm run in 0.16 M Tris-HCl, pH 8.5, at 5.0 ml/hour) of the VIP iodination product (as Table I) with a large amount of added cold VIP. The eluted radioactive product is shown as the solid line and cold VIP as the dashed line. The second peak of radioactivity bound over 90% to VIP antiserum, with a blank of 5%, and was employed thereafter as the radioimmunoassay label. The first peak was ^{125}I.

ion-exchange chromatography of the product successfully separates iodinated from noniodinated VIP (Figure 2). Thus, a label with theoretical maximum specific activity is obtained which is at the same time highly purified and free of any degradation products. This material is very stable on storage and can be used for as long as six months. The limiting factor is the decay of the ^{125}I whereby a steady reduction in the specific activity occurs, necessitating longer and longer sample counting time. Prevention of chemical damage to the VIP is aided by storage, well diluted in a proteinaceous solution (2% albumin), below $-20°C$.

Other techniques for purifying labeled VIP have also been successfully applied. Fahrenkrug and Schaffalitzky de Muckadel (1977) have utilized gel filtration on an 11 × 550 mm column of Sephadex G-50 superfine, eluting at 12 ml/hour at 4°C with 0.25 M ammonium acetate, pH 6.5, containing 72.5 μmole BSA per liter. Ebeid *et al.* (1976) have used Whatman CF 1 columns for purification. After removal of unreacted iodide by washing with 0.3 M phosphate, pH 7.5, iodinated VIP was eluted with phosphate buffer containing 12.5% bacitracin.

D. Assay Procedure

Although a number of different assay schedules are possible (for example, quick incubation to achieve rapid but less accurate results or small volume assays for use with limited sized samples), the following procedure has been found to be the most generally useful for assay of human plasma VIP. Duplicate tubes are set up containing a total volume of 800 μl of which 200 μl is plasma (standard or unknown) and the remainder 50 mmole/l phosphate buffer, pH 7.0, containing 1% albumin and 1000 KIU/ml aprotinin (Trasylol). Antibody at a final dilution of 1 : 400,000 and label, (1.0 fmole ^{125}I-VIP per tube), diluted in this buffer, are added in a volume of 100 μl each. Every assay contains control tubes without antibody, tubes with excess antibody, and tubes containing either one-half or two times the amount of VIP label as a check on its specific activity. Control VIP-free plasma, prepared by affinity chromatography using VIP antiserum coupled to cyanogen bromide Sepharose beads (Parmacia Ltd), is run at regular intervals throughout each assay to check for any assay drift. Standards (0.1 to 50 fmole/tube) are made up in the same control, VIP-free plasma. Lyophilized vials, containing 1.0 pmole of porcine VIP standard to make a new disposable stock solution for each assay, were originally prepared by weighing fresh pure porcine VIP kindly provided by Professor V. Mutt. The assay is set up on 4°C cooling trays, and the unknown samples rapidly thawed and maintained at 4°C in order to minimize proteolytic degradation of VIP. Maximum sensitivity is obtained by incubation for at least four days at 4°C. No advantage has been seen with late addition of the label.

E. Separation Procedure

Addition of a charcoal suspension provides cheap and reliable separation of antibody-bound from free radioactive VIP. The exact amount of charcoal required per tube varies with the preparation used, and, therefore, a bulk quantity should be purchased and tested as depicted in Figure 3. It can be seen there is a wide plateau area in which an error in the amount of charcoal added makes very little difference to the percentage of hormone bound. We routinely use 26 mg/tube of Norit GSX charcoal (Hopkins and Williams Ltd). This is made up as a 200-ml suspension in 0.05 M Veronal buffer, pH 8, of charcoal (10.4 gm), and 10 ml VIP-free plasma is added as a precoating agent. After stirring vigorously for 30 minutes at 4°C, 0.5 ml is rapidly added to each test tube with an automatic pipette. The assay tubes are then vigorously shaken, and, after a five-minute incubation period, the charcoal is separated by centrifugation. The supernatant and precipitate are both measured, and the supernatant is expressed as a percentage of the whole. This avoids any significant effect of small errors in

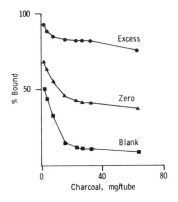

Figure 3. Effect of varying additions of charcoal in the assay separation procedure on values of assay blank, zero, and excess.

the original radioactive VIP addition and prevents any slow changes in counter efficiency from affecting the answer.

F. Sample Preparation

VIP is rapidly destroyed by proteolytic enzymes, possessing two separate double basic amino acid sequences (see Figure 1) which are particularly favored for attack by trypsin-like enzymes. In addition, it possesses methionine, which makes it sensitive to oxidative damage, and two asparagines, which may be deamidated. Further, VIP is rapidly absorbed onto active surfaces, particularly when these are negatively charged. Thus, considerable care is required in sample preparation. For blood, in which a high concentration of proteins are present to reduce surface phenomenon, the main problem is prevention of proteolysis. Thus, the sample is taken directly into aprotinin (1000 KIU/ml blood), heparinized with 10 U/ml, and rapidly centrifuged. The plasma, which should be free of hemoglobin, since this indicates red cell destruction and release of proteolytic enzymes, is best frozen at $-20°C$ within 15 minutes of venipuncture. It may then be stored at this temperature for several months without obvious loss of hormonal activity. The act of thawing and freezing, however, seems to produce significant losses, and samples which have undergone this process several times may show a greatly diminished VIP content. For international transport of samples, we have found the most satisfactory method is prolonged lyophilization of 1.0-ml aliquots. The reduction of the moisture content to an extremely low level is important, since it greatly increases stability. The samples, when sealed *in vacuo*, remain stable at room temperature for some weeks or even months. In a series of 20 samples so treated and stored at 25°C for 30 days, the mean VIP level was compared with duplicate samples which were never thawed until both were assayed. The mean loss was only 10%. Tissue extracts appear more stable at a pH between 2 and 4, when surface absorption phenomenon are perhaps also less troublesome, but storage at low temperatures is also advisable. VIP is thermostable, at least at the temperature of boiling water, and thus heating tissues to 100°C is effective in destroying proteolytic enzymes without loss of VIP and forms a useful initial extraction step.

III. ASSAY CHARACTERISTICS

A. Specificity

None of the antisera so far raised show any cross-reaction with other members of the hormone group, e.g., secretin, glucagon, and GIP. If a crude gut extract is subject to gel chromatography, only a single peak of VIP immunoreactivity is noted (Figure 4). This elutes in the same position as the pure VIP to which the antibodies were raised. Thus, there appears to be no cross-reaction with any other peptide present in the gut. In brain extracts, however, a small peak of high molecular weight VIP immunoreactivity is noted, and this might either be VIP adherent to a larger molecule, big VIP analogous to proinsulin, high molecular weight artifactual interference with the assay, or possibly it may be another peptide which cross-reacts in the assay. The amounts present, however, are extremely small and would not appear to affect the validity of assay results.

The accuracy of radioimmunoassay results is not only affected by possible cross-reaction with other peptides of similar constitution but also by nonspecific effects. It is well known, for example, that high concentrations of salts or urea will nonspecifically uncouple antibody–antigen combinations and so produce erroneous radioimmunoassay results. These nonspecific assay artifacts can be investigated by use of specific immunoabsorbance (affinity chromatography). High-titer VIP antisera are coupled to a solid phase, for example, cyanogen bromide–Sepharose beads (Pharmacia Ltd). The techniques for attraction of Sepharose and antibody conjugation are described in Chapter 30. These solid-phase antibody preparations must not release the antibody even in minute amounts or themselves absorb further material, because both situations interfere with the analysis of the

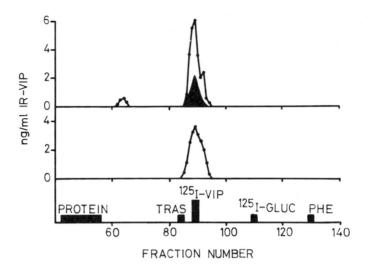

Figure 4. Elution pattern of immunoreactive VIP extracted from porcine brain (top) and gastrointestinal tract (gallbladder) (middle) run on a 1 × 90 cm Sephadex G-50 column. The position of molecular size markers is shown in the bottom panel and porcine VIP as the shaded area in the top panel.

results. Cyanogen bromide–Sepharose bead antibodies fulfill these criteria, provided they are washed immediately before use and the amount of antibody bound is not too large. The unknown sample is divided into four portions. The first (A) acts as control, and the second (B) is treated with the specific VIP immunoabsorbent. The third (C) is treated with an identically prepared immunoabsorbent but prepared with antisera to another hormone. A considerable quantity of cold VIP is added to the fourth sample (D), and this is also treated with the specific VIP immunoabsorbent. With a high-capacity bead preparation, the treatment time of the unknown sample is only 15–30 minutes with gentle mixing. The volume of each aliquot may be 1.0 ml or less, and 10 μl of antibody beads will be adequate to remove all VIP. In a typical experiment, in which nonspecific interference is minimal, samples B and D will read zero, having been successfully cleared of all VIP, while samples A and C will give identical readings of the true VIP content. The specific VIP immunoabsorbent beads are also used to prepare the reference VIP-free control plasma for use in the routine radioimmunoassay.

It is important to ascertain which part of the VIP molecule provides the antigenic site. Major assay problems may arise if the antisera react avidly with VIP degradation fragments. It has been shown for other hormones that radioimmunoassay and bioassay values may coincide very well during the initial release of a hormone following a stimulus but during later measurements of VIP removal from the circulation, large discrepancies may occur. Thus, the radioimmunoassay shows a much slower rate of hormone removal than the bioassay. This is explained by the presence of nonbiologically active circulating hormone fragments which register in some radioimmunoassays as whole active hormone, although they are not detected by the bioassay. It is obviously preferable to choose antisera which react only with the whole molecule and which are influenced little by the presence of fragments. Fragment testing of two VIP antisera is shown in Figure 5. Antiserum V9, which we routinely use in our assay, shows no reaction at concentrations likely to be met physiologically with either VIP fragment 1–22 or 18–28 (Figure 5). The use of such antisera is preferable, since they are therefore less likely to be significantly influenced by biologically inactive VIP fragments.

B. Sensitivity and Reproducibility

Using antiserum V9 and the assay protocol described above, differences between two single unknown plasma samples of 1.5 pmole/liter can be detected with 95% confidence. The antibody titer is adjusted to give 50% ^{125}I-VIP binding at the zero point (about 1 : 400,000 dilution). The smallest amount of ^{125}I-VIP is added which we can comfortably

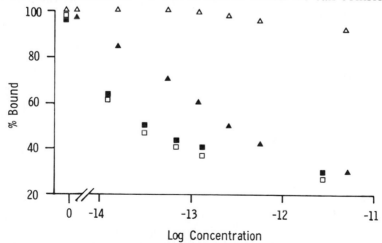

Figure 5. Displacement curves of whole VIP (squares) and VIP fragment 18-28 (triangles) against antiserum V9 (open symbols) and V25 (closed symbols). The vertical axis shows the percent of zero point binding. (VIP fragments kindly provided by Professors Bodanszky and Yanaihara.)

count. This is usually about 0.5 to 1.0 fmole (2.0 pg) per tube. Thus, a label specific activity of 400 μCi/μg (1.3 mCi/mole) yields between 500 and 1000 cpm, depending on counter efficiency. Under these conditions, addition of an unknown plasma containing 15 pmole/liter causes the percent bound to drop to 30% from an assay zero of 50%. At this part of the standard curve, the standard deviation for a single answer is about 1%, and thus samples 2% apart can be distinguished with p less than 0.05. Error increases as the antibody binding of label moves away from the 50% point, so that if more label is added it is wise to increase the amount of antibody to maintain the assay zero binding at about 50%. Clearly, assay sensitivity could be increased by use of the more avid antibody or by decreasing the assay error. The intraassay variation is about 10%, whereas the interassay variation is somewhat greater at around 20–25%.

C. Plasma Values

The basal human plasma VIP concentration is very low, at about 5.0 pmole/liter. In a recent series of 110 healthy subjects, the fasting VIP ranged between less than 1.0 and 21 pmole/liter with a mean of 2.1 and a mode of 1.5 pmole/liter. No change was seen after ingestion of a meal, and the level was unaltered in patients receiving various hormone infusions, calcium infusion, and intravenous nutrition. The level was not elevated in patients with uncomplicated hepatic cirrhosis, mild renal failure, or other gastrointestinal diseases such as ulcerative colitis. In a series of 40 patients with pancreatic tumors producing watery diarrhea, the plasma VIP level was always above 65 pmole/liter and in some patients exceeded 1000 pmole/liter. Following treatment with the drug streptozotocin, plasma VIP greatly decreased, and in patients whose symptoms disappeared the level fell below 65 pmole/liter. Treatment with steroids, however, which also diminished the diarrhea, did not greatly reduce the plasma VIP level. In a series of 400 other patients with various types of diarrhea sent to us for exclusion of a VIP-producing tumor, the VIP level was always below 30 pmole/liter.

IV. CONCLUSION

The radioimmunoassay for VIP may be performed in a quite conventional manner and has no special technical difficulties. The sensitivity of the present assay system, however, only appears capable of measuring tissue extracts and elevated levels of plasma VIP. The detection of subnormal levels is still not possible.

REFERENCES

Barbezat, G. O., and Grossman, M. I. (1971). Intestinal secretion: Stimulation by peptides. *Science* 174, 422–423.

Bloom, S. R., and Iversen, J. (1976). The influences of gut hormones on glucagon and insulin release. *Metab., Clin. Exp.* 25, 1457–1458.

Bloom, S. R., and Polak, J. M. (1975). The role of VIP in pancreatic cholera. *In* "Gastrointestinal Hormones" (J. C. Thompson, ed.), pp. 635–642. Univ. of Texas Press, Austin.

Bloom, S. R., Polak, J. M., and Pearse, A. G. E. (1973). Vasoactive intestinal peptide and watery diarrhoea syndrome. *Lancet* 2, 14–16.

Bodanszky, M., Klausner, Y. S., and Said, S. I. (1973). Biological activities of synthetic peptides corresponding to fragments of and to the entire sequence of the vasoactive intestinal peptide. *Proc. Natl. Acad. Sci. U.S.A.* 70, 382–384.

Bryant, M. G., Bloom, S. R., Polak, J. M., Albuquerque, R. H., Modlin, I., and Pearse, A. G. E. (1976). Possible dual role for vasoactive intestinal peptide as gastrointestinal hormone and neurotransmitter substance. *Lancet* 1, 991–993.

Ebeid, A. M., Murray, P., Hirsch, H., Wesdorp, R. I. C., and Fischer, J. E. (1976). Radioimmunoassay of vasoactive intestinal peptide. *J. Surg. Res.* 20, 355–360.

Fahrenkrug, J., and Schaffalitzky de Muckadell, O. (1977). Radioimmunoassay of vasoactive intestinal polypeptide in plasma. *J. Lab. Clin. Med.* 89, 1379–1388.

Giachetti, A., Rosenberg, R. N., and Said, S. I. (1976). Vasoactive polypeptide in brain synaptosomes. *Lancet* 2, 741–742.

Kraft, A. R., Thompkins, R. K., and Zollinger, R. M., (1970). Recognition and management of the diarrhoeal syndrome caused by nonbeta islet cell tumours of the pancreas. *Am. J. Surg.* 119, 163–170.

Larsson, L.-I., Fahrenkrug, J., Schaffalitzky de Muckadell, O., Sundler, F., and Hakanson, R. (1976). Localization of vasoactive intestinal polypeptide (VIP) to central and peripheral neurones. *Proc. Natl. Acad. Sci. U.S.A.* 73, 3197–3200.

Said, S. I., and Mutt, V. (1970). Polypeptide with broad biological activity: Isolation from small intestine. *Science* 169, 1217–1218.

Said, S. I., and Mutt, V. (1972). Isolation from porcine-intestinal wall of a vasoactive octacosapeptide related to secretin and to glucagon. *Eur. J. Biochem.* 28, 199–204.

Schwartz, C. J., Kimberg, D. V., Sheerin, H. E., Field, M., and Said, S. I. (1974). Vasoactive intestinal peptide stimulation of adenylate cyclase and active electrolyte secretion in intestinal mucosa. *J. Clin. Invest.* 54, 536–544.

Verner, J. V., and Morrison, A. B. (1974). Endocrine pancreatic islet disease with diarrhoea. Report of a case due to diffuse hyperplasia of nonbeta islet tissue with a review of 54 additional cases. *Arch. Intern. Med.* 133, 492–500.

Villar, H. V., Fender, H. R., Rayford, P. L., Bloom, S. R., Ramus, N. I., and Thompson, J. C. (1976). Suppression of gastrin release and gastric secretion by gastric inhibitory polypeptide (GIP) and vasoactive intestinal polypeptide (VIP). *Ann. Surg.* 184, 97–102.

28

Motilin

JILL R. DRYBURGH AND JOHN C. BROWN

I. INTRODUCTION

Instillation of fresh pig pancreatic juice into the duodena of dogs was found to stimulate motor activity in the extrinsically denervated or transplanted pouch of the stomach. The effect could be mimicked if alkali (0.3 M Tris buffer, pH 9.5) was the perfusate (Brown *et al.*, 1966). The question of the existence of some humoral agent, released from the duodenal mucosa upon elevation of the pH of duodenal contents, led to the isolation and purification of motilin from hog duodenal mucosa. This peptide contains 22 amino acid residues and bears no struc-

567

Methods of Hormone Radioimmunoassay, Second Edition

tural resemblance to any of the presently known and characterized gastrointestinal peptides. Its structure is as follows:

Phe-Val-Pro-Ile-Phe-Thr-Tyr-Gly-Glu-Leu-Gln-Arg-
Met-Gln-Glu-Lys-Glu-Arg-Asn-Lys-Gly-Gln

The radioimmunoassay was developed in order to determine if motilin was, in fact, the agent released upon alkalinization of the duodenum. Its use naturally extends to investigation of its physiologic role in man.

II. METHOD OF RADIOIMMUNOASSAY

A. Nature and Source of Antigen

Natural porcine motilin was extracted from hog duodenal and jejunal mucosa as described by Brown *et al.* (1972), in the laboratories of V. Mutt, Karolinska Institute, Stockholm, and J. C. Brown, University of British Columbia, Vancouver. Homogeneity of the final product, designated M5, was established by polyacrylamide gel electrophoresis, high-voltage electrophoresis at pH 6.5, and amino acid analyses of the individual fractions in the last purification stage and was confirmed by determination of the amino acid sequence (Brown *et al.*, 1973). M5 was used throughout the radioimmunoassay for immunization, iodination, and preparation of standards.

B. Production and Characterization of Antisera

1. Immunization

Antibodies to motilin have been raised in both guinea pigs and rabbits, M5 being the immunogen. The best results were obtained if at least one immunization was performed with the peptide conjugated to a large molecular weight protein, prior to emulsification with complete Freund's adjuvant.

In a typical conjugation reaction, 1.0 mg motilin in 0.2 ml deionized water, 20 μl ^{125}I-motilin containing 100,000 cpm, 1.0 mg bovine serum albumin in 0.1 ml water, and 10.0 mg 1-ethyl-3-(-3-diethyl-aminopropyl)carbodiimide in 0.1 ml water were mixed and stirred for 60 minutes. The conjugated material was collected by separation on a Sephadex G-25 column using 0.2 M acetic acid as the eluant. The degree of conjugation was monitored both by the added trace label and with high-voltage electrophoresis at pH 6.5.

The animals were initially immunized with 50 μg M5 in deionized water, emulsified with an equal volume of complete Freund's adjuvant. Each animal received 0.5 ml of this emulsion in several sites, the guinea pigs being injected subcutaneously in the lower abdomen and inner thigh, the rabbits intradermally in the suprascapular region. Two weeks later the animals received 100 μg M5, conjugated with bovine serum albumin by the carbodiimide method of Goodfriend *et al.* (1964), followed four weeks later with an identical immunization. The guinea pigs were bled by cardiac puncture and the rabbits from the marginal ear vein 10–12 days after this injection, and any animal not producing antisera of reasonable titer was discarded. The remaining animals were reinforced with boosters of 50 μg nonconjugated material in complete Freund's adjuvant at three- to six-month intervals, bled monthly, and discarded if the antisera titer showed signs of diminishing.

2. Characterization

Serial dilutions of antisera were incubated with ^{125}I-motilin under routine assay conditions (see Section III,D). The curves obtained in such experiments indicated the best antisera dilutions for the assay, i.e., those dilutions which will bind 50% of the labeled antigen (Figure 1).

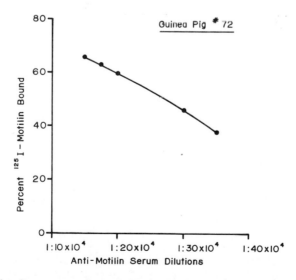

Figure 1. A binding curve of serial dilutions of an anti-motilin serum. In routine assays, the $1:17 \times 10^4$ dilution would be used, i.e., that dilution producing 50% binding of the tracer.

3. Storage

Antisera suitable for radioimmunoassay were aliquotted in appropriate volumes, i.e., 200–500 μl, and lyophilized for storage at $-20°C$. When needed, an aliquot was reconstituted in diluent buffer to give a 1 : 10 dilution, and stored frozen in 100-μl aliquots. The shelf life of the lyophilized serum was at least three years; the frozen diluted antiserum was viable for several months.

C. Preparation and Purification of ¹²⁵I-Motilin

The isotope of choice is ¹²⁵I (100 mCi/ml). The chloramine-T method of Hunter and Greenwood (1963), with slight modifications, has repeatedly produced a stable ¹²⁵I-motilin with a specific activity in the range 250–450 mCi/mg. The lactoperoxidase method (Miyachi *et al.*, 1972) was also applied successfully and is used as the method of choice by Bloom *et al.* (1976). Motilin was not as readily damaged by exposure to the oxidizing agent as some of the other gastrointestinal peptides, e.g., glucagon, gastric inhibitory polypeptide, and vasoactive intestinal peptide, and withstood exposure to chloramine-T for up to two minutes with no evidence of peptide fragmentation when checked by polyacrylamide gel electrophoresis.

1. Iodination

This procedure has been described fully by Dryburgh and Brown (1975). The peptide, chloramine-T, and sodium metabisulfite were weighed out and diluted appropriately in 0.2 M sodium phosphate buffer, pH 7.5, just prior to use. The reaction was performed in a siliconized 10 × 75 mm glass tube.

Pure motilin was aliquotted in 2.0–4.0-μg quantities, lyophilized, and stored under nitrogen. To 2.0 μg M5 in 50 μl phosphate buffer was added Na¹²⁵I (1.0 mCi in 10 μl). Chloramine-T (40 μg in 10 μl phosphate buffer) was added with vigorous bubbling, and after 15 seconds the reaction was terminated by the addition of sodium metabisulfite (100 μg in 20 μl phosphate buffer).

2. Purification

Separation of ¹²⁵I-motilin was accomplished by gel filtration on Sephadex G-25 (fine). The reaction mixture was transferred immediately to a 0.9 × 30 cm column and eluted with 0.1 M formic acid containing 0.5% bovine serum albumin and 2% Trasylol. Nonspecific binding (NSB) was measured across the ¹²⁵I-motilin peak by immediate addition to a suitable label dilution of dextran-coated charcoal and separation of bound and free portions as described in detail in Section II,D. The pooling and use of only the lowest NSB fractions effectively remove the di- or triiodinated peptide from the monoiodinated form. The chosen tubes were pooled, diluted with 0.1M formic acid containing 0.5% bovine serum albumin and 2% Trasylol, and aliquotted in siliconized tubes so that each tube contains 2×10^6 cpm in 2.0 ml. The label was stored at $-20°C$ and can be used without further repurification for three months.

The specific activity of the label was not tested after every iodination but was checked at intervals by preparing standard curves with (a) constant label and increasing dilutions of unlabeled motilin, and with (b) increasing concentrations of labeled motilin only. If the binding kinetics of the antiserum were identical for labeled and unlabeled peptide, the scales can be adjusted so that the curves are superimposable (Figure 2). The number of counts that must be added to produce the same displacement as a standard amount of cold motilin may be read directly from the curve and converted to mCi/mg peptide. The specific activity of labeled motilin averages 300–400 mCi/mg.

D. Assay Procedure

1. Conditions of Incubation

The diluent buffer, 0.04 M sodium phosphate buffer, pH 6.5, containing 5% charcoal-extracted aged human plasma and 0.25% Trasylol, was used for making all dilutions and for correcting the final incubation volume to 1.0 ml. The composition of the incubation volume was as follows: 100 μl ^{125}I-motilin containing 5000 cpm, 100 μl standard motilin (range 12.5–400 pg), or 50–200 μl test serum, or 100 μl control (porcine motilin made up to 100 pg/100 μl in diluent buffer) 100 μl antiserum at an appropriate dilution, i.e., 1 : 8000 (GP.75) or 1 : 10,000 (R.Mo7), and diluent buffer to a final volume of 1.0 ml.

The assay was set up in siliconized 10×75 mm glass culture tubes, which were vortexed gently and incubated at 4°C for 48–72 hours. NSB tubes, without antiserum, were included for the standard curve, internal controls, and each group of sera from one subject.

2. Separation of Bound and Free ^{125}I-Motilin

Although other more specific methods of separation of bound and free portions do exist, including Sepharose-bound antibody (which is dealt with briefly in Section IV), the original technique used

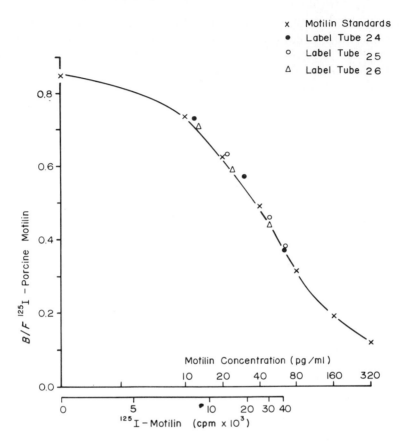

Figure 2. Standard curve to motilin (×——×) in comparison with label fractions 24 (●), 25 (○), and 26 (△). Dilutions of each fraction from 8×10^3 to 40×10^3 cpm were added, and the dilution of fraction 26 containing 25×10^3 cpm was fitted to the standard curve, the other fractions fitting accordingly.

was absorption of the free label onto dextran-coated charcoal; this has continued to be used routinely, since it produces reliable and reproducible results and is the least expensive in materials.

Sodium phosphate buffer (0.04 M, pH 6.5) containing 0.25% Trasylol was cooled to 4°C; dextran T-70 (Pharmacia Ltd., Uppsala, Sweden) and charcoal (carbon decolorizing C-170, Fisher Scientific Ltd., Fair Lawn, New Jersey) were added with gentle mixing to give a final concentration of 2.5 mg charcoal and 0.5 mg dextran per 200 μl buffer. The dextran-coated charcoal suspension was prepared at least 30 minutes before use and the tubes were centrifuged at 2800 rpm for 20 minutes immediately after the addition of 200 μl of this suspension.

The supernatants were discarded and the tube containing the charcoal pellet, i.e., the free labeled polypeptide, was counted in an automatic gamma counter. All results are expressed as percent bound, after correction for nonspecific binding.

E. Handling of Biological Samples

Plasma and serum can be assayed interchangeably. At dilutions of 1 : 3 to 1 : 10, there have been no serious plasma or serum problems.

Tissue extracts can be prepared by quick boiling of tissue in water for ten seconds, followed by homogenization in and extraction with ten volumes of 0.5 M acetic acid. After filtration or centrifugation until clear, the extract should be diluted in deionized water and lyophilized.

III. EVALUATION OF THE RADIOIMMUNOASSAY

A. Sensitivity and Precision

The concentrations of porcine motilin (M5) in the standard range were 12.5–400 pg per ml. Antisera from guinea pig 75 or rabbit Mo7 were used at final dilutions of 1 : 80,000 or 1 : 100,000, respectively. At these dilutions, both antisera record a 10% inhibition of binding from the zero condition for the addition of 12.5 pg motilin per tube.

Reproducibility of the assay system has been checked by assaying serum samples from two dogs on two separate occasions. Sera from one experiment were diluted 10% with Trasylol, while the other sera were stored without dilution. All samples were kept at −20°C between assays. The results (Figure 3), showed that Trasylol appeared to be unnecessary for the storage of motilin. Only one sample, from the Trasylol-treated batch of sera, lay outside the 25% limit. Recovery of added motilin has averaged 100 ± 14%.

Peak immunoreactive-motilin samples from these same two experiments, one obtained after exogenous intravenous administration of motilin and the other after endogenous motilin released by intraduodenal infusion of alkali, were serially diluted and assayed. The results could be fitted to the standard curve.

B. Standardization

Interassay variability was compared by routinely including an internal control in each assay. The control solution was motilin made

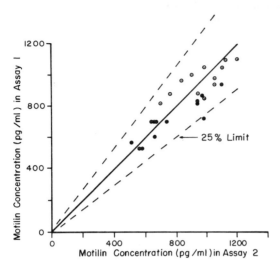

● Serum Samples, 10% Trasylol
Dates 6/24 ,   7/9

○ Serum Samples, No Trasylol
Dates 6/24 ,   7/9

Figure 3.   Reproducibility of motilin determinations on serum samples stored between assays at −20°C, with (●) or without (○) dilution with Trasylol. Only one sample showed more than 25% difference on reassay.

up in 0.04 M phosphate buffer, pH 6.5, containing 0.5% bovine serum albumin with 2% Trasylol to contain 100 pg motilin per 100 μl. The control solutions were aliquotted in approximately 1.0-ml portions in polyethylene Eppendorf tubes and stored at −20°C. After an aliquot was thawed, any remaining solution was discarded. The variability of this measure was 110 ± 23 pg, and any assay in which these limits were not met was questionable.

Standards were prepared from 1.0-μg aliquots of M5, lyophilized, and stored at −20°C. At monthly intervals, an aliquot was diluted with assay diluent buffer to a concentration of 80 ng/ml, divided into Eppendorf tubes, and frozen. Thawed standards were discarded after use.

C. Specificity and Affinity of Antisera

Comparative immunoreactivities of gastric inhibitory polypeptide, natural porcine secretin, synthetic glucagon, synthetic human gastrin (SHG 15-Leu), and 10% cholecystokinin–pancreozymin versus ^{125}I-motilin are shown in Figure 4. No significant cross-reactivity could be detected with up to 10 ng of each peptide. Although not shown in the figure, vasoactive intestinal peptide did not cross-react with the motilin antibody.

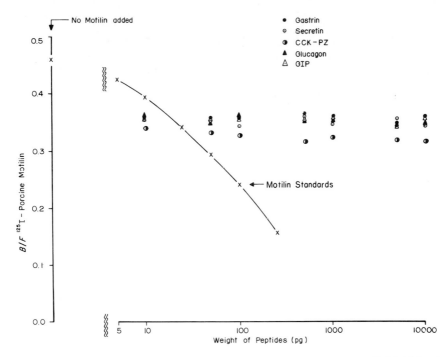

Figure 4. Comparative immunoreactivities of motilin, synthetic gastrin (SHG 15-Leu), synthetic glucagon, natural porcine secretin, cholecystokinin–pancreozymin (10% pure), and natural porcine gastric inhibitory polypeptide.

The affinity constant of each antiserum has been obtained by plotting the normal standard curve as a Scatchard plot (Figure 5) and measuring K, the slope of the line. From a series of such estimations, an index of the affinity of binding between the antigen and antibody for all motilin antisera may be obtained. This confirmed the correct choice of antiserum for routine assay purposes and gives a measure of the maintenance of titer and affinity of an antiserum between successive bleedings. The K values for antisera GP75 and Mo7 are 1.2×10^{14} and 8.0×10^{14}, respectively.

D. Physiological Observations

Pure natural porcine motilin administered intravenously in doses of 1.0 μg/kg/hour has been shown to stimulate motor activity in the gastric fundus, gastric antrum, and duodenum in dogs. No effect on gastric acid production was noted, although pepsin secretion was in-

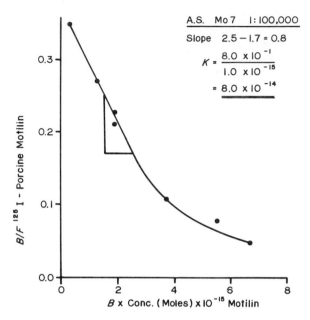

Figure 5.   Standard curve for motilin antiserum rabbit Mo7, at a dilution of $1 : 10 \times 10^4$, presented as a Scratchard plot, in which the affinity constant K is given by the slope of the line.

creased. The peak level of circulating immunoreactive motilin (IR-motilin) achieved in this manner (850 ± 85 pg/ml, S.E.M.) was comparable to that released endogenously upon instillation of alkali into the duodenum (860 ± 106 pg at six minutes), and had similar effects on gastric and duodenal motor activity.

Jennewein *et al.* (1975) investigated the effects of intravenous administration of natural motilin, either as a single shot of 30 ng/kg or as an infusion of 100 ng/kg/hour, on lower esophageal sphincter pressure (LESP) in dogs. Motilin was found to induce low frequency activity in the LESP in phase with the activity stimulated in the fundus and antrum.

The fasting serum levels of IR-motilin in both dogs and humans were in the range 200–350 pg per ml. To date, no physiologic secretagogue for motilin has been demonstrated in humans, and no elevation of IR-motilin levels has been associated with the well-documented response of increased LESP in response to gastric alkalinization in man (Castell and Levine, 1971; Picker and Brenner, 1972; Kline *et al.*, 1975).

IV. AFFINITY CHROMATOGRAPHY

A. Application to Radioimmunoassay

Motilin antiserum was coupled to cyanogen bromide-activated Sepharose 4B by the method of Cuatrecasas *et al.* (1968). Sepharose B was activated in the hood by addition of an equal volume of cold deionized distilled water and 100 mg cyanogen bromide per gram of Sepharose dissolved in water just prior to addition. Sodium hydroxide (4 N) was added until the pH stabilized between 10.5 and 11. The material was filtered on a Buchner filter, washed with 0.1 M NaHCO$_3$, and stored at 4°C for up to one week. Coupling was accomplished by mixing equal volumes of activated Sepharose, 0.1 M NaHCO$_3$, and antiserum (to a final antiserum concentration of 30 μl/gm of Sepharose). The mixture was stirred at 4°C for 24 hours, after which it was washed with 20 volumes of cold deionized water on a Buchner filter and stored at 4°C. Serial dilutions of the coupled ligand were incubated with ^{125}I-motilin, and the dilution curve obtained gives an index of the amount required to bind 50% of the label (cf. normal antiserum dilution curves). When this volume of Sepharose-bound antibody was used in a slightly modified radioimmunoassay, the sensitivity of the upper portion of the curve was slightly increased, but there was no significant improvement over dextran-coated charcoal for the separation of bound and free portions.

B. Application to Purification of Label and Motilin in Sera and Extracts

Small columns of Sepharose 4B coupled to motilin antisera were prepared in Pasteur pipettes with a bed volume of 1.0 ml. The columns were well equilibrated with 0.04 M phosphate-buffered saline (PBS), pH 6.5, and a sample of labeled motilin containing 50,000 cpm applied in the equilibrating buffer. Of the initial material, 80% remained bound. The labeled motilin was eluted from the column with 0.2 M acetic acid, and 72% of the absorbed material was recovered. Stronger acid or the addition of 6 M guanidine would probably increase this recovery.

In similar fashion 4.0 ng pure motilin in charcoal-extracted plasma was applied to a column, and radioimmunoassay was used to monitor the recovery of motilin after elution with acetic acid. Of the 83% motilin initially absorbed, 100% was recovered.

The starting material in the purification of motilin is a side fraction in the purification of secretin, designated presekretin (Brown *et al.*, 1971). The original purification procedure, which involved five stages of column chromatography, was monitored using the chronic dog preparation as a bioassay for motor stimulating activity and resulted in a pure material. When presekretin was applied to a column of Sepharose 4B–antibody, the absorbed portion, which was 90–100% recovered, represented approximately 5% of the total, and its homogeneity can be checked by electrophoresis on polyacrylamide gel. This represented a great improvement in the efficiency of the purification process, both in time and material.

REFERENCES

Bloom, S. R., Mitznegg, P., and Bryant, M. G. (1976). Measurement of human plasma in motilin. *Scand. J. Gastroenterol.* **11**, Suppl. 39, 47–52.
Brown, J. C., Johnson, L. P., and Magee, D. F. (1966). Effect of duodenal alkalinization on gastric motility. *Gastroenterology* **50**, 333–339.
Brown, J. C., Mutt, V., and Dryburgh, J. R. (1971). The further purification of motilin, a gastric motor activity stimulating polypeptide from the mucosa of the small intestine of hogs. *Can. J. Physiol. Pharmacol.* **49**, 399–405.
Brown, J. C., Cook, M. A., and Dryburgh, J. R. (1972). Motilin, a gastric motor activity stimulating polypeptide: Final purification, amino acid composition, and C-terminal residues. *Gastroenterology* **62**, 401–404.
Brown, J. C., Cook, M. A., and Dryburgh, J. R. (1973). Motilin, a gastric motor activity stimulating polypeptide: The complete amino acid sequence. *Can. J. Physiol. Pharmacol.* **51**, 533–537.
Castell, D. O., and Levine, S. M. (1971). Lower esophageal sphincter response to gastric alkalinization. A new method for the treatment of heartburn with antacids. *Ann. Intern. Med.* **74**, 223–227.
Cuatrecasas, P., Wilchek, M., and Anfinsen, C. B. (1968). Selective enzyme purification by affinity chromatography. *Proc. Natl. Acad. Sci. U.S.A.* **61**, 636–643.
Dryburgh, J. R., and Brown, J. C. (1975). Radioimmunoassay for motilin. *Gastroenterology* **68**, 1169–1176.
Goodfriend, T. L., Levine, L., and Fasman, G. D. (1964). Antibodies to bradykinin and angiotensin: A use of carbodiimides in immunology. *Science* **144**, 1344–1346.
Hunter, W. M., and Greenwood, F. C. (1963). Preparation of ^{131}I-labelled human growth hormone of high specific activity. *Biochem. J.* **89**, 114–123.
Jennewein, H. M., Hummelt, H., Siewert, R., and Waldeck, F. (1975). The motor-stimulating effect of natural motilin on the lower esophageal sphincter, fundus, antrum and duodenum in dogs. *Digestion* **13**, 246–250.
Kline, M. M., McCallum, R. W., Curry, N., and Sturdevant, R. A. L. (1975). Effect of

gastric alkalinization on lower esophageal sphincter pressure and serum gastrin. *Gastroenterology* **68**, 1137–1139.

Miyachi, Y., Vaituikaitis, J. L., Nieschlag, E., and Lipsett, M. B. (1972). Enzymatic radioiodination of gonadotropins. *J. Clin. Endocrinol. Metab.* **34**, 23–28.

Picker, B. B. S., and Brenner, G. G. (1972). The effect of intragastric aluminum hydroxide on lower oesophageal sphincter pressures. *S. Afr. Med. J.* **216**, 1387–1389.

Schubert, H., and Brown, J. C. (1974). Correction to the amino acid sequence of porcine motilin. *Can. J. Biochem.* **52**, 7–8.

29

Bombesin-Like Peptides

JOHN H. WALSH AND HELEN C. WONG

I. INTRODUCTION

Bombesin is a tetradecapeptide amide, isolated from the skin of the frog, *Bombina bombina,* by Erspamer and co-workers. It is the most potent known stimulant of gastrin release and also causes release of cholecystokinin and pancreatic polypeptide when administered parenterally into mammals. Bombesin also has a direct effect on the pancreas *in vitro,* causing stimulation of enzyme secretion. Other biologic effects of bombesin include increase in blood pressure, stimulation of smooth muscle contraction, antidiuresis, hyperglycemia, and lowering of body temperature following intracisternal administration. It is not known whether any of these pharmacologic actions has a physiologic counterpart due to the release of mammalian bombesin-like peptides, and the presence of such peptides has not been established with certainty. Immunofluorescence studies have revealed en-

581

Methods of Hormone Radioimmunoassay, Second Edition
Copyright © 1979 by Academic Press, Inc.
All rights of reproduction in any form reserved. ISBN 0-12-379260-6

docrinelike cells with bombesin-like immunoreactivity in the stomach and intestine of man and other mammals. Preliminary data also have been obtained which indicate that bombesin-like material can be extracted from the gastrointestinal tract of mammals.

The structure of bombesin is shown in Table I. The C-terminal nonapeptide amide fragment of bombesin (B-9) retains full biologic activity, but the octapeptide has only minimal activity. For convenience, we frequently use the abbreviation B-14 to designate the tetradecapeptide amide. B-14 contains no tyrosine residue, but the synthetic analog ^{1}Tyr-bombesin decapeptide amide (Tyr-B-10) has been prepared for use in radioiodination. The molecular weights, molar extinction coefficients at 280 nm, and the factors used for conversion of A_{280} of peptide solutions into concentrations in μg/ml or nmole/ml also are presented in the table.

Bombesin is related structurally to several other peptides that have been identified in frogs or mammals (Table I). The frog peptides alytesin, ranatensin, and litorin share a number of pharmacologic properties with bombesin. Two mammalian peptides, both of which have

Table I   Bombesin and Related Peptides[a]

Bombesin peptides	1	2	3	4	5	6	7	8	9	10	11	12	13	14
B-14	Glp-	Gln-	Arg-	Leu-	Gly-	Asn-	Gln-	Trp-	Ala-	Val-	Gly-	His-	Leu-	Met- NH₂
B-9						Asn-	Gln-	Trp-	Ala-	Val-	Gly-	His-	Leu-	Met- NH₂
Tyr-B-10					Tyr-	Asn-	Gln-	Trp-	Ala-	Val-	Gly-	His-	Leu-	Met- NH₂
Related frog peptides														
Alytesin	Glp-	Gly-	Arg-	Leu-	Gly-	Thr-	Gln-	Trp-	Ala-	Val-	Gly-	His-	Leu-	Met- NH₂
Ranatensin		Glp-	Val-	Pro-	Gln-	Trp-	Ala-	Val-	Gly-	His-	Phe-	Met- NH₂		
Litorin			Glp-	Gln-	Trp-	Ala-	Val-	Gly-	His-	Phe-	Met- NH₂			
Related mammalian peptides														
Substance P	Arg-	Pro-	Lys-	Pro-	Gln-	Gln-	Phe-	Phe-	Gly-	Leu-	Met-	NH₂		
VIP	-Tyr-	Thr-	Arg-	Leu-	Arg-	Lys-	Gln-	Met-	Ala-	Val-	Lys-	Lys-	Tyr-	Leu-
	(10)													(23)

				Factor[c]	
Peptide	MW	E_{280}[b]	μg/ml	nmole/ml
Bombesin (B-14)	1620	5377	301	186
Bombesin nonapeptide (B-9)	1054	5377	196	186
^{1}Tyr-bombesin decapeptide (Tyr-B-10)	1218	6884	177	145

[a] Residues set in italic type indicate identities with bombesin molecule.
[b] E_{280}, Extinction coefficient at 280 nm based on Trp = 5377 and Tyr = 1507.
[c] Multiply absorbance at 280 nm by factor to obtain concentration in indicated units.

been found in both gut and brain tissues, also have some structural similarity with bombesin. Neither of these peptides, substance P and vasoactive intestinal peptide (VIP), is known to cause release of gastrin. The chemical structure of mammalian bombesin-like peptide(s) has not been determined.

II. METHOD OF RADIOIMMUNOASSAY

A. Source of Peptides

The synthetic bombesin peptides B-14, B-9, Tyr-B-10, litorin, and eledoisin were gifts of Dr. Roberto de Castiglione, Section Head of Chemical Research, Farmitalia, Milan, Italy. These peptides were prepared by classical peptide synthetic techniques. Shorter fragments of bombesin were synthesized for studies of structure–activity relationships, but the supply of these peptides appears to have been exhausted. We are not aware of alternate sources of these peptides. Although it would be desirable to have pure or synthetic mammalian bombesin peptides for use as immunogens and assay standards, such peptides are not available at the present time.

B. Preparation of Antigen

We have produced antibodies to bombesin by immunization of animals with B-14 or B-9 conjugated to heterologous serum albumin. The carbodiimide reaction has been used most often for the conjugation procedure, although B-9 also has been conjugated using glutaraldehyde as a coupling reagent.

B-14 was dissolved in 40% methanol in water adjusted to pH 3.5, then the pH was brought to 7.5 by addition of NaOH. The conjugation mixture contained 3.0 ml B-14 solution (1160 nmole), 2.0 mg (32 nmole) purified bovine serum albumin in 2 ml 0.05 M Na phosphate buffer, pH 6.7, and 20 mg (118 μmole) 1-ethyl-3-(3-dimethylaminopropyl)carbodiimide in phosphate buffer. The mixture was stirred overnight at 22°C, and was then centrifuged to remove a white precipitate. Unreacted B-14 and carbodiimide were removed by dialysis against 0.15 M NaCl for 48 hours. The original molar ratios of reactants were approximately 32 : 1 : 3700 (B-14 : BSA : carbodiimide) and the efficiency of conjugation was found to be approximately 32% as determined by measurement of absorbance at 280 nm before and after dialysis with correction for absorbance of albumin.

C. Immunization of Animals

New Zealand white rabbits were immunized by multiple intradermal injections at intervals of six to ten weeks. Emulsions were prepared from equal parts of conjugated antigen and complete Freund's adjuvant. Each rabbit received 2.0 ml of the emulsion, containing approximately 30–50 nmole B-14 divided into 30–40 sites at each injection. We have not attempted to immunize other types of animals. Useful antibodies were obtained in only one of six rabbits immunized during one immunization program, but in eight of nine rabbits immunized in a second group. The reasons for the marked difference in success rates were not obvious. Antibodies usually were first detected after the second or third immunization.

D. Characterization of Antibody

Antibody titers were defined as the final dilution of serum that would bind 50% of labeled Tyr-B-10 added in a concentration of 1000 cpm/ml (approximately 10 fmole/ml) after incubation at 4°C for 48 hours. Titers obtained with several rabbits ranged between 1 : 100 and 1 : 100,000. The most useful antibody, 1078, was used in a final concentration of 1 : 30,000–1 : 80,000.

Antibodies were characterized for sensitivity and specificity. Sensitivity was expressed as the final concentration of peptide that caused 50% inhibition of initial B/F ratio (ID_{50}). As expected, sensitivity could be altered by varying the conditions of incubation, including specific activity of labeled Tyr-B-10, antibody dilution, and incubation time. Under optimal conditions, the ID_{50} for antibody 1078 for B-14 was 15–20 pmole/liter. The sensitivity of other bombesin antibodies, when B-14 was used as the standard, ranged from 50 to 1200 pmole/liter.

The specificity of antibody 1078 is indicated in Figure 1. Three bombesin peptides with identical C-terminal structure (B-14, B-9, and Tyr-B-10) demonstrate almost identical inhibitory potency. C-terminal specificity is expected in this system, since the labeled Tyr-B-10 would not be expected to bind to N-terminal bombesin antibodies. The Leu-Met-NH$_2$ C-terminal dipeptide region appears to have special importance, since substitution of Phe for Leu in litorin leads to a 500-fold reduction in immunochemical potency. Substance P, which contains the terminal Leu-Met-NH$_2$ configuration, has weak immunopotency (approximately 1 : 10,000) compared with the bombesin peptides. Eledoisin, which is structurally related to substance P but has less chemical identity with bombesin, has minimal cross-

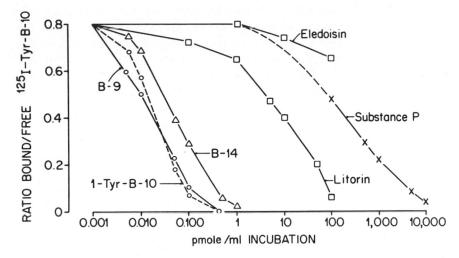

Figure 1.   Inhibition of binding of ^{125}I-Tyr-B-10 to bombesin antibody 1078 produced by varying concentrations of peptides structurally related to bombesin.

reactivity. No inhibition of binding was found with VIP, gastrin, secretin, or cholecystokinin at concentrations of 1.0 nmole/ml.

E. Radioiodination

Since bombesin contains no tyrosine residue, the synthetic Tyr-B-10 peptide is very satisfactory for labeling. Attempts to label B-9 by the Bolton–Hunter conjugation technique have been unsuccessful in our laboratory. The iodination reaction is carried out in a shielded radioactive hood at 20°–22°C. The following reagents are added in order to a small glass test tube: 50 μl 0.25 M Na phosphate buffer, pH 7.4, 0.9 nmole Tyr-B-10 in 20 μl 50% ethanol, 1.0 mCi (0.58 nmole) Na ^{125}I in 10 μl solvent, and 143 nmole chloramine-T in 20 μl phosphate buffer. After a reaction time of 15 seconds, 526 nmole sodium metabisulfite is added in 20 μl phosphate buffer.

The iodination mixture then is applied to a 1.0 × 10 cm Sephadex G-10 column prepared in 3% acetic acid containing 0.2% bovine serum albumin and fractions of 1.0 ml are obtained. Enough fractions are collected to include both the labeled peptide and free iodide. Radioactivity is measured in each tube in order to estimate percent incorporation of radioiodide into the peptide. The peptide peak should contain 70–90% of total radioactivity. The peak tube from the G-10 column then is applied to a 1.0 × 100 cm column of Sephadex G-50

SF and eluted with 0.02 M barbital buffer, pH 8.4, containing 0.2% bovine serum albumin. This step permits partial separation of labeled from unlabeled Tyr-B-10 as shown in Figure 2. The iodinated peptide elutes slightly behind the noniodinated peptide, and both substances elute later than the salt peak. The initial G-10 column removes free iodide, which also would elute in the same region. Use of barbital buffer for the second step produces somewhat better separation of labeled and unlabeled peptide than is obtained when acetic acid is used for elution.

Specific activity of the labeled peptide can be assessed by performing label inhibition curves with material obtained from various regions in the peak of radioactivity obtained from the Sephadex G-50 column. Serial twofold dilutions are made so that the final concentration in the radioimmunoassay tubes ranges from 1000 to 64,000 cpm/ml. The concentration of labeled peptide, expressed as cpm/ml, required to produce 50 per inhibition of initial B/F ratio is compared with the concentration of unlabeled Tyr-B-10 required to produce equal inhibition when the incubation mixture contains 1000 cpm/ml of

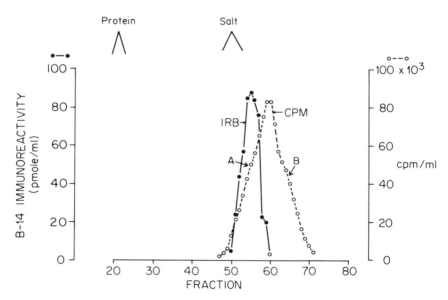

Figure 2. Partial separation of radioiodinated Tyr-B-10 from unlabeled peptide by gel filtration on Sephadex G-50 SF column, 1.0 × 100 cm, eluted with 0.02 M Veronal buffer containing 0.2% protein. In this experiment, unlabeled Tyr-B-10 was mixed with the protein peak obtained from Sephadex G-10. Specific activity of the labeled material obtained from point A was much lower than specific activity of material obtained from point B.

high specific activity labeled peptide. Such tests of specific activity have revealed that labeled peptide obtained from the ascending slope of the G-50 elution (marked A in Figure 2) has a specific activity of only 30–60 cpm/fmole, while labeled peptide from the descending slope (marked B on Figure 2) has a specific activity as high as 2500 cpm/fmole. Since some compromise between the highest specific activity and adequate yield must be made, we usually pool all tubes from the descending slope on G-50 for use in the radioimmunoassay. When it is desirable to maximize assay sensitivity, tubes can be selected only from the midportion of the descending slope in order to achieve greatest specific activity. Labeled peptide retains immunoreactivity for at least six weeks when stored frozen at −40°C or colder.

F. Preparation of Samples for Radioimmunoassay

At the present time, our bombesin radioimmunoassay has not been successful in demonstrating circulating bombesin-like immunoreactivity in mammals, a finding which may reflect the relatively poor sensitivity of the assay. There is a significant inhibitory effect produced by serum protein that leads to apparent bombesin-like immunoreactivity of 100–200 pmole/liter in serum samples assayed at 1 : 10 final dilution. However, when standard curves are prepared with charcoal-extracted serum (see below) or serum which has been treated with bombesin antibody coupled to Sepharose beads, the apparent activity disappears. Furthermore, if the same serum sample is assayed before and after treatment by affinity chromatography to remove bombesin-like immunoreactivity, no differences in apparent concentration can be detected. This method removes bombesin-like material which is extracted from gut tissues and added to serum almost quantitatively.

The bombesin radioimmunoassay has been used successfully to measure bombesin-like immunoreactivity in extracts prepared from the gut and brain of mammals and frogs and from the skin of certain frogs. The most efficient extraction method appears to be homogenization and boiling for 15 minutes in 3% acetic acid. Such extraction is two to three times more efficient than boiling water or methanol. Strong acid produces some inhibition in the radioimmunoassay system, so that concentrated extracts must either be neutralized or lyophilized before assay. Alternatively, the same concentration of acetic acid present in the extracts being tested can be used in preparation of the standard curve.

G. Assay Procedure

Standard B-14 and B-9 solutions are stored in aliquots containing 100 nmole/liter peptide in 0.15 M NaCl and are stored at $-70°C$. The standard solution is diluted 1 : 10, 1 : 100, and 1 : 1000 immediately prior to assay. Standard curves are prepared by pipetting 200, 100, 50, and 20 μl of each standard solution into duplicate tubes with a Micromedic automatic pipettor and adjusting the final volume to 1000 μl by addition of an appropriate amount of standard diluent consisting of 0.02 M sodium barbital buffer containing 0.2% plasma protein solution and 0.02% sodium azide. The final incubation volume is 2.0 ml, so the range covered by the standard curve is 1–1000 pmole/liter with two points of overlap (10 and 100 pmole/liter) to test the accuracy of dilution of the standard solution. Unknown solutions are added in volumes of 20 to 200 μl, depending on the expected concentration of bombesin-like immunoreactivity present and may be prediluted when necessary. The final volume of unknown solutions also is brought to 1.0 ml by addition of standard diluent. Labeled Tyr-B-10 is diluted in standard diluent to contain 2000 cpm per 0.8 ml and is added as a second step along with 0.2 ml diluted antibody, prepared at a concentration ten times higher than the desired final concentration, through parallel delivery pumps.

Tubes are incubated for 24–72 hours at 4°C. The optimal incubation time is determined empirically for each antibody. Separation of bound and free labeled peptide is performed with dextran-coated charcoal. The separation mixture contains 20 mg activated charcoal, 20 mg dextran, and 20 μl plasma in a final volume of 0.2 ml. Tubes should be kept on ice during the separation procedure. After thorough mixing, the tubes are centrifuged at 3000 rpm for 15 minutes and the supernatant solutions are removed by pouring off into separate tubes. Both bound (supernatant) and free (pellet) are counted for two to five minutes, depending on the accuracy desired, and the calculations of unknown concentrations are performed by standard methods.

H. Purification by Affinity Chromatography

The technique of affinity chromatography is useful for concentrating small concentrations of bombesin-like immunoreactive material in tissue extracts, for demonstrating the specificity of inhibitory substances found in extracts, and for preparation of serum and other solutions free of bombesin-like material. It is an especially useful technique for determining whether apparent bombesin-like material identified in protein-rich tissue extracts is due to a specific peptide or due to nonspecific inhibition of the antigen–antibody reaction by protein or other substances present in the extracts.

Sepharose 4B beads preconjugated with CNBr are purchased from Pharmacia Fine Chemicals (catalog No. 74301). The beads are washed extensively with 3 liters $0.003 M$ HCl and 1.5 liters $0.1 M$ NaCl–$0.14 M$ NaHCO₃ by gentle suction filtration. An original aliquot of 6.0 gm of beads is suspended in a final volume of 40 ml NaCl–NaHCO₃ buffer. γ-Globulin is prepared from a suitable antiserum by ammonium sulfate precipitation. To 3.0 ml antibody, add 1.0 ml saturated ammonium sulfate slowly with continuous stirring in an ice bath. Let the mixture stand for ten minutes in the cold, and then centrifuge for five minutes at 2000 rpm. Discard the fibrinogen precipitate. To the supernatant add 1.0 ml saturated ammonium sulfate with continuous stirring to produce a final solution which is 40% saturated. After allowing to stand for ten minutes in ice, centrifuge at 2000 rpm for ten minutes and reserve the precipitated γ-globulin. The precipitate is dissolved in 1.0 ml distilled water and dialyzed for 24 hours against two changes of NaCl–NaHCO₃ buffer. The γ-globulin dialysate is added to the washed beads and agitated gently by rotation for 24 hours in an Ehrlenmeyer flask with a siliconized ground glass stopper. The bead–antibody conjugate then is washed with alternating 1.0 liter volumes 0.1 M acetic acid–1 M NaCl, pH4, and 0.1 M NaHCO₃–1.0 M NaCl, pH8, and is suspended in 1.0 l 1 M glycine for three hours to saturate any unreacted CNBr binding sites. The suspension finally is washed with 3.0 liter $0.1 M$ NaHCO₃–$0.14 M$ NaCl and stored in a final volume of 50 ml of this buffer containing 1 : 10,000 Merthiolate at 4°C.

In this system, in a typical experiment, a 100-μl bead suspension bound 50% of added labeled Tyr-B-10 in five minutes and 80% in 60 minutes at room temperature. Addition of graded concentrations of B-14 resulted in competitive displacement of labeled Tyr-B-10 (Figure 3). The concentration of B-14 that was 50% bound to beads was approximately 12 pmole, representing a capacity of approximately 2.0 nmole/ml of original antiserum. These experiments were done batchwise in test tubes. The efficiency of binding is improved somewhat by use of beads in a short column. It is apparent that the binding capacity of such beads is sufficient for extraction of picomole quantities of bombesin-like peptides from serum or tissue extracts but is not sufficient for large-scale purification of such peptides. The bombesin bound to these beads can be recovered quantitatively either by boiling in water or by incubating with acid.

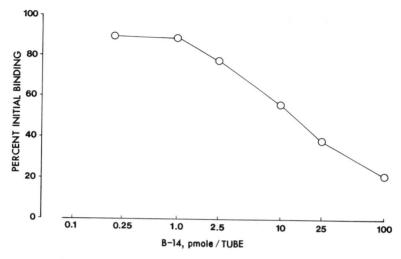

Figure 3. Binding of ^{125}I-Tyr-B-10 to affinity chromatography beads prepared with bombesin antiserum in the presence of graded concentrations of unlabeled bombesin. Each incubation tube contained 15,000 cpm labeled bombesin (150–200 fmole), 100 μl beads (representing 6.0 μl original antibody) and the indicated amount of bombesin in a final volume of 1.0 ml. Incubation was carried out for 40 min at 20°C with gentle agitation, and the beads were separated from the liquid by centrifugation. Binding in the absence of added bombesin was 66%, of which 8% could be explained by trapping of liquid in the beads.

III. BOMBESIN-LIKE MATERIAL IN TISSUES

Although bombesin-like immunoreactivity has not been identified with certainty in plasma, it has been identified in tissues obtained from a number of mammals, including dog, hog, human, rabbit, and rat. The total amount of immunoreactivity recovered has been low, 1–10 pmole/gm tissue in gastric mucosa and lesser amounts in other tissues. It is not clear whether the relatively low bombesin-like immunoreactivity measured in tissue extracts reflects inefficient extraction by boiling water, poor cross-reactivity of mammalian bombesin-like immunoreactivity with the frog bombesin radioimmunoassay, or whether it is a true reflection of the amount of peptide present. Characterization of the immunoreactive material obtained from dog stomach mucosa by Sephadex G-50 gel filtration reveals that it has a larger apparent molecular weight than synthetic bombesin or bombesin-like immunoreactivity extracted from the skin of *Rana pipiens* (Figure 4). The biologic activity and other properties of this material have not yet been characterized. Bombesin-like immunoreactivity also has been iden-

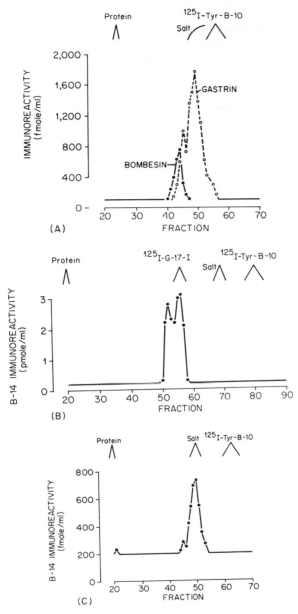

Figure 4.   Gel filtration elution pattern of bombesin-like immunoreactivity obtained by chromatography on Sephadex G-50 SF column, 1.0 × 100 cm, eluted with 0.02 M Veronal buffer containing 0.2% protein. (A) Boiling water extract of dog fundus mucosa. (B) Rechromatography of dog fundus extract after concentration by affinity chromatography. (C) Boiling water extract of *Rana pipiens* skin.

tified in lesser concentrations in a number of other dog tissues, including the intestinal mucosa, liver, spleen, and brain. Concentration of these extracts by affinity chromatography and liberation of the extracted bombesin-like material from affinity beads with boiling water produced almost identical estimates of tissue bombesin-like immunoreactivity. The apparent widespread distribution of the immunoreactive material in dog tissues is unexplained and may reflect the presence of this material in nerves as well as in gut mucosal cells. Inhibition curves performed with bombesin-like immunoreactivity prepared by affinity concentration were roughly parallel with the inhibition curve produced by B-14 standard, suggesting chemical similarity among the substances. Boiling water extracts of beads which had not been reacted with tissue extracts failed to liberate measurable bombesin-like immunoreactivity (Figure 5).

There are several immediate problems which need to be solved in order to apply the radioimmunoassay of bombesin to physiologic studies. The sensitivity of the assay needs to be improved and the problem of nonspecific serum interference must be solved in order to determine circulating concentrations of bombesin-like immunoreactivity and to characterize mechanisms for release of bombesin-like immunoreactivity into the circulation. The bombesin-like immunoreactivity present in tissue extracts needs to be characterized further and prepared in highly purified form, and the complete structure needs to be determined. If mammalian bombesin-like im-

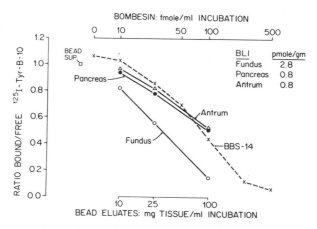

Figure 5. Inhibition curves produced by bombesin and by graded amounts of extracts of dog fundus mucosa, antrum mucosa, and pancreas after concentration by affinity chromatography. Failure of boiling water supernatant of affinity beads alone to produce inhibition is indicated in the upper left.

munoreactivity differs significantly from bombesin, it may be necessary to immunize animals with this material in order to obtain antibodies of sufficient avidity and specificity for successful radioimmunoassay. When these conditions have been satisfied, it may be possible to determine whether or not circulating bombesin has a physiologic role in regulation of release of gastrin or some other physiologic function.

REFERENCES

Anastasi, A., Erspamer, V., and Bucci, M. (1972). Isolation and amino acid sequences of alytesin and bombesin, two analogous active tetradecapeptides from the skin of European discoglossid frogs. *Arch. Biochem. Biophys.* **148**, 443–446.

Basso, N., Lezoche, F., Materia, A., Giri, S., and Speranza, V. (1975a). Effect of bombesin on extragastric gastrin in man. *Am. J. Dig. Dis.* **20**, 923–927.

Basso, N., Giri, S., Improta, G., Lezoche, E., Melchiorri, P., Percoco, M., and Speranza, V. (1975b). External pancreatic secretion after bombesin infusion in man. *Gut* **16**, 994–998.

Basso, N., Lezoche, E., Giri, S., Percoco, M., and Speranza, V. (1977). Acid and gastrin levels after bombesin and calcium infusion in patients with incomplete antrectomy. *Am. J. Dig. Dis.* **22**, 125–128.

Bertaccini, G. (1976). Active polypeptides of nonmallian origin. *Pharmacol. Rev.* **28**, 127–177.

Bertaccini, G., Impicciatore, M., Molina, E., and Zappia, L. (1974). Action of bombesin on human gastrointestinal motility. *Rend. Gastro-Enterol.* **6**, 45–51.

Broccardo, M., Falconieri Erspamer, G., Melchiorri, P., Negri, L., and de Castiglione, R. (1975). Relative potency of bombesin-like peptides. *Br. J. Pharmacol.* **55**, 221–227.

Brown, M., Rivier, J., and Vale, W. (1977). Bombesin: Potent effects on thermoregulation in the rat. *Science* **196**, 998–1000.

Caprilli, R., Melchiorri, P., Improta, G., Vernia, P., and Frieri, G. (1975). Effects of bombesin and bombesin-like peptides on gastrointestinal myoelectric activity. *Gastroenterology* **68**, 1228–1235.

Corraziari, E., Torsoli, A., Melchiorri, P., and Delle Fave, G. F. (1974). Effect of bombesin on human gallbladder emptying. *Rend. Gastro-Enterol.* **6**, 52–54.

Deschodt-Lanckman, M., Robberecht, P., De Neef, P., Lammens, M., and Christophe, J. (1976). In vitro action of bombesin and bombesin-like peptides on amylase secretion, calcium efflux, and adenylate cyclase activity in the rat pancreas: A comparison with other secretagogues. *J. Clin. Invest.* **58**, 891–898.

Erspamer, V., and Melchiorri, P. (1973). Active polypeptides of the amphibian skin and their synthetic analogues. *Pure Appl. Chem.* **35**, 463–494.

Erspamer, V., and Melchiorri, P. (1975). Actions of bombesin on secretions and motility of the gastrointestinal tract. *In* "Gastrointestinal Hormones" (J. C. Thompson, ed.), p. 575. Univ. of Texas Press, Austin.

Erspamer, V., Improta, G., Melchiorri, P., and Sopranzi, N. (1974). Evidence of cholecystokinin release by bombesin in the dog. *Br. J. Pharmacol.* **52**, 227–232.

Impicciatore, M., Debas, H., Walsh, J. H., Grossman, M. I., and Bertaccini, G. (1974). Release of gastrin and stimulation of acid secretion by bombesin in dog. *Rend. Gastro-Enterol.* **6**, 99–101.

Konturek, S. J., Krol, R., and Tasler, J. (1976). Effect of bombesin and related peptides on the release and action of intestinal hormones on pancreatic secretion. *J. Physiol. (London)* **257**, 663–672.

Pearse, A. G. E., Polak, J. M., and Bloom, S. R. (1977). The newer gut hormones. Cellular sources, physiology, pathology, and clinical aspects. *Gastroenterology* **72**, 746–761.

Polak, J. M., Bloom, S. R., Hobbs, S., Solcia, E., and Pearse, A. G. E. (1976). Distribution of a bombesin-like peptide in human gastrointestinal tract. *Lancet* **1**, 1109–1110.

Walsh, J. H., and Holmquist, A. L. (1976). Radioimmunoassay of bombesin peptides: Identification of bombesin-like immunoreactivity in vertebrate gut extracts. *Gastroenterology* **70**, 948.

30

Bile Acids

LAURENCE M. DEMERS

I. INTRODUCTION

Bile acids are present in most body fluids in complex mixtures, with the highest concentrations found in bile. There are four major bile acids, cholic acid, chenodeoxycholic acid, deoxycholic acid, and lithocholic acid, as well as several other minor bile acids usually found in minute concentrations. Bile acids usually exist conjugated at the carboxyl group with either glycine or taurine, but may also be conjugated with glucuronide or sulfate esters at the hydroxyl groups on bile

595

Methods of Hormone Radioimmunoassay, Second Edition

acids. In infants less than three months of age, bile acids are conjugated primarily to taurine; in older children and adults, bile acids are conjugated with a ratio of glycine : taurine. Thus, measurement of bile acids presents a complicated picture, considering the number and type of bile acids present in urine, serum, bile, and feces. In addition, bile acids are present in varied physical states depending on the type of body fluid. In serum, they are found bound to protein, in urine they are in solution, while in stools they are usually precipitated.

Until recently, the measurement of bile acids in serum, urine, or bile was achieved only through gas–liquid chromatography (GLC) (Van Berge Henegegouwen *et al.*, 1974). This involved elaborate extraction procedures and solvolysis in preparation for GLC measurements. Although identification of the four major bile acids was possible by GLC, only the determination of total bile acid levels was obtainable, and one could not differentiate between the conjugated and free (unconjugated) bile acid forms present in serum, urine, or bile. An extension of the GLC approach has been developed using combined gas chromatography–mass spectrometry (Elliot, 1973). This technique has proved to be an effective means of identifying a wide variety of unknown bile acids and provides more sensitivity than the conventional GLC method. This method, however, cannot distinguish free from conjugated forms of bile acids and is as tedious as it is costly to perform.

Another analytical procedure used to determine bile acid levels in biologic fluids is based on an enzymatic technique (Barnes, 1976). However, this procedure, like GLC, can only determine total bile acid concentrations. This technique utilizes hydroxysteroid dehydrogenase, which catalyzes the oxidation of the 3α-hydroxyl group of bile acids to a 3-ketone in the presence of an accompanying reduction of NAD to NADH. This reaction can be followed spectrophotometrically. However, due to the low concentrations of bile acids usually found in serum, the relatively low sensitivity of this procedure precludes valid determinations of bile acid levels in serum from normal individuals.

A breakthrough in methodology for bile acid measurements occured with the introduction of radioimmunoassay for serum bile acid determinations (Simmonds *et al.*, 1973; Demers and Hepner, 1976a; Murphy *et al.*, 1974). This technique provides the sensitivity needed to determine bile acids in serum in normal individuals and provides the specificity needed to allow for the differentiation of free from conjugated forms in serum, urine, and bile. Some laboratories have antibodies that will allow for measurement of total conjugated bile acids (glycine plus taurine conjugates), while other laboratories have more specific antibodies which can be used to assay only glycine-conjugated forms of the four major bile acids. To date, there have been no reports of taurine conjugate-specific radioimmunoassay systems for bile acids.

Bile acid measurements in serum by radioimmunoassay have already made striking advances possible in the area of understanding hepatobiliary disease and the dynamics of bile acid metabolism in the enterohepatic circulation. Indeed, in studies reported on 38 patients with chronic active hepatitis (Korman *et al.*, 1974), fasting serum bile acids proved to be a more sensitive indicator of activity of liver disease than the conventional tests of liver function, including bilirubin, alkaline phosphatase, aspartate transaminase, and proteins. When patients relapsed, a rise in serum bile acids preceded changes in transaminase activity by several weeks. Of greater significance was the observation that serum bile acids were elevated before any histologic changes were evident.

In another report on 40 patients with liver cancer (Demers and Hepner, 1976b), 25% of patients with histologically diagnosed hepatomas had an elevated serum bile acid level as the only detectable biochemical abnormality. Thus in biochemically silent liver disease, as judged by conventional liver function tests, serum bile acid measurements by radioimmunoassay have proved to be of significant value in diagnosing the presence and nature of liver disease.

II. METHODS OF RADIOIMMUNOASSAY

A. Preparation of Reagents and Samples

1. Sources of Bile Acid and Bile Acid Conjugates

Relatively pure major bile acids and bile acid conjugates can be obtained from Calbiochem (La Jolla, California), Sigma Chemical Company (St. Louis, Missouri), and P.L. Biochemicals, Inc. (Milwaukee, Wisconsin). Before use as standards, bile acids should be further purified using thin-layer chromatography on silicic acid plates with the solvent system of isoamyl acetate, propionic acid, n-propanol, water (40:30:40:10). Iodine crystal vaporization is used to visualize the plates once separation has been achieved. With this system, R_f values are cholylglycine 0.34, chemodeoxycholylglycine 0.49, deoxycholylglycine 0.50, sulfolithocholyglycine 0.71. More recently

(Demers *et al.*, 1978), high-pressure liquid chromatography has been used successfully to purify the commercially purchased bile acids using the following flow system: for the glycine derivatives, a solvent system of methanol, 0.15 M KH$_2$PO$_4$, isopropanol, 70 : 25 : 5, apparent pH 3.1 with a flow of 0.5 ml/minute, pressure 2400 psi, using column ES Chromegabond C-18 5 μl (Waters Associates) at a wavelength of 210 nm, 0.425 mA, and a chart speed of 1.0 cm/minute; for the taurine derivatives, the same system was utilized except for a solvent ratio of 60 : 33 : 7 and pressure of 2750 psi.

2. Preparation of Standards

Pure bile acid standards are initially dissolved in absolute ethanol to give a concentration of 800 nmole/ml. From this working stock a standard of 8.0 nmole/ml is prepared by diluting 100 μl of the 800 nmole/ml stock with 9.9 ml ethanol. To prepare standards for assay, 100 μl working stock standard (8.0 nmole/ml) is diluted with 900 μl 0.85% saline, pH 7.4, containing 1% bovine γ-globulin and 4% bovine serum albumin to give an assay standard of 80 pmole/100 μl. This standard is serially diluted in 1% bovine γ-globulin and 4% bovine serum albumin to obtain standards of 40, 20, 10, and 5.0 pmole/100 μl for use in the assay. Sets of working stock standard (8.0 nmole/ml) are prepared for up to three months and stored frozen in 100-μl aliquots at $-20°C$ for assay.

3. Production of Antibodies

In our laboratory, antibodies were raised against the glycine conjugates of cholic, chenodeoxycholic, deoxycholic, and sulfolithocholic acids by covalently coupling bovine serum albumin to the bile acids using the carbodiimide reaction.

a. Immunogen Preparation. Ten milligrams of the purified bile acid (as the sodium salt) in 0.8 ml ethanol is combined with 16 mg fatty acid-free bovine serum albumin in 7.2 ml distilled deionized water. With constant stirring, 8.0 mg carbodiimide [1-ethyl-3(3-dimethylaminopropyl)carbodiimide hydrochloride] is then added. The total mixture is then vortex-mixed and allowed to stand at room temperature for 24 hours. After equilibration at room temperature, the mixture is extensively dialyzed against phosphate-buffered physiologic saline (10 mmole phosphate per liter, pH 7.4) at 4°C for 72 hours. A small amount of radiolabeled bile acids (3000 cpm) can be added to the original reaction mixture to determine the extent of conjugation to bovine serum albumin. Using this technique, 30–35% of the bile acids becomes linked covalently to BSA. One-half-milliliter aliquots of the dialyzed conjugate preparation are stored at −20°C for subsequent injection into rabbits.

   b. **Immunization and Bleeding Schedule.** Adult New Zealand rabbits are injected with 0.5 ml of the conjugate preparation (3.0–4.0 mg) that has been emulsified with 0.5 ml of complete Freund's adjuvant (Difco Laboratories, Detroit, Michigan). The injections are made subcutaneously at multiple sites into the dorsal skin once a week for four weeks and then at monthly intervals as booster injections. Rabbits are bled from the marginal ear vein after one month and then ten days after each monthly injection. The resulting antiserum collected following centrifugation is then lyophilized and stored at −70°C. For use, 50 mg lyophilized powder is combined with 10 ml 0.01 M phosphate buffer to represent a 1 : 10 dilution. Diluted aliquots for assay use are prepared from this and frozen at −20°C, and thawed just prior to use.

   c. **Other Methods for Producing Bile Acid Antibodies.** Antiserum to conjugates of cholic acid that cross-react with glycine and taurine have been prepared by Murphy et al. (1974) using the mixed anhydride technique of Erlanger et al. (1957). These investigators used an absorption step to remove albumin antibodies present in their antiserum prior to use.

B. Radiolabeled Bile Acid Sources

   The four major bile acids (cholic acid, chenodeoxycholic acid, deoxycholic acid, and lithocholic acid) either free or conjugated to glycine, are readily available as tritium-labeled compounds from New England Nuclear (Waltham, Massachusetts) with specific activities ranging from 1.0–25 Ci/mmole. In addition, taurocholic acid labeled with tritium is also available from New England Nuclear as stock material. When purchased, trace material should be subjected to thin-layer chromatography similar to that for the standard material for additional purification prior to use.

   Stock solutions of trace material are kept in ethanol. For use in the immunoassay, an aliquot is evaporated under nitrogen and then diluted with 0.01 M phosphate-buffered saline (PBS), pH 7.4, to yield a radioactivity concentration of 10,000 cpm per 100 μl. A parallel dilution is made directly into a scintillation vial and the counts are checked in a liquid scintillation counter prior to each assay run.

   Recently, an iodinated trace of glycocholic acid was prepared by

Spenney *et al.* (1977). They linked histamine to cholylglycine using the carbodiimide reaction and then iodinated the cholylglycyl–histamine complex with Na^{125}I using the chloramine-T reaction. They achieved an iodination preparation which approximated 2000 Ci/mmole.

The cholylglycylhistamine was synthesized by stirring 10 mmole each of cholyglycine, N-hydroxysuccinide, and 1-ethyl-3-(3-diethylaminepropyl)carbodiimide in 75 ml N,N-dimethylformamide (DMF) for 90 minutes at 23°C. Ten millimoles of histamine dihydrochloride and triethylamine were suspended in 25 ml DMF, added to the active bile salt ester, and the reaction was allowed to proceed for 120 minutes. After addition of 100 ml water, the pH was adjusted to 10–11 with concentrated NaOH for 60 minutes, to pH 5 with HCl, and then the material was purified by ion-exchange chromatography. A 20-gm Dowex 50W-X8 cation exchange column was washed with ethanol and benzene and equilibrated with DMF–water, 1:1, at pH 5.0. After application of the product to the column, the column was washed with 50 ml DMF–water and 100 ml absolute ethanol. The cholylglycylhistamine was eluted with ethanol-NH$_3$, 85:15, collecting 3.0-ml aliquots. The appropriate fractions were dried using rotary vaporization and then vacuum for 18 hours and the compound was crystallized as a hydrochloride by addition of HCl.

Iodination was performed by reacting 50 nmole cholylglycyl–histamine in 10 μl of a 20% ethanolic aqueous solution, 10 μl 0.5 M phosphate buffer, pH 7.4, 2 mCi Na^{125}I, and 35 μg chloramine-T in 10 μl 0.5 M phosphate for 30 seconds. The reaction was stopped by adding 250 μg sodium metabisulfite in 100 μl 0.5 M phosphate and 2.0 ml 0.01 M phosphate buffer, pH 7.4. Purification of the iodinated product was carried out in two steps, ion-exchange and thin-layer chromatography. The iodination reaction mixture was applied to a 0.7 × 3.0 cm Amberlite XAD-2 column containing 1.0 gm resin. The column was washed with 3.0 ml 0.01 M phosphate buffer and then water until the iodide was totally eluted. The labeled bile acid was eluted with absolute ethanol, and was then dried to a volume of 0.1 ml under N$_2$. This material was then applied to a silica gel sheet using authentic unlabeled cholylglycylhistamine as a marker. The chromatogram was developed in a solvent system consisting of ethyl acetate–benzene–methanol–triethylamine (50:25:25:10). Appropriate spots were scraped off the chromatogram and the labeled bile salt derivatives were eluted using absolute ethanol.

Abbott Laboratories (North Chicago, Illinois) have recently disclosed the availability of commercial reagents for the radioimmunoassay of glycocholic and the sulfated form of glycolithocholic acid. These reagents include an iodinated bile acid trace preparation.

C. Characterization of Antiserum

1. Titer

The titer of the bile acid antiserum used for the assay is a function of the separation technique used to separate antibody-bound from free trace, as well as the nature of the trace, whether labeled with tritium or ^{125}I. Under normal circumstances, a reasonable titer of antiserum has been achieved for the bile acids studied to date within six to eight months following initiation of the immunization schedule. Antibodies have been produced of sufficient titer to allow for use in radioimmunoassay.

Two types of separation techniques have been employed for these assays, ammonium sulfate precipitation of the antibody–bile acid complex and polyethylene glycol (PEG) precipitation. A saturated ammonium sulfate solution (Amersham Searle, ultra pure) is prepared by adding 500 gm to 500 ml of distilled water followed by addition of salt until proper sedimentation of crystals indicates saturation has been achieved. A working solution of 60% ammonium sulfate is then prepared and used in the assay to separate antibody-bound from free tracer. Although effective, this separation technique has some inherent drawbacks which affect the precision of the results. Improved reproducibility can be achieved with the use of polyethylene glycol for the separation step. This procedure is also more amenable to an automated pipetting unit than the ammonium sulfate procedure and does not have the reagent-to-reagent variability that may exist with different preparations of saturated ammonium sulfate. An 18% solution of polyethylene glycol 6000 prepared in 0.85% saline is used to effect separation.

2. Specificity

The specificity of each bile acid antiserum is checked by performing cross-reactivity studies with various types of free and conjugated bile salts as well as other molecules that structurally resemble the bile acids. The specificity of any one antiserum prepared even from the same conjugate pool will vary from animal to animal and from one bleeding to the next, so that it is imperative to characterize the titer and specificity of each bleeding. In addition, some antisera will not

Table I   Cholyglycine Antiserum Specificity

Compound	Relative cross-reaction (%)
Cholylglycine	100
Cholyltaurine	18
Cholic acid	8.0
Chenodeoxycholylglycine	4.0
Chenodeoxycholic acid	4.0
Deoxycholylglycine	1.0
Deoxycholic acid	<0.1
Lithocholic acid	<0.1
Lithocholylglycine	3.0
Sulfolithocholylglycine	1.0
Chenodeoxycholytaurine	<0.2
Deoxycholyltaurine	<0.1
Lithocholyltaurine	<0.1
Cortisol	<0.1
Cholesterol	<0.1
Estrogen	<0.1
Testosterone	<0.3
Progesterone	<0.3

distinguish between taurine and glycine conjugates, and, thus, in this situation the assay will determine total conjugated bile acids.

The relative specificities of the four major bile acid antisera preparations from our laboratory are shown in Tables I–IV. Relative cross-reactivity is expressed in percentage as the mass required to displace 50% of bound radiolabeled bile acid from its respective antibody. The specificity is sufficient not to warrant a sample extraction or isolation by chromatography prior to performing the radioimmunoassay. As noted, there is a small degree of cross-reactivity by the taurine-conjugated bile acids with the glycine-conjugated bile acid antibody.

Table II   Chenodeoxycholylglycine Antiserum Specificity

Compound	Relative cross-reaction (%)
Chenodeoxycholylglycine	100
Chenodeoxycholytaurine	8.0
Chenodeoxycholic acid	0.3
Lithocholyltaurine	0.3
Lithocholylglycine	0.3
Cholyltaurine	<0.1
Lithocholic acid	<0.1
Deoxycholylglycine	<0.1
Deoxycholic acid	<0.1
Deoxycholyltaurine	<0.1

Table III   Deoxycholylglycine Antiserum Specificity

Compound	Relative cross-reaction (%)
Deoxycholylglycine	100
Deoxycholic acid	16
Deoxycholyltaurine	<0.1
Lithocholic acid	<0.1
Lithocholylglycine	<0.1
Sulfolithocholylglycine	<0.1
Chenodeoxycholic acid	<0.1

Table IV   Sulfolithocholylglycine Antiserum Specificity

Compound	Relative cross-reaction (%)
Sulfolithocholylglycine	100
Lithocholylglycine	6.0
Chenodeoxycholylglycine	0.4
Cholylglycine	<0.1
Deoxycholylglycine	<0.1
Lithocholic acid	<0.1
Sulfodeoxycholic	5.0
Sulfochenodeoxycholylglycine	1.0

D. Preparation of Serum Samples for Radioimmunoassay

Blood samples are collected in glass test tubes with the serum taken off following centrifugation. The major bile acids are normally present in serum in micromolar concentrations. Patient samples must be diluted to accommodate assay at the picomole level. These dilutions range from 1 : 3 to 1 : 50, depending on the patient source and whether the patient has active liver disease. Urine and bile are handled identically. Dilutions are achieved with 0.01 M phosphate-buffered saline containing 1% bovine γ-globulin and 4% human serum albumin, pH 7.4.

E. Radioimmunoassay Procedure

Separate homologous radioimmunoassays are performed for each bile acid.

1. Radioimmunoassays are performed in duplicate, in 12 × 75 mm acid-washed disposable test tubes. Samples, total counts, and blanks are run in duplicate.

2. Standards of cholylglycine, chenodeoxycholylglycine, deoxy-cholylglycine, and sulfolithocholylglycine are added in duplicate in 0.1-ml aliquots in amounts ranging from 5.0 to 120 pmole to prepare radioimmunoassay standard curves.

3. Pipette 100 μl of unknowns into labeled test tubes in duplicate in dilutions ranging from three- to fifty-fold.

4. Pipette 100 μl bile acid antiserum diluted in buffer to a concentration at which 50% of the radiolabeled bile acid is bound (1 : 500 to 1 : 2000) to all tubes except the total count and blank tubes.

5. Pipette 100 μl radiolabeled bile acids (2–3 pg) with radioactivity equivalent to approximately 10,000 cpm into each tube including blank and total count tubes.

6. Gently vortex all tubes and allow reaction to equilibrate, first at 42°C for 60 minutes, then at 4°C for 18–24 hours when the ammonium sulfate separation procedure is used. With the polyethylene glycol separation technique, equilibration can be attained within one hour at 37°C.

7. Following the equilibration period, the separation step is performed: (a) For ammonium sulfate—Keeping the tubes in ice, add 1.0

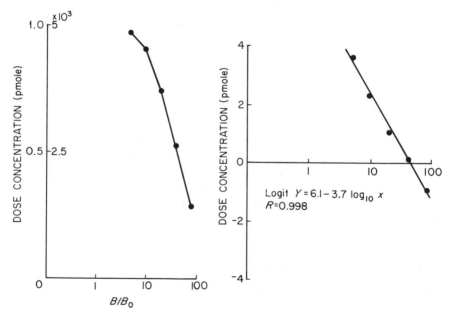

Figure 1. Standard curve for radioimmunoassay of glycocholic acid. Curve on left represents B/B_0 plotted versus log dose concentration. Curve on right reflects a logit transformation of B/B_0 versus log dose concentration.

ml of a 60% ammonium sulfate solution to all tubes except total count tubes. The mixture is vortex-mixed, allowed to stand on ice for ten minutes, and then centrifuged at 4°C for 20 minutes at 2000 rpm. The supernate containing the free radiolabeled bile acid is then decanted directly into scintillation vials containing 10 ml aqueous counting scintillant ("ACS," Amersham/Searle, Arlington Heights, Illinois). (b) For polythylene glycol separation—Pipette 0.5 ml PEG solution into all tubes except total count tubes. Mix well for five seconds and centrifuge in a 4°C refrigerated centrifuge for 15 minutes at 2500 rpm. Decant supernate containing the free radiolabeled bile acid into scintillation vials containing 10 ml of "ACS."

8. Radioactivity is determined in a suitable counter with an efficiency of at least 30%. Both separation techniques yield samples with some degree of quenching. This quenching is fairly constant; therefore, quench correction is unnecessary.

9. Quantitation of data and calculation of bile acid concentrations are determined using a logit plot with linear regression analysis. A typical standard curve for one of the bile acids is shown in Figure 1. This figure shows a characteristic standard curve of B/B_0 (counts bound for an arbitrary dose relative to that for second dose) and a logit transformation for the particular bile acid.

III. VALIDATION OF ASSAY

Assay sensitivity, precision, and accuracy studies have been performed on all four major bile acids. As a prototype of the validation results obtained for all bile acids studied, these data will be depicted for glycocholic acid using the PEG mode of separation.

A. Reproducibility of Standard Curves

Standard curves were performed on 14 different days with two different lots of reagents. Mean values and standard deviations of the percent bound ($B/B_0 \times 100$) for each standard were calculated and are depicted in Figure 2.

B. Sensitivity

As shown by the data for the standard curve, as little as 5.0 pmole of each standard bile acid can displace significant amounts of tracer at an antibody titer binding 50% of labeled bile acid.

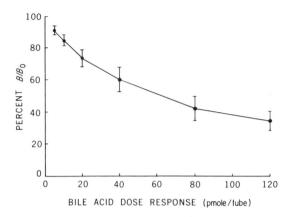

Figure 2. Reproducibility of standard curves. Each point represents the mean and S.D. of B/B_0 for 14 standard curves.

C. Precision

Intraassay precision was examined by performing ten replicates of serum pools at three different concentrations within the same assay. Mean, standard deviation, and coefficient of variation data for these studies are listed in Table V.

D. Analytical Recovery

The accuracy of the bile acid radioimmunoassay was determined by performing recovery studies of bile acids added to bile acid-free serum. Bile acid-free serum is prepared by adding 50 mg washed and dried charcoal (Norit A) for each milliliter of normal rabbit serum to be extracted. The charcoal mixture is vortexed, allowed to stand for 15 minutes at room temperature, and then centrifuged at 2000 rpm for 20 minutes. The supernatant is then siphoned off with a Pasteur pipette, filtered through a Millipore system (45 minutes), and then diluted 1 : 2 for use with phosphate-buffered saline.

Table V   Intraassay Precision of Glycocholic Acid

Matrix	Mean (pmole/tube)	S.D.	Coefficient of variation (%)
Serum intraassay	24.08	2.9	12.4
Serum intraassay	33.14	2.5	7.4
Serum intraassay	62.44	4.1	6.2

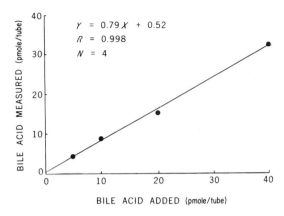

Figure 3. Recovery of bile acid (glycocholic) added to bile acid-free serum. Average recovery of bile acid was 85%.

In Figure 3 is depicted a representative recovery study following the addition of known amounts of glycocholic acid to the bile acid-free serum and then reassay by radioimmunoassay. The average recovery of bile acid was 85%. Measured and expected bile acid values agreed well ($r = 0.998$) and gave a linear relationship between the amount added and the amount measured by radioimmunoassay.

E. Parallelism

A necessary condition for assay specificity is parallelism. This is particularly important for the bile acid radioimmunoassays in which dilutions of patient serum are necessary in order to obtain values that

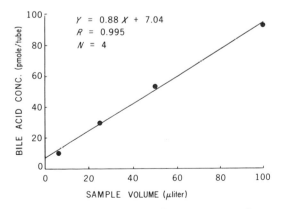

Figure 4. Parallelism of serum bile acid radioimmunoassay for glycocholic acid.

fall within the limits of the picomole standard curve. As shown in Figure 4, assaying serial dilutions of a high serum bile acid pool gave a linear relationship between the bile acid concentrations measured and the concentrations used in the assay. Linear regression analysis yielded a slope of 0.876 with a correlation of 0.995. Over the ranges of bile acids investigated, good parallelism was achieved.

IV. NORMAL VALUES AND CONCENTRATIONS OF THE INDIVIDUAL BILE ACIDS IN SERUM IN VARIOUS STATES OF HEPATOBILIARY DISEASE

The clinical relevance of determining the individual bile acids by radioimmunoassay is currently being explored in several institutions across the country and in industry, where manufacturers are developing the reagents for commercial availability in kits. For the bile acid radioimmunoassays developed to date, there is good correlation between determinations made by immunoassay and those using the con-

Table VI   The Effects of Feeding on Serum Bile Acid Levels (μmole/liter) in Man

State	No.	CG[a]	CDG[a]	DG[a]	SLCG[a]
Fasting	22	0.35 ± 0.29[b]	0.27 ± 0.9	0.048 ± 0.014	0.10 ± 0.03
Postprandial	21	0.97 ± 0.33[c]	0.41 ± 0.14[c]	0.058 ± 0.011	0.14 ± 0.04

[a] CG, cholylglycine; CDG, chenodeoxycholylglycine; DG, deoxycholylglycine; and SLCG, sulfolithocholylglycine.

[b] Mean ± S.D.

[c] Significant at $P < 0.05$ from fasting level.

Table VII   Serum Bile Acids in Hepatobiliary Disease[a]

Patients	No.	CG[b] (μmole/ liter)	CDG[b] (μmole/ liter)	DG[b] (μmole/ liter)	SLCG[b] (μmole/ liter)
Controls	302	0.24 ± 0.19[c]	0.22 ± 0.20	0.11 ± 0.10	0.33 ± 0.26
Cirrhosis	61	7.0 ± 3.5	8.4 ± 4.1	0.41 ± 0.05	3.32 ± 1.6
Hepatitis	29	18.7 ± 7.6	6.6 ± 7.1	0.26 ± 0.07	4.61 ± 1.1
Cholestasis	22	24.6 ± 1.2	15.20 ± 1.50	0.12 ± 0.67	1.76 ± 1.23
Liver cancer	40	94.1 ± 44.2	0.91 ± 0.11	0.16 ± 0.04	1.92 ± 0.63

[a] Results are expressed in micromoles of glycine-conjugated bile acids per liter of serum.

[b] CG, cholylglycine; CDG, chenodeoxycholylglycine; DG, deoxycholylglycine; and SLCG, sulfolithocholylglycine.

[c] Mean ± S.D.

ventional gas–liquid chromatography method. In the serum of normal individuals, fasting levels of the four major bile acids are relatively low, rarely exceeding 1.0 μM; these levels can be increased two- to threefold in normal patients by the ingestion of a meal (Table VI) (Hepner and Demers, 1977; Schalm *et al.*, 1977).

When patients with hepatobiliary diseases are studied, the serum bile acid level becomes significantly raised above control, with several hundredfold elevations seen in certain bile acids in cases of liver cancer and hepatitis (Demers and Hepner, 1976b). Table VII lists serum bile acid values in control patients with no evidence of liver disease and in patients with various forms of hepatobiliary disease.

ACKNOWLEDGMENTS

The expert technical assistance of Dennis D. Derck and Linda Ebright as well as the typing assistance of Carol Rohrer are gratefully acknowledged.

REFERENCES

Barnes, P. J. (1976). Progress in the enzymatic assay of bile acids and stools. *Am. Lab.*, 67–73.

Demers, L. M., and Hepner, G. W. (1976a). Radioimmunoassay of bile acids in serum. *Clin. Chem.* **22**, 602–606.

Demers, L. M., and Hepner, G. W. (1976b). Levels of immunoreactive glycine conjugated bile acids in hepatobiliary disease. *Am. J. Clin. Pathol.* **66**, 65–73.

Demers, L. M., Paul, E., Buchmsky, M., and Derck, D. (1978). Separation of glycine and taurine by high pressure liquid chromatography. *Clin. Chem.* **24**, 1051.

Elliot, W. H. (1973). Bile acids. *In* "Biochemical Applications of Mass Spectrometry" (G. L. Waller, ed.), p. 291. Wiley (Interscience), New York.

Erlanger, B. F., Borek, F., Beiser, S. M., and Lieberman, S. (1957). Steroid protein conjugates. *J. Biol. Chem.* **228**, 713–727.

Hepner, G. W., and Demers, L. M. (1977). Dynamics of the enterohepatic circulation of the glycine conjugates of cholic, chenodeoxycholic, deoxycholic and sulfolithocholic acid in man. *Gastroenterology* **72**, 499–501.

Korman, M. G., Hofmann, A. F., and Summerskill, W. H. J. (1974). Assessment of activity of chronic active liver disease. Serum bile acids compared with conventional tests and histology. *N. Engl. J. Med.* **290**, 1399–1402.

Murphy, G. M., Edkins, S. M., Williams, J. W., and Catty, D. (1974). The preparation and properties of an antiserum for the radioimmunoassay of serum conjugated cholic acid. *Clin. Chim. Acta* **54**, 81–89.

Schalm, S. W., van Berge Henegouwen, G. P., Hofmann, A. F., Cowen, A. E., and Turcotte, J. (1977). Radioimmunoassay of bile acids: Development, validation, and preliminary application of an assay for conjugates of chenodeoxycholic acid. *Gastroenterology* **73**, 285–290.

Simmonds, W. J., Korman, M. G., Go, W. W. L., and Hoffmann, A. F. (1973). Radioimmunoassay of conjugated cholyl bile acids in serum. *Gastroenterology* **65,** 705–711.

Spenney, J. G., Johnson, B. J., Hirschowitz, B. I., Mihas, A. A., and Gibson, R. (1977). An ^{125}I radioimmunoassay for primary conjugated bile salts. *Gastroenterology* **72,** 305–311.

Van Berge Henegegouwen, G. P., Ruben, A., and Brandt, K. H. (1974). Quantitation analysis of bile acids in serum and bile using gas–liquid chromatography. *Clin. Chim. Acta* **54,** 249–261.

PANCREATIC HORMONES

31

Insulin, Proinsulin, and C-Peptide

J. I. STARR, D. L. HORWITZ, A. H. RUBENSTEIN, AND M. E. MAKO

I. INTRODUCTION

The introduction of radioimmunoassay in 1959 provided scientists with a sensitive and reproducible method for the study of hormone

613

Methods of Hormone Radioimmunoassay, Second Edition
Copyright © 1979 by Academic Press, Inc.
All rights of reproduction in any form reserved. ISBN 0-12-379260-6

regulation and clinicians with the diagnostic capability of evaluating endocrine abnormalities associated with hyper- and hyposecretion. Originally introduced by Yalow and Berson (1960) for the measurement of plasma insulin, this technique is presently used for the detection of minute amounts of other hormones as well as biologically active substances including enzymes and drugs. A detailed historical account of the development of the method has been published (Yalow and Berson, 1971a) and the subject has been critically reviewed on a number of occasions (Kirkham and Hunter, 1971; Berson and Yalow, 1964, 1968b).

Radioimmunoassay methods rapidly gained popularity because of the many problems inherent in the biologic assay systems which were initially used for measuring the concentration of circulating hormones. In the case of insulin, these included the rat diaphragm (Vallance-Owen and Hurlock, 1954) and fat pad (Sheps et al., 1960) methods. The specificity of the techniques was subsequently improved by measuring glucose uptake or utilization in the presence and absence of anti-insulin serum (Froesch et al., 1963), but they still lacked reproducibility and sensitivity. Despite these difficulties, the unresolved dilemma concerning the nature of circulating insulinlike activity (ILA) has provided a rational basis for continuing investigations using these methods. For this purpose, the use of isolated fat cells derived from rat adipose tissue seems to have significant advantages over other methods.

The immunologic heterogeneity of circulating parathormone was observed as early as 1967–1968 (Berson and Yalow, 1968a), but the significance of this finding and its implications for other hormones were not generally appreciated. The subsequent identification of proinsulin, the biosynthetic precursor of insulin, in blood and urine (Roth et al., 1968; Rubenstein et al., 1968) provided a logical basis for the existence of heterogeneity and prompted the more detailed characterization of other circulating hormones. Multiple forms of plasma glucagon, growth hormone, parathyroid hormone, gastrin, ACTH, and vasopressin have subsequently been described, but the relationship of these circulating peptides to biosynthetic precursors is still uncertain in many instances.

In this chapter, we shall outline the methods used in our laboratory to measure insulin, proinsulin, and C-peptide in blood and urine and comment upon the advantages and disadvantages of alternative techniques. In addition, the procedure for separating proinsulin from insulin and some aspects of the problem of the heterogeneity of circulating hormones will be described.

II. METHODS OF RADIOIMMUNOASSAY

A. Source of Hormone

The hormone concentration in an unknown sample is calculated by comparing its immunochemical reactivity with that of standard solutions containing measured amounts of hormone. A prerequisite for any assay is the demonstration that the plasma and standard hormone compete identically with the tracer for antibody-binding sites, so that the concentration of the unknown sample falls linearly with dilution. Although crystalline insulins from most species have nearly identical biologic potencies, their immunologic reactivities may differ significantly. The standards should thus be prepared from the same species as the unknown samples. In the case of insulin, investigators are particularly fortunate to have the assistance of a number of companies which are involved in the commercial production of the hormone for diabetic patients. Highly purified crystalline insulin is readily available from these sources. Recently, their preparations have been further purified to yield monocomponent (Novo Company, Copenhagen) or single-component (Eli Lilly Company, Indianapolis, Indiana) insulin, which is essentially free of proinsulin, insulin aggregates, and other minor components that cocrystallize with insulin. Alternatively, insulin may be extracted and purified from the pancreas of the particular species under investigation.

Because most antisera raised against porcine insulin react identically with the human and porcine hormone, either may be used as standard for the measurement of the circulating hormone in man. Insulins are defined in international bioassay units on the basis of potency, one unit being the activity contained in 0.04167 mg of the Fourth International Standard Preparation, which contains almost equal proportions of bovine and porcine insulin. In the dry state, these preparations are stable for long periods of time, but have been noted to deteriorate during storage in solution and with repeated freezing and thawing.

We are currently using as our standard a preparation of human insulin (Lot 258-1064B-27; 26.9 U/mg) provided by the Eli Lilly Company, Indianapolis, Indiana. However, with regard to proinsulin, a human preparation is not readily available, and its lack has resulted in serious problems in the precise quantitation of this polypeptide. The need for a human proinsulin standard is particularly urgent because porcine (and bovine) proinsulin does not react similarly to the human peptide and, thus, cannot be used in its place, as in the case of insulin. Moreover, the comparative reaction of different insulin antisera with insulin and proinsulin varies, and it is, therefore, unsatisfactory to measure proinsulin in terms of an insulin standard. A small amount of human proinsulin has recently been purified from twice crystallized insulin (kindly provided by the Novo Company, Copenhagen) by gel filtration on Sephadex G-50 and gradient elution chromatography on DEAE-cellulose (Oyer et al., 1971). The proinsulin was characterized by NH$_2$-terminal analysis and polyacrylamide electrophoresis, in which it had the same R_f as labeled human proinsulin prepared by in vitro incubation of slices from an islet cell adenoma. Since the quantity of proinsulin was limited, it was further characterized after labeling with ^{131}I. The iodinated proinsulin migrated as a single component on paper electrophoresis in 20% acetic acid–8.0 M urea, and after incubation for 30 minutes at 37°C with trypsin (2.5 μg/ml), was converted to a product which had the same elution volume on Sephadex G-50 as insulin. Aliquots of this preparation have been distributed to investigators to standardize their assay.

B. Immunization

In 1959, Berson and Yalow showed that guinea pig antisera reacted strongly with human insulin. At the same time, Morse (1959), working in their laboratory, demonstrated that antisera raised in rabbits were not very sensitive for the human hormone. These findings, together with the observations that insulin antibodies which developed in man following treatment with beef–pork insulin mixtures reacted more strongly with the bovine than porcine hormone led these workers to raise antisera for use in immunoassays by immunizing guinea pigs with porcine insulin (Yalow and Berson, 1961, 1971a). Since that time, most investigators have successfully used guinea pig anti-porcine insulin systems. Crude preparations are not necessarily poor immunogens and on occasion may possibly prove to be superior to the purified antigen (Yalow and Berson, 1971a). Crystalline, Lente, PZI, NPH, or regular pork insulin (available for therapeutic purposes) and other preparations have all been used successfully. However, the identification of significant impurities in crystalline insulin preparations has led to a reevaluation of the inherent immunogenicity of this peptide. Studies by Schlichtkrull et al. (1972) and Root et al. (1972) have demonstrated that certain higher molecular weight components which cocrystallize with insulin may be largely responsible for antibody stimulation, and that highly purified insulin preparations are less immunogenic. It should be noted that their investigations were concerned with rabbits and diabetic patients and the results may not be applicable to guinea pigs.

There have been few studies comparing different schedules and methods for raising antisera. Various immunization procedures have been suggested by Parker (1971), Boyd *et al.* (1969), Odell *et al.* (1971), Vaitukaitis *et al.* (1971), and Nixon and Cargille (1971). An excellent study of the immune response of guinea pigs to insulin has been published by Makulu and Wright (1971). These authors investigated the role of the frequency of injections, bacterial adjuvants, insulin dose, and species on insulin antibody production. In addition, the fate of the circulating antibodies in actively and passively immunized animals and the suppression of antibody production by antimetabolic drugs and prednisolone were determined. It should be remembered that there is a limit to the total dose of insulin which can be injected with safety at any one time, because of the risk of precipitating severe hypoglycemia and death in the guinea pigs (Moloney and Goldsmith, 1957). To avoid this hazard, Makulu and Wright (1971) advocate using a very viscous emulsion of lanolin and heavy mineral oil as the vehicle for the insulin. The advantages of various adjuvants have also been reviewed by Pope (1966), Wright and Norman (1966), and Wright *et al.* (1968). Although insulin antibody complexes are usually soluble, Heinzel *et al.* (1971) have recently shown that if the insulin is chelated into large soluble aggregates with glutaraldehyde, it will form precipitating complexes with antibodies raised to the native protein. It is thus probable that the absence of an insoluble immunoprecipitate in the reaction between insulin and insulin antibodies even at high concentrations is due to the molecular size or other properties of insulin itself rather than to unusual features in the antibodies which it elicits.

For immunization (Makulu and Wright, 1971), 5 mg porcine insulin should be dissolved in 7 ml of 0.3% (w/v) phenol acidified to pH 2.3 with dilute acetic acid and 3 ml *H. pertussis* vaccine (Lilly). The aqueous phase is thoroughly emulsified with 10 ml of mineral oil and lanolin (7 ml heavy mineral oil and 3 ml lanolin, mixed at 60°–90°C, and cooled). Guinea pigs should receive 2 ml of emulsion subcutaneously at 3-week intervals.

Antisera suitable for use in the immunoassay are now available from a number of commercial firms.

C. Characterization of Antiserum

The theoretical basis underlying immunoassays has been discussed in detail using the interactions of insulin and its antibodies as examples. The energy requirements which permit the detection of those concentrations of insulin found in plasma, and the cross-reactions of different species of insulin with various antisera have also been described (Berson and Yalow, 1959). As with other antisera, those of insulin are characterized in terms of their titer, affinity, and specificity.

The optimal titer for use in the radioimmunoassay is determined by incubating serial dilutions of the antiserum with labeled insulin (Figure 1) and noting the dilution which binds approximately 50% of the tracer (a bound : free ratio of 1 : 1). In general, this concentration will give an optimal ratio of sensitivity and precision in a radioimmunoassay (Odell *et al.*, 1971). Most insulin antisera can be used at a final concentration of 1 : 10,000 or greater; consequently, there is no shortage of this material. The affinity of the antibodies is expressed in terms of their equilibrium constants or k values. From a practical point of view, this is reflected in the steepness of the slope of the dose–response curve and the smallest quantity of hormone detectable. Since the fasting concentration of plasma insulin ranges between 1.0 and 20 μU/ml, and sample volumes of 0.1 ml (or 0.2–0.4 ml in samples with low insulin concentrations) are usually assayed, sensitivities in the order of 20 pg are desirable. However, the introduction of methods to measure proinsulin and insulin in column fractions after gel filtration of small quantities of serum has necessitated the use of assays with greater sensitivity.

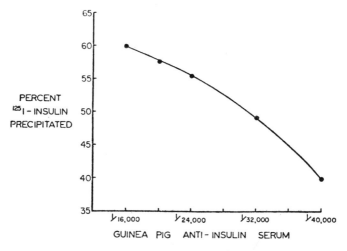

Figure 1. A typical binding curve of serial dilutions of an anti-insulin serum. To set up an assay, one would use a 1 : 30,000 dilution of this antiserum to obtain 50% binding of the tracer in the zero dose tube.

Prior to the discovery of proinsulin and its related forms, no circulating substances which resembled insulin immunologically had been identified. The A and B chains do not react with insulin antibodies, and there is no evidence for other immunologically reactive degradation products in plasma. Since, to date, there are no antisera specific for proinsulin, the choice of an insulin antiserum will depend upon whether one wishes to measure mainly insulin or both proinsulin and insulin in the insulin immunoassay. The rationale for this choice lies

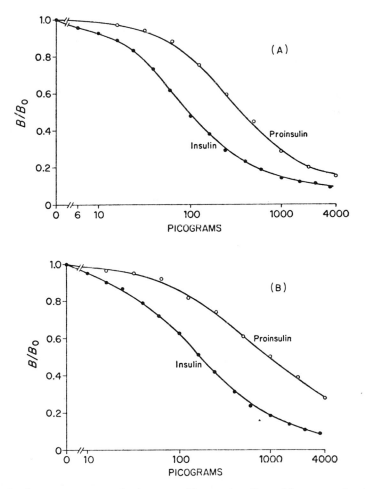

Figure 2. Immunoassay standard curves of human insulin and human proinsulin. The upper set of curves (A) represents an insulin antiserum that reacts with the two peptides to give almost parallel displacement curves. The lower figure (B) shows displacement curves with nonparallel displacement using a different insulin antiserum in the assay.

in the observation that some insulin antisera react more strongly with proinsulin (when compared to insulin) than others and will, therefore, be more suitable for the latter purpose. An additional factor that should be considered is the comparative displacement slopes of insulin and its precursor. These vary with different antisera, but it is obviously advantageous to select an antiserum which gives parallel curves with standards of human insulin and proinsulin (Figure 2).

D. Preparation of Radioactive Ligand

Although the iodine monochloride (McFarlane, 1958), peroxidase (Lambert *et al.*, 1972), and electrolytic (Glover *et al.*, 1967) methods have been used to iodinate insulin, the chloramine-T method developed by Hunter and Greenwood (1962) is still the most popular. The modification of this latter method which has been introduced by Frechet *et al.* (1971) has resulted in an improvement in immunochemical characteristics of the labeled insulin and enhanced its stability in storage. We now use this method for iodinating insulin, proinsulin, C-peptide, and other peptides and have been impressed with its flexibility and reproducibility. Either ^{131}I or ^{125}I may be used for iodination, and the relative merits of the two isotopes will be found in a discussion by Freedlender (1969). This laboratory has obtained ^{125}I from Union Carbide (New York) and Industrial Nuclear (St. Louis, Missouri), but there now seems to be little difference among the isotope preparations available from different commercial sources. Insulin and proinsulin can be iodinated by the same technique, but ^{125}I-insulin is used as the tracer in the radioimmunoassay measurement of human insulin and proinsulin.

Method

The following method is used for labeling insulin. The following reactants are mixed in a small (2-ml) conical shaped tube.

> Na^{125}I, 2.5–5.0 mCi, 0.005 ml
> Sodium phosphate buffer, pH 7.4 (0.3 *M*), 0.05 ml
> Insulin (5.0 μg) in phosphate buffer, 0.01 ml
> Chloramine-T (33 μg/ml), 0.02 ml

The hormone and chloramine-T are weighed and diluted to the required concentration immediately before use. The reaction is allowed to proceed for three minutes with vigorous shaking. Sodium metabisulfite (200 μg/ml), 0.0005 ml, is then added and is followed by 2.5% albumin in phosphate buffer (0.1 ml).

A small column (2.5 ml in the barrel of a 3.0-ml disposable syringe) containing cellulose powder (Whatman, standard grade) packed over a Pyrex wool plug is used to adsorb the undamaged iodinated protein while permitting the damaged fractions and iodide to pass through. This is accomplished by placing the iodination mixture on the column (prewetted with phosphate buffer), followed by a wash of 4.0 to 5.0 ml albumin-free phosphate buffer, 0.3 M, pH 7.4. Thereafter, the labeled insulin is eluted into separate tubes using 0.6-ml volumes of 12.5% albumin in phosphate buffer (total of eight tubes). Each aliquot is collected separately and diluted in borate–albumin (0.5%) buffer and, after counting, the peak tubes are selected for use in the immunoassay. The ^{125}I-insulin in these tubes is then diluted further in the assay buffer and frozen in aliquots at −20°C until required. The preferred percentage iodination in our procedure is 40–60%, and the degree of labeling is less than one iodine atom per molecule insulin. The specific activity of the ^{125}I-insulin is in the range of 150 to 220 mCi/mg.

We have checked the integrity of the labeled preparation on Bio-Gel P-30 columns equilibrated in 6.0 M urea–3.0 M acetic acid and found more than 99% of the radioactivity eluting in the insulin region of the column (Figure 3). Csorba and Gattner (1970) have shown that even lightly iodinated insulin preparations contain a proportion of aggregated dimers and cross-linked molecules. The biologic activity of these abnormal forms is more markedly reduced than their immunoreactivity. The stability of radioiodinated insulin obtained from commercial sources and a description of some of the factors affecting its immunologic competence during storage have been investigated by van Orden (1972), and recommendations which may prolong its integrity have been made. Other methods, such as dialysis, gel filtration, gel electrophoresis, and ion-exchange chromatography, have been used for separating the labeled hormone from unreacted iodide and damaged products.

A comparison of the iodine monochloride and chloramine-T methods of iodinating ox insulin was made by Glover et al. (1967). These investigators pointed out some of the factors influencing the small-scale iodination of proteins and suggested methods to improve the reliability of the process and minimize chemical change in the product. In particular, the importance of using the minimum concentration of chloramine-T required for efficient iodination was pointed out. A useful method for the standardization of the chloramine-T method has been described by Hunter (1970). The potential (EMF) of the reaction mixture is monitored and used to determine the minimum amount of chloramine-T required for acceptable iodination.

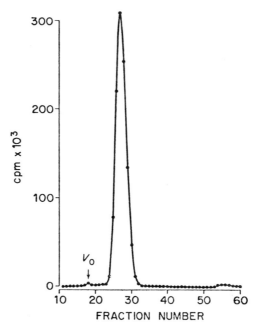

Figure 3.   Radioactivity eluting from a Bio-Gel P-30 column equilibrated in 6.0 M urea-3.0 M acetic acid to which an aliquot of freshly iodinated pork insulin has been applied. More than 99% of the radioactivity elutes in a single peak with very small amounts in the void volume and in the salt peak.

The assessment of the immunoreactivity of the iodinated preparation is checked in two ways. If one wishes to keep the antibody dilution constant, one can vary the number of counts per tube and determine the quantity of tracer that will give the required binding (e.g., 45–55%) in the zero tubes. Alternatively, the number of counts can be kept constant and the antibody dilution can be varied. We have preferred the former method, especially when two antigens such as proinsulin and insulin are used as standards in the same assay.

The relationship between the degree of iodination of insulin and its biologic, electrophoretic, and immunologic properties has been investigated by Izzo et $al.$ (1964) and Brunfeldt et $al.$ (1968). The distribution of the ^{125}I between the four tyrosyl residues can be determined by separating the two chains by paper electrophoresis after oxidative sulfitolysis. The chains may then be cleaved by chymotrypsin (A chain) and trypsin (B chain). Most radioactivity is found as monoiodotyrosine on the tyrosyl residue A-19.

E. Preparation of Sample for Immunoassay

1. Blood

Insulin and proinsulin are stable in blood at room temperature or 4°C for a number of hours. No special precautions are thus necessary in collecting samples or their preparation for assay. Plasma and serum have been stored at −20°C for prolonged periods of time without significant loss of immunoreactive insulin or proinsulin.

Although we prefer to assay serum, plasma is equally acceptable. Henderson (1970) has reported that the concentration of insulin in heparinized plasma is higher than in serum, but it is likely that this is due to an effect of heparin in the immunoassay. Heparin is a strong polyanion and may inhibit the reaction between antigen and antibody (Yalow and Berson, 1971b). This effect is dose dependent and is seldom a problem if the concentration of heparin in the samples is kept at low levels. Heparin may also influence the insulin value by affecting the precipitation reaction in the double antibody radioimmunoassay.

2. Urine

Samples should be collected in bottles containing albumin (to a final concentration of 0.2 to 0.5 %) and kept at −4°C until processed. Although Ørskov and Johansen (1972) recommended dialysis of the urine in 10-mm (8/32) Visking membranes against the immunoassay buffer for 24 hours, this may not be necessary providing that the pH is adjusted to approximately 7.0, the insoluble material is removed by centrifugation, and the volume assayed is sufficiently small (Rubenstein *et al.*, 1967).

3. Preparation of Samples for Measurement of Proinsulin and Insulin

Although it would be advantageous to measure human proinsulin and its intermediate fractions by direct immunoassay in unextracted serum, this has not been possible. The reasons lie in the cross-reactivity of proinsulin with insulin, on the one hand, and the C-peptide, on the other. Since all three of these peptides have been identified in the circulation, a preliminary step is required in order to separate them from one another. The most commonly used approach has involved gel filtration of serum followed by measurement of the column fractions in the insulin immunoassay. In our initial studies, we extracted insulin and proinsulin from serum into acid ethanol and separated the two peptides by gel filtration on a Bio-Gel P-30 column equilibrated in 3.0 M acetic acid (Melani *et al.*, 1970a). The initial reason for choosing this technique was the reluctance to gel-filter serum in neutral or alkaline buffers in which polymerization or aggregation of insulin might occur. In fact, this does not appear to be a problem. Another advantage is the ability to extract large volumes of serum and still separate the hormones on relatively small columns. Furthermore, it is easier to characterize the separated proinsulin and insulin under these conditions when most of the other serum proteins have been removed. The most obvious disadvantages of the method are the length of time required for the procedure and the limitation on the number of samples that can be analyzed by one laboratory.

Roth and co-workers (1968) have separated proinsulin and insulin on 1.0×50 cm columns of Sephadex G-50, fine, equilibrated in a

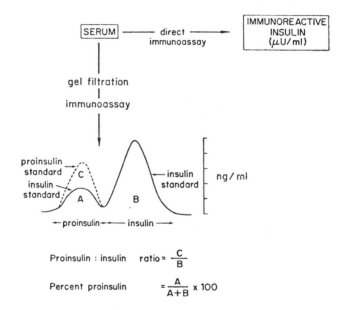

Figure 4.   A schematic flow diagram for the measurement of proinsulin and insulin in serum. Serum is measured directly in the immunoassay [immunoreactive insulin (IRI)]. It is then gel filtered to separate the proinsulin and insulin, and each fraction is assayed in the insulin radioimmunoassay. The early eluting peak (proinsulin-like component) is read off the human proinsulin standard (curve C), if one is available, or alternatively the insulin standard (curve A). The late peak (insulin) is measured against the insulin standard (curve B). The sum of the individual fractions in each peak (corrected for volume) is the proinsulin and insulin concentration, respectively. The relationship between proinsulin and insulin has been expressed in two ways: the proinsulin to insulin ratio, with each read off its appropriate standard; and the percentage proinsulin, where both peptides have been read off the insulin standard.

Veronal buffer (0.05 M, pH 8.6) to which human serum albumin (2.5 mg/ml), rabbit fraction II (0.1 mg/ml) and toluene are added. One or two milliliters of serum is applied directly to the column, fraction sizes of 1.0 to 1.5 ml are collected, and 0.4- to 0.8-ml aliquots are taken for immunoassay. We have modified this method to use a column of Bio-Gel P-30, equilibrated in the immunoassay buffer (boric acid 8.25 gm, sodium hydroxide 2.7 gm, bovine albumin fraction V 5 gm in 950 ml deionized water; adjust pH to 8.0 with concentrated hydrochloric acid, and bring volume to 1.0 liter). Fractions can be collected directly into the immunoassay tubes, thus obviating the need for further pipetting at this stage. The void volume is determined by the elution position of ^{125}I-albumin, or blue dextran 2000, while the salt peak is marked by $Na^{125}I$. The column is calibrated with tracers of ^{125}I-proinsulin and ^{125}I insulin. Because certain preparations of these labeled hormones may not elute identically with the native proteins, it may be preferable to determine the characteristics of the column by assaying the elution position of unlabeled insulin (2.0 ng) and proinsulin (2.0 ng).

When serum is directly applied to the columns, essentially complete recoveries have been obtained. In order to calculate the absolute level of proinsulin and insulin, fractions of the earlier eluting peak are read from a human proinsulin standard, while those comprising the second peak are measured against a human insulin standard (Figure 4). Since the supply of human proinsulin is limited at present, it may be necessary to express the values of proinsulin in terms of the insulin standard. Although the absolute concentration of proinsulin will usually be underestimated by this procedure, comparison of the levels obtained in different laboratories will be possible.

F. Assay Procedure

1. Preparation of Standards

Pork or human insulin and human proinsulin standards, 0–100 μU or 0–4 ng, are prepared from a concentrated stock solution which is stored in aliquots at $-20°C$. After thawing, the solution may be kept for approximately one week at 4°C, after which it should be discarded. The final concentrations of standard for both insulin and proinsulin (0–100 μU or 0–4.0 ng per tube) may be made by serial dilution, but it is preferable to prepare individual concentrations from the stock solution by measuring different volumes with a set of preset Hamilton syringes with Chaney adapters. An informative discussion regarding the stability and potential problems of insulin standards can be found in Section IV of "Radioimmunoassay Methods" by Kirkham and Hunter (1971). Certainly meticulous attention should be paid to the stability of the preparation in various solutions, the avoidance of bacterial contamination and enzymatic degradation, and the optimal storage temperature.

2. Method and Separation Technique

The procedure used in our laboratory (Tables I and II) is based on the double antibody precipitation method described by Morgan and Lazarow (1963) and modified by Soeldner and Slone (1965) and Welborn and Fraser (1965). The volume for the antibody reaction is 1.2 ml and the incubation period is 72 hours at 4°C. The time necessary for equilibration of the reactants is initially determined by separating the bound and free labeled insulin by chromatoelectrophoresis on Whatman 3MM paper.

The second antibody reaction involves the addition of serum from rabbits (or sheep, goats, etc.) immunized against guinea pig globulin (or whole serum) to precipitate the soluble insulin–antibody complex. Since the insulin antiserum is diluted into the range of 10^{-4} to 10^{-6}, additional carrier guinea pig serum must be added to ensure reliable and complete precipitation. The precipitate and supernatant can be separated in a number of ways, but centrifugation is probably the easiest and most widely used technique. Although we decant the supernatant, it can be aspirated to decrease contamination of the

Table I   Assay Method

Step	Amount (ml)
A. In 10×75 or 12×75 mm disposable glass culture tubes	
1. Serum	0.01–0.4
or standard	0–1.0
2. Buffer to total	1.0
3. ^{125}I-insulin diluted in the assay buffer to contain the desired cpm	0.1
4. Anti-insulin serum diluted in the assay buffer	0.1
B. Incubate at 4°C for 72 hours	
C. Add	
5. Normal guinea pig serum diluted in the assay buffer	0.1
6. Rabbit (or sheep or goat) anti-guinea pig serum (or globulin) diluted in the assay buffer	0.1
D. Incubate at 4°C for 72 hours	
E. Centrifuge at 4°C at 2000 rpm for 20 to 25 minutes	
F. Decant or aspirate supernatant	
G. Count precipitate for sufficient time to get at least 10,000 counts in the zero dose tubes	

Table II   Typical Assay Flow Sheet

Tube No.	Sample	Volume buffer (ml)	Volume sample (ml)	Pork ^{125}I-insulin (ml)	Anti-insulin serum (ml)
1–4	Nonspecific binding	1.1	0	0.1	0
5–10	Zero dose	1.0	0	0.1	0.1
Human insulin standard (2.4 μU/ml)					
11, 12	0.12 μU	0.95	0.05	0.1	0.1
13, 14	0.24 μU	0.9	0.1	0.1	0.1
15, 16	0.48 μU	0.8	0.2	0.1	0.1
17, 18	0.72 μU	0.7	0.3	0.1	0.1
19, 20	1.2 μU	0.5	0.5	0.1	0.1
Human insulin standard (97 μU/ml)					
21, 22	2.4 μU	0.975	0.025	0.1	0.1
23, 24	4.85 μU	0.95	0.05	0.1	0.1
25, 26	9.7 μU	0.9	0.1	0.1	0.1
27, 28	19.4 μU	0.8	0.2	0.1	0.1
29, 30	48.5 μU	0.5	0.5	0.1	0.1
31, 32	97 μU	0	1.0	0.1	0.1
Standard sera					
33, 34	1–low	0.9	0.1	0.1	0.1
35, 36	2–medium	0.9	0.1	0.1	0.1
37, 38	3–high	0.9	0.1	0.1	0.1
Samples	GTT Reg. No. 1377				
39, 40	Fasting	0.9	0.1	0.1	0.1
41, 42	30 minutes	0.9	0.1	0.1	0.1
43, 44	60 minutes	0.9	0.1	0.1	0.1
45, 46	90 minutes	0.9	0.1	0.1	0.1
47, 48	120 minutes	0.9	0.1	0.1	0.1

counting tubes. The precipitate alone, or both the precipitate and supernatant, are counted.

The advantages of this method lie in its simplicity, in the clean separation of free from bound hormone that is achieved, and its ready adaptability to other assay systems (Daughaday and Jacobs, 1971). However, unless one is aware of the problems which may be encountered, there is a danger that a false sense of security may prevail. Among the common difficulties that occur are the variable interfering effects of human serum on the precipitation reaction, the necessity to determine the optimal concentrations of precipitating antibody and carrier, and the inability to recognize damage to the tracer during the first antibody incubation. It should be stressed that each batch of reagents used in the precipitation reaction may differ, and every laboratory should check and standardize their own materials.

A number of suggestions have been made to ensure full precipitation. Welborn and Fraser (1965) have used trace amounts of labeled guinea pig γ-globulin to monitor precipitation in the presence and absence of human serum. We routinely use this technique to determine the optimal concentrations of new batches of carrier and precipitating sera (Figure 5). Prolonging the second antibody incubation period (Soeldner and Slone, 1965; Welborn and Fraser, 1965), decreasing the volume of serum, addition of heparin (Welborn and Fraser, 1965) or EDTA (Morgan *et al.*, 1964), purification of the reagents, and preprecipitation of the guinea pig antiserum (Hales and Randle, 1963) have all been tried, with variable success. It should also be noted that human serum may occasionally increase immunoprecipitation when compared with the results in buffer alone. Burr and associates (1969) described this phenomenon in sheep anti-rabbit γ-globulin systems, and we and others (Brunfeldt and Jorgensen, 1967) have shown that it may occur with rabbit anti-guinea pig sera as well. This effect will result in certain sera having negative insulin values.

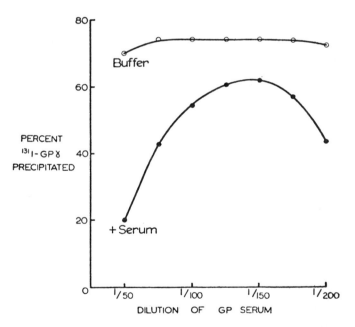

Figure 5.   To determine the optimal concentration of carrier serum for full precipitation, a rapid (nine hours) incubation with second antibody and tracer-radioiodinated guinea pig γ-globulin under assay conditions is undertaken. The peak precipitation with serum under these conditions is the optimal ratio. Repeating this with 24-, 48-, and 72-hour incubations can then be carried out to determine the length of incubation needed for complete precipitation in both buffer and serum tubes.

Little in the way of special equipment is required for the insulin assay. However, the introduction of semiautomated methods using the micromedic autodispenser have been extremely useful and have led to significant improvements in speed and reproducibility.

III. VERIFICATION OF ASSAY DATA

A. Validity

The insulin assay has been repeatedly validated by demonstrating that the endogenous hormone in serum and urine, and human insulin standards react identically with insulin antisera. Exogenous insulin added to samples is fully recovered, and the concentration in unknown samples falls linearly with dilution so that the curve is superimposable on that of the standards. Assay of fractions in the insulin region of the column following gel filtration of sera results in values comparable to those obtained by the direct measurement of the samples. Similar procedures have been used to characterize circulating proinsulin. In assays using porcine ^{125}I-insulin and an antiserum against porcine insulin, serial dilutions of serum proinsulin, isolated by gel filtration, showed immunologic identity with a human pancreatic proinsulin standard. Tryptic digestion of serum proinsulin converted it to products indistinguishable from insulin and desoctapeptide insulin.

Sonksen and co-workers (1971) have pointed out that there is excellent agreement between the antibody-suppressible insulin values measured by the rat epididymal fat pad bioassay method and the radioimmunoassay. The close relationship was evident in fasting and post-stimulated sera taken from healthy subjects, and patients with diabetes and acromegaly. It is of considerable interest that the only discrepancies were found in patients suffering from islet cell tumors, who, in retrospect, probably had high proportions of circulating proinsulin. In the bioassay system, proinsulin has very low activity, thus accounting for the lower concentrations measured by this method.

B. Calculation of Results and Statistical Analyses

Results can be calculated by plotting the points of the standard curve against the dose on semilog paper and fitting the curve by hand; the samples can then be read off this curve. However, many satisfactory computer programs have been developed for automation of these calculations. Most use the logit–log transformation for linearizing the

QUALITY CENTRAL DATA

	CURRENT VALUE	MEAN	STANDARD DEVIATION	MEAN +2SD	MEAN -2SD	RANGE HIGH	LOW
DOSE, 50% DISPLACEMENT	4.950	3.775	.657	4.738	2.764	4.950	2.657
SLOPE LN(X) VS. LOGIT(Y)	-1.1715	-.9714	.0601	-.8312	-1.915	-.956	-1.1715
RESIDUAL VARIANCE	4.074	1.1934	.7535	2.7034	-.3135	4.074	.2774
PERCENT BINDING 0 DOSE	.4562	.775	.0310	.5013	.437	.5664	.233
TOTAL COUNTS	16731	14297	4625	23927	4667	26245	6223
STANDARD SERUM 5	31.019	17.635	3.932	25.499	9.771	31.019	4.554
STANDARD SERUM 4	104.576	74.173	11.403	100.054	55.272	104.576	53.317
STANDARD SERUM 2	64.242	47.051	5.245	57.541	36.562	64.242	34.900
STANDARD SERUM 1	29.693	18.096	1.543	21.961	14.211	22.235	13.747

H DOSE, 50% DISP. L I   O
H SLOPE L I   O
H RESIDUAL VARIANCE L I   O
H PERCENT BINDING L I   O
H TOTAL COUNTS L I   O

H STANDARD SERUM 5 L I   O
H STANDARD SERUM 3 L I   O
H STANDARD SERUM 2 L I   O
H STANDARD SERUM 1 L I   O

QUALITY CENTRAL DATA

	CURRENT VALUE	MEAN	STANDARD DEVIATION	MEAN +2SD	MEAN -2SD	RANGE HIGH	LOW	
DOSE, 50% DISPLACEMENT	4.950	3.775	.657	4.738	2.764	4.950	2.657	DANGER
SLOPE LN(X) VS. LOGIT(Y)	-1.1715	-.9714	.0601	-.8312	-1.915	-.956	-1.1715	DISASTER
RESIDUAL VARIANCE	4.074	1.1934	.7535	2.7034	-.3135	4.074	.2774	DISASTER
PERCENT BINDING 0 DOSE	.4562	.775	.0310	.5013	.437	.5664	.233	
TOTAL COUNTS	16731	14297	4625	23927	4667	26245	6223	
STANDARD SERUM 5	31.019	17.635	3.932	25.499	9.771	31.019	4.554	DISASTER
STANDARD SERUM 4	104.576	74.173	11.403	100.054	55.272	104.576	53.317	DANGER
STANDARD SERUM 2	64.242	47.051	5.245	57.541	36.562	64.242	34.900	DISASTER
STANDARD SERUM 1	29.693	18.096	1.543	21.961	14.211	29.693	13.747	DISASTER

standard curve. Programs for desk-top computers are available through individual manufacturers and a sample program for large digital computers can be obtained from the NIH (McBride and Rodbard, 1971).

The most common parameters used for assessing radioimmunoassays are the least detectable dose and the intraassay and interassay coefficients of variation. Automation of assay computations using a digital computer has greatly facilitated the calculations and rapidly provided measurements of accuracy, precision, and sensitivity for each assay. We have used the equations developed by Rodbard (1971) and Feldman and Rodbard (1971), and have modified the NIH program "Radioimmunoassay Processing Report NIH RIA 71–2" to calculate the assay and intrassay characteristics and include a quality control subroutine which gives the interassay comparisons of these parameters. The points that are monitored include the total counts per assay tube, percent binding at the zero dose, slope of the logit–log transformation of the standard curve, dose giving 50% displacement, residual variance, and values of at least three standard sera. Each of these parameters is compared to the previous values and a sequential plot of the data is made, so that trends may be readily detected (Figure 6). Our intraassay coefficient of variation for single replicates is approximately 3% in the mid range of the standard curve and the interassay coefficient of variation is about 12%. This latter figure is reduced to between 8 to 10% when data from a single technician are used.

C. Normal Values

After an overnight fast, insulin levels in healthy subjects range from 1.0 to 20 μU/ml. There is some variability from assay to assay, the double antibody method tending to give lower values. Soeldner and Slone (1965) found a mean concentration of 8.44 ± 0.35 μU/ml in 75 normal subjects, while Welborn and co-workers (1966) reported a similar mean value and pointed out that the values were log-normally distributed. The fasting level falls further with prolonged starvation.

Figure 6. Sample output from our quality control subroutine. (Top) Usual assay with each of the control parameters listed and compared with the historical data. This is followed by a plot of each of these parameters chronologically to detect any trends. (Bottom) The quality control listing of an unacceptable assay with significant errors. The program has flagged all parameters outside two standard deviations from the mean of the historical values. "Danger" indicates that the current value is between two and three standard deviations from the mean. "Disaster" indicates that the current value is greater than three standard deviations from the mean.

Higher values are found in obese subjects, acromegalics, patients with Cushing's syndrome, dystrophia myotonica, the third trimester of pregnancy, and in islet cell tumors, while children tend to have lower levels.

The serum insulin concentrations rise four- to tenfold after the ingestion of 100 gm oral glucose, attain their maximum values at 30 to 60 minutes, and thereafter gradually fall to the fasting level or below at two to four hours. During intravenous glucose tolerance tests, peak levels were reached at one to two minutes ($72 \pm 14 \mu$U/ml) and returned to control values by 60–120 minutes (Soeldner and Slone, 1965). The insulin response to glucagon, tolbutamide, arginine, leucine, and other stimuli has also been measured. However, it is advisable to establish normal values for each test in individual laboratories.

Fasting proinsulin levels (read from a human proinsulin standard) in normal subjects range between 0.05 and 0.5 ng/ml, representing 5–48% of the insulin concentration (Melani *et al.*, 1970a). In studies using a human insulin standard for measurement of both proinsulin and insulin, the percentage contribution of proinsulin to the total serum immunoreactive insulin concentration in healthy subjects was 5–22%. After oral glucose, the levels of proinsulin rose slowly and peaked later than insulin. When expressed as a percentage of the total serum insulin concentration, a decline from the fasting value was observed during the first 15–60 minutes (Gorden and Roth, 1969). Thereafter, proinsulin contributed an increasing amount to the immunoreactive insulin level. Although abnormalities in the proinsulin concentration or the ratio of insulin to proinsulin have been described in a number of pathologic states (chronic renal failure, hypokalemia, familial hyperproinsulinemia, severe diabetes), markedly elevated levels are most frequently observed in patients with beta cell tumors (Rubenstein *et al.*, 1972).

IV. PROBLEMS RELATED TO THE MEASUREMENT OF INSULIN AND PROINSULIN

Under most circumstances, plasma proinsulin is present in relatively small amounts, and does not appreciably affect the absolute values of immunoreactive insulin measured against a human insulin standard. There are, however, occasions when proinsulin comprises the major component of circulating insulin. Because proinsulin reacts considerably less well than insulin with insulin antibodies, the concentration of "immunoreactive insulinlike material" will be markedly underestimated in the direct assay of these plasma samples.

After separating proinsulin from insulin by gel filtration, most investigators have expressed proinsulin and insulin as a percentage of the total insulinlike immunoreactivity in plasma. Certain problems are inherent in this approach. Because of the limited availability of human proinsulin, most investigators have measured the individual fractions of both the proinsulin and insulin peaks against a standard of human insulin. The total immunoreactivity in all the fractions is summed, and the percentage in each peak is calculated. Furthermore, the absolute concentration of the proinsulin peak has been determined by multiplying its percentage by the total plasma insulin concentration, which is also assayed against the human insulin standard (Figure 4). The potential errors in this method are given below:

1. The total insulinlike immunoreactivity (proinsulin and insulin) determined by direct immunoassay of plasma against an insulin standard is underestimated because proinsulin and its intermediates usually react less well than insulin with insulin antibodies.

2. The proinsulin peak, separated by gel filtration, may be underestimated for the same reason.

3. The sum of immunoreactivity (read from an insulin standard) in the proinsulin plus insulin peaks is derived from the addition of heterogeneous nonidentically reacting components.

Measurement of the proinsulin peak against a standard of human proinsulin has partly solved this difficulty. Under these circumstances, it has seemed appropriate to express the concentration of proinsulin (in the early eluting peak) as a percentage of the insulin concentration (in the second peak) rather than as a percentage of the combined immunoreactivity in the two peaks. It should be noted, however, that if intermediate forms are present in plasma, and if their reaction is different from that of proinsulin, then the absolute concentration of proinsulin read from this standard may be incorrect.

V. OTHER RADIOIMMUNOASSAYS AVAILABLE

There are numerous alternative methods available for the measurement of insulin. Most vary in terms of the methods of separating the antibody-bound from free antigen. Among the techniques which have been successfully used are chromatoelectrophoresis, gel filtration, precipitation with sodium sulfite or ethanol, enzymatic hydrolysis of the unbound hormone with activated ficin, and solid-phase adsorption of the antigen with charcoal, talc, or microgranules of silica (QUSO). Insulin has also been measured by the immunoradiometric assay described by Addison and Hales (1971) in which labeled antibodies were used. Each of these methods has advantages and disadvantages, which should be carefully considered before a final choice for a particular laboratory is made.

Another method for separating insulin from proinsulin has been described by Kitabchi and his co-workers (1971; Duckworth and Kitabchi, 1972). These investigators have used an enzyme which is relatively specific for the proteolytic degradation of insulin, but not proinsulin. Measuring samples in an insulin assay before and after incubation with this enzyme [insulin-specific protease (ISP)] should enable one to determine the relative concentrations of the two peptides. The accuracy of this method is limited, however, especially at low serum immunoreactive insulin concentrations, because the degradation of insulin is generally incomplete. This may be due, in part, to the presence of noncompetitive inhibitors of the enzyme in plasma (Cresto et al., 1974; Starr et al., 1975).

VI. RADIOIMMUNOASSAY FOR HUMAN C-PEPTIDE

Equimolar amounts of C-peptide and insulin are produced in the pancreatic beta cells when proinsulin is cleaved in the secretory granules (Clark et al., 1969). The C-peptide is not degraded in the beta cell and is secreted together with insulin into the circulation (Rubenstein et al., 1969). Since C-peptide does not cross-react with insulin, a separate system is needed for its measurement. A number of radioimmunoassays for human C-peptide have now been described (Melani et al., 1970b; Kaneko et al., 1974; Heding, 1975).

A. Assay Procedure

1. Standards

A suitable standard may be prepared by extraction of C-peptide from human pancreas obtained at autopsy (Oyer et al., 1971). The C-peptide is purified by paper electrophoresis and ion-exchange chromatography. C-peptide may also be synthesized by solid-phase methods (Yanaihara et al., 1972). Although synthesis appears to be an easier method of obtaining the C-peptide, the standard curves obtained from natural pancreatic human C-peptide and synthetic human C-peptide are not identical. For this reason, we have preferred using the naturally occurring peptide as the standard in our assay. Because there are marked variations in the sequences of C-peptides from the different species (Steiner *et al.*, 1972), a homologous assay must be used. Human C-peptide is commercially available from Calbiochem.

2. Antiserum

Antiserum to human C-peptide has been prepared in both guinea pigs and rabbits by immunization with the C-peptide covalently linked to albumin (Melani *et al.*, 1970b). Conjugation has been performed by incubating 3.0 mg human C-peptide, 1.5 mg rabbit serum albumin, and 1-ethyl-3-(3-diethylaminopropyl) carbodiimide HCl (400 mg/ml) in the presence of trace amounts of ^{131}I-tyrosine C-peptide. A change in the elution position of the radioactive label after gel filtration on Bio-Gel P-30 confirmed conjugation of C-peptide to albumin. After purification on Sephadex G-10, the conjugate was emulsified with complete Freund's adjuvant for immunization. Animals received the equivalent of 0.35 mg C-peptide in each of four immunizations at two to three-week intervals; the animals were bled ten days after the third and fourth immunizations (Melani *et al.*, 1970b). For immunization, it has been most feasible to use synthetically prepared C-peptide rather than that obtained by extraction from human pancreas because of the large amounts of C-peptide needed. Antibodies raised against these synthetic C-peptides have been quite satisfactory in practice (Faber *et al.*, 1976).

3. Preparation of Radioactive Ligand

Since human C-peptide does not contain tyrosine, it must be tyrosylated prior to iodination. Human C-peptide (0.5 mg) was dissolved in 0.15 ml 0.0025 *N* HCl and 0.15 ml 0.01 *M* phosphate, pH 7.6. *N*-Carboxytyrosyl anhydride (Cyclo Chemical Co.) was added (2 mg in 0.1 ml dioxane) and incubated for 16 hours at 2°C. After centrifugation to remove any precipitate, the supernatant was dissolved in 0.8 ml of 3 *M* acetic acid and purified on a 1.0 × 50 cm Bio-Gel P-30 column. Fractions containing tyrosylated C-peptide were pooled, concentrated, and made up to 100 µg/ml in 0.075 *M* Veronal buffer, pH 8.6 (Melani *et al.*, 1970b). As an alternative to this, the C-peptide has been synthesized with a tyrosine incorporated at either terminus (Yanaihara *et al.*, 1972). This material appears to be equally satisfactory when stored in the lyophilized state, but iodination of peptide that had been stored in solution did not provide as satisfactory a label. The iodination procedure itself is similar to that described for insulin, except that the iodination mixture is purified by gel filtration on a 0.8×10 cm column of Bio-Gel P-30 equilibrated in borate buffer. In the final step of the iodination procedure, instead of adding 2.5% albumin to the mixture, 100 μl assay buffer (borate buffer with 0.5% bovine serum albumin) is added.

4. Assay Procedure

The method of assay is similar to that used for insulin, except, for convenience, we have used a final volume for the first incubation of 1.0 ml instead of 1.2 ml. The appropriate dilution of antiserum is determined in a manner similar to that used for the insulin assay. We have been using a rabbit anti-human C-peptide antiserum, and, therefore, for the precipitation step, we add a sheep anti-rabbit γ-globulin serum and normal rabbit serum as carrier. The incubations, separations, and calculations are similar to the insulin assay. Done in this way, the C-peptide radioimmunoassay is sensitive to 75 pg/tube.

B. Interpretation of the Assay Data

Insulin does not cross-react in the C-peptide assay. Proinsulin reacts about one-fifth to one-fifteenth as well as C-peptide on a weight basis, depending on the antiserum used. Since proinsulin is present at only 10–20% of the level of C-peptide in normal serum, it contributes less than 4% to the C-peptide immunoreactivity (CPR) in healthy subjects. Consequently, extraction and gel filtration of samples are not necessary for measurement of C-peptide in normal serum. However, in serum from insulin-treated diabetic patients, the situation is more complicated. These patients develop insulin-binding antibodies, which also bind endogenously secreted proinsulin. Because of this binding, the amount of proinsulin in the blood can be substantially increased, at times accounting for as much of 90% of total C-peptide immunoreactivity. In this situation, we have found it useful to separately measure the "free" C-peptide, which is conveniently determined by precipitating antibody-bound proinsulin with polyethylene glycol (PEG). In order to perform this procedure, 0.3 ml 25% aqueous PEG (Carbowax 6,000) solution, chilled to 4°C, is added to 0.3 ml serum, mixed vigorously, and centrifuged at 4°C. The supernatant is assayed for C-peptide in the usual manner. This method has given highly satisfactory results (Kuzuya et al., 1977b).

The C-peptide assay is complicated further by the recent discovery of heterogeneity in circulating C-peptide. Also, we have shown that the C-peptide concentration may not be stable during storage (Kuzuya *et al.*, 1977a) and that different antisera may react differently with the fragments formed. Thus, it is apparent that any antiserum must be characterized carefully before being used to establish an immunoassay for this peptide.

C. Urine C-Peptide

Determination of C-peptide in urine has the potential advantage of being able to give an integrated measure of beta cell secretory function over a given period of time. Furthermore, it is useful when frequent blood sampling is not feasible, such as in small children. In addition, the amount of proinsulin excreted in the urine is very small, and antibody-bound proinsulin is not filtered and does not appear in the urine. Therefore, interference by proinsulin does not need to be considered in interpreting the results of the urinary C-peptide assay. Assay of urinary C-peptide has been demonstrated to be a useful quantitative procedure (Horwitz *et al.*, 1977). The method is the same as that used for assay of serum. Because the concentration of C-peptide is much higher in urine than it is in serum, it is often possible to assay as little as 10 μl urine. For urine samples with low concentrations of C-peptide, volumes up to 200 μl may be used without invalidating the assay. Because as much as 5% of the C-peptide secreted by the pancreas appears in the urine, compared to only 0.1% of the secreted insulin, it is more accurate to quantitate beta cell function by measurement of urinary C-peptide rather than insulin. The C-peptide clearance has been shown to be independent of creatinine clearance over a range of 2.0–190 ml/min. Therefore, urinary C-peptide measurement can be used even in patients with impaired renal function (Horwitz *et al.*, 1977).

D. Clinical Applications

C-peptide levels correlate with those of insulin in the serum of normal subjects when measured in both portal and peripheral blood. C-peptide has, therefore, been used as an alternative measure of beta cell function (Block *et al.*, 1972; Horwitz *et al.*, 1976). Normal values depend upon the antiserum used. Fasting concentrations range from 1.0 to 2.0 ng/ml (0.3–0.7 pmole/ml) and a four- to six-fold increase is seen after the administration of glucose. C-peptide determinations are a useful measure of endogenous beta cell function in insulin-requiring diabetic patients (Block *et al.*, 1972). The clinical indications for

Table III   Clinical Indications for C-Peptide Measurement

Hypoglycemic states
 1. Diagnosis of insulinoma (or ? beta cell hyperplasia) in insulin-requiring diabetics
 2. Diagnosis of insulinoma (suppression test)
 3. Diagnosis of surreptitious injection of insulin
Euglycemic state
 1. Demonstration of remission phase or recovery from diabetes
Hyperglycemic states
 1. Follow-up evaluation after pancreatectomy
 2. Evaluation of the brittle diabetic

measuring C-peptide have been reviewed and are summarized in Table III (Horwitz *et al.*, 1976).

REFERENCES

Addison, G. M., and Hales, C. N. (1971). The immunoradiometric assay. *In* "Radioimmunoassay Methods" (K. E. Kirkham and W. M. Hunter, eds.), pp. 447–466. Churchill, London.

Berson, S. A., and Yalow, R. S. (1959). Recent studies on insulin binding antibodies. *Ann. N.Y. Acad. Sci.* **82**, 338–344.

Berson, S. A., and Yalow, R. S. (1964). Immunoassay of protein hormones. *In* "The Hormones" (G. Pincus, K. V. Thimann, and E. B. Astwood, eds.), Vol. 4, pp. 557–630. Academic Press, New York.

Berson, S. A., and Yalow, R. S. (1968a). Immunochemical heterogeneity of parathyroid hormone. *J. Clin. Endocrinol. Metab.* **28**, 1037–1047.

Berson, S. A., and Yalow, R. S. (1968b). Principles of immunoassay of peptide hormones in plasma. *In* "Clinical Endocrinology" (E. B. Astwood and C. E. Cassidy, eds.), Vol. 2, pp. 699–720. Grune and Stratton, New York.

Block, M. B., Mako, M. E., Steiner, D. F., and Rubenstein, A. H. (1972). Circulating C-peptide immunoreactivity: Studies in normals and diabetic patients. *Diabetes* **21**, 1013–1026.

Boyd, G. W., Adamson, A. R., Fiz, A. E., and Peart, W. S. (1969). Radioimmunoassay determination of plasma-renin activity. *Lancet* **1**, 213–218.

Brunfeldt, K., and Jorgensen, K. R. (1967). Some factors of significance in the double antibody immunoassay of insulin. *Acta Endocrinol. (Copenhagen)* **54**, 347–361.

Brunfeldt, K., Hansen, B. A., and Jorgensen, K. R. (1968). The immunological reactivity and biological activity of iodinated insulin. *Acta Endocrinol. (Copenhagen)* **57**, 307–329.

Burr, I. M., Grant, P. C., Sizonenko, S. L., Kaplan, S. L., and Grumbach, M. M. (1969). Some critical factors in double antibody radioimmunoassay systems utilizing sheep anti-rabbit precipitated sera for measurement of human serum LH, FSH, HGH. *J. Clin. Endocrinol. Metab.* **29**, 948–956.

Clark, J. L., Cho, S., Rubenstein, A. H., and Steiner, D. F. (1969). Isolation of a proinsulin connecting peptide fragment (C-peptide) from bovine and human pancreas. *Biochem. Biophys. Res. Commun.* **35**, 456–461.

Cresto, J. C., Lavine, R. L., Fink, G., and Recant, L. (1974). Plasma proinsulin: Comparison of insulin specific protease and gel filtration assay. *Diabetes* **23**, 505–511.

Csorba, T. R., and Gattner, H. G. (1970). Cross-linking of insulin induced by iodination. *Horm. Metab. Res.* **2**, 305–306.

Daughaday, W. H., and Jacobs, L. S. (1971). Methods of separating antibody-bound from free antigen. *In* "Principles of Competitive Protein-Binding Assays" (W. D. Odell and W. H. Daughaday, eds.), pp. 303–316. Lippincott, Philadelphia, Pennsylvania.

Duckworth, W. C., and Kitabchi, A. E. (1972). Direct measurement of plasma proinsulin in normal and diabetic subjects. *Am. J. Med.* **53**, 418–424.

Faber, O. K., Markussen, J., Naithani, J. K., and Binder, C. (1976). Systemic production of antisera to synthetic C-peptide of human proinsulin. *Hoppe-Seyler's Z. Physiol. Chem.* **357**, 751–757.

Feldman, H., and Rodbard, D. (1971). Mathematical theory of radioimmunoassay. *In* "Principles of Competitive Protein-Binding Assays" (W. D. Odell and W. H. Daughaday, eds.), pp. 158–199. Lippincott, Philadelphia, Pennsylvania.

Frechet, P., Roth, J., and Neville, D. M. (1971). Monoiodoinsulin: Demonstration of its biological activity and binding to fat cells and liver membranes. *Biochem. Biophys. Res. Commun.* **43**, 400–408.

Freedlender, A. E. (1969). Practical and theoretical advantages for the use of I^{125} in radioimmunoassay. *Protein Polypeptide Horm., Proc. Int. Symp., 1968.* Excerpta Med. Found. Int. Congr. Ser. No. 161, Part 2, pp. 351–353.

Froesch, E. R., Burgi, H., Ramsier, E. B., Bally, P., and Labhart, A. (1963). Antibody-suppressible and non-suppressible insulin-like activities in human serum and their physiological significance: An insulin assay with adipose tissue of increased precision and specificity. *J. Clin. Invest.* **42**, 1816–1834.

Glover, J. S., Salter, D. N., and Shepperd, B. P. (1967). A study of some factors that influence the iodination of ox insulin. *Biochem. J.* **103**, 120–128.

Gorden, P., and Roth, J. (1969). Plasma insulin: Fluctuations in the "big" insulin component in man after glucose and other stimuli. *J. Clin. Invest.* **48**, 2225–2234.

Hales, C. N., and Randle, P. J. (1963). Immunoassay of insulin with insulin-antibody precipitate. *Biochem. J.* **88**, 137–146.

Heding, L. G. (1975). Radioimmunological determination of human C-peptide in serum. *Diabetologia* **11**, 541–548.

Heinzel, W., Grimminger, H., and Kallee, E. (1971). Precipitating insulin–anti-insulin complexes. *Diabetologia* **7**, 204–205.

Henderson, J. R. (1970). Serum insulin or plasma insulin. *Lancet* **2**, 545–546.

Horwitz, D. L., Kuzuya, H., and Rubenstein, A. H. (1976). Circulating serum C-peptide. *N. Engl. J. Med.* **295**, 207–209.

Horwitz, D. L., Rubenstein, A. H., and Katz, A. I. (1977). Quantitation of human pancreatic beta cell function by immunoassay of C-peptide in urine. *Diabetes* **26**, 30–35.

Hunter, R. (1970). Standardization of the chloramine-T method of protein iodination. *Proc. Soc. Exp. Biol. Med.* **133**, 989–992.

Hunter, W. M., and Greenwood, F. C. (1962). Preparation of iodine[131] labelled growth hormone of high specific activity. *Nature (London)* **194**, 495–496.

Izzo, J. L., Roncone, A., Izzo, M. J., and Bale, W. F. (1964). Relationship between degree of iodination of insulin and its biological, electrophoretic, and immunochemical properties. *J. Biol. Chem.* **239**, 3749–3754.

Kaneko, T., Oka, II., Munemura, M., Oda, T., Yamashita, K., Suzuki, S., Yanaihara, N., Hashimoto, T., and Yanaihara, C. (1974). Radioimmunoassay of human proinsulin

C-peptide using synthetic human connecting peptide. *Endocrinol. Jpn.* **21**, 141–145.

Kirkham, K. E., and Hunter, W. M., eds. (1971). "Radioimmunoassay Methods." Churchill, London.

Kitabchi, A. E., Duckworth, W. C., Brush, J. S., and Heinemann, M. (1971). Direct measurement of proinsulin in human plasma by the use of an insulin-degrading enzyme. *J. Clin. Invest.* **50**, 1792–1799.

Kuzuya, H., Blix, P. M., Horwitz, D. L., Rubenstein, A. H., Steiner, D. F., Binder, C., and Faber, O. (1977a). Heterogeneity of circulating C-peptide. *J. Clin. Endocrinol. Metab.* **44**, 952–962.

Kuzuya, H., Blix, P. M., Horwitz, D. L., Steiner, D. F., and Rubenstein, A. H. (1977b). Determination of free and total insulin and C-peptide in insulin-treated diabetics. *Diabetes* **26**, 22–29.

Lambert, B., Sutter, B. C. J., and Jacquimin, C. (1972). Effect of iodination on the biological activity of insulin. *Horm. Metab. Res.* **4**, 149–151.

McBride, L., and Rodbard, D. (1971). "Radioimmunoassay Data Processing," Rep. No. NIH-RIA-71-2. US Department of Commerce, National Technical Information Service, Springfield, Virginia.

McFarlane, A. S. (1958). Efficient trace labelling of proteins with iodine. *Nature (London)* **182**, 53–55.

Makulu, D. R., and Wright, P. (1971). Immune response to insulin in guinea pigs. *Metab., Clin. Exp.* **20**, 770–781.

Melani, F., Rubenstein, A. H., and Steiner, D. F. (1970a). Human serum proinsulin. *J. Clin. Invest.* **49**, 497–507.

Melani, F., Rubenstein, A. H., Oyer, P. E., and Steiner, D. F. (1970b). Identification of prosinulin and C-peptide in human serum by a specific immunoassay. *Proc. Natl. Acad. Sci. U.S.A.* **67**, 148–155.

Moloney, P. J., and Goldsmith, L. (1957). On the antigenicity of insulin. *Can. J. Biochem. Physiol.* **35**, 79–92.

Morgan, C. R., and Lazarow, A. (1963). Immunoassay of insulin: Two antibody system. Plasma insulin levels of normal, subdiabetic and diabetic rats. *Diabetes* **12**, 115–126.

Morgan, C. R., Sorensen, R. L., and Lazarow, A. (1964). Studies of an inhibitor of the two antibody system. *Diabetes* **13**, 1–5.

Morse, J. H. (1959). Rapid production and detection of insulin-binding antibodies in rabbits and guinea pigs. *Proc. Soc. Exp. Biol. Med.* **101**, 722–725.

Nixon, W. E., and Cargille, C. M. (1971). Binding of tracer FSH, LH, GH and TSH by anti-FSH sera prepared by several immunization regimens. *J. Lab. Clin. Med.* **78**, 949–956.

Odell, W. D., Abraham, G. E., Skowsky, W. R., Hescox, M. A., and Fisher, D. A. (1971). Production of antisera for radioimmunoassays. *In* "Principles of Competitive Protein-Binding Assays" (W. D. Odell and W. H. Daughaday, eds.), pp. 57–76. Lippincott, Philadelphia, Pennsylvania.

Ørskov, H., and Johansen, K. (1972). Immunological measurements of urinary insulin for the evaluation of insulin production. *Acta Endocrinol. (Copenhagen)* **71**, 697–708.

Oyer, P. E., Cho, S., Peterson, J., and Steiner, D. F. (1971). Studies on human proinsulin: Isolation and amino acid sequence of the human pancreatic C-peptide. *J. Biol. Chem.* **246**, 1375–1386.

Parker, C. W. (1971). Nature of immunological responses and antigen-antibody interaction. *In* "Principles of Competitive Protein-Binding Assays" (W. D. Odell and

W. H. Daughaday, eds.), pp. 25–48. Lippincott, Philadelphia, Pennsylvania.

Pope, C. G. (1966). The immunology of insulin. *Adv. Immunol.* **5**, 209–244.

Rodbard, D. (1971). Statistical aspects of radioimmunoassays. *In* "Principles of Competitive Protein-Binding Assays" (W. D. Odell and W. H. Daughaday, eds.), pp. 204–253. Lippincott, Philadelphia, Pennsylvania.

Root, M. A., Chance, R. E., and Galloway, J. A. (1972). Immunogenicity of insulin. *Diabetes* **21**, Suppl. 2, 657–660.

Roth, J., Gorden, P., and Pastan, I. (1968). "Big insulin:" A new component of plasma insulin detected by immunoassay. *Proc. Natl. Acad. Sci. U.S.A.* **61**, 138–145.

Rubenstein, A. H., Lowy, C., and Fraser, T. R. (1967). Radioimmunoassay for insulin in urine. *Diabetologia* **3**, 453–459.

Rubenstein, A. H., Cho, S., and Steiner, D. F. (1968). Evidence for proinsulin in human urine and serum. *Lancet* **1**, 1353–1355.

Rubenstein, A. H., Clark, J. L., Melani, F., and Steiner, D. F. (1969). Secretion of proinsulin C-peptide by pancreatic β cells and its circulation in blood. *Nature (London)* **224**, 697–699.

Rubenstein, A. H., Block, M. B., Starr, J., Melani, F., and Steiner, D. F. (1972). Proinsulin and C-peptide in blood. *Diabetes* **21**, Suppl. 2, 661–672.

Schlichtkrull, J., Branke, J., Christiansen, A. H., Hallund, O., Heding, L. G. and Jørgensen, K. R. (1972). Clinical aspects of insulin-antigenicity. *Diabetes* **21**, Suppl. 2, 649–656.

Sheps, M. C., Nickerson, R. J., Dagenais, Y. M., Steinke, J., Martin, D. B., and Renold, A. E. (1960). Measurement of small quantities of insulin-like activity using rat adipose tissue. *J. Clin. Invest.* **39**, 1499–1510.

Soeldner, J. S., and Slone, D. (1965). Critical variables in the radioimmunoassay of serum insulin using the double antibody technic. *Diabetes* **14**, 771–779.

Sonksen, P. H., Ellis, J. P., Marcuson, R., Rutherford, A., Nussey, I. D., and Nabarro, J. D. N. (1971). *In* "Radioimmunoassay Methods" (K. E. Kirkham and W. M. Hunter, eds.), pp. 584–588. Churchill, London.

Starr, J. I., Juhn, D. J., Rubenstein, A. H., and Kitabchi, A. E. (1975). Degradation of insulin in serum by insulin specific protease. *J. Lab. Clin. Med.* **86**, 631–636.

Steiner, D. F., Kemmler, W., Clark, J. L., Oyser, P. E., and Rubenstein, A. H. (1972). The biosynthesis of insulin. *In Handb. Physiol., Sect. 7: Endocrinol.* **1**, 175–198.

Vaitukaitis, J., Robbins, J. B., Nieschlag, E., and Ross, G. T. (1971). A method for producing specific antisera with small doses of immunogen. *J. Clin. Endocrinol. Metab.* **33**, 988–991.

Vallance-Owen, J., and Hurlock, B. (1954). Estimation of plasma insulin by rat diaphragm method. *Lancet* **1**, 68–72.

van Orden, D. (1972). Factors affecting the stability of radioiodinated insulin during storage. *J. Lab. Clin. Med.* **79**, 470–479.

Welborn, T. A., and Fraser, R. T. (1965). The double-antibody immunoassay of insulin. *Diabetologia* **1**, 211–218.

Welborn, T. A., Rubenstein, A. H., Haslam, R., and Fraser, R. T. (1966). The normal insulin response to glucose. *Lancet* **1**, 280–284.

Wright, P. H., and Norman, L. L. (1966). Some factors affecting insulin antibody production in guinea pigs. *Diabetes* **15**, 668–674.

Wright, P. H., Makulu, D. R., and Posey, I. J. (1968). Guinea pig anti-insulin serum; adjuvant effect of *H. pertussis* vaccine. *Diabetes* **17**, 513–516.

Yalow, R. S., and Berson, S. A. (1960). Immunoassay of endogenous plasma insulin in man. *J. Clin. Invest.* **39**, 1157–1175.

Yalow, R. S., and Berson, S. A. (1961). Immunologic specificity of human insulin: Application to immunoassay for insulin. *J. Clin. Invest.* **40**, 2190–2198.

Yalow, R. S., and Berson, S. A. (1971a). Introduction and general considerations. *In* "Principles of Competitive Protein-Binding Assays" (W. D. Odell and W. H. Daughaday, eds.), pp. 1–21. Lippincott, Philadelphia, Pennsylvania.

Yalow, R. S., and Berson, S. A. (1971b). Problems of validation of radioimmunoassays. *In* "Principles of Competitive Protein-Binding Assays" (W. D. Odell and W. H. Daughaday, eds.), pp. 374–400. Lippincott, Philadelphia, Pennsylvania.

Yanaihara, N., Hashimoto, T., Yanaihara, C., Sakagami, M., and Sakura, N. (1972). Synthesis of polypeptides related to porcine proinsulin. *Diabetes* **21**, Suppl. 2, 476–485.

32

Glucagon

VIRGINIA HARRIS, GERALD R. FALOONA, AND
ROGER H. UNGER

I. INTRODUCTION

Glucagon, a 29 amino acid peptide hormone, is secreted by the α cells of the islets of Langerhans. Recently, α cells have been found in the fundus and duodenum of dogs (Sasaki *et al.*, 1975; Baetens *et al.*, 1976), and humans (Sasagawa *et al.*, 1974). In 1923, glucagon was named as the hyperglycemic factor in crude insulin extracts by Murlin and co-workers and was then all but ignored until 1953, when it was purified by Staub *et al.* Four years later, Bromer *et al.* (1957) determined its amino acid sequence (see Chapter 27). Glucagon's status as a

643

Methods of Hormone Radioimmunoassay, Second Edition

hormone remained in doubt until the development of radioimmunoassays provided a means of measuring glucagon in plasma and established the hormone's role as a component in a bihormonal system of metabolic regulation.

Berson and Yalow (1959) were the first to introduce the technique of radioimmunoassay with their radioimmunoassay of insulin. The first report of a radioimmunoassay for glucagon (Unger et al., 1959) came shortly thereafter, but the development of a sensitive and specific means of measuring the concentration of glucagon in peripheral plasma required several additional years of work, for reasons detailed below.

II. SPECIAL PROBLEMS ENCOUNTERED IN THE MEASUREMENT OF PLASMA GLUCAGON BY RADIOIMMUNOASSAY

A. Cross-Reactivity with Nonpancreatic Glucagon-Like Immunoreactivity (GLI)

Orci et al. (1968), Polak et al. (1971), and Larsson and co-workers (1975) all have demonstrated the presence of α-like cells in the stomach, duodenum, and jejunum believed to be the source of glucagon-like immunoreactivity (GLI). Under normal circumstances and in the presence of adequate quantities of insulin, glucagon activity derived from the extrapancreatic α cells constitutes only a tiny portion of the immunoreactive glucagon pool (Unger et al., 1977). However, after nonphysiologic stimulation, such as after the infusion of arginine, extrapancreatic glucagon levels are increased (Muñoz-Barragan et al., 1976). Furthermore, in insulin deprivation either by total pancreatectomy (Blazquez et al., 1976) or after treatment with alloxan (Blazquez et al., 1977), the gastric fundus appears to be an important source of plasma immunoreactive glucagon, at least in the dog.

Unger (1976) distinguished glucagon-like immunoreactivity from pancreatic–gastrointestinal glucagon on the basis of molecular weight of the predominant form (2900 versus 3485 daltons), isoelectric point (>10 versus 6.2), and decreased glycogenolytic and adenylate cyclase-stimulating activity. GLI appears to circulate in considerably higher concentrations than authentic pancreatic (or gastrointestinal glucagon). Thus, a major obstacle in the development of a radioimmunoassay for plasma glucagon was the production of a suitable antiserum capable of measuring small quantities of glucagon in the presence of greater amounts of glucagon-like peptides of enteric origin.

B. Proteolytic Degradation of Glucagon by Plasma

Glucagon is highly susceptible to the normal proteolytic activity of plasma. Mirsky *et al.* (1959) reported that human plasma degraded ^{131}I-glucagon, and it was later recognized by Unger *et al.* (1963) that degradation of tracer during its incubation with plasma in the glucagon radioimmunoassay could give rise to spuriously high values.

The discovery that Trasylol, a proteolytic inhibitor, could prevent detectable degradation of labeled glucagon during a four-day incubation with human plasma (Eisentraut *et al.*, 1968) apparently solved the problem of incubation damage. Since degradation of endogenous glucagon can occur in the preparation of plasma samples prior to assay, Trasylol should also be added to blood at the time of collection (Aguilar-Parada *et al.*, 1969; Heding, 1971).

Ensinck and co-workers reported in 1972 that benzamidine, a less expensive proteolytic inhibitor, prevented glucagon degradation by human plasma and could replace Trasylol as a radioimmunoassay reagent. We have only recently begun to use benzamidine in the collection of samples, and thus far have found no evidence that it interferes in other radioimmunoassay systems.

C. Heterogeneity of Plasma Glucagon

A number of investigators (Valverde *et al.*, 1974, 1975, 1976; Kuku *et al.*, 1976a,b) have reported the presence of four separate molecular forms of circulating glucagon in man and dog. Plasma from blood containing EDTA and 500 U Trasylol (2.0 ml) was chromatographed on 1.0×50 cm columns of Bio-Gel P-30 at 10 ml/hour eluting with 0.2 M glycine containing 0.25% HSA and 1% normal sheep serum. The four forms include: (1) big plasma glucagon, a macromolecule with a molecular weight of about 60,000; (2) proglucagon, a relatively inert molecule (Rigopoulou *et al.*, 1970) with a molecular mass of approximately 9000 daltons, which can be converted to biologically active glucagon by trypsinization and separation from a carboxyl-terminal fragment (O'Connor and Lazarus, 1976); (3) true glucagon; and (4) a small peak of immunoreactive material with a molecular mass of 2000 daltons. Since these molecular forms cross-react with most antiglucagon antisera, the molecular heterogeneity complicates interpretation of glucagon radioimmunoassay data.

III. METHODS OF RADIOIMMUNOASSAY

A. Source of Hormone

Highly purified crystalline glucagon can be obtained from Eli Lilly (Indianapolis, Indiana) and NOVO Laboratories (Copenhagen, Denmark). We use crystalline glucagon (Lilly Lot No. 258D301384) for radioimmunoassay standards and iodination and a less purified glucagon from NOVO for immunogen preparations.

Beef and pork glucagon have identical structures (Bromer *et al.*, 1971). The amino acid composition and probably the sequence of rat, rabbit, and human glucagons are identical (Sundby and Markussen, 1971, 1972; Thomsen *et al.*, 1972). This identity among every mammalian species studied thus far indicates a conservation of structure suggesting a highly specific structural requirement for biologic activity (Bromer *et al.*, 1972) and permits plasma samples from any number of species to be radioimmunoassayed with a single reference standard.

B. Preparation of Antibodies

Glucagon, like most other small peptides, is by itself a poor immunogen. It is clear, however, that the immunogenicity and the resultant antibody-binding capacity and affinity for glucagon are greatly increased by chemically coupling or adsorbing it to larger molecules (Heding, 1972). Assan *et al.* (1965) demonstrated that the adsorption of glucagon to polyvinylpyrrolidone (PVP) prior to emulsification with adjuvant greatly increased antibody production in rabbits.

The production of specific antisera cannot be attributed to any special method of immunization, since numerous rabbits immunized in an identical manner have yielded nonspecific antiserum.

1. Preparation of Immunogen

The method of immunization that we have used since 1967 is based on that of Assan *et al.* (1965). Ten milligrams of glucagon (Eli Lilly Company or Novo Industries) is dissolved in 1.0 ml of the diluting fluid which accompanies each ampoule and is then transferred to another vial. The ampoule is rinsed with another milliliter of diluting fluid, and this is added to the first milliliter. Three milliliters of a 25% solution of PVP (MW ~ 40,000) is added and after thorough mixing the glucagon–PVP solution is incubated for one hour at 4°C. At the end of the hour, 5.0 ml Freund's adjuvant is added (complete Freund's for the first few injections and incomplete for all subsequent injections), and the suspension is emulsified by vigorous shaking or by repeated aspiration through a 20-gauge needle. The emulsion contains one milligram of glucagon per milliliter.

Rabbits initially receive a total of one to two mg of glucagon injected subcutaneously into the hip or thigh region at two-week intervals for three to six months.

Blood is obtained by cardiac puncture at the end of the initial series. If an appreciable amount of glucagon antibodies has been produced, a second series of three to four injections is given, and the rabbits are bled at two- to four-week intervals for several months. One to two booster injections are given every six months, and the bleeding schedule is resumed.

Each drawing of antiserum is stored at $-20°C$, and thawing and refreezing do not seem to affect the antiserum.

2. Other Methods of Immunization

Grey and associates (1970) reported the production of high-affinity antibodies by coupling glucagon to hemocyanin. This antiserum apparently neutralized glucagon *in vivo*. Cuatrecasas and Illiano (1971) reported high-affinity antibodies using a glucagon–poly-L-lysine conjugate. The specificity of these antisera for pancreatic glucagon has not been reported.

Of other methods of immunization attempted, Heding (1972) has had the most success with glucagon coupled to glucagon, and an alum-precipitated egg albumin mixture (Unger and Eisentraut, 1967; Heding, 1972) produced the most specific antiserum (G58) yet produced in this laboratory.

3. Screening of Antisera

The vast majority of antiglucagon sera are unsuitable for measuring pancreatic glucagon in plasma either because of a lack of affinity, a lack of specificity, or both. The procedure which follows is used to screen antiglucagon sera for possible use in a radioimmunoassay. The incubation conditions and charcoal separation techniques are exactly the same as those used in routine immunoassays (15 pg ^{125}I-glucagon, 1000 U Trasylol in a final volume of 1.2 ml).

First, the percentage binding of ^{125}I-glucagon is determined for 10^2-, 10^3-, 10^4-, and 10^5-fold dilutions of antisera. From these data, a suitable dilution can be selected for determining a standard curve which binds approximately 50% of the tracer. The shape of the standard curve is a measure of the affinity of the antisera and, therefore, the potential sensitivity of the radioimmunoassay. Antisera of high and moderate affinity are checked for specificity. The specificity of the antisera is checked by measuring the GLI content of gut extracts and several plasma samples of predictable pancreatic and enteroglucagon content, i.e., dog plasma after intraduodenal glucose or arginine infusion, depancreatized dog plasma, and normal human plasma.

In order to distinguish pancreatic-like glucagon from GLI and to be considered specific for glucagon, an antiserum should (a) react weakly or not at all with extracts of jejunum, (b) show proportional dilution of plasma glucagon immunoreactivity, (c) show a decrease rather than a rise in immunoreactivity at all times after an oral glucose load, and (d) give near zero readings for totally depancreatized animals.

C. Sources and Purification of ^{125}I-Glucagon

[125]I-Glucagon can readily be prepared using the technique of Greenwood *et al.* (1963) or it can be purchased from Nuclear Medical Laboratory (Dallas, Texas), New England Nuclear (Boston, Massachussetts), or Cambridge Nuclear (Billerica, Massachusetts). The specific activity is usually greater than 400 μCi/μg and minimal amounts of damaged glucagon and free ^{125}I are present initially.

Upon receipt, an aliquot of ^{125}I-glucagon is diluted for use in the immunoassay and the remainder is stored in 1.0-ml aliquots at $-20°C$ in glass tubes. The material is purified every two weeks by gel filtration.

Using the ^{125}I-glucagon from Nuclear Medical Laboratory, we have found that it is unnecessary to repurify the hormone. In the event that repurification should become necessary, the following method is employed. A 1.0-ml sample is loaded on a 0.9 × 52 cm Sephadex G25 column previously equilibrated with 0.2 M glycine, pH 8.8, containing 0.5% human albumin. After a 10-ml void volume, 1.0-ml fractions are collected in tubes containing 1000 U Trasylol. The peak tubes, usually numbers 6–9, are pooled and stored in 0.5-ml aliquots at $-20°C$. The glucagon concentration is calculated based on the assumption that 100% of the protein is eluted uniformly in the ^{125}I-glucagon peak of eluates. This assumption normally tends to slightly overestimate the concentration of ^{125}I-glucagon protein.

The integrity of the ^{125}I-glucagon is measured by electrophoresis using Toyo paper strips and by binding to an excess of glucagon antibodies. Electrophoresis is carried out for one hour at 720 V using 0.05 M sodium barbital buffer, pH 8.4. Radioactivity which migrates further than one inch from the zone of origin is considered to be damaged ^{125}I-glucagon.

In freshly purified preparations, only 1–4% damage is observed, and greater than 90% of the radioactivity is bound by an excess of glucagon antibodies. However, appreciable deterioration occurs after three to four weeks.

Other methods of purification include absorption and elution from cellulose (Lawrence, 1966); salting out, dissolving the salt cake in serum, and extracting with ethanol (Heding, 1971); and ion-exchange chromatography (Jørgensen and Larsen, 1972). Heding (1971) observed a remarkable stability of purified ^{125}I-glucagon stored in 80% ethanol.

D. Preparation of Standards

A desiccated sample of 2.5–5.0 mg of highly purified crystalline glucagon is weighed out and dissolved in 0.02 N HCl to exactly 0.50 mg/ml and then diluted to 10 μg/ml with assay diluent (0.2 M glycine, pH 8.8, containing 0.25% albumin and 1% normal sheep serum). The concentration of the 0.50 mg/ml solution in 0.02 N HCl should be checked by measuring its absorption at 278 nm. This should be 1.055 O.D. Subsequent volumetric dilutions of the 10 μg/ml solution are made with assay diluent to the desired concentrations of standards. Sets of standards for each assay system are stored up to three months at $-20°$C, and each set is thawed once and then discarded.

Most crystalline glucagon preparations contain about 10% mono-desamidoglucagon and trace amounts of didesamidoglucagon. The deamidation is believed to be random among the glutamine residues and is most probably an artifact of the extraction and purification procedures (Bromer et al., 1972).

E. Preparation of Plasma Samples

Blood samples are collected in glass tubes which contain 1.2 mg sodium EDTA and 500–1000 U of Trasylol for each milliliter of blood to be collected. Benzamidine at a final concentration of 0.03 M can be substituted for the Trasylol. The blood samples should be kept in an ice bath until the time of centrifugation, which is for 30 minutes at 2000 rpm at 4°C. The plasma is then transferred to glass test tubes and stored at $-20°$C. Storage for several months does not appear to be associated with any loss of glucagon immunoreactivity. However, repeated thawing and refreezing do seem to lead to a loss in immunoreactivity. At the time of assay, the samples are thawed and brought to room temperature, mixed by inverting several times, and centrifuged at 4°C for 15 minutes at 2000 rpm.

F. Radioimmunoassay Technique

1. Incubation Conditions

The conditions of incubation for the glucagon radioimmunoassay (total volume, temperature, duration, amount of tracer, amount of Trasylol, choice of diluent or buffer, and volume of plasma) used in this laboratory have been modified over the years in an effort to improve the sensitivity and reliability of the assay. We are currently using the following conditions.

a. Assay Diluent. All radioimmunoassay reagents are diluted with 0.2 M glycine, pH 8.8, containing 0.25% human albumin and 1% normal sheep serum. Both the albumin and sheep serum should be checked for proteolytic activity and glucagon content.

b. Trasylol (Aprotinin). This should be considered an essential reagent for the radioimmunoassay of glucagon and can be purchased from FBA Pharmaceuticals (New York). Trasylol (1000 U) should be added to each incubation tube and it can be added with the ^{125}I-glucagon to avoid additional pipetting. Occasionally, a larger amount of Trasylol is needed for plasma containing high levels of proteolytic activity, such as is found in some patients with pancreatitis.

c. Duration and Temperature of Incubation. All pipetting is performed at room temperature and all incubations are for four days at 4°C. We have found that efforts to decrease the incubation time result in loss of sensitivity of the assay. Most other assays allow at least four days to reach equilibrium (Luyckx, 1972; Assan *et al.*, 1967). Heding (1971) preincubates standards and samples with antiserum before the addition of tracer and reduces the incubation time to less than two days.

d. Typical Incubation Mixtures. The amounts of tracer and the dilution of antiserum are varied according to the desired sensitivity of the assay. In experiments in which a rise in glucagon is anticipated, the system contains 15 pg ^{125}I-glucagon, final (30K) antiserum dilution of 1 : 40,000, and 0.2 ml either standard or plasma. In experiments in which a suppression of glucagon is expected, the sensitivity of the assay is increased by decreasing the amount of tracer to 7.5 pg, increasing the 30K antiserum dilution to 1 : 60,000, and increasing the volume of plasma to 0.5 ml. Both systems include 1000 U of Trasylol, and the total volume of both incubation mixtures is 1.2 ml.

The assay for GLI uses the following system: 25 pg ^{125}I-glucagon, 0.05 ml of standard or plasma, and a final dilution of 78J antiserum of 1 : 1500 or MP-1 antiserum of 1 : 1000. The system uses 250 U Trasylol in a total volume of 0.3 ml.

Extra tubes of tracer or tracer plus Trasylol should be pipetted for all assays. These serve as counting standards or total count tubes and eliminate the need, after separation, to count both the free and bound tubes.

2. Separation Technique

As with most radioimmunoassays, there is a large variety of methods that can be used to separate free from antibody-bound glucagon, including cellulose powder (Nonaka and Foà, 1969) or ethanol precipitation (Heding, 1971). We use a modification of the dextran-coated charcoal technique introduced by Herbert *et al.* (1965). In our hands, it is relatively simple and at least as accurate and reproducible as other methods.

Equal volumes of a 1.0% activated charcoal (Norit A) and a 0.50% solution of dextran T-70, each in 0.2 M glycine, pH 8.8, are mixed at room temperature and stirred for at least 15 minutes prior to its addition to the incubation tube. In the more sensitive assay described above, 0.5 ml sheep serum is added to each of the tubes containing standards or diluted plasma, and 0.5 ml assay diluent is added to each unknown plasma tube in order to make the protein concentration nearly identical in all tubes before the addition of the charcoal–dextran mixture.

Under constant stirring, 0.5 ml of the charcoal–dextran mixture is added to each of the incubation tubes in a 4°C water bath. The tubes are mixed by shaking and incubated for 45 minutes at 4°C. The tubes are then centrifuged at 4°C for 15 minutes at 2000 rpm. The supernatants are aspirated with a Pasteur pipette, and the charcoal pellets containing the free hormone are counted. The coefficient of variation for the separation technique is <1%.

G. Results of Glucagon Radioimmunoassay

1. Sensitivity

The standard error or sensitivity of the method described is <1% bound calculated from typical standard curve data or from groups of

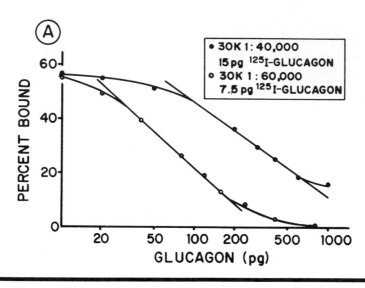

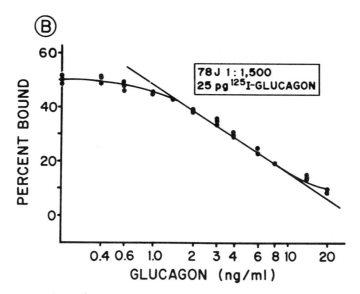

Figure 1. (A) and (B) Typical calibration curves in glucagon radioimmunoassays.

unknowns using antiserum 30K. This represents <5 pg/ml glucagon in the range where most values are read. The average coefficient of variation between triplicates is <1%. Typical standard curves are shown in Figure 1.

2. Circulating Glucagon Levels

Plasma concentrations of glucagon reported in the literature have varied widely, mainly because of the variable cross-reactivity of different antisera to extrapancreatic GLI. The downward trend over the years has resulted from the use of more specific antisera.

In a recent group of 59 normal human subjects, the plasma concentration of glucagon after an overnight fast ranged from 30 to 210 pg/ml and averaged 75 ± 4 (SEM) pg/ml using antiserum G-58. Pek and associates (1972) reported a mean concentration of 84 pg/ml in normal subjects. In their studies of 32 normals, Kuku and colleagues (1976a) noted an average fasting glucagon level of 113 ± 9 pg/ml.

Valverde and associates (1976) reported normal $(n = 10)$ plasma levels of each of the molecular forms of glucagon as: big plasma glucagon 113 ± 79 pg/ml, proglucagon 11 ± 16 pg/ml, authentic glucagon 31 ± 29 pg/ml, and small glucagon immunoreactive fraction 26 ± 18 pg/ml.

Elevated plasma glucagon levels have been reported in patients with hyperglycemic diabetes, chronic renal failure, and glucagonoma. However, the pattern of elevations of the molecular forms in these three clinical entities is quite different. In diabetes (mean levels 1525 ± 578 pg/ml) the authentic glucagon levels are increased, whereas in chronic renal failure (mean basal level 540 ± 40 pg/ml), the predominant elevation is in proglucagon (Kuku et al., 1976a,b). In a patient with a glucagonoma (total plasma glucagon 2600 pg/ml), Valverde et al. (1976) noted enormous elevations in both the 9000- and 3500-dalton molecules.

REFERENCES

Aguilar-Parada, E., Eisentraut, A. M., and Unger, R. H. (1969). Effects of starvation on plasma pancreatic glucagon in man. *Diabetes* **18**, 717–723.

Assan, R., Rosselin, G., Drouet, J., Dolais, J., and Tchobroutsky, G. (1965). Glucagon antibodies. *Lancet* **2**, 590–591.

Assan, R., Rosselin, G., and Dolais, J. (1967). Effets sur la glucagonémie des perfusions et ingestions d'acide amines. *In* "Journees annuelles de diabetologie de l'Hotel-Dieu," pp. 25–41. Medicales Flammarion, Paris.

Baetens, D., Rufener, C., Srikant, C. B., Dobbs, R. E., Unger, R. H., and Orci, L. (1976). Identification of glucagon-producing cells (A-cells) in dog gastric mucosa. *J. Cell Biol.* **69**, 455–464.

Berson, S. A., and Yalow, R. S. (1959). Recent studies on insulin-binding antibodies. *Ann. N.Y. Acad. Sci.* **82**, 388–444.

Blazquez, E., Muñoz-Barragan, L., Patton, G. S., Orci, L., Dobbs, R. E., and Unger, R. H. (1976). Gastric A cell function in insulin-deprived depancreatized dogs. *Endocrinology* **99**, 1182–1188.

Blazquez, E., Muñoz-Barragan, L., Patton, G. S., Dobbs, R. E., and Unger, R. H. (1977). Demonstration of gastric glucagon hypersecretion in insulin-deprived alloxan-diabetic dogs. *J. Lab. Clin. Med.* **89**, 971–977.

Bromer, W. W., Sinn, L., Behrens, O. K., and Staub, A. (1957). The amino acid sequence of glucagon. III. The hydrolysis of glucagon by trypsin. *J. Am. Chem. Soc.* **79**, 2801–2805.

Bromer, W. W., Boucher, M. E., and Koffenberger, J. E. (1971). Amino acid sequence of bovine glucagon. *J. Biol. Chem.* **246**, 2822–2827.

Bromer, W. W., Boucher, M. E., Patterson, J. M., Pekar, A. H., and Frank, B. H. (1972). Glucagon structure and function. I. Purification and properties of bovine glucagon and monodesimidoglucagon. *J. Biol. Chem.* **247**, 2581–2585.

Cuatrecasas, P., and Illiano, G. (1971). Production of anti-glucagon antibodies in poly-L-lysine "responder" guinea pigs. *Nature (London), New Biol.* **230**, 60–61.

Eisentraut, A. M., Whissen, N., and Unger, R. H. (1968). Incubation damage in the radioimmunoassay for human plasma glucagon and its prevention with "Trasylol." *Am. J. Med. Sci.* **255**, 137–142.

Ensinck, J. W., Shepard, C., Dudl, R. J., and William, R. H. (1972). Use of benzamidine as a protelytic inhibitor in the radioimmunoassay of glucagon in plasma. *J. Clin. Endocrinol. Metab.* **35**, 463–467.

Greenwood, F. C., Hunter, W. M., and Glover, J. S. (1963). The preparation of ^{131}I-labeled human growth hormone of high specific radioactivity. *Biochem. J.* **89**, 114–123.

Grey, N., McGuigan, J. E., and Kipnis, D. M. (1970). Neutralization of endogenous glucagon by high titer glucagon antiserum. *Endocrinology* **86**, 1383–1388.

Heding, L. G. (1971). Radioimmunological determination of pancreatic and gut glucagon in plasma. *Diabetologia* **7**, 10–19.

Heding, L. G. (1972). Immunologic properties of pancreatic glucagon: Antigenicity and antibody characteristics. *In* "Glucagon: Molecular Physiology, Clinical and Therapeutic Implications" (P. Lefebvre and R. H. Unger, eds.), Chapter 12, pp. 187–200. Pergamon, Oxford.

Herbert, V., Lau, K. S., Gottlieb, C. W., and Bleicher, S. J. (1965). Coated charcoal immunoassay of insulin. *J. Clin. Endocrinol. Metab.* **25**, 1375–1384.

Jørgensen, K. R., and Larsen, U. D. (1972). Purification of ^{125}I-glucagon by anion exchange chromatography. *Horm. Metab. Res.* **4**, 223–224.

Kuku, S. F., Jaspan, J. B., Emmanouel, D. S., Zeidler, A., Katz, A. I., and Rubenstein, A. H. (1976a). Heterogeneity of plasma glucagon. *J. Clin. Invest.* **58**, 742–750.

Kuku, S. F., Zeidler, A., Emmanouel, D. S., Katz, A. I., and Rubenstein, A. H. (1976b). Heterogeneity of plasma glucagon: Patterns in patients with chronic renal failure and diabetes. *J. Clin. Endocrinol. Metab.* **42**, 173–176.

Larsson, L. I., Holst, J., Hakanson, R., and Sundler, F. (1975). Distribution and properties of glucagon immunoreactivity in the digestive tract of various mammals: An immunohistochemical and immunochemical study. *Histochemistry* **44**, 281–290.

Lawrence, A. M. (1966). Radioimmunoassayable glucagon levels in man; effects of starvation, hypoglycemia, and glucose administration. *Proc. Natl. Acad. Sci. U.S.A.* **55**, 316–320.

Luyckx, A. (1972). Immunoassays for glucagon. *In* "Glucagon: Molecular Physiology, Clinical and Therapeutic Implications" (P. Lefebvre and R. H. Unger, eds.), Chapter 19, pp. 285–298. Pergamon, Oxford.

Mirsky, A., Perisutti, G., and Davis, N. C. (1959). The destruction of glucagon by the blood plasma from various species. *Endocrinology* **64**, 992–1001.

Muñoz-Barragan, L., Blazquez, E., Patton, G. S., Dobbs, R. E., and Unger, R. H. (1976). Gastric A cell function in normal dogs. *Am. J. Physiol.* **231**, 1057–1061.

Murlin, J. R., Clough, H. D., Gibbs, C. B. F., and Stokes, A. M. (1923). Aqueous extract of pancreas. I. Influence on the carbohydrate metabolism of depancreatized animals. *J. Biol. Chem.* **56**, 253–296.

Nonaka, K., and Foà, P. P. (1969). A simplified glucagon immunoassay and its use in a study of incubated pancreatic islets. *Proc. Soc. Exp. Biol. Med.* **130**, 330–336.

O'Connor, K. J., and Lazarus, N. R. (1976). The purification and biological properties of pancreatic big glucagon. *Biochem. J.* **156**, 265–277.

Orci, L., Pictet, R., Forssmann, W. G., Renold, A. E., and Rouiller, C. (1968). Structural evidence for glucagon producing cells in the intestinal mucosa of the rat. *Diabetologia* **4**, 56–67.

Pek, S., Fajans, S. S., Floyd, J. C., Knopf, R. F., and Conn, J. W. (1972). The role of glucagon in the worsening of the diabetic state by infection. *Diabetes* **21**, Suppl. 1, 324.

Polak, J. M., Bloom, S., Coulling, I., and Pearse, A. G. E. (1971). Immunofluorescent localization of enteroglucagon cells in the gastrointestinal tract of the dog. *Gut* **12**, 311–318.

Rigopoulou, D., Valverde, I., Marco, J., Faloona, G. R., and Unger, R. H. (1970). Large glucagon immunoreactivity in extracts of pancreas. *J. Biol. Chem.* **245**, 496–501.

Sasagawa, T., Kobayashi, S., and Fujita, T. (1974). Electron microscope studies on the endocrine cells of the human gut and pancreas. *In* "Gastro-Entero-Pancreatic Endocrine System. A Cell Biological Approach" (T. Fujita, ed.), pp. 17–38. Igaku Shoin, Ltd., Tokyo.

Sasaki, H., Rubalcava, B., Baetens, D., Blazquez, E., Srikant, C. B., Orci, L., and Unger, R. H. (1975). Identification of glucagon in the gastrointestinal tract. *J. Clin. Invest.* **56**, 135–145.

Staub, A., Sinn, L., and Behrens, O. K. (1953). Purification and crystallization of hyperglycemic glycogenolytic factor (HGF). *Science* **117**, 628–629.

Sundby, F., and Markussen, J. (1971). Isolation, crystallization, and amino acid composition of rat glucagon. *Horm. Metab. Res.* **3**, 184–187.

Sundby, F., and Markussen, J. (1972). Rabbit glucagon: Isolation, crystallization, and amino acid composition. *Horm. Metab. Res.* **4**, 56.

Thomsen, J., Kristiansen, K., and Brunfeldt, K. (1972). The amino acid sequence of human glucagon. *FEBS Lett.* **21**, 315–319.

Unger, R. H. (1976). Diabetes and the alpha cell. *Diabetes* **25**, 136–151.

Unger, R. H., and Eisentraut, A. M. (1967). Glucagon. *In* "Hormones in Blood" (C. H. Gray and A. L. Bacharach, eds.), 2nd ed., Chapter V, pp. 83–128. Academic Press, New York.

Unger, R. H., Eisentraut, A. M., McCall, M. S., Keller, S., Lanz, H. C., and Madison, L. L. (1959). Glucagon antibodies and their use for immunoassay of glucagon. *Proc. Soc. Exp. Biol. Med.* **102**, 621–623.

Unger, R. H., Eisentraut, A. M., and Madison, L. L. (1963). The effects of total starvation upon the levels of circulating glucagon and insulin in man. *J. Clin. Invest.* **42,** 1031–1039.

Unger, R. H., Raskin, P., Srikant, C. B., and Orci, L. (1977). Glucagon and the A cells. *Recent Prog. Horm. Res.* **33,** 477–517.

Valverde, I., Villanueva, M. L., Lozano, I., and Marco, J. (1974). Presence of glucagon immunoreactivity in the globulin fraction of human plasma ("Big Plasma Glucagon"). *J. Clin. Endocrinol. Metab.* **39,** 1020–1028.

Valverde, I., Dobbs, R. E., and Unger, R. H. (1975). Heterogeneity of plasma glucagon immunoreactivity in normal, depancreatized, and alloxan diabetic dogs. *Metab., Clin. Exp.* **24,** 1021–1028.

Valverde, I., Lemon, H. M., Kessinger, A., and Unger, R. H. (1976). Distribution of plasma glucagon immunoreactivity in a patient with a suspected glucagonoma. *J. Clin. Endocrinol. Metab.* **42,** 804–808.

33

Human Pancreatic Polypeptide (HPP) and Bovine Pancreatic Polypeptide (BPP)

RONALD E. CHANCE, NANCY E. MOON, AND
MELVIN G. JOHNSON

I. INTRODUCTION

Human pancreatic polypeptide (HPP) was isolated in our laboratory in 1970 as a side product from studies that were designed to isolate human proinsulin. We soon realized, however, that HPP is a homolog of avian pancreatic polypeptide (APP) (Kimmel *et al.*, 1968), and that both polypeptides are potential candidate hormones (Lin and Chance, 1974). At the same time, we also isolated bovine pancreatic polypeptide (BPP) while purifying insulin and glucagon (Chance and Jones, 1974) and subsequently determined that the amino acid se-

Methods of Hormone Radioimmunoassay, Second Edition
Copyright © 1979 by Academic Press, Inc.

Table I   Structure of HPP and Related Homologs[a]

	1	2	3	4	5	6	7	8	9
	Ala-	Pro-	Leu-	Glu-	Pro-	Val-	Tyr-	Pro-	Gly-
	10	11	12	13	14	15	16	17	18
	Asp-	Asn-	Ala-	Thr-	Pro-	Glu-	Gln-	Met-	Ala-
	19	20	21	22	23	24	25	26	27
	Gln-	Tyr-	Ala-	Ala-	Asp-	Leu-	Arg-	Arg-	Tyr-
	28	29	30	31	32	33	34	35	36
	Ile-	Asn-	Met-	Leu-	Thr-	Arg-	Pro-	Arg-	Tyr-NH$_2$

		Amino acid at position			
		2	6	11	23
Species differences compared to HPP					
Human	(HPP)	Pro	Val	Asn	Asp
Bovine	(BPP)		Glu		Glu
Ovine	(OPP)	Ser	Glu		Glu
Porcine	(PPP) ⎫				
Canine	(CPP) ⎭			Asp	Glu

[a] R. E. Chance, M. G. Johnson, J. A. Hoffmann, W. E. Jones, and J. E. Koffenberger, Jr. (unpublished data). Position 6 in BPP and OPP is Glu instead of Gln and position 11 is Asn instead of Asp as reported earlier (Floyd *et al.*, 1977).

quences of HPP and BPP, as well as several of the other mammalian polypeptide counterparts, are nearly identical (Table I). The primary structure of APP, on the other hand, differs from the mammalian polypeptides at more than half of the 36 positions (Kimmel *et al.*, 1975).

The physiologic function of this newly recognized hormone is unknown. Hazelwood *et al.* (1973) observed that APP is a powerful gastric stimulant when injected into chickens, and studies in our laboratory (Lin and Chance, 1972, 1974; Lin *et al.*, 1977) indicated that BPP has a wide spectrum of pharmacologic actions on the gastrointestinal tract, the most notable being suppression of cholecystokinin-induced pancreatic enzyme secretion in dogs.

The hormonal status of HPP and related homologs has been strengthened by numerous immunocytochemical studies using the BPP and HPP antisera described below in Section II,B. Larsson *et al.* (1975) noted that HPP cells are endocrinelike cells present in human pancreatic islets but distinct from A, B, and D cells. Further studies indicate that HPP cells occur in both the islet periphery and throughout the exocrine parenchyma (Gersell *et al.*, 1976; Heitz *et al.*, 1976; Larsson *et al.*, 1976a; Polak *et al.*, 1976; Bergstrom *et al.*, 1977; Gepts *et al.*, 1977; Pelletier and Leclerc, 1977).

The use of a sensitive radioimmunoassay for plasma HPP has

provided additional insights into the role of HPP in health and disease. Plasma HPP levels are significantly increased after a protein-rich meal (Floyd *et al.*, 1975, 1976, 1977; Adrian *et al.*, 1976, 1977; Schwartz *et al.*, 1976), and elevated plasma levels often occur in diabetics (Floyd *et al.*, 1976, 1977) and patients with islet cell tumors (Adrian *et al.*, 1976; Floyd *et al.*, 1976, 1977; Larsson *et al.*, 1976b).

A radioimmunoassay for APP has also been reported (Langslow *et al.*, 1973), and Kimmel and Pollock (1975) have noted that plasma APP levels respond dramatically to a protein meal. However, we will restrict our discussion to the mammalian hormones, since there is little if any cross-reactivity between the avian and mammalian polypeptide assays (Figure 1) (Langslow *et al.*, 1973). The purpose of this discussion is to describe the HPP radioimmunoassay as used in our laboratory and to mention pertinent modifications suggested to us by other investigators.

II. METHODS OF RADIOIMMUNOASSAY

A. Source of BPP and HPP

Both BPP and HPP are isolated from acid–alcohol extracts of pancreas using multiple gel filtration and ion-exchange chromatographic steps (Chance and Jones, 1974; R. E. Chance, M. G. Johnson, J. A. Hoffmann, W. E. Jones, and J. E. Koffenberger, Jr., unpublished data; Floyd *et al.*, 1977). Highly purified preparations of BPP and its porcine counterpart (PPP) are available upon request from the Lilly Research Laboratories, Indianapolis, Indiana, for use in animal or *in vitro* experiments only. Small amounts of HPP are available for radioimmunoassay standards as described below.

B. Immunization and Selection of Antibodies

Antibodies against BPP and HPP were raised in New Zealand white rabbits according to the following general schedule of injections. Each animal received a primary immunization consisting of 1.0 mg of immunogen dissolved in 0.6 ml distilled water and emulsified with 0.6 ml complete Freund's adjuvant (Difco Laboratories, Detroit, Michigan) and injected at different sites (0.3 ml in each hind footpad, 0.2 ml subcutaneously, 0.2 ml intramuscularly). A booster immunization was given one month later using 0.4 mg immunogen dissolved in 0.3 ml distilled water and emulsified with 0.3 ml incomplete Freund's adjuvant (Difco) and administered at multiple sites (0.1 ml in each hind footpad, 0.2 ml subcutaneously, and 0.2 ml intramuscularly). Similar booster immunizations were repeated at 6–12-month intervals.

The rabbits were bled at one- or two-week intervals following each booster immunization, and the antisera were titered using either the ethanol assay or the double antibody assay described in Section II,F. One of the four rabbits immunized with BPP developed a particularly high-titer antiserum two to six weeks after the first booster injection. These antisera (Lilly Lot Nos. 615-R110-146-5 and 615-R110-146-6) have been particularly useful for immunocytochemical studies and are also useful in radioimmunoassays at high dilution. When this rabbit was boosted one year later the antiserum collected at three weeks (Lilly Lot No. 615-R110-146-10) was found to be useful in the radioimmunoassay at a working dilution of 1 : 400,000 (50% binding).

The development of an acceptable HPP antiserum took longer, with only one of six animals responding with a good antiserum after either the second or third booster immunization. For example, the working dilutions necessary to bind 60% of the ^{125}I-HPP were as follows: (a) first booster (7–13 week bleedings) − 1 : 3000; (b) second booster (week 4 bleeding) − 1 : 80,000; (c) third booster (week 4 bleeding) − 1 : 120, 000; (d) fourth booster (2–4 week bleedings) − 1 : 70,000.

The antiserum collected after the third booster (Lilly Lot No. 615-1054B-249-19) is the main antiserum we and many other investigators use for the HPP radioimmunoassay. It is useful at working dilutions ranging from 1 : 50,000 to 1 : 200,000.

The antisera are stored at −20°C. To avoid repeated freezing and thawing we prepare several diluted aliquots (1 : 1000) of the main antisera using a phosphate–albumin buffer (0.04 M sodium phosphate, pH 7.4, 0.1% human serum albumin, 0.0242% Merthiolate). It is also a good practice to lyophilize several small aliquots of the most valuable antisera and store them in an alternate freezer to avoid catastrophic losses due to freezer malfunctions. Lyophilized samples are stable and can be shipped to other investigators without refrigeration. We routinely lyophilize 10 μl antiserum together with 1.0 mg human serum albumin. The albumin may not be necessary, but it serves as a convenient carrier protein and does not interfere in subsequent radioimmunoassays.

C. Radioiodination of BPP and HPP

We use a modification of the Hunter and Greenwood technique (1962) for radioiodinating BPP and HPP. A survey of fourteen other investigators conducting the HPP radioimmunoassay indicates that all are also using some variation of the chloramine-T labeling procedure, although each laboratory has evolved its own specific modification as a result of experience with other polypeptide hormones, such as gastrin, GIP, VIP, insulin, glucagon, etc. We use the following procedure in collaboration with Dr. Martha Bhatti of the Lilly radiolabeling laboratory. Freshly weighed BPP is dissolved in 0.25 M phosphate buffer, pH 7.5, and stored at $-20°C$ in plastic vials (5.0 μg in 100 μl per vial) and thawed just prior to labeling, which is conducted at 25°C in the plastic storage vial. One millicurie of ^{125}I-labeled sodium iodide (1.0–2.0 μl) is added followed by 10 μg of a fresh solution of chloramine-T dissolved in 20 μl 0.25 M phosphate buffer, pH 7.5. The reaction mixture is shaken gently for 15 seconds followed by the addition of 250 μl distilled water, 10 μg sodium metabisulfite in 20 μl water, and finally 250 μl of an albumin-containing buffer (0.05 M phosphate, pH 7.5, 0.1 M NaCl, 1% bovine serum albumin).

D. Purification and Characterization of Labeled Tracer

The freshly labeled BPP is immediately purified by gel filtration on a 0.9 × 50 cm column of Sephadex G-50 (superfine) equilibrated and run in phosphate–albumin buffer at 25°C. Fractions of about 0.5 ml are collected into glass tubes, and 10-μl aliquots are counted for one minute. A small radioactive peak is observed at the void volume ($\sim$12 ml). The peak of ^{125}I-BPP elutes at $\sim$25 ml, and the iodide peak elutes at $\sim$35 ml. The specific activity of the labeled hormone prepared under these conditions is $\sim$150 μCi/μg. We obtain the purified label from the ascending portion of the main peak, as we and others (e.g., Schwartz *et al.*, 1978) believe that better binding to the antisera is obtained when fractions ahead of the peak fraction are used in the assay. The appropriate fraction (usually two tubes prior to the peak) is diluted with a phosphate–albumin–Merthiolate buffer (0.04 M phosphate, pH 7.5, 0.1% human serum albumin, and 0.0242% Merthiolate) to give $\sim$3000 cpm per 0.1 ml and stored in aliquots at $-20°C$ and thawed only for use in the radioimmunoassay. We and other investigators have found the label to be stable at least four to six weeks.

Polyacrylamide gel electrophoresis (PAGE) is an additional purification step that can be used to separate unlabeled from labeled pancreatic polypeptide (BPP or HPP), thereby increasing the specific activity of the radioactive hormone preparation (Marco *et al.*, 1978). In most cases, however, this procedure is not necessary, since the Sephadex-purified preparation mentioned above usually provides sufficient assay sensitivity, particularly when used in conjunction with the disequilibrium incubation procedure (see Section II,F).

The PAGE purification procedure is also useful for determining the heterogeneity of the radioactive hormone preparation and has been used in our laboratory to characterize the iodinated products. In this procedure, $10\,\mu$Ci labeled PP (BPP or HPP) from the appropriate G-50 Sephadex fraction mentioned above is diluted with 2.0 ml 7 M urea (pH 3 with HCl) and used immediately or stored in 0.5-ml aliquots at $-20°C$. The electrophoretic separation is conducted essentially according to Davis (1964) using 10% acrylamide gels (6 × 55 mm) crosslinked with 0.1% bisacrylamide and polymerized in a pH 8.7 Tris–HCl buffer (0.38 M) with ammonium persulfate as the catalyst. Approximately 50 μl of the urea solution containing the labeled polypeptide is applied to each of several gels, and the electrophoresis is conducted for 15 minutes at 1.0 mA per gel, then 2.0 mA per gel for 105 minutes using a pH 8.4 Tris–borate buffer (0.05 M).

The resulting radioactive profiles for ^{125}I-BPP and ^{125}I-HPP, which are determined by counting 2.0-mm slices from one of the gels, are slightly different, since BPP has an approximate charge of minus one and HPP is essentially uncharged at pH 8.4. The main peak of ^{125}I-BPP has a R_f of about 0.5 as compared to 0.3 for ^{125}I-HPP. The labeled hormones are extracted from the appropriate gel slices using a phosphate–albumin–Merthiolate buffer (0.04 M phosphate, pH 7.5, 0.1% human serum albumin, and 0.0242% Merthiolate). Approximately 70% of the radioactivity is extracted after stirring for 3 hours at 4°C in sufficient buffer to give ~3000 cpm per 0.1 ml. Aliquot fractions are stored up to six weeks at $-20°C$ and thawed only prior to use in the assay.

In addition to the main peak mentioned above, we often find other minor radioactive peaks along with some presumably free iodide in the anodic electrode buffer (1.0–10% of the total depending upon age of preparation). These peaks presumably are various iodinated isomers. For example, the labeled BPP preparation usually contains a minor component immediately cathodic to the major ^{125}I-BPP peak. We resolve these two peaks by using longer gels (80 mm) and a longer electrophoresis time (1.0 mA per gel for 15 minutes followed by 2.0 mA for 180 minutes). In studies designed to characterize each peak, we found by use of tryptic peptides that the minor peak was probably monoiodinated BPP labeled at Tyr^{27} and that the major peak was diiodinated BPP labeled at Tyr^{36}-NH$_2$. These conclusions were reached by comparing the R_f's of BPP (0.55), monodesamido-BPP (0.76), the minor peak (0.60), and the major peak (0.73) and assuming a full negative charge for a diiodinated tyrosine. Our preliminary studies indicate that the diiodinated BPP labeled at Tyr^{36}-NH_2 works better in the radioimmunoassay than the monoiodinated BPP labeled at Tyr^{27}. A similar observation was made by J. R. Kimmel (personal communication) using ^{125}I-labeled avian pancreatic polypeptide (APP) in an APP radioimmunoassay.

E. Preparation and Storage of Standards

1. HPP

Standard samples of HPP are prepared from a highly purified HPP preparation (Lilly Lot No. 615-1054B-200). Approximately 0.3 mg is dissolved in 1.0 ml 0.3 M acetic acid, and the protein concentration is determined by optical density measurements at 276 nm ($E_{1cm}^{0.1\%}$ = 1.42). Appropriate serial dilutions are made from an aliquot of this primary stock solution using a pH 7.4 phosphate buffer described by Heding (1971) (0.04 M sodium phosphate, 0.1 M NaCl, 0.1% human scrim albumin, and 0.0242% Merthiolate). These HPP standards ranging from 1.0 pg/ml to 0.1 μg/ml appear to be quite stable, as we have stored them at 4°C for as long as two years without noticeable loss in immunopotency. They can also be stored at −20°C, but should not be frozen and thawed more than once. We recommend that several sets of the various HPP standard concentrations be pipetted into assay tubes (0.1 ml per tube) in advance of the assay and stored at either 4° or −20°C.

The remainder of the primary HPP stock solution is divided into 1.0-μg aliquots and lyophilized with 1.0 mg human serum albumin per aliquot to prevent HPP absorption to glass. Each batch of lyophilized standards is assayed repeatedly to establish the immunopotency relative to the primary standard, since apparently some loss (10–20%) occurs during the lyophilization step.

2. BPP

Stock solutions of highly purified BPP (Lilly Lot No. 615-D63-166-1) are prepared essentially as described for HPP above except that the extinction coefficient ($E_{1cm}^{0.1\%}$) at 276 nm is 1.41. The primary HPP and BPP standards prepared in this manner are often used in the same assay to monitor assay consistency. See Section III for a comparison of HPP and BPP standards in both homologous and heterologous assays.

F. Incubation and Separation Procedures

We use two different assay methods that are based on different procedures for separating antibody-bound and free hormone. The ethanol separation method (Heding, 1971), as the name implies, involves precipitation of the antibody–antigen complex with ethanol. This assay is used to determine relative antibody titers, integrity of labeled antigen, and hormone concentrations in pancreatic tissue extracts. The double antibody separation method (Morgan and Lazarow, 1963) involves precipitation of the antibody–antigen complex with a second antibody. This assay is used to determine serum or plasma levels of HPP, since it gives less nonspecific binding of labeled antigen.

1. Ethanol Assay

Each assay tube contains a final volume of 0.3 ml consisting of the following components: (a) 0.1 ml standard or test sample, (b) 0.1 ml diluted antiserum, and (c) 0.1 ml labeled antigen. After an appropriate incubation period as discussed below, 1.6 ml 96% ethanol is added and the precipitated antibody–antigen complex is collected by centrifugation. Following are many of the specific details of this assay procedure. The standard or test sample is contained in a pH 7.4 phosphate buffer (0.04 M sodium phosphate, 0.1 M NaCl, 0.1% human serum albumin, 0.0242% Merthiolate), and the antiserum is diluted to a predetermined concentration with the same buffer. For example, the anti-HPP serum (Lilly Lot No. 615-1054B-248-19) used in a homologous HPP assay illustrated in Figure 1 was used at a working dilution of 1 : 70,000. Thus, the final dilution was 1 : 210,000. A similar displacement curve was obtained in a homologous BPP assay using anti-BPP serum (Lilly Lot No. 615-R110-146-10) at a working dilution of 1 : 300,000. The labeled antigen, ^{125}I-BPP or ^{125}I-HPP, is used in a pH 7.4 phosphate buffer that lacks NaCl (see Section II,D). The approximate amount of radioactivity in this solution is 3000 cpm per 0.1 ml.

All three components of the assay can be incubated simultaneously (equilibrium assay), or the labeled antigen can be added at some time after the antigen–antibody complex has formed (disequilibrium assay). In the equilibrium type of assay, we obtain optimal results by incubating for three to five days at 4°C, although similar results are obtained with a shorter incubation period (two to three hours at 37°C followed by 16 hours at 4°C). This shorter incubation is satisfactory for determining cross-reaction among various species of the hormone, approximate antibody titers of new antisera, and the integrity of the labeled hormone preparation; it is not recommended when the test sample

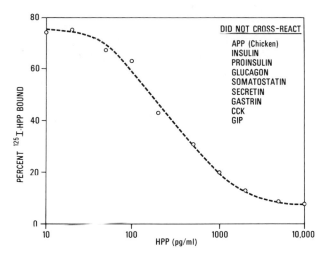

Figure 1. Standard curve for highly purified HPP (Lilly Lot No. 615-1054B-200) obtained in a homologous HPP assay under equilibrium incubation conditions (four days at 4°C) using the ethanol separation method (see Section II,F) and a final dilution of rabbit anti-HPP serum (Lilly Lot No. 615-1054B-248-19) of 1 : 210,000. Each point on the curve is an average of three assay tubes. A comparable curve was obtained in the double antibody assay in which the final dilution of antiserum was 1 : 400,000. A similar curve was also obtained in a homologous BPP assay under equilibrium assay conditions as above using highly purified BPP, ^{125}I-BPP, and rabbit anti-BPP serum (Lilly Lot No. 615-R110-146-10) at a final dilution of 1 : 900,000 for the ethanol assay and 1 : 3,000,000 for the double antibody assay. The following hormones did not cross-react in these assays when tested at the following concentrations: APP, 0.1 μg/ml; insulin, 0.1 μg/ml; proinsulin, 100 μg/ml; glucagon, 0.1 μg/ml; somatostatin, 100 μg/ml; secretin, 19 μg/ml; gastrin, 4 μg/ml; CCK, 38 μg/ml; GIP, 10 μg/ml; and VIP, 100 μg/ml.

contains potential enzymes that might degrade the labeled hormone. The displacement curve illustrated in Figure 1 resulted from an equilibrium assay incubated at 4°C for 4 days.

The assay sensitivity can be increased by use of a disequilibrium assay (Gingerich *et al.,* 1978). In this procedure we incubate the test sample and antiserum for three to five days at 4°C followed by the addition of the labeled hormone for an additional 16–24 hours at 4°C. The antibody-bound hormone is precipitated by the addition of 1.6 ml 96% ethanol to each tube. After standing at 25°C for ten minutes, the tubes are centrifuged 20 minutes at 2000 rpm at 4°C. Both the supernatant and precipitate are counted for five minutes, and the percent of labeled hormone bound by the antibody is calculated and plotted as in Figure 1. Nonspecific binding in this assay is about 8–10%.

Two assay controls that do not contain test sample are included in the assay. One control has the standard dilution of antiserum (i.e., 1 : 70,000 if anti-HPP serum as above) and the other has a lesser dilution of antiserum (1 : 1000). The percent of labeled hormone bound by the higher antibody concentration is usually >95% when the labeled hormone is purified by both gel filtration and polyacrylamide gel electrophoresis (see Section II,D). On the other hand, the percent binding is usually about 90% when the labeled hormone is purified only by gel filtration. When the binding falls below 80%, the labeled hormone is usually less effective and a new preparation is needed.

2. Double Antibody Assay

Each assay tube contains a total volume of 1.0 ml consisting of the following components: (a) 0.1 ml standard (see Section II,E,1) plus 0.7 ml of the pH 7.4 phosphate buffer with NaCl (0.04 M sodium phosphate, 0.10 M NaCl, 0.1% human serum albumin, 0.0242% Merthiolate) or 0.8 ml plasma or serum diluted at least 1 : 4 in the same buffer; (b) 0.1 ml diluted antiserum (see Section II,B) contained in the above phosphate buffer without NaCl; and (c) 0.1 ml labeled antigen (3000 cpm) diluted with the phosphate buffer without NaCl (see Section II,D). As in the ethanol assay above, either an equilibrium or a disequilibrium incubation procedure can be used. However, better sensitivity is achieved by the disequilibrium method, which involves incubation of test sample and antibody for three to five days at 4°C followed by the addition of the labeled antigen for an extra day at 4°C. In the equilibrium method, all three components are incubated together for three to five days at 4°C. A displacement curve similar to the one shown in Figure 1 was obtained in our studies using an equilibrium assay (four days at 4°C) and the anti-HPP serum (Lilly Lot No. 615-1054B-248-19) at a working dilution of 1 : 40,000 or a final dilution of 1 : 400,000. Several investigators have used this antiserum in similar assay systems at final dilutions ranging from 1 : 400,000 to 1 : 2,000,000, depending upon the sensitivity required. Increased assay sensitivity can be achieved with the higher antibody dilution. Also, as mentioned above, the assay sensitivity can be increased by use of the disequilibrium incubation method. The working dilution for the anti-BPP serum (Lilly Lot No. 615-1054B-146-10) in this assay system is 1 : 300,000 to give a displacement curve similar to Figure 1 for a homologous BPP assay. However, this antiserum is essentially untested for use in assaying HPP in human plasma.

The antibody-bound hormone is precipitated by addition of goat anti-rabbit γ-globulin (Antibodies, Inc., Davis, California). We add 0.2 ml normal rabbit serum (diluted 1 : 50 with the phosphate buffer without NaCl) and 0.2 ml goat anti-rabbit γ-globulin serum (diluted 1 : 10 with the phosphate buffer without NaCl) and incubate one to two days at 4°C, although the precipitation is nearly complete after eight hours. The precipitate is collected by centrifugation, and both the precipitate and supernatant are counted for five minutes. The percent of labeled hormone bound by the antibody is calculated and plotted as in Figure 1. The same assay controls described for the ethanol assay are used in the double antibody assay also.

Normal fasting plasma (or serum) levels of HPP determined by this procedure appear to be ~50 pg/ml for young adults, a level which agrees with the results of Floyd *et al.* (1977). These investigators also use a double antibody assay with a pH 8.6 barbital buffer (J. C. Floyd, Jr., personal communication). They also observed that fasting plasma HPP levels increase significantly with age (Floyd *et al.*, 1977). Quantitative plasma HPP determinations may differ slightly from laboratory to laboratory, depending upon whether homologous or heterologous assays are employed (see Section III).

III. HOMOLOGOUS AND HETEROLOGOUS ASSAYS

Ideally, each species of pancreatic polypeptide (PP) would be determined with a homologous assay, but this is often not practical or even possible due to insufficient hormone reagents. In the case of HPP, we initially supplied a few investigators with anti-HPP serum and highly purified HPP for both radiolabeling and standards (see Floyd *et al.*, 1977; Adrian *et al.*, 1976). However, the popularity of this assay grew rapidly, and we soon realized that our supply of highly purified HPP (Lilly Lot No. 615-1054B-200) would not suffice for both radiolabeling and standards. Therefore, we have encouraged the use of BPP for the labeled tracer in conjunction with the HPP antiserum and HPP standards in a heterologous-type assay. Generally, the heterologous HPP assay has been satisfactory, although there may be some sacrifice in assay sensitivity; also, basal plasma HPP levels may be slightly higher by this type of assay (J. C. Floyd, Jr., personal communication; A. I. Vinik, personal communication). However, the decreased sensitivity can be overcome by using the disequilibrium incubation procedure.

Another type of heterologous assay that may be a promising alternative for assaying plasma HPP involves the use of anti-BPP serum, ^{125}I-BPP, and HPP standards. Both Schwartz *et al.* (1978) and G. Boden (personal communication) report excellent results with such an assay.

We have not examined all the various combinations and permutations of reagents available for the five mammalian PP's listed in Table I. However, we have conducted numerous studies with both HPP and BPP antisera, and have obtained the following results. In a homologous HPP assay such as illustrated in Figure 1, the cross-reactivity of each of the other four mammalian PP's (BPP, CPP, OPP, PPP) was about 70% of the HPP standard. On the other hand, in a heterologous HPP assay in which ^{125}I-BPP was used, CPP, HPP, and PPP all cross-reacted about 70% as well as BPP. Although the OPP was not tested, we would expect it to behave like BPP due to the structural similarity between the two molecules (Table I). All of these comparisons were made with PP sample solutions that were assigned concentrations on the basis of optical density measurements (see Section II,E). In a homologous BPP assay, we have observed that CPP, HPP, and PPP all cross-react approximately ~50% as well as BPP. G. Boden (personal communication) has similarly noted the same degree of cross-reactivity with HPP and PPP using the homologous BPP assay. Thus, for accurate results, it is important to include the proper PP standard for each species.

Although the assays mentioned above have been used successfully to determine plasma and serum levels of HPP and CPP, they have not been very helpful in measuring the pancreatic polypeptide counterpart hormone in rats and mice (Y. C. Patel, personal communication; T. W. Schwartz, personal communication; N. S. Track, personal communication). Our studies with rat pancreatic extracts suggest that the failure to measure rat PP conclusively in the plasma may be due to a low degree of cross-reactivity in these assays, possibly due to a significantly different amino acid sequence.

The cross-reactivity of several other polypeptide hormones was examined in both the BPP and HPP assays (see legend of Figure 1). No reactivity was detected with avian pancreatic polypeptide (APP), porcine insulin, porcine proinsulin, porcine glucagon, synthetic ovine somatostatin, porcine secretin, porcine gastrin, porcine cholecystokinin (CCK), gastric inhibitory polypeptide (GIP), and porcine vasoactive intestinal polypeptide (VIP). These studies were confirmed by Schwartz *et al.* (1978). Adrian *et al.* (1976) extended this list to include porcine motilin, which also did not cross-react in the HPP radioimmunoassay.

IV. ALTERNATE METHODS

The radioimmunoassay for HPP is still relatively new, and although it appears to work well under the conditions outlined above, assays can always be improved in terms of sensitivity and reliability. The procedures outlined above were essentially adapted from assays operational in our laboratory for insulin and related substances. Similarly, other investigators have used these PP reagents in their own existing assays with excellent results. Undoubtedly, the HPP assay could be patterned after any of a number of polypeptide hormone assays described in other chapters throughout this volume. For example, Villanueva *et al.* (1977) and T. M. O'Dorisio (personal communication) use the pH 8.8 glycine buffer that was originally designed for use in the glucagon radioimmunoassay (Faloona and Unger, 1974). Many investigators use essentially the conditions for the gastrin assay, namely, a pH 8.6 barbital buffer (Schwartz *et al.*, 1978; J. H. Walsh, personal communication), similar to that described by Jaffe and Walsh (1974).

HPP and BPP are easily labeled with the conventional chloramine-T procedure. Here again, there appears to be considerable flexibility in the conditions used, since a survey of 14 laboratories indicated that successful labeling was achieved using 0.5 to 5.0 μg of hormone and chloramine-T levels ranging from <1.0 to 20 μg. Likewise, reaction times ranged from 15 seconds to three minutes. Purification of the labeled hormone is most often by molecular sieve chromatography on columns of Sephadex G-50 (superfine). However, T. M. O'Dorisio (personal communication) successfully purified ^{125}I-BPP on a fibrocellulose column, and D. J. Byrnes (personal communication) used carboxymethyl-Sephadex chromatography as used for purifying ^{125}I-secretin (Byrnes and Marjason, 1976). The QAE–Sephadex method for purifying ^{125}I-glucagon (Jørgensen and Larsen, 1972) is used successfully by S. S. Schwartz (personal communication) and by K. H. Gabbay (personal communication) to purify ^{125}I-BPP. Villanueva *et al.* (1977) use either Bio-Gel P-30 or Sephadex G-100 molecular sieve chromatography.

The most popular procedure for separating antibody-bound HPP is the double antibody method, as it is usually the most specific (A. H. Rubenstein, personal communication) and gives the lowest nonspecific binding. The dextran–charcoal method (Schwartz *et al.*, 1976, 1978) is also used frequently, as is a polyethylene glycol (PEG) method (N. S. Track, personal communication; A. I. Vinik, personal communication). This latter investigator found that the PEG procedure works better with our pH 7.4 phosphate buffer assay than with a pH 8.6 barbital buffer assay.

Plasma (or serum) HPP is remarkably stable, thus eliminating the need for a broad-spectrum protease inhibitor such as Trasylol (J. C. Floyd, Jr., personal communication), although it should be noted that

Villaneuva *et al.* (1977) observed heterogeneous HPP immunoreactivity in plasma. Also, it should be mentioned that plasma obtained from patients who have received insulin may have antibodies against BPP and/or PPP (Bloom *et al.*, 1976; Floyd *et al.*, 1977). Such antibodies may contribute to false high plasma HPP levels. Undoubtedly, there will be additional problems of this type to be considered as investigators gain experience with the HPP radioimmunoassay in studying the role of this newly recognized hormone in health and disease.

ACKNOWLEDGMENTS

We thank Mrs. Lillian Witter for typing assistance and Drs. W. W. Bromer and Mary A. Root of the Lilly Research Laboratories for helpful suggestions on the development of the radioimmunoassays. We also thank the following investigators for sharing unpublished results and valuable suggestions: Drs. S. Bloom, G. Boden, D. Byrne, J. Floyd, K. Gabbay, R. Gingerich, B. Gonen, J. Hansky, J. Kimmel, G. Lundqvist, J. Marco, T. O'Dorisio, Y. Patel, A. Rubenstein, T. Schwartz, S. Schwartz, I. Taylor, N. Track, A. Vinik, and J. Walsh.

REFERENCES

Adrian, T. E., Bloom, S. R., Bryant, M. G., Polak, J. M., Heitz, P., and Barnes, A. J. (1976). Distribution and release of human pancreatic polypeptide. *Gut* **17**, 940–944.
Adrian, T. E., Bloom, S. R., Besterman, H. S., Barnes, A. J., Cooke, T. J. C., Russell, R. C. G., and Faber, R. G. (1977). Mechanism of pancreatic polypeptide release in man. *Lancet* **1**, 161–163.
Bergstrom, B. H., Loo, S., Hirsch, H. J., Schutzengel, D., and Gabbay, K. H. (1977). Ultrastructural localization of pancreatic polypeptide in human pancreas. *J. Clin. Endocrinol. Metab.* **44**, 795–798.
Bloom, S. R., Adrian, T. E., Mitchell, S. J., Barnes, A. J., and Kohner, E. M. (1976). Dirty insulin, a stimulant to autoimmunity. *Diabetologia* **12**, 381 (abstr.).
Byrnes, D. J., and Marjason, J. P. (1976). Radioimmunoassay of secretin in plasma. *Horm. Metab. Res.* **8**, 361–365.
Chance, R. E., and Jones, W. E. (1974). Polypeptides from bovine, ovine, human, and porcine pancreas. U.S. Patent 3,842,063.
Davis, B. J. (1964). Disc electrophoresis. II. Method and application to human serum proteins. *Ann. N.Y. Acad. Sci.* **121**, 404–427.
Faloona, G. R., and Unger, R. H. (1974). Glucagon. *In* "Methods of Hormone Radioimmunoassay" (B. M. Jaffe and H. R. Behrman, eds.), pp. 317–330. Academic Press, New York.
Floyd, J. C., Jr., Chance, R. E., Hayashi, M., Moon, N. E., and Fajans, S. S. (1975). Concentrations of a newly recognized pancreatic islet polypeptide in plasma of healthy subjects and in plasma and tumors of patients with insulin-secreting islet-cell tumors. *Clin. Res.* **23**, 535A.
Floyd, J. C., Jr., Fajans, S. S., and Pek, S. (1976). Regulation in healthy subjects of the secretion of human pancreatic polypeptide, a newly recognized pancreatic islet polypeptide. *Trans. Assoc. Am. Physicians* **89**, 146–158.

Floyd, J. C., Jr., Fajans, S. S., Pek, S., and Chance, R. E. (1977). A newly recognized pancreatic polypeptide; plasma levels in health and disease. *Recent Prog. Horm. Res.* 33, 519–570.

Gepts, W., DeMey, J., and Marichal-Pipeleers, M. (1977). Hyperplasia of "pancreatic polypeptide"—cells in the pancreas of juvenile diabetics. *Diabetologia* 13, 27–34.

Gersell, D. J., Greider, M. H., and Gingerich, R. L. (1976). Cellular localization of pancreatic polypeptide in the human and canine pancreas. *Diabetes* 25, Suppl. 1, 364.

Gingerich, R. L., Lacy, P. E., Chance, R. E., and Johnson, M. G. (1978). Regional pancreatic concentration and *in vitro* secretion of canine pancreatic polypeptide, insulin and glucagon. *Diabetes* 27, 96–101.

Hazelwood, R. L., Turner, S. D., Kimmel, J. R., and Pollock, H. G. (1973). Spectrum effects of a new polypeptide (third hormone?) isolated from the chicken pancreas. *Gen. Comp. Endocrinol.* 21, 485–497.

Heding, L. G. (1971). Radioimmunological determination of pancreatic and gut glucagon in plasma. *Diabetologia* 7, 10–19.

Heitz, P., Polak, J. M., Bloom, S. R., and Pearse, A. G. E. (1976). Identification of the D₁-cell as the source of human pancreatic polypeptide (HPP). *Gut* 17, 755–758.

Hunter, W. M., and Greenwood, F. C. (1962). Preparation of iodine-131 human growth hormone of high specific activity. *Nature (London)* 194, 495–496.

Jaffe, B. M., and Walsh, J. H. (1974). Gastrin and related peptides. *In* "Methods of Hormone Radioimmunoassay" (B. M. Jaffe and H. R. Behrman, eds.), pp. 251–273. Academic Press, New York.

Jørgensen, K. H., and Larsen, U. D. (1972). Purification of ¹²⁵I-glucagon by anion exchange chromatography. *Horm. Metab. Res.* 4, 223–224.

Kimmel, J. R., and Pollock, H. G. (1975). Factors affecting blood levels of avian pancreatic polypeptide (APP), a new pancreatic hormone. *Fed. Proc., Fed. Am. Soc. Exp. Biol.* 34, 454.

Kimmel, J. R., Pollock, H. G., and Hazelwood, R. L. (1968). Isolation and characterization of chicken insulin. *Endocrinology* 83, 1323–1330.

Kimmel, J. R., Hayden, L. J., and Pollock, H. G. (1975). Isolation and characterization of a new pancreatic polypeptide hormone. *J. Biol. Chem.* 250, 9369–9376.

Langslow, D. R., Kimmel, J. R., and Pollock, H. G. (1973). Studies of the distribution of a new avian pancreatic polypeptide and insulin among birds, reptiles, amphibians and mammals. *Endocrinology* 93, 558–565.

Larsson, L.-I., Sundler, F., and Håkanson, R. (1975). Immunohistochemical localization of human pancreatic polypeptide (HPP) to a population of islet cells. *Cell Tissue Res.* 156, 167–171.

Larsson, L.-I., Sundler, F., and Håkanson, R. (1976a). Pancreatic polypeptide—a postulated new hormone: Identification of its cellular storage site by light and electron microscopic immunocytochemistry. *Diabetologia* 12, 211–226.

Larsson, L.-I., Schwartz, T., Lundqvist, G., Chance, R. E., Sundler, F., Rehfeld, J. F., Grimelius, L., Fahrenkrug, J., Schaffalitzky de Muckadell, O., and Moon, N. (1976b). Occurrence of human pancreatic polypeptide in pancreatic endocrine tumors. *Am. J. Pathol.* 85, 675–684.

Lin, T.-M., and Chance, R. E. (1972). Spectrum gastrointestinal actions of a new bovine pancreas polypeptide (BPP). *Gastroenterology* 62, 852.

Lin, T.-M., and Chance, R. E. (1974). Bovine pancreatic polypeptide (BPP) and avian pancreatic polypeptide (APP). *Gastroenterology* 67, 737–738.

Lin, T.-M., Evans, D. C., Chance, R. E., and Spray, G. F. (1977). Bovine pancreatic peptide: Action on gastric and pancreatic secretion in dogs. *Am. J. Physiol.* **232,** E311-E315 or *Am. J. Physiol.: Endocrinol. Metab. Gastrointest. Physiol.* **1,** E311-E315.

Marco, J., Hedo, J. A., and Villanueva, M. L. (1978). Control of pancreatic polypeptide secretion by glucose in man. *J. Clin. Endocrinol. Metab.* **46,** 140–145.

Morgan, C. R., and Lazarow, A. (1963). Immunoassay of insulin: Two antibody system. Plasma insulin levels of normal, subdiabetic and diabetic rats. *Diabetes* **12,** 115–126.

Pelletier, G., and Leclerc, R. (1977). Immunohistochemical localization of human pancreatic polypeptide (HPP) in the human endocrine pancreas. *Gastroenterology* **72,** 569–571.

Polak, J. M., Bloom, S. R., Adrian, T. E., Heitz, P., Bryant, M. G., and Pearse, A. G. E. (1976). Pancreatic polypeptide in insulinomas, gastrinomas, vipomas, and glucagonomas. *Lancet* **1,** 328–330.

Schwartz, T. W., Rehfeld, J. F., Stadil, F., Larsson, L.-I., Chance, R. E., and Moon, N. (1976). Pancreatic-polypeptide response to food in duodenal-ulcer patients before and after vagotomy. *Lancet* **1,** 1102–1105.

Schwartz, T. W., Holst, J. J., Fahrenkrug, J., Jensen, S. L., Nielsen, O. V., Rehfeld, J. F., Schaffalitzky de Muckadell, O. B., and Stadil, F. (1978). Vagal, cholinergic regulation of pancreatic polypeptide secretion. *J. Clin. Invest.* **61,** 781–789.

Villanueva, M. L., Hedo, J. A., and Marco, J. (1977). Heterogeneity of pancreatic polypeptide immunoreactivity in human plasma. *FEBS Lett.* **80,** 99–102.

STEROID HORMONES

34

Plasma Estradiol, Estrone, Estriol, and Urinary Estriol Glucuronide

RAY HANING, GAYLE P. ORCZYK, BURTON V. CALDWELL, AND HAROLD R. BEHRMAN

I. PLASMA ESTRADIOL, ESTRONE, AND ESTRIOL

A. Introduction

A radioimmunoassay for estrogen, as well as other steroid hormones, has depended primarily upon the availability of methods for preparing steroid–protein conjugates which, when injected into the host, would result in the production of steroid-specific antibodies. Over the past 20 years, most studies concerning the covalent linking of low molecular weight, nonimmunogenic compounds (e.g., estrogen) to an antigen

675

Methods of Hormone Radioimmunoassay, Second Edition

(e.g., bovine serum albumin) have been carried out by two research groups. Both were successful in preparing conjugates that elicit steroid-specific antibodies (Lieberman *et al.*, 1959; Goodfriend and Sehon, 1970).

Among the earliest estrogen radioimmunoassay procedures published were the solid-phase method of Abraham (1969), the double antibody assay of Niswender and Midgley (1970; see also Midgley *et al.*, 1969), the method of Jiang and Ryan (1969), in which separation of free and bound hormone was accomplished either by ammonium sulfate, Dowex-1 resin, or dextran-coated charcoal, and the method of Mikhail *et al.* (1970), in which polymerized estrogen antibodies were used.

Recently, the production of highly specific antisera has permitted assay of estradiol without prior chromatographic isolation of the hormone (England *et al.*, 1974; Korenman *et al.*, 1974) and, in one case, without extraction from the plasma as well (Jurjens *et al.*, 1975). Purification procedures are still required for radioimmunoassay of estrogens other than estradiol, and these procedures have also been improved in terms of convenience and efficiency (Kushinsky and Anderson, 1974; Carstensen and Bäckström, 1976). Modifications of the original estrogen radioimmunoassay include separation of bound from free steroid by gel filtration (Franek and Hruska, 1976) or polyethylene glycol (Schiller and Brammall, 1974) and the use of ^{125}I-estrogen as a radioligand (Lindberg and Edqvist, 1974; Barnard *et al.*, 1975). Such modifications have led to the establishment of a more rapid, inexpensive, and sensitive radioimmunoassay.

The estrogen radioimmunoassay to be described herein is based on the methods described by Hotchkiss *et al.* (1971) and Behrman *et al.* (1971) in which dextran-coated charcoal is employed for separation of antibody-bound from free steroid. Tritiated estradiol is used as the radioligand, and the three estrogens that are measured (estrone, estradiol, and estriol) are isolated by column chromatography on Sephadex LH-20.

B. Previous Assay Methods

Biologic assay for estrogens include that described by Allen and Doisey (1923), a procedure which depends on alterations in the appearance of the vaginal smear of the castrate mouse, and that of Astwood (1938), an assay which depends on the increase in uterine weight of immature rats. Estrogen can be quantified by gas–liquid chromatography, by colorimetric or fluorometric determination, or indirectly by measuring the rate of reaction of certain estrogen-sensitive enzymes (see O'Donnell and Preedy, 1967, for review). A double isotope derivative method for estrogen measurement has also been developed (Svendsen and Sorensen, 1964; Baird and Guevara, 1969). The best sensitivity (low nanogram range) can be achieved by using fluorometry or the double isotope derivative method; the lower limits of other methods are 0.2–0.3 μg. All of the above methods have been limited by their lack of sensitivity and the necessity for extensive purification of the samples prior to quantitation.

Competitive protein-binding assays of estrogen have been carried out using a preparation of receptor protein present in the supernatant fraction of homogenized uteri of certain animals (Corker *et al.*, 1970; Korenman *et al.*, 1970). Using rabbit uterine cytosol, Corker *et al.* (1970) have measured plasma estradiol-17β during the normal menstrual cycle and have reported values similar to those obtained by radioimmunoassay or the double isotope derivative method. Both the protein-binding and radioimmunoassay methods are far more sensitive than any of those techniques previously mentioned and, thus, provide sufficient sensitivity to measure the low picogram quantities of estrogen that are present in samples of two to three milliliters of plasma.

Although both the binding protein and the antiserum used for estrogen determinations are highly specific for estrogen, some preliminary isolation is necessary when either method is used for individual evaluation of estrone, estradiol, and estriol levels. Therefore, neither method is superior in terms of rapidity or ease in measuring the three classic estrogens. However, unlike uterine cytosol preparations, estrogen antiserum does not bind synthetic estrogen. Hence, endogenous estrogen levels of patients receiving synthetic estrogen treatment can easily be measured by radioimmunoassay. Another advantage to measuring estrogen by radioimmunoassay is the stability of the antiserum and the ease with which it can be obtained. The antiserum can be purchased from the following suppliers: Calbiochem, San Diego, California; New England Nuclear Biomedical Assay Laboratories, Worcester, Massachusetts; and Research Plus Laboratories, Denville, New Jersey. Antiserum is prepared by the investigator by immunization of rabbits or sheep with a commercially available estrogen–BSA conjugate (Steroloids, Wilton, New Hampshire). In either case, large quantities of the antiserum can be stored frozen as a concentrate or as a lyophilized preparation for extended periods of time. Repeated use of the same antiserum is advantageous, since it permits assay reproducibility over a number of years.

C. Methods for Radioimmunoassay

1. Source of Hormone

Estradiol-17β obtained from Sigma Chemical, St. Louis, Missouri, is dissolved in the minimum volume of warmed acetone (40°C, added dropwise) and then allowed to recrystallize overnight at 4°C. A stock estradiol solution (10 mg recrystallized estradiol-17β in 10 ml benzene–absolute ethanol, 9 : 1) is serially diluted with absolute ethanol to a concentration of 1.0 pg/μl. The standard curve is composed of 10-, 25-, 50-, 75-, 100-, 150-, and 200-μl aliquots removed in duplicate from this final (1.0 pg/μl) solution. Similar standard solutions of estriol and estrone can be prepared. All solutions of unlabeled steroids made up in organic solvents are stored at -20°C to minimize evaporation.

An alternate procedure for preparation of the standard curve can also be used. A series of stock solutions are prepared by dissolving 10, 25, 50, 75, 100, and 150 pg of the purified estradiol, estrone, or estriol in 0.1 ml of either a 0.01 M potassium phosphate buffer, pH 7.4, containing 1.0 mM EDTA, 0.01% Thimerosal, 0.9% NaCl, and 0.1% Difco gelatin (hereafter designated PBS + 0.1% gel) or a 0.01 M sodium phosphate buffer, pH 7.2, containing 0.9% NaCl, 0.1% Na azide, and 0.1% bovine γ-globulin fraction II. Although both buffers are satisfactory, the sodium phosphate buffer system containing γ-globulin instead of gelatin resembles the normal plasma sample more closely and is, therefore, at least theoretically, better suited for use as an assay blank. Standard stock solutions can be stored at 4°C. Using this method, no preliminary drying down of standards is necessary, and, because the standard solutions are made in buffer, there is less chance of concentration of the standard due to solvent evaporation over time. However, this method requires addition of 0.1 ml of buffer solution to each unknown tube so that the volume in every assay tube is equalized prior to addition of antiserum and trace.

The investigator who would measure the elevated blood and/or urinary levels of estriol during pregnancy should note that adjustment of the standard curve might be necessary. Standard estriol concentrations ranging from 100 pg to 2.5 ng have been prepared and successfully employed for determination of estriol during pregnancy. An alternative to adjusting the standard curve would be to extract an aliquot of sample previously diluted with buffer such that the unknown estriol reading will fall in the range of the 10–200 pg standard curve.

2. Preparation of Immunogen and Immunization Schedule

The antiserum used in our laboratory for estrogen determination was originally prepared at the Worcester Foundation for Experimental Biology. The procedure has previously been reported (Tillson *et al.*, 1970; Thorneycroft *et al.*, 1970). Estradiol-17β hemisuccinate was coupled to purified bovine serum albumin (BSA) according to the method of Lieberman *et al.* (1959). Three milligrams of the conjugate was dissolved in 3.0 ml 0.9% saline emulsified in 3.0 ml complete Freund's adjuvant. This preparation was divided into equal parts, and sheep were injected subcutaneously in five separate sites which were located near the axillary and pelvic lymph nodes. The animals were injected once a week for six weeks and were given monthly boosters thereafter. The highest antibody titers were noted 10–14 days following each booster injection.

3. Characterization of Antiserum

The estrogen antiserum was removed of anti-BSA antibodies by precipitation with BSA in borate buffer as described by Thorneycroft *et al.* (1970). It was then diluted 1 : 5 with the sodium phosphate buffer described previously and stored frozen. In our hands, this antiserum when diluted 1 : 150,000 binds approximately 50% of the tritiated estradiol added. We have found it convenient to dilute the antiserum 1 : 100 with PBS + 0.1% gel and to freeze small aliquots of this preparation for storage. The antiserum is highly specific for estrogens; it will not cross-react with neutral steroids up to a concentration of 1.0 μg. Figure 1 shows the cross-reactivity of the three estrogens when tested with batch SLC-10C of the estrogen antiserum described herein. We have found our antiserum to bind almost equally with estrone and to have a cross-reaction with estriol of approximately 10%[i]. Therefore, using this same antiserum, independent quantification of each of these three estrogenic hormones can be achieved using tritiated estradiol as the labeled trace (see Section I,C,4) and the specific chromatographic fraction obtained as described in Section I,C,5.

4. Source of Label

2,4,6,7-^{3}H-Estradiol (specific activity equals 100 Ci/mM) obtained from New England Nuclear, Boston, Massachusetts (Net-317), is diluted first to a concentration of 25 μCi/ml with benzene : absolute ethanol (9 : 1) and, using an aliquot of this solution, diluted to 5.0 μCi/ml with absolute ethanol. Both solutions are stored at −20°C. Aliquots of the 5.0 μCi/ml solution are dried under nitrogen and redis-

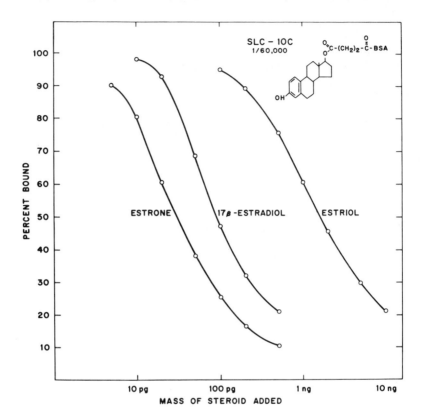

Figure 1. Cross-reactivity of anti-estradiol antiserum with estradiol, estrone, and estriol. Reproduced from Speroff *et al*: (1972) with the permission of the publisher.

solved in PBS + 0.1% gel such that two working solutions of tritiated estradiol are available, one having a concentration of 1000 cpm/25 μl and another having a concentration of 10,000 cpm/100 μl. Working solutions of 6,7-³H-estriol (New England Nuclear; Net-169; specific activity 40–50 Ci/mM) and 2,4,6,7-³H-estrone (New England Nuclear; Net-319; specific activity 100 Ci/mM) are made similarly in buffer at a concentration of 1000 cpm/25 μl. If all three estrogens are to be measured, 25 μl (approximately 1000 cpm) each of tritiated estradiol, estrone, and estriol is added to each plasma sample prior to extraction to assess procedural losses. At the same time, 25-μl aliquots taken from each tritiated steroid solution are also added to scintillation vials so as to obtain a total count for calculation of percentage recovery. On the average, a 75–85% recovery is obtained for each estrogen.

5. Preparation of Sample

After addition of the tritiated estrogens for recovery calculation, the sample is extracted twice by shaking for 15 minutes with 4.0 ml of fresh diethyl ether. Separation of phases is completed each time by a five-minute centrifugation at 2000 rpm. The ether extracts are pooled by removing the upper layer with a Pasteur pipette and transferring it each time to a conical centrifuge tube. The pooled extracts are dried under a stream of nitrogen in a 37°C water bath. After concentrating the extract by washing the sides of the tube twice with ethanol and twice drying the ethanol, the extract is subjected to chromatographic separation on a column of Sephadex LH-20 (Pharmacia Fine Chemicals, Piscataway, New Jersey).

One procedure for column chromatography of the estrogens is carried out as follows. Glass columns (1.0 × 16 cm, Macalaster-Bicknell, New Haven, Connecticut) are rinsed with methanol, fitted with a piece of GF/A Whatman glass–fiber filter paper, and packed with a slurry of 0.9 gm Sephadex LH-20 in 3.0–5.0 ml benzene : methanol (90 : 10). The column is rinsed with 8.0 ml of the eluting solvent, isooctane : benzene : methanol (62 : 20 : 18), and a second piece of glass–fiber filter paper is placed on top of the Sephadex LH-20. To the dry sample tube, 0.2 ml eluting solvent is added and the tube is gently vortexed. The redissolved sample is applied to the column with a Pasteur pipette. A second rinse of the sample tube with 0.1 ml eluting solvent is used to complete the transfer of sample to the column. Successive elution with 4.0, 3.0, 3.5, 4.5, and 7.0 ml of isooctane : benzene : methanol (62 : 20 : 18) permits the isolation of estrone, estradiol, and estriol in fractions 2, 3, and 5, respectively, as shown on the flow sheet (Figure 2). It should be noted that the column should be allowed to run dry (stop dripping) prior to each solvent addition. Separation of the estrogens is illustrated in Figure 3.

6. Assay Procedure

The eluates obtained after chromatography are collected in scintillation vials, evaporated to dryness, and redissolved in 2.0 ml ethanol. Aliquots equivalent to 10 and 40% of the 2.0 ml are transferred to 12 × 75 mm disposable culture tubes (Scientific Products, McGaw Park, Illinois) and dried under nitrogen in a 37°C water bath. The 1.0 ml remaining in the scintillation vial is dried, redissolved in 10 ml Aquasol (New England Nuclear), and counted by liquid scintillation spectrometry for calculation of percentage recovery.

Following volume equalization of unknown assay tubes with 0.1 ml

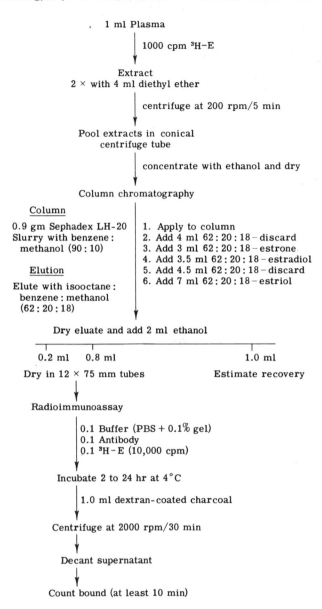

Figure 2.   Flow sheet for estrogen radioimmunoassay.

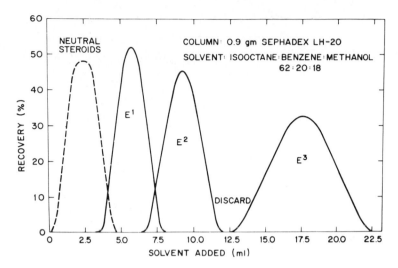

Figure 3. Chromatographic separation of estrone, estradiol, and estriol from a plasma sample on Sephadex LH-20 columns.

PBS + 0.1% gel, 0.1 ml antibody is added, the antibody having been diluted with buffer such that approximately 50% binding will be achieved (usually 1 : 150,000). After shaking by vortex, 0.1 ml tritiated estradiol (approximately 10,000 cpm) is added to each tube. The tubes are vortexed and allowed to incubate at 4°C for two to 24 hours.

Along with the standard and unknown assay tubes, we routinely run in duplicate a set of tubes prepared for determination of nonspecific binding, a determination which permits evaluation of the efficiency of the charcoal separation procedure, and antibody binding, which provides a check on the antibody stability. The tubes are prepared as follows:

"0-0-0" tubes—To obtain total cpm of ^{3}H-estradiol
    0.2 ml PBS + 0.1% gel
    0.1 ml ^{3}H-estradiol (10,000 cpm)
"0-0" tubes—To observe nonspecific binding by subjecting to charcoal separation
    0.2 ml PBS + 0.1% gel
    0.1 ml ^{3}H-estradiol (10,000 cpm)
"0" tubes—To obtain percentage binding of ^{3}H-estradiol by antibody
    0.1 ml PBS + 0.1% gel
    0.1 ml antibody (diluted in buffer for 50% binding)
    0.1 ml ^{3}H-estradiol (10,000 cpm)

7. Separation Technique and Calculations

A stock solution of dextran-coated charcoal containing 0.25% Dextran T-70 and 2.5% Norit A is prepared in 0.1 M potassium phosphate buffer, pH 7.4. At the time that separation of the free from bound steroid is to be carried out, the stock solution is diluted 1 : 10 with 0.01 M PBS + 0.1% gel. Note that, when in use, both solutions are constantly mixed on a magnetic stirrer so that the charcoal is maintained in suspension. The separation procedure is carried out as given below:

1. Add 0.1 ml PBS + 0.5% gel to all tubes.
2. Vortex.
3. Add 1.0 ml PBS + 0.1% gel to "0-0-0" tubes.
4. Add 1.0 ml diluted dextran-coated charcoal solution (0.025% Dextran T-70 and 0.25% Norit A) to all remaining tubes.
5. Vortex.
6. Allow 15 minutes for equilibration.
7. Centrifuge 30 minutes at 2000 rpm.
8. Decant resulting supernatant fraction into 10 ml of Aquasol and shake vial.
9. Count by liquid scintillation spectrometry for 10 minutes or until 10,000 cpm have accumulated.

The amount of estrogen in each unknown is calculated from the standard curve, which is plotted in a linear manner by applying logit transformation. A computer program, based on that described by Rodbard and Lewald (1970), is used for automatic calculation. Unknown values are corrected for losses during extraction and isolation as determined by percentage recovery of the tritiated estrogen(s) added to the plasma sample.

D. Characteristics of the Radioimmunoassay

1. Variation

A typical standard curve for estradiol-17β using this assay method has been shown by Behrman *et al.* (1971). The curve was run in triplicate, and the coefficient of variation between replicates was found to range from 1.0 to 5.5%. The coefficient of variation between replicate samples in the 50 and 100 pg range was found to be between 12 and 16%.

To validate the assay procedure, it is suggested that known amounts of the hormone are added to buffer or a previously determined plasma sample and measured. Values within 15% of the amount added have been considered acceptable for validation of the assay (Auletta *et al.*, Chapter 36, this volume.)

To determine reliability between assays, it is recommended that estimation of estrogen in a sample taken from the same plasma pool is performed with each assay. The coefficient of variation should not exceed 15% (Chapter 36, this volume). Also, in each assay, a buffer or water blank is usually run to determine whether or not nonspecific factors are present which falsely elevate values.

2. *Sensitivity*

The method described here is sufficiently sensitive to detect 10 pg of estrogen as indicated by significant displacement of ^{3}H-estradiol by this concentration of cold steroid. However, the level of estrogen in the sample that can be measured reliably must ultimately be established by the investigator. This limit of sensitivity of the assay is usually defined as two times the standard deviation of the blank determination. Certainly, factors such as sensitivity and precision of the standard curve and accuracy and reproducibility of low estrogen measurements should also be considered when assessing assay sensitivity.

3. *Normal Estrogen Levels*

The mean levels of estradiol measured in plasma from over 200 women during the menstrual cycle are shown in Table I. The determinations were made using a technique which can reliably measure 25 pg of estradiol per milliliter of plasma sample. Plasma levels of estriol during pregnancy are summarized in Table II.

Table I   Plasma Estradiol during the Normal Menstrual Cycle

Day of collection	Mean estradiol concentration (pg/ml)
Days 1–10 (follicular phase)	50 or below
Days 10–12	100–500
Days 12–14 (ovulatory peak)	350–600
Days 14–28 (luteal phase)	200–400

Table II   Levels of Estriol during Pregnancy

Weeks of pregnancy	Estriol (ng/ml)
20–29	2–3
30–33	3–6
34–38	4–10
38–41	8–16

II. URINARY ESTRIOL GLUCURONIDE

A. Introduction

The utility of direct radioimmunoassay of estriol-16α(β-D-glu-curonide) in diluted pregnancy urine for monitoring estriol production in pregnancy is well established (Davis and Loplaux, 1975; Di-Pietro, 1976; Adlercreutz *et al.*, 1976; Soares *et al.*, 1976). Recently, the sensitivity of the method has been extended to the range necessary for monitoring Pergonal induction of ovulation (Haning *et al.*, 1977b). These reports followed less specific radioimmunoassays for estriol in urine with (Goebelsmann *et al.*, 1972; Anderson and Goebelsmann, 1972) and without hydrolysis (Gurpide *et al.*, 1971). Direct assay of conjugates in urine eliminates the necessity for hydrolysis, and the conjugates make excellent haptens (Kellie *et al.*, 1972).

Estriol-16α(β-D-glucuronide) represents 70% of conjugated estriol in term pregnancy urine, while estriol-3(β-D-glucuronide), estriol-3-sulfate-16α(β-D-glucuronide), and estriol-3-sulfate represent the remaining 13, 12, and 5%, respectively (Young *et al.*, 1976).

Estriol-3-sulfate-16-glucuronide is the predominant conjugate in maternal pregnancy plasma. The renal clearances of the various conjugates, as well as plasma and urinary concentrations, have been extensively evaluated (Young *et al.*, 1976).

Bell has demonstrated that estriol is the major urinary estrogen excreted during the ovulatory phase in the cycling woman. Estriol comprised 50% of the mean total urinary estrogens excreted, with estrone and estradiol being 35 and 15%, respectively. This proportion was demonstrated to vary from 44% at minimum levels to 61% at maximum levels of estrogen production (Loraine and Bell, 1963).

Because of its rapidity and simplicity, the radioimmunoassay has currently replaced the fluorometric assay at the Yale Gynecology Endocrine Laboratory for pregnancy on a seven-days-a-week basis. It is hoped that with further evaluation to establish normal ranges in induction of ovulation, the assay will also serve for monitoring induction of ovulation with human menopausal gonadotropins (Haning *et al.*, 1977b).

B. Previous Assay Methods

The assay of urinary estrogen is based on two major principles, the colorimetric/fluorometric and the gas chromatographic methods. The colorimetric and fluorometric methods stem from the observations of

Kober (1931) and Brown (1955). Estrogens produce intense fluorescence in sulfuric acid. Ittrich (1960) devised techniques to gain specificity and to suppress the blank. The gas chromatographic method (Adlercreutz, 1971; Larsen, 1971) depends on derivative formation and measurement of peak height or area under the curve. The specificity of the method stems from separation from other materials on the column. Both methods require hydrolysis of urinary conjugates either with acid (Brown and Blair, 1950) or various enzyme preparations (Rahman, 1972; Larsen, 1971). The fluorometric methods measure total estrogens unless separation is obtained through extraction or chromatography. The direct radioimmunoassay methods have been developed to circumvent the work and slowness inherent in the older methods.

C. Methods for Radioimmunoassay

1. Source of the Hormone

Estriol-16α(β-D-glucuronide) and the various estrogens and conjugates needed for checking cross-reactions are available commercially from Sigma Chemical, St. Louis, Missouri.

2. Preparation of the Immunogen

The conjugates of estriol-16α(β-D-glucuronide) may be produced to keyhole limpet hemocyanin or bovine serum albumin. Estriol-16α(β-D-glucuronide) is not readily soluble in dioxane. This requires modification of the method of Erlanger et al. (1957). Accordingly, the details of the techniques are presented as reported by Haning et al. (1977b).

a. Synthesis of Estriol-16α(β-D-glucuronide)—Keyhole Limpet Hemocyanin Conjugate. Tri-N-butylamine (2.6 ml) and isobutylchlorocarbonate (1.42 ml) (Eastman Kodak, Rochester, New York) are each individually diluted to 10 ml with dimethylformamide (SpectrAR, Mallinckrodt Chemical Works, St. Louis, Missouri). Estriol-16α(β-D-glucuronide) (25 mg) (53.6 μmole) containing trace amounts of label is dried *in vacuo* and dissolved in 0.2 ml dimethylformamide. One-tenth milliliter (109 μmole) of the solutions of tri-N-butylamine and isobutylchlorocarbonate is then added in rapid succession, and the resulting reaction mixture is refrigerated 20 minutes at 4°C (mixture A). Keyhole limpet hemocyanin (Calbiochem, San Diego, California) (25 mg) is dissolved in 2.2 ml deionized water in a 15-ml conical glass centrifuge tube. Two-tenths milliliter of 1.0N NaOH, 2.2 ml dimethylformamide, and mixture A are added in rapid succession to the vortexed solution. The mixture is allowed to stand at 20°C overnight and dialyzed exhaustively and lyophilized.

b. Synthesis of Estriol-16α(β-D-glucuronide)—Bovine Serum Albumin Conjugate. Crystalline bovine serum albumin (25.5 mg) (Miles Laboratories, Kankahee, Illinois) (0.364 μmole), is dissolved in 0.6 ml deionized water. Twenty-five microliters of 1.0 N NaOH and 600 μl dimethylformamide are added in rapid succession (solution A). Fifteen milligrams of estriol-16α(β-D-glucuronide) (32.2 μmole) containing trace amounts of ³H-estriol-16α(β-D-glucuronide) is dried *in vacuo* in a 10 × 75 mm glass test tube, dissolved in 0.2 ml dimethylformamide, and chilled to 4°C. Eight microliters of Tri-N-butylamine (33.5 μmole) and 4.0 μl isobutylchloroformate (30.4 μmole) are added in rapid succession, and the resultant mixture is mixed immediately with solution A and allowed to stand for 70 minutes. The material is dialyzed exhaustively and lyophilized.

Synthesis of the estriol-16α(β-D-glucuronide)–keyhole limpet hemocyanin conjugate as described above resulted in 14% incorporation of radioactivity. The bovine serum albumin conjugate procedure results in 54% incorporation. Thus, it appears possible to achieve a more efficient incorporation into bovine serum albumin than into keyhole limpet hemocyanin and yet maintain solubility of the conjugate. However, for radioimmunoassay purposes, the most important parameter of a conjugate is its antigenicity. The antigenicity of the conjugates has not been properly compared. Both have been capable of inducing antibody responses. DiPietro (1976) has reported the successful use of A ring conjugates.

3. Immunization Schedule

Adult ewes are immunized with the keyhole limpet hemocyanin conjugate or the bovine serum albumin conjugate. The conjugate is dissolved in 1.0 mg/ml 0.1 M sodium phosphate buffer, pH 7.6, and stored at −20°C in 1.0-ml aliquots. A 1.0-ml aliquot is thawed, mixed with 4.0 ml of complete Freund's adjuvant, and then injected among four subcutaneous sites near the shoulders and hips. The animals are injected every two weeks and bled from the jugular vein at monthly intervals prior to immunization. Antibodies should appear within two months. There is marked variation between animals.

4. Characterization of Antiserum

a. Cross-Reactions. Estrone, estradiol, estriol, and the various glucuronides are first dissolved in dimethylformamide as in preparation of the standard curve and then diluted in appropriate tenfold dilutions in deionized water. The steroid sulfates are dissolved primarily in deionized water prior to preparation of the dilutions. The serial tenfold dilutions for all substances cover the range from 10 to 10^5 ng/ml. The serial dilutions are used to prepare standard curves for each cross-reacting substance analogous to the regular standard curve. For a single antiserum bleeding, all curves were prepared at one time and cross-reactions were determined in one assay using the same stock for all reagents. The routine standard curve of estriol-16α(β-D-glucuronide) is run in the same assay for comparison. To demonstrate nonlinearity, curves may be constructed by plotting percent cross-reaction versus percent displacement (Haning et al., 1977a).

The plots of percent cross-reaction versus percent displacement from B_0 constructed as previously reported (Haning *et al.*, 1977a) are presented for antiserum No. 142·6·1·76 in Figure 4. The data from which Figure 4 was constructed are presented in Table III, along with cross-reactions at 50% displacement. Our antiserum cross-reacts highly with estriol and to a small extent with estrone. The remaining cross-reactions are much smaller.

b. Titer. The titer of antiserum No. 142·6·1·76 was 1:12,500 in our system. However, titer reflects only the number of binding sites per milliliter. The use of 50,000 cpm of ^{3}H-estriol-16α(β-D-glucuronide) allows rapid counting and requires the use of relatively larger numbers of binding sites. Haning *et al.* (1977b) also produced a large pool of titer 1:300 which is equally satisfactory for use in the assay. Five milliliters of 1:1000 titer antiserum can provide 5×10^4 tubes, about a 1-year supply for an active laboratory doing about 100 samples per week.

5. Source of the Label

^{3}H-Estriol-16α(β-D-glucuronide) may be obtained from Amersham-Searle, Arlington Heights, Illinois.

6. Preparation of Samples

Twenty-four hour urine specimens are collected without preservative and refrigerated. The volume of each specimen is measured and

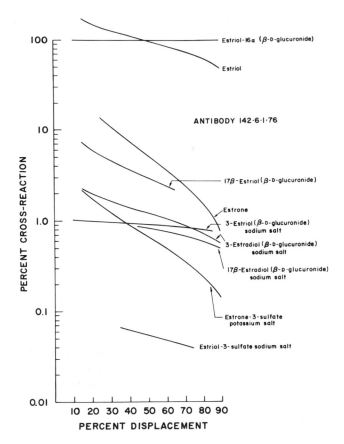

Figure 4.   Cross-reaction as a function of percent displacement from antibody 142.6.1.76. (Reproduced from Haning *et al.*, 1977b, with permission of the publisher.)

an aliquot is taken for determination of creatinine content. Urine (1/1000 of the total volume) is diluted to 10 ml in deionized water (Hydroservice and Supplies, Durham, North Carolina) (dilution 1). A further 1 : 100 dilution in deionized water is then prepared for pregnancy urine (dilution 2). When specimens are known to be other than 24-hour collections, an appropriate correction is made at the time of preparation of dilution 1 (e.g., for an 8-hour collection, $\frac{3}{1000}$ of the total volume is diluted to 10 ml). Thus, 0.1 ml of dilution 1 represents 10^{-5} of the 24-hour specimen and 0.1 ml of dilution 2 represents 10^{-7} of the 24-hour specimen.

Table III Analysis of Antiserum[a]

Compound	MW	A	B	% Cross-reaction at 50% displacement	Molar % cross reaction
Estriol-16α(β-D-glucuronide)	464.5	0.212415392	−1.031734712	100	100
Estrone	270.4	1.70531849	−0.540823379	14.11	8.12
Estradiol	272.4			$<1.23 \times 10^{-3}$	$<0.72 \times 10^{-3}$
Estriol	288.4	0.164977833	−0.772017718	99.22	61.59
Estradiol-3-(β-D-glucuronide) sodium salt	470.5	3.463124836	−0.751319048	1.22	1.24
Estradiol-17β(β-D-glucuronide) sodium salt	470.5	4.155918043	−0.831363990	0.83	0.84
Estradiol-3-sulfate-17β(β-D-glucuronide) dipotassium salt	604.8			$<1.23 \times 10^{-3}$	$<1.60 \times 10^{-3}$
Estriol-3-(β-D-glucuronide) sodium salt	486.5	4.670796928	−0.950441709	0.90	0.94
Estriol-17β(β-D-glucuronide)	464.5	2.496002522	−0.671402527	2.98	2.98
Estriol-3-sulfate sodium salt	390.4	6.028501403	−0.779728697	0.05	0.04
Estrone-3-sulfate potassium salt	388.6	3.075375630	−0.590669744	0.67	0.56

[a] Animal No. 142: 6/1/76; titer = 1 : 12,500, Mass for logit = 0, Displacement = 1.23 ng.

7. Reagents and Buffers

a. Buffer G. Bovine γ-globulin fraction II (Schwarz-Mann, Orangeburg, New York) (1.0 gm/liter), 0.538 gm/liter $NaH_2PO_4 \cdot H_2O$, 1.635 gm/liter $Na_2HPO_4 \cdot 7 H_2O$, 1.0 gm/liter NaN_3, and 9.0 gm/liter NaCl, are dissolved in deionized water.

b. Dextran-Coated Charcoal. Charcoal, (0.5 gm/200 ml) and 0.05 gm/200 ml Dextran T-70 (Pharmacia Uppsala, Sweden), are suspended and dissolved, respectively, in buffer G in 200-ml batches.

c. ^{3}H-Estriol-16α(β-D-glucuronide) Solution for Radioimmunoassay. ^{3}H-Estriol-16α(β-D-glucuronide) $(1 \times 10^8$ cpm) in ethanol is taken to dryness under air and dissolved in 200 ml buffer G.

d. Standard for Estriol-16α(β-D-glucuronide). Estriol-16α(β-D-glucuronide) 1.0–3.0 mg is weighed on a microanalytical balance, dissolved in 0.2 ml dimethylformamide, and diluted to 100 ml with deionized water. A 1.0 μg/ml stock solution is then prepared in deionized water and stored at $-20°$C in 5.0-ml aliquots.

e. Standard Curve. Each week, primary dilutions from the 1.0 μg/ml stock are prepared containing 200, 100, 50, 20, 10, 5, 2, and 1.0 ng/ml in deionized water. Sixteen 0.1-ml aliquots of each dilution are prepared in 10 × 75 mm glass culture tubes and stored at $-20°$C. Each day, two tubes of each dilution are thawed and used for assay.

f. Antibody Dilution for Radioimmunoassay. The antibody serum is diluted in Buffer G so that 0.1 ml diluted antiserum added to 0.1 ml deionized water and 0.1 ml ^{3}H-estriol-16α(β-D-glucuronide) solution result in binding of 50% of the counts.

8. Assay and Separation Techniques

a. Assay. The assay is prepared in 10 × 75 mm glass culture tubes as in Table IV. The tubes are vortexed briefly and incubated for one hour at 4°C.

b. Separation Techniques and Calculation: Buffer or dextran-coated charcoal are then added where indicated (Table IV) within 2.5 minutes. The tubes are allowed to stand for 7.5 minutes from the start of

Table IV   Preparation of the Assay[a]

	^{3}H-E$_3$Gluc	Water	Standard	Urine	Antibody	Buffer G	Charcoal
Background	0	0.1	0	0	0	1.2	0
Total count	0.1	0.1	0	0	0	1.1	0
0-AB	0.1	0.1	0	0	0	0.1	1
B$_0$	0.1	0.1	0	0	0.1	0	1
Standards	0.1	0	0.1	0	0.1	0	1
Urine	0.1	0	0	0.1	0.1	0	1

[a] ^{3}H-E$_3$Gluc, ^{3}H-estriol-16α(β-D-glucuronide) solution for radioimmunoassay; water, deionized water; standard, thawed prepared standard for radioimmunoassay; urine, either dilution 1 or dilution 2 of the 24-hr urine depending on whether Pergonal or pregnancy urine is being used; charcoal, dextran-coated charcoal suspension; 0-AB, no antibody control; B$_0$, tube for binding with no added estriol glucuronide.

dextran-coated charcoal addition and centrifuged for five minutes at 1000 g. The contents of each tube are decanted into counting vials, and 10 ml ACS (Amersham-Searle, Arlington Heights, Illinois) counting solution is added. The samples are counted for two minutes or 10^4 counts in a liquid scintillation spectrometer with punched paper tape printout. The data are analyzed by computer program using the logit/log transformation of Feldman and Rodbard (1971). All urine specimens are run in triplicate.

D. Characteristics of the Radioimmunoassay

1. Variation

Five different dilutions of a single sample were prepared on each of six days. Each dilution was run as a typical urine specimen (in triplicate) and the mean was computed. The 30 means for the urine specimen were then subjected to one-way analysis of variance to compute the intraassay and interassay variations and the corresponding standard deviations and coefficients of variation. Sample mean equals 41.5 mg/24 hours, intraassay standard deviation equals 3.92, coefficient of variation equals 9.5%, interassay standard deviation equals 3.0, and coefficient of variation equals 7.25%.

2. Sensitivity and Specificity

The slope of the dose–response curve was −1.03 with midrange of the assay (mass for logit = 0 displacement) of 0.9 ng. The least detectable concentration (two standard deviations from the mean B_0) was 0.23 ng. The specificity of the assay depends entirely on the specificity of the antiserum and on the relative concentrations of the cross-reacting substances (Figure 4). The cross-reacting substances will have a greater effect when the estriol concentration is lower as can be seen from the figure.

The recovery of estriol-16α(β-D-glucuronide) from male urine was evaluated both in the pregnancy range and in the range found during Pergonal induction of ovulation (Figures 5 and 6). Estriol-16α(β-D-glucuronide) (2.3 mg) was dissolved in 23 ml of a male urine pool (100 mg/liter). Dilutions of 50 and 10 mg/liter and 200, 100, and 50 μg/liter were prepared using the male urine pool as diluent. The urines were then assayed in duplicate as samples assuming a total volume of 1000 ml and a 24-hour collection. Dilution 1 was used in the microgram range and dilution 2 was used in the milligram range. The results were analyzed by regression analysis. In the pregnancy range: Found

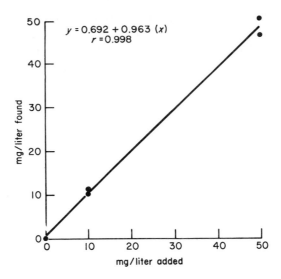

Figure 5. Estriol-16α(β-D-glucuronide) radioimmunoassay mass recovery experiment in the pregnancy range (Reproduced from Haning *et al.*, 1977b, with permission of the publisher.)

= 0.6917 + 0.96259x, added mg/liter r = 0.998. In the Pergonal range: Found = 1.572 + 1.10203x, added μg/liter, r = 0.997.

3. Normal Estrogen Levels

a. **Evaluation of the Radioimmunoassay for Urinary Estriol.** The radioimmunoassay method was evaluated by simultaneous determina-

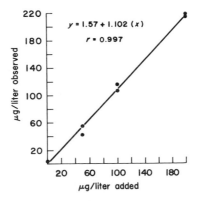

Figure 6. Estriol-16α(β-D-glucuronide) radioimmunoassay mass recovery experiment in the Pergonal range. (Reproduced from Haning *et al.*, 1977b, with permission of the publisher.)

tion of estriol in 127 consecutive samples by radioimmunoassay and by the standard method used in the Yale Gynecology Endocrine Laboratory. The standard method is a fluorometric technique involving ammonium sulfate precipitation followed by acid hydrolysis and estrogen determination by the method of Brown (1955) as modified by Ittrich (1960). Correction for losses in precipation was based on recovery of counts of ^{3}H-estradiol-17β(β-D-glucuronide) added to the initial aliquot of urine. These data are presented in Figure 7. Analysis of the data as suggested by Rodbard (Davis and Loriaux, 1975), using the $\log_e$ transformation of all data to correct the heterogeneity of variance gave the following results: $y = \log_e$ (fluorometric data), $x = \log_e$ (radioimmunoassay data): $y = 0.534 + 0.857x$ (y on x), $y = -1.32 + 1.41x$ (x on y), $r = 0.78$ for both regressions. Computation of the line bisecting the

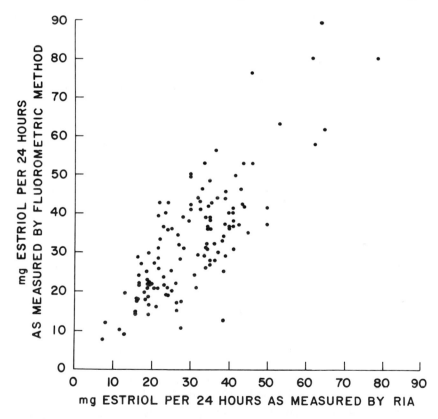

Figure 7. Untransformed pregnancy urinary estriol data, fluorometric versus radioimmunoassay estriol-16α(β-D-glucuronide) outputs. (Reproduced from Haning *et al.*, 1977b, with permission of the publisher.)

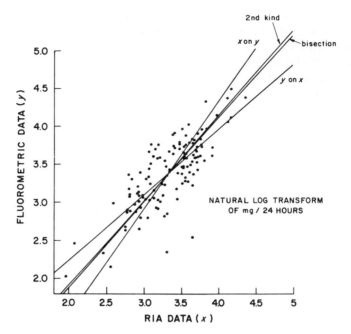

Figure 8.   Normal log transformation of urinary estriol data from Figure 5 [fluorometric versus radioimmunoassay measurements of estriol-16α(β-D-glucuronide)]. (Reproduced from Haning *et al.*, 1977b, with permission of the publisher.)

two regressions gives the equation: $y = 0.266 + 1.097x$. Computation using the formula for regression of the "second kind" yields the formula $y = 0.376 + 1.130x$ (Figure 8). These slopes are not significantly different from 1. Accordingly, following Rodbard, the mean $\log_e$ of the ratio fluorometric result/radioimmunoassay result was computed to be 0.05691 ± 0.2571 S.E. This results in the equation fluorometric determination = $(1.059 \pm 0.027$ S.E.) × radioimmunoassay determination or radioimmunoassay determination = $(0.945 \pm 0.024$ S.E.) × fluorometric determination. This indicates that the two assays were essentially giving identical results and that no change in normal values was necessary.

b. Plasma Estradiol versus Urinary Estriol for Monitoring Induction of Ovulation with Pergonal. Twenty-four hour urine collections were obtained from volunteers who were undergoing induction of ovulation with Pergonal monitored by the plasma estradiol concentration. The urine collections were timed to end the morning when a plasma estradiol level was scheduled to be drawn so that the correla-

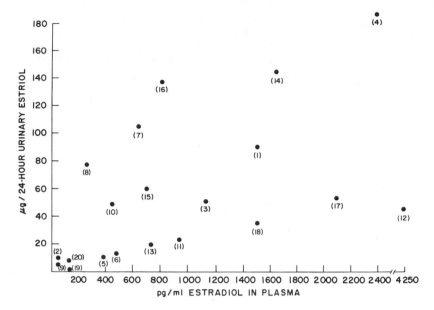

Figure 9.   Urinary estriol-16α(β-D-glucuronide) as a function of plasma estradiol at the termination of the 24-hour collection. The numbers with points represent serial sample numbers for clinical correlations as more data is available. (Reproduced from Haning *et al.*, 1977b, with permission of the publisher.)

tion of the two values could be studied. These data are presented in Figure 9. Because of increasing variation with larger estrogen values, log transformation of the data was performed. Evaluation of the correlation coefficient on the transformed data demonstrated a statistically significant correlation between plasma estradiol and urinary estradiol-16α(β-D-glucuronide): $r = 0.625$ ($p < 0.01$). A further clinical study has demonstrated that an estriol glucuronide window of 40 to 100 μg/day corresponds approximately to a plasma estradiol window of 1000 to 2000 pg/ml on the morning of the 5 to 9 PM hCG injection in Pergonal induction of ovulation. Timing of the hCG injections is critical in using plasma or urine windows for monitoring Pergonal induction of ovulation (Haning *et al.*, 1978).

REFERENCES

Abraham, G. E. (1969). Solid-phase radioimmunoassay of estradiol-17β. *J. Clin. Endocrinol. Metab.* **29**, 866–870.

Adlercreutz, H. (1971). Evaluation of gas–liquid chromatographic techniques for the estimation of oestrogens. *Clin. Chim. Acta* **34**, 231–240.

Adlercreutz, H., Lehtinen, T., Tikkanen, M. (1976). Preliminary studies on the determination of estriol-16α-glucuronide in pregnancy urine by direct radioimmunoassay without hydrolysis. *J. Steroid Biochem.* **7**, 165.

Allen, E., and Doisey E. A. (1923). On ovarian hormone. Preliminary report on its focalization, extraction, and partial purification, and action in test animals. *J. Am. Med. Assoc.* **81**, 819–821.

Anderson, D. W., and Goebelsmann, U. (1972). Estriol in pregnancy. I. A radioimmunoassay for urinary estriol. *Am. J. Obstet. Gynecol.* **112**, 802.

Astwood, E. B. (1938). A six-hour assay for quantitative determination of estrogen. *Endocrinology* **23**, 25–31.

Baird, D. T., and Guevara, A. J. (1969). Concentration of unconjugated estrone and estradiol in peripheral plasma in nonpregnant women through the cycle, castrate, and post-menopausal women and in men. *J. Clin. Endocrinol. Metab.* **29**, 149–156.

Barnard, G. J. R., Hennam, J. F., and Collins, W. P. (1975). Further studies on radioimmunoassay systems for plasma estradiol. *J. Steroid Biochem.* **6**, 107–116.

Behrman, H. R., Yoshinaga, K., Wyman, H., and Greep, R. O. (1971). Effects of prostaglandin on ovarian steroid secretion and biosynthesis during pregnancy. *Am. J. Physiol.* **221**, 189–193.

Brown, J. B. (1955). A chemical method for the determination of oestriol, oestrone, and oestradiol in human urine. *Biochem. J.* **60**, 185.

Brown, J. B., and Blair, H. A. F. (1950). The hydrolysis of conjugated oestrone, estradiol-17β, and oestriol in human urine. *J. Endocrinol.* **17**, 411–424.

Carstensen, J., and Bäckström, T. (1976). A paper chromatographic saturation analysis method for measuring estradiol, testosterone and 5α-dihydrotestosterone from the same sample. *J. Steroid Biochem.* **7**, 145–149.

Corker, C. S., Exley, D., and Naftolin, F. (1970). Assay of 17β-oestradiol by competitive protein binding methods. *Proc. 2nd Symp. Steroid Assay by Protein Binding*, Karolinska Institutet, Stockholm, pp. 305–319.

Davis, S. E., and Loriaux, D. L. (1975). A simple specific assay for estriol in maternal urine. *J. Clin. Endocrinol. Metab.* **40**, 895.

DiPietro, D. L. (1976). Assay of estriol-16α[β-D-glucuronide] in pregnancy urine with a specific antiserum. *Am. J. Obstet. Gynecol.* **125**, 841.

England, B. G., Niswender, G. D., and Midgley, A. R., Jr. (1974). Radioimmunoassay of estradiol-17β without chromatography. *J. Clin. Endocrinol. Metab.* **38**, 42–50.

Erlanger, B. F., Borek, F., Beiser, S. M., and Lieberman, S. (1957). Steroid protein conjugates. I. Preparation and characterization of conjugates of bovine serum albumin with testosterone and with cortisone. *J. Biol. Chem.* **288**, 713.

Feldman, H., and Rodbard, D. (1971). Mathematical theory of radioimmunoassay. *In* "Principles of Competitive Protein-Binding Assays" (W. D. Odell and W. H. Daughaday, eds.), pp. 158–203. Lippincott, Philadelphia, Pennsylvania.

Franek, M., and Hruska, K. J. (1976). Separation of free and protein-bound ligands in the radioimmunoassay by gel filtration-centrifugation. *J. Chromatogr.* **119**, 167–172.

Goebelsmann, U., Thorneycroft, I. H., Nakamura, R. M., and Mishell, D. R., Jr. (1972). Estriol in pregnancy. I. A radioimmunoassay for urinary estriol. *Am. J. Obstet. Gynecol.* **112**, 802.

Goodfriend, T. I.., and Sehon, A. (1970). Early approaches to production analysis and use of steroid-specific antisera. *In* "Immunologic Methods in Steroid Determination" (F. G. Perón and B. V. Caldwell, eds.), Chapter 2, pp. 15–39. Appleton, New York.

Gurpide, E., Giebenhain, T., Seng, L., and Kelley, W. G. (1971). Radioimmunoassay for estrogens in human pregnancy urine, plasma, and amniotic fluid. *Am. J. Obstet. Gynecol.* **109**, 897.

Haning, R. V., Kieliszek, F., Alberino, S., and Speroff, L. (1977a). A radioimmunoassay for 13,14-dihydro-15-ketoprostaglandin $F_{2\alpha}$ with chromatography and internal recovery standard prostaglandins. *Prostaglandins* **13**, 445–477.

Haning, R. V., Satin, K. P., Lynsky, M., and Speroff, L. (1977b). A direct radioimmunoassay for estriol-16-glucuronide in urine for monitoring pregnancy and induction of ovulation. *Am. J. Obstet. Gynecol.* **128**, 793–802.

Haning, R. V., Levin, R., Behrman, H., Kase, N., and Speroff, L. (1978). Evaluation of the 1000–2000 pg/ml ovulation window and comparison of plasma estradiol and urinary estriol glucuronide determinations for monitoring menotropin induction of ovulation. *Am. J. Obstet. Gynecol.* In press.

Hotchkiss, J., Atkinson, L. E., and Knobil, E. (1971). Time course of serum estrogen and luteinizing hormone (LH) concentrations during the menstrual cycle of the rhesus monkey. *Endocrinology* **89**, 177–183.

Ittrich, G. (1960). Untersuchungen über die extraktion des roten Kober-Farbstoffs durch organische Lösungmittel zur Ostrogen bestimmung im Harn. *Acta Endocrinol. (Copenhagen)* **35**, 34.

Jiang, N., and Ryan, R. J. (1969). Radioimmunoassays for estrogens: A preliminary communication. *Mayo Clin. Proc.* **44**, 461–465.

Jurjens, H., Pratt, J. J., and Woldring, M. G. (1975). Radioimmunoassay of plasma estradiol without extraction and chromatography. *J. Clin. Endocrinol. Metab.* **40**, 19–25.

Kellie, A. E., Samuel, V. K., Riley, W. J., and Robertson, D. M. (1972). Steroid glucuronoside–BSA complexes as antigens: The radioimmunoassay of steroid conjugates. *J. Steroid Biochem.* **3**, 275.

Kober, S. (1931). Eine koloriemtrische Bestimmung des Brunsthormons (Menformon). *Biochem. Z.* **239**, 209–212.

Korenman, S. G., Tulchinksy, D., and Eaton, L. W., Jr. (1970). Radioligand procedures for estrogen assay in normal and pregnancy plasma. *Acta Endocrinol. Suppl.* **147**, 291–304.

Korenman, S. G., Stevens, R. H., Carpenter, L. A., Robb, M., Miswender, G. D., and Sherman, B. M. (1974). Estradiol radioimmunoassay without chromatography: Procedure, validation and normal values. *J. Clin. Endocrinol. Metab.* **38**, 718–720.

Kushinsky, S., and Anderson, M. (1974). A non-chromatographic radioimmunoassay of estrone and estradiol-17β in serum. *Steroids* **23**, 535–548.

Lieberman, S., Erlanger, B. F., Bieser, S. M., and Agate, F. J., Jr. (1959). Steroid–protein conjugates: Their chemical, immunochemical and endocrinological properties. *Recent Prog. Horm. Res.* **15**, 165–200.

Larsen, A. E. (1971). Gas chromatographic analysis of estrogen and progesterone metabolites in human pregnancy urine. *Am. J. Med. Technol.* **37**, 279–291.

Lindberg, P., and Edqvist, L. E. (1974). The use of 17β-oestradiol-6-(O-carboxymethyl) oxime-^{125}I-tyramine as tracer for the radioimmunoassay of 17β-oestradiol. *Clin. Chim. Acta* **53**, 169–174.

Loraine, J. A., and Bell, E. T. (1963). Hormone excretion during the normal menstrual cycle. *Lancet* **1**, 1340–1342.

Midgley, A. R., Jr., Niswender, G. D., and Sri Ram, J. (1969). Hapten-radioimmunoassay: A general procedure for estimation of steroidal and other haptenic substances. *Steroids* **13**, 731–737.

Mikhail, G., Wu, C. H., Ferin, M., and Vande Wiele, R. L. (1970). Radioimmunoassay of plasma estrone and estradiol. *Steroids* **15**, 333–352.

Niswender, G. D., and Midgley, A. R., Jr. (1970). Hapten-radioimmunoassay for steroid hormones. *In* "Immunologic Methods in Steroid Determination" (F. G. Perón and B. V. Caldwell, eds.), Chapter 8, pp. 149–173. Appleton, New York.

O'Donnell, V. J., and Preedy, J. R. K. (1967). The oestrogens. *In* "Hormones in Blood" (C. H. Gray and A. L. Bacharach, eds.), Chapter IV, pp. 109–186. Academic Press, New York.

Rahman, M. (1972). A rapid colorimetric method for oestriol assay in pregnancy urine. *Clin. Chim. Acta* **39**, 287–291.

Rodbard, D., and Lewald, J. E. (1970). Computer analysis of radioligand assay and radioimmunoassay data. *Acta Endocrinol. Suppl.* **147**, 79–103.

Schiller, H. S., and Brammall, M. A. (1974). A radioimmunoassay of plasma estradiol-17β with the use of polyethylene glycol to separate free and antibody-bound hormone. *Steroids* **24**, 665–678.

Soares, J. R., Zimmermann, E., and Gross, S. J. (1976). Direct radioimmunoassay of 16-glucosiduronate metabolites of estriol in human plasma and urine. *FEBS Lett.* **61**, 263.

Speroff, L., Caldwell, B. V., Brock, W. A., Anderson, G. G., and Hobbins, J. C. (1972). Hormone levels during prostaglandin $F_{2\alpha}$ infusion for therapeutic abortion. *J. Clin. Endocrinol. Metab.* **34**, 531–536.

Svendsen, R., and Sorenson, B. (1964). The concentration of unconjugated oestrone and 17β-oestradiol in plasma during pregnancy. *Acta Endocrinol. (Copenhagen)* **47**, 237–244.

Thorneycroft, I. H., Tilson, S. A., Abraham, G. E., Scaramuzzi, R. J., and Caldwell, B. V. (1970). Preparation and purification of antibodies to steroids. *In* "Immunologic Methods in Steroid Determination" (F. G. Perón and B. V. Caldwell, eds.), Chapter 4, pp. 63–86. Appleton, New York.

Tillson, S. A., Thorneycroft, I. H., Abraham, G. F., Scaramuzzi, R. J., and Caldwell, B. V. (1970). Solid-phase radioimmunoassay of steroids. *In* "Immunologic Methods in Steroid Determination" (F. G. Perón and B. V. Caldwell, eds.), Chapter 7, pp. 127–147. Appleton, New York.

Young, B. K., Jirku, H., Kadner, S., and Levitz, M. (1976). Renal clearances of estriol conjugates in normal pregnancy at term. *Am. J. Obstet. Gynecol.* **126**, 38.

35

Progesterone and 20α-Dihydroprogesterone

GAYLE P. ORCZYK, MARTIN HICHENS, GLEN ARTH,
AND HAROLD R. BEHRMAN

I. INTRODUCTION

Early measurement of progesterone was based on biologic assays, the endpoints of which included either maintenance of pregnancy or cytologic and/or biologic changes in the uteri of various test animals. Such bioassays lack specificity, since several progestational compounds produce effects similar to progesterone itself. Also, because the relative response to progesterone and progestinlike compounds varies greatly in different tests and in different animal species, bioassay methods present difficulties in terms of obtaining reliable measurements (see van der Molen and Aakvaag, 1967). Among the physicochemical methods for progesterone quantitation are

701

spectrophotometric and fluorometric methods, which, with modification (Heap, 1964), have been reported to offer sensitivity on the order of 0.01 μg; the double isotope derivative method, the sensitivity of which has been shown to be 0.0025–0.0050 μg/10 ml plasma sample Riondel et al., 1965), and gas–liquid chromatography, which has a sensitivity similar to the double isotope method, have been used to estimate small amounts of progesterone in peripheral blood (van der Molen and Groen, 1965). Since none of these methods is specific for progesterone, numerous purification procedures (e.g., solvent extraction, paper and/or thin-layer chromatography) must be performed prior to estimation. For a complete review of these methods, their modifications, and the sensitivity, accuracy, and precision that they offer, the reader is referred to the review by van der Molen and Aakvaag (1967).

The application of Murphy's (1967) competitive protein-binding technique for the measurement of progesterone (Neill et al., 1967) has provided a most sensitive and specific assay. However, the corticosteroid-binding protein used in this procedure binds other steroids as well. Therefore, the method requires at least one thin-layer or paper chromatographic step for prior purification of the sample. Two protein-binding assays not requiring prior sample purification by thin-layer chromatography have been reported, but one results in loss of sensitivity (Johansson, 1969) and the other requires a number of solvent extraction procedures for sample purification (Lurie and Patterson, 1970).

The earliest radioimmunoassay procedures for progesterone also required sample purification. Abraham and associates (1971) prepared antiserum to a conjugate consisting of the 21-hemisuccinate derivative of 11-deoxycortisol coupled to human serum albumin. After an ether extraction and chromatography on a celite microcolumn, progesterone was quantitated by a radioimmunoassay method in which dextran-coated charcoal was used for separation of antibody-bound from free steroid. Another progesterone radioimmunoassay method employing precipitation by ammonium sulfate for the separation procedure has been described by Furuyama and Nugent (1971). The antiserum used was produced by immunizing with progesterone-3-carboxymethyl-oxime–bovine serum albumin, and progesterone was isolated from hexane extracts by Al_2O_3 microcolumn chromatography. Highly specific progesterone antiserum has been obtained by linking progesterone (at carbon-11) to bovine serum albumin, using either 11α-hydroxyprogesterone hemisuccinate (Spieler et al., 1972; Youssefnejadian et al., 1972; DeVilla et al., 1972; Bodley et al., 1972) or the chlorocarbonate derivative of 11-hydroxyprogesterone (Niswender and Midgley, 1970). Use of such antiserum permits direct measurement of progesterone in ether extracts, since cross-reaction by other steroids in the extract has been shown to be minimal.

Human plasma progesterone levels measured by two radioimmunoassay procedures employing highly specific antiserum as well as one utilizing less specific antiserum and a chromatographic purification procedure are shown in Table I. The assays described here require no prior purification of the sample, because highly specific antibodies are used. The conjugate required for production of such antibody can be purchased from Steraloids (Pawling, New York).

Numerous refinements and modifications of the progesterone radioimmunoassay have been made in an attempt to increase the convenience and rapidity of the procedure while decreasing its cost. Such recent innovations as the synthesis and utilization of ^{125}I-labeled progesterone as radioligand (Scarisbrick and Cameron, 1975), combined

Table I Human Plasma Progesterone Levels Measured by Radioimmunoassay

Source	Progesterone concentration (ng/ml ± SD)	Reference
Female cycle		DeVilla et al. (1972)
Days 2–10	0.50 ± 0.44	
Days 19–23	12.10 ± 4.81	
Postmenopausal cycle	0.25 ± 0.09	DeVilla et al. (1972); Youssefnejadian et al. (1972)
Days 1–14	0.555 ± 0.265[a]	
	0.424 ± 0.187[b]	
Days 14–end	7.70 ± 2.49[a]	
	7.70 ± 1.90[b]	
Pregnancy		Youssefnejadian et al. (1972)
12 weeks–term	144 ± 66[a]	
	104 ± 55[b]	
Cycle		Abraham et al. (1971)
Follicular phase	0.545 ± 0.103	
Midluteal phase	8.561 ± 4.661	
Pregnancy		Abraham et al. (1971)
16–18 weeks	48.4 ± 18	
28–30 weeks	98.0 ± 28	
38–40 weeks	178.5 ± 48	
Male	0.26 ± 0.08	DeVilla et al. (1972);
	0.495 ± 0.132[a]	Youssefnejadian et al. (1972)
	0.230 ± 0.068[b]	

[a] Without chromatography.
[b] With chromatography.

radioimmunoassay of several steroids in one milliliter of plasma (Abraham *et al.*, 1975), and separation of bound from free progesterone by Millipore filtration (Batra, 1976) have contributed to the establishment of more efficient assays.

II. METHODS OF RADIOIMMUNOASSAY

A. Source of Hormone

Crystalline progesterone and 20α-dihydroprogesterone (Sigma Chemical, St. Louis, Missouri) can be used to prepare a series of stock solutions made in 95% ethanol at concentrations of 10, 25, 50, 75, 100, and 200 ng/ml. From these solutions 10-μl aliquots can be removed and dried in assay tubes for preparation of a standard curve ranging from 0.1 to 2.0 ng.

The progesterone and 20α-dihydroprogesterone standard curves can also be prepared in a potassium phosphate buffer (0.01 M, pH 7.4) containing 0.001 M EDTA, 0.01% Thimerosol, 0.9% NaCl, and 0.1% Difco gelatin (hereafter referred to as PBS + 0.1% gel). This is the preferred procedure in our laboratory, since the problem of concentration of the standard solutions due to solvent evaporation over time is eliminated, as well as the problem associated with solubilization of steroid into the radioimmunoassay reaction mixture, particularly at the higher concentrations. Since steroids are not readily soluble in aqueous media, the method requires initial verification of the standard concentrations. This is determined on the basis of solubilization of labeled steroid in buffer. To do this, crystalline progesterone (100 μg) and 20α-dihydroprogesterone (100 μg) dissolved in ethanol are added to a small vial containing approximately 3000 cpm of 1,2-^{3}H-progesterone or 1,2-^{3}H-20α-dihydroprogesterone (New England Nuclear, Boston, Massachusetts) (40–50 Ci/mM). After the contents of the vial have evaporated to dryness, 5.0 ml PBS + 0.5% Difco gelatin are added, and the vial is gently vortexed for five minutes. The counts per minute of an aliquot removed 24 hours later can be used to estimate the percentage recovery of redissolved steroid and, thereby, to establish the concentration of the stock solution (we observe nearly 100% recovery of steroid in buffer at this concentration). The stock solution is then adjusted to a concentration of 20 μg/100 ml PBS + 0.1% gel and diluted with PBS + 0.1% gel to make a series of standards containing 100, 250, 500, 750, 1000, and 2000 pg/0.1 ml.

B. Preparation and Characterization of Immunogen

The progesterone conjugate was prepared by coupling 11α-hydroxyprogesterone hemisuccinate to bovine serum albumin by the active ester method (Anderson *et al.*, 1964). The procedure was carried out as follows: Solutions of 11α-hydroxyprogesterone (215 mg/2.0 ml), dicyclohexyldicarbodiimide (DCDI; 113 mg/1.0 ml), and N-hydroxysuccinimide (NHS; 57.5 mg/1.0 ml) were prepared in dry dioxane. After successive addition of the NHS and DCDI to the steroid derivative, the dicyclohexyl urea was allowed to settle out of the mixture for two hours at room temperature or for 24 hours at 4°C. The urea was removed by filtration, and of the solution of active ester plus the dioxane washings (total volume, 8.0 ml), 6.4 ml was used for coupling to bovine serum albumin (BSA). The active ester was added dropwise to a solution of BSA (500 mg per 10 ml 0.2 M phosphate buffer) with mixing at room temperature. The pH was maintained at 8 to 8.5, and water was added simultaneously with the later dioxane additions to prevent precipitation of the conjugate. The complete mixture was stirred for one hour, after which it was diluted with water and dialyzed against multiple changes of distilled water.

The product was assessed by measuring the optical density at 243 nm against a blank of unconjugated BSA at the same concentration and using the absorbance of 11α-hydroxyprogesterone (E_m = 16,600) to calculate the steroid content of the conjugate. Two separate preparations were calculated to contain 25 and 27 moles of progesterone per mole protein, representing approximately 45% utilization of the steroid.

The 20α-dihydroprogesterone active ester was prepared in the same manner and conjugated to BSA with results essentially similar to those seen with the progesterone conjugate.

C. Immunization Schedule

Male rabbits (New Zealand white) were injected initially with 1.5 mg of conjugate dissolved in 0.5 ml of 0.9% saline emulsified in 0.5 ml of complete Freund's adjuvant. One-half of the preparation was injected subcutaneously in the back of the neck; the other half was injected intradermally in six separate sites on the back. Monthly boosters of 0.5–1.0 mg of conjugate were injected in incomplete Freund's adjuvant.

D. Characterization of Antibody

The progesterone antibody was titered using both ammonium sulfate precipitation and dextran-coated charcoal (see below) for separation of free and bound antibody. Using the ammonium sulfate method, the concentration of antibody required for 50% binding was found to be approximately five times less than that required for 50% binding when charcoal was used. However, when antibody concentrations were adjusted for each separation method such that 50% binding would result, standard curves were similar. We regularly use the charcoal separation method, and to eliminate variation due to stripping, a 15-minute incubation period is used following addition of charcoal.

The antibody has an average affinity constant of 8×10^8 to 10×10^8 liters/mole and is highly specific for progesterone. The cross-reactivity of various steroids was calculated, and these are shown for the progesterone antiserum in Table II and for the 20α-dihydroprogesterone antiserum in Table III.

Cross-reaction was determined by calculating the ratio of concentration of unlabeled progesterone (e.g., for the progesterone antiserum) to the test steroid concentration (expressed as a percentage) necessary to produce 50% displacement of the labeled progesterone from the antibody. Both antibodies were highly specific for the steroid used for immunization (see Tables II and III).

Small aliquots of the antibody are stored frozen at a dilution of 1 : 10. For radioimmunoassay, the progesterone antibody is diluted 1 : 1000

Table II   Cross-Reactivity of Progesterone Antiserum to Various Steroids

Steroid	Cross-reactivity(%)[a]
Progesterone	100
20α-Dihydroprogesterone	0.10
17α-Hydroxyprogesterone	0.09
Cortisol	<0.02
Deoxycorticosterone	1.54
Testosterone	<0.02
Dihydrotestosterone	<0.02
Pregnenolone	<0.05
Estradiol-17β	<0.02
Estrone	<0.02
Estriol	<0.02

[a] Based on the ratio of mass of steroid to the mass of progesterone required for 50% displacement ($\times 100$) of labeled progesterone from the antibody.

Table III Cross-Reactivity of 20α-Dihydroprogesterone Antiserum to Various Steroids

Steroid	Cross-reactivity(%)[a]
20α-Dihydroprogesterone	100
17α-Hydroxyprogesterone	0.01
Progesterone	0.40
Pregnenolone	<0.01
Cortisol	<0.01
Deoxycorticosterone	0.05
Testosterone	0.01
Dihydrotestosterone	<0.01
Androstenedione	<0.01
Dehydroepiandrosterone	<0.01
Estradiol	<0.01
Estrone	<0.01
Estriol	<0.01

[a] Based on the ratio of mass of steroid to mass of 20α-dihydroprogesterone required for 50% displacement ($\times 100$) of labeled 20α-dihydroprogesterone from the antibody.

in PBS + 0.1% gel and added in a volume of 0.1 ml to achieve approximately 50% binding. The 20α-dihydroprogesterone antibody is diluted 1:3000. The limit of the sensitivity of the standard curve is 100 pg for progesterone and 50 pg for the 20α-dihydroprogesterone antibody.

E. Source of Label

1,2-³H-Progesterone and 1,2-³H-20α-dihydroprogesterone (specific activity 40–50 Ci/mM) can be purchased from New England Nuclear, Boston, Massachusetts. Approximately 10,000,000 cpm of labeled steroid is removed from the original container and evaporated to dryness in a 150-ml flask.

Five milliliters of PBS + 0.5% gel is added to the flask, which is gently shaken. The volume is brought to 100 ml by addition of 95 ml of PBS + 0.1% gel, and the resulting solution is used as a stock for both recovery and assay trace. The recovery ³H-steroid is added to each sample prior to extraction in a volume of 30 to 50 μl (approximately 3000–5000 cpm). At the same time, an equal volume of the labeled steroid is added to a scintillation vial containing 10 ml Aquasol (New England Nuclear) so that a total count can be obtained for calculation of percentage recovery. When performing the radioimmunoassay, tritiated steroid is added to each assay tube in a volume of 0.1 ml (approximately 10,000 cpm).

F. Preparation of Samples

1. Extraction

Conical glass-stoppered centrifuge tubes (12–50 ml depending on sample size) are rinsed twice with redistilled petroleum ether. Plasma samples, generally 0.25–2.0 ml depending on animal species, sex, and reproductive state, are added to the centrifuge tubes, and approximately 3000–5000 cpm (30–50 μl) of tritiated progesterone is added to correct for procedural losses. (^{3}H-Progesterone may be used to assess recovery for both steroids.)

The samples are extracted once with ten volumes of petroleum ether. The tubes are sealed with polyethylene stoppers and shaken while positioned horizontally in an Eberbach reciprocating shaker (280 excursions/minute) for 30 minutes. Following phase separation by a five-minute centrifugation at 2000 rpm, eight volumes of the petroleum ether are removed and transferred to a disposable round-bottom glass tube. The petroleum ether is evaporated to dryness under nitrogen in a 37°C water bath, and the extract is concentrated by twice rinsing the sides of the tube with small volumes of petroleum ether (0.2 ml), evaporating off the solvent each time.

If no column chromatography is anticipated, the concentrated extracts are redissolved in buffer by adding 1.0 ml PBS + 0.1% gel. The tubes are gently mixed with a Vortex and stored at 4°C overnight. Because of the insolubility of progesterone in aqueous media, we have tested the efficacy of a number of buffer preparations in providing the highest progesterone recovery. Solutions of PBS containing 0.1 or 0.5% gelatin, 0.1% bovine serum albumin, or 0.1% rabbit γ-globulin were tested and found to be equally effective. Although any one of the buffer systems described did not seem to enhance progesterone solubilization, we did find that the volume of buffer and the relationship of the volume of buffer to the surface area of the glass were critical factors in this regard. Detergents or acetone were also found not to be useful because they interfered with the antibody binding. Therefore, we strongly recommend using round-bottom tubes and concentrating the extract prior to buffer addition. The overnight extraction method described above provides a progesterone recovery ranging from 55 to 65%.

2. Column Chromatography

Although it is not necessary for our technique, if necessary, the extract can be further purified on a Sephadex LH-20 column in a manner originally described by Carr *et al.* (1971) and modified by Macdonald *et al.* (1973). Three milliliters of benzene : methanol (90 : 10) containing 0.8 gm Sephadex LH-20 (Pharmacia Fine Chemicals, Piscataway, New Jersey) is transferred to a disposable 10-ml serological pipette (broken off at the 2.0-ml mark) which has previously been fitted with a glass wool plug and rinsed with 5.0 ml of the benzene : methanol solution. The packed column is rinsed with 5.0 ml of the eluting solvent, isooctane : benzene : methanol (90 : 5 : 5), and the dried petroleum ether extract is applied in 0.2 ml of the eluting solvent with a Pasteur pipette. A second 0.2 ml of eluting solvent is used to rinse the tube and to complete the application of the extract. The first three milliliters of eluting solvent allowed to run through the column is discarded; it contains neutral lipids. The second three-milliliter fraction (ml 4–6) contains the progesterone. This eluate is collected in a round-bottom glass tube, evaporated to dryness, concentrated with ether, and redissolved in 1.0 ml PBS + 0.1% gel. Recovery of tritiated progesterone after such purification is approximately 40–50%. If purification of the ^{3}H-progesterone used for recovery and radioimmunoassay is necessary, the above column chromatographic procedure can be used.

G. Assay and Separation Procedures

In addition to the standard and sample tubes, six assay tubes, two labeled "0-0-0" (total cpm), two labeled "0-0" (nonspecific binding), and two labeled "0" (initial binding of antigen by antibody) are prepared. The nonspecific binding tube permits the evaluation of the charcoal separation procedure, and the antiserum-binding tube permits a check on the stability of the antibody. Steps (1) through (5) of the following procedure can be performed at room temperature. Separation steps are carried out at 4°C. The identical procedure is used to assay both progesterone and 20α-dihydroprogesterone. The following procedure is described for progesterone.

1. Antiserum (0.1 ml) (previously diluted to obtain 50% binding-1 : 1000 with our antiserum), is added to all radioimmunoassay tubes except tubes "0-0-0" and "0-0."

2. PBS + 0.1% gel (0.2 ml) is added to the "0-0-0" and "0-0" tubes; 0.1 ml PBS + 0.1% gel is added to the "0" tubes.

3. For the standard curve, 0.1 ml of each of the standard solutions of progesterone (described in Section II,A) is added in duplicate to the radioimmunoassay tubes.

4. Aliquots of the samples to be quantitated for progesterone are added in duplicate in volumes of 0.05 and 0.1 ml. It is important that the volume of the reaction mixture of tubes containing 0.05 ml of sample be adjusted with an additional 0.05 ml of PBS + 0.1% gel. For determination of progesterone loss during extraction, purification, and buffer solubilization, a 0.1-ml aliquot of sample is also removed at this time and counted in 10 ml of Aquasol.

5. All tubes are vortexed and incubated for 30 minutes at room temperature.

6. ^{3}H-Progesterone (0.1 ml) containing approximately 10,000 cpm is added to all tubes. Tubes are then vortexed and incubated at 4°C for 12 to 24 hours.

7. All tubes receive 0.1 ml PBS containing 0.5% gelatin and are mixed by Vortex.

8. Diluted charcoal solution (1.0 ml) is added to all tubes except the "0-0-0" tubes, which receive 1.0 ml PBS + 0.1% gel. All tubes are vortexed and incubated for 15 minutes at 4°C. A stock solution of dextran-coated charcoal composed of 0.25% Dextran T-70 and 2.5% activated Norit A in 0.1 M potassium phosphate buffer, pH 7.4, is diluted 1 : 10 with 0.01 M PBS + 0.1% gel immediately before use. Both charcoal suspensions are constantly mixed on a magnetic stirrer.

9. The tubes are centrifuged at 3000 rpm for ten minutes.

10. Each supernatant fraction is decanted into a scintillation vial containing 10 ml of Aquasol; the vials are shaken and counted for ten minutes or until 10,000 cpm have accumulated.

A computer program (Rodbard and Lewald, 1970) which uses logit and log transformations and linear regression analysis is used for automated calculation of the progesterone in each unknown. Correction for procedural losses is accomplished by calculation of the percentage recovery of tritiated progesterone added to each plasma sample.

III. SENSITIVITY AND PRECISION

A typical progesterone standard curve representing the mean of five standard curves each run in duplicate is shown in Figure 1. The limit of the sensitivity of our assay by applying the definition of two times

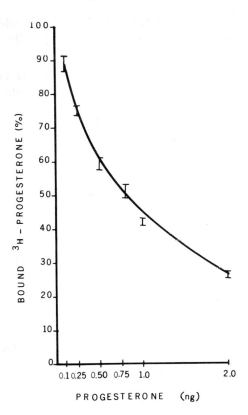

Figure 1. Standard curve for progesterone radioimmunoassay; figure represents the mean of five duplicate standard curves.

the standard deviation of the blank determination results in a reliable quantitation of at least 200 pg progesterone and 100 pg 20α-dihydroprogesterone per milliliter of plasma.

To test the precision and accuracy of the assay, we have measured replicates of buffer samples containing 20 ng progesterone ($n = 5$) and sheep plasma samples containing 10 ng progesterone ($n = 5$). Progesterone measurements in the 20-ng buffer samples averaged 18.80 ± 0.60 (± SEM); those in the 10-ng plasma samples averaged 10.04 ± 0.14. The percentage coefficient of variation between 10- and 20-ng replicates was found to be 3.1 and 7.1%, respectively. For the 20α-dihydroprogesterone assay, the interassay and intrassay coefficients of variation were 12 and 8%, respectively.

To determine the reliability between assays, it is recommended that estimation of progesterone and 20α-dihydroprogesterone in a sample taken from the same plasma pool be performed with each assay. Also in each assay, a buffer or water blank is run to determine whether or not nonspecific factors which produce falsely elevated values are present. To validate the assay and check its accuracy and precision, it is suggested that known amounts of the hormone be added to a number of buffer or plasma blanks and measured repeatedly.

Loraine and Bell (1971) have discussed the limits of variation regarded as satisfactory for quantitative methods. We consider a coefficient of variation of less than 15% acceptable for inter- and intraassay variation.

REFERENCES

Abraham, G. E., Swerdloff, R., Tulchinsky, D., and Odell, W. D. (1971). Radioimmunoassay of plasma progesterone. *J. Clin. Endocrinol. Metab.* **32**, 619–624.

Abraham, G. E., Manlimos, F. S., Solis, M., Garza, R., and Maroulis, G. B. (1975). Combined radioimmunoassay of four steroids in one ml of plasma. I. Progestins. *Clin. Biochem.* **8**, 369–373.

Anderson, G. W., Zimmerman, J. E., and Callahan, F. M. (1964). The use of esters of N-hydroxy succinimide in peptide synthesis. *J. Am. Chem. Soc.* **86**, 1839–1842.

Batra, S. (1976). New simplified procedures for the determination of progesterone by competitive protein binding and radioimmunoassay. *J. Steroid Biochem.* **7**, 131–134.

Bodley, F. H., Chapdelaine, A., Flickinger, G., Mikhail, G., Yaverbaum, S., and Roberts, K. D. (1972). A highly specific radioimmunoassay for progesterone using antibodies covalently linked to acrylamine-glass particles. *Steroids* **21**, 1–16.

Carr, B. R., Mikhail, G., and Flickinger, G. L. (1971). Column chromatography of steroids on Sephadex LH-20. *J. Clin. Endocrinol. Metab.* **33**, 358–360.

DeVilla, G. O., Jr., Roberts, K., Wiest, W. G., Mikhail, G., and Flickinger, G. (1972). A specific radioimmunoassay of plasma progesterone. *J. Clin. Endocrinol. Metab.* **35**, 458–460.

Furuyama, S., and Nugent, C. A. (1971). A radioimmunoassay for plasma progesterone. *Steroids* **17**, 633–674.

Heap, R. B. (1964). A flourescence assay of progesterone. *J. Endocrinol.* **30**, 293–305.

Johansson, E. D. B. (1969). Progesterone levels in peripheral plasma during the luteal phase of the normal human menstrual cycle measured by a rapid competitive protein binding technique. *Acta Endocrinol. (Copenhagen)* **61**, 592–606.

Loraine, J. A., and Bell, E. T. (1971). "Hormone Assays and Their Clinical Application," 3rd ed. Williams & Wilkins, Baltimore, Maryland.

Lurie, A. O., and Patterson, R. J. (1970). Progesterone in nonpregnancy plasma. An assay method for the clinical chemistry laboratory. *Cin. Chem.* **16**, 856–860.

Macdonald, G. J., Yoshinaga K., and Greep, R. O. (1973). Progesterone values in monkeys near term. *Am. J. Phys. Anthropol.* **38**, 201–206.

Murphy, B. E. P. (1967). Some studies of the protein-binding of steroids and their application to the routine micro and ultramicro measurement of various steroids in body fluids by competitive protein binding radioassay. *J. Clin. Endocrinol. Metab.* **27**, 973–990.

Neill, J. D., Johansson, E. D. B., Datta, J. K., and Knobil, E. (1967). Relationship between the plasma levels of luteinizing hormone and progesterone during the normal menstrual cycle. *J. Clin. Endocrinol. Metab.* **27**, 1167–1173.

Niswender, G. D., and Midgley, A. R., Jr. (1970). Hapten-radioimmunoassay for steroid hormones. *In* "Immunologic Methods in Steroid Determination" (F. G. Perón and B. V. Caldwell, eds.), Chapter 8, pp. 149–173. Appleton, New York.

Riondel, A., Tait, J. F., Tait, S. A. S., Gut, M., and Little B. (1965). Estimation of progesterone in human peripheral blood using 35S-thiosemicarbazide. *J. Clin. Endocrinol. Metab.* **25**, 229–242.

Rodbard, D., and Lewald, J. E. (1970). Computer analysis of radioligand assay and radioimmunoassay data. *Proc. 2nd Symp. Steroid Assay by Protein Binding*, pp. 79–103. Karolinska Institute, Stockholm.

Scarisbrick, J. J., and Cameron, E. II. D. (1975). Radioimmunoassay of progesterone: comparison of [1,2,6,7-3H$_4$]-progesterone and progesterone-^{125}I-iodohistamine radioligands. *J. Steroid Biochem.* **6**, 51–56.

Spieler, J. M., Webb, R. L., Saldarini, R. J., and Coppola, J. A. (1972). A radioimmunoassay for progesterone. *Steroids* **19**, 751–762.

van der Molen, H. J., and Aakvaag, A. (1967). Progesterone. *In* "Hormones in Blood" (C. H. Gray and A. L. Bacharach, eds.), Chapter VI, pp. 221–303. Academic Press, New York.

van der Molen, H. J., and Groen, D. (1965). Determination of progesterone human peripheral blood using gas-liquid chromatography with electron capture detection. *J. Clin. Endocrinol. Metab.* **25**, 1625–1639.

Youssefnejadian, E., Florensa, E., Collins, W. P., and Sommerville, I. F. (1972). Radioimmunoassay of plasma progesterone. *J. Steroid Biochem.* **3**, 893–901.

36

Androgens: Testosterone and Dihydrotestosterone

FREDERICK J. AULETTA, BURTON V. CALDWELL,
AND GERALD L. HAMILTON

I. INTRODUCTION

Indirect measurement of androgenic function by quantitating urinary 17-ketosteroids is time-consuming and is rather nonspecific. The measurement of androgens in peripheral plasma has been limited, until recently, to laboratories using rather sophisticated techniques such as double isotope derivative methods (Bardin and Lipsett, 1967). Following the same procedures used for the development of radioimmunoassays for estrogens (Hotchkiss *et al.*, 1971; Wu and Lundy, 1971), investigators soon turned to generating antibodies to testosterone and described several assay systems for the measurement of

715

this steroid in peripheral plasma (Furuyama *et al.*, 1970; Coyotupa *et al.*, 1972; Ismail *et al.*, 1972; Bartke *et al.*, 1973). These techniques are rapid, specific, and reliable. The purpose of this chapter is to present our method for the extraction, chromatographic separation, and quantitative determination of testosterone and dihydrotestosterone (DHT) as used in research studies and for the evaluation of clinical samples. We will present, in complete detail, all of the steps required to validate an assay and to establish this procedure in any laboratory possessing the suitable antibody.

II. METHOD OF RADIOIMMUNOASSAY

A. Preparation of Testosterone–Protein Conjugate and Immunization Procedure

To induce the antibody used in our laboratory, the immunizing conjugate was prepared by the covalent binding through the 3-oxime linkage of testosterone with bovine serum albumin as previously reported by Erlanger *et al.* (1957). This conjugation reaction is difficult and requires chemical expertise. BSA–testosterone conjugates are commercially available from Steroids, Inc., Pawling, New York, and the use of these conjugates is suggested. Rabbits are immunized once a week for four weeks with 1.0 ml (1.0 mg) of conjugate divided into four subcutaneous injection sites as an emulsion with saline and complete Freund's adjuvant 1 : 1. Monthly boosters are administered without Freund's adjuvant. Animals are bled seven to ten days later. This procedure should yield antibodies useful for the radioimmunoassay of testosterone. Suitable antibodies are also available commercially from Calbiochem Co., San Diego, California.

B. Characterization of Antiserum

1. Titer and Affinity

The titer and affinity of any antiserum set the practical limits for its use in any assay system. The principal factor associated with titer is the number of assays which can be performed with a given supply. However, the degree to which the antiserum can be diluted also may be important in that with increasing dilution of the antibody, the extraneous proteins are also diluted, usually beyond any significant level, yielding a reasonably purified solution of highly specific antibody. It is often possible to increase the apparent titer of a given antiserum by preliminary treatment with a dextran-coated charcoal solution. When charcoal is stirred for 6–12 hours in the antiserum (500 mg/100 ml) most of the endogenous steroid is "stripped" from the antibody so that the titer may increase two- to fivefold.

The affinity of the antiserum usually dictates the procedure employed for the separation of free from antibody-bound steroid. A double antibody system, or other procedures which remove the antibody-bound fraction, can be used with antiserum of poor affinity. However, dextran-coated charcoal or procedures which remove the free fraction of the equilibration reaction can only be employed with high-affinity antiserum. The reason for this fact can be better appreciated by referring to the equilibrium reaction below:

$$Ab + {}^3H\text{-}T \leftrightarrows Ab\text{--}{}^3H\text{-}T$$

It can be seen that procedures which remove the bound fraction (Ab–^{3}H-T) leave only the free (^{3}H-T) remaining, and no further reaction can occur (antibody is limited in this reaction and is virtually all removed by precipitation with second antibody). On the other hand, procedures which remove only the free steroid (^{3}H-T) allow a new equilibrium to be established as the antibody-bound steroid is released. In high-affinity antiserum, this is not a serious problem; however, each antiserum must be carefully evaluated to determine whether this "stripping" action of dextran-coated charcoal may be a limitation. It will be noted that in the present assay system an equilibrium period of 15 minutes is proposed in order to minimize the "stripping" action of the charcoal.

2. Specificity

The specificity of any antisera dictates the chromatographic procedures which are necessary to ensure specificity in the assay. The testosterone antisera (used in this method) showed a high degree of specificity for both testosterone and DHT (Figure 1) with a 2% cross-reaction with androstenedione. Since there are no anti-DHT antibodies, and the anti-testosterone antisera cannot distinguish well between DHT and testosterone, the chromatographic procedure used in this assay was developed primarily to separate testosterone and DHT (Figure 2). This separation procedure allows the measurement of DHT and testosterone in separate chromatographic samples using the same antisera.

The specificity of any antiserum prepared from the same conjugate may vary from animal to animal and from bleeding to bleeding; there-

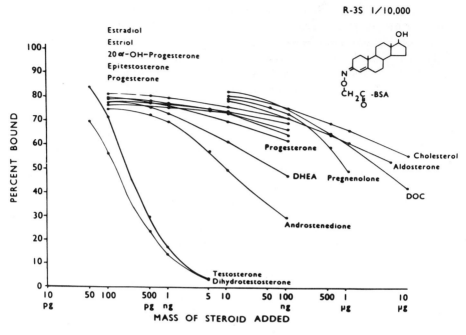

Figure 1.   Cross-reactions of various steroids showing displacement curves compared against testosterone. ³H-Testosterone was used as the tracer. See text for details.

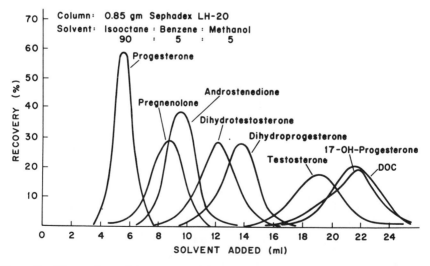

Figure 2.   Chromatographic separation of neutral steroids on Sephadex LH-20 column. See text for details.

fore, it is essential to characterize and recheck each bleeding for specificity.

C. Extraction

In devising a method for the extraction and chromatography of steroids, there are four objectives which should be considered. The procedure should be efficient (65–75% recovery of both testosterone and DHT through the method), specific, reproducible, and reasonably rapid and simple.

Figure 3 shows the flow sheet for the extraction, chromatography, and assay of testosterone and DHT.

For the extraction from small amounts of blood the following steps should be followed:

1. To a 10-ml extraction tube, add approximately 1000 cpm of tritium-labeled testosterone and/or DHT, whichever is to be measured. The tracer should be added in 0.1 ml of buffer G ($0.15\,M$ NaCl, $0.1\,M$ phosphate, pH 7.4, containing 0.1% γ-globulin).

2. Add plasma (0.2 ml for male, 1.0 ml for female) to the extraction tube and gently shake to ensure solubility of tracer androgen.

3. Extract the sample vigorously with 4.0 ml of anhydrous ether (for 60 seconds) and centrifuge the tube at 1200 g for five minutes. Repeat the extraction with 4.0 ml anhydrous ether and centrifugation.

4. Pool the ether extracts in a conical centrifuge tube and dry under air.

5. Concentrate the androgen samples by washing the walls of the centrifuge tube with 1.0 ml of ether. Evaporate.

D. Column Chromatography

The major factor in chromatography is the complete separation of testosterone and DHT from the remaining neutral steroids; this, however, is normally a function of the specificity of the antisera. The best method of accomplishing group separation was found to be the Sephadex LH-20 "minicolumns." This proved to be the best method because it was rapid, reliable, and gave good separation, good efficiency of recovery, and most important did not produce a "blank" in the radioimmunoassay method. (Figure 2 shows the elution pattern for the separation of the neural steroids.)

1. Sephadex LH-20 (0.85 gm; 100 mesh, Mallinckrodt) is slurried in solvent I (benzene : methanol, 85 : 15) and pipetted into a 1.0 × 16

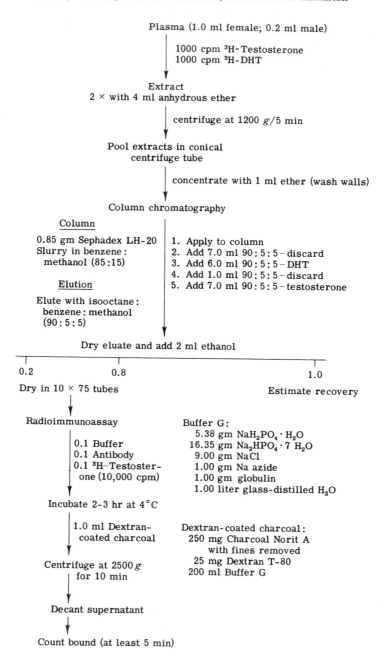

Figure 3.   Flow sheet for radioimmunoassay of androgens.

cm glass column Brock mini-columns, Macalaster-Bicknell, New Haven, Connecticut) plugged with a circle of GF/A Whatman glass-fiber filter paper, which had been previously rinsed with methanol.

2. After all of solvent I has passed through the column, add approximately 8 ml of solvent II (isooctane : benzene : methanol, 90 : 5 : 5) and allow it to rinse through the column to saturate the Sephadex; a second circle of glass-fiber filter paper is then positioned at the top of the Sephadex.

3. To the pooled extracts in the centrifuge tube add 0.2 ml solvent II, vortex (10–15 seconds), and apply to top of Sephadex column. Repeat using 0.2 ml solvent II, and allow the column to run dry.

4. The elution and collecting pattern can be seen in the following tabulation:

Volume solvent II added (ml)	Total solvent added (ml)	Fraction[a]
7.0	7.0	Discard
6.0	13.0	DHT
1.0	14.0	Discard
7.0	21.0	Testo

[a] Collection of DHT and testosterone (Testo) should be made in scintillation vials.

5. All recoveries will be in the 65–85% range.

E. Assay Incubation

1. The radioimmunoassay is performed in 10×75 mm glass disposable culture tubes. Stock solutions of DHT and testosterone, 1.0 mg/ml in ethanol, are dried, taken up in buffer G, and are aliquoted in duplicate through a concentration of 0.01 to 1.0 ng in 0.1 ml (standard curve) including a water blank and plasma pool. For testosterone radioimmunoassay, testosterone serves as standard; DHT determinations are based on DHT standards.

2. The DHT and the testosterone fractions from the column are dried and dissolved in 2.0 ml of 100% ethanol and 0.2 and 0.8 ml are aliquoted into 10×75 mm disposable culture tubes and dried.

3. The remaining 1.0 ml of each is dried and counted for recovery (after the assay has been counted to ensure the samples are within the range of the standard curve).

4. When all sample tubes are dried, 0.1 ml of buffer G is added to each tube.

5. Anti-testosterone antiserum (0.1 ml in buffer G, diluted so that

maximum dilution used at 50% binding) and approximately 10,000 cpm of ^{3}H-T 40–60 Ci/mM, in 0.1 ml of buffer G are then added to each tube in both testosterone and DHT assays to bring the final volume to 0.3 ml. ^{3}H-DHT is not used in DHT assays because it is available only with much lower specific activity than is ^{3}H-testosterone.

6. Vortex for 15 to 20 seconds to ensure thorough mixing and allow to equilibrate at 4°C for two to three hours.

7. After incubation, 1.0 ml dextran-coated charcoal (see Figure 3) is added within 45 seconds (vortex 2–3 seconds).

8. After 15 minutes of equilibrium (from first tube in which charcoal was added) centrifuge at 2500 g for ten minutes.

9. The supernatant is decanted directly into scintillation vials and 10 ml of Aquasol (New England Nuclear) is added.

10. Radioactivity is determined with 30% efficiency on a Packard Tricarb Scintillation Counter, Model 3375.

11. Quantitations of samples are determined using a logit plot with linear regression analysis (Figure 4). The equation for determination of logit values is $L = \ln(p/100p)$ where p = total count bound (sample) $\times$ 100/total counts bound (blank).

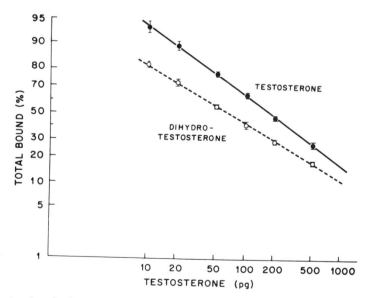

Figure 4. Standard curves for testosterone and dihydrotestosterone using a logit transformation of the data as described in the text.

III. VALIDATION OF ASSAY

Figure 4 shows a logit transformation of a typical standard curve for DHT and testosterone. The normal range of linearity for both these steroids is between 10 and 500 pg. As can be seen by the standard deviation the variation of less than 10% can be achieved at any point along the curve.

The principal procedure for the validation of any assay involves the addition of known amounts of the substance to be measured to a previously determined plasma sample. Tables I and II show the results of such a procedure for varying amounts of testosterone and dihydrotestosterone added to a low-level plasma pool. Acceptable values for this type of procedure should be within 15% of the expected amount.

Once the procedure described above has been successfully achieved, the next step is to determine the intraassay reliability. This is accomplished by repeated estimation of a plasma pool sample. Again the coefficient of variation should not exceed 15%. The interassay reliability should be continually assessed by measuring the same plasma pool with every assay; values should fall within the 15% limit of varia-

Table I   Radioimmunoassay of Known Amounts of Testosterone Added to Plasma

Testosterone added (ng)	N	Plasma volume (ml)	Plasma level of testosterone measured[a] mean ± SD (ng)
0.00	4	0.4	0.0212 ± 0.0069
0.50	5	0.4	0.4826 ± 0.0786
1.00	5	0.4	1.0864 ± 0.1885
5.00	4	0.4	5.0375 ± 0.1995

[a] Corrected for recovery; uncorrected for plasma endogenous level. Total mean ± SD: 86.40 ± 9.21% for recovery.

Table II   Radioimmunoassay of Known Amounts of DHT Added to Plasma

DHT added (ng)	N	Plasma volume (ml)	Plasma level of DHT measured[a] mean ± SD (ng)
0.00	4	0.4	0.0005 ± 0.0006
0.50	5	0.4	0.4354 ± 0.0701
1.00	5	0.4	1.0466 ± 0.0722
5.00	5	0.4	4.8342 ± 0.1109

[a] Corrected for recovery; uncorrected for plasma endogenous level. Total mean ± SD: 77.42 ± 11.86% for recovery.

tion. It is also advisable to measure either a "blank" plasma or water with each assay to ensure that no extraneous factors may be contributing to the values obtained. When all of these conditions are met, the investigator can be reasonably assured that the assay is reliable and reproducible.

IV. NORMAL VALUES

These assays are currently being employed in this laboratory for the evaluation of gonadal function in men and women and as an aid in the diagnosis of hirsutism. Figure 5 shows values of testosterone and DHT in normal females during the menstrual cycle and menopause. Figure 6 shows these steroid levels in different age males.

Figure 7 shows the testosterone levels before and after treatment with oral progestational agents in hirsute women. As can be seen, the levels decreased from a pretreatment mean of 1.0 ng/ml to 0.2 ng/ml after treatment. This decrease was consistent with chemical findings with decreased hirsutism.

As more information about levels of testosterone and dihydrotestosterone become available in endocrine dysfunction, it is probable that the assay will find greater use in clinical evaluations.

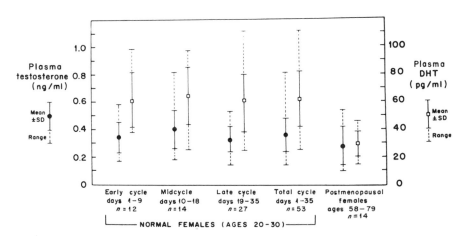

Figure 5. Normal values for testosterone and dihydrotestosterone in women at different times of the estrous cycle using the method described herein.

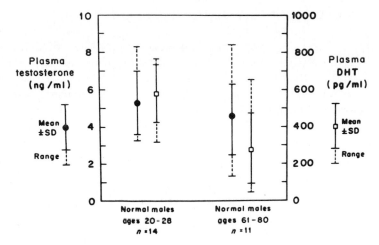

Figure 6.   Plasma testosterone and dehydrotestosterone in men.

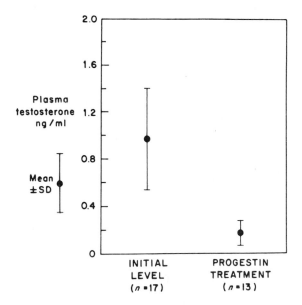

Figure 7.   Plasma testosterone in hirsute women before and after treatment with progestational agents. (Reproduced from Speroff *et al.*, 1973, with permission of the publishers.)

V. OTHER ANDROGENS—ANDROSTENEDIONE

As determined by other means, androstenedione circulates in plasma in significant concentrations; in males they average 0.6–0.9 ng/ml, while in women they average 1.0–3.0 ng/ml (Eberlein *et al.*, 1967). The low degree of androstenedione cross-reactivity with our anti-testosterone antibodies precludes their use in androstenedione radioimmunoassay. Jeffcoate (1971) has described an androstenedione radioimmunoassay, but further evaluation of the importance of this androgen depends on the development of specific techniques by other investigators interested in androgenic function.

REFERENCES

Bardin, C. W., and Lipsett, M. B. (1967). Estimation of testosterone and androstenedione in human peripheral plasma. *Steroids* 9, 71–84.

Bartke, A., Steel, R. E., Musto, N., and Caldwell, B. V. (1973). Fluctuations in plasma testosterone levels in adult male rats and mice. *Endocrinology* 92, 1223–1228.

Coyotupa, J., Parlow, A. F., and Abraham, G. E. (1972). Simultaneous radioimmunoassay of plasma for testosterone and dihydrotestosterone. *Anal. Lett.* 5, 329–337.

Eberlein, W. R., Winter, J., and Rosenfeld, R. L. (1967). The androgens. *In* "Hormones in the Blood" (C. II. Grey and A. L. Bachrach, eds.), pp. 187–220. Academic Press, New York.

Erlanger, B. F., Borek, F., Beiser, S. M., and Lieberman, S. (1957). Steroid–protein conjugates. 1. Preparation and characterization of conjugates of bovine serum albumin with testosterone and with cortisone. *J. Biol. Chem.* 228, 713–727.

Furuyama, S., Mayes, D. M., and Nugent, C. A. (1970). A radioimmunoassay for plasma testosterone. *Steroids* 16, 415–428.

Hotchkiss, J., Atkinson, L. E., and Knobil, E. (1971). Time course of serum estrogen and luteinizing hormone during the menstrual cycle of the rhesus monkey. *Endocrinology* 89, 177–183.

Ismail, A. A. A., Niswender, G. D., and Midgley, A. R. (1972). Radioimmunoassay of testosterone without chromatography. *J. Clin. Endocrinol. Metab.* 34, 177–184.

Jeffcoate, S. L. (1971). A Radioimmunoassay for testosterone, androstenedione, and other 3-oxo-4-unsaturated steroids. *J. Endocrinol.* 49, 2–3.

Speroff, L., Glass, R. H., and Kase, N. G. (1973). "Clinical Gynecologic Endocrinology and Infertility," p. 66. Williams & Wilkins, Baltimore, Maryland.

Wu, C.-H., and Lundy, L. E. (1971). Radioimmunoassay of plasma estrogens. *Steroids* 18, 91–111.

37

Radioiodinated Steroid Hormones—General Principles

KENT PAINTER AND GORDON D. NISWENDER

I. INTRODUCTION

Current radioimmunoassay methods for the quantification of steroid hormones are based on the pioneering studies of Erlanger *et al.* (1958), who first described the synthesis of steroid–protein conjugates for use as immunogens. In 1969, antibodies were first used for the quantification of testosterone (Niswender and Midgley, 1969) and estradiol (Abraham, 1969; Midgley *et al.*, 1969), and numerous assays for steroid hormones followed. Many of the initial radioimmunoassays for steroid hormones utilized commercially available tritiated steroids. However, the early work of Oliver *et al.* (1968) with digitoxin indicated that haptens could be conjugated to tyrosine moieties, which can be radioiodinated. Subsequently, many radioimmunoassays were de-

Methods of Hormone Radioimmunoassay, Second Edition

Table I   A Partial Listing of γ-Labeled Steroid Radioimmunoassays

Steroid	Reference
Cortisol	Malvano *et al.* (1973), Chambers *et al.* (1975, p. 177), Fahmy *et al.* (1975), Hasler *et al.* (1976)
Estradiol	Niswender *et al.* (1970), Comoglio *et al.* (1974), England *et al.* (1974), Lindberg *et al.* (1974), Edwards *et al.* (1974), Hunter *et al.* (1975)
Estrone	Niswender *et al.* (1970), Kato *et al.* (1974)
Progesterone	Niswender *et al.* (1970), Niswender (1973), Cameron *et al.* (1975)
Testosterone	Midgley *et al.* (1970), Cameron *et al.* (1974), Edwards *et al.* (1974)

veloped utilizing radioiodinated steroid derivatives (Table I). In this chapter we review previous developments, general principles, and the current status of radioimmunoassay techniques using radioiodinated steroid hormones.

II. ADVANTAGES AND DISADVANTAGES OF RADIOIODINATED STEROIDS

With the exception of phenolic estrogens, it is not practical to radioiodinate steroid molecules directly. Therefore, these compounds must be conjugated to moieties, such as tyramine, tyrosine, histamine, and histidine, which can be easily radioiodinated. There are a number of advantages for the utilization of a radioiodinated form of steroid for radioimmunoassays. The primary impetus for research in this area was to gain increased sensitivity due to the high specific activity that could be obtained with these compounds. A comparison of specific activities, half-lives, and typical mass added to each assay tube for common isotopes is listed in Table II. Radioiodinated forms of steroid hormones permit the use of considerably less mass of radioactive antigen, resulting in a more sensitive assay system if the affinity of the antibody is not a limiting factor. The decreased mass of radioactive steroid also results in a saving of antiserum, since less antibody is needed for each assay tube. The higher specific activity of the radioiodinated steroid allows the addition of more counts per minute (i.e., 30,000 to 60,000 cpm) to each assay tube, thereby reducing the counting time necessary to obtain reliable counting statistics. The use of radioiodinated steroid hormones allows more economical counting

Table II   A Comparison of the Utility of Common Radionuclides for the Radioimmunoassay of Steroid Hormones

Nuclide	^{14}C	^{3}H	^{125}I	^{131}I	^{75}Sc
Half-life	5,600 years	12.3 years	60 days	8.1 days	120 days
Decay mode	Beta	Beta	X-ray	Beta, gamma	Gamma
Counting method	LSC[a]	LSC	LSC, SS[b]	LSC, SS	SS
Counting efficiency (%)	90	30	70	90	85
S_{max}(Ci/mA)[c]	0.062	29	2,160	16,000	1,100
Commercial isotopic abundance (%)	100	100	100	20	3
No. radioactive atoms/molecule	1.0	4.0	1.0	1.0	1.0
S_p(Ci/mmole)[d]	0.062	174	2,160	3,200	40
Tracer mass per 10,000 cpm (pg)[e]	2.4×10^5	40	0.89	0.53	40
Count loss (one month) (%)	0	0	29	92	15

[a] LSC, liquid scintillation counting.

[b] SS, solid (NaI) well crystal scintillation counting.

[c] S_{max}, theoretical maximum specific activity per atom replaced.

[d] S_p, practical specific activity (accounting for number of atoms/molecule; isotopic abundance).

[e] The calculation of tracer mass assumes 10,000 cpm are required for totals, and takes into account the number of atoms per molecule labeled, commercial isotopic abundance, and counting efficiency.

by eliminating the necessity of transfer to a separate vial and the addition of scintillation fluid. Finally, in assays in which it is necessary to monitor procedural losses, use of tritiated steroids for this purpose does not influence quantification of the radioiodine by gamma counting.

There are also several disadvantages to the use of radioiodinated steroids. The chemistry necessary to synthesize these compounds can be quite complex. Due to the relatively short half-life of radioiodine, the derivatives must be radioiodinated frequently, but once radioiodinated, these compounds appear quite stable (Niswender, 1975). Although assays employing radioiodinated steroids are generally more sensitive, in many cases the increased sensitivity may be of no real advantage or may be a disadvantage.

A more serious problem, bridge binding, is frequently observed when radioiodinated analogs are used. If one prepares an immunogen through an intermediate identical to the radioiodinated derivative, the antiserum can recognize the linking moiety or chemical bridge between hapten and histamine or tyrosine analog. The result can be a system in which the antibody binds the radioiodinated steroid analog with much greater affinity than the unmodified steroid. Therefore, the addition of steroid will not inhibit the binding of the radioactive analog, and the laws of mass action no longer apply (Niswender, 1975; Hunter *et al.*, 1975). This problem can usually be solved by changing the chemical derivative used for conjugation to tyrosine methyl ester (TME) or histamine (i.e., if the antibody is made to estradiol-11β-succinyl–BSA, then use an estradiol-11α-succinyl–TME (Figure 1), or if the antibody is made to progesterone-11α-carbonyl–BSA, then use a progesterone-11α-succinyl–TME (Figure 2).

A second approach may be used to solve the problem. The antibody and standard or sample are allowed to react for a substantial period of time, and the radioiodinated steroid is added for a short time (5–15 minutes). Separation of antibody-bound from free radioactivity is effected rapidly (Figure 1). Under these conditions, the radioiodinated steroid binds to the unbound antibody sites, but does not displace the bound steroid originating from the samples or standards. Such procedures, referred to as nonequilibrium or sequential addition assays,

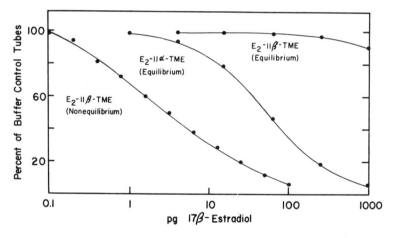

Figure 1. Standard inhibition curves obtained using an antiserum produced against estradiol-17β,11α-succinyl–BSA. Up to 1.0 ng of standard estradiol-17β was not able to compete with estradiol-17β,11α-succinyl–^{125}I-TME when the radioiodinated analog and the estradiol-17β were added at the same time (equilibrium assay conditions). However, when the standard estradiol-17β was allowed to react with the antibody for at least two hours and the estradiol-17β,11α-succinyl–^{125}I-TME was added and allowed to react for only 15 minutes (nonequilibrium assay conditions), the resultant assay was very sensitive. Under these conditions it is necessary that radioactive steroid bound to antibody be separated from free radioactive steroid very rapidly (dextran-coated charcoal, polyethylene glycol). Standard estradiol-17β was able to compete effectively with estradiol-17β, 11α-succinyl–^{125}I-TME for binding to the antibody.

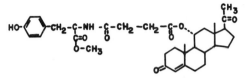

PROGESTERONE-11α-CHLOROCARBONATE-TME

PROGESTERONE - 11α-HEMISUCCINATE - TME

(a)

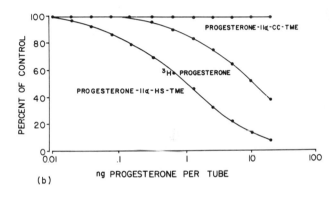

(b)

Figure 2. (a) The structures of two progesterone–tyrosine methyl ester derivatives. (b) A comparison of standard inhibition curves obtained using three different radioactive forms of progesterone in combination with an antiserum prepared against progesterone-11α-carbonyl-BSA.

have been used for a long time to increase the sensitivity of radioimmunoassays for protein hormones.

Although this chapter will concentrate on the use of ^{125}I, two other γ-labeled nuclides have been used in radioimmunoassay. Labeling with ^{131}I has been employed by methodologies analogous to the ^{125}I technique. However, ^{131}I is of little practical value due to its short (8.1 days) half-life; ^{125}I has a 60-day half-life, which reduces the necessity for frequent radioiodinations. Although the theoretical maximum specific activity of ^{131}I is approximately seven times greater than ^{125}I, the commercial isotopic abundance of ^{131}I is rarely above 20% (Table

II). Since ^{125}I is available in almost isotopically pure form, the resulting specific activities are very similar. For the above reasons, ^{131}I has not been generally applied to radioimmunoassays for steroid hormones. Selenium-75 has also been used (Chambers *et al.*, 1975), but its use also is limited due to low commercial isotopic enrichment. Further limitations include laborious syntheses and the toxicity of selenium and its nonradioactive daughter, arsenic.

The number of radioiodinated steroid analogs available commercially is increasing rapidly, thus eliminating the major disadvantages associated with the use of these compounds. For laboratories routinely radioiodinating protein hormones, radioiodinated steroids are easily integrated into the schedule once the precursor has been synthesized and a suitable purification scheme has been devised.

III. PREPARATION OF THE STEROID ANALOGS FOR RADIOIODINATION

Erlanger *et al.* (1967) reviewed methods of coupling haptens to proteins which involve the synthesis of a reactive intermediate. These intermediates can also be conjugated to a variety of molecules for radioiodination (Figure 3). Although the examples shown relate to steroids, similar techniques have been applied to amino acids, peptides, nucleic acids, cyclic nucleotides, and drugs.

Progesterone analogs can be prepared from commercially available 11α-hydroxyprogesterone, as shown in Figure 3. Since the precursor contains only one hydroxyl group in the C ring, the reaction is quantitative with no undesirable by-products. Cortisol (Figure 3) is an example of a more involved synthesis in which selective reaction conditions are employed due to the existence of three hydroxyl groups and two keto groups (Hasler *et al.*, 1976). Derivatization conditions must be employed which selectively produce cortisol-3-carboxymethyl oxime, followed by condensation with histidine methyl ester.

IV. RADIOIODINATION OF STEROID HORMONES

A. Direct Radioiodination Methods

After the steroid derivative has been synthesized, it may be radioiodinated by direct or indirect methods. The most popular

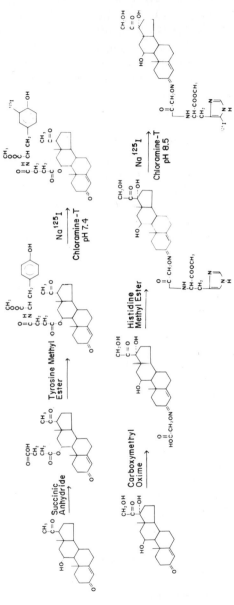

Figure 3. A schematic representation of the reaction sequence for the preparation of radioiodinated progesterone-11α-succinyl tyrosine methyl ester (above) and cortisol-3-carboxymethyl oxime histidine methyl ester (below).

method is the direct chloramine-T procedure (Midgley *et al.*, 1971) modified from the original method of Greenwood *et al.* (1963). This procedure has been used extensively for many steroids; however, it cannot be used for estrogens which contain an easily radioiodinated phenolic A ring. Due to the dimension of the iodine atom, which is approximately the same as the A ring in estrogens, direct addition of iodine to the A ring results in a preparation which is sterically hindered from binding to most anti-estrogen antibodies. This problem can usually be avoided by employing indirect radioiodination procedures, using a procedure, such as adsorption or ion exchange chromatography, which separates the different radioiodinated species and using the radioactive steroid which retains its ability to bind to antibody, or synthesis of an analog which contains a component such as N,N-dimethyl-p-phenylenediamine, which radioiodinates approximately 2000 times more easily than the phenolic A ring in estrogens. However, spontaneous deiodination is a problem with N,N-dimethyl-p-phenylenediamine compounds unless stored in chloroform.

B. Indirect Radioiodination Methods

Recently, methods have been developed whereby reactive derivatives of tyrosine, tyramine, histamine, and histidine are radioiodinated, purified, and then reacted with the steroid derivative (indirect radioiodination methods). One method is based upon the Bolton–Hunter procedure (Bolton and Hunter, 1973) for radioiodinating labile proteins. Using this procedure, a succinimidyl tyrosine or similar analog is radioiodinated by the chloramine-T procedure and reacted directly with compounds containing an amine group. The advantages of the procedure are that redox reagents are not in contact with sensitive steroidal compounds, and a single radioiodination can be performed to produce a sensitive reactive radioiodinated species which will react with any protein or amine-containing hapten by simply mixing in water at room temperature. Recently, compounds similar in concept to the Bolton–Hunter reagent have been described (Wood *et al.*, 1975).

Nars and Hunter (1973) have described an indirect mixed anhydride procedure for coupling radioiodinated histamine to estrogens which contain phenolic A rings. An example of this procedure is shown in Figure 4.

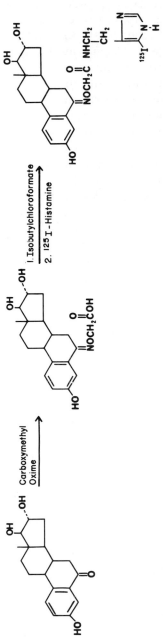

Figure 4. A schematic representation of the reaction sequence for the indirect radioiodination of estriol by the preparation of estriol-6-carboxymethyl oxime ^{125}I-histamine.

V. PURIFICATION OF RADIOIODINATED STEROID HORMONES

Following direct radioiodination procedures there is a mixture of free radioiodine, unreacted steroid precursor, and monoiodinated and diiodinated forms of radioactive analog present in the reaction mixture. To achieve maximal specific activity, the nonradioactive steroid and free radioiodine must be separated from the radioiodinated analog. Ion exchange or gel filtration chromatography, polyacrylamide gel electrophoresis, and thin-layer chromatography are commonly employed for this purpose (Hasler *et al.*, 1976; Hunter *et al.*, 1975; Niswender, 1973).

In the radioiodination of histamine and tyrosine analogs, mono- and diiodinated products are frequently formed. It is often desirable to purify and utilize one of these products. For radioimmunoassays performed directly on serum, the monoiodinated analogs are usually preferred, since they bind less avidly to serum proteins than the diiodo analogs. However, the diiodinated derivative will result in a twofold greater specific activity, which may be desirable in situations requiring sensitivity. Monoiodo and diiodo analogs can be separated using ion exchange or thin-layer chromatography. When indirect radioiodination procedures are used, it is necessary to separate the unreacted steroid derivative, the unreacted radioactive tyrosine or histamine derivative, free radioiodine, and the radioactive steroid analog. This can be accomplished using procedures similar to those described for direct radioiodination techniques.

VI. DEVELOPMENT AND/OR ADAPTATION OF RADIOIMMUNOASSAY PROCEDURES

Any research or clinical laboratory which uses radioimmunoassay procedures must demonstrate that the assay reliably measures the hormone to be quantified. This is true regardless of whether the reagents are produced within the laboratory or are provided from other sources. Even the performance of a commercial kit should be carefully checked before it is used for routine procedures. One of the most important decisions to be made in the development of radioimmunoassays for steroid hormones is the selection of a method for separation of antibody-bound and free radioactivity. The ideal method should provide a clean separation and be unaffected by serum or other nonspecific interferences in the reaction mixture. In addition, the method should be rapid, simple, reproducible, and inexpensive. The methods of separation most commonly employed are solid-phase antibodies (Abraham, 1969; Mikhail et al., 1970), solid-phase adsorption of antibody (Moore and Axelrod, 1972; Bodley et al., 1973; Bizollon et al., 1974), solid-phase adsorption of antigen (Herbert et al., 1965), chemical precipitation of antigen–antibody complexes (Mayes et al., 1970; Desbuquois and Aurbach, 1971), and immunoprecipitation of antigen–antibody complexes (Niswender, 1973; England et al., 1974). The advantages and disadvantages of each of these procedures have been reviewed (Niswender et al., 1975a).

Specificity of a radioimmunoassay, the characteristic which ultimately determines its usefulness, may be defined as the freedom from interference by substances other than the steroid intended to be measured. The specificity of antisera against steroids is dependent upon the site through which the steroid molecule is conjugated to protein (Niswender et al., 1975b; Niswender, 1973). To assess the specificity of an antiserum, the first step is to determine the ability of related steroidal compounds to inhibit the binding of the radioactive steroid to antibody. The final test of specificity is to demonstrate close agreement between estimates of steroid content in various samples by radioimmunoassay and by totally different well-established procedures, such as gas–liquid chromatography or double isotope derivative techniques. This agreement should exist in a reasonable number of samples obtained from subjects in a variety of physiological states. Alternatively, when double isotope derivative or gas–liquid chromatographic procedures are not available or practical, it is possible to compare radioimmunoassay estimates before and after chromatographic purification of the steroid in the sample. However, it should be obvious that this procedure is only as reliable as the purification technique employed and that proof of specificity is necessary for each class of samples to be analyzed, i.e., sera from males, females, pregnant females, and tissue extracts. A radioimmunoassay which is valid for quantification of progesterone in extracts of luteal tissue is not necessarily valid for quantification of progesterone in serum from midluteal phase females or males.

Due to the presence of proteins which bind steroids and interfere with the binding of steroid to the antisera, it has not been feasible until recently to quantify steroid hormones in unextracted serum, even in the presence of high-affinity antibodies. Therefore, it has been necessary to extract the steroid from the sample, most commonly by the use of organic solvents. This procedure eliminates proteins, and with careful choice of extraction solvents it can also rid the sample of other substances which have the potential to interfere with the assay. For example, petroleum ether extraction of a sample for progesterone gives an extract that is not only free of binding protein but also is relatively free of other steroids. Numerous solvents have been used to extract steroid hormones, with the final choice depending upon the identity of the steroid the laboratory conducting the assay. To monitor extraction efficiency and chromatographic purification procedures, tritiated steroid hormones are usually added to each sample. The recovery of the tritiated steroid is used to correct the final values obtained by radioimmunoassay. Since most steroids have a limited solubility in water, recovery estimates should be made after solubilization of the extract in the aqueous assay buffer. Aliquots from the same aqueous solution should be pipetted for radioimmunoassay and for recovery determinations at the same time. For steroid hormones which are present in minute quantities in biological samples (i.e., estrogens and aldosterone), it is necessary that the mass of radioactivity added for recoveries be minimized and that, if necessary, the final sample estimate be corrected for this mass.

Recently a new procedure has been employed for cortisol (Hasler *et al.*, 1976), which is present in serum in high concentrations. This procedure involves the use of subtilisin, a proteolytic enzyme, to hydrolyze interfering proteins in serum followed by heat denaturation of the enzyme and assay of the sample.

After proof of the specificity of a radioimmunoassay system, evaluation of other parameters is necessary to describe its performance. The sensitivity of the assay can be defined as the least amount of hormone that can be reliably distinguished from no hormone. Precision may be defined as the extent to which a given set of measurements of the same sample agree with the mean, usually expressed as a coefficient of variation following repeated estimations of the hormone concentration of the same sample in the same assay (intraassay variation) and repeated estimates in different assays (interassay variation). Precision in any radioimmunoassay varies at different levels along the standard inhibition curve (Midgley *et al.*, 1971).

The accuracy of a radioimmunoassay system is the degree to which the assay estimate agrees with the actual quantity of steroid hormone in the sample. To evaluate accuracy, recovery of known quantities of steroid from biological samples which represent a wide range of physiological conditions must be demonstrated. These procedures have been discussed elsewhere (Midgley *et al.*, 1971).

Finally, a major stumbling block to the routine use of radioimmunoassay procedures for steroid hormones has been the identification and solution of problems relating to blanks. Blanks may result from interference with the binding of radioactive steroid to antibody by nonspecific or contaminating substances or by substances which interfere with the method used to separate antibody-bound radioactive from free steroid. Blanks may originate from any of the reagents or apparatus used for pipetting, extraction, purification, or quantification of steroid. Correction of radioimmunoassay values for blanks is not satisfactory, although commonly practiced. It is very likely that blank values vary from sample to sample and cannot be estimated precisely in each sample. Unless the blank produces inhibition curves in the radioimmunoassay that are parallel to those obtained with the standard, they cannot legitimately be subtracted. Therefore, the only meaningful solution of blank problems is to eliminate them or reduce them to insignificant levels. Precautionary measures which have generally proved useful in eliminating or reducing blanks have been discussed (Niswender *et al.*, 1975a).

VII. SUMMARY

The use of γ-labeled steroids for radioimmunoassays is becoming widespread. The advantages of greater sensitivity, simplified economical counting, improved precision, high antiserum dilutions, and adaptability to routine clinical procedures have sparked renewed interest in the development of novel radioimmunoassay procedures. With the commercial availability of a wide variety of radioiodinated steroid derivatives, the major problem of synthesis and radiolabeling of these compounds will be eliminated.

REFERENCES

Abraham, G. E. (1969). Solid-phase radioimmunoassay of estradiol-17β. *J. Clin. Endocrinol. Metab.* **29**, 866–870.
Bizollon, C. A., Riviere, J., Franchimont, P., Faure, A., and Claustrat, B. (1974). Solid-phase radioimmunoassay of plasma aldosterone. *Steroids* **23**, 809–819.
Bodley, F. H., Chapdelaine, A., Flickinger, G., Mikhail, G., Yaveerbaum, C., and Roberts, K. D. (1973). A highly specific radioimmunoassay for progesterone using antibodies covalently linked to acrylamide-glass particles. *Steroids* **21**, 809–819.
Bolton, A. E., and Hunter, W. M. (1973). The labelling of proteins to high specific radioactivities by conjugation to a ^{125}I-containing acylating agent. *Biochem. J.* **133**, 529–539.
Cameron, E. H. D., Scarisbrick, J. J., Morris, S. E., Hillier, S. G., and Read, G. (1974).

Some aspects of the use of ^{125}I-labelled ligands for steroid radioimmunoassay. *J. Steroid Biochem.* **5**, 749–756.

Cameron, E. H. D., Scarisbrick, J. J., Morris, S. E., and Read, G. (1975). ^{125}I-Iodohistamine derivatives as tracers for the radioimmunoassay of progesterone. *In* "Steroid Immunoassay" (E. H. D. Cameron, S. G. Hillier, and K. Griffiths, eds.), pp. 153–176 Alpha Omega Alpha Publ., Cardiff, Wales.

Chambers, V. E. M., Glover, J. S., and Tudor, R. (1975). [^{75}Se]-radioligands in steroid immunoassay. *In* "Steroid Immunoassay" (E. H. D. Cameron, S. G. Hillier, and K. Griffiths, eds.), pp. 141–152. Alpha Omega Alpha Publ., Cardiff, Wales.

Comoglio, S., Saracco, B., and Rosa, U. (1974). Preparation of 17β-oestradiol-6-(O-carboxymethyl) oxime [^{125}I]-tyramine for oestradiol radioimmunoassay. *J. Nuclear Biol. Med.* **18**, 98–103.

Desbuquois, B., and Aurbach, G. D. (1971). Use of polyethylene glycol to separate free and antibody found hormones in radioimmunoassays. *J. Clin. Endocrinol. Metab.* **33**, 732–738.

Edwards, R., Gilby, E. D., and Jeffcoate, S. L. (1974). Iodine-125 tracers in steroid radioimmunoassay. *In* "Radioimmunoassay and Related Procedures in Medicine," Vol. 2, pp. 31–40. I.A.E.A., Vienna.

England, B. G., Niswender, G. D., and Midgley, A. R., Jr. (1974). Radioimmunoassay of estradiol-17β without chromatography. *J. Clin. Endocrinol. Metab.* **38**, 42–50.

Erlanger, B. F., Borek, F., Beiser, S. M., and Lieberman, S. (1958). Preparation and characterization of conjugates to bovine serum albumin with testosterone and cortisone. *J. Biol. Chem.* **228**, 713–727.

Erlanger, B. F., Beiser, S. M., Borek, F., Edel, F., and Lieberman, S. (1967). The preparation of steroid-protein conjugates to elicit antihormonal antibodies. *In* "Methods in Immunology and Immunochemistry" (C. A. Williams and M. W. Chase, eds.), pp. 144–150. Academic Press, New York.

Fahmy, D., Read, G., and Hillier, S. G. (1975). Radioimmunoassay for cortisol: Comparison of H^3-, Se^{75}-, and J^{125} labeled ligands. *J. Endocrinol.* **65**, 45P–46P.

Greenwood, F. C., Hunter, W. M., and Glover, S. J. (1963). The preparation of ^{131}I-labelled human growth hormone of high specific activity. *Biochem. J.* **89**, 114–123.

Hasler, M., Painter, K., and Niswender, G. (1976). A rapid iodine-125 cortisol radioimmunoassay employing enzymatic denaturation of serum binding proteins. *Clin. Chem.* **22**, 1850–1854.

Herbert, V., Law, K. S., Gottlieb, C. W., and Bleicher, S. J. (1965). Coated charcoal immunoassay of insulin. *J. Clin. Endocrinol. Metab.* **25**, 1375–1384.

Hunter, W. M., Nars, P. W., and Rutherford, F. J. (1975). Preparation and behaviour of ^{125}I-labeled radioligands for phenolic and neutral steroids. *In* "Steroid Immunoassay" (E. H. D. Cameron, S. G. Hillier, and K. Griffiths, eds.), pp. 141–152. Alpha Omega Alpha Publ., Cardiff, Wales.

Kato, H., Ito, T., Kido, Y., and Torigoe, T. (1974). Preparation of ^{125}I-labeled estrone-trityrosine methyl ester. *Horm. Metab. Res.* **6**, 334–335.

Lindberg, P., and Edqvist, L.-E. (1974). The use of 17β-oestradiol-6-(O-carboxy-methyl) oxime-[^{125}I] tyramine as trace for the radioimmunoassay of 17β-oestradiol. *Clin. Chim. Acta* **53**, 169–174.

Malvano, R., Dotti, C., and Grosso, P. (1973). ^{125}I-Labelled cortisol-TME for competitive protein binding. *Clin. Chim. Acta* **47**, 167–173.

Mayes, D., Furuyama, S., Kem, D. C., and Nugent, C. A. (1970). A radioimmunoassay for plasma aldosterone. *J. Clin. Endocrinol. Metab.* **30**, 682–685.

Midgley, A. R., Jr., Niswender, G. D., and Ram, S. (1969). Hapten radioimmunoassay: A general procedure for the estimation of steroidal and other haptenic substances. *Steroids* **13**, 731–737.

Midgley, A. R., Jr., and Niswender, G. D. (1970). Radioimmunoassay of steroids. *Acta Endocrinol. (Copenhagen)* Suppl. 147, 320–331.

Midgley, A. R., Jr., Niswender, G. D., Gay, V. L., and Reichert, L. E., Jr. (1971). Use of antibodies for characterization of gonadotropins and steroids. *Recent Prog. Horm. Res.* **27**, 235–286.

Mikhail, G., Chung, H. W., Ferin, M., and Vande Wiele, R. L. (1970). Radioimmunoassay of plasma estrogens: Use of polymerized antibodies. *In* "Immunologic Methods in Steroid Determination" (F. G. Perón and B. V. Caldwell, eds.), pp. 113–126. Appleton, New York.

Moore, P. H., and Axelrod, L. R. (1972). A solid-phase radioimmunoassay for estrogen by estradiol-17β antibody covalently bound to a water insoluble synthetic polymer (Ensacryl AA). *Steroids* **20**, 188–212.

Nars, P. W., and Hunter, W. M. (1973). A method for labelling oestradiol-17β with radioiodine for radioimmunoassays. *J. Endocrinol.* **57**, 157–158.

Niswender, G. D. (1973). Influence of site of conjugation on the specificity of antibodies to progesterone. *Steroids* **22**, 413–424.

Niswender, G. D. (1975). Discussion. *In* "Steroid Immunoassay" (E. H. D. Cameron, S. G. Hillier, and K. Griffiths, eds.), pp. 165–167. Alpha Omega Alpha Publ., Cardiff, Wales.

Niswender, G. D., and Midgley, A. R., Jr. (1969). Hapten-radioimmunoassay for testosterone. *Proc. 51st Annu. Meet., Am. Endocr. Soc.* Abstract 22.

Niswender, G. D., and Midgley, A. R., Jr. (1970). Hapten-radioimmunoassay of steroids. *In* "Immunologic Methods in Steroid Determination," (F. G. Perón, and B. V. Caldwell, eds.), pp. 149–173, Appleton-Century-Crofts, New York.

Niswender, G. D., Akbar, A. M., and Nett, T. M. (1975a). Use of specific antibodies for quantification of steroid hormones. *In* "Methods in Enzymology" (B. W. O'Malley and J. G. Hardman, eds.), Vol. 36, pp. 16–34. Academic Press, New York.

Niswender, G. D., Nett, T. M., Meyer, D. L., and Hagerman, D. D. (1975b). Factors influencing the specificity of antibodies to steroid hormones. *In* "Steroid Immunoassays" (E. H. D. Cameron, S. G. Hillier, and K. Griffiths, eds.), pp. 61–66. Alpha Omega Alpha Publ., Cardiff, Wales.

Oliver, G. C., Jr., Parker, B. M., Brasfield, D. L., and Parker, C. W. (1968). The measurement of digitoxin in human serum by radioimmunoassay. *J. Clin. Invest.* **47**, 1035–1042.

Wood, F. T., Wu, M. M., and Gerhart, G. C. (1975). The radioactive labeling of proteins with an iodinated amidination reagent. *Anal. Biochem.* **69**, 339–349.

38

Mineralocorticoids: Aldosterone, Deoxycorticosterone, 18-Hydroxydeoxycorticosterone, and 18-Hydroxycorticosterone

GORDON H. WILLIAMS AND
RICHARD H. UNDERWOOD

I. INTRODUCTION

The chemist's ability to measure accurately the levels of steroids in biologic fluid has improved considerably since the early 1930's, when the only assays available were crude bioassays. The initial assays for

743

Methods of Hormone Radioimmunoassay, Second Edition
Copyright © 1979 by Academic Press, Inc.
All rights of reproduction in any form reserved. ISBN 0-12-379260-6

mineralocorticoid activity utilized changes in the level of sodium and/or potassium excretion by adrenalectomized dogs (Hartman and Spoor, 1940; Harrop *et al.*, 1936; Thorn and Engel 1938) or rats (Wirtz, 1950). These, however, only gave a gross estimation of the amount of mineralocorticoid present in the extract. In 1947, Dorfman *et al.* suggested that the excretion of radioactive sodium by adrenalectomized animals could be the basis of a more sensitive assay. Simpson and Tait (1952) extended this method to include alterations in the radioactive excretion of both ^{24}Na and ^{42}K. A number of other modifications have been suggested but most have been dependent on a change in the ratio of sodium to potassium excretion. The sensitivity of the assay was probably best achieved with adrenalectomized rats, in which levels as low as 0.01 μg/animal could be detected.

In the late 1950's and early 1960's, after the isolation and characterization of aldosterone by Simpson *et al.* (1954), a number of physicochemical assays were developed based on the physical and chemical properties of this compound. Most procedures used a chromatographic purification step with actual quantification by spectrophotometry. The reaction of the α-ketol side chain in the aldosterone molecule with a tetrazolium reagent to produce a formazan absorbing at 510 nm was utilized in methods for measuring the hormone (Mader and Buck, 1952; Nowaczynski *et al.*, 1955). However, the specificity of this method was intrinsically low because of the presence of other groupings which may also reduce the tetrazolium salt. Another technique was the development of soda fluorescence by steroids containing a 3-oxo-4-ene group when reacted with alkali and irradiated with ultraviolet light. This had greater sensitivity and specificity than the formazan derivative method. Finally, in the mid-1960's, more precise and specific assays using radioactively labeled reagents were developed by a number of laboratories. Using these techniques, a radioactive-labeled standard aldosterone, i.e., tritium, was used for estimating losses during the purification steps, and a reagent with a different radioactive label, i.e., carbon-14, was used to react with aldosterone. By double isotope counting, and knowing the specific activity of the labeled reagent, the amount of aldosterone could be estimated and appropriately corrected for procedural losses. Kliman and Peterson (1960) applied this technique using ^{14}C-acetic anhydride to measure aldosterone in urine and also adrenal venous samples. In 1967, two different groups using a similar technique published methods for the measurement of aldosterone in peripheral plasma (Brodie *et al.*, 1967; Coghlan and Scoggins, 1967). These methods had several potential advantages over previous methods but also some disadvantages. The advantages were the almost limitless potential sensitivity depending only on the specific activity of the labeled reagent. Values as low as 50 pg were measurable. The estimation was unaffected by losses in the procedure after the indicator was added, since these were corrected. The purity of the derivative could be tested by surveying the isotope ratios. The disadvantages were that the method had little intrinsic specificity, since any compound containing free hydroxyl groups could react with the labeled reagents. It was also expensive and required specialized skill and equipment. The inherent difficulty of this procedure is apparent when one considers that there was a great deal of interest to measure plasma aldosterone levels in the mid- to late 1960's; yet fewer than half a dozen laboratories published data obtained by double isotope derivative techniques.

In parallel with the improvement in methodology related to the measurement of aldosterone has been the rapid advance of techniques used to measure polypeptide hormones. A breakthrough occurred in the late 1950's, when Berson and Yalow (1959) published their methods for measuring insulin levels by radioimmunoassay. At about the same time, Goodfriend and Sehon (1958) and Lieberman *et al.* (1959) developed techniques to raise antibodies against steroids by first coupling the steroid to a carrier protein. Ten years later, this information was applied to the measurement of aldosterone in peripheral plasma (Mayes *et al.*, 1970). Since that time, several other methods have been developed for the measurement of plasma aldosterone (e.g., Bayard *et al.*, 1970; Ito *et al.*, 1972; Underwood and Williams, 1972; Farmer *et al.*, 1973; Martin and Nugent, 1973) and one for 11-deoxycorticosterone (Arnold and James, 1971) by radioimmunoassay. Two detailed methods for the measurement of 18-hydroxydeoxycorticosterone (18-OH-DOC) have been reported (Chandler *et al.*, 1976; Williams *et al.*, 1976) and a method has been described in brief by Edwards *et al.* (1974). One method has been published for 18-hydroxycorticosterone (18-OH-B) (Martin *et al.*, 1975). This chapter will briefly review the features of these methods and will present a more detailed account of one. With this technique, aldosterone, DOC, 18-OH-DOC, and 18-OH-B are extracted, purified by paper chromatography, and measured independently with steroid-specific antibodies and homologous tritiated steroid markers.

II. METHODS OF RADIOIMMUNOASSAY

Aldosterone, DOC, 18-OH-DOC, and 18-OH-B are all derived from the adrenal cortex. Aldosterone is exclusively derived from the outer cell layer (glomerulosa) of the adrenal cortex. DOC, 18-OH-DOC, and 18-OH-B are produced by both glomerulosa and fasciculata layers. The hormones have the same structure in animals and man.

Antibodies to aldosterone and aldolactone described in this chapter were made by Haning and co-workers at the Worcester Foundation; antibodies to aldosterone are now available from the National Institute of Arthritis and Metabolic Diseases. Antibodies to DOC described were produced by Dr. Guy Abraham, University of California at Los Angeles, California. Antibodies to 18-OH-DOC and 18-OH-B were prepared as described.

A. Immunogen Preparation

The most important ingredient in an accurate radioimmunoassay system is an antibody that is specific for the substance to be measured and binds it with a high affinity so that small amounts of the substance can be measured. Aldosterone and deoxycorticosterone, like other steroids, present a unique problem not shared by larger polypeptide hormones in that they are not inherently antigenic. Aldosterone is made antigenic by covalently linking it to an appropriate protein carrier. The most stable linkage is a peptide bond and, therefore, the hydroxyl and keto groups in the steroid molecule first must be changed into carboxyl groups which can then react with free amino groups on the carrier protein. There are three general procedures used, i.e., the formation of an oxime derivative of a keto group, conversion of a hydroxyl group to a hemisuccinate, or conversion of a hydroxyl group to a chlorocarbonate (Figure 1). In preparing steroid derivatives, one must consider the structure of the steroid to be measured in relationship to other steroids that may be present in the biologic fluid. For example, one could make a derivative of aldosterone by linking it through the 21-position or the 3-position. However, if linked through the 3-position, specificity of the configuration of the A ring will be lost, and if linked at the other end of the molecule, specificity for the D ring will be lost. On the other hand, if the protein is conjugated to aldosterone through the 6-position, leaving both ends of the molecule exposed, a more specific antibody would theoretically be produced.

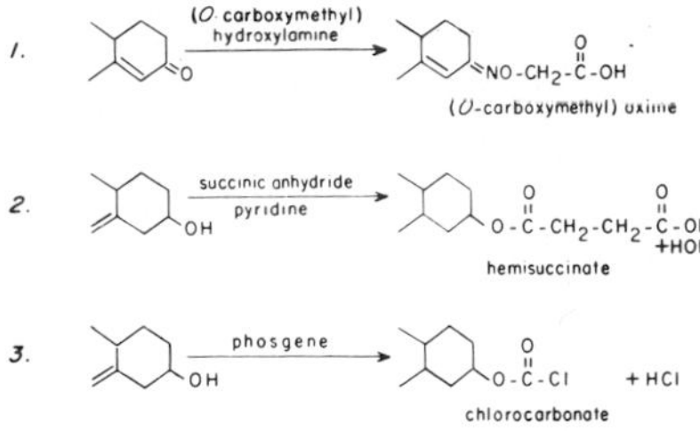

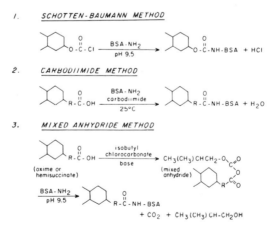

Figure 1. Preparation of steroid intermediates for conjugation. (Reproduced from Williams and Underwood, 1973, with permission of the publishers.)

B. Preparation of Steroid Conjugates

There are three methods commonly used to conjugate the steroid derivative to a protein (Figure 2). The most commonly used one is the mixed anhydride method, in which the oxime or hemisuccinate of the steroid is reacted in the presence of isobutyl chlorocarbonate to form the mixed anhydride of the steroid; the mixed anhydride will then react with free amino groups on the protein molecule. Alternatively, carbodiimide could be used for the condensation, or if the chlorocarbonate derivative had been formed, the Schotten–Baumann method is used. The number of steroid molecules incorporated is dependent on the number of free amino groups available for condensation. For

Figure 2. Methods for preparing steroid–protein conjugates. (Reproduced from Williams and Underwood, 1973, with permission of the publisher.)

example, bovine serum albumin has 60 free amino groups, 59 on lysine residues, and one at the N-terminal end of the molecule. In our experience, if less than ten molecules of steroid have been incorporated into each protein molecule, a relatively poor antiserum is produced (Haning *et al.*, 1972). Therefore, it is advisable to use a molar excess of steroid to protein of 40–80 to 1.0, and to determine the level of incorporation in the conjugate prior to immunization. The degree of steroid incorporation is evaluated by dissolving known amounts of conjugate in 0.05 M Tris, pH 8.4, and by measuring absorbancy around 240 nm ($E_m = 16,000$).

Aldosterone 18,21-dihemisuccinate was prepared by reacting 50.4 mg aldosterone and 50 mg succinic anhydride in 2.5 ml pyridine for 18 hours. The pyridine was removed under vacuum and the remaining oil was dissolved in 30 ml methylene chloride and 10 ml water. Purification was achieved by extraction into 0.25 M NaHCO$_3$ (6 ml 3×), acidification by the addition of 4.0 ml 5 N HCl, and reextraction into methylene chloride (20 ml 3×). The product was further purified by liquid–liquid partition chromatography on a 2.0 × 60 cm column of celite (400 ml ethanol, 125 ml water, 375 ml acetic acid, and 3000 ml benzene). The fractions containing aldosterone 18,21-dihemisuccinate were dried under vacuum (Haning *et al.*, 1972).

Aldosterone 18,21-dihemisuccinate was covalently conjugated to BSA by incubation (41 : 1 aldosterone hemisuccinate–BSA mole ratio) with equimolar amounts of isobutyl chlorocarbonate and tri-*n*-butylamine to react all carboxyl groups. The conjugate was dialyzed against distilled water, lyophilized, and made up to 1.7 mg/ml in 0.1 M phosphate, pH 7.6 (Haning *et al.*, 1972).

The 18-OH-DOC lactone was prepared by oxidizing 20 mg 18-OH-DOC with 0.8 ml periodic acid containing 0.1 N periodic acid in a 2% pyridine solution in water overnight at 24°C in the dark. The periodic acid solution was extracted with methylene chloride and the methylene chloride washed with 0.25 N NaHCO$_3$ to remove etioacids (Williams *et al.*, 1972). A 50-μg aliquot of this solution was submitted to paper chromatography in the Bush 3 system (Skellysolve–benzene–methanol–water, 650 : 300 : 400 : 100). A single spot was detected by uv and soda fluorescence with an R_f of 0.42. No other products were detected on the paper chromatogram. The 18-OH-DOC lactone solution was quantitated by measurement in a uv spectrophotometer, λ_{max} 241 nm, E_m 16,000. The oxime derivative of 18-OH-DOC lactone was prepared using carboxymethoxylamine by the method of Erlanger *et al.* (1957). In brief, 25 mg 18-OH-DOC was refluxed for two hours with a threefold excess of carboxymethoxylamine in 20 ml ethanol and 20 ml pyridine, and $KHCO_3$ was added to make the solution alkaline. The aqueous solution was then extracted with methylene chloride and the aqueous phase was adjusted to pH 2.0 with concentrated HCl and stirred. The white flocculent precipitate which formed was dissolved by shaking with methylene chloride, and the methylene chloride extract was washed with hydrochloric acid and water and taken to dryness. The 18-OH-DOC lactone oxime was crystallized from ethyl acetate, mp 210° (decomp), λ_{max} 250 nm.

The BSA conjugate of the 18-OH-DOC lactone oxime was prepared

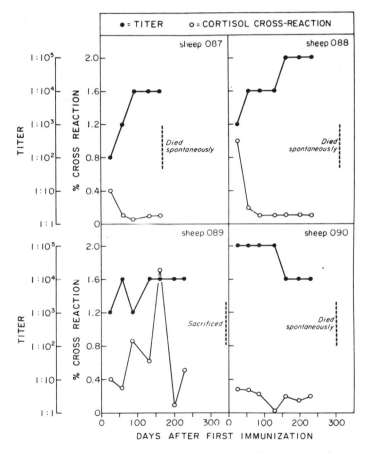

Figure 3. Evolution of titer and percentage molar cross-reaction with cortisol of aldosterone-binding antibodies as a function of time in four sheep immunized with aldosterone 18,21-dihemisuccinate–bovine serum albumin conjugate.

by the method described above for preparing the BSA conjugate of aldosterone-18,21-dihemisuccinate.

A variety of animals, such as rabbits, guinea pigs, goats, and sheep, have been used to raise antibodies to steroid hormones. Most studies indicate that there is little inherent advantage of one animal over another as far as antibody response is concerned. The choice is, therefore, in part dependent on the previous experience of the investigator, the size of animal facilities, and the availability of various animals. We have used the sheep almost exclusively for our studies for two reasons: first, they are large animals, so that with each bleeding 250–300 ml of blood can be obtained. Therefore, if a particular bleeding has a significant titer of a very good antibody, there is a great deal of antisera available. Second, we have the facilities to keep these large animals. Other large animals could be used; however, the sheep in our experience is the most docile.

Most investigators have emulsified their antigen in complete Freund's adjuvant prior to injection. Injection techniques vary greatly. We inject intradermally into eight to twenty different sites. Others have used multiple injections subcutaneously into lymph nodes or into foot pads. The frequency of immunizations and the timing of the immunization to bleeding have also varied. Our technique is to immunize biweekly for six weeks, 1.7 mg per immunization, then at monthly intervals (Haning *et al.*, 1972). Forty sheep have been immunized using this technique. Significant titers have occurred in all but one sheep. Figure 3 illustrates the evolution of titer and specificity in sheep immunized against the 18,21-dihemisuccinate of aldosterone conjugated to bovine serum albumin. While significant titers occurred in all sheep, there was considerable individual variation for both titer and cross-reaction.

C. Characterization of Antibodies

The most important characteristics of an antibody are affinity constant, titer, and cross-reactivity.

1. Affinity Constant

The affinity constant of an antibody is an index of the affinity of binding between antigen and antibody. If the experimental results of a dose–response curve are graphed as a Scatchard plot, $R = K (Q - B)$, where R = bound/free ratio, Q is the concentration of unbound antigen, and K is affinity constant, then the slope of the line will be $-K$, and Q will be the intercept on the abscissa. Thus, K can be determined directly from a plot of experimental results. A value for K can also be calculated when the bound/free ratio is 1.0. When a hapten H is bound to an antibody B, then at equilibrium applying the law of first-order mass action, we have [Eq. (1)]:

$$K = \frac{[HB]}{[H][B]} \tag{1}$$

At half-saturation of antibody binding sites, i.e., when the ratio of bound/free is 1.0, then $[HB] = [B]$ and $K = 1/[H]$. Using this formula, the K values for the antibodies were: aldosterone, 2.0×10^{11}, aldolactone, 4.7×10^{9}, DOC, 1.3×10^{10}, 18-OH-DOC, 9.2×10^{10}, and 18-OH-B, 1.2×10^{10} liters/mole, respectively.

2. Titer

Titer is the extent to which the antiserum can be diluted while still exhibiting a degree of binding sufficient for setting up a standard curve. The dilution of an antibody that gives a 1 : 1 ratio for bound/unbound radioactively labeled antigen is generally accepted as giving optimal conditions for sensitivity and precision in radioimmunoassay Odell *et al.* (1971). Dilutions for optimally sensitive curves are: aldosterone, 1 : 10^6, aldolactone, 1 : 300,000, DOC, 1 : 100,000, 18-OH-DOC, 1 : 300,000, and 18-OH-B, 1 : 280,000. Standard curves are shown in Figure 4.

3. Cross-Reaction

The percentages of cross-reaction of various steroids with the antibodies are shown in Table I. The results are calculated on a weight to weight basis from the amount of standard aldosterone, aldolactone, and DOC, and the amount of the other steroids that produce a 40% decrease in the binding of ^{3}H-aldosterone and ^{3}H-18-OH-DOC lactone, 20% decrease for ^{3}H-aldolactone, and a 25% decrease for ^{3}H-DOC with their respective antibodies. The aldosterone and aldolactone antibodies were very similar in their cross-reactions with other steroids. Both antibodies exhibited less than 0.1% cross-reaction with all the steroids tested except DOC, which showed a 0.2% cross-reactivity. The cross-reactivity of the aldolactone and aldosterone antibodies with aldosterone and aldolactone were 11.4 and 18.1%, respectively. The DOC antibody exhibited greater affinity for progesterone than DOC as illustrated by its 120% cross-reaction, and almost equal affinity for 17α-hydroxyprogesterone (90% cross-reactivity). Cross-reactions with the other C-17,21-dihydroxysteroids tested (cortisol, corticosterone, and cortisone) were 6, 8, and 3%, respectively.

Table I Percent Cross-Reaction of Aldosterone, Aldolactone, and Deoxycorticosterone Antibodies with Other Steroids[a,b]

Antibody	Aldo	Aldo-lactone	DOC	Prog.	18-OH-DOC	B	E	18-OH-B	F	T	17β	17α-OH-Prog.
Aldosterone	100	18.1	0.20	0.10	0.10	0.08	0.03	0.03	0.01	0	0	—
DOC	0.06	0.03	100	120	0.16	8	3	0.05	6	0.04	0	96
Aldolactone	11.4	100	0.03	0.05	<0.10	<0.01	<0.02	0.02	<0.01	<0.01	<0.01	0.02
18-OH-DOC lactone	<0.01	0.30	0.05	0.03	0.50	0.02	<0.01	0.13 (lactone 61.0)	<0.01	0.10	—	<0.01

[a] Data calculated on a weight to weight basis.

[b] Aldo, aldosterone; Aldolactone, aldosterone lactone; DOC, deoxycorticosterone; Prog., progesterone; 18-OH-DOC, 18-hydroxydesoxycorticosterone; B, corticosterone; E, cortisone; 18-OH-B, 18-hydroxycorticosterone; F, cortisol; T, testosterone; E-17β, 17β-estradiol; 17-OH-Prog., 17-hydroxyprogesterone.

However, cross-reactions with both the C-21, 18-dihydroxy, and C-17 steroids tested were 0.06% or less, except 0.16% with 18-OH DOC. The 61% cross-reactivity of the 18-OH-DOC antibody with 18-OH-B enabled this antibody to be used for the measurement of 18-OH-B as well as 18-OH-DOC.

D. Preparation and Sources of Radioactive Ligand

1,2-^{3}H-Aldosterone, aldosterone-γ-etiolactone, deoxycorticosterone, all 40–60 Ci/mmole, were purchased from New England Nuclear, Boston, Massachusetts, and were tested for purity by paper chromatography in the systems benzene–methanol–water, $2:1:1$ ($R_f = 0.27$); cyclohexane–benzene–methanol–water, $5:2:5:1$, and Skellysolve–benzene–methanol–water, $2:1:4:1$ ($R_f = 0.48$), respectively. When the tritiated steroids were found to be >98% pure, they were used without further purification. If more than 2% impurities were present, then the steroids were purified before use in the respective paper chromatographic systems. ^{3}H-18-OH-DOC and ^{3}H-18-OH-B were obtained from the Amersham-Searle and were submitted to paper chromatography in a Bush 5 solvent system, benzene–methanol–water, $1:1:1$, prior to further utilization. The specific activity of ^{3}H-18-OH-DOC was estimated at 29 Ci/mmole by radioimmunoassay. A scan of this paper indicated two peaks, the major one accounting for 96% of the radioactivity migrated at the same R_f as nonradioactive 18-OH-DOC. ^{3}H-18-OH-B, 41 Ci/mmole, was found to be >95% pure by paper chromatography and was used without further purification. Lactones were prepared by oxidizing ^{3}H-18-OH-B and ^{3}H-18-OH-DOC with periodic acid solution (Williams et al., 1972). The ^{3}H-18-OH-DOC lactone was purified by paper chromatography in the Bush 3 solvent system. A scan of the chromatogram indicated a single peak of radioactivity with an R_f of 0.42. This was eluted with methanol and stored for further use. It was stable for up to six months at 4°C. The ^{3}H-18-OH-B lactone was purified by paper chromatography in a cyclohexane–benzene–methanol–water system ($500:200:500:100$).

E. Preparation of Sample for Radioimmunoassay

1. Materials

Toluene: (A.R.), Fisher Chemical
Methylene chloride, benzene, and methanol, spectroquality: Matheson, Coleman, and Bell

Whatman No. 1 filter paper, washed with benzene, then methanol 48 hours each, in a Soxhlet extraction apparatus: No. JE-5700 Scientific Glass Apparatus

Borate buffer solution: 8.25 gm boric acid (A.R. J.T. Baker Chemical Co.) and 2.7 gm sodium hydroxide are dissolved in 500 ml glass-distilled water. HCl is added to give pH 8.0, then the mixture is diluted to 1000 ml with water.

Bovine serum albumin: fraction V from bovine plasma No. 2296, Armour Pharmaceutical.

Plastic cups and caps: 3.0 ml autoanalyzer polystyrene cups with conical tip No. 137-0066 fitted with polystyrene caps No. 534-0000, Technicon.

PCS: (scintillation solubilizer fluid) Amersham-Searle.

Polyethylene radioactivity counting vials: Walter Sarstedt, No. 50/16L, 146.

Dextran-coated charcoal solution: 1.25 gm charcoal (Matheson, Coleman and Bell) and 125 mg dextran 80 (Pharmacia Fine Chemicals) added to 500 ml borate buffer solution, stored at 4°C.

Steroids: Aldosterone, DOC (Sigma Chemical), and aldosterone-γ-lactone (Ikapharm, Ramat-Gan, Israel) were used without further purification. 18-OH-DOC (Steraloids) 18-OH-B (Ikapharm, Ramat-Gan, Israel) were used to prepare the lactone derivatives.

2. Extraction

a. **Plasma** (Underwood and Williams, 1972). ^{3}H-Aldosterone or ^{3}H-DOC (3000 dpm), or 1500 dpm ^{3}H-18-OH-DOC or ^{3}H-18-OH-B in 0.05 ml ethanol is added directly to 1.0–4.0 ml human peripheral plasma in a 25-ml glass stoppered tube. Sodium hydroxide (0.2 ml, 0.1 N) is then added and the plasma, if less than 4.0 ml is used, is made up to a total volume of 4.0 ml with water and extracted with 10 ml ice-cold methylene chloride. The extract is washed twice with 2.0 ml of water, transferred to a 25-ml round-bottom flask, and taken to dryness (*in vacuo*, 55°C). Prior to chromatography, the 18-OH-DOC and 18-OH-B extracts are lactonized by adding 0.8 ml of 0.1 N periodic acid in a 2% pyridine solution of water for 18 hours at 24°C in the dark. The periodic acid solution is then extracted with methylene chloride, and the methylene chloride is partitioned with 0.25 N sodium bicarbonate and then dried (*in vacuo*, 55°C). All extracts are then submitted to paper chromatography as described below.

b. **Urine** (Rayfield *et al.*, 1973). Following the intravenous injection of 10 μCi of ^{3}H-aldosterone into a subject, 5.0 ml of the 24-hour urine output is made up to 10 ml with water and extracted with twice its volume of methylene chloride. The methylene chloride layer is discarded, and the urine is brought to pH 1.0 by adding 5.0 N HCl and left for 24 hours at 24°C. The urine is neutralized with 1.25 N NaOH and extracted with three times its volume of methylene chloride. If only the excretion rate is to be measured, no ^{3}H-aldosterone is injected into the patient prior to the 24-hour urine collection, but 3000 dpm ^{3}H-aldosterone is added to the urine aliquot after the methylene chloride extraction and immediately before pH 1.0 hydrolysis to act as an internal indicator to correct for losses during the procedure. The methylene chloride extract is dried (*in vacuo*, 55°C) and submitted to paper chromatography.

c. **Tissue** (Williams *et al.*, 1972). Aldosterone in tissue is measured as the lactone. After incubation of rat glomerulosa tissue, an aliquot of the incubation medium is extracted with methylene chloride. The extract is partitioned between cyclohexane and 20% ethanol–water. The ethanol–water solution is extracted with methylene chloride, and the methylene chloride extract is taken to dryness (*in vacuo*, 55°C) and lactonized as described above. After oxidation, the periodic acid solution is extracted with methylene chloride and the methylene chloride is washed with 0.25 N sodium bicarbonate to remove etioacids.

3. Paper Chromatography

The use of unwashed filter paper resulted in high blank values. Thus, the filter paper is cut to give paper chromatograms, 16 cm wide and 55 cm long, and vertically cut to give five strips approximately three cm wide. These are then washed with benzene and methanol 48 hours each in a large Soxhlet extraction apparatus. The dried extracts are applied to the three inner strips on the chromatogram, each with 1.0 × 0.2, 1.0 × 0.1 washes of methanol–methylene chloride, 1:1. Approximately 40,000 dpm of ^{3}H-aldosterone, ^{3}H-DOC, ^{3}H-aldolactone, ^{3}H-18-OH-DOC lactone, or ^{3}H-18-OH-B lactone to act as a chromatography standard are applied to the left and right outer strips in 0.02 ml methanol–methylene chloride, 1:1. The paper chromatograms are equilibrated and developed in the following systems: aldosterone (benzene–methanol–water, 2:1:1) Bush 5, equilibrated 16 hours, run seven hours ($R = 0.27$); DOC (heptane–methanol–water, 1:4:1) Bush A, equilibrated five hours, run 36 hours (DOC runs 13 cm); aldolactone, 18-OH-DOC lactone, 18-OH-B lactone, (cyclohexane–

benzene–methanol–water, 500 : 200 : 500 : 100) equilibrated five hours, run 12–14 hours (aldolactone runs 16 cm, 18-OH-DOC lactone six cm, and 18-OH-B lactone 29 cm).

Following chromatography, each outer strip is scanned to detect the tritiated chromatography standard. Areas on the three inner sample strips are cut level with the ^{3}H standard and eluted with methanol. An aliquot of each eluate is taken for radioactivity assay. This is for recovery determination (recovery for all five compounds averages 55%) in measurements of the mineralocorticoids in plasma, aldosterone excretion rate (AER) in urine, and for calculating the specific activity of urinary aldosterone in the determination of aldosterone secretion rate (ASR). The methanol extracts are taken to dryness in a glass scintillation counting vial (*in vacuo*, 55°C), and 2.0 ml borate buffer containing 0.5% BSA is added. An appropriately sized aliquot, either 0.2 ml (10%), 0.3 ml (15%), or 0.4 ml (20%), is transferred to a 7.0-ml plastic counting vial and made up to a total volume of 0.5 ml with additional borate buffer containing 0.5% BSA. One milliliter of borate buffer is then added followed by 4.0 ml PCS, the vial is capped and the contents are thoroughly mixed by shaking. The tritium is assayed in a liquid scintillation counter.

F. Assay

1. Preparation of Antibody Binding Solution

a. Stock Solution. The original serum containing the antibody is diluted 100-fold by mixing with normal sheep serum and then divided into 0.1-ml aliquots in plastic vials and stored deep frozen at −15°C. Fifty milliliters of borate buffer is added to a 0.1-ml aliquot to give a dilution of the antibody of 1 : 50,000. This is poured into a 100-ml round bottom flask containing ^{3}H-aldosterone, ^{3}H-aldolactone, ^{3}H-DOC, [3]H-18-OH-DOC lactone, or [3]H-18-B lactone, thoroughly shaken, and stored at 4°C. (The amount of each ^{3}H-steroid added to the flask is calculated from the amount required in the binding solution described below.)

b. Binding Solution. The stock solution is diluted with 0.5% bovine serum albumin in borate buffer solution at pH 8.0 to give concentrations of 1 : 1,000,000 of aldosterone antibody, 1 : 300,000 for aldolactone antibody, 1 : 100,000 for DOC antibody, 1 : 300,000 for 18-OH-DOC antibody, and 1 : 280,000 for 18-OH-B antibody and concentrations of 10,000 dpm ^{3}H-aldosterone, 20,000 dpm ^{3}H-aldolactone,

10,000 dpm ^{3}H-DOC, and 5000 dpm ^{3}H-18-OH-DOC lactone or ^{3}H-18-OH-B lactone per 0.1 ml, respectively.

2. Assay Performance

a. **Standard Curve and Sample Preparation.** Independent assays are done for each steroid. Standard solutions in borate buffer containing 0.5% BSA are prepared containing (in 0.1 ml) 0, 10, 20, 50, 100, and 200 pg aldosterone or 18-OH-DOC lactone; 0, 12.5, 25, 50, 100, 200, and 400 pg aldolactone; 0, 20, 50, 100, 200, and 400 pg DOC; and 25, 50, 100, 250, 500 pg 18-OH-B. These solutions are stored at 4°C. Duplicate 0.1-ml aliquots of standard solutions, and duplicate aliquots (0.1–0.4 ml) of the unknown samples (eluted from the paper chromatograms and made up in 2.0 ml borate buffer containing 0.5% BSA) are transferred to plastic cups and the volume is adjusted, if necessary, to a total of 0.4 ml by adding borate buffer containing 0.5% BSA. One-tenth milliliter of the binding solution is added to two empty cups, labeled AB$_1$, and AB$_2$, and 0.4 ml borate buffer containing 0.5% BSA is added to each one. All samples are incubated at 4°C for 48 hours.

b. **Separation of Free from Antibody-Bound Steroid.** After incubation, the cups are placed in a deep freeze (-15°C) for ten minutes, transferred immediately to a 4°C cold room where (within a period of one minute) 1.0 ml dextran-coated charcoal solution is added to each cup, except the cups labeled AB$_1$ and AB$_2$. After a total operating period of five minutes in the cold room, the samples are placed in a deep freeze for four minutes, then immediately centrifuged at 4000 rpm for five minutes (except AB$_1$ and AB$_2$ to each of which 1.0 ml of borate buffer is added).

The clear supernatant liquid, which contains the ^{3}H-steroid bound to antibody, is decanted into a 7.0-ml plastic radioactivity counting vial, 4.0 ml PCS scintillation solution is added the vials are capped and thoroughly shaken, and every sample is counted for a total of 4000 counts in a liquid scintillation counter.

3. Calculation of the Amount of Steroid (Aldosterone, 18-OH-DOC, 18-OH-B, Aldolactone, DOC) in the Samples

a. **Hand Calculation.** The cpm tritium in cups AB$_1$ and AB$_2$ represents the total amount of ^{3}H-steroid present in the volume of binding solution added to every cup in a particular assay for binding. The percentage of ^{3}H-steroid bound to the antibody in a cup is given in Eq. (2).

$$[(\text{cpm }^3\text{H sample})/(\text{cpm }^3\text{H in AB})] \times 100 \tag{2}$$

The duplicate values for a particular sample are averaged.

b. Standard Curve. A curve is drawn with the standard amount of steroid plotted along the abscissa and the percentage bound ^{3}H-steroid on the ordinate. Typical standard curves for aldosterone, aldolactone, and DOC are shown in Figure 4.

c. Steroid in Samples. The recovery of the ^{3}H-steroid added initially is first determined and the cpm of this ^{3}H indicator present in the aliquot taken for binding is calculated. This amount of ^{3}H counts per minute for each sample is added to the ^{3}H counts per minute in the AB sample, and the amount is used as the "AB" figure in the formula [Eq. (3)]:

$$\text{Percentage }^3\text{H-steroid bound} = \frac{\text{cpm }^3\text{H sample}}{\text{cpm }^3\text{H in "AB"}} \times 100 \tag{3}$$

The amount of steroid equivalent to the percentage ^{3}H-steroid bound in a sample is then read directly from the appropriate standard curve. The value is then corrected for recovery of ^{3}H-steroid added initially as indicator.

d. Computed Calculation. Schulster *et al.* (1970) have previously described a mathematical model for converting the standard protein-binding curve for corticosterone into a linear relationship. In brief, the value F/B_c is plotted against mass of standard steroid where

$$F/B_c = (T - B)/(B - B_{HM}) \tag{4}$$

and F = dpm ^{3}H-steroid free, B = dpm ^{3}H-steroid bound, T = total dpm ^{3}H-steroid added, i.e., AB + "AB," B_{HM} = dpm ^{3}H-steroid bound when a large excess of inert steroid is present. Using this relationship, a computer program was devised which calculated the standard curve, determined the mass of the unknown sample from the curve, subtracted the mass of indicator in the sample, and corrected for aliquots and recovery. Values are now determined using this program and a PDP 10 computer.

4. Calculation of ASR and AER

The secretion rate and excretion rate of aldosterone in micrograms per day are calculated from the Eqs. (5) and (6):

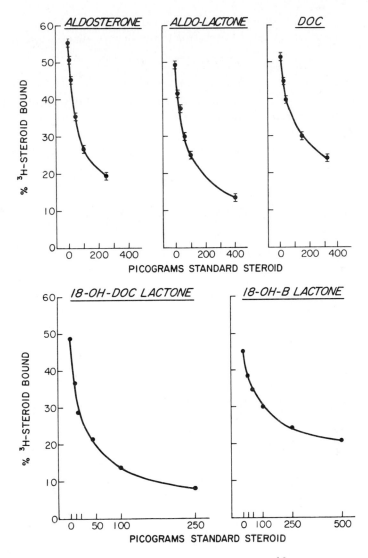

Figure 4. Typical standard radioimmunoassay curves using aldosterone antisera $(1:10^6$ dilution), aldolactone antisera $(1:300,000$ dilution), DOC antisera $(1:100,000$ dilution), 18-OH-DOC antisera $(1:300,000$ dilution), and 18-OH-B antisera $(1:280,000$ dilution).

$$\text{ASR} = \frac{\text{dpm } ^3\text{H-aldo injected into subject}}{\text{specific activity of metabolite in 24-hour urine (dpm}/\mu\text{g)}} \quad (5)$$

$$\text{AER} = \frac{(M \times 100 \times 100 \times TV)}{(10^6 \times F \times R \times V)} \quad (6)$$

where M = mass in picograms of aldosterone in the aliquot taken for binding, F = percent of purified extract taken for binding, R = percent of recovery of the ^{3}H-aldo added as internal indicator, V = volume in milliliters of urine extracted, and TV = total volume of 24-hour urine collected.

III. EVALUATION OF THE RADIOIMMUNOASSAY

A. Comparison of Radioimmunoassay and Double Isotope Derivative Methods

The aldosterone secretion rate in 20 patients and the aldosterone in 20 samples of tissue incubation media and in 11 samples of human peripheral plasma were measured by both radioimmunoassay and double isotope derivative techniques. The results are shown in Table II. The results obtained by the two methods are in excellent agreement. The mean values were not significantly different from each

Table II   Comparison of Aldosterone Measured in Plasma, Aldosterone, and Aldosterone Secretion Measured as Aldolactone in Rat Glomerulosa Tissue Incubation Medium, and Determinations in Patients by Radioimmunoassay (RIA) and Double Isotope Derivative Analysis (DID)

Sample number	RIA assay	DID analysis	Percentage difference
Plasma (ng/100 ml)			
1	8.1	7.0	16
2	3.7	3.8	3
3	11.3	14.0	19
4	14.0	11.0	27
5	17.7	25.0	29
6	50.0	54.0	7
7	86.0	78.0	10
8	86.0	100.0	14
9	43.0	44.0	2
10	40.0	38.0	5
11	217.0	190.0	14
Mean	52.4	51.3	13.2 ± 9.1 (SD)

Table II (*Continued*)

Sample number	RIA assay	DID analysis	Percentage difference
Incubation medium (ng)			
1	106	95	10
2	132	167	27
3	365	448	21
4	840	829	1
5	92	90	2
6	147	131	11
7	29	31	7
8	46	51	11
9	71	55	22
10	38	32	16
11	57	51	10
12	45	51	13
13	64	77	20
14	350	300	14
15	460	450	2
16	740	602	19
17	4450	3560	20
18	1100	929	15
19	372	492	32
20	244	268	10
Mean	487	436	14.2 ± 8.2 (SD)
Secretion rate (μg/day)			
1	549	574	4.6
2	712	864	21.3
3	712	712	0
4	812	806	0.7
5	618	665	7.6
6	1050	1225	16.7
7	942	1087	15.4
8	564	411	27.1
9	836	638	23.7
10	508	610	20.0
11	759	622	18.1
12	1689	1437	14.9
13	1842	2192	19.0
14	617	664	7.6
15	190	194	2.1
16	355	486	36.9
17	770	604	22.7
18	730	880	20.5
19	2173	2118	2.5
20	812	806	0.7
Mean	862	880	14.1 ± 10.4 (SD)

other and agreed to within 10%. The absolute percentage difference was between 13 and 14%.

B. Specificity, Sensitivity, Precision

The specificity of these methods is determined from the extent of cross-reaction of the antibody with other steroids and by the values obtained by processing an extract of water or adrenalectomized plasma through the method. The cross-reaction on a percentage (w/w) basis with other steroids is shown in Table I and has been discussed earlier. The mean blank value for each method was less than the sensitivity of the particular method. Sensitivity was defined as twice the standard deviation of zero point, i.e., the smallest amount significantly different from zero. In ten consecutive experiments, the mean value of the percentage binding of ^{3}H-aldosterone to the antibody in the absence of aldosterone was 65.7 ± 2.2 (S.D.) ± 3.3% (coefficient of variation). Thus, the sensitivity of the method is 2–3 pg. For DOC, the value was 4.0 pg, 6.0 pg for the aldolactone method, and 2.0 pg for the 18-OH-DOC and 18-OH-B methods.

The precision of the methods is indicated by the standard deviation of the mean value obtained in replicate measurements on a plasma or urine sample. For example, the mean plasma value for aldosterone was 6.6 ± 0.68 S.D. ± 10.3% (coefficient of variation), and the coefficient of variation on ten replicate aldosterone secretion determinations on a urine sample was 10.4%.

IV. PROBLEMS RELATED TO MEASURING MINERALOCORTICOIDS

The major problem in measuring these steroids is related to their low concentrations in peripheral plasma and the difficulty of obtaining a sufficiently low methodology blank. Because an extraction and separation procedure has been necessary in all reported assays of these hormones, methodologic blanks may be either nonspecific or aldosterone or deoxycorticosterone that has inadvertently strayed into the method. The nonspecific blank is usually related to impurities in the solvents used for extraction or elution or in the chromatography system. In the assays described earlier, we have found that by washing the paper for 24 to 48 hours with the solvent used in the chromatography system the nonspecific blank can be almost entirely eliminated. The specific blank, i.e., the presence of stray aldosterone or deoxycorticosterone, may be more elusive, but most can be eliminated by scrupulous cleanliness when dealing with the paper and extraction apparatus. Wherever possible, we have utilized disposable equipment so that any stray steroid would be eliminated. A major source of inert aldosterone may come from the markers used in the paper chromatography system. If microgram amounts of steroid, sufficient for detection by ultraviolet absorption, are used as chromatography markers, then a significant blank (between 20 and 50 pg) has been found. This presumably comes from this inert marker which is in a concentration one to five millionfold greater than that in the sample. To eliminate this problem, tritiated aldosterone is used as the indicator and the position of the steroid is determined by scanning the paper for the tritium peak.

V. OTHER RADIOIMMUNOASSAY METHODS

Several methods have been published for measurement of plasma levels of aldosterone by radioimmunoassay (e.g., Mayes *et al.*, 1970; Bayard *et al.*, 1970; Ito *et al.*, 1972). The method of Bayard *et al.* (1970) is similar to the one described here with the exception that Florisil is used to separate the bound from free steroid. The method described by Ito *et al.* (1972) used a Sephadex LH-20 column rather than a paper chromatogram to purify and, therefore, is more rapid. Finally, Mayes *et al.* (1970) used paper chromatography followed by a silica gel column and have, therefore, the most complicated of those methods presently available. The method of Ito *et al.* (1972) is the simplest but is not readily applicable to the measurement of several steroids simultaneously from the same aliquot of plasma.

The radioimmunoassay method for plasma deoxycorticosterone by Arnold and James (1971) is essentially the same as the present method except a Bush 3 system is used and the paper is eluted through a silica gel column similar to that used by Mayes *et al.* (1970) for aldosterone. Separation of bound from free in the Arnold–James method is achieved by ammonium sulfate precipitation of the bound form rather than dextran-coated charcoal adsorption of the free form.

Finally, Farmer *et al.* (1972) have described a rapid aldosterone radioimmunoassay that can be applied to unchromatographed urine or plasma. Their method uses the aldosterone lactone antibody similar to that described in the present chapter for urine and tissue extract. If reliable, this would be more rapid than any of the assays previously developed. However, in our experience, while the 18-hydroxycorticosterone or 11-deoxy-18-hydroxycorticosterone does not significantly cross-react with the lactone antibody, because in the oxidation step these, as well as 18-hydroxy-11-dehydrocorticosterone, are converted into γ-lactones, a significant cross-reaction may occur. Because the plasma level of 18-hydroxycorticosterone is greater than aldosterone, a significant error in the estimation of aldosterone may occur. In order to eliminate these cross-reacting lactones, a chromatographic step would be essential. Chandler *et al.* (1976) and Edwards *et al.* (1974) have each published a method for measuring 18-OH-DOC. Both methods employ lactone formation, and the sensitivities and specificites are similar to those of the method described. Also, the extent of cross-reactivity of the antibody with other steroids requires that a chromatographic purification step be done before measurement.

A method with similar precision and sensitivity for the measurement of 18-OH-B has been reported by Martin *et al.* (1975). Antibody to 18-OH-B was produced in the rabbit by administration of 18-OH-B lactone 3-monooxime–BSA. It is noteworthy that the antiserum has a 100% cross-reactivity with 18-OH-DOC lactone. However, a paper chromatographic purification step ensures that the latter steroid is resolved from the 18-OH-B lactone before assay.

VI. NEWER DEVELOPMENTS

Now that methods are available for assaying all the mineralocorticoids, the major need is for the production of more specific antibodies. If an antibody could be developed with adequate minimum, or preferably zero, cross-reactivity with the other mineralocorticoids, the chromatographic purification step could be eliminated and the assay time thus considerably shortened. To date, this has proved to be difficult, due to the close structural characteristics of the mineralocorticoids within themselves and with a number of the other steroids which are present in much greater concentrations in peripheral plasma. In contrast, in urine with the built-in specificity of the pH 1.0 conjugate of aldosterone, it is achievable. While the measurement of mineralocorticoids by radioimmunoassay is certainly more precise and sensitive than by double isotope techniques, the ability to measure them directly in plasma, as is possible for insulin and growth hormone, has not yet been realized.

REFERENCES

Arnold, M. L., and James, V. H. T. (1971). Determination of deoxycorticosterone in plasma: Double isotope and immunoassay methods. *Steroids* 18, 789–891.

Bayard, F., Beitins, I. Z., Kowarski, A., and Migeon, C. J. (1970). Measurement of plasma aldosterone by radioimmunoassay. *J. Clin. Endocrinol. Metab.* 31, 1–6.

Berson, S. A., and Yalow, R. S. (1959). Recent studies on insulin-binding antibodies. *Ann. N.Y. Acad. Sci.* 82, 338–344.

Brodie, A. H., Shimizu, N., Tait, S. A. S., and Tait, J. F. (1967). A method for the measurement of aldosterone in peripheral plasma using ³H-acetic anhydride. *J. Clin. Endocrinol. Metab.* 27, 997–1012.

Chandler, D. W., Tuck, M. L., and Mayes, D. M. (1976). The measurement of 18-hydroxy-11-deoxy corticosterone in human plasma by radioimmunoassay. *Steroids* 27, 235–246.

Coghlan, J. P., and Scoggins, B. A. (1967). Measurement of aldosterone in peripheral blood of man and sheep. *J. Clin. Endocrinol. Metab.* 27, 1470–1486.

Dorfman, R. I., Potts, A. M., and Feil, M. L. (1947). Studies on the bioassay of hormones: The use of radiosodium for the detection of small quantities of desoxycorticosterone. *Endocrinology* 41, 464–469.

Edwards, C. R. W., Biglieri, E. G., Martin, V. I., Taylor, A. A., and Bartter, F. C. (1974). The development of radioimmunoassays for 18-hydroxycorticosterone and 18-hydroxydeoxycorticosterone. *J. Clin. Endocrinol. Metab.* 63, 29–30.

Erlanger, B. F., Borek, F., Beiser, S. M., and Lieberman, S. (1957). Steroid protein conjugates. I. Preparation and characterization of conjugates of bovine serum albumin with testosterone and with cortisone. *J. Biol. Chem.* 228, 713–722.

Farmer, R. W., Roup, W. G., Jr., Pellizzari, E. D., and Fabre, L. F., Jr. (1972). A rapid aldosterone radioimmunoassay. *J. Clin. Endocrinol. Metab.* 34, 15–22.

Farmer, R. W., Brown, D. H., Howard, P. Y., and Fabre, L. F., Jr. (1973). A radioimmunoassay for plasma aldosterone without chromatography. *J. Clin. Endocrinol. Metab.* 36, 460–465.

Goodfriend, L., and Sehon, A. H. (1958). Preparation of an estrone-protein conjugate. *Can. J. Biochem. Physiol.* 36, 1177–1184.

Haning, R., McCracken, J., Cyr, M. St., Underwood, R., Williams, G., and Abraham, G. (1972). The evolution of titer and specificity of aldosterone binding antibodies in hyperimmunized sheep. *Steroids* 20, 73–88.

Harrop, G. A., Nicholson, W. M., and Strauss, H. (1936). Studies on the suprarenal cortex. V. The influence of the cortical hormone upon the excretion of water and electrolytes in the suprarenalectomized dog. *J. Exp. Med.* 64, 233–251.

Hartman, F. A., and Spoor, H. J. (1940). Cortin and the Na factor of the adrenal. *Endocrinology* 26, 871–876.

Ito, T., Woo, J., Haning, R., and Horton, R. (1972). A radioimmunoassay for aldosterone in human peripheral plasma including a comparison of alternate techniques. *J. Clin. Endocrinol. Metab.* 34, 106–112.

Kliman, B., and Peterson, R. E. (1960). Double isotope derivative assay of aldosterone in biological extracts. *J. Biol. Chem.* 235, 1639–1648.

Lieberman, S., Erlanger, B. F., Bieser, S. M., and Agate, F. J., Jr. (1959). Steroid-protein conjugates: Their chemical, immunochemical and endocrinological properties. *Recent Prog. Horm. Res.* 15, 165–196.

Mader, W. J., and Buck, R. R. (1952). Colorimetric determination of cortisone and related ketol steroids. *Anal. Chem.* **24**, 666–667.

Martin, B. T., and Nugent, C. A. (1973). A non-chromatographic radioimmunoassay for plasma aldosterone. *Steroids* **21**, 169–180.

Martin, V. I., Edwards, C. R. W., Biglieri, E. G., Vinson, G. R., and Bartter, F. C. (1975). The development and application of a radioimmunoassay for 18-hydroxycorticosterone. *Steroids* **26**, 591–604.

Mayes, D., Furuyama, S., Kem, D. C., and Nugent, C. A. (1970). A radioimmunoassay for plasma aldosterone. *J. Clin. Endocrinol. Metab.* **30**, 682–685.

Nowaczynski, W. J., Goldner, M., and Genest, J. (1955). Microdetermination of corticosterioids with tetrazolium derivatives. *J. Lab. Clin. Med.* **45**, 818–821.

Rayfield, E. J., Rose, L. I., Dluhy, R. G., and Williams, G. H. (1973). Aldosterone secretory and glucocorticoid excretory responses to alpha 1–24 ACTH (Cortrosyn) in sodium-depleted normal man. *J. Clin. Endocrinol. Metab.* **36**, 30–35.

Schulster, D., Tait, S. A. S., Tait, J. F., and Mrotek, J. (1970). Production of steroids by *in vitro* superfusion of endocrine tissue. III. Corticosterone output from rat adrenals stimulated by adrenocorticotropin or cyclic 3′, 5′-adenosine monophosphate and the inhibitory effect of cycloheximide. *Endocrinology* **86**, 487–502.

Simpson, S. A., and Tait, J. F. (1952). A quantitative method for the bioassay of the effect of adrenal cortical steroids on mineral metabolism. *Endocrinology* **50**, 150–161.

Simpson, S. A., Tait, J. F., Wettstein, A., Neher, R., von Euq, J., Schindler, O., and Reichstein, T. (1954). Adrenal cortex compounds and related substances. XCI. The isolation and properties of aldosterone. *Helv. Chim. Acta* **37**, 1163–1200.

Thorn, G. W., and Engel, L. L. (1938). The effect of sex hormones on the renal excretion of electrolytes. *J. Exp. Med.* **68**, 299–312.

Underwood, R. H., and Williams, G. H. (1972). The simultaneous measurement of aldosterone, cortisol and corticosterone in human peripheral plasma by displacement analysis. *J. Lab. Clin. Med.* **79**, 848–862.

Williams, G. H., and Underwood, R. H. (1973). Radioimmunoassay of steroid hormones. IV. Congress of ALASBIMN, Santiago, Chile, 1973. *Rev. Med. Nucl.* **5**, 85.

Williams, G. H., McDonnell, L. M., Tait, S. A. S., and Tait, J. F. (1972). The effect of medium composition and *in vitro* stimuli on the conversion of corticosterone to aldosterone in rat glomerulosa tissue. *Endocrinology* **91**, 948–960.

Williams, G. H., Braley, L. M., and Underwood, R. H. (1976). The regulation of plasma 18-hydroxy-11-deoxycorticosterone in man. *J. Clin. Invest.* **58**, 221–227.

Writz, H. (1950). Der Einfluß von Desoxycorticosteron und 11-Dehydro-17-hydroxycorticosteron auf das Plasma-natrium adrenalektomerter Ratten. *Helv. Physiol. Acta* **8**, 186–194.

39

Glucocorticoids: Cortisol, Cortisone, Corticosterone, Compound S, and Their Metabolites

P. VECSEI

I. INTRODUCTION

Interest in the radioimmunoassay of glucocorticoids did not arise until after development of the radioimmunoassay of aldosterone (Mayes *et al.*, 1970). The protein-binding assays, described first by Murphy *et al.* in 1963 for the determination of plasma cortisol, seemed to make elaboration of this kind of assay unnecessary. The principle of

Methods of Hormone Radioimmunoassay, Second Edition
Copyright © 1979 by Academic Press, Inc.
All rights of reproduction in any form reserved. ISBN 0-12-379260-6

the protein-binding assay was adapted later for determination of corticosterone (Newsome *et al.*, 1972; Nowaczynski *et al.*, 1972; Spät and Jozan, 1972) and of compound S (Spark, 1971). Protein-binding assays are practical enough to meet most requirements of clinical and research laboratories; however, the radioimmunoassay of glucocorticoids has some advantages over the protein-binding methods, i.e., higher sensitivity, greater specificity, and long-term usefulness of the same antibody preparation.

At the time we first reported on the radioimmunoassay of cortisol and corticosterone in March 1972 (Vecsei *et al.*, 1972a), other groups were also working on this problem, as was revealed by later publications (Underwood and Williams, 1972; Ruder *et al.*, 1972; Richardson and Schulster, 1972; Abraham *et al.*, 1972; Gross *et al.*, 1972; Tait *et al.*, 1972). At the end of 1972, the paper of Mahajan *et al.* provided the first description of the radioimmunoassay of compound S. In 1973, Srivastava *et al.* described the radioimmunoassay of cortisone.

Several other reports have been published since then. This chapter will deal with the progress that has been made in the production of antibodies, the improvement and simplification of techniques, and new applications. In addition, the radioimmunoassays of the glucocorticoid metabolites, tetrahydrocortisol (THF), tetrahydrocortisone (THE), tetrahydrocorticosterone (THB), and tetrahydro-compound S (THS) will also be described.

II. METHODS OF RADIOIMMUNOASSAY

A. Production of Antibodies

1. Antigen and Technique of Immunization

Presented in Table I are data on the antigens used for immunization against cortisol, cortisone, corticosterone, compound S, and their metabolites. The main aim of using different types of antigens was to obtain antibodies with better specificity. Techniques for the preparation of oxime and hemisuccinate derivatives and their conjugation to serum proteins are described in detail in Chapters 35 and 38.

For immunization of rabbits, 1.0 mg (for sheep, use 3.0 mg) of the antigen was dissolved in 1.0 ml 0.9% NaCl solution and emulsified with 1.0 ml Freund's adjuvant. This suspension was given intramuscularly to rabbits in the gluteal area and to sheep in the pectoral musculature. Identical injections were repeated at intervals of two to four

Table I   Antigens Used for Immunization[a]

Antigen types	References
Cortisol	
21-Hemisuccinate	Vecsei et al. (1972a, b, d); Ruder et al. (1972)
3-Oxime-21-acetate	Cook et al. (1973)
3-Oxime	Dash et al. (1975); Fahmy et al. (1975)
3,20-Dioxime	P. Vecsei (unpublished)
6α- or 6β-Hemisuccinoxy-	Nishina et al. (1974)
Cortisone	
21-Hemisuccinate	Srivastava et al. (1973)
Corticosterone	
21-Hemisuccinate	Underwood and Williams (1972); Vecsei et al. (1972a, b); Tait et al. (1972)
3-Oxime	Vetter et al. (1974)
3,20-Dioxime	P. Vecsei (unpublished)
Compound S	
21-Hemisuccinate	Mahajan et al. (1972); Vielhauer et al. (1974)
3-Oxime	Nishina et al. (1974); Thomas et al. (1976)
6α- or 6β-Hemisuccinoxy-	Nishina et al. (1974)
THF, THE, THB, and THS	
20-Oxime	Will et al. (1975); Vecsei et al. (1976); Vielhauer et al. (1976)
21-Hemisuccinate[b]	Will (1975a)

[a] Colburn (1975) used antibody raised with prednisolone-3-oxime for cortisol radioimmunoassay.

[b] Only for THF and THE.

weeks. At the end of the third month, we obtained antibodies in some of the rabbits, but it required prolonged immunization until the ninth to fourteenth month in order to develop higher titers. Ruder et al. (1972) have reported production of antibody against cortisol in rabbits immunized by multiple intradermal injections using a total of 50 μg antigen. The details of the intradermal immunization technique have been reported by Vaitukaitis et al. (1971).

It is difficult to obtain exact information on the efficiency of immunization. Table II presents data on our corresponding results. It is obvious that the efficiency is influenced by the animals used (unclarified genetic factors) and by the composition of the antigens. Vetter et al. (1974a) reported that the optimal antibody response could be achieved when 15 aldosterone molecules are linked to one protein (rabbit

Table II   Titers Obtained in Our Laboratory

Steroid	Type of antigen	Species	Number of animals	Titer
Cortisol	21-Hemisuccinate	Sheep	12	1 : 1800–1 : 7400
Cortisol	21-Hemisuccinate	Rabbit	20	1 : 170–1 : 33,000
Cortisol	3-20-Dioxime	Rabbit	4	1 : 270–1 : 850
Cortisol-21-acetate	3-Oxime	Rabbit	4	1 : 600–1 : 850
Compound S	21-Hemisuccinate	Sheep	2	1 : 30,000–1 : 58,000
Compound S	21-Hemisuccinate	Rabbit	13	1 : 280–1 : 170,000
Compound S	3-Oxime	Rabbit	5	1 : 700–1 : 34,000
Corticosterone	21-Hemisuccinate	Sheep	3	1 : 1200–1 : 37,000
Corticosterone	21-Hemisuccinate	Rabbit	13	1 : 100–1 : 32,000
Corticosterone	3-20-Dioxime	Rabbit	7	1 : 800–1 : 6000
THF	21-Hemisuccinate	Rabbit	4	1 : 450–1 : 5500
THF	20-Oxime	Rabbit	7	1 : 4800–1 : 35,000
THE	21-Hemisuccinate	Rabbit	4	1 : 26,000–1 : 140,000
THE	20-Oxime	Rabbit	6	1 : 3500–1 : 90,000
TH-Corticosterone	20-Oxime	Rabbit	5	1 : 300–1 : 19,000
TH-Compound S	20-Oxime	Rabbit	10	1 : 1450–1 : 12,000

serum albumin) molecule. No comparative figures have yet been published on similar patterns of glucocorticoid antigens. It is very probable, however, that an optimum exists.

2. Biologic Effects of Immunization

In the first series of immunizations, abscesses appeared after six months in some rabbits immunized against cortisol and corticosterone and in animals immunized simultaneously against cortisol, corticosterone, deoxycorticosterone, and aldosterone. In some rabbits, muscle weakness, occasional paralysis, and an increasing inability to take food and water were observed. This syndrome, which may have been facilitated by the abscesses, is a symptom complex resembling hypercorticism. In these animals, elevation of plasma cortisol and corticosterone (Figure 1) and hypokalemia were observed, and the sera were often lipemic. However, in later series of immunization of rabbits and sheep, similar symptoms were not present, but elevation of plasma cortisol and corticosterone was seen. The reason for the irregular appearance of symptoms as described above is not known.

We are aware of no report of symptoms of hyper- or hypocorticism, although different corticoids have been used by various workers for immunization. Fleischer et al. (1967) have noted increased blood ACTH levels in patients with ACTH antibodies after ACTH treatment, but none of them developed signs of adrenal hyperfunction. On

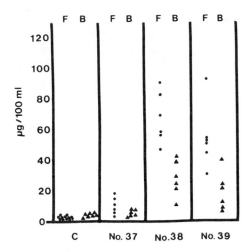

Figure 1. Plasma cortisol (F) and corticosterone (B) levels measured in control rabbits (C, rabbits treated with Freund's adjuvant without antigen and untreated animals) and in rabbits No. 37, 38, and 39. For data obtained in other animals see Gless *et al.* (1973, 1974). Titers: No. 37 = 1 : 500–1 : 2400; No. 38 = 1 : 11,000–1 : 20,000; No. 39 = 1 : 8200–1 : 29,000.

the other hand, immunization against testosterone, estrogens, and progesterone has evoked biologic effects, i.e., signs of hypofunction. Similar observations were also made after successful immunization against vasopressin, thyrotropin, etc. (Morton and Waite, 1972; Beall *et al.*, 1973; Raziano *et al.*, 1972; Nieschlag *et al.*, 1975; Csapo *et al.*, 1975). Figure 1 shows the correlation between the success of immunization and the elevation of plasma corticoids. In rabbits with high titers (No. 38 and 39) excessively elevated plasma cortisol and corticosterone levels were observed; in rabbit No. 37 with a moderate immune response, a relatively small increase in plasma corticoids was found. Nishina *et al.* (1974) immunized rabbits with cortisol-3-oxime antigens. They found only a moderate elevation in mean plasma cortisol concentrations up 5.8 μg/100 ml. It is not clear whether the difference between the data of Nishina *et al.* (1974) and ours is due to the different type of antigen used or to the different efficiency of immunization.

The elevation in plasma cortisol and corticosterone concentrations may have been evoked at least partly by the stimulation of the adrenals that is caused by binding of corticosteroids to the antibodies, thereby preventing a negative feedback effect on the secretion of ACTH. Both

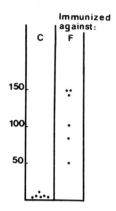

Figure 2.   Plasma ^{3}H-cortisol concentrations after intravenous injection of 4.5×10^6 to 6.25×10^6 cpm 1,2-^{3}H-cortisol in control rabbits (C) and in rabbits immunized against cortisol (F). The measurements were carried out 150 minutes after the injection of the radioactive steroid. The disappearance of tritiated corticosterone, deoxycorticosterone, and aldosterone from the blood of rabbits immunized against the corresponding steroids was also found to be delayed.

the presence and the degree of binding could be demonstrated by the delayed disappearance of ^{3}H-cortisol from the blood of the immunized rabbits (Figure 2).

The measurement of free biologically relevant steroid levels is made difficult by technical problems due to the high percentage of bound steroids in the immunized animals (Hillier *et al.*, 1975). However, an elevation of the free plasma steroid concentration could also be demonstrated in sheep immunized against aldosterone (Vielhauer *et al.*, 1976b). As opposed to other corticosteroids, aldosterone is only bound to plasma proteins to the extent of 30–40%.

It is not known to what extent the elevation in circulating corticoids was due to the stimulation of adrenal function. The involvement of adrenal function was indicated by histologic findings (Nieschlag *et al.*, 1975). The reaction of plasma cortisol and corticosterone levels to exogenous ACTH was exaggerated (Gless *et al.*, 1974).

B. Antibody

1. Assay and Separation Techniques

Table III shows details of the radioimmunologic reaction as performed in our laboratory. The bottom of the same table also contains data on the materials used. Most of the methods and the materials are

Table III   Details of Radioimmunologic Technique

Steps
1. 0.1 ml [1,2-³H]cortisol (or corticosterone)[a] solution (3–5000 cpm [0.05 M borate buffer (pH 8) with 0.1% lysozyme]
2. 0.1 ml solution with unknown amounts of cortisol (or corticosterone) (5% ethanol solution)
3. 0.5 ml solution with cortisol (or corticosterone) antibodies (0.05 M borate buffer with 0.1% lysozyme)
4. Incubation, 4°C, two hours
5. Separation of the protein-bound and -unbound radioactivity with dextran-coated charcoal
6. Measurement of the protein-bound radioactivity

Materials
Test tubes: polystyrene tubes (length: 40 mm, diameter: 10 mm) with Lupolene caps (Strömberg & Co., Langenfeld)
Pipettes: Eppendorf pipettes with "one way" tips
Lysozyme: Serva, Heidelberg
Human serum γ-globulin (used in the preparation of the dextran-coated charcoal): "Forschungs-Gamma-Globulin," Deutsche Kabi GmbH, Munich.
Dextran-coated charcoal: One volume activated charcoal solution (5.0 gm Norit A, Serva, Heidelberg, in 80 ml, pH 8.0, 0.05 M borate buffer containing 0.6% human γ-globulin) plus six volumes dextran solution (100 mg dextran T-70, Pharmacia, Uppsala) dissolved in 80 ml γ-globulin buffer solution, stirred for ten minutes prior to use. The volume used is 0.1 ml.

[a] An improvement in the sensitivity of the radioimmunologic-reaction may be possible through the use of corticosteroids with very high specific radioactivity. We have tried to apply [1,2,6,7-³H]corticosterone, and obtained a greater degree of sensitivity. However, the 1,2,6,7-derivative was found not to be stable enough, at least under our circumstances.

used commonly in the steroid and radioimmunologic laboratories, with two exceptions:

a. For the technique of separating free from protein-bound radioactivity, we have applied the method of Poulsen (1969) used for the determination of angiotensin II. Dextran-coated charcoal (0.1 ml) was transferred to disposable caps and the caps were placed on tubes which were then inverted simultaneously and shaken.

b. We have introduced a decantation device (Figure 3), enabling us to carry out the decantation of the protein-bound corticosteroid radioactivity simultaneously (Ballman and Vecsei, 1973).

Most authors have used dextran-coated charcoal for separation of protein-bound radioactivity (Ruder et al., 1972; Underwood and Williams, 1972; Richardson and Schulster, 1972; Abraham et al., 1972;

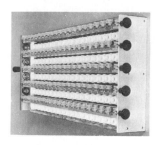

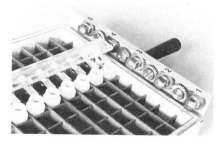

Figure 3.   One part of the decantation equipment. One hundred samples can be decanted at the same time.

Tait *et al.*, 1972). Foster and Dunn (1974) have applied hemoglobin-coated charcoal; Lee and Schiller (1975) used polyethylene glycol; Nabors *et al.* (1974), Mahajan *et al.* (1972), and Colburn (1975) used the double antibody technique. Gomez-Sanchez *et al.* (1975), however, preferred the use of a saturated solution of ammonium sulfate for precipitation of the protein-bound radioactivity. Rolleri *et al.* (1976) used antibodies bound to CNBr-activated cellulose as a solid-phase radioimmunoassay for the estimation of cortisol. As another solid-phase technique, antibodies covalently coupled to the surface of nylon were used in our laboratory for the radioimmunoassay of THF and THE (Vecsei *et al.*, 1975). However, the latter technique did not give satisfactory results for the cortisol assay. One advantage to the solid-phase assay is that it can be performed at room temperature. Several commercial firms offer cortisol radioimmunoassay kits based on the coated tube technique. The same method was described also by Comoglio and Celada (1976).

Hunter *et al.* (1975) have used ^{125}I-labeled cortisol. Chambers *et al.* (1975) used ^{75}Se-labeled cortisol instead of ^{3}H-labeled material. Fahmy *et al.* (1975) compared the cortisol radioimmunoassay techniques with ^{3}H, ^{125}I, and ^{75}Se labeling. In the case of one particular antibody, ^{3}H-cortisol was the best label, being the most sensitive and specific. For the assays of other glucocorticoids and glucocorticoid metabolites, only ^{3}H-labeled steroids have been used.

An enzyme immunoassay for the estimation of cortisol has been presented by Comoglio and Celada (1976). *Escherichia coli* β-galactosidase was used as a marker.

2. *Sensitivity of the Radioimmunologic Reaction*

Figure 4 shows a typical calibration curve for the cortisol radioimmunoassay (Vecsei *et al.*, 1972d). The linear part of the curve starts at 25 pg. Corresponding values for the corticosterone and compound S assays are 20 and 30 pg, respectively. No major variation was observed in sensitivity of the cortisol assay and the slope of the calibration curve

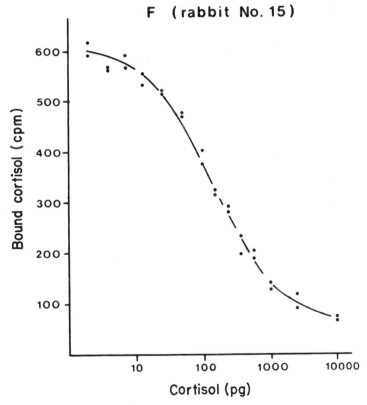

Figure 4. Calibration curve, obtained with different amounts of unlabeled cortisol. Length of incubation: two hours at 4°C.

using the same antibody for five years. Lysozyme, gelatin, and bovine serum albumin functioned equally well in the assay buffer.

3. Specificity of the Radioimmunologic Reaction

Table IV shows cross-reaction values of cortisol antibodies. The same values in the protein-binding assay (Murphy, 1975) are entered for comparison. In other sections of the table, the cross-reactions of cortisone, corticosterone, compound S, and corticosteroid metabolite antisera are shown. The cross-reactions of some antisera raised with 3-oxime antigens are lower than the cross-reactions of 21-hemisuccinate antisera. However, the figures indicate that the specificity depends not only on the type of antigen used but also on the technical details, such as the type and quality of the protein dissolved in the incubation fluid (Table V).

Variations in cross-reaction can be caused by the batch of protein used in the assay. For instance, the human γ-globulin preparation delivered in the summer of 1971 evoked a significant increase in cross-reaction of the cortisol antibody with compound S that probably was due to transcortin impurity.

C. Preparation of Biological Samples for Radioimmunoassay

1. Plasma Samples

Table VI indicates the steps for extraction of plasma cortisol (Vecsei et al., 1972d). Abraham et al. (1972) have also used alcohol extraction, without addition of ^{3}H-cortisol to the samples to measure loss during extraction. However, we have observed certain variations in the recovery figures. Ruder et al. (1972) used dichloromethane extraction without additional separation. Foster and Dunn (1974) as well as Klemm and Gupta (1975) have introduced a thermodestruction step to remove transcortin (based on a procedure published by Murphy et al. in 1963) and an additional radioimmunoassay of cortisol without further procedure. Foster and Dunn (1974) submitted the prediluted plasma samples to 100°C for ten minutes and Klemm and Gupta (1975) to 60°C for 60 minutes. We submitted plasma samples prediluted 1 : 50–1 : 100 to 70°C for 60 minutes, followed by a short cooling at room temperature and then incubation according to the description in Table III. There was excellent correlation between these values and those estimated after alcohol extraction.

Table IV Cross-Reactions of Anti-glucocorticoid Antibodies

	Cross-reaction values (%)					
	Vecsei et al. (1972d)[a]	Ruder et al. (1972)[a]	Abraham et al. (1972)[a]	Dash et al. (1975)[b]	Murphy et al. 1977 Transcortin preparations	
					Human	Horse
a. Cortisol antibodies						
Cortisol	100	100	100	100	100	100
Compound S	10	100	9.0	3.8	22	28
21-Deoxycortisol	100[c]	100		3.7	60	71
Corticosterone	1.4	46	5.0	12.5	83	30
DOC	0	46	1.0	0.06	68	42
17-OH-Progesterone		56	2.5	0.06	74	22
6-β-Cortisol				0.05		
Prednisolone				28.5		

	Cross-reaction value (%) Srivastava et al. (1973)[a]
b. Cortisone antibodies	
Cortisone	100
Cortisol	0.68
Compound S	0.66
Corticosterone	1.15
DOC	0.88
17-OH-Progesterone	0.75

(Continued)

Table IV (Continued)

c. Corticosterone antibodies

	Vecsei et al. (1972a,b)[a]	Underwood and Williams (1972)[a]	Cross-reaction values (%) Richardson and Schuster (1972)[a]	P. Vecsei (unpublished)[a]
Corticosterone	100	100	100	100
Aldosterone	0.36	0.30	1.7	
18-OH-Corticosterone	0.1	0.02		
Deoxycorticosterone	16.8	4.7	7.5	5.6
18-OH-Deoxycorticosterone	1.2	0.05		
Cortisol	0.46	0.50	1.0	1.2
Cortisone		0.03	1.0	
Compound S	5.6			0.3
11-Dehydrocorticosterone			0.1	
11-OH-Progesterone	4.2			
Progesterone	5.9	3.5	10.2	
17-OH-Pregnenolone			1.0	
Pregnenolone			1.0	
Testosterone		0		
Estradiol		0		
Aldadiene	2.9			

d. Compound S antibodies

	Nishina et al. (1974)[e]	Mahajan et al. (1972)[a]	P. Vecsei (unpublished)[b]	Vielhauer et al. (1974)[a]
Compound S	100	100	100	100
17-Hydroxyprogesterone	0.2	100	10	21
11-Deoxycorticosterone	4.2	7.1		5.7
Progesterone		5.7		
Testosterone		3.1		
Cortisol	1.0	1.7	1.18	1.83
Aldosterone		0.1		0
Corticosterone	0.07	<0.01	0	0.16
Dehydroepiandrosterone		<0.01		
17β-Estradiol		<0.01		

e. THE, THF, THB; and THS antibodies

	Will et al. (1975a,b and 1977)			M. Mok and P. Vecsei (unpublished)	Vecsei et al. (1976); Kohl et al. (1978)
	THE	THE	THF	THS	THB
Tetrahydro-cortisol (THF)	0.76	8.9	100	0.01	0.7
Tetrahydrocortisone (THE)	100	100	0.32	<0.01	0
Tetrahydrocorticosterone (THB)	<0.01	0.8	1.5	0.01	100
Tetrahydro-11-dehydrocorticosterone (THA)					0.3
Tetrahydrodeoxycortisol (THS)	0.31	3.1	3.97	100	0.6
5α-Dihydrocortisol (DHF)	<0.01	<0.01	0.05		
5α-Dihydrocortisone (DHE)	<0.01	0.2	<0.01		
5β-Dihydrocortisol (DHF)	<0.01	<0.01	8.18		
5β-Dihydrocortisone (DHE)	1.1	0.69	0.02		
5β-Dihydrocorticosterone (DHB)					1.14
allo-Tetrahydrocortisone (allo-THE)	0.3	0.16	<0.01		
allo-Tetrahydrocorticosterone (allo-THB)	<0.1	<0.1	1.5		0.53
allo-Tetrahydrodeoxycortisol (allo-THS)	<0.1	<0.1	3.97	0.27	0
Cortisol (F)	<0.01	<0.01	0.13		0
Cortisone (E)	<0.01	<0.01	<0.01		
Corticosterone (B)	<0.01	<0.01	<0.01		
THF-3-glucuronide	<1.0		3.8	0	0
THF-21-glucuronide	12.5		100	0.8	1.1
THE-3-glucuronide	<1.0		0	0	4.8
THE-21-glucuronide	100		0	0	0
THB-3-glucuronide	0		0	0	0.2
THB-21-glucuronide	0		15.8	0	39.0
THS-3-glucuronide				0	0
THS-21-glucuronide				60.0	0
THAld-3-glucuronide					0

[a] Antigen: 21-hemisuccinate.
[b] Antigen: 3-oxime.
[c] Recent observation.
[d] Antigen: 3, 20-oxime.
[e] Antigen: 6α-hemisuccinoxy.
[f] Antigen: 20-oxime.

Table V   Influence of the Protein in the Incubation Fluid on Cross-Reactions with Cortisol Antibody[a]

Protein in the incubation fluid	Corticosterone	Compound S
Human γ-globulin	35.4	13.3
Bovine serum albumin	4.6	16.5
Lysozyme	5.3	8.5
Gelatin	11.6	15.8
Gelatin (dried-dissolved)	1.4	10.0

[a] Values are given in percent.

Table VI   Extraction of the Plasma Samples for Cortisol Radioimmunoassay[a]

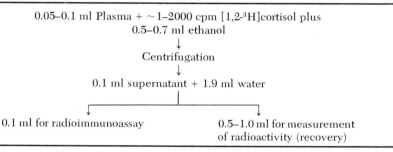

0.05–0.1 ml Plasma + ~1–2000 cpm [1,2-³H]cortisol plus
0.5–0.7 ml ethanol
↓
Centrifugation
↓
0.1 ml supernatant + 1.9 ml water
|
0.1 ml for radioimmunoassay   0.5–1.0 ml for measurement
                                      of radioactivity (recovery)

[a] From Vecsei et al. (1972d).

The procedure of Rolleri et al. (1976) is very simple. They reported an assay based on the estimation of cortisol without any procedure other than dilution of samples with a pH 3.5 buffer solution. The radioimmunoassay was carried out using antibodies coupled to CNBr-activated cellulose at room temperature. It is likely that these authors used antibodies of very high affinity. The incubation performed at room temperature and at pH 3.5 made the binding of cortisol to transcortin relatively weak.

The flow sheet in Table VII shows the steps for extraction of plasma corticosterone as performed in our laboratory. Gomez-Sanchez et al. (1975) have also estimated corticosterone without chromatography in rat serum after methanol inactivation of transcortin. Underwood and Williams (1972), Roy et al. (1973), and Nabors et al. (1974) were forced to use a chromatographic separation for human plasma, as were Gross et al. (1972) in rat experiments.

The procedure for the preparation of plasma samples for the radioimmunoassay of compound S is very similar to that shown for plasma corticosterone in Table VII (Vielhauer et al., 1974). The most

Table VII   Extraction of the Plasma Samples for Corticosterone Radioimmunoassay

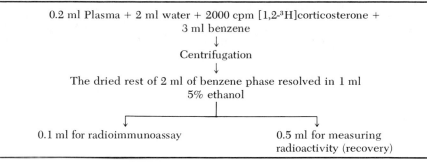

0.2 ml Plasma + 2 ml water + 2000 cpm [1,2-³H]corticosterone +
3 ml benzene
↓
Centrifugation
↓
The dried rest of 2 ml of benzene phase resolved in 1 ml
5% ethanol

| 0.1 ml for radioimmunoassay | 0.5 ml for measuring radioactivity (recovery) |

important difference is that carbon tetrachloride is used for extraction instead of benzene. Mahajan *et al.* (1972), Connel and Linfoot (1973), and Kao *et al.* (1975) have used dichloromethane, while Lee and Schiller (1975) utilized carbon tetrachloride for extraction, without additional chromatographic separation. Schöneshöfer *et al.* (1976) reported on the chromatographic separation of compound S prior to radioimmunoassay. Obviously, the extraction and isolation procedure depends on the specificity of antibody as well as on the aim of compound S assay. Authors who use the assay of compound S only for evaluation of metyrapone test can be satisfied with a less specific technique (Mahajan *et al.*, 1972).

2. Urine Samples

For separation of free urinary cortisol, Ruder *et al.* (1972) introduced, in addition to the dichloromethane extraction, a thin-layer chromatography step using a developing solvent mixture of dichloromethane–methanol–water, 100:6:0.3 (R_f = 0.12). Deck *et al.* (1976) have extracted samples with 20 ml dichloromethane. After washing the organic phase with 5.0 ml each of 0.1 N NaOH, 0.1 N acetic acid, and water, the extracts were chromatographed on the above system. Fahmy *et al.* (1975) have claimed that the specificity of the cortisol antibody permitted the routine estimation of urinary free cortisol without incorporating a chromatographic step.

For estimation of cortisol metabolites the following procedures were introduced (Will *et al.*, 1975a, 1977): (a) estimation of the sum of unconjugated THF and THF-21-glucuronide in highly diluted (1:300) unprocessed human urine, (b) a similar estimation for THE and THE-21-glucuronide, and (c) estimation of THF and THE after β-glucuronidase (Ketodasc) treatment and dilution (1:300). After dilution, 0.1-ml samples are submitted to incubation with corresponding ^{3}H-labeled material according to the description in Table III.

For tetrahydrocorticosterone (THB) and tetrahydro compound S (THS) assay, two different techniques have been introduced (Vielhauer *et al.*, 1976a; Vecsei *et al.*, 1976; Kohl *et al.*, 1978; M. Mok and P. Vecsei, unpublished data). Screening techniques were carried out similar to procedures (a) and (b) for THF and THE (see above) as well as radioimmunoassay after chromatographic separation. For the latter purpose a 2.0–10 ml urine sample was treated with β-glucuronidase (Ketodase), extracted with dichloromethane, and subjected to paper chromatography in benzene–heptane–methanol–water, 30 : 70 : 60 : 40, to isolate THB or in a propylene glycol–toluene system to isolate THS. Values obtained in the screening technique were significantly correlated with the results of the chromatographic method (Vielhauer *et al.*, 1976a; Vecsei *et al.*, 1976; Kohl *et al.*, 1978; M. Mok and P. Vecsei, unpublished data).

3. Amniotic Fluid

Since the first publication of Liggins and Howle (1972) it has been assumed that respiratory distress syndrome (RDS) of premature newborn children results from an insufficiency of fetal cortisol production followed by a retardation of lung development. On the basis of this theory, the use of corticoids (β-methasone methylprednisolone) was introduced as a method for prevention of this syndrome. Fencl and Tulchinsky (1975) have estimated the cortisol concentrations in amniotic fluid as a procedure to determine the fetal cortisol production. They estimated cortisol concentrations by radioimmunoassay after an alcohol extraction of amniotic fluid. Aderjan *et al.* (1977) have compared cortisol radioimmunoassays in amniotic fluid using different preparations, alcohol and dichloromethane extraction, and simple dilution (1 : 50). The best correlation between the age of pregnancy and between amniotic fluid cortisol concentrations was found after simple dilution.

III. EVALUATION OF RADIOIMMUNOASSAY DATA

A. Extraction Procedure

A previous extraction with CCl_4, benzene, or heptane did not influence plasma cortisol values after either ethanol or dichloromethane extraction.

The reliability of the ethanol extraction was also checked by chromatographic analysis. In this test, human plasma was extracted with ethanol and the extract was chromatographed. The chromatography paper strip was cut into pieces of 10–20 mm, and aliquots of the eluate of each section of paper were submitted to measurement of radioactivity and radioimmunoassay (Figure 5). A good correlation was observed between the radioactivity (originating from 1,2-³H-cortisol added to the plasma sample prior to the extraction) and the radioimmunologic activity. The radioimmunologic analysis of the chromatograms enable us to check for possible cross-reaction with unknown or exogenous materials, such as exogenous steroids and their metabolites.

In the case of corticosterone radioimmunoassay (apart from the rare exception in certain types of AGS), a previous extraction did not influence the values determined from benzene extraction. However, the use of ethanol or dichloromethane instead of benzene occasionally resulted in an increase in the values. The extraction procedure for the corticosterone radioimmunoassay has also been checked by means of a chromatographic analysis (Figure 6).

According to a chromatographic analysis (Vielhauer *et al.*, 1974), although 17-OH-progesterone has relatively high cross-reactivity, it

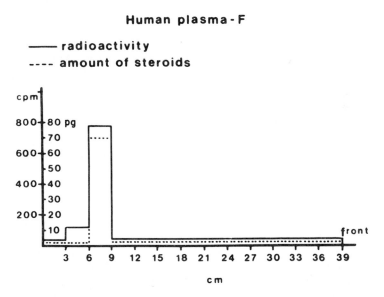

Figure 5. Radioimmunologic analysis of the chromatogram of the ethanol extract (see Table VI) from a human plasma sample. (Chromatographic system, benzene–isooctane–methanol–water, 80 : 20 : 55 : 45.)

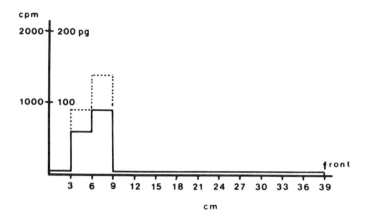

Figure 6. Radioimmunologic analysis of the chromatogram of the benzene extract (see Table VII) from a rat plasma sample. (Chromatographic system, benzene–*n*-heptane–methanol–water, 60 : 40 : 70 : 30.)

did not significantly interfere with compound S radioimmunoassay performed by CCl₄ extraction. Using the crude dichloromethane extract of plasma samples for compound S radioimmunoassay, Mahajan *et al.* (1972) also found that additional chromatography in one or two systems did not alter significantly the plasma compound S values determined after metyrapone treatment. Using compound S antibodies raised with the 3-oxime antigen, we have not seen differences in the plasma compound S concentrations when the values were compared with those estimated using a 21-hemisuccinate antiserum (the specificity figures are shown in Table IV). However, lower compound S values were estimated with 3-oxime antibody in plasma samples of pregnant women.

Immunochromatographic analyses were also carried out to check the usefulness of THF, THE, THB, and THS antibodies. These studies have indicated that in unprocessed urine samples or in *n*-butanol extracts, radioimmunologic reactions could be obtained only in eluates of areas of chromatography paper with glucuronides of the corresponding tetrahydro derivatives or with the corresponding tetrahydrosteroids. When the analysis was performed after previous β-glucuronidase treatment, the paper areas containing THF, THE, THB and THS, respectively, were found to be immunoreactive.

B. Results of Glucocorticoid Radioimmunoassay

1. *Cortisol*

Results of the plasma cortisol assay in human blood are shown in Figure 7. The range of normal values obtained in our laboratory is similar to the data given in the literature (e.g., Fraser and James, 1968; Spark, 1971). The values obtained from patients with Addison's disease are very low or unmeasurable. After dexamethasone treatment and in pituitary insufficiency, very low levels were measured, supporting the specificity of the radioimmunoassay. As expected, ACTH caused an increase in the plasma cortisol concentrations. The average normal plasma 8 A.M. cortisol value was published by Ruder *et al.* (1972) as 12.8 ± 4.1 μg/100 ml. The same value was reported by Abraham *et al.* (1972) as 8.0 ± 1.4 μg/100 ml, by Foster and Dunn (1974) as 13.1 ± 1.05 μg/100 ml, by Dash *et al.* (1975) as 17.7 ± 5.0 μg/100 ml, and by Rolleri *et al.* (1976) as 12.6 ± 4.1 μg/100 ml. The urinary free cortisol value reported by Ruder *et al.* (1972) was 43 ± 15 μg/24 hours, which is in agreement with the findings of Murphy (1968) and

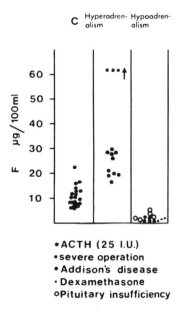

● ACTH (25 I.U.)
▪ severe operation
● Addison's disease
· Dexamethasone
○ Pituitary insufficiency

Figure 7. Concentration of cortisol (F) in human plasma. C, control; ACTH, one or two hours after 25 I.U., intravenous; dexamethasone, ten hours after 2.0–4.0 mg dexamethasone.

Hsu and Bladsoe (1970) using protein binding assay. The normal values of Deck *et al.* (1975, 1976) are very similar to the values of Ruder *et al.* (1972).

2. *Cortisone*

The mean normal value found by Srivastava *et al.* (1973) was 2.6 ± 0.5 μg/100 ml.

3. *Corticosterone*

Figure 8 details human plasma corticosterone values. The range we have found with the radioimmunoassay procedure is comparable to data reported by Fraser and James (1968) and by Peterson and Pierce (1960). However, Newsome *et al.* (1972) and Nowaczynski *et al.* (1972), using a protein-binding assay, and Underwood and Williams (1972) and Nabors *et al.* (1974), using a radioimmunoassay, have determined lower concentrations. Especially low normal plasma concentrations were published by Roy *et al.* (1974). In the paper by Nabors *et al.*, the normal values for males were significantly lower than those for females. The reason for the differences in the normal values found by different authors is unexplained. It is possible that the control values may have been influenced by diet, postural factors, etc.

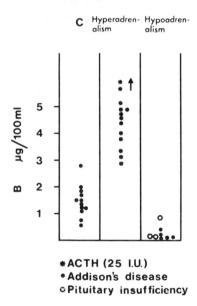

Figure 8.   Concentration of corticosterone in human plasma. C, control; ACTH, one or two hours after 25 I.U. intravenous.

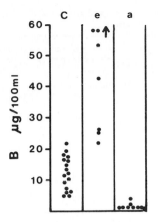

Figure 9.   Concentration of corticosterone in rat plasma. C, control; e, ether stress; a, 24 hours after adrenalectomy.

Figure 9 shows rat plasma corticosterone values determined in our laboratory. These values agree with those formerly published by us using another method (Vecsei, 1962) and after the same handling of the animals. Using our corticosterone antibody, Hilfenhaus (1976) found in rats under extreme stress-free circumstances, 1.0–2.0 μg/100 ml plasma corticosterone in the morning and 15–20 μg/100 ml in the late afternoon. The daily maximum level of corticoid is in the late afternoon in rats.

4. Compound S

Vielhauer *et al.* (1974) have reported normal compound S levels in human plasma samples of 0.147 ± 0.044 μg/100 ml. In Addison's disease, the concentration of compound S was decreased, and in Cushing's syndrome it was partly elevated. When normal persons have taken 30 mg/kg metyrapone per os at 12 midnight the plasma compound S values determined eight hours later were found to be 8.99 ± 2.19 μg/100 ml (range 5.8–12.9). The reaction to metyrapone was depressed after hypophysectomy or in hypopituitarism. The normal values of Lee and Schiller (1975), Kao *et al.* (1975), and Schöneshöfer *et al.* (1976) were similar or somewhat higher. The values of Mahajan *et al.* (1972), determined after metyrapone administration, were in the range similar to those found by Vielhauer *et al.* (1976a).

Table VIII   Daily Excretion of Tetrahydrocortisol (THF), Tetrahydrocortisone (THE), and Tetrahydrocorticosterone (THB)

	Human urine concentrations	
	Urine after β-glucuronidase[a]	Untreated urine
THE		
Normal[b]	$3.9 \pm 1.6\, n = 19$	$2.0 \pm 1.0\, n = 146$
Hypercorticism	$24.3 \pm 6.8\, n = 13$	$11.9 \pm 7.8\, n = 13$
Hypocorticism	$1.3 \pm 0.5\, n = 5$	$0.6 \pm 0.22\, n = 5$
THF		
Normal[b]	$3.76 \pm 1.5\, n = 19$	$1.63 \pm 0.7\, n = 152$
Hypercorticism	$25.5 \pm 6.2\, n = 13$	$19.6 \pm 5.3\, n = 13$
Hypocorticism	$0.5 \pm 0.2\, n = 5$	$0.4 \pm 0.23\, n = 5$
THB		
Normal[c]	$324.4 \pm 71.7\, n = 10$	$523.5 \pm 99.8\, n = 10$
Hypercorticism	$1.691.4 \pm 426.2 n = 11$	$1.286.3 \pm 277.6\, n = 11$
Hypocorticism	$11.50 \pm 39.2\, n = 6$	$131.8 \pm 53.6\, n = 6$

[a] The THB estimation was accomplished with an additional chromatography step (Kohl et al., 1978).

[b] Mean ± S.D. (mg/24 hr).

[c] Mean ± S.D. (μg/24 hr).

5. THF, THE, THS, and THB

Table VIII shows THF, THE, and THB-glucuronide values in normal human urines and in hyper- and hypocorticism (Will et al., 1975a,b; Vecsei et al., 1976; Will et al., 1977). A highly significant correlation could be obtained between THB-glucuronide and THB values estimated after chromatographic isolation.

The THS-glucuronide values were found to be elevated to a high degree after metyrapone administration (13.9 ± 5.6 μg/ml urine versus 0.19 ± 0.11 μg/ml without metyrapone). The urine collection was carried out eight to ten hours after metyrapone treatment (Vielhauer et al., 1976a; M. Mok and P. Vecsei, unpublished data).

C. Recovery, Accuracy, and Precision

With the extraction of water, the blank values in the cortisol radioimmunoassay were zero (Vecsei et al., 1972d). The overall recovery of tritiated cortisol added to plasma samples was 70–80%. The recovery of known amounts of unlabeled cortisol added to water was 94.4 ± 2.6% (n = 34). The intraassay error was 12.4 ± 1.4% (n = 37) and the interassay error was 16.0 ± 1.9% (n = 36). Since 1972, the reproducibility figures for our assay have improved. Good reproducibility has also been obtained by other authors [e.g., 8.5% intraassay error and 5.7% interassay error by Dash *et al.* (1975)].

The water blank values of our corticosterone assay were zero. The overall recovery of the ^{3}H-corticosterone added to the plasma samples prior to the extraction was 50–70%. The recovery of known amounts of corticosterone was 96 ± 2.7% ($n = 49$). Interassay error was 14.3 ± 3.2% ($n = 20$).

One can say that the accuracy and precision of the radioimmunoassay of glucocorticoids (cortisol, corticosterone, and compound S) are as good as those of the protein-binding assay. The same conclusion can also be drawn from the publications of Ruder *et al.* (1972), Underwood and Williams (1972), and Mahajan *et al.* (1972). The corresponding figures for the THF, THE, THB, and THS assays are also in a similar order of magnitude (Will *et al.*, 1977; Vielhauer *et al.*, 1976a; Vecsei *et al.*, 1976; Kohl *et al.*, 1978; M. Mok and P. Vecsei, unpublished data).

IV. OTHER USES FOR CORTISOL AND CORTICOSTERONE ANTIBODY

The high cross-reaction values of some of cortisol antibodies with compound S (e.g., Ruder *et al.*, 1972; Farmer and Pierce, 1974) raise the possibility of measuring this steroid with the cortisol antibody after a separation either with chromatography or with differential extraction, e.g., with CCl_4. No such attempt has been made. However, Roy *et al.* (1974) have used a nonspecific cortisol antiserum to estimate corticosterone isolated by celite microcolumn chromatography.

The corticosterone antibody could be used for estimation of greater amounts of 18-OH-deoxycorticosterone and 18-OH-corticosterone. This was revealed by the radioimmunologic analysis of chromatogram strips of the dichloromethane extract of incubation fluid from surviving adrenal slices in rat experiments (Figure 10). Schöneshöfer *et al.* (1976) separated a γ-globulin fraction with high affinity to 18-OH-deoxycorticosterone from a corticosterone antiserum raised in our laboratory and used it for estimation of 18-OH-deoxycorticosterone in human plasma samples.

V. GENERAL DISCUSSION

The radioimmunoassay of cortisol represents a substantial improvement in the determination of this corticosteroid, both for clinical

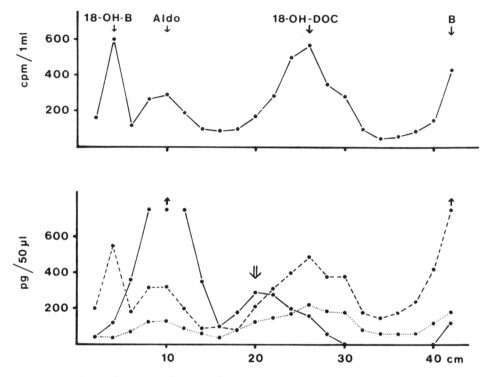

Figure 10. Radioimmunologic analysis of the chromatogram (propylene glycol–toluene system) of the extract from the incubation fluid of rat adrenals. The incubation was carried out in the presence of [1,2-³H]deoxycorticosterone. Top: radioactive steroid fractions formed by the adrenal tissue. 18-OH-B, 18-OH-corticosterone; Aldo, aldosterone; 18-OH-DOC, 18-OH-deoxycorticosterone; B, corticosterone. ●———●, Immunoactivity measured with aldosterone antibody (see the description of Vecsei *et al.,* 1972c). ●----●, Immunoactivity measured with corticosterone antibody. ●·····●, Immunoactivity measured with deoxycorticosterone antibody (Vecsei *et al.,* 1972b). ⇓, Unidentified steroid with substantial reaction with the aldosterone antibody.

and research uses. The method is very simple, rapid, and provides several advantages over the protein-binding assays. These advantages are even greater for the assays of cortisone, corticosterone, compound S, and tetrahydrocorticosteroid metabolites.

A. Sensitivity

The radioimmunoassay of cortisol is more sensitive than the protein-binding assay. This advantage is not very decisive in everyday clinical practice because of the relatively high cortisol content of random plasma samples. However, this great sensitivity can play a role in cases in which the low concentration of cortisol or the limited amount of the sample challenges the determination.

The radioimmunoassay of cortisol after simple dilution with or without heating permits us to assay 1.0–$5.0\,\mu l$ of plasma taken from a finger prick by glass capillaries. It is possible to perform serial cortisol estimations in newborns and in amniotic fluid samples. The radioimmunoassay is useful for measuring plasma cortisol concentrations in species with low plasma cortisol levels, such as rabbits.

B. Specificity

The cortisol radioimmunoassay is of relatively high specificity. In humans, the presence of corticosterone and compound S cannot cause significant interference, even if their concentrations are elevated. Considering the cross-reactions, the reliability of the radioimmunoassay is greater than that of the protein-binding assay, which has very high cross-reaction with corticosterone and compound S. Murphy (1975) has proposed the use of a horse plasma transcortin preparation instead of human transcortin for the protein-binding assay of cortisol; horse transcortin is more specific and has a higher affinity for cortisol than the human. However, specificity similar to the better radioimmunoassays could still not be achieved by this measure. As exceptions, the cross-reactions with 21-deoxycortisol and 21-deoxycortisone should be considered. They are very high in most radioimmunoassays as well as in protein-binding assays.

In situations with extremely high concentrations of plasma compound S, such as in 11-hydroxylase deficiency, after the administration of metyrapone, or in the presence of elevated plasma levels of 21-deoxycortisol and 21-deoxycortisone, as in forms of AGS with 21-hydroxylase deficiency, a chromatographic step or separation by differential extraction is essential. Such methods were described for the protein-binding assay, e.g., previous extractions with benzene, CCl_4, and hexane–CCl_4 mixtures (Murphy, 1975).

Several authors reported on comparative studies between radioimmunoassay and protein-binding assay of cortisol (Garza and Abraham, 1972; Farmer and Pierce, 1974). In general, the radioimmunoassay values show a good correlation with those of protein-binding assay. However, systematic divergences could be seen in very different degrees. On the basis of the known cross-reaction figures and the known concentration of plasma steroids, no explanation for such differences can be found. The same problem exists, when one compares the very different normal values found by different groups.

The cross-reaction figures for glucocorticoid hormones are higher than those established for the mineralocorticoids, aldosterone, deoxycorticosterone, 18-OH-deoxycorticosterone (Chapter 38). However, it is possible that using different types of antigens, such as 11, 16, 17, and 19 derivatives, higher specificity might be achieved in the future. When comparing the specificity of radioimmunoassay and protein binding assays, the advantage of higher specificity is even greater for corticosterone and compound S.

Comparative studies estimating THF and THE as well as the glucuronides of these cortisol metabolites have shown a significant correlation with 17-ketogenic steroids and total corticoid estimations (Will *et al.*, 1975a; Will *et al.*, 1977). The specificity and the simplicity of these urinary radioimmunoassays indicate that they may replace the above-mentioned assays for routine clinical tests.

For THB and THS estimations, only very sophisticated methods were available until now. The radioimmunoassay for these glucocorticoid metabolites, both the screening assay estimating THB- and THS-glucuronides in unprocessed urine, and the assay after one chromatography step, make a more frequent assay of these corticosteroid metabolites possible.

REFERENCES

Abraham, G. E., Buster, J. E., and Teller, R. C. (1972). Radioimmunoassay of plasma cortisol. *Anal. Lett.* **5**, 757–766.

Aderjan, R., Lorenz, U., Rauh, W., Vecsei, P., and Rüttgers, H. (1977). Determination of cortisol, cortisol-metabolites corticosterone and aldosterone in human amniotic fluid. *J. Steroid Biochem.* **8**, 525–528.

Ballmann, F., and Vecsei, P. (1973). German registered design No. 7223441.

Beall, G. N., Chopra, I. J., Solomon, D. H., Pierce, J. G., and Cornell, J. S. (1973). The effects on rabbits of immunization with bovine thyroid-stimulating hormone and its subunits. *J. Clin. Invest.* **52**, 2986–2992.

Chambers, V. E. M., Glover, J. S., and Tudor, R. (1975). (Se^{75})-Radioligands in steroid radioimmunoassay. *Steroid Immunoassay, Proc. Tenovus Workshop, 5th, 1974*, pp. 177–182.

Colburn, W. A. (1975). Radioimmunoassay for cortisol using antibodies against prednisolone conjugated at the 3-position. *J. Clin. Endocrinol. Metab.* **41**, 868–875.

Comoglio, S., and Celada, F. (1976). An immuno-enzymatic assay of cortisol using *E. coli* β-galactosidase as label. *J. Immunol. Methods* **10**, 161–170.

Connel, G. M., and Linfoot, J. A. (1973). Radioimmunoassay of plasma deoxycortisol. *Endocrinology* **92**, Suppl. A.

Cook, I. F., Rowe, P. H., and Dean, P. D. G. (1973). Investigations into the immune response to steroid conjugates using corticoids as a model. I. A specific cortisol antibody. *Steroids Lipids Res.* **4**, 302–309.

Csapo, A., Dray, F., and Erdos, T. (1975). The biological effects of injected antibodies to estradiol-17β and to progesterone in pregnant rats. *Endocrinology* 97, 603–614.

Dash, R. J., England, B. G., Midgley, A. R., and Niswender, G. D. (1975). A specific, non-chromatographic radioimmunoassay for human plasma cortisol. *Steroids* 26, 647–661.

Deck, K., Eberlein, L., Vetter, H., and Hillen, H. (1976). Die Bestimmung von freiem Cortisol im Urin. *Dtsch. Med. Wochenschr.* 101, 818–821.

Fahmy, D., Read, G., and Hillier, S. G. (1975). Radioimmunoassay for cortisol: Comparison of H³-, Se⁷⁵- and J¹²⁵-labeled ligands. *J. Endocrinol.* 65, 45P-46P.

Farmer, R. W., and Pierce, C. E. (1974). Plasma cortisol determination: Radioimmunoassay and competitive protein binding compared. *Clin. Chem.* 20, 411–414.

Fencl, M., and Tulchinsky, D. (1975). Total cortisol in amniotic fluid and fetal lung maturation. *N. Engl. J. Med.* 292, 133–136.

Fleischer, N., Abe, K., Liddle, G. W., Orth, D. N., and Nicholson, W. E. (1967). ACTH antibodies in patients receiving depot porcine ACTH to hasten recovery from pituitary-adrenal suppression. *J. Clin. Invest.* 46, 196–204.

Forster, L. B., Dunn, R. T. (1974). Single antibody technique for radioimmunoassay of cortisol in unextracted serum or plasma. *Clin. Chem.* 20, 365–368.

Fraser, R., and James, V. H. T. (1968). Double isotope assay of aldosterone, corticosterone, and cortisol in human peripheral plasma. *J. Endocrinol.* 40, 59–72.

Garza, R., and Abraham, G. E. (1972). Comparison between two assays for plasma cortisol. *Anal. Lett.* 5, 767–771.

Gless, K. H., Vecsei, P., Hanka-Posztoky, M., and Knorr, E. (1973). Plasma corticoids in rabbits immunized against various adrenal steroids. *Naunyn-Schmiedeberg's Arch. Pharmacol.* 277, Suppl., 22.

Gless, K. H., Hanka, M., Vecsei, P., and Gross, F. (1974). Hypercorticism in rabbits immunized against corticosteroids. *Acta Endocrinol. (Copenhagen)* 75, 342–349.

Gomez-Sanchez, C., Murry, B. A., Kem, D. C., and Kaplan, N. M. (1975). A direct radioimmunoassay of corticosterone in rat serum. *Endocrinology* 96, 796–799.

Gross, H. A., Ruder, H. J., Brown, K. S., and Lipsett, M. B. (1972). A radioimmunoassay for plasma corticosterone. *Steroids* 20, 681–695.

Hilfenhaus, M. (1976). Circadian rhythm of plasma renin activity, plasma aldosterone and plasma corticosterone in rats. *Int. J. Chronobiol.* 3, 213–229.

Hillier, S. G., Groom, G. V., Boyns, A. R., and Cameron, E. H. D. (1975). The active immunisation of intact adult rats against steroid-protein conjugates: Effects on circulating hormone levels and related physiological processes. *Steroid Immunoassay, Proc. Tenovus Workshop, 5th, 1974* pp. 97–110.

Hsu, T. H., and Bledsoe, T. (1970). Measurement of urinary free corticoids by competitive protein-binding radioassay in hypoadrenal states. *J. Clin. Endocrinol. Metab.* 30, 443–448.

Hunter, W. M., Nars, P. W., and Rutherford, F. J. (1975). Preparation and behaviour of I¹²⁵-labelled radioligands for phenolic and neutral steroids. *Steroid Immunoassay, Proc. Tenovus Workshop, 5th, 1974* pp. 141–152.

Kao, M., Voina, S., Nichols, A., and Horton, R. (1975). Parallel radioimmunoassay for plasma cortisol and 11-deoxycortisol. *Clin. Chem.* 21, 1644–1647.

Klemm, W., and Gupta, D. (1975). A routine method for the radioimmunoassay of plasma cortisol without chromatography. *In* "Radioimmunoassay of Steroid Hormones VII" (D. Gupta, ed.), pp. 143–151. Verlag Chemie, Weinheim.

Kohl, K.-H., Gless, K.-H., Abdelhamid, S., Penke, B., and Vecsci, P. (1978). Radioimmunoassay of tetrahydrocoticosterone (THB) in human urine. *Acta Endocrinol. (Copenhagen)* **88**, 139–148.

Lee, L., and Schiller, H. S. (1975). Nonchromatographic radioimmunoassay of plasma 11-deoxycortisol, for use in the metyrapone test, with polyethylene glycol as the precipitant. *Clin. Chem.* **21**, 719–724.

Liggins, G. C., and Howle, R. N. (1972). A controlled trial of antepartum glucocorticoid treatment for prevention of the respiratory distress syndrome in free nature infants. *Pediatrics* **50**, 515–525.

Mahajan, D. K., Wahlen, J. D., Tyler, F. H., and West, C. D. (1972). Plasma 11-deoxycortisol radioimmunoassay for metyrapone tests. *Steroids* **20**, 609–620.

Mayes, D., Furuyama, S., Kem, D. C., and Nugent, C. A. (1970). A radioimmunoassay for plasma aldosterone. *J. Clin. Endocrinol. Metab.* **30**, 682–685.

Morton, J. J., and Waite, M. A. (1972). The possible relationship between the affinity of argininevasopressin antibodies and the degree of polyuria and polydipsia in activily immunized rabbits. *J. Endocrinol.* **54**, 523–524.

Murphy, B. E. P. (1968). Clinical evaluation of urinary cortisol determinations by competitive protein binding. *J. Clin. Endocrinol. Metab.* **28**, 343–348.

Murphy, B. E. P. (1975). Non-chromatographic radiotransinassay for cortisol: Application to human adult serum, umbilical cord serum, and amniotic fluid. *J. Clin. Endocrinol. Metab.* **41**, 1050–1057.

Murphy, B. E. P., Engelberg, W., and Pattee, C. J. (1963). Simple method for the determination of plasma corticoids. *J. Clin. Endocrinol. Metab.* **23**, 293–300.

Nabors, C. J., West, C. D., Mahajan, D. K., and Tyler, F. H. (1974). Radioimmunoassay of human plasma corticosterone: Method, measurement of episodic secretion and adrenal suppression and stimulation. *Steroids* **23**, 363–378.

Newsome, H. H., Jr., Clements, A. S., and Borum, E. H. (1972). The simultaneous assay of cortisol, corticosterone, 11-desoxy-cortisol, and cortisone in human plasma. *J. Clin. Endocrinol. Metab.* **34**, 473–483.

Nieschlag, E., Kley, H. K., and Usadel, K. H. (1975). Production of steroid antisera in rabbits. *Steroid Immunoassay, Proc. Tenovus Workshop, 5th 1974* pp. 87–96.

Nishina, T., Tsuji, A., and Fukushima, D. K. (1974). Site of conjugation of bovine serum albumin to corticosteroid hormones and specificity of antibodies. *Steroids* **24**, 861–874.

Nowaczynski, W., Küchel, O., and Genest, J. (1972). Aldosterone, deoxycorticosterone, and corticosterone metabolism in benign essential hypertension. *In* "Hypertension '72" (J. Genest and E. Koiw, eds.), pp. 244–254. Springer-Verlag, Berlin-Heidelberg-New York.

Peterson, R. E., and Pierce, C. E. (1960). The metabolism of corticosterone in man. *J. Clin. Invest.* **39**, 741–757.

Poulsen, K. (1969). Radioimmunoassay for angiotensin II to be used in direct conjunction with renin assay. *Scand. J. Lab. Invest.* **24**, 285–290.

Raziano, J., Ferin, M., Raymond, L., and Vande Wiele, R. (1972). Effects of antibodies to estradiol-17β and to progesterone on nidation and pregnancy in rats. *Endocrinology* **90**, 1133–1138.

Richardson, M. C., and Schulster, D. (1972). Corticosteroidogenesis in isolated adrenal cells: Effect of adrenocorticotrophic hormone, adenosine 3′,5′-monophosphate and β^{1-24}-adreno-cortriphotropic hormone diazotized to polyacrylamide. *J. Endocrinol.* **55**, 127–139.

Rolleri, E., Zannino, M., Orlandini, S., and Malvano, R. (1976). Direct radioimmunoassay of plasma cortisol. *Clin. Chim. Acta* **66**, 319–330.

Roy, S. K., Garza, R., Maroulis, G., and Abraham, G. E. (1974). Radioimmunoassay of Plasma Corticosterone. *Anal. Lett.* **7**, 109–114.

Ruder, H. J., Guy, R. L., and Lipsett, M. B. (1972). A radioimmunoassay for cortisol in plasma and urine. *J. Clin. Endocrinol. Metab.* **35**, 219–224.

Schöneshöfer, M., Halim, W. R., and Penke, B. (1976). Characterization of an 18-OH-deoxycorticosterone binding antiserum. *Acta Endocrinol. (Copenhagen), Suppl.* **202**, 71–73.

Spark, R. F. (1971). Measurement of serum 11-deoxycortisol and cortisol after metyrapone. *Ann. Intern. Med.* **75**, 717–723.

Spät, A., and Jozan, S. (1972). Competitive protein binding assay of corticosterone. *J. Steroid Biochem.* **3**, 755–759.

Srivastava, L. S., Werk, E. E., Thrasher, K., Sholiton, L. J., Kozera, R., Nolten, W., and Knowles, H. C. (1973). Plasma cortisone concentration as measured by radioimmunoassay. *J. Clin. Endocrinol. Metab.* **36**, 937–943.

Tait, S. A. S., Tait, J. F., and Bradley, J. E. S. (1972). The effect of serotonin and potassium on corticosterone and aldosterone production by isolated zona glomerulosa cells of the rat adrenal cortex (1972). *Aust. J. Exp. Biol. Med. Sci.* **50**, 833–846.

Thomas, S. J., Wilson, D. W., Pierrepoint, C. G., Cameron, E. H. D., and Griffiths, K. (1976). Measurement of cortisol, cortisone, 11-deoxycortisol, and corticosterone in foetal sheep plasma during the perinatal period. *J. Endocrinol.* **68**, 181–189.

Underwood, R. H., and Williams, G. H. (1972). The simultaneous measurement of aldosterone, cortisol, and corticosterone in human peripheral plasma by displacement analysis. *J. Lab. Clin. Med.* **79**, 848–862.

Vaitukaitis, J., Robbins, J. B., Nieschlag, E., and Ross, G. T. (1971). A method for producing specific antisera with small doses of immunogen. *J. Clin. Endocrinol. Metab.* **33**, 988–991.

Vecsei, P. (1962). Verhalten des Corticosterongehaltes im peripheren Blut weisser Ratten nach Formolbehandlung. *Endokrinologie* **42**, 154–157.

Vecsei, P., Akangbou, C., Joumaah, A., and Sallum, N. I. (1972a). Studies on antibodies against corticoid hormones. *Acta Endocrinol. (Copenhagen)* **69**, Suppl. 159, 33.

Vecsei, P., Joumaah, A., Sallum, N. I., and Akangbou, C. (1972b). Studies of antibodies against cortisol, corticosterone and desoxycorticosterone. *Excerpta Med. Found. Int. Congr. Ser.* **256**, 388.

Vecsei, P., Penke, B., and Joumaah, A. (1972c). Radioimmunoassay of free aldosterone and of its 18-oxoglucuronide in human urine. *Experientia* **28**, 622–624.

Vecsei, P., Penke, B., Katzy, R., and Baek, L. (1972d). Radioimmunological determination of plasma cortisol. *Experientia* **28**, 1104–1105.

Vecsei, P., Schäfer, A., Faulstich, M., Vielhauer, W., Will, H., and Kapp, S. (1975). Radioimmunoassay of aldosterone and other corticoids by means of nylon-bound antibodies. *Clin. Chem.* **21**, 1022.

Vecsei, P., Kohl, K. H., Mok, B., Pallai, P., Penke, B., Vielhauer, W., and Will, H. (1976). Antibodies against tetrahydro-11-deoxycortisol (THS), tetrahydrocorticosterone (THB), and tetrahydroaldosterone (THAld). *Proc. Int. Congr. Endocrinol., 5th, 1976* Abstract pp. 373–374.

Vetter, W., Armbruster, H., Tschudi, B., and Vetter, H. (1974a). Production of antisera specific to aldosterone: Effect of hapten density and of carrier proteins. *Steroids* **23**, 741–756.

Vetter, W., Vetter, H., Diethelm, U., Armbruster, H., and Siegenthaler, W. (1974b). Antisera specific to corticosterone. *J. Steroid Biochem.* **5**, 303.

Vielhauer, W., Gless, K. H., and Vecsei, P. (1974). Radioimmunoassay of 11-deoxycortisol in human plasma. *Acta Endocrinol. (Copenhagen), Suppl.* **184**, 65.

Vielhauer, W., Mok, M., von Mittelstaedt, G., Gless, K. H., and Vecsei, P. (1976a). Estimation of THS (tetrahydro-11-deoxycortisol) and THS-glucuronide-equivalents after the metyrapone test by radioimmunoassay and comparison with plasma 11-deoxycortisol concentrations. *Acta Endocrinol. (Copenhagen), Suppl.* **202**, 74–75.

Vielhauer, W., Vecsei, P., Rosmalen, F., and Gless, K. H. (1976b). Effects of active immunization against aldosterone on free and total plasma aldosterone. *Proc. Int. Congr. Endocrinol., 5th, 1976* p. 83.

Will, H. (1975a). "Solid phase" and "liquid phase" Radioimmunoassay zur Bestimmung von Tetrahydrocortisol, Tetrahydrocortison und deren Glucuronidäquivalente. Thesis for title Diplom Biology. University of Heidelberg, Heidelberg.

Will, H., Vecsei, P., Vielhauer, W., Penke, B., and Pallai, P. (1975b). Studies with tetrahydrocortisol (THF), tetrahydrocortisone (THE), and tetrahydrodesoxycortisol (THS) antibodies. *Acta Endocrinol. (Copenhagen), Suppl.* **193**, 124.

Will, H., Aderjan, R., Winkler, T., Penke, B., and Vecsei, P. (1977). Radioimmunoassays of tetrahydrocortisone and tetrahydrocortisol in human urine. *Acta Endocrinol. Copenhagen* **86**, 369–379.

40

Arthropod Molting Hormones

ERNEST S. CHANG AND JOHN D. O'CONNOR

I. INTRODUCTION

In order to increase in size, arthropods must replace a small confining exoskeleton with a larger one and subsequently grow to fill it. This periodic shedding of the old exoskeleton is accomplished by molting, which is the external manifestation of discontinuous growth in arthropods. The regulation of the molting process is effected by variations in the circulating titers of β-ecdysone (**VIII**). It appears clear now that the ecdysial glands of arthropods (the Y organ of crustaceans and

797

Methods of Hormone Radioimmunoassay, Second Edition

the prothoracic gland of insects) synthesize and secrete α-ecdysone (**I**), which is hydroxylated to its active form, β-ecdysone, by a number of systemic tissues (King *et al.*, 1974; Chang and O'Connor, 1977; King and Siddall, 1969; Chang *et al.*, 1976b). Thus, prior to each molt, the circulating levels of β-ecdysone increase dramatically, thereby inducing the ecdysial events (Bollenbacher *et al.*, 1975).

II. QUANTIFICATION OF ECDYSTEROIDS

Until recently, the quantitative measurement of either the circulating levels of α- and β-ecdysone or tissue concentrations has been ac-

(**I**) α-ecdysone
(**II**) α-ecdysone-2,3-acetonide
(**III**) α-ecdysone-2,3-acetonide-22-hemisuccinate
(**IV**) α-ecdysone-2,3-acetonide-22-hemisuccinate methyl ester
(**V**) α-ecdysone 22-hemisuccinate
(**VI**) α-ecdysone 22-hemisuccinate methyl ester
(**VII**) Triol nucleus
(**VIII**) β-ecdysone
(**IX**) β-ecdysone-carboxymethoxyamine

complished largely by use of the bioassay (Kaplanis *et al.*, 1966; Williams, 1968; Fraenkel and Zdarek, 1970). Although the sensitivity of such assays varied between 5.0 and 10 ng, the necessity for replicate samples at various dilutions mandated that a significant number of organisms be pooled for each data point. Consequently, single organisms could not be followed throughout a molting cycle. Recently, a number of gas–liquid chromatographic (GLC) techniques have been developed which permit the separation and quantification of picomolar amounts of α- and β-ecdysone (Ikekawa *et al.*, 1972; Borst and O'Connor, 1974; Morgan and Poole, 1976). Such GLC techniques require the derivatization of the sample with a trimethylsilylating reagent. The requirement that the sample be highly purified prior to such derivatization severely limits the number of samples that can be run within a reasonable time period. Although some of the difficulties associated with silylation can be avoided by use of a coupled GLC–mass spectrometer, the expense in setting up this technique is such that mass fragmentography is not readily available to most laboratories for routine analyses. Other methods of detecting ecdysteroids, such as high-pressure liquid chromatography, coupled to a uv detector, have the limitation inherent in the extinction coefficient of the ecdysone in question ($\epsilon = 12,400$ for α-ecdysone in ethanol at 242 nm).

Thus, the above techniques are either relatively insensitive, tedious, and therefore not conducive to large sample numbers, or very expensive to set up (or all three of the above). In contrast, the radioimmunoassay is highly sensitive, relatively selective, inexpensive, and compatible with large sample numbers.

III. COMPARISON OF AVAILABLE RADIOIMMUNOASSAYS FOR ECDYSTEROIDS

The initial radioimmunoassay for ecdysone was reported by Borst and O'Connor (1972; see Table I). The carboxymethyloxime (CMO) derivative of β-ecdysone (**IX**) was conjugated to bovine serum albumin, suspended in complete Freund's adjuvant, and injected into rabbits. The resulting antiserum required 1.5 ng unlabeled β-ecdysone and 4.8 ng unlabeled α-ecdysone to achieve 50% inhibition of bound radioactivity (^{3}H-β-ecdysone) in the ammonium sulfate pellet. The radioligand in these initial assays had a specific activity of 6.0 Ci/mmole. However, the availability of ^{3}H-α-ecdysone with a specific activity of 68 Ci/mmole improved the lower limit of sensitivity from 200 to 25 pg of β-ecdysone.

Table I Summary of Radioimmunoassays for Ecdysteroids

Antigen	50% Inhibition (pmole) β	α	$\beta/\alpha_{50\%}$	Radioligand	50% Inhibition other ecdysteroids (pmole)	Reference
β-Ecdysone-6-carboxymethyl oxime–BSA 3.3 haptens per molecule BSA $\overset{\parallel}{N}$—O—CH$_2$—COOH	3.1	10.3	1:3.3	[^{3}H]β-Ecdysone (6 Ci/mmole)		Borst and O'Connor (1972)
Same as above R—O—$\overset{\text{O}}{\overset{\parallel}{C}}$—CH$_2CH_2$—COOH	2.5	3.1	1:1.3	[^{3}H]β-Ecdysone	Inokosterone: 4.0; Ponasterone A: 22.6; 22,25-Dideoxy-α-ecdysone: >23; 3-OH-Cholestan-6-one: >23; Cholesterol: >23	Borst and O'Connor (1974)
Mixture of the 2,3,22-N-hydroxysuccinimide esters of β-ecdysone–HSA 20 haptens per molecule HSA R—O—$\overset{\text{O}}{\overset{\parallel}{C}}$—CH$_2CH_2$—$\overset{\text{O}}{\overset{\parallel}{C}}$—O—N	4.6	90.0	1:19.6	[^{3}H]β-Ecdysone (6 Ci/mmole)	5-β-OH-β-Ecdysone: 7.5; Inokosterone: 18.0; Makisterone A: 31.0; 2,3,22-Triacetate-α-ecdysone: >100; 3β, 20,22-Trihydroxy-5α-cholestane: >100	Lauer et al. (1974)
Succinic acid esters of β-ecdysone at undetermined positions–HSA 11 haptens per molecule HSA R—O—$\overset{\text{O}}{\overset{\parallel}{C}}$—CH$_2CH_2$—COOH	3.2	3.2	1:1	[^{125}I]Succinyl-β-ecdysone-tyrosine methyl ester	Cholesterol: >1500	De Reggi et al. (1975)
β-Ecdysone-6-carboxymethyl oxime–BSA 20 haptens per molecule BSA	0.15	0.15–0.75	1:1–1:5	[^{125}I]β-Ecdysone–CMO-tyramine (400 Ci/mmole)		Porcheron et al. (1976)
α-Ecdysone-22-hemisuccinate–thyroglobulin 140 haptens per molecule thyroglobulin —O—$\overset{\text{O}}{\overset{\parallel}{C}}$—CH$_2CH_2$COOH	1.0	0.15	6.7:1	[^{3}H]α-Ecdysone (68 ci/mole)	2-Deoxy-β-ecdysone: 28.0; Ponasterone A: 0.86; Inokosterone: 0.79; Cyasterone: 0.79; 5-β-OH-β-Ecdysone: 13.3; 22-Iso-α-Ecdysone: 0.3; 2β,3β,14α-Trihydroxy-5β-cholest-7-en-6-one: 3.3	Horn et al. (1976)

Subsequently, a more detailed account of this radioimmunoassay has been published in which the authors described an antiserum which possesses similar affinities for α- and β-ecdysone. Such a property makes this antiserum extremely useful for the determination of total molting hormone activity, since it has been shown that the predominant ecdysteroids of arthropods are α- and β-ecdysone (Horn, 1971; Chang *et al.*, 1976b). The ratio of the amounts of unlabeled β- and α-ecdysone that, respectively, inhibit the binding of the radiolabeled ecdysteroids by 50% ($\beta/\alpha_{50\%}$) was 0.8 for the antiserum. It was also seen that other ecdysone analogs, such as ponasterone A (25-deoxy-β-ecdysone) or inokosterone (20,26 dihydroxy-α-ecdysone), required about seven and 13 times as much steroids to elicit similar 50% inhibition of binding (Figure 1).

Although additional radioimmunoassays have been reported (De Reggi *et al.*, 1975; Lauer *et al.*, 1974; Porcheron *et al.*, 1976; Horn *et al.*, 1976), the initial antiserum has found the widest use. It has been used to identify the titers of ecdysone in last larval instar cockroach homogenates (Borst and O'Connor, 1974), late developmental stages of *Drosophila melanogaster* (Borst *et al.*, 1974; Hodgetts *et al.*, 1977), adult mosquitoes (Schlaeger *et al.*, 1974), third larval instar

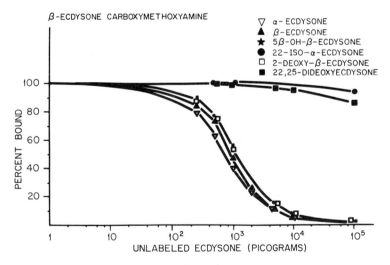

Figure 1. Competitive binding curves for the β-ecdysone-CMO antiserum (Borst and O'Connor, 1974). The cross-reactivities of the various ecdysteroids were determined by adding increasing amounts of unlabeled steroid in the presence of 12,000 dpm of [23,24-³H]α-ecdysone (specific activity equals 68 Ci/mmole). The antiserum concentration was 0.75% with a total serum concentration of 3.0% in the first incubation volume. The ordinate indicates the percent of radioactivity bound by the antiserum.

Manduca sexta (Bollenbacher *et al.*, 1975), crab hemolymph following molt induction (Chang *et al.*, 1976a), crabs following leg autotomy (McCarthy and Skinner, 1977), and ecdysone secretion by the crab Y organ during the normal molt cycle (Chang, 1978). In addition, it has been useful in monitoring the recovery of various ecdysteroids during the multiple chromatographic steps involved in the purification of the secretory form of the hormone from endocrine tissue, e.g., the insect prothoracic gland (King *et al.*, 1974; Borst and Engelmann, 1974), the dipteran ring gland (Bollenbacher *et al.*, 1976), the adult mosquito ovary (Hagedorn *et al.*, 1975), and the crab Y organ (Chang and O'Connor, 1977).

Using the *N*-hydroxysuccinimide ester of β-ecdysone conjugated to human serum albumin, a relatively insensitive antiserum was obtained that was specific for β-ecdysone (Lauer *et al.*, 1974); 50% inhibition was obtained with 2.1 ng β-ecdysone and with 47 ng α-ecdysone, a $\beta/\alpha_{50\%}$ of approximately 0.05. Other ecdysones hydroxylated at the C-20 position, such as 5-β-hydroxy-β-ecdysone, inokosterone, and ponasterone A, also displayed a greater affinity for the antisera than did α-ecdysone. Applications employing this antiserum have not yet been published.

In an attempt to increase the sensitivity of radioimmunoassays for ecdysteroids, De Reggi *et al.* (1975) constructed a succinyltyrosine methylester of β-ecdysone and labeled it with ^{125}I. These authors were able to detect less than 10 pg of either β- or α-ecdysone using such a ligand in conjunction with an antiserum produced in response to a succinylated β-ecdysone conjugate. However, the 50% inhibition level for their antiserum was similar to that initially reported by Borst and O'Connor (i.e., 1.5 ng), and the $\beta/\alpha_{50\%}$ was 1.0. Unlike the previously described assays in which ammonium sulfate was added to the incubation mixture in order to precipitate the bound hormone, these authors (De Reggi *et al.*, 1975) utilized equilibrium dialysis to separate the bound from the free hormone. This latter antiserum has been used to measure ecdysone levels in third instar and pupating *Drosophila melanogaster* (De Reggi *et al.*, 1975), oocytes of *Bombyx mori* (Legay *et al.*, 1976), hemolymph of larval and pupal *Bombyx* and *Philosamia* (Calvez *et al.*, 1976), hemolymph of the crab *Carcinus maenas* (Lachaise *et al.*, 1976), tissues of queens of the termite *Macrotermes bellicosus* (Bordereau *et al.*, 1976), and during the ovarian cycle of *Locusta migratoria* (Lageux *et al.*, 1976, 1977).

Porcheron *et al.* (1976) also used the carboxymethyloxime derivative of β-ecdysone conjugated to BSA as an antigen. Their radioligand, however, was the β-ecdysone–CMO–tyramine derivative labeled with ^{125}I to a specific activity of 400 Ci/mmole. These authors were able to achieve 50% inhibition of label binding with only 70 pg of unlabeled β-ecdysone. The $\beta/\alpha_{50\%}$ varied from 1.0 to 0.2, depending upon the lot of antiserum used. This radioimmunoassay has been used to measure ecdysone levels in the hemolymph and Y organs of both normal and parasitized crabs (Andrieux *et al.*, 1976).

The most recent anti-ecdysone antiserum has been developed by Horn *et al.* (1976). After the 2- and 3-hydroxyl groups of α-ecdysone were first protected via the acetonide, the 22-hydroxyl group was succinylated. In contrast to the previously described antigens, this derivative was conjugated to a protein larger than albumin, so that a greater number of haptens could be attached per protein molecule. It was calculated that 140 haptens per thyroglobulin molecule (compared to 20 or less in the previous antigens) had been attached, and presumably this resulted in the higher binding constant of 7.0×10^9 liters/mole for α-ecdysone.

Additionally, this antigen elicited an antiserum showing a high degree of specificity for the tetracyclic nucleus (**VII**) of ecdysone. Substitutions in the ring structure, e.g., 5-β-hydroxy-β-ecdysone or 2-deoxy-β-ecdysone, result in a 13- or 28-fold decrease in sensitivity

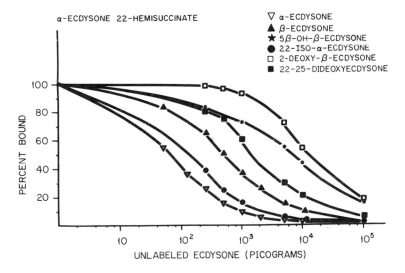

Figure 2. Competitive binding curves for the α-ecdysone 22-hemisuccinate–thyroglobulin antiserum (Horn *et al.*, 1976). The cross-reactivities of various ecdysteroids were determined as in Figure 1. The antiserum concentration was 0.04% with a total serum concentration of 3.0% in the final incubation volume.

compared to β-ecdysone. Side chain modifications, as seen in inokosterone, cyasterone, 22-iso-α-ecdysone, or $2\beta,3\beta,14\alpha$-trihydroxy-5β-cholest-7-en-6-one, result in significant yet relatively minor variations in the standard curve (Figure 2). The $\beta/\alpha_{50\%}$ is 7.0. When this antiserum is used in conjunction with an antiserum having a $\beta/\alpha_{50\%}$ equal to unity [such as the one described by Borst and O'Connor (1974)], the quantitative and qualitative analysis of α- and β-ecdysone mixtures in biological samples can be quickly ascertained (see Section V).

IV. PROTOCOL

A. Antigen Preparation

1. β-Ecdysone-CMO–BSA.

β-Ecdysone (40 mg) was derivatized in 5.0 ml of a 4% solution of carboxymethoxyamine (CMA) in pyridine at 40°C overnight. The derivatization process was followed by TLC analysis. Purification of the resultant oxime derivative (β-ecdysone-CMO) was done on preparative TLC plates (20 × 20 cm, 0.5 mm thick) and the band corresponding to the derivative was scraped and eluted with ethanol. A second TLC purification was often necessary to increase the purity of the product. Yields were approximately 60%. This derivative was characterized by TLC (methanol–chloroform, 2:3, R_f = 0.11; methanol–chloroform, 1:1, R_f = 0.16; corresponding values for β-ecdysone are 0.40 and 0.55, respectively), uv (maximal in methanol 252 nm, ϵ_M = 18,900; for β-ecdysone, corresponding values are 242–243 nm and 12,800, respectively), and ir spectroscopy, gas chromatography, and mass spectroscopy.

A mixed anhydride of β-ecdysone-CMO was formed by mixing 20 mg β-ecdysone-CMO and 50 μl tributylamine in 400 μl methanol (Erlanger *et al.*, 1967). Isobutylchloroformate (32 μmole) was added and the mixture was incubated for 30 minutes. The resultant mixed anhydride was reacted with 32 mg bovine serum albumin in 6.6 ml of a 1:1 solution of dioxane–water to which 300 μl 0.5 N NaOH had been added. The reaction proceeded for five hours at 4°C with frequent mixing, after which the mixture was dialyzed overnight against running distilled water and then lyophilized. Characterization was done by uv spectrometry. A hapten to carrier ratio of 3.3 was obtained.

Milligram quantities of antigen were suspended in 0.9% NaCl solution and then mixed with an equal volume of complete Freund's adjuvant. Three New Zealand white rabbits were injected with the antigen both subcutaneously and intramuscularly. A booster injection of 1.0 mg antigen followed five weeks after the initial injection and again one to two weeks before some of the bleedings. This serum was collected at different intervals from a peripheral artery of the ear, stored overnight at 4°C to allow clot retraction, and the clear yellow supernatant was collected and frozen in 2-ml aliquots.

2. α-Ecdysone 22-hemisuccinate–thyroglobulin

a. 2β,3β-isopropylidenedioxy-α-ecdysone (II)

i. Unlabeled material. Phosphomolybdic acid (14.7 mg) was added to 225 mg α-ecdysone (I) dissolved in 50 ml reagent agrade acetone, and the mixture was stirred at room temperature for 30 minutes. The solution was then concentrated on a rotary evaporater to 2.0 ml, and 50 ml water and 2.0 mg potassium hydrogen carbonate were added. This mixture was extracted with ethanol–chloroform (1 : 1). The chloroform layer was washed with water and evaporated to dryness and the residue was chromatographed on silica gel (152 mg). Crystallization of the main fraction from ethyl acetate afforded the pure acetonide (II), mp 251°–253°C.

ii. Labeled material. Radioactive α-ecdysone, stored as a solution in ethanol–benzene, was added to α-ecdysone (1.0 mg) and the acetonide was prepared as above. Chromatography afforded peak fractions (~0.6 mg, 11.5×10^6 cpm).

b. 2β,3β-Isopropylidene-α-ecdysone 22-Hemisuccinate (III).

Dry tetrahydrofuran (100 ml) and pyridine (600 μl) were added to the α-ecdysone (162 mg) and radioactive α-ecdysone (0.5 mg, 6.6×10^6 cpm) acetonides in a 250-ml flask fitted with a serum cap under argon and containing a magnetic stirrer. The mixture was cooled to 0°C. Succinyl chloride (400 μl) was added and the mixture was stored overnight at 4°C. Water was added and the tetrahydrofuran was evaporated. The residue was extracted with chloroform, evaporated to dryness, and chromatographed on silica gel. The peak fractions (194 mg) were combined and crystallized, mp 160°–170°C. To characterize this acid, a 10-mg portion was methylated with diazomethane to give the chloroform-soluble methyl ester (IV).

c. α-Ecdysone 22-Hemisuccinate (V).

2β,3β-Isopropylidene-α-ecdysone 22-hemisuccinate (193 mg) in 100 ml tetrahydrofuran and 10 ml of 1.0 *M* aqueous hydrochloric acid was allowed to stand at room temperature for 6.5 hours. Ammonium hydroxide solution (100 ml, 0.05 *M*) was added. The tetrahydrofuran was then evaporated off and the aqueous residue was extracted twice with 100 ml chloroform–ethanol (3 : 1). The combined extracts after washing with water were evaporated to dryness and the residue (169 mg) was chromatographed on silica gel using chloroform–ethanol–acetic acid (89 : 10 : 1). The peak fractions were collected and recrystallized from ethyl acetate, mp 158°–163°C. To characterize the acid, a portion was methylated with diazomethane. Crystallization from ethyl acetate afforded the methyl ester (**VI**), mp 161°–164°C.

d. Conjugation of α-Ecdysone 22-Hemisuccinate to Thyroglobulin. A chilled solution of α-ecdysone hemisuccinate (7.8 mg, 2.7×10^5 cpm) in 300 μl pyridine–water (1 : 1) was added to a vial in an ice bath containing 1-ethyl-3(3-dimethylaminopropyl)-carbodiimide hydrochloride (51.5 mg, Sigma Chemical) and rinsed in with 30 μl pyridine–water (1 : 3). The mixture was gently agitated until the carbodiimide dissolved, about one minute. Thyroglobulin (9.9 mg, bovine type I, Sigma Chemical) dissolved in 250 μl of water was then added, and the mixture was rotated slowly for three minutes and allowed to stand overnight at room temperature. The mixture was dialyzed in a 7.0-mm dialysis tube that was initially filled with 2.0 ml of water and was suspended overnight in water and then washed in 30% aqueous pyridine. The reaction mixture was quantitatively transferred to the dialysis tube with 30% pyridine and dialyzed against a fixed volume (100 ml) of stirred 30% aqueous pyridine which was changed at daily intervals. The rate of dialysis was monitored by counting aliquots of the dialysis fluid. The amounts of free α-ecdysone 22-hemisuccinate dialyzed out per day was rapid at first but continued slowly even after five days (1920, 166, 57, 39, and 23 cpm/ml). An examination of the material dialyzed on the last day confirmed it to be unchanged α-ecdysone 22-hemisuccinate. For the purpose of raising antibodies it is not essential to have the antigen completely free of ecdysone 22-hemisuccinate, and the material after two to three days of dialysis was considered satisfactory for this purpose. The contents of the dialysis tube were transferred to a vial and lyophilized at low pressure.

e. Determination of the Number of Haptens per Molecule of Protein. To determine the number of haptens per molecule of protein, 1.15-mg aliquots of the dialysis tube contents (total weight 800 to 900 mg) were counted using Soluene 100 (Packard Instrument) as a solubilizer. Quenching ($\sim 13\%$) was determined by adding weighed amounts of labeled α-ecdysone of known specific activity. The final value for the amount of radioactivity due to bound α-ecdysone 22-hemisuccinate ($\sim 4.0 \times 10^4$ cpm) was obtained by subtracting from the value of the total amount of radioactivity ($\sim 4.4 \times 10^4$ cpm) the value for the amount of radioactivity due to undialyzed free α-ecdysone 22-hemisuccinate ($\sim 0.4 \times 10^4$ cpm). This latter value was obtained by interpolation of values for α-ecdysone 22-hemisuccinate dialyzed out with time. From these data, it was calculated that about 140 haptens were bound to each molecule of thyroglobulin.

f. **Antisera.** Milligram quantities of the lyophilized conjugate were suspended in 300 μl water and briefly sonicated. This solution was then diluted with two volumes of incomplete Freund's adjuvant and mixed vigorously. Each of five New Zealand white rabbits was then injected subcutaneously along the back with 0.8 to 1.0 mg of the α-ecdysone–thyroglobulin conjugate. Booster injections consisting of 0.4 mg of conjugate in incomplete Freund's adjuvant were administered to two of the rabbits 12 weeks after the initial injections. Sera from the rabbits were collected for a period of 17 weeks at approximately ten-day intervals. Bleedings were taken from the ear by venipuncture, and after initial coagulation at room temperature, they were stored overnight at 4°C to allow for adequate clot retraction. The supernatants were then removed, Merthiolate (1 : 10,000 dilution) was added as an antibacterial agent, and the sera were stored in 2.0-ml aliquots at 0°C.

B. Assay Tubes

Disposable culture tubes (Kimble No. 73500) are used throughout this assay. Depending upon the vendor, the 6 × 50 mm assay tubes may not accept a total volume of 600 μl. In that case, appropriate volume adjustments should be made when the liquid scintillation cocktail is added.

C. Sample Preparation

1. Hemolymph

Ten microliters of fresh hemolymph from either insect or crustacean sources can be added directly to 100 μl borate buffer containing the radioligand (see Section D) without any pretreatment whatsoever. Fresh hemolymph sample volumes greater than 10 μl should be avoided since they can result in an inability to pellet the antibody–hapten reactants in a centrifugal field at the termination of the reaction.

2. Tissue Sources

Isolated tissues or whole organisms should be extracted in a final concentration of 80% ethanol (v/v). The insoluble material can then be removed by filtration or centrifugation. Varying amounts of the clarified supernatant (filtrate) can be added to the incubation tube and the solvent can be removed under a gentle stream of nitrogen.

3. Standards

A standard curve is generated by adding to a series of incubation tubes concentrations of α- or β-ecdysone from 25 pg to 4.0 ng. The general series used in this laboratory is 25, 50, 125, 250, 500, 1000, 2000, and 4000 pg. The concentrations of the standards are determined by appropriate dilutions of a stock (normally 50 ng/ml) whose concentration is routinely determined spectrophotometrically at 242 nm. The various standards are added to the incubation tubes in ethanol and the solvent is removed under a stream of N_2. In addition, a standard blank (i.e., with control serum) is incubated so that background may be subtracted.

D. Incubation

To the aqueous hemolymph or to the dry tissue extract or the standards is added 100 μl borate buffer (0.1 M boric acid, 0.1 M sodium tetraborate, 0.075 M NaCl, pH 8.4) containing approximately 12,000 dpm ^{3}H-α-ecdysone (68 Ci/mmole, courtesy of Dr. David King, Zoecon Corporation, Palo Alto, California). The tubes are mixed to allow adequate equilibration of labeled and unlabeled ecdysone.

Next, 100 μl of a 1.2% anti-β-ecdysone-CMO antiserum solution in borate buffer is added to the incubation resulting in a final concentration of 0.6% antiserum. In the case of the antiserum raised against the 22-hemisuccinate of α-ecdysone, the final concentration of antiserum is 0.04%. In both cases, however, a final total serum concentration of 3% is maintained by the addition of control rabbit serum to the antiserum dilutions. This facilitates pellet formation at the termination of the incubation. Following addition of the antiserum, the tubes are mixed thoroughly and allowed to incubate for three to four hours at room temperature or overnight at 4°C.

E. Termination of Incubation

If not already at 4°C, the tubes are allowed to cool to this temperature, at which all subsequent steps of the assay are conducted. The incubation is terminated by precipitation of the antibody–hapten complex upon the addition of 200 μl saturated ammonium sulfate. After 20 minutes, the samples are centrifuged for 15 minutes at 500 rpm (4800 g) (HS-4 rotor DuPont Co. equipped with four 24-place buckets).

After the supernatants are removed by vacuum aspiration, the pellets are washed with 400 μl 50% saturated ammonium sulfate in borate buffer. The washed pellets are centrifuged as before. Following removal of the supernatants, the pellets are ready for counting.

F. Liquid Scintillation Spectrometry

The pellets are dissolved first in 25 μl water and then 600 μl of an efficient aqueous cocktail such as Aquasol (New England Nuclear) is added. After mixing, the assay tubes are placed into 10 × 50 mm glass shell vial inserts, which are then placed into standard scintillation vials.

G. Data Reduction

Standard curves are constructed as illustrated in Figures 1 and 2. Maximal binding of the radioligand to antibodies occurs in that tube to which only labeled ligand and antiserum have been added. Addition of cold ligand displaces the label in the manner illustrated in Figures 1 and 2. Prior to plotting, all the values were corrected for instrument and operational background by subtracting the value of the blank tube (i.e., the tube to which tritiated ligand plus control serum was added and subsequently carried through the additional steps of the assay). The values for the unkowns can be read directly from the curves. Once the equation solving the shape of the standard curve has been obtained, the data reduction can easily be computerized using APL 360 (Iverson, 1962).

If a mixture of both α- and β-ecdysone is present in the sample, then either a chromatographic separation followed by radioimmunoassay of the separated components or a dual antisera determination should be performed to quantitate the separated moieties.

V. DUAL ANTISERA DETERMINATIONS

As mentioned above, antisera differing in their $\beta/\alpha_{50\%}$ can be used to determine quantitatively the individual amounts of α- and β-ecdysone in a sample. The data can be obtained in either of two ways. First, a series of standard curves can be generated by assaying various dilutions of mixtures of α- and β-ecdysone ranging from 0% α with 100% β to 100% α with 0% β. These mixtures are then assayed in a standard manner using the antiserum with a high $\beta/\alpha_{50\%}$ (Horn et al., 1976), and the percent bound is plotted as a function of total amount of standard ecdysone (α plus β) initially present. These standard curves would then generate a family of curves as shown in Figure 3.

Parallel dilutions of the unknown samples would then be individually assayed using both the α-ecdysone-specific (Horn et al., 1976) and nonspecific (Borst and O'Connor, 1974) antisera. The former assay would give the percent bound for each dilution, whereas the latter assay would indicate the combined mass of ecdysones present. With the two sets of values for each dilution, it would then be possible to match the resulting curve with the family of standard mixtures to determine the fraction of α- and β-ecdysone in the sample.

Alternatively, a computer-generated equation has been derived from the family of standard mixture curves. The equation is

$$y = \frac{10^4}{100 + x^{[\alpha^{(1.3966-1.04745\alpha)}]}}$$

where y is the percent bound determined with the α-ecdysone-specific antiserum, x is the total radioimmunoassay activity of the sample in nanograms determined by the nonspecific antiserum, and α is the fraction of α-ecdysone in the sample (where α-plus β-ecdysone is assumed to equal one).

As seen in Figure 3, a small amount of α-ecdysone in the mixture results in a substantial displacement of the standard curve from the 100% β-ecdysone curve, a displacement which is understandable since the α-ecdysone-specific antiserum shows a much higher affinity for α- than β-ecdysone. Therefore, the usable range of mixtures of β-ecdysone : α-ecdysone is from 100 : 0 to about 60 : 40. Fortuitously,

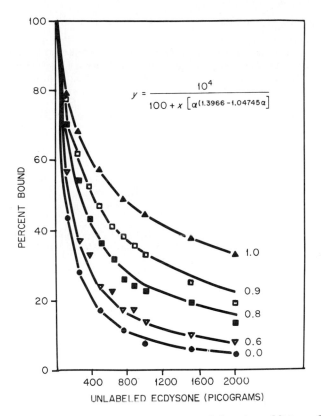

$$y = \frac{10^4}{100 + x\left[\alpha^{(1.3966 - 1.04745\alpha)}\right]}$$

Figure 3. Standard competition curves generated by the addition of increasing amounts of unlabeled α- and β-ecdysone mixtures in the presence of 12,000 dpm [23,24-^{3}H]α-ecdysone (specific activity equals 68 Ci/mmole) using the anti-α-ecdysone 22-hemisuccinate–thyroglobulin antiserum. Fractions to the right of the curves indicate the amount of β-ecdysone in the unlabeled mixture. The symbols represent experimentally derived values, whereas the curves have been computer-generated by the equation shown (see text for explanation).

this is the range in which the two molting hormones have predominantly been found in nature (Bollenbacher *et al.*, 1975; Chang *et al.*, 1976a).

This laboratory is currently investigating the use of this technique to monitor the ecdysone ratios during the different developmental stages of insects and crustaceans. After this work was begun, an analogous report appeared for the assay of mixtures of testosterone and 5α-dihydrotestosterone (Llewelyn *et al.*, 1976).

ACKNOWLEDGMENTS

We thank Ms. Becky A. Sage for valuable technical assistance and Ms. June Baumer for the computer analysis of the dual antisera determinations. The work described from our laboratory was generously supported by Grant NS 08990 from the National Institutes of Health and Grant PCM 73-01592 AO1 from the National Science Foundation.

REFERENCES

Andrieux, N., Porcheron, P., Berreur-Bonnenfant, J., and Dray, F. (1976). Determination du taux d'ecdysone au cours du cycle d'intermue chez le crabe *Carcinus moenas;* comparison entre individus sains et parasités par *Sacculina carcini. C. R. Hebd. Seances Acad. Sci.* **283,** 1429–1432.

Bollenbacher, W. E., Vedeckis, W. V., Gilbert, L. I., and O'Connor, J. D. (1975). Ecdysone titers and prothoracic gland activity during the larval–pupal development of *Manduca sexta. Dev. Biol.* **44,** 46–53.

Bollenbacher, W. E., Goodman, W., Vedeckis, W. V., and Gilbert, L. I. (1976). The *in vitro* synthesis and secretion of α-ecdysone by the ring glands of the fly, *Sarcophaga bullata. Steroids* **27,** 309–324.

Bordereau, C., Hirn, M., Delbecque, J.-P., and De Reggi, M. (1976). Presence d'ecdysones chez un insecte adulte: La reine du termite. *C. R. Hebd. Seances Acad. Sci.* **282,** 885–888.

Borst, D. W., and Engelmann, F. (1974). *In vitro* secretion of α-ecdysone by prothoracic glands of a hemimetabolous insect, *Leucophaea maderae. J. Exp. Zool.* **189,** 413–419.

Borst, D. W., and O'Connor, J. D. (1972). Arthropod molting hormone: Radioimmune assay. *Science* **178,** 418–419.

Borst, D. W., and O'Connor, J. D. (1974). The trace analysis of ecdysones by gas-liquid chromatography, radioimmunoassay and bioassay. *Steroids* **24,** 637–656.

Borst, D. W., Bollenbacher, W. E., O'Connor, J. D., King, D. S., and Fristrom, J. W. (1974). Ecdysone levels during metamorphosis of *Drosophila melanogaster. Dev. Biol.* **39,** 308–316.

Calvez, B., Hirn, M., and De Reggi, M. (1976). Ecdysone changes in the haemolymph of two silkworms (*Bombyx mori* and *Philosamia cynthia*) during larval and pupal development. *FEBS Lett.* **71,** 57–61.

Chang, E. S. (1978). Identification, quantification, and metabolism of crustacean molting hormones. Ph.D. Thesis, University of California, Los Angeles.

Chang, E. S., and O'Connor, J. D. (1977). Secretion of α-ecdysone by crab Y-organs *in vitro. Proc. Natl. Acad. Sci. U.S.A.,* **74,** 615–618.

Chang, E. S., Sage, B. A., and O'Connor, J. D. (1976a). The characterization of circulating ecdysone titers in the crab, *Pachygrapsus crassipes. Colloq. Int. C. N. R. S.* **251,** 263–271.

Chang, E. S., Sage, B. A., and O'Connor, J. D. (1976b). The qualitative and quantitative determinations of ecdysones in tissues of the crab, *Pachygrapsus crassipes,* following molt induction. *Gen. Comp. Endocrinol.* **30,** 21–33.

De Reggi, M. L., Hirn, M. II., and Delaage, M. A. (1975). Radioimmunoassay of ecdysone. An application to *Drosophila* larvae and pupae. *Biochem. Biophys. Res. Commun.* **66,** 1307–1315.

Erlanger, B. F., Bieser, S. M., Borek, F., Edel, F., and Libermann, S. (1967). *Methods Immunol. Immunochem.* **1,** 144.

Fraenkel, G., and Zdarek, J. (1970). The evaluation of the "*Calliphora* test" as an assay for ecdysone. *Biol. Bull. (Woods Hole, Mass.)* **137,** 138–150.

Hagedorn, H. H., O'Connor, J. D., Fuchs, M. S., Sage, B., Schlaeger, D. A., and Bohm, M. K. (1975). The ovary as a source of α-ecdysone in an adult mosquito. *Proc. Natl. Acad. Sci. U.S.A.* **72,** 3255–3259.

Hodgetts, R. B., Sage, B., and O'Connor, J. D. (1977). Ecdysone titers during postembryonic development of *Drosophila melanogaster. Dev. Biol.* **60,** 310–317.

Horn, D. H. S. (1971). The ecdysones. *In* "Naturally Occurring Insecticides" (M. Jacobson and D. G. Crosby, eds.), pp. 333–459. Dekker, New York.

Horn, D. H. S., Wilkie, J. S., Sage, B. A., and O'Connor, J. D. (1976). A high affinity antiserum specific for the ecdysone nucleus. *J. Insect Physiol.* **22,** 901–905.

Ikekawa, N., Hattori, F., Rubio-Lightbourn, J., Miyazaki, H., Ishibashi, M., and Mori, C. (1972). Gas chromatographic separation of phytoecdysones. *J. Chromatogr. Sci.* **10,** 233–242.

Iverson, K. E. (1962). "A Programming Language." Wiley, New York.

Kaplanis, J. N., Tabor, L. A., Thompson, M. J., Robbins, W. E., Shortino, T. J. (1966). Assay for ecdysone (molting hormone) activity using the house fly *Musca domestica. Steroids* **8,** 625–631.

King, D. S., and Siddall, J. B. (1969). Conversion of α-ecdysone to β-ecdysone by crustaceans and insects. *Nature (London)* **221,** 955–56.

King, D. S., Bollenbacher, W. E., Borst, D. W., Vedeckis, W. V., O'Connor, J. D., Ittycheriah, P. I., and Gilbert, L. I. (1974). The secretion of α-ecdysone by the prothoracic glands of *Manduca sexta in vitro. Proc. Natl. Acad. Sci. U.S.A.* **71,** 793–796.

Lachaise, F., Lagueux, M., Feyereisen, R., and Hoffmann, J. A. (1976). Métabolisme de l'ecdysone au cours du développment de *Carcinus maenas* (Brachyura, Decapoda). *C. R. Hebd. Seances Acad. Sci.* **283,** 943–946.

Lagueux, M., Hirn, M., De Reggi, M., and Hoffmann, J. A. (1976). Taux des ecdystéroides et dévelopement ovarïen chez les femelles adultes de *Locusta migratoria. C. R. Hebd. Seances Acad. Sci.* **282,** 1187–1190.

Lagueux, M., Hirn, M., and Hoffmann, J. A. (1977). Ecdysone during ovarian development in *Locusta migratoria. J. Insect Physiol.* **23,** 109–119.

Lauer, R. C., Solomon, P. H., Nakanishi, K., and Erlanger, B. F. (1974). Antibodies to the insect moulting hormone β-ecdysone. *Experientia* **30,** 560–562.

Legay, J.-M., Calvez, B., Hirn, M., and De Reggi, M. (1976). Ecdysone and oocyte morphogenesis in *Bombyx mori. Nature (London)* **262,** 489–490.

Llewelyn, D. E. H., Hillier, S. G., and Read, G. F. (1976). The use of multivariable standard curves in the radioimmunoassay of testosterone and 5α-dihydrotestosterone. *Steroids* **28,** 339–348.

McCarthy, J. F., and Skinner, D. M. (1977). Proecdysial changes in serum ecdysone titers, gastrolith formation, and limb regeneration following molt induction by limb autotomy and/or eyestalk removal in the land crab, *Gecarcinus lateralis. Gen. Comp. Endocrinol.* **33,** 278–292.

Morgan, E. D., and Poole, C. F. (1976). The extraction and determination of ecdysones in arthropods. *Adv. Insect Physiol.* **12,** 17–62.

Porcheron, P., Fourcrier, J., Gros, C., Pradelles, P., Cassier, P., and Dray, F. (1976). Radioimmunoassay of arthropod moulting hormone: β-ecdysone antibodies production and ^{125}I-iodinated tracer preparation. *FEBS Lett.* **61**, 159–162.

Schlaeger, D. A., Fuchs, M. S., and Kang, S. H. (1974). Ecdysone-mediated stimulation of dopa decarboxylase activity and its relationship to ovarian development in *Aedes aegypti. J. Cell Biol.* **61**, 454–465.

Williams, C. M. (1968). Ecdysone and ecdysone-analogues: Their assay and action on diapausing pupae of the cynthia silkworm. *Biol. Bull. (Woods Hole, Mass.)* **134**, 344–355.

UTERINE AND PLACENTAL HORMONES

41

Specific Human Chorionic Gonadotropin Assay

JUDITH L. VAITUKAITIS

I. INTRODUCTION

Human chorionic gonadotropin (hCG) is a glycoprotein hormone composed of a protein core with branched carbohydrate side chains. It shares extensive structural homology with human luteinizing hormone (hLH) (Bahl *et al.*, 1973; Closset *et al.*, 1973; Morgan *et al.*, 1973a). Both hCG and hLH have indistinguishable biologic and immunologic activities in most assay systems. Human chorionic gonadotropin is normally synthesized and secreted by syncytiotrophoblastic cells of the normal placenta; human luteinizing hormone is normally synthesized and secreted by cells of the anterior pituitary. Both hCG and hLH share common quaternary structures characterized by two dissimilar α and β subunits; the subunits are not covalently linked (Bellisario *et al.*, 1973; Carlsen *et al.*, 1973; Morgan *et al.*, 1973a). The primary amino acid sequences of the α subunits of LH and hCG are essentially identical (Bellisario *et al.*, 1973; Sairam *et al.*, 1972) and

Methods of Hormone Radioimmunoassay, Second Edition
Copyright © 1979 by Academic Press, Inc.

accounts for the extensive immunologic cross-reactivity observed among the human glycoprotein hormones (Vaitukaitis and Ross, 1972). The β subunits of those two hormones also share extensive structural homology. Of the 115 amino acid residues of hLH-β, approximately 80% are identical with those found in hCG-β (Closset *et al.*, 1973; Morgan *et al.*, 1973a). On the other hand, the β subunit of hCG contains a unique carboxyl terminus grouping of 28–30 amino acids not found in LH nor any other glycoprotein hormone (Morgan *et al.*, 1973a; Carlsen *et al.*, 1973).

Most clinical radioimmunoassays published to date cannot selectively detect hCG in samples containing both LH and hCG in the same sample. Trophoblastic tumors, as well as a wide variety of nontrophoblastic tumors, secrete hCG (Braunstein *et al.*, 1973b; Rosen *et al.*, 1975). In some cases, the level is too low to be certain whether hCG, LH, or both are present in sera samples by conventional radioimmunoassays, which cannot discriminate between LH and hCG. Consequently, an assay which selectively measures hCG in sera

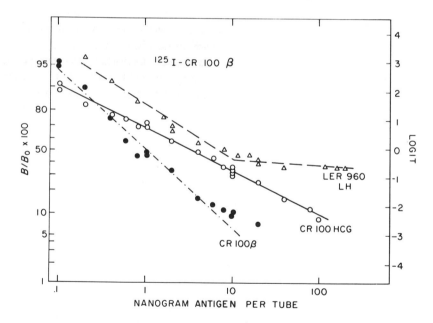

Figure 1.   Dose–response curves for highly purified hCG-β (CR100-β), highly purified hCG (CR100-hCG), and highly purified human pituitary LH (LER 960) run in a homologous hCG-β radioimmunoassay system. The dose–response curves for hCG and LH have significantly different slopes. (Reproduced from Vaitukaitis *et al.*, 1971, with permission of the publisher.)

samples containing both hCG and LH constitutes an effective tool for early diagnosis and follow-up of individuals with tumors secreting hCG. In addition, selective hCG measurement allows diagnosis of pregnancy as early as eight to ten days after ovulation (Catt *et al.*, 1975; Braunstein *et al.*, 1973a). Conventional pregnancy tests, using hemagglutination inhibition techniques, are 100-fold less sensitive than the specific hCG radioimmunoassay.

Initial studies characterizing hCG-β antisera showed that intact hCG and native hLH behaved differently in conventional double antibody radioimmunoassays using anti-hCG-β sera (Vaitukaitis *et al.*, 1971; Vaitukaitis and Ross, 1972). Figure 1 depicts dose–response curves for hCG and hLH in a homologous hCG-β assay system. The dose–response curves of native hCG and LH were significantly different, suggesting that an antiserum to hCG-β may be sufficiently sensitive and specific to selectively measure hCG in plasma or serum samples containing both hCG and hLH (Vaitukaitis *et al.*, 1972; Vaitukaitis and Ross, 1974). The development and validation of a specific hCG assay system are described herein.

II. METHOD OF RADIOIMMUNOASSAY

A. Generation of Specific Antisera

Highly purified hCG-β may be obtained commercially or it may be obtained from the National Pituitary Agency if it is to be used for clinical research. Native hCG may be dissociated into its respective α and β subunits by techniques that have been well worked out (Bahl *et al.*, 1973; Canfield *et al.*, 1971; Morgan *et al.*, 1973b). Antisera to isolated hCG-β may be generated in New Zealand white rabbits. It has been ascertained empirically that a minimum dose of 50 μg hCG-β is needed to generate antibody with a single immunizing dose (Vaitukaitis *et al.*, 1971; Vaitukaitis and Ross, 1974). An emulsion is prepared using equal volumes of complete Freund's adjuvant (Difco) and 0.15 M NaCl. Each animal is immunized with 2.0 ml of an emulsion containing equal volumes of complete Freund's adjuvant (Difco) and 0.15 M NaCl, 50 μg hCG-β, and an additional 5.0 mg dried tubercle bacilli (heat-killed, Difco). The emulsion, prepared with a high-speed homogenizer, is then injected intradermally over 30 to 50 sites of each animal which has had its back and proximal limbs previously shaved of fur. Two to three days prior to injecting the emulsion, the animal may be injected with 0.5 ml crude *Bordetella pertussis* vaccine. Antibody usually becomes detectable four to five weeks after the primary

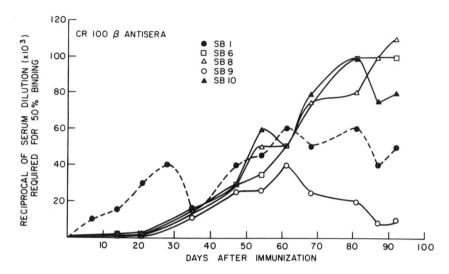

Figure 2. Antibody titers of four rabbits following a 50-µg primary immunizing dose of highly purified hCG-β and a booster injection of 20 µg in an animal (------) initially immunized with 20 µg hCG-β six weeks previously. A minimum of three weeks was needed before significant titer of antibody was detected in the four animals receiving a primary immunization with hCG-β. In the animal which received a booster injection with 20 µg hCG-β, significant antibody became detectible within one week of reimmunization. (Reproduced from Vaitukaitis *et al.*, 1971, with permission of the publisher.)

immunizing series of injections. Figure 2 shows the antibody titer of several animals immunized with hCG-β. If no antibody is detectable by six weeks, the animals should be reimmunized with one-half to one-fourth of the initial immunizing dose (12–25 µg) of hCG-β and the animals bled one week later by either central ear artery puncture or peripheral vein vacuum collection. The serum should be separated from cells and a preservative, such as thiomersal or sodium azide, added before storing the sera at −16°C. Antisera obtained over several weeks and having comparable sensitivity and specificity may be pooled.

B. Characterization of Antibody

The antibody is then titered with iodinated hCG-β and the final tube dilution of antisera needed to yield a starting $(B - N)/(T - N) \times 100$ (B = bound counts, T = total counts, N = nonspecific counts trapped in pellet) of 30–40% is ascertained. That dilution of antibody is then used to check the sensitivity of the antisera for measuring native hCG.

Operationally this is done by constructing dose–response curves for hCG with each antiserum. There is no relationship between sensitivity and titer. In essence, an antiserum with a high titer may not be the most sensitive antiserum, and, consequently, one needs to empirically check each antibody for sensitivity. Those antisera proved to be sufficiently sensitive are then subjected to further testing.

To check antisera for sufficient specificity for hCG, one constructs dose–response curves for both hCG and hLH. Again, there is no way to predict which antisera will be sufficiently sensitive and specific; consequently, this must be ascertained empirically. One selects an antiserum which appears to be sufficiently sensitive and specific and then subjects it to further testing. One must be certain that high physiologic concentrations of LH do not give false positive specific hCG assay results. Serum samples selected from patients with known high circulating LH concentrations are subjected to the "specific hCG" assay. The desired endpoint is no significant inhibition of samples containing high LH concentrations in that assay system. Figure 3

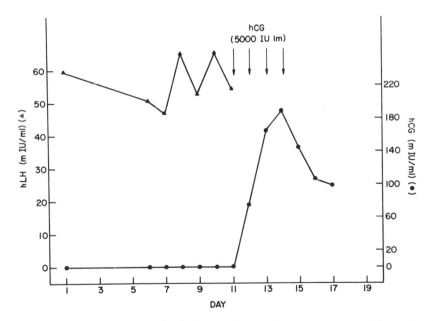

Figure 3. Plasma hLH (▲) values determined by a radioimmunoassay which could not discriminate between hCG and hLH and plasma hCG (●) values obtained in a specific hCG radioimmunoassay system. Plasma samples were obtained from a castrate male before and after exogenous hCG administration. Only after exogenous hCG administration was there any detectible hCG in peripheral blood.

depicts results of a series of samples obtained from a single subject whose circulating LH concentrations had undergone wide fluctuation. When those same samples were subjected to the specific hCG assay system, no significant inhibition was detected. Additional validation is required, since some antisera are sensitive to nonspecific plasma protein effects. For the specific hCG assay system, this can best be checked by adding varying volumes of serum not containing hCG to assay tubes containing antibody, iodinated hCG-β, and buffer, and by observing whether increasing volumes of blank sera decrease binding in those assay tubes. Since those serum samples contain no hCG, any inhibition could be attributable to nonspecific serum protein effects. When this maneuver was carried out for the specific hCG assay system described here, significant nonspecific protein effects were observed (Vaitukaitis et al., 1972). However, the nonspecific effects were obviated by adding a constant volume of serum to all assay tubes, including nonspecific (N), maximum binding tubes (B_0), and each tube of the standard curve. The nonspecific serum effects were dose dependent in terms of the volume of serum added, and, consequently, a fixed volume of serum must be added to all assay tubes. Most hCG-β antisera checked to date have been sensitive to nonspecific protein effects.

C. Preparation of Labeled Hormone

Highly purified hCG or hCG-β may be iodinated with modification of a chloramine-T method of Greenwood et al. (1963) or by a lactoperoxidase method (Miyachi et al., 1972) catalyzed by hydrogen peroxide. Both techniques are more than satisfactory for conventional radioimmunoassays. Human chorionic gonadotropin or its β subunit may be labeled with Na^{125}I or Na^{131}I. Since ^{125}I has a significantly longer half-life (59 days) versus that for ^{131}I (8 days), it is probably to one's advantage to use carrier-free Na^{125}I for radioimmunoassay techniques in general. Iodination of hCG is rather straightforward and can be carried out as follows. The iodination procedure must be carried out in a well-ventilated shielded hood, preferably in an isolated laboratory area. To conserve highly purified ligand for labeling, it is probably best to aliquot 1.0–5.0 μg hCG or hCG-β, diluted in distilled water, in separate reaction vessels (12 × 75 mm glass or plastic tubes) and store in a frozen state. At the time of iodination, one of the tubes can be removed and the reagents are added to the test tube containing the aliquoted hormone or subunit. Repeated freeze–thaw cycles may denature the protein to be radiolabeled and should be avoided.

1. *Chloramine-T Procedure*

The chloramine-T iodination procedure is carried out as follows:

a. To the reaction tube containing hCG or hCG-β, add 30–50 μl 0.5 M NaHPO$_4$, pH 7.5.

b. Add 0.5–1.0 mCi Na^{125}I. The radionuclide is usually dissolved in 0.01 N NaOH. However, some distributors of radioactive iodide do not carefully control the normality of the NaOH, and, consequently, the concentration of NaOH may be significantly higher. The buffering capacity of 0.5 M NaHPO$_4$ will correct for those errors in most cases.

c. To initiate the iodination reaction, add 10 μl (25 μg) chloramine-T. The tube is gently shaken initially and allowed to stand for 30–60 seconds. In general, the longer the reaction time, the higher the specific activity attained. The chloramine-T should be diluted in 0.01 M NaHPO$_4$, pH 7.5, containing 0.15 M NaCl (PBS).

d. Add sodium metabisulfite (50–70 μg/20 μl) to the reaction mixture. The sodium metabisulfite should be diluted in PBS.

e. Apply the reaction mixture to the top of either a Sephadex G-75 or BioGel P-60 column, previously washed with 1.0 ml 2% BSA and equilibrated with PBS. Half milliliter fractions are collected into tubes containing a drop (60–100 μl) of 2% BSA in PBS. The organic iodide will elute first as a radioactive peak, separate from the inorganic iodide. Specific activities can be calculated, assuming that the number of counts transferred is directly proportional to the amount of hormone transferred from the reaction vessel to the column and that an insignificant amount of labeled hormone adsorbs to the column bed. Using a simulated ^{125}I standard (^{129}I), one can approximate the specific activity of the newly labeled polypeptide. Alternatively, one can ascertain the mass of ^{125}I-labeled hormone by using an assay system with ^{131}I-labeled hormone and vice versa. A calibrated source of ^{125}I is needed to accurately ascertain the amount of radioactivity present.

2. *Lactoperoxidase Method*

The lactoperoxidase method of iodination may be carried out as follows:

a. 1.0–5.0 μg of hormone is dissolved in 20 μl of distilled water and placed in the bottom of a 12 × 75 mm test tube.

b. Add 50 μl 0.5 M morpholinoethane sulfonic acid (MES), pH 6.0.

c. Add 1.0 μg lactoperoxidase (5 μl).

d. Add 1.0 mCi Na^{125}I to the reaction tube.

e. The chemical reaction is initiated by adding 100 ng H_2O_2 in 10 μl 0.01 M MES, pH 6.0. The reagents are allowed to react for five minutes and an additional 100-ng aliquot of H_2O_2 is added and allowed to react for an additional 5 minutes. If a lower specific activity is desired, only one addition of H_2O_2 is used.

f. At the termination of the reaction time, the organic and inorganic $Na^{125}I$ is separated by gel filtration through either Sephadex G-75 or Bio-Gel P-60 columns.

3. Iodination Check

After the hormone is labeled, the immunoreactivity of the labeled preparations may be checked by using an excess of first antibody in order to ascertain the maximum number of counts that are immunoprecipitable. Because an excess of antibody is used, the reaction time is shortened considerably and usually takes two to three hours to reach equilibrium. One need not use a specific antibody for this procedure. An acceptable range of immunoreactivity can be empirically ascertained so that assay results are more likely to be within acceptable quality control limits. In our laboratory, when 80% or more of the counts are immunoprecipitable with excess first antibody, labeled hCG or hCG-β are sufficiently immunoreactive to consistently yield radioimmunoassay with less than 10% intraassay and less than 20% interassay variation.

4. Batch Cleanup Techniques for Iodinated Polypeptides

In general, labeled hCG or hCG-β may be used for assays for two weeks after carrying out the iodination procedure. With time after labeling, the level of immunoreactivity will progressively decrease. One can use batch cleanup methods to remove free iodide, damaged hormone, or both. This is best done as follows:

1. Add an aliquot of labeled hormone to 2.0 ml of 2% bovine serum albumin in PBS. Add a sufficient number of counts for the size of the assay to be run, remembering that approximately 25% of the counts added will be removed with this procedure.

2. Add 300–400 mg Dowex-I Ag-10 (Bio-Rad).

3. Vortex the contents of the tube for a few seconds.

4. Centrifuge for five minutes at 2500 rpm. The supernatant is removed and diluted for assay.

An alternative method for further purifying the labeled sialylated glycoprotein is to use a minicolumn of agarose–concanavalin A (Pharmacia). This is carried out as follows:

1. Make 2.0-ml bed of concanavalin A–Sepharose 4B in a Pasteur pipette, plugged with a small glass bead.
2. Equilibrate with ten volumes of PBS.
3. Apply labeled hormone.
4. Wash column with ten volumes of PBS to get rid of free ^{125}I and hormonal fragments.
5. Elute immunoreactive ^{125}I-hCG or β with 0.2 M methyl-α,D-glycopyranoside, collecting 1.0-ml fractions.
6. Pool fractions with highest number of counts and dilute for assay.

The agarose–concanavalin A column can be used as the primary separation technique after having carried out the iodination procedure. If that procedure is used, then one would have to assay the ^{125}I preparation in an ^{131}I assay system and ascertain the amount of radioactivity present relative to a calibrated standard in order to calculate the specific activity of the labeled glycoprotein eluted from the concanavalin A–Sepharose column. In our laboratory, we try to keep the specific activity between 50 and 120 μCi/μg for hCG and its subunits. If the specific activity is greater than that, then the immunoreactivity decreases rapidly after radiolabeling and intra- and interassay variations increase markedly.

D. Assay Procedure

The specific hCG assay used in our laboratory is performed as follows. Tubes used for assay are 12 × 75 mm glass disposable tubes with uniform dimensions and lead content. Since ^{125}I is of lower energy than ^{131}I, it is imperative to assure uniformity of the assay tubes so that quenching is uniform throughout. The assay buffer is 0.01 M NaHPO$_4$, 0.15 M NaCl, pH 7.5, containing 2.5 vol% carrier normal rabbit serum and 0.1% sodium azide as a preservative. The reaction volume of each assay tube is 1.0 ml. The first four tubes of the assay are control tubes for nonspecific binding (N), and each contains 500 μl of PBS containing 2.5 vol% normal rabbit serum, 100 μl 0.1 M disodium EDTA, pH 7.5, 200 μl adult male serum, and 200 μl iodinated hCG in PBS. The second four tubes are designated maximum binding tubes, B_0, and each of these four tubes contains 300 μl buffer, 100 μl EDTA, 200 μl normal human male serum, 200 μl antibody to hCG-β, and 200 μl ^{125}I-HCG or ^{125}I-hCG-β containing approximately 15,000–20,000 cpm. Nine separate concentrations of hCG in replicate comprise the standard curve. The amounts of hCG in replicate are as follows: 6.0, 4.0,

2.0, 1.0, 0.6, 0.4, 0.2, 0.1, 0.05 ng per tube. Each standard curve tube contains 200 μl normal human male serum, as well as 200 μl antibody, 200 μl trace, 100 μl EDTA, and sufficient PBS containing 2.5 vol% normal rabbit serum to make the reaction mixture to 1.0 ml. Each unknown sample is added in 200-μl volumes. If sufficient hCG is present, such that the value would be off the dose–response curve, then serial 1 : 10 dilutions of the sample should be added to the assay tubes; however, 200 μl human male serum should be added to assure that each assay tube within the assay contains a constant volume of serum in order to obviate nonspecific protein effects.

After all the assay tubes are set up, each tube is gently vortexed and subsequently incubated at 37°C for two hours, and then transferred to 4°C for a minimum of 15 hours. The antigen and antibody are at equilibrium by the end of this time; for convenience, the tubes may be incubated for an additional 24–48 hours before adding second antibody. Sufficient second antibody is added to cause maximum precipitation of the rabbit γ-globulin. A large amount of carrier normal rabbit serum (2.5 vol%) is used so that clearly visible pellets result after centrifuging the tubes. The second antibody reaction is at equilibrium within four hours of having added the second antibody. If one chooses to use less carrier normal rabbit serum to conserve second antibody, then a longer incubation time is required for the second antibody reaction to reach equilibrium. To separate bound from free hCG, the assay tubes are centrifuged at 4°C for 20 minutes at 2500 rpm. At the end of that time, the supernatants are aspirated and the pellets are counted. The pellets contain the antibody-bound hormone.

E. Assay Calculation

The resulting dose–response curve is then plotted, and unknowns may be interpolated either from the dose–response curve visually or the data subjected to computerized programs as designed by Rodbard (1974) and others.

In order to obviate false positive results because of freeze–thaw cycles of unknown samples and to obviate false positives created by technical handling, and possibly low but normal hCG secretion, a cutoff point of 75% on the dose–response curve is used in the specific hCG assay system. The point of 75% binding $(B\text{-}N)/(B_0\text{-}N)$ is usually equivalent to 0.2 ng per tube or 1.0 ng/ml of an unknown sample if 200 μl is assayed. Highly purified hCG has an immunoreactivity of approximately 5 mIU/ng in terms of the Second International Standard hCG.

F. Interpretation of Results

In some cases, hCG, as well as free hCG-β or altered forms of hCG, may be secreted by tumors; consequently, samples containing free hCG-β and other altered forms of hCG will fail to dose out in a parallel fashion with highly purified hCG in the specific hCG assay system. When the latter is observed, it is the first clue to look for altered forms of hCG and its subunits. All tumors ectopically secreting hCG also secrete free subunits of hCG (Vaitukaitis, 1973). Men and women normally do not have detectable immunoreactive hCG in peripheral blood; however, a few patients with inflammatory bowel disease, or patients with duodenal or gastric ulcers, have been found to have low but significant levels of immunoreactive hCG in peripheral blood (Vaitukaitis et al., 1976). If one can rule out the preceding diagnoses, as well as pregnancy, then hCG present in excess of 1.0 ng/ml is pathologic, and the presence of a tumor should be suspected. With this assay system, hCG first becomes detectable approximately eight to nine days after initiation of implantation (Catt et al., 1975; Braunstein et al., 1973a), several days before expected time of menses. Trophoblastic tumors, as well as tumors ectopically secreting hCG, should be considered.

Tumors of the gastrointestinal tract, especially adenocarcinomas of the stomach, hepatomas, and adenocarcinomas of the pancreas, are most commonly associated with ectopic hCG secretion. Among those disorders, as many as one-third of patients will have significant levels of circulating hCG (Braunstein et al., 1973b). In fact, some patients will have levels of circulating hCG in excess of those encountered in the first trimester of pregnancy, when hCG levels may be as high as 150 IU/ml. Rarely are tumors ectopically secreting hCG associated with circulating hCG levels in excess of 100 IU/ml. Moreover, in spite of markedly elevated circulating levels of hCG, patients usually have no clinical manifestations of the excess circulating hCG. Prepubertal boys may present with signs of precocious puberty if an hCG-secreting tumor is present (Vaitukaitis, 1974). Gynecomastia has been described in men with gonadotropin-secreting lung tumors, melanomas, and adrenal tumors (Vaitukaitis, 1974).

This assay system has come to be known as the "beta-hCG assay." That term is misleading, since most persons then conclude that hCG-β only is being measured. The assay as performed has a higher affinity for hCG than hCG-β. However, if both were present, both would be detected in the radioimmunoassay. Since hCG has a plasma half-life of 24 to 36 hours and hCG-β a plasma half-life of 12 to 14 minutes

(Braunstein *et al.*, 1972), hCG is the predominant circulating form found in serum of patients having hCG-secreting tumors.

ACKNOWLEDGMENT

Supported in part by NIH Grants RR-533 and GRS-57-228.

REFERENCES

Bahl, O. P., Carlsen, R. B., Bellisario, R., and Swaminathan, N. (1973). Human chorionic gonadotropin-amino acid sequence of the α and β subunits. *Biochem. Biophys. Res. Commun.* **48**, 416–422.

Bellisario, R., Carlsen, R. B., and Bahl, O. P. (1973). Human chorionic gonadotropin linear and amino acid sequence of the α subunit. *J. Biol. Chem.* **248**, 6796–6809.

Braunstein, G. D., Vaitukaitis, J. L., and Ross, G. T. (1972). The *in vivo* behavior of human chorionic gonadotropin after dissociation into subunits. *Endocrinology* **91**, 1030–1036.

Braunstein, G. D., Grodin, J. M., Vaitukaitis, J., and Ross, G. T. (1973a). Secretory rates of human chorionic gonadotropin by normal trophoblast. *Am. J. Obstet. Gynecol.* **115**, 447–450.

Braunstein, G. D., Vaitukaitis, J. L., Carbone, P. P., and Ross, G. T. (1973b). Ectopic production of human chorionic gonadotropin by neoplasms. *Ann. Intern. Med.* **78**, 39–45.

Canfield, R. E., Morgan, R. J., Kammerman, S., Bell, J. J., and Agosto, G. M. (1971). Studies of human chorionic gonadotropin. *Recent Prog. Horm. Res.* **27**, 121–164.

Carlsen, R. B., Bahl, O. P., and Swaminathan, N. (1973). Human chorionic gonadotropin. Linear amino acid sequence of the β subunit. *J. Biol. Chem.* **248**, 6810–6827.

Catt, K. J., Dufau, J. L., and Vaitukaitis, J. L. (1975). Appearance of hCG in pregnancy plasma following the initiation of implantation of the blastocyst. *J. Clin. Endocrinol. Metab.* **40**, 537–540.

Closset, J., Hennen, G., and Lequin, R. M. (1973). Luteinizing hormone: The amino acid sequence of the β subunit. *FEBS Lett.* **29**, 97–100.

Greenwood, F. C., Hunter, W. L., and Glover, J. J. (1963). The preparation of ^{131}I-labeled growth hormone of high specific activity. *Biochem. J.* **89**, 114–123.

Miyachi, Y., Vaitukaitis, J. L., Nieschlag, E., and Lipsett, M. B. (1972). Enzymatic radio-iodination of gonadotropins. *J. Clin. Endocrinol. Metab.* **34**, 23–28.

Morgan, F. J., Birken, S., and Canfield, R. E. (1973a). Human chorionic gonadotropin: A proposal for its amino acid sequence. *Mol. Cell Biochem.* **2**, 97–99.

Morgan, F. J., Canfield, R. E., Vaitukaitis, J. L., and Ross, G. T. (1973b). The preparation and characterization of the subunits of human chorionic gonadotropin (hCG). *In* "Methods in Investigative and Diagnostic Endocrinology" (S. Berson and R. Yalow, eds.), Vol. 2B, Part 3, pp. 733–742. North-Holland Publ., Amsterdam.

Rodbard, D. (1974). Statistical quality control and routine data processing for radioimmunoassays and immunoradiometric assays. *Clin. Chem.* **20**, 1255–1270.

Rosen, S. W., Weintraub, B. D., Vaitukaitis, J. L., Sussman, H. H., Hershman, J. M., and Muggia, F. M. (1975). Placental proteins and their subunits as tumor markers. *Ann. Intern. Med.* **82**, 71–83.

Sairam, M. R., Papkoff, H., and Li, C. H. (1972). Human pituitary interstitital cell stimulating hormone: Primary structure of the α subunit. *Biochem. Biophys. Res. Commun.* **48**, 530–537.

Vaitukaitis, J. L. (1973). Immunologic and physical characterization of human chorionic gonadotropin (hCG) secreted by tumors. *J. Clin. Endocrinol. Metab.* **37**, 505–514.

Vaitukaitis, J. L. (1974). Human chorionic gonadotropin as a tumor marker. *Ann. Clin. Lab. Sci.* **4**, 276–280.

Vaitukaitis, J. L., and Ross, G. T. (1972). Antigenic similarities among the human glycoprotein hormones and their subunits. *In* "Gonadotropins" (B. Saxena, H. Gandy, and C. Beling, eds.), pp. 435–447. Wiley, New York.

Vaitukaitis, J. L., and Ross, G. T. (1974). Subunits of human glycoprotein hormones— Their immunologic and biologic behavior. *Isr. J. Med. Sci.* **10**, 1280–1287.

Vaitukaitis, J. L., Robbins, J. B., Nieschlag, E., and Ross, G. T. (1971). A method for producing specific antisera with small doses of immunogen. *J. Clin. Endocrinol. Metab.* **33**, 988–991.

Vaitukaitis, J. L., Braunstein, G. D., and Ross, G. T. (1972). A radioimmunoassay which specifically measures human chorionic gonadotropin in the presence of human luteinizing hormone. *Am. J. Obstet. Gynecol.* **113**, 751–758.

Vaitukaitis, J. L., Ross, G. T., Braunstein, G. D., and Rayford, P. L. (1976). Glycoprotein hormones and their subunits: Basic and clinical studies. *Recent Prog. Horm. Res.* **32**, 289–331.

42

Radioimmuno- and Radioreceptor Assays of Placental Lactogens

BUDDHA P. ROY AND HENRY G. FRIESEN

Methods of Hormone Radioimmunoassay, Second Edition
Copyright © 1979 by Academic Press, Inc.
All rights of reproduction in any form reserved. ISBN 0-12-379260-6

I. INTRODUCTION

Human placental lactogen (hPL) was the first among the family of placental lactogens to be purified. Since the development of the radioimmunoassay for hPL more than ten years ago, placental lactogens have been identified in 12 other species, representing three different orders of mammals. Although different modifications of the radioimmunoassay technique continue to be described, the principle of the system and the results obtained by using this method have not changed significantly during this period. In the techniques which are described, hPL is used as the model unless otherwise stated.

In recent times, the most important development concerning prolactin and placental lactogen measurement has been the establishment of radioreceptor assays (RRA), which are extremely sensitive and which, unlike radioimmunoassays, are not species specific. While radioreceptor assays may be applied to blood samples for ordinary clinical purposes, the radioreceptor assay in no way replaces radioimmunoassays. Radioreceptor assays have been particularly useful in the identification of newer placental lactogens from various species.

Descriptions of the different methods of assaying placental lactogens, along with the merits and shortcomings of the techniques involved, are considered in this chapter. The variations in concentrations of human placental lactogen in blood during pregnancy are summarized briefly.

A. Historical Background

The major impetus to the study of human placental lactogen came from Josimovich and McLaren (1962). They noted that a lactogenic substance which cross-reacted weakly with antisera to human growth hormone (hGH) was present in the human placenta and in peripheral and retroplacental serum of pregnant women. Although the discovery of human placental lactogen (hPL) stirred much interest, a placental luteotropin was first reported in the rat in 1938 by Astwood and Greep. In 1961, Fukushima and Ito and Higashi (1961) reported on the isolation of a human placental factor with lactogenic–somatotropic activity, and shortly thereafter Josimovich and McLaren (1962) identified hPL. Subsequently, Kaplan and Grumbach (1965) and Friesen (1965a,b) exploited the immunological cross-reaction between human placental extracts and antisera to hGH to purify hPL. Methods for the extraction and purification of hPL in pure form were necessary in order to develop radioimmunoassays for clinical use and also to elucidate the chemistry of hPL. Josimovich and McLaren (1962) and Friesen (1965a) used fresh or frozen placentas ground to powder in dry ice as the tissue source for extraction. A more suitable method was developed subsequently, using a side fraction obtained during the purification of γ-globulin from placental extracts as the starting material (Friesen, 1965a,b; Florini et al., 1966). With this procedure, large amounts of hPL were obtained which made clinical studies of hPL feasible, permitting the development of radioimmunoassays and ultimately providing sufficient material for amino acid sequence analysis.

B. Comparative Chemistry of Human Placental Lactogen (hPL) and Human Growth Hormone (hGH)

Human placental lactogen is a single chain polypeptide. Its molecular weight, amino acid composition, and amino acid sequence are similar to those of hGH. It consists of 191 amino acids with two intrachain disulfide bonds.

Comparison of the complete amino acid sequence of hPL and hGH shows that 80% of the amino acids in corresponding positions are identical amino acid pairs or related through highly favored codon substitutions (Niall et al., 1971, 1973; Niall, 1972; Li et al., 1971; Sherwood, 1967; Sherwood et al., 1971). There is a somewhat greater degree of identity at the carboxy-terminus, although the chemical similarity is a feature of the entire polypeptide chain. Homologies between hPL, hGH, and ovine prolactin also are evident but less striking. A most significant aspect of the chemistry of these molecules is the internal homology of hPL, hGH, and ovine prolactin, consisting of four peptides each approximately 20 amino acid residues in length (Niall et al., 1971; Niall, 1972). It is possible that the three hormones may have arisen through successive duplication of the original structural cistron. It is more likely that the primitive polypeptide which existed may have been similar to prolactin, since the latter is found throughout the vertebrate phylum, with growth hormone and placental lactogen probably evolving at a later stage.

C. Big Placental Lactogen

A macromolecular form of human placental lactogen (hPL) has been found in extracts of human placenta and in sera from pregnant women. The chromatographic behavior of this substance suggests it has a higher molecular weight than the major form of hPL in the circulation (Schneider *et al.*, 1974). It has been suggested that the big hPL is not an artifact of extraction and purification and that it is not a simple aggregate because of its stability in the presence of urea or guanidine. Schneider *et al.* (1975), using affinity chromatography, have recently purified big hPL and determined its molecular weight as 45,000 on SDS-gel. Upon reduction with mercaptoethanol, a single band with molecular weight of 23,000 was noted. This result indicates that big hPL is composed of two peptide chains which are likely to be identical, since reduction leads to a single band with approximately half the original molecular weight. It seems likely that, like other big hormones of the growth hormone–prolactin family, big hPL is a disulfide-linked dimer and not really a precursor of hPL such as proinsulin or proparathyroid hormone. Physiologic significance of the high molecular form of hPL has yet to be determined. In addition to the heterogeneity of the molecular size of hPL in the circulation, several studies have demonstrated the synthesis of pro-hPL. Using mRNA isolated from human placentas and wheat germ translational systems, a protein of MW 25,000 is synthesized which cross-reacts with antiserum to hPL (Boime *et al.*, 1976).

D. Biologic Actions of Placental Lactogens

Some of the biologic actions of lactogenic hormones (prolactin and hPL) that have been reported are summarized in Table I. Even though many biologic effects of placental lactogens have been well documented, no primary action of the hormone has been defined. The two well-known actions of the lactogenic hormones are (1) stimulation of mammary gland development (Forsyth, 1974) and (2) lactogenesis, i.e., initiation of lactation. In large doses, placental lactogen has also been reported to possess growth-promoting actions (Kaplan and Grumbach, 1965). The role of placental lactogens on the maintenance of luteal function is well known in rats (Matthies, 1967; Linkie and Niswender, 1973). Lactogenic hormones are also known to affect glycogen levels, free fatty acid synthesis, RNA synthesis, blood glucose, osmoregulation, ion transport, blood volume, and cardiac output (Elghamry *et al.*, 1966; Chen *et al.*, 1972; Wang *et al.*, 1972; Mainoya, 1975; Lockett, 1965; Lawson and Gala, 1974; Hanwell and Linzell, 1972).

The term "human placental lactogen" will be used throughout this chapter. Other names assigned to this hormone include chorionic

Table I   Actions of Lactogenic Hormones[a]

Action	Target organ
Mammogenesis	Mammary gland
Lactogenesis	Mammary gland
Growth	Epiphyseal cartilage, body weight gain
Somatomedin production	Liver
Maintenance of luteal function	Corpus luteum
Luteolysis	Corpus luteum
Stimulation of male secondary sex organ	Prostate, seminal vesicles
Glycogenolysis	Liver
Increase FFA	Mammary gland, liver
RNA synthesis	Liver, mammary gland
Reduction of blood glucose	Blood
Increased fluid and ion transport	Intestine
Osmoregulation	Intestine
Elevation of cardiac output	Heart
Reduction of blood volume	Circulatory system
Modulation of hormone receptors for estrogens	Liver, mammary tumor, uterus
Modulation of hormone receptors for lactogenic hormones	Liver, mammary tumor, prostate, testis, pigeon crop sac
Modulation of hormone receptors for LH	Ovary

[a] From Kelly (1977).

growth hormone prolactin (CGP), purified placental protein (PPH), and human chorionic somatomammotropin (hCS) (Li *et al.*, 1968).

II. RADIOIMMUNOASSAY

There is no one satisfactory bioassay for measuring hPL in blood, although the method used for measuring prolactin could be used (Kleinberg and Frantz, 1971; Turkington, 1971; Lowenstein *et al.*, 1971). The principle of competitive inhibition, which forms the basis of any radioimmunoassay (RIA), is summarized in Scheme 1 for human placental lactogen.

Many investigators have reported on the development of radioimmunoassays for hPL. The following are among those groups which have provided clinically useful RIA's: Grumbach and Kaplan (1964), Frantz *et al.* (1965), Beck *et al.* (1965), Spellacy *et al.*, (1966), Samaan *et al.* (1966), Sciarra *et al.*, (1968), Josimovich *et al.*, (1970), and

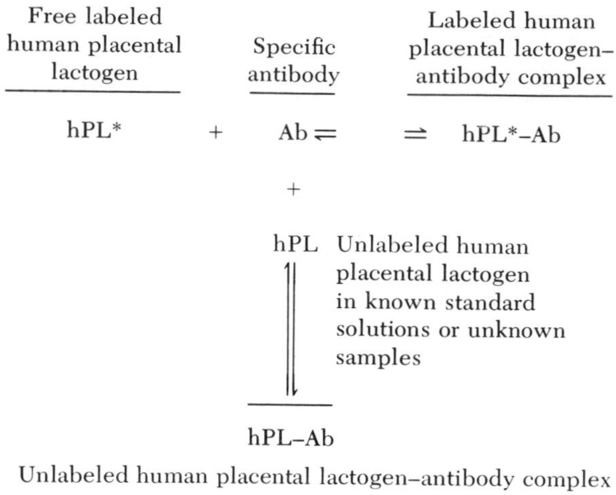

Free labeled human placental lactogen	Specific antibody	Labeled human placental lactogen–antibody complex

hPL*   +   Ab ⇌   ⇌   hPL*–Ab

$+$

hPL Unlabeled human placental lactogen in known standard solutions or unknown samples

$\Updownarrow$

hPL–Ab

Unlabeled human placental lactogen–antibody complex

Scheme 1

Letchworth *et al.* (1971). A description of the method used in our laboratory is given below.

A. Preparation of Buffers

1. *Phosphate-Buffered Saline (0.01 M PBS)*

NaCl, 8.77 gm, $Na_2HPO_4 \cdot 7H_2O$, 2.33 gm, $NaH_2PO_4 \cdot H_2O$, 0.18 gm, and sodium azide (as preservative), 0.10 gm, is added to dissolve the reagents in 1.0 liter distilled water. The pH is then adjusted, if necessary, to 7.4 by dropwise addition of 1.0 M NaOH. The buffer is stored at 4°C.

2. *Phosphate-Buffered Saline and Bovine Serum Albumin (BSA), 0.01 M PBS with 2.5% BSA*

Twenty-five grams of BSA is dissolved in 1.0 liter of the above-mentioned PBS buffer. The pH should then be rechecked when the albumin is completely dissolved.

3. *Phosphate Buffer, 0.5 M, pH 7.6*

$NaH_2PO_4 \cdot 7H_2O$ (6.9 gm) is dissolved in 100 ml water; 13.4 gm $Na_2HPO_4 \cdot 7H_2O$ is dissolved in 100 ml water. The monobasic buffer is added to the dibasic buffer until the pH is 7.6 (approximately ratio 1 : 9, monobasic : dibasic).

B. Standard hPL Preparation

A comparison of results of the measurement of serum hPL concentrations by different laboratories has been hampered by the fact that no appropriate International Reference Preparation is yet available. Highly purified human placental lactogen (hPL) can be obtained from the National Institutes of Health, National Institute of Arthritis, Metabolic and Digestive Diseases, and the Division of Biological Standards, Medical Research Council, London, England.

Highly purified hPL (lyophilized powder) is weighed on a microbalance and then dissolved in $0.05\,M$ NH_4HCO_3. If there is any difficulty in dissolving it, a drop of $0.01\,N$ NaOH may be added. The solution is diluted with $0.05\,M$ NH_4HCO_3, and this produces a stock solution containing 200 μg hPL per milliliter that must be kept at $-20°C$. In order to minimize thawing and refreezing, the solution is divided into small aliquots.

The stock hPL solution is diluted with $0.01\,M$ PBS containing 2.5% BSA to produce standards for the assay, and these are also divided into 0.5-ml aliquots and kept at $-20°C$.

C. Iodination of Human Placental Lactogen

Carrier-free $Na^{125}I$ in NaOH is used for the iodination of hPL. Either of two methods, chloramine-T (Hunter and Greenwood, 1962; Greenwood et al., 1963) or lactoperoxidase (Thorell and Johansson, 1971) can be used to prepare ^{125}I-hPL. The procedure used here is slightly modified from the originally described method and is outlined below.

1. Chloramine-T Method

The reaction is conducted in a 12×75 mm glass test tube. Reagents at room temperature are added to the test tube in the following order: hPL, 5.0 μg in 25 μl $0.05\,M$ NH_4HCO_3, $Na^{125}I$ 1.0 mCi in 25 μl (buffered with $0.5\,M$ sodium phosphate at pH 7.6, and chloramine-T, 25 μl of 4.0 mg/ml solution. The reagents are mixed gently by shaking the tube and the reaction is allowed to occur for 30 seconds. The addition of 100 μl of sodium metabisulfite (2.5 mg/ml in $0.01\,M$ phosphate buffer, pH 7.4) followed by 100 μl potassium iodide (10 mg/ml) and 2.0 ml $0.01\,M$ PBS with 2.5% BSA terminates the reaction.

Next, all of the reaction mixture is applied to a 2×50 cm column of Sephadex G-100 pretreated with 1.0 ml 2.5% BSA and equilibrated with $0.01\,M$ PBS, pH 7.4. Fractions of approximately 1.0 ml in tubes containing 0.2 ml 2.5% BSA in 0.01 M PBS are collected. The relative radioactivity of the fractions is measured by a Geiger counter. It is usually possible to distinguish three peaks of radioactivity that appear in the following sequence: (1) the damaged (aggregated) material, (2) the usable ^{125}I-hPL, and (3) the free iodide.

2. Lactoperoxidase Method

In this iodination procedure, sodium azide is not used in buffers as preservative because azides are inhibitors of lactoperoxidase. Combine the following reagents in a 12×75 mm glass tube at room temperature: 0.05 M phosphate buffer, pH 7, 25 μl; hPL, 5.0 μg in 25 μl of 0.05 M NH$_4$HCO$_3$; Na^{125}I, 1.0 mCi in 25 μl (buffered with 0.5 M phosphate buffer pH 7.6); and lactoperoxidase (1.0 mg/ml solution in 0.05 M phosphate buffer, pH 7), 5.0 μl.

Hydrogen peroxide (30%) is diluted 1 : 15,000 in H$_2$O and 5.0 μl of the diluted H$_2$O$_2$ is used. The reagents are mixed by flicking the tube gently for five minutes. A second 5.0 μl of diluted H$_2$O$_2$ is added after three to five minutes. The reaction is stopped by the addition of 1.0 ml protein-free 0.01 M PBS, pH 7.4, or 25 mM Tris-HCl, pH 7.6. The entire reaction mixture is then applied to a 2×50 cm column of Sephadex G-100 that has been pretreated with 1.0 ml 2.5% BSA. Fractions are collected in the same way as for the chloramine-T method, with the use of either PBS or Tris-HCl as the column buffer.

The desired peak tubes from the gel filtration column are collected and then stored at $-20°$C. The shelf life of iodinated hPL is usually about three weeks. The initial specific activity is about 100 μCi/μg hPL.

D. Testing the Iodoinated Placental Lactogen

A convenient test of the iodinated hPL employs charcoal treated with dextran to separate bound and free hormone. The preparation is prepared by stirring together the following reagents for one to two hours: 1.25 gm charcoal (Norit-A), 0.125 gm Dextran T-250 (Pharmacia), and 100 ml sodium phosphate buffer, 0.15 M, pH 7.4. The next step is to incubate 0.1 ml ^{125}I-hPL (diluted with 0.01 M PBS, pH 7.4, containing 0.5% BSA to give about 60,000 cpm/0.1 ml) with 0.6 ml 0.5% BSA in 0.01 M PBS, pH 7.4, in duplicate tubes; this is called the "tracer test." Two additional tubes containing 0.1 ml ^{125}I-hPL, 0.5 ml 0.5% BSA in 0.01 M PBS, pH 7.4, and 0.1 ml antibody in excess (e.g., 1 : 200 dilution) are then set up. For this purpose, it is not necessary to use the highest quality antiserum. The period of incubation is 24 hours at 4°C. The dextran–charcoal suspension is vigorously stirred while withdrawing 1.0-ml aliquots, and this suspension is added to each test tube. The contents are mixed several times during a 20-minute period at room temperature followed by centrifugation for 30 minutes at 3000 rpm. The supernatant is decanted and the pellets are counted for ^{125}I-hPL. If the iodinated hPL is satisfactory, more than 90% will have bound to the charcoal in the tubes which contained no antibody and less than 20% in the tubes which contained excess antibody. It should be noted that the buffer for this test contains only 0.5% BSA, since high concentrations of protein inhibit the binding of iodinated hPL to charcoal.

Usually, this tracer test is performed on several gel filtration fractions around the selected peak. Those containing satisfactory ^{125}I-hPL can be pooled for use in the assay itself.

E. Production of Antisera to hPL

Human placental lactogen is dissolved in $0.05\,M$ NH_4HCO_3, diluted with saline to produce a concentration of 0.5 mg/ml; 0.5–1.0 ml of this is emulsified with an equal volume of complete Freund's adjuvant. The latter is injected intradermally on the back of rabbits or in the foot pads. The usual schedule is three to four injections at 14-day intervals. The animals receive booster injections every four to six weeks. About 50% of the rabbits are likely to produce satisfactory antisera, and the antisera can be harvested by bleeding the rabbit from an ear vein after six weeks. Blood (10–20 ml) is removed and allowed to clot at room temperature. The serum is separated by centrifugation and stored in 1.0-ml aliquots at $-20°C$. It is possible to obtain additional antiserum every four to six weeks.

The antiserum from each bleeding of an animal is tested to determine the optimal dilution to be used in an assay. Dilutions of antisera ranging from 1 : 100 to 1 : 100,000 or greater are made in $0.01\,M$ PBS, pH 7.4, with 2.5% BSA. The assay is set up in a manner similar to a regular radioimmunoassay (see details below) with the exception that 0.1 ml of each dilution of antiserum is tested in duplicate tubes. The percentage of iodinated hPL bound at each concentration of antiserum is then determined. By repeating the above procedure and including 0.05 ml of unlabeled hPL in the minimum concentration at which it is desired to measure, final selection of an appropriate dilution of the antiserum can be made. Figure 1 illustrates a typical dose–response curve, i.e., a plot of dilution of anti-human hPL against percent of radioiodinated hPL bound which is used to determine the best antiserum dilution for routine radioimmunoassay of hPL. The dilution of

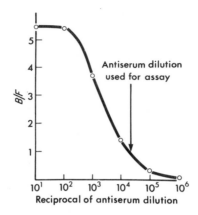

Figure 1.   Antiserum dilution curve. Reciprocal of antiserum dilution on the abscissa is plotted against antibody-bound ^{125}I-hPL on the ordinate.

antisera is chosen so that it gives a ratio of bound : free ^{125}I-hPL of 1 : 1, e.g., the dilution required to bind 50% of the radiolabeled antigen. The chosen dilution will give an optimal ratio of sensitivity and precision.

F. Separation of Free and Bound hPL

After a period of incubation of the labeled and unlabeled hormone with the specific antibody, the antibody-bound and free labeled hormone are separated.

Several different methods have been developed for the separation of bound and free hormone. In general, these methods are based upon: (1) adsorption of free tracer, e.g., ion exchange, charcoal, silica, talc; (2) precipitation of bound tracer, e.g., double antibody, salt precipitation, solvent fractionation; (3) differential migration of bound and free tracer, e.g., chromatography, electrophoresis, chromatoelectrophoresis, gel filtration.

Double Antibody Method

In the double antibody method, the reaction of protein hormones with their specific antibodies in dilute solution results in the formation of a soluble complex. The soluble complex can then be precipitated by a second antibody obtained from an animal of different species than was used in the immunization with the hormone. In practice, for example, anti-rabbit γ-globulin is the second antibody and is prepared by immunizing sheep. The optimal concentration of sheep anti-rabbit γ-globulin to be used in the assay is determined in the following way.

The assay is set up as usual but the first antibody (rabbit anti-hPL) is used in high concentration (e.g., 1 : 200 dilution) in every tube. All dilutions consist of 0.01 M PBS containing 2.5% BSA. Following the initial period of incubation (12–18 hours), 0.1 ml normal rabbit serum (1 : 200 or 1 : 300) plus serial dilutions (i.e., 1 : 1 to 1 : 64) of second antibody is added to each tube; these mixtures are then incubated for a 24-hour period. The iodinated hormone in the precipitates is counted. The greatest dilution of the second antibody that precipitates 80% or more of the iodinated hPL is used in subsequent experiments.

G. Variations in Methodology

The most important difference between the many published accounts of variations in methodology for radioimmunoassays of hPL is probably the choice of method for separating bound from free hormone Examples of different separation techniques are shown in Table II. The double antibody and dextran–charcoal methods are the most popular today, since both allow easy handling of large numbers of assay tubes. In Letchworth's assay (Letchworth *et al.*, 1971), a high concentration of antibody and labeled hormone is used to ensure equilibration within 10–15 minutes and this eliminates the need for a plasma dilution step. Two volumes of ethanol are used to separate the bound from free hormone, a reaction which occurs within ten minutes.

The advantages of using an antibody in high concentration include: (1) assays can be completed within one hour, because the reagents come to equilibrium quickly, and (2) large amounts of ^{125}I-hPL may be

Table II Different Methods of Separating Bound from Free Hormone

References	Method
Grumbach and Kaplan (1964)	Chromatoelectrophoresis
Frantz *et al.* (1965)	Chromatoelectrophoresis
Beck *et al.* (1965)	Second antibody
Samaan *et al.* (1966)	Second antibody
Spellacy *et al.* (1966)	Second antibody
Sciarra *et al.* (1968)	Dextran–charcoal
Saxena *et al.* (1968)	Dextran–charcoal
Leake and Burt (1969)	Solid-phase radioimmunoassay
Genazzani *et al.* (1969)	Second antibody
Josimovich *et al.* (1970)	Dextran-charcoal
Haour (1971)	Dioxane
Lectchworth *et al.* (1971)	Ethanol
Gardner *et al.* (1974)	Solid-phase radioimmunoassay

used, specific activity need not be high, and statistically accurate counts can be gathered over a short time. Steep slope of the resulting standard curve allows optimal precision. The disadvantage of using high concentrations of antibody is the high demand for antiserum. The use of ethanol for separating bound from free hormone has the advantages of low cost, speed, and reproducibility.

Another reliable method of separating bound from free antigen is the use of antibodies coupled to a solid phase. A number of different solid phases include: linked dextran (Wide and Porath, 1966), agarose (Hart, 1972), styrene derivatives (Catt *et al.*, 1966), polystyrene tubes (Catt *et al.*, 1970), and paper discs (Ceska and Lundkvist, 1972). Techniques for coupling of antibody include diazotization (Catt *et al.*, 1966), physical adsorption (Catt *et al.*, 1970), the use of isothiocyanates (Wide and Porath, 1966), and cyanogen halides (Wide, 1969). Few detailed comparisons have been made between the operation of solid-phase and soluble systems in a radioimmunoassay. Major advantages of the solid-phase technique are: (1) universal applicability, (2) separation can be carried out quickly, and (3) separation of antibody-bound and free antigen is virtually complete, as opposed to many other procedures of separation. The disadvantages include: (1) the loss of a considerable proportion of antibody during initial coupling reaction, (2) during incubation, the tubes must be continuously mixed, and (3) reduced sensitivity in the assay system indicates a reduction in the apparent affinity constant of the antibody after coupling. When the achievement of high sensitivity is not a requirement and the supply of antiserum is abundant, the solid phase antibodies were felt to be of the greatest value.

The use of ^{125}I (Leake and Burt, 1969) has replaced ^{131}I (Grumbach and Kaplan, 1964) for radioactive labeling. The advantage is a longer half-life and longer useful shelf life of the iodinated hormone.

Variables which may influence the assay include: differences in the buffer used, concentration of BSA, incubation time, volume, and proportion of serum in the reaction mixture. Hormone-free serum is added to all tubes containing standards. Serum may cause nonspecific reduction of binding of ^{125}I-hPL to antibody, a phenomenon which is ascribed to nonspecific binding of the label to serum globulins and results in a spuriously high value in a double antibody assay. Therefore, serum should preferably be diluted as much as 1:20 in the assay.

Variations in methodology offer advantages or disadvantages in terms of speed, sensitivity, and convenience. Yet most of the methods remain quite adequate for clinical purposes, for which it is more important to establish long-term quality control and to define carefully the range of values in different situations than to strive for speed or supersensitivity.

H. Calculation of Results

The standard curve is drawn by plotting bound ^{125}I-hPL (cpm) against the concentration of hormone. Unknown values can be read through the use of interpolation. Rodbard and Lewald (1970) have proposed a very useful analytic procedure employing a computer to perform linear regression analysis of the data after logarithmic or logit transformation. It is vital to check the values of pools included in each assay; if not satisfactory, the assay must be discarded. The reason for performing the assay and the requirements demanded may determine what constitutes a satisfactory pool value. When five separate pools are used, the estimates of values in two or more pools should not deviate by more than 20% from the mean estimates of those pool values that have been derived from previous assays, especially when values in the clinically important range are measured.

I. The Radioimmunoassay of hPL in Serum Samples

The assay is conducted in 12×75 mm glass test tubes, which are numbered and placed in racks. All standard and sample tubes are arranged in duplicate, and serum pools in each assay act as quality controls. PBS ($0.01\,M$), containing 2.5% BSA, is used to make all dilutions of samples, sera, and iodinated hPL. To each tube the following reagents are added in order: 0.5 ml 2.5% BSA in $0.01\,M$ PBS, 0.05 ml standard (0–16 ng/ml), serum sample or serum pool, 0.1 ml first antibody at optimal dilution (1 : 150,000), and 0.1 ml ^{125}I-hPL (about 30,000 cpm). The tubes are incubated for 72 hours at 4°C. Then to each is added the following: 0.1 ml second antibody at appropriate dilution and 0.1 ml normal rabbit serum (1 : 200). The tubes are incubated an additional 24 hours at 4°C, then are centrifuged at $2000\,g$ for 30 minutes, decanted, and drained before counting the pellets for ^{125}I-hPL in an automatic gamma counter.

III. RADIORECEPTOR ASSAYS FOR hPL

A. General Principles

Studies on membrane receptors have revealed specific binding sites on target cell membranes for almost all peptide hormones, but the

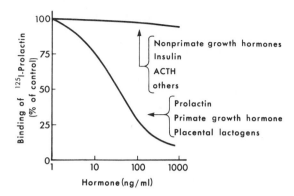

Figure 2. The specificity of prolactin receptors from mammary glands. Nonprimate growth hormones and other hormones do not bind to receptor sites but prolactin, hGH, and placental lactogen bind about equally. (Reproduced from Shiu and Friesen, 1976a, with permission of the publisher.)

functional role of these hormone binding sites or receptors has yet to be defined (Cuatrecasas, 1974).

The mammary gland is considered as a primary target for prolactin, and, therefore, a study on prolactin receptors was undertaken by Shiu and Friesen (1974a,b, 1976a,b) on mammary glands of pregnant rabbits. The study demonstrated specific binding of ^{125}I-prolactin in tissue slices or in subcellular particles enriched in plasma membranes. Only peptide hormones with prolactinlike actions in the rabbit have the capacity to compete with ^{125}I-prolactin (Figure 2); this fact shows the specificity of the binding of ^{125}I-prolactin. Hormones, such as human growth hormone and many placental lactogens, also exhibit prolactinlike actions. It is presumed that they act on the mammary glands by interacting with the same set of receptors. The prolactin receptor is often referred to as a lactogen receptor, since all the hormones mentioned above are known as lactogens.

The interaction of polypeptide hormones with their receptors on target cell plasma membranes has been used to develop radioligand assays. It has also been used for hPL and other placental lactogens. Radioactively labeled placental lactogen is allowed to react with a suitable receptor in the presence of varying quantities (standards and unknowns) of unlabeled hormone. The proportion of radioactive hormone that is bound to the receptor is reduced in the presence of increasing concentrations of unlabeled hormone. It is possible to construct a standard curve of the fraction bound as a function of hormone concentration (similar to a radioimmunoassay standard curve) by separating membrane-bound and free components and measuring the radioactivity associated with the receptors. The bound and free hormone can be separated by centrifugation if particulate or whole cell tissue preparations of the receptor are used.

Radioimmunoassay depends upon binding of hormone by an antibody which may be directed against any part of the hormone molecule. On the other hand, the receptor–hormone interaction is thought to involve the biologically active site of the hormone molecule. Thus, the measure of a hormone by radioreceptor assay provides a more accurate index of biologic potency. It leads to different patterns of cross-reactivity between varying species of hormones and receptors that depend on the bioactivity of the hormone in the species from which the receptor is obtained.

A receptor assay in one sense is like an *in vitro* bioassay because it involves binding of the hormone to a cell or a cell membrane preparation. As the result of a hormone–receptor interaction, a product may be generated and if easily measured, can be used as a bioassay; or one can also utilize the binding of a radioactively labeled hormone to the receptor and measure the degree of competitive binding in the presence of unlabeled hormone. This constitutes a radioreceptor assay.

A schematic representation of the competition between ^{125}I-labeled and unlabeled lactogen for binding to the specific receptor is shown in Scheme 2. The extent of inhibition of the binding of labeled hormone is a direct function of the amount of unlabeled hormone present.

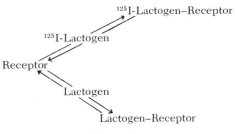

Scheme 2

In Figure 3 is shown the interaction of three different species of placental lactogen (PL_1, PL_2, and PL_3) with rabbit mammary, rat liver, and rat ovary membrane preparations. PL_2, which is most potent in rat liver membrane preparation, is least active in rat ovary, but PL_3 shows maximum activity in rat ovary and minimum in rabbit mammary and rat liver. Similar kinds of differences in activity may be observed when lactogens are assayed in biologic systems. Despite their chemical similarities, it is possible that the receptors which mediate the hor

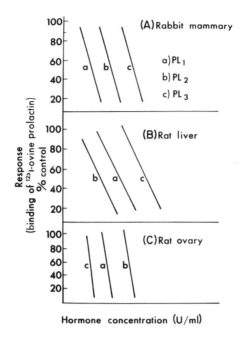

Figure 3.   Dose–response curves for three hypothetical placental lactogen preparations (PL_1, PL_2, PL_3) using three membrane preparations (A) rabbit mammary (B) rat liver, and (C) rat ovary. The competitive displacement curves of placental lactogens from three species are indicated. The rank order of potency of the preparations may vary depending on the membrane preparation used. Thus when rabbit mammary membranes are used PL_1 (curve a) is the most potent, whereas in the case of membranes from rat ovary PL_3 (curve c) is the most potent.

monal action of lactogens bind lactogens with different affinities, thus accounting for different potency estimates when several assays are used.

B. Techniques of Radioreceptor Assay for Placental Lactogen

The radioreceptor assay method consists of the following steps:
1. Preparation of rabbit mammary gland receptors.
2. Preparation of lactogen standard.
3. Iodination of ovine prolactin or hPL.
4. The radioreceptor assay of lactogens in serum.
5. Calculation of results.

1. Preparation of Rabbit Mammary Gland Receptors

Mammary glands of 25- to 30-day pregnant female New Zealand white rabbits are used as the source of receptors since these glands have been found to show a greater degree of specific binding of placental lactogen than those of both males and nonpregnant females (Kelly *et al.*, 1974). After the animals are killed with intravenous Nembutal, mammary glands are removed and are either frozen or kept at 4°C if processed immediately. The glands are cut into small pieces and washed in ice-cold 0.3 M sucrose and then homogenized in five volumes (v/w) of 0.3 M sucrose with a Brinkman Polytron PT-10 at maximum speed for a one-minute period. The homogenate is centrifuged for 15 minutes at 15,000 g at 4°C; then, the supernatant fraction is recentrifuged for one hour at 100,000 g at 4°C. Shiu and Friesen (1974a) have shown that the 100,000 g pellet contains the highest proportion of the binding sites for placental lactogen (Figure 4). This pellet is suspended in 25 mM Tris-HCl buffer, pH 7.6 (containing 10 mM MgCl₂ but no BSA) with a few strokes of a 15 ml Pyrex glass hand homogenizer; 1.0 ml of buffer is used for each gram of whole mammary gland being processed. This particulate receptor concentrate is stored at −20°C, and when required it is thawed and rehomogenized with a few strokes in a hand homogenizer. Specific binding in the radioreceptor assay is linear when receptor is used in a range of 100–400 μg of receptor protein per assay tube (0.1 ml). In the assay, the receptor suspension is used after dilution; this may be done either (1) according to protein content to yield a final concentration of 1.0–4.0 mg/ml [the

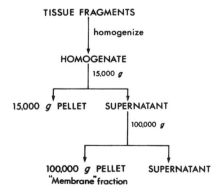

Figure 4. A schematic outline of rabbit mammary receptor preparation. For details, see text.

protein is measured in 10-μl aliquots of the receptor concentrate by the method of Lowry *et al.* (1951)], or (2) by testing different dilutions to find the smallest amount of receptor which binds approximately 10–15% of labeled oPRL or hPL under standard assay conditions.

2. Buffers 25 mM Tris–HCL, pH 7.6, with 0.1% BSA and 10 mM Mg

The reagents (Tris, 3.03 gm, and $MgCl_2 \cdot 6H_2O$, 2.3 gm) are dissolved in distilled water; the pH is adjusted to 7.6 by adding in 10–15 ml 6.0 N HCl, and the final volume is made up to 1.0 liter. One gram of bovine serum albumin (BSA) is dissolved in the buffer, and once again the pH is checked. During preparation of the particulate receptor concentrate, the same buffer without BSA is used, and the same buffer with BSA is used to terminate the incubation. For preparation of the standards, this Tris–BSA buffer *without* $MgCl_2$ is used.

3. Preparation of Lactogen Standard

Although purified hPL as used for radioimmunoassay is also suitable for radioreceptor assays, ovine prolactin (oPRL) is routinely used as the standard for the lactogen radioreceptor assay in this laboratory. Since the radioreceptor assay is not species specific and is sensitive to lactogenic activity, other lactogenic hormones, such as hGH and hPRL, may be used; for the same reasons, oPRL, hGH, or hPL may be used as tracers in this radioreceptor assay. Ovine prolactin is preferred because it is readily available and a stock of 200 μg/ml is prepared in 0.05 M NH_4HCO_3. Exposure of the oPRL to NaOH should be avoided since this may reduce its potency. Dilution of this stock with Tris-HCl buffer (25 mM, pH 7.6, with 0.1% BSA and no $MgCl_2$) produces standards for the radioreceptor assay with a range of values from 5.0 to 2000 ng/ml.

4. Iodination of Ovine Prolactin

The lactoperoxidase method described in the section on radioimmunoassay is also used for iodination using $Na^{125}I$. Since oPRL iodinated by the chloramine-T method does not bind well to the receptors, which presumably fail to recognize even mildly damaged hormone, this method is not satisfactory. ^{125}I-oPRL prepared by the lactoperoxidase method has a shelf life of two to three weeks; it is kept in aliquots frozen at $-20°C$ and thawed only once immediately prior to use.

The appropriate peak fractions of ^{125}I-oPRL from the gel filtration step are tested directly against a receptor using incubation conditions as described below. These conditions are the same as for the routine radioreceptor assay. The ability of the tracer to bind to receptor and to be displaced by unlabeled oPRL is determined; 50×10^3 to 100×10^3 cpm of ^{125}I-oPRL in 0.1 ml 25 mM Tris–HCl buffer, pH 7.6, 10 mM MgCl$_2$, and 0.1% BSA are incubated with 200 μg (protein) particulate receptor (a) in the absence of unlabeled hPL, (b) in the presence of 10 ng, (100 ng/ml standard), and (c) in the presence of 200 ng (2000 ng/ml standard) unlabeled oPRL.

5. The Radioreceptor Assay of Placental Lactogens in Serum

A series of 12×75 mm plastic or glass tubes containing 25 μl of either standard oPRL solutions or unknown sera is set up according to the protocol given below. Standards of oPRL are used at concentrations of 0, 5.0, 10, 20, 30, 50, 80, 100, 200, 300, 500, 1000, and 2000 ng/ml; to each standard tube is added 25 μl of serum from a nonpregnant woman with no appreciable lactogens (hGH, hPL, hPRL) detected by radioimmunoassay. Each standard and unknown is set up in duplicate. In each assay are included several tubes with reference pool sera to act as quality controls.

To a series of 12×75 mm plastic or glass tubes, reagents are added in the order shown in the tabulation below.

Reagent	Experimental sample	Standard curve
Buffer (ml)	0.275	0.250
Standard/serum sample (ml)	0.025 serum sample	0.025 standard
Control serum (ml)	Nil	0.025
Receptor (ml)	0.1	0.1
Tracer (ml)	0.1	0.1

The concentrations of the standards range from 5.0 to 2000 ng/ml. When nonserum samples are assayed, 0.1 ml of sample or standard is used with no need to compensate for nonspecific effects by introduction of control sera (Figure 5).

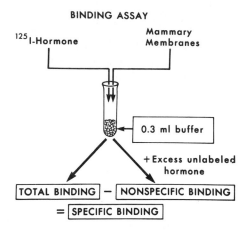

Figure 5. The method used in determining specific binding of ^{125}I-labeled hormone from measurements of total and nonspecific binding is diagrammatically represented (Reproduced from Posner, 1975, with permission of the publisher.)

6. *Calculation of Results*

The ^{125}I-oPRL or ^{125}I-hPL cpm bound is plotted as a function of the concentration of oPRL or hPL on semilogarithmic graph paper to produce a standard curve in similar fashion to that of radioimmunoassay. The concentrations of hPL as total lactogen in the unknown samples are estimated by interpolation. It is also possible, with the aid of a small computer, to perform linear regression analysis on the data after logarithmic or logit transformation; the unknown values are obtained by using the line with the best fit. The poor values are checked and unsatisfactory assays are discarded.

IV. APPLICATIONS OF RADIOIMMUNOASSAY AND RADIORECEPTOR ASSAYS

A. Comparison of Immuno- and Receptor Assays

Radioimmunoassays for lactogens are available to date from only a few species and in most circumstances could only be developed when the purified hormones became available to raise antibodies. The radioreceptor assay is an alternate method with important advantages in measuring prolactin and other lactogenic hormones.

The radioreceptor assay, simple to perform and widely applicable, enables researchers to identify and quantitate many new lactogens which in the past could only be detected by difficult, time-consuming, and insensitive bioassays. Using bioassays, a number of investigators suggested the existence of placental lactogens in several species (Avcrill *et al.*, 1950; Matthies, 1967; Buttle *et al.*, 1972; Forsyth, 1972; Kohmoto and Bern, 1970; Talamantes, 1973). For example, radioreceptor assay has facilitated the purification of lactogens from sheep, rats, goats, and cows (Bolander and Fellows, 1976; Parke and Forsyth, 1975; Chan *et al.*, 1976; Robertson and Friesen, 1975), and it can be predicted that it will have a wide application particularly in the area of research on placental hormones.

Radioreceptor assay is useful because it serves as a complimentary assay system to radioimmunoassays as well as to bioassays for prolactin and placental lactogen. Since the assay is not species specific, it can be used to study the biology of prolactin and placental lactogen in many species and is of particular use in situations in which radioimmunoassays are not available. In general, radioreceptor assay is a satisfactory technique for measurement of prolactin, hGH, and hPL in tissue extracts, column fractions, and pure and crude preparations of prolactin. For inter- and intraassays, the coefficient of variation tends to be 5–15% and is always below 30% if the assays have been properly performed.

Radioreceptor assay cannot be considered as a true bioassay, yet it does detect prolactin and lactogens that are bioassayable. Prolactin and lactogen levels in serum samples obtained from individuals under most clinical conditions determined by radioimmunoassay are similar to those levels determined by radioreceptor assay; this implies that lactogens detected by radioimmunoassay under these conditions are also biologically active.

B. Cautionary Notes

Radioreceptor assay has a few shortcomings, such as detecting other peptide hormones which are also lactogenic, i.e., hGH and hPRL. If the concentrations of two or more of these hormones are sufficiently high in the same sample, then interference would occur and the value obtained for any one hormone would be the sum of all. In practice, however, the concentration of hGH is normally less than 5.0 ng/ml, and hPL is absent unless the samples are taken from pregnant subjects in whom, for example, mean concentrations of hPL and hPRL in late pregnancy might be 5000 and 200 ng/ml, respectively, and radioreceptor assay would not distinguish the two. Nonprimate GH's, however, are not lactogenic and cannot be detected by the assay; hence, the presence of GH in samples from these species will not affect the assay. Therefore, cross-interference from other hormones need not necessarily be a problem in many of the assays that are performed.

The nonspecific interference of serum in the radioreceptor assay is a significant problem. On assaying serum samples, it was observed that serum depresses the binding of ^{125}I-prolactin to receptors. Incorrect values would result if a standard curve obtained in the absence of serum were used to read the prolactin or lactogen values for the unknown serum samples (See Figure 6) (Shiu, 1974).

The standard curves obtained when 0.025 ml of sera from control sources was introduced into each assay tube are shown in Figure 7A (Shiu, 1974), and there is a significant lowering of the initial binding by sera. Different batches of sera from the same species may vary a great deal in their effects on the assay; therefore, a batch of serum should preferably be tested before use, and, when measuring unknown serum samples from one species, control serum obtained from the same species should be added to the prolactin or lactogen standards. When the assay was set up, satisfactory and reproducible standard curves were obtained (Figure 7A).

Because the sample size of the prolactin and lactogen standards was 0.025 ml, the sensitivity of the assay became 10–25 ng/ml, compared to a threshold of 5.0 ng/ml when 0.10 ml of nonserum sample was used. The inset in Figure 7A shows that results obtained when a patient's serum sample containing 1080 ng/ml prolactin (determined by

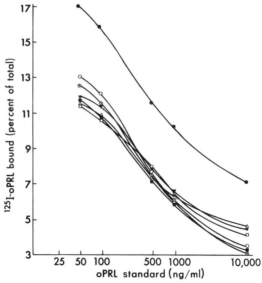

Figure 6. Illustration showing the effect of sera on the radioreceptor assay in which 25 μl serum and 25 μl prolactin standard solution were used. The rat serum was obtained from normal males. No serum added, ●; human serum, ○; rat serum, ⊙; dog serum, ▼; mouse serum, ×; monkey serum, △; rabbit serum, □.

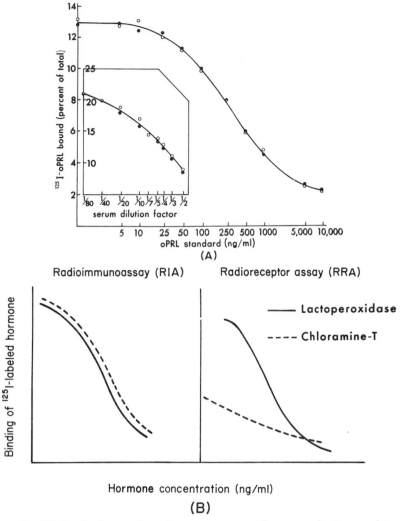

Figure 7. (A) Standard curve for radioreceptor assay of serum prolactin was obtained when serum from a hypophysectomized rat was used in the incubations, O; standard curve obtained when human serum from a hypopituitary patient was used in the incubation, ●. For details see text. The inset illustrates the serial dilution of a human serum sample (obtained from a patient with pituitary tumor) with a prolactin content of 1080 ng/ml as determined by radioimmunoassay (●) and the serial dilution of a hypophysectomized rat serum sample with ovine prolactin added to give a concentration of 1000 ng/ml (O). (B) The figure illustrates schematically that ^{125}I-labeled human placental lactogen iodinated using either chloramine-T or lactoperoxidase is suitable in a radioimmunoassay. In a radioreceptor assay, however, the product obtained with the chloramine-T method is unsuitable. Similarly some standards may be satisfactory in a radioimmunoassay whereas in a receptor assay they prove unsatisfactory.

radioimmunoassay) was serially diluted and tested in receptor assay; the binding of ^{125}I-oPRL was inhibited in a manner parallel to that observed when similarly diluted hypophysectomized rat serum received additions of oPRL in concentrations up to 1000 ng/ml. Therefore, it is valid to introduce control serum into the prolactin and lactogen standards for the measurement of prolactin and lactogen concentrations in serum samples. The nature of the factor(s) that causes serum effects has not been discovered; however, the inhibiting factor(s) was eluted in the void volume upon gel filtration of the serum. This suggests that the factor(s) is quite likely a large molecule. Further studies are required to verify this (Shiu, 1974).

Another shortcoming of radioreceptor assay is its lack of adequate sensitivity in measuring prolactin and hPL concentrations in all serum samples. In one laboratory, the intraassay coefficient of variation for the radioreceptor assay for serum samples ranged from 6 to 20%, and the interassay coefficient of variation was 14–45%, depending on the actual values to be determined. For radioimmunoassay, corresponding values were 5–10% and 10–20%, respectively. Hence, the variability of the radioreceptor assay is at least twice that of radioimmunoassay.

It is worth mentioning here that in a radioreceptor assay the method of iodination of prolactin or lactogens is very important. We have found that ^{125}I-labeled hormone prepared by the chloramine-T method binds poorly to the mammary membrane receptor (Figure 7B), leading to erroneous estimates of hormone concentration in unknown samples or misleading information about the lactogen receptor. For example, Etzrodt *et al.* (1976) concluded that in a rat liver membrane preparation there is a binding site for growth hormone and not for prolactin; Posner *et al.* (1974), on the other hand, identified principally prolactin-binding sites in rat liver membrane preparations. One of the explanations for this discrepancy could be that the unlabeled prolactin used by Etzrodt *et al.* (1976) for displacement of the tracer may have been chemically pure and adequate for radioimmunoassay but biologically inactive and, as a result, causing no displacement of the labeled hormone.

As more and more research on hormones is being done with receptor assays, it is important that any agency which distributes hormones should clearly mention the suitability, adequacy, and potency of a preparation in terms of classic bioassays as well as for radioimmunoassay and radioreceptor assay. For example, one preparation may have a specific activity of 2.0 U/mg by radioimmunoassay but only 0.2 U/mg by receptor assay. Either the unlabeled or labeled hormone may be unsuitable for receptor assay. In Figure 7B the point is made that a

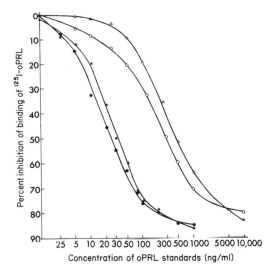

Figure 8. Illustrates the comparison of sensitivities of the radioreceptor assay using particulate and soluble receptor preparations. Standard curves were obtained in the presence or absence of serum. For details see text. Standard curve obtained with the use of particulate receptor preparation: in the absence of serum, O; and in the presence of serum, △. Standard curves obtained with the use of soluble receptor preparation in the absence of serum, ●, and in the presence of serum, ▲.

labeled hormone preparation, while satisfactory in a radioimmunoassay, may be unsuitable in a receptor assay.

C. Possible Modification of Standard Conditions

Due to the higher binding affinity of the solubilized prolactin receptor using Triton X-100 (Shiu, 1974), improved sensitivity of the radioreceptor assay is anticipated and has been observed (Figure 8). In radioimmunoassay, it is normal to use an amount of antiserum that will bind 50% or less of the added labeled hormone in order to improve sensitivity. A similar approach was explored using the soluble receptor. A gradual improvement in receptor assay sensitivity results from serial dilutions of receptor protein (Shiu, 1974). Rodbard *et al.* in 1971, proved that greater sensitivity was effected by delayed addition of the labeled hormone. Using the soluble receptor preparation, different strategies in combination complement one another and greatly improve the sensitivity of radioreceptor assay. The limit of detection decreased from 10–25 ng/ml to 1.0–2.5 ng/ml of prolactin in serum and the usable range of the assay was reduced to 50–80 ng/ml from 500–

1000 ng/ml. It is feasible to use soluble receptors to develop radioreceptor assays for prolactin as well as lactogens with a sensitivity comparable to that of radioimmunoassay.

D. Measurement of hPL in Blood during Pregnancy

Human placental lactogen (hPL) is synthesized by the syncytiotrophoblast of the placenta in large and increasing amounts during pregnancy. Since its half-life is about 25 minutes, its measurement in maternal serum should provide a sensitive indication of placental biosynthetic function. Careful investigation of hPL levels in expectant mothers, particularly those at high risk, coupled with intensive antepartum care may reduce perinatal mortality and morbidity.

Frantz et al. (1965), Samaan et al. (1966), and Chard (1975) have reported that hPL levels in blood rise steadily throughout pregnancy and reach a maximum in the third trimester (Figure 9). In plasma, hPL levels in women during labor have been found to be anywhere from 4.0–16 μg/ml (Frantz et al., 1965). During the third trimester, the levels range from 4.0–9.0 μg/ml. A mean value of 3.3 μg/ml serum at term was verified by Samaan et al. (1966). The hPL level is much higher in the maternal circulation than in the fetal circulation (Grumbach and Kaplan, 1964; Samaan et al. (1966). In 1966, Samaan et al. found no significant changes in the hPL levels in serum during intravenous glucose tolerance tests, insulin tolerance tests, or in relation to food and exercise.

Several studies have been carried out in patients with threatened abortion (Genazzani et al., 1969, 1971, 1972; Saxena et al., 1969). The hPL assays done in the first and second trimesters distinguished those patients who required hospital care, and those whose pregnancies were not in immediate danger. A normal pattern of increasing serum hPL levels correlated with a normal successful pregnancy; low and decreasing hPL levels tended in the majority of cases to correlate with abortion (Spona and Janisch, 1971). In late pregnancy, there seems to be a poor correlation between hPL levels and fetal distress in many cases (Singer et al., 1970). There is a gradual decrease of circulating maternal hPL following antepartum fetal death (Spellacy et al., 1970; Samaan et al., 1969).

Studies of diabetic pregnancies have shown seemingly contradictory results. Although some studies report no significant difference between the serum hPL levels in this group and those in uncomplicated pregnancies (Samaan et al., 1969; Josimovich et al., 1970), other studies have found much greater day-to-day fluctuations in the diabe-

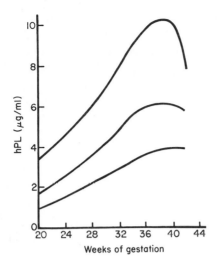

Figure 9. Illustrates the range of circulating hPL levels in normal pregnancy ±2 S.D. The distribution around the mean is skewed. (Reproduced from Chard, 1975, with permission of the publisher.)

tic patient than is normally expected (Spona and Janisch, 1971). In cases showing no evidence of placental dysfunction, there was a higher range of hPL levels than in normal pregnancies; in cases with placental insufficiency, the levels were significantly lower. Hence, it was concluded that the interpretation of results in diabetic pregnancies depends on a knowledge of the hPL levels that are normally associated with this complication. The considerable overlap between groups with and without placental dysfunction emphasizes the need for serial assays at frequent intervals (Ursell *et al.*, 1973).

Several studies have indicated that cases of toxemia can be associated with decreased levels of hPL at all stages of pregnancy. The hPL levels were low in the majority of cases which resulted in fetal death (Josimovich *et al.*, 1970: Spellacy *et al.*, 1971; Letchworth and Chard, 1972a).

There is controversy about the significance of hPL as an indicator of retarded fetal growth (Spellacy *et al.*, 1966; Singer *et al.*, 1970). In a study in which pregnancies resulted in small-for-dates babies, single hPL measurements were performed at different stages in each of the pregnancies; low, normal, and high levels were found in five, eight, and two cases, respectively (Josimovich *et al.*, 1970). In several studies, there was a positive correlation with fetal birth weight when hPL levels were assayed ten days before birth. After 36 weeks of gestation, during the last trimester (Seppälä and Ruoslahti, 1970; Letchworth et al., 1971; Spellacy et al., 1971), subnormal weight correlated with lower than normal serum hPL levels (Saxena et al., 1969).

According to two studies, there is no significant difference between hPL levels in cases of prolonged pregnancy not demonstrating the postmaturity syndrome and those of normal pregnancies. However, in prolonged pregnancies with evidence of fetal distress, significant decreases in hPL levels were reported prior to labor (Genazzani et al., 1971).

A study by Keller et al. (1971) of patients judged to have normal and abnormal fetal–placental function concluded that maternal serum hPL measurements correctly predicted fetal–placental distress in all cases, but suggested that 35% of those classified normal may have had unrevealed fetal–placental distress. Spellacy et al. (1972), with his serial measurements on women with complications of pregnancy, concluded that hPL assays did not help determine patients needing biophysical monitoring. However, Letchworth and Chard (1972b) claimed that fetal distress during or immediately after labor could be predicted in a proportion of patients by serial measurements of maternal hPL.

Thus far, reports have revealed a greater correlation between maternal hPL levels and fetal viability in early pregnancy than in the last trimester. The measurements of hPL seem to be of little value in the latter stage, particularly in diabetic pregnancies.

In pregnancies complicated with toxemia, hPL assays appear to give a satisfactory index of fetal–placental distress, especially when serial measurements are made. However, Spellacy et al. (1972) claim that there is still no convincing evidence that the clinical application of hPL assays improves perinatal survival.

Despite extensive clinical investigation, it is not clearly established whether hPL is a useful diagnostic parameter in assessing placental function in patients with a high risk of fetal death during pregnancy. It still must be demonstrated that induction of labor or Cesarean section in patients in whom concentrations of hPL are low would significantly lower perinatal mortality. Only when this evidence is available can it be said that hPL is a useful clinical tool in the management of high-risk pregnant patients.

E. Placental Lactogens in Different Species

As already mentioned, radioreceptor assays have several advantages over bioassays; namely, they are easier to perform, more sensitive, quantitative, less expensive, and most importantly, they are not species specific.

Human and monkey placental lactogens (hPL and mPL) are fairly well defined. The advent of rabbit mammary gland receptor assays developed in our laboratory (Shiu *et al.*, 1973) for prolactin or placental lactogen and rabbit liver receptor for growth-hormone-like activity (Tsushima and Friesen, 1973) has greatly aided research on placental lactogens. Using these assays, the identification and quantitation of placental lactogens in the circulation of a large number of species from primates and nonprimates have been accomplished (Table III) (Kelly *et al.*, 1973; Kelly, 1977). Prolactinlike and growth-hormone-like activities in serum and in placental extracts quantitated for nine species by the use of two receptor assays (Kelly *et al.*, 1976) are shown in

Table III   Distribution of Placental Lactogens[a]

Species	Qualitative	Quantitative	Purified[b]
Human	Pigeon crop sac, *in vivo* rat mouse mammary culture growth promoting	RIA, RRA	Josimovich and MacLaren (1962); Friesen (1965a,b)
Monkey	Pigeon crop sac growth promoting	RIA, RRA	Shome and Friesen (1971)
Baboon	Mouse mammary culture luteotropic	RIA	Josimovich *et al.* (1973)
Cow	Mouse mammary culture	RRA, RIA	Bolander and Fellows (1976)
Sheep	Mouse mammary culture	RRA, RIA	Fellows *et al.* (1974); Martal and Djiane (1975); Chan *et al.* (1976)
Deer	Mouse mammary culture	—	—
Guinea Pig	Mouse mammary culture	—	—
Chinchilla	Mouse mammary culture	—	—
Hamster	Mouse mammary culture	RRA	—
Rat	Pigeon crop sac, *in vivo* rat mouse mammary culture luteotropic, growth promoting	RRA	Robertson and Friesen (1975)
Mouse	*In vivo* mouse mouse mammary culture luteotropic	RRA	—

[a] From Kelly (1977).

[b] The authors listed in this column have reported on the purification of the various species of placental lactogens.

Table IV   Lactogen and Growth-Hormone-like Activities (GHLA) in Serum and Placental Extracts[a,b]

Species	Day of pregnancy	Serum (ng/ml)		Placenta (μg/gm of wet weight of tissue)	
		Lactogenic	GHLA	Lactogenic	GHLA
Monkey	170	45,000	45,000	100.0	100.0
Human	270	5,000	200	200.0	5.0
Guinea pig	49	2,500	—	1.0	1.0
Hamster	14	2,500	—	22.0	—
Sheep	140	2,000	700	200.0	200.0
Goat	148	1,200	1,200	75.0	55.0
Rat	12	1,200	—	11.0	—
	18	800	—	45.0	—
Mouse	11	1,200	—	27.0	—
	18	1,200	—	90.0	—
Cow	270	50	50	30.0	50.0

[a] Modified from Kelly et al. (1976).

[b] The values in this table represent mean peak values observed at the indicated day of pregnancy at which serum (plasma) or placental tissue samples were examined. Samples were removed and stored for varying periods of time prior to assay. Variations in the absolute value of PL (placental lactogen) or GHLA (growth-hormone-like activity) activity depend on the stage of pregnancy at which the samples were obtained.

Table IV. In general, the concentration of placental lactogen in serum measured by radioreceptor assay begins to rise at or before midpregnancy and either remains elevated until term (hamster, goat, sheep, monkey, human), gradually declines after reaching peak concentrations just beyond midpregnancy (guinea pig), or shows two peaks of activity (mouse, rat). The serum placental lactogen concentration in different species ranges from less than 200 ng/ml in the cow to 45,000 ng/ml in the monkey. The plasma concentrations of growth-hormone-like activity were similar to placental lactogen levels, except in human and monkey. The maximum concentrations of these hormones in placental extracts varies from 1.0 μg/gm in guinea pigs to 200 μg/gm in sheep, and the ratio of lactogen to growth-hormone-like activities varies among species, both in serum and in placental extracts.

V. SUMMARY

The development of a specific radioimmunoassay for the human placental lactogen has produced extensive data on serum levels of placental lactogen. The significance of such data to improvement in clinical practice of obstetrics has yet to be proved. With the advent of radioreceptor assay for prolactin and placental lactogen, research in the field of placental lactogen has progressed rapidly. A dozen or so newer placental lactogens have been identified in various species, and studies on the role of these placental lactogens should serve to clarify their importance to maternal adaptations of pregnancy as well as to fetal growth and development.

ACKNOWLEDGMENTS

We acknowledge the secretarial assistance of Miss Nikki Ryan. This research was supported by grants from the Medical Research Council of Canada and from the NIH, the National Institute Child Health and Human Development.

REFERENCES

Astwood, E. B., and Greep, R. O. (1938). A corpus luteum stimulating substance in the rat placenta. *Proc. Soc. Exp. Biol. Med.* **38**, 713–716.

Averill, S. C., Ray, E. W., and Lyons, W. R. (1950). Maintenance of pregnancy in hypophysectomized rats with pacental implants. *Proc. Soc. Exp. Biol. Med.* **75**, 3–6.

Beck, P., Parker, M. L., and Daughaday, W. H. (1965). Radioimmunological measurement of human placental lactogen in plasma by double antibody method during normal and diabetic pregnancies. *J. Clin. Endocrinol. Metab.* **25**, 1457–1462.

Boime, I., McWilliam, S. D., Szczesna, E., and Camel, M. (1976). Synthesis of human placental lactogen messenger RNA as a function of gestation. *J. Biol. Chem.* **251**, 820–825.

Bolander, F. F., and Fellows, R. E. (1976). Purification and characterisation of bovine placental lactogen. *J. Biol. Chem.* **251**, 2703–2708.

Buttle, H. L., Forsyth, I. A., and Knaggs, G. S. (1972). Plasma prolactin measured by radioimmunoassay and bioassay in pregnant and lactating goats and the occurrence of a placental lactogen. *J. Endocrinol.* **53**, 483–491.

Catt, K. J., Niall, H. D., and Tregear, G. W. (1966). Solid phase radioimmunoassay of human growth hormone. *Biochem. J.* **100**, 31–33.

Catt, K. J., Tregear, G. W., Burger, H. G., and Skermer, C. (1970). Antibody-coated tube method for radioimmunoassay of human growth hormone. *Clin. Chim. Acta* **27**, 267–279.

Ceska, M., and Lundkvist, U. (1972). A new and simple radioimmunoassay method for the determination of IgE. *Immunochemistry* **9**, 1021–1030.

Chan, J. S. D., Robertson, H. A., and Friesen, H. G. (1976). Purification and characterization of ovine placental lactogen. *Endocrinology* **98**, 65–76.

Chard, T. (1975). Monitoring the fetoplacental unit—the placenta. *Postgrad. Med. J.* **51**, 221–226.

Chen, H. W., Hamer, D. H., Helinger, H. J., and Meir, H. (1972). Stimulation of hepatic RNA synthesis in dwarf mice by ovine prolactin. *Biochim. Biophys. Acta* **287**, 90–97.

Cuatrecasas, P. (1974). Membrane receptors. *Annu. Rev. Biochem.* **43**, 169–214.

Elghamry, M. I., Said, A., and Elmougy, S. A. (1966). The effect of lactogenic hormone on liver glycogen and blood glucose in ovariectomized mice. *Naturwissenschaften* **53**, 530.

Etzrodt, H., Musch, K. A., Schleyer, M., and Pfeiffer, E. F. (1976). Growth hormone radioligand assay unresponsive to human prolactin. *J. Clin. Endocrinol. Metab.* **42**, 1184–1187.

Fellows, R. E., Hurley, T., Maurer, W., and Handwerger, S. (1974). Isolation and chemical characterization of ovine placental lactogen. *Endocrinology, Suppl.* Abstr. A-113.

Florini, J. R., Tonelli, G., Breuer, C. P., Coppola, J., Ringler, J., and Bell, P. H. (1966). Characterization and biological effects of purified placental protein (PPH). *Endocrinology* **79**, 692–708.

Forsyth, I. A. (1972). Use of a rabbit mammary gland organ culture system to detect lactogenic activity in blood. *In* "Lactogenic Hormones." *Ciba Found. Symp.* **102**, 151–168.

Forsyth, I. A. (1974). The comparative study of placental lactogenic hormones, a review *In* "Lactogenic Hormones, Fetal Nutrition and Lactation" (J. B. Josimovich, M. Reynolds, and E. Cobo, eds.), Vol. 2, pp. 49–67. Wiley, New York.

Frantz, A. G., Rabkin, M. T., and Friesen, H. (1965). Human placental lactogen in choriocarcinoma of the male. *J. Clin. Endocrinol. Metab.* **25**, 1136–1215.

Friesen, H. G. (1965a). Purification of a placental factor with immunological and chemical similarity to human growth hormone. *Endocrinology* **76**, 369–381.

Friesen, H. G. (1965b). Further purification and characterization of a placental protein with immunological similarity to human growth hormone. *Nature (London)* **208**, 1214–1215.

Fukushima, M. (1961). Studies on somatotropic hormone in gynecology and obstetrics. *Tohoku J. Exp. Med.* **74**, 161–174.

Gardner, J., Bailey, G., and Chard, T. (1974). Observations on the use of solid-phase coupled antibodies in the radioimmunoassay of hPL. *Biochem. J.* **137**, 469–476.

Genazanni, A. R., Casoli, M., Aubert, M. L., Fioretti, P., and Felber, J. P. (1969). Use of human placental lactogen radioimmunoassay to predict outcome in cases of threatened abortion. *Lancet* **2**, 1385–1387.

Genazzani, A. R., Cocola, F., Casoli, M., Mello, G., Scarselli, E. G., Neri, P., and Fioretti, P. (1971). Human chorionic somatomammotrophin radioimmunoassay in evaluation of placental function. *J. Obstet. Gynaecol. Br. Commonw.* **78**, 577–589.

Genazzani, A. R., Cocola, F., Neri, P., and Fioretti, P. (1972). Human chorionic somatomammotropin (HCS) plasma levels in normal and pathological pregnancies and their correlation with the placental function. *Acta Endocrinol. (Copenhagen)*, Suppl. **167**, 3–39.

Greenwood, F. C., Hunter, W. M., and Glover, J. S. (1963). The preparation of ^{131}I-labelled human growth hormone of high specific radioactivity. *Biochem. J.* **89**, 114–123.

Grumbach, M. M., and Kaplan, S. L. (1964). On the placental origin and purification of chorionic "growth hormone-prolactin" and its immunoassay in pregnancy. *Trans. N.Y. Acad. Sci.* **27**, 167–188.

Hanwell, A., and Linzell, J. L. (1972). Elevation of the cardiac output by prolactin and growth hormone in rats. *J. Endocrinol.* **53,** lvii.

Haour, F. (1971). A rapid radioimmunoassay of human chorionic somatomammotropin (hCS or hPL) using dioxan. *Horm. Metab. Res.* **3,** 131–132.

Hart, I. C. (1972). A solid phase radioimmunoassay for ovine and caprine prolactin using Sepharose 6B: Its application to the measurement of circulation levels of prolactin before and during parturition in the goat. *J. Endocrinol.* **55,** 51–62.

Hunter, W. M., and Greenwood, F. C. (1962). Preparation of iodine-[131]labelled human growth hormone of high specific activity. *Nature (London)* **194,** 495–496.

Ito, U., and Higashi, K. (1961). Studies on the prolactin-like substance in human placenta. II. *Endocrinol. Jpn.* **8,** 279–287.

Josimovich, J. B., and MacLaren, J. A. (1962). Presence in the human placenta and term serum of a highly lactogenic substance immunologically related to pituitary growth hormone. *Endocrinology* **71,** 209–220.

Josimovich, J. B., Kosor, B., Bocella, L., Mintz, D. H., and Hutchinson, D. L. (1970). Placental lactogen in maternal serum as an index of fetal health. *Obstet. Gynecol.* **362,** 244–250.

Josimovich, J. B., Levitt, M. J., and Stevens, V. C. (1973). Comparison of baboon and human placental lactogens. *Endocrinology* **93,** 242–244.

Kaplan, S. L., and Grumbach, M. M. (1965). Serum chorionic growth hormone prolactin and serum pituitary growth hormone in mother and fetus at term. *J. Clin. Endocrinol. Metab.* **25,** 1370–1374.

Keller, P. J., Baertschi, U., Bader, P., Gerber, C., Schmid, J., Soltermann, R., and Kopper, E. (1971). Biochemical detection of foeto-placental distress in risk pregnancies. *Lancet* **2,** 729–731.

Kelly, P. A. (1977). Secretion and biological effects of placental lactogens. *Proc. Int. Congr. Endocrinol., 5th, 1976* Excerpta Med. Found. Int. Congr. Ser. No. 402, pp. 298–302.

Kelly, P. A., Shiu, R. P. C., Friesen, H. G., and Robertson, H. A. (1973). Placental lactogen levels in several species throughout pregnancy. *55th Annu. Meet. Endocr. Soc.* Abstract No. 370 P.A. 233.

Kelly, P. A., Robertson, H. A., and Friesen, H. G. (1974). Temporal pattern of placental lactogen and progesterone secretion in sheep. *Nature (London)* **248,** 435–437.

Kelly, P. A., Tsushima, T., Shiu, R. P. C., and Friesen, H. G. (1976). Lacogenic and growth hormone-like activities in pregnancy determined by radioreceptor assays. *Endocrinology* **99,** 765–774.

Kleinberg, D. L., and Frantz, A. G. (1971). Human prolactin, measurement in human plasma by *in vitro* bioassay. *J. Clin. Invest.* **50,** 1557–1568.

Kohmoto, K., and Bern, H. A. (1970). Demonstration of mammotrophic activity of the mouse placenta in organ culture and by transplantation. *J. Endocrinol.* **48,** 99–107.

Lawson, D. M., and Gala, R. R. (1974). The influence of surgery, time of day, blood volume reduction and anaesthetics on plasma prolactin in ovariectomized rats. *J. Endocrinol.* **62,** 75–83.

Leake, N. H., and Burt, R. L. (1969). Solid phase radioimmunoassay of human placental lactogen. *Obstet. Gynecol.* **34,** 471–477.

Letchworth, A. T., and Chard, T. (1972a). hPL levels in pre-eclampsia. *J. Obstet. Gynaecol. Br. Commonw.* **79,** 680–683.

Letchworth, A. T., and Chard, T. (1972b). hPL as a screening test for foetal distress and neonatal asphyxia. *Lancet* **1,** 704–706.

Letchworth, A. T., Boardman, R. J., Bristow, C., Landon, J., and Chard, T. (1971). A rapid semi-automated method for the measurement of human chorionic somatomammotrophin. The normal range in the third trimester and its relation to fetal weight. *J. Obstet. Gynaecol. Br. Commonw.* **78**, 542–548.

Li, C. H., Grumbach, M. M., Kaplan, S. L., Josimovich, J. B., Friesen, H., and Catt, K. J. (1968). Human chorionic somatomammotropin (HCS), proposed terminology for designation of a placental hormone. *Experientia* **24**, 1188.

Li, C. H., Dixon, J. S., and Chung, D. (1971). Primary structure of the human chorionic somatomammotropin (HCS) molecule. *Science* **173**, 56–57.

Linkie, D. M., and Niswender, G. (1973). Characterisation of rat placental luteotropin: Physiological and physiochemical properties. *Biol. Reprod.* **8**, 48–57.

Lockett, M. F. (1965). A comparison of the direct renal actions of pituitary growth and lactogenic hormones. *J. Physiol. (London)* **181**, 192–199.

Loewenstein, J. E., Mariz, I. K., Peake, G. T., and Daughaday, W. H. (1971). Prolactin bioassay by induction of N-acetyllactosamine synthetase in mouse mammary gland explant. *J. Clin. Endocrinol. Metab.* **33**, 217–224.

Lowry, O. H., Rosebrough, N. J., Farr, A. L., and Randall, R. J. (1951). Protein measurement with the Folin Phenol reagent. *J. Biol. Chem.* **193**, 265–275.

Mainoya, J. R. (1975). Effects of bovine growth hormone, human placental lactogen and ovine prolactin on intestinal fluid and ion transport in the rat. *Endocrinology* **95**, 1165–1170.

Martal, J., and Djiane, J. (1975). Purification of a lactogenic hormone in sheep placenta. *Biochem. Biophys. Res. Commun.* **65**, 770–778.

Matthies, D. L. (1967). Studies of the luteotropic and mammotropic factor found in trophoblast and maternal peripheral blood of the rat in midpregnancy. *Anat. Rec.* **159**, 55–67.

Niall, H. D. (1972). The chemistry of the human lactogenic hormones. *Prolactin Carcinog., Proc. Tenovus Workshop, 4th, 1972* pp. 13–20.

Niall, H. D., Hogan, M. L., Sauer, R., Rosenblum, Y., and Greenwood, F. C. (1971). Pituitary and placental lactogenic and growth hormones: Evolution from a primordial gene reduplication. *Proc. Natl. Acad. Sci. U.S.A.* **68**, 866–869.

Niall, H. D., Hagan, M. L., Tregear, G. W., Segré, G. V., Hwang, P., and Friesen, H. G. (1973). The chemistry of growth hormone and the lactogenic hormones. *Recent Prog. Horm. Res.* **29**, 387–416.

Parke, L., and Forsyth, I. A. (1975). Assay of lactogenic hormones using receptors isolated from rabbit liver. *Endocr. Res. Commun.* **2**, 137–149.

Posner, B. I. (1975). Polypeptide hormone receptors: Characteristics and applications. *Can. J. Physiol. Pharmacol.* **53**, 689–703.

Posner, B. I., Kelly, P. A., Shiu, R. P. C., and Friesen, H. G. (1974). Studies of insulin, growth hormone, and prolactin binding. Tissue distribution species variation and characterization. *Endocrinology* **95**, 521–531.

Robertson, M. C., and Friesen, H. G. (1975). Purification and characterization of rat placental lactogen. *Endocrinology* **95**, 621–629.

Rodbard, D., and Lewald, J. E. (1970). Computer analysis of radioligand assay and radioimmunoassay data. *Acta Endocrinol. (Copenhagen), Suppl.* **147**, 79–103.

Rodbard, D., Ruder, H. J., Vaitukaitis, J. and Jacobs, H. S. (1971). Mathematical analysis of kinetics of radioligand assays: Improved sensitivity obtained by delayed addition of labeled ligand. *J. Clin. Endocrinol. Metab.* **33**, 343–355.

Samaan, N. A., Yen, S. S. C., Friesen, H., and Pearson, O. H. (1966). Serum placental lactogen levels during pregnancy and in trophoblastic disease. *J. Clin. Endocrinol. Metab.* **26**, 1303–1308.

Samaan, N. A., Bradbury, J. T., and Goplerud, C. P. (1969). Serial hormone studies in normal and abnormal pregnancy. *Am. J. Obstet. Gynecol.* **104**, 781–794.

Saxena, B. N., Refetoff, S., Emerson, K., and Selenkow, H. A. (1968). A rapid radioimmunoassay for human placental lactogen application to normal and pathologic pregnancies. *Am. J. Obstet. Gynecol.* **101**, 874–885.

Saxena, B. N., Emerson, K., and Selenkow, H. A. (1969). Serum placental lactogen (HPL) levels as an index of placental function. *N. Engl. J. Med.* **281**, 225–231.

Schneider, A. B., Kowalski, K., and Sherwood, L. M. (1974). Large molecular weight form of human placental lactogen (hPL) in placental extracts and serum. *Clin. Res.* **22**, 600A.

Schneider, A. B., Kowalski, K., and Sherwood, L. M. (1975). "Big" human placental lactogen: Disulfide-linked peptide chains. *Biochem. Biophys. Res. Commun.* **64**, 717–724.

Sciarra, J. J., Sherwood, L. M., Varma, A. A., and Lundberg, W. B. (1968). Human placental lactogen (hPL) and placental weight. *Am. J. Obstet. Gynecol.* **101**, 413–418.

Seppälä, M., and Ruoslahti, E. (1970). Serum concentration of human placental lactogenic hormone (HPL) in pregnancy complications. *Acta Obstet. Gynecol. Scand.* **49**, 143–147.

Sherwood, L. M. (1967). Similarities of the chemical structure of human placental lactogen and human growth hormone. *Proc. Natl. Acad. Sci. U.S.A.* **58**, 2307.

Sherwood, L. M., and Handwerger, S. (1969). Correlations between structure and function of human placental lactogen and human growth hormone. *In* "Fifth Rochester Trophoblast Conference" (C. Lund and J. W. Choate, eds.), pp. 230–255. Rochester Univ. Press, Rochester, New York.

Sherwood, L. M., Handwerger, S., McLaurin, W. D., and Launer, M. (1971). Amino acid sequence of human placental lactogen. *Nature (London), New Biol.* **233**, 59–61.

Shiu, R. P. C. (1974). The properties and purification of a prolactin receptor and the development of a radioreceptor assay for lactogenic hormones. Ph.D. Thesis, McGill University, Montreal.

Shiu, R. P. C., and Friesen, H. G. (1974a). Properties of a prolactin receptor from the mammary gland. *Biochem. J.* **140**, 310–311.

Shiu, R. P. C., and Friesen, H. G. (1974b). Solubilization and purification of a prolactin receptor from the rabbit mammary gland. *J. Biol. Chem.* **249**, 7902–7911.

Shiu, R. P. C., and Friesen, H. G. (1976a). Studies on prolactin receptors. *In* "Basic Applications and Clinical Uses of Hypothalamic Hormones" (A. L. Charro Salgado, R. Firandez Durango, and J. G. Lopez del Camp, eds.), pp. 53–57.

Shiu, R. P. C., and Friesen, H. G. (1976b). Prolactin receptor. *In* "Molecular Biology Series" (M. Bletcher, ed.), Vol. 9, Part II, pp. 565–595. Dekker, New York.

Shiu, R. P. C., Kelly, P. A., and Friesen, H. G. (1973). Radioreceptor assay for prolactin and other lactogenic hormones. *Science* **18**, 968–971.

Shome, B., and Friesen, H. G. (1971). Purification and characterization of monkey placental lactogen. *Endocrinology* **89**, 631–641.

Singer, W., Desjardins, P., and Friesen, H. G. (1970). Human placental lactogen: An index of placental function. *Obstet. Gynecol.* **36**, 222–237.

Spellacy, W. N., Carlson, K. L., and Birk, S. A. (1966). Dynamics of human placental lactogen. *Am. J. Obstet. Gynecol.* **96**, 1164–1173.

Spellacy, W. N., Teoh, E. S., and Buhi, W. C. (1970). Human chorionic somatomammotrophin levels prior to fetal death in high risk pregnancies. *Obstet. Gynecol.* **35**, 685 and 694.

Spellacy, W. N., Teoh, E. S., Buhi, W. C., Birk, S. A., and McCreary, S. A. (1971). Value of human chorionic somatomammotrophin in managing high risk pregnancies. *Am. J. Obstet. Gynecol.* **109**, 588–598.

Spellacy, W. N., Buhi, W. C., Birk, S. A., and Holsinger, K. K. (1972). Human placental lactogen levels and intra-partum fetal distress: Meconium stained amniotic fluid, fetal heart rate patterns and Apgar scores. *Am. J. Obstet. Gynecol.* **114**, 803–811.

Spona, J., and Janisch, H. (1971). Serum placental lactogen (HPL) as index of placental function. *Acta Endocrinol. (Copenhagen)* **68**, 401–412.

Talamantes, F., Jr. (1973). Mammotropic activity of chinchilla, hamster and rat placentae. *55th Annu. Meet. Endocr. Soc.* Abstract No. 454 P. A-275.

Thorell, J. I., and Johansson, B. G. (1971). Enzymatic iodination of polypeptides with ^{125}I to high specific activity. *Biochim. Biophys. Acta* **251**, 363–369.

Tsushima, T., and Friesen, H. G. (1973). Radioreceptor assay for growth hormone. *J. Clin. Endocrinol. Metab.* **37**, 334–337.

Turkington, R. W. (1971). Measurement of prolactin activity in human serum by induction of specific milk proteins in mammary gland in vitro. *J. Clin. Endocrinol. Metab.* **33**, 210–216.

Ursell, W., Brudenell, M., and Chard, T. (1973). Placental lactogen levels in diabetic pregnancy. *Br. Med. J.* **2**, 80–82.

Wang, D. Y., Hallowes, R. C., Bealing, J., Strong, C. R., and Dils, R. (1972). The effect of prolactin and growth hormone on fatty acid synthesis by pregnant mouse mammary gland in organ culture. *J. Endocrinol.* **53**, 311–321.

Wide, L. (1969). Radioimmunoassays employing immunosorbents. *Acta Endocrinol. (Copenhagen), Suppl.* **142**, 207–218.

Wide, L., and Porath, J. (1966). Radioimmunoassay of proteins with the use of sephadex-coupled antibodies. *Biochim. Biophys. Acta* **130**, 257–260.

43

Radioimmunoassay of Human Chorionic Thyrotropin

JEROME M. HERSHMAN AND AKIRA HARADA

I. INTRODUCTION

A. Biologic Characterization

Human chorionic thyrotropin (hCT) is a polypeptide found in normal human placentas that has thyroid-stimulating activity in the mouse TSH bioassay (Hennen *et al.*, 1969; Hershman and Starnes, 1969). This biologic activity is neutralized by antibodies to both human and bovine TSH (Hershman and Starnes, 1969). In a radioimmunoassay for bovine TSH, there was parallel cross-reaction of hCT and bovine TSH. The most highly purified hCT had thyrotropic activity of 1000 mU/mg (Hershman and Starnes, 1971a), 358 mU/mg (Hen-

867

Methods of Hormone Radioimmunoassay, Second Edition
Copyright © 1979 by Academic Press, Inc.
All rights of reproduction in any form reserved. ISBN 0-12-379260-6

nen *et al.*, 1969), and 125 mU/mg (Tojo *et al.*, 1973). Based on gel filtration, its molecular size is similar to pituitary thyrotropin, approximately 25,000.

B. hCG as a Thyrotropin

There is a second placental thyrotropin. In 1963, Odell *et al.* reported thyrotropic activity in choriocarcinoma tissue. Thyrotropic activity was extracted from the trophoblastic tumor or serum of women who had hyperthyroidism accompanying a hydatidiform mole or choriocarcinoma (Hershman *et al.*, 1970; Hershman and Higgins, 1971; Hershman, 1972). This thyroid stimulator was not hCT, human pituitary TSH, or the long-acting thyroid stimulator of Graves' disease. In 1967, Burger reported that crude preparations of chorionic gonadotropin had thyrotropic activity in a TSH bioassay. Recent work has shown that the thyrotropin in throphoblastic tissue and the serum of patients with hydatidiform mole or choriocarcinoma and hyperthyroidism is chorionic gonadotropin (hCG) (Kenimer *et al.*, 1975; Cave and Dunn, 1976). Highly purified hCG has intrinsic thyroid stimulating activity (Nisula *et al.*, 1974; Kenimer *et al.*, 1975).

C. Placental and Serum Content of hCT

Extraction of batches of placentas showed that placental content of hCT averaged 160 mU/placenta in one study (Hennen *et al.*, 1969) and 645 mU/placenta in another study (Hershman and Starnes, 1969). However, extraction of 15 individual full-term placentas revealed considerable variation in hCT content, which ranged from 3.0 to 18,500 mU/500 gm placenta; most placentas contained about 10 mU (Hershman and Starnes, 1971b). Of 15 placentas obtained at 51 to 133 days of gestation, only two contained more than 5.0 mU hCT (Hershman *et al.*, 1974).

Data on the concentration of hCT in serum are conflicting. Hennen *et al.* (1969) found concentrations of 80–1300 μU/ml early in pregnancy; in contrast, we found that hCT concentrations did not exceed 35 μU/ml and were usually less than 2.0 μU/ml (Hershman and Starnes, 1971b; Hershman *et al.*, 1975). Tojo *et al.* (1973) reported that hCT concentrations increased with the duration of pregnancy and were 12–50 μg/ml in late pregnancy; based on their biologic activity of 125 mU/mg, hCT concentration would then be 1500–6250 μU/ml, an extremely high value which should be readily detectable in bioassays.

The physiologic role of the placental thyroid stimulators, hCT and hCG, in the control of thyroid function during pregnancy is still unclear. Recent data with a sensitive TSH radioimmunoassay show that the serum concentration of pituitary TSH (hTSH) is inversely related to the concentration of hCG (Braunstein and Hershman, 1976). Early in pregnancy, when hCG is high, hTSH is relatively low, but it is still detectable.

D. Rationale for hCT Radioimmunoassay

In our studies and in those of Hennen *et al.* (1969), hCT cross-reacted very well with various antisera to bovine TSH in homologous radioimmunoassays for bovine TSH. Thus, antisera to bovine TSH and highly purified bovine TSH comprise the essential reagents for a sensitive radioimmunoassay for hCT. To provide adequate specificity, the bovine TSH radioimmunoassay for hCT must discriminate against both human pituitary TSH and hCG because these two hormones would also be present in serum or tissue extracts containing hCT. We shall describe our current assay for hCT using a sensitive homologous radioimmunoassay for bovine TSH.

II. TECHNIQUE OF hCT RADIOIMMUNOASSAY

A. Materials

WHO International Standard bovine TSH (National Institute for Biological Standards and Control, Holly Hill, London) was used as standard. Highly purified bovine TSH (40 U/mg) was generously provided by Dr. John G. Pierce of the University of California, Los Angeles, and was used for radioiodination. The anti-bovine TSH antiserum was raised in rabbits repeatedly immunized with 1.0 U of impure bovine TSH (4.0 U/mg) in Freund's adjuvant (see Chapter 14). $Na^{125}I$ was purchased from Amersham-Searle, bovine serum albumin (fraction V) (BSA) from Armour Pharmaceutical Co., and human serum albumin (fraction V) (HSA) from Miles Laboratories. A serum pool free of hCT for addition to the standard curve was obtained from healthy male volunteers. Antibody to normal rabbit γ-globulin (fraction II, Pentex) was obtained from female goats repeatedly immunized with this preparation. Other materials were reagent grade from ordinary commercial sources.

B. Radioiodination and Purification of Bovine TSH

Bovine TSH (bTSH) was labeled with ^{125}I by the method of Greenwood *et al.* (1963) with slight modification. Two micrograms of Pierce bTSH (20 μl), approximately 1.0 mCi Na[125]I (10 μl), 0.5 M sodium phosphate, pH 7.5 (50 μl), and 12 μg chloramine-T (20 μl) were mixed and reacted for 20 seconds. Then, 30 μg sodium metabisulfite (50 μl) was added to stop the reaction. The reaction mixture was then applied to a 0.8 × 25 cm column of Sephadex G-50 that was previously equilibrated with 2% BSA, 0.05 M phosphate–0.15 M NaCl buffer, pH 7.5, and eluted with the phosphate–saline buffer. Fractions of 15 drops (~1.0 ml) were collected and the radioactivity was counted; fractions from the first peak (protein) were pooled, diluted with 2% BSA–phosphate–saline, and stored at −70°C in small aliquots. ^{125}I-bTSH was purified just before being used in the radioimmunoassay by gel filtration on a 1.0 × 120 cm column of Ultrogel AcA 44 (LKB) which was also previously equilibrated with 2% BSA–phosphate–saline buffer and eluted with phosphate–saline buffer. Figure 1 shows the rechromatography of ^{125}I-bTSH on Ultrogel AcA 44 and B_0/T of each protein fraction.

C. Anti-bovine TSH Antiserum

Anti-bTSH antiserum (R_1E) at the dilution of 1 : 100 is stored at −70°C, and before being used is diluted to 1 : 40,000 with 0.1 M EDTA in assay buffer (see below).

Figure 2 shows the cross-reactivity of R_1E with hCG, human pituitary TSH (hTSH), and partially purified hCT (specific activity 1000 mU/mg). This antibody does not react with hCG. Its cross-reaction with hTSH is very weak.

D. Details of the Assay

Figure 3 shows the assay procedure schematically. The working buffer consists of 0.25% HSA, 0.02% Merthiolate in 0.05 M phosphate–0.15 M NaCl, pH 7.5. ^{125}I-bTSH, bTSH standards, normal rabbit serum, and anti-rabbit γ-globulin goat antiserum (Ab_2) were diluted with working buffer. Antibody R_1E was diluted with 0.1 M EDTA in working buffer.

For a more sensitive assay, a nonequilibrium method was used. Two hundred microliters of bTSH standard (0.05–20 μU), 200 μl of hCT-free serum pool, 100 μl anti-bovine TSH R_1E (1 : 40,000), and 400 μl working buffer [or 200 μl of unknown serum sample, 100 μl R_1E

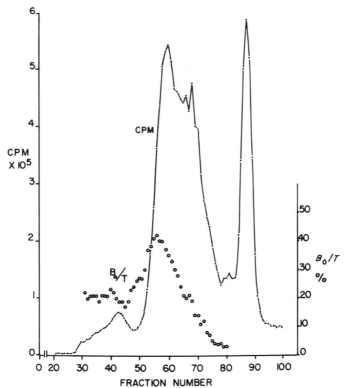

Figure 1. Elution pattern of ^{125}I from Ultrogel AcA 44 column. Each fraction No. 31–80 was diluted with working buffer to approximately 10,000 cpm/100 μl and incubated with R_1E (1 : 40,000) for three days; B_0/T is represented as open circles.

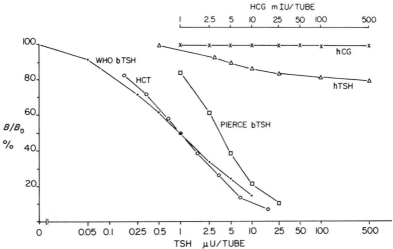

Figure 2. Cross-reaction of anti-bTSH antiserum (R_1E) with WHO Standard bTSH, partially purified hCT, purified bTSH (Pierce), purified hTSH, and purified hCG (upper scale).

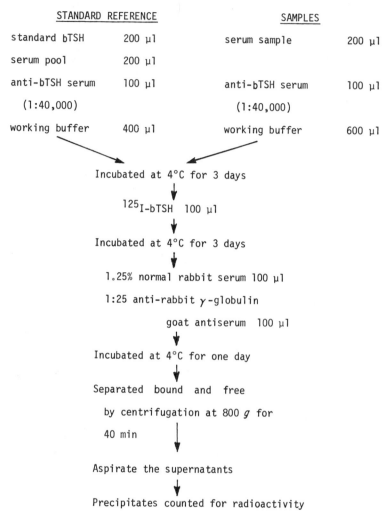

Figure 3.   Scheme of assay procedure for hCT.

(1 : 40,000), and 600 μl working buffer] were incubated at 4°C for three days. Then 100 μl ^{125}I-bTSH (approximately 10,000 cpm/100 μl) was added and incubated for an additional three days. Then, 100 μl 1.25% normal rabbit serum and 100 μl second antibody (1 : 25) were added and incubated for one day. The precipitate was centrifuged in a refrigerated centrifuge, the supernatant was aspirated, and the precipitate was counted. The results were analyzed with a computer program.

III. RESULTS AND INTERPRETATION

Even though the assay sensitivity has been improved recently so that hCT can be detected in serum in a concentration as low as 0.5 μU/ml, most pregnancy sera do not contain detectable hCT. Detectable concentrations with this assay have generally been only 0.5–1.5 μU/ml. If highly purified bTSH had been used as the standard rather than the International bTSH reference standard, the results would have been several-fold higher because the curve for purified bTSH is shifted to the right of the International bTSH standard (Figure 2).

Other explanations for the low serum values may reside in limitations of the present antiserum to bTSH, nonspecific effects of serum on the assay, or other methodologic problems. However, bioassay of pregnancy samples with a very sensitive bioassay suggests that high hCT values are not likely to be found.

Radioimmunoassay of hCT in acetone-precipitated placental powders gave values of 10–40 μU hCT/gm powder. Based on these data, placental content of hCT is only 0.3–0.7 mU in most placentas. Additional work is necessary to quantify hCT secretion and establish its role as a thyroid stimulator. At the present time, the radioimmunoassay of hCT is mainly a research tool and does not have direct clinical application.

ACKNOWLEDGMENT

Supported by Veterans Administration Medical Research Funds and United States Public Health Service Grant HD-7181.

REFERENCES

Braunstein, G. D., and Hershman, J. M. (1976). Comparison of serum pituitary and chorionic gonadotropin concentrations throughout pregnancy. *J. Clin. Endocrinol. Metab.* **42**, 1123–1126.

Burger, A. (1967). Studies on a thyroid stimulating factor in urinary chorionic gonadostrophin preparations. *Acta Endocrinol* (Kbh) **55**, 587–599.

Cave, W. T., Jr., and Dunn J. T. (1976). Choriocarcinoma with hyperthyroidism: Probable identity of the thyrotropin with human chorionic gonadotropin. *Ann. Intern. Med.* **85**, 60–63.

Greenwood, F. C., Hunter, W. M., and Glover, J. S. (1963). The preparation ^{131}I-labelled human growth hormone of high specific activity. *Biochem. J.* **89**, 114–123.

Hennen, G., Pierce, J. G., and Freychet, P. (1969). Human chorionic thyrotropin: Further characterization and study of its secretion during pregnancy. *J. Clin. Endocrinol. Metab.* **29**, 581–594.

Hershman, J. M. (1972). Hyperthyroidism induced by trophoblastic thyrotropin. *Mayo Clin. Proc.* **47**, 913–918.

Hershman, J. M., and Higgins, H. P. (1971). Hydatidiform mole—a cause of clinical hyperthyroidism: Report of two cases with evidence that the molar tissue secreted a thyroid stimulator. *N. Engl. J. Med.* **284**, 573–577.

Hershman, J. M., and Starnes, W. R. (1969). Extraction and characterization of a thyrotropic material from the human placenta. *J. Clin. Invest.* **48**, 932–929.

Hershman, J. M., and Starnes, W. R. (1971a). Placental content and characterization of human chorionic thyrotropin. *J. Clin. Endocrinol. Metab.* **32**, 52–58.

Hershman, J. M., and Starnes, W. R. (1971b). Big and little placental thyrotropins: Interconversion and function. *Program 53rd Meet. Endocr. Soc.* p. A-131.

Hershman, J. M., Higgins, H. P., and Starnes, W. R. (1970). Differences between thyroid stimulator in hydatidiform mole and human chorionic thyrotropin. *Metab., Clin. Exp.* **19**, 735–744.

Hershman, J. M., Starnes, W. R., Kenimer, J. G., and Patillo, R. A. (1974). Human chorionic thyrotropin. *Endocrinol., Proc. Int. Congr., 4th, 1972* Excerpta Med. Found. Int. Congr. Ser. No. 273, pp. 682–687.

Hershman, J. M., Kenimer, J. G., Higgins, H. P., and Patillo, R. A. (1975). Placental thyrotropins. *In* "Perinatal Thyroid Physiology and Disease" (D. A. Fisher and G. N. Burrow, eds.), pp. 11–20. Raven Press, New York.

Kenimer, J. G., Hershman, J. M., and Higgins, H. P. (1975). The thyrotropin in hydatidiform moles is human chorionic gonadotropin. *J. Clin. Endocrinol. Metab.* **40**, 482–491.

Nisula, B. C., Morgan, F. J., and Canfield, R. E. (1974). Evidence that chorionic gonadotropin has intrinsic thyrotropic activity. *Biochem. Biophys. Res. Commun.* **59**, 86–91.

Odell, W. D., Bates, R. W., Rivlin, R. S., Lipsett, M. B., and Hertz, R. (1963). Increased thyroid function without clinical hyperthyroidism in patients with choriocarcinoma. *J. Clin. Endocrinol. Metab.* **23**, 658–664.

Tojo, S., Kanazawa, S., Nakamura, A., Kitagaki, S., and Mochizuki, M. (1973). Human chorionic TSH (hCTSH, hCT) during normal or molar pregnancy. *Endocrinol. Jpn.* **20**, 505–516.

44

Relaxin

O. DAVID SHERWOOD

I. INTRODUCTION

Relaxin is a polypeptide hormone which is produced in the ovaries and/or reproductive tracts of many species during pregnancy. Relaxin has relaxative effects on the pelvic joints of estrogen-primed guinea pigs and mice and also inhibits the spontaneous contractions of the uterine myometrium of guinea pigs, mice, and rats (Hall, 1960). It is these two effects of relaxin that are used as endpoints for the commonly employed relaxin bioassays (Steinetz et al., 1969). Relaxin bioassays have proved to be useful for the measurement of relaxin activity within tissue extracts of the reproductive tract and also for the identification of relaxin activity within the blood during mid- to late pregnancy in female pigs (Belt et al., 1971), guinea pigs (Zarrow, 1947), rabbits (Marder and Money, 1944), and human beings (Zarrow

Methods of Hormone Radioimmunoassay, Second Edition

et al., 1955). However, these bioassay methods lack both the sensitivity and precision required for accurate determinations of relaxin levels within the peripheral circulation throughout pregnancy. For example, the widely used direct measurement mouse pubic symphysis bioassay requires a minimum of approximately 100 ng of highly purified porcine relaxin and is characterized by coefficients of variation which range from approximately 30 to 40%. The limitations associated with relaxin bioassays and also the lack of pure relaxin preparations have long hindered efforts to understand better the physiological significance of this hormone.

Recently, Sherwood and O'Byrne (1974) reported a method for the isolation of highly purified porcine relaxin and the subsequent development of a sensitive and specific radioimmunoassay for this hormone (Sherwood *et al.*, 1975a). This chapter presents a detailed account of the methodology employed for both the development and for the routine use of this porcine relaxin radioimmunoassay. The levels of relaxin immunoactivity within pig plasma throughout pregnancy and at parturition are also presented.

II. METHOD OF RADIOIMMUNOASSAY

A. Source of Relaxin

Sherwood and O'Byrne (1974) reported a method for the isolation of highly purified porcine relaxin from the ovaries of pregnant pigs. Frozen sow ovaries (1.0 kg) were homogenized and extracted with acid–acetone (0.15 N HCl–70% acetone). After centrifugation at 1500 g for 15 minutes, the extract was precipitated by adding five volumes of acetone at −15°C. The precipitate was dissolved and chromatographed on a 9.4 × 115 cm column of Sephadex G-50 fine in 0.2 M ammonium acetate, pH 6.8, at 4°C. Collecting 6.0-ml fractions, the relaxin activity was confined to tubes 180–240. This fraction was further purified on a 2.5 × 27 cm column of carboxymethyl cellulose in 0.08 M ammonium acetate–acetic acid, pH 5.5. After the unabsorbed protein was eluted, a linear gradient of equilibrating buffer plus NaCl with an increasing concentration of 20 mM per 48 ml was applied to the column. Three contiguous preparations of relaxin, designated CM-B, CM-a, and CM-a', were eluted from the carboxymethyl cellulose column with the linear gradient of sodium chloride. Biological and physicochemical analyses showed no clear differences among the three relaxin preparations. Each contains 2500 to 3000 U* of biological activity, and their molecular weights of approximately 6000, isoelectric points of approximately pH 10.6, and amino acid contents are nearly identical to one another. All three relaxin preparations lack the amino acids tyrosine and histidine, which normally incorporate iodine when the conventional method of Hunter and Greenwood (1962) is employed for radioiodination. These three highly purified microheterogeneous preparations of relaxin were used for the development of the relaxin radioimmunoassay and are collectively designated native relaxin. Native relaxin was used for the preparation of antiporcine relaxin sera, for preparation of polytyrosyl-relaxin, and as the porcine relaxin standard.

B. Preparation of Antisera

1. First Antisera: Rabbit Anti-porcine Relaxin Sera

Porcine relaxin antigen was prepared by emulsifying 5.0 mg native relaxin in 2.5 ml 0.9% saline and 2.5 ml complete Freund's adjuvant. Four adult male New Zealand white rabbits were initially immunized with 1.0 mg native relaxin at biweekly intervals by intradermal injections into three or four sites in the medial aspect of the thigh. After two months, 1.0 mg native relaxin was administered intramuscularly at biweekly intervals for an additional two months in 1.0 ml 0.9% saline. Seven days after the ninth injection of porcine relaxin, 50 ml blood was removed from each rabbit by cardiac puncture.

The rabbit anti-porcine relaxin sera were tested for immunopotency by preparing serial dilutions of each antiserum, ranging from 1:200 to 1:40,000 in a solution containing 0.14 M sodium chloride and 0.01 M sodium phosphate at pH 7.0 (PBS) and 1% ovalbumin. The dilution of each of the four anti-porcine relaxin sera, which bound 50% of the precipitable radioiodinated relaxin employed within each reaction tube, was determined. These dilutions were determined as described in Section II,E except that 500 μl of PBS–1% ovalbumin which contained no relaxin was employed. The four rabbits injected with native relaxin over a four-month period produced anti-porcine relaxin sera suitable for use in the relaxin radioimmunoassay at final dilutions rang-

---

* Biological activity of relaxin preparations expressed relative to Warner–Lambert Relaxin Reference Standard W1164, 48 E 2103a which by definition contains 1000 U of relaxin activity per milligram.

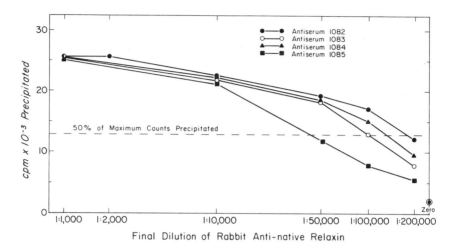

Figure 1.   Titration curve of four rabbit anti-porcine relaxin antisera. The counts precipitated are the means of four observations at each dilution of the antisera.

ing from 1 : 50,000 to 1 : 200,000 (Figure 1). Antiserum from rabbit 1082 is routinely employed for the porcine relaxin radioimmunoassay.

2. Second Antisera: Sheep Anti-rabbit γ-Globulin

Rabbit γ-globulin antigen was prepared by emulsifying 10 mg rabbit γ-globulin (fraction II, Nutritional Biochemical) in 1.25 ml 0.9% saline and 0.5 ml complete Freund's adjuvant. Adult male sheep were injected with 10 mg rabbit γ-globulin at biweekly intervals. The antigen was injected subcutaneously into the four axillary regions and in the neck. After five or six immunizations, 500 ml of blood was removed from the jugular vein. The anti-rabbit γ-globulin sera were tested for immunopotency by preparing serial dilutions of each antiserum ranging from 1 : 2 to 1 : 128 in PBS-1% ovalbumin.

C. Preparation of Polytyrosyl-Relaxin

Conventional techniques employed for the radioiodination of polypeptide hormones incorporate radioactive iodine into residues of tyrosine and histidine. Porcine relaxin lacks both of these amino acids, and, as expected, initial efforts to radioiodinate native relaxin according to the commonly used procedure of Hunter and Greenwood (1962) were not successful (Figure 2B).

Tyrosine was covalently bound to amino groups of native relaxin by an amide bond employing the reagent N-carboxy-L-tyrosine anhydride

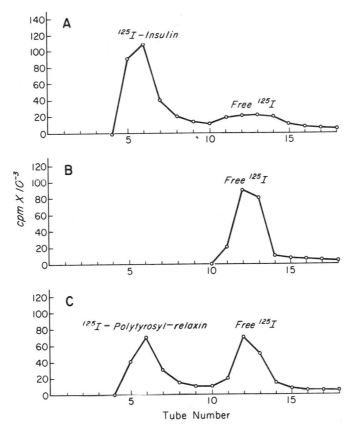

Figure 2. Radioactive ^{125}I elution profiles from BioGel P-6 columns after the modified radioiodination procedure of Hunter and Greenwood (1962) was employed with (A) insulin, (B) native relaxin, and (C) polytyrosyl-relaxin. (Reproduced from Sherwood *et al.*, 1975a, with permission of the publisher.)

according to a modification of the procedure described by Becker and Stahmann (1953) for the preparation of polypeptidyl proteins. Twenty-five milligrams of native relaxin was dissolved in 10 ml $0.1 M$ phosphate buffer at pH 7.52. The solution was cooled to 4°C and stirred rapidly during the addition of 8.32 mg N-carboxy-L-tyrosine anhydride. The resulting suspension was maintained at 4°C with constant stirring for 24 hours, then centrifuged at 60,000 g for one hour at 4°C to remove the precipitate. The supernatant was dialyzed for seven days at 4°C against distilled water. The polytyrosyl-relaxin was dried by lyophilization and stored at −5°C. The protein yield of the product designated polytyrosyl-relaxin was determined to be 14.4 mg by means of the biuret reaction (Gornall *et al.*, 1949). Amino acid analysis indicated native relaxin incorporated 1.67 mole of tyrosine per mole of native relaxin. Mouse interpubic ligament bioassays (Steinetz *et al.*, 1969) showed that polytyrosyl-relaxin was as biologically active as native relaxin (Sherwood *et al.*, 1975a). The use of *N*-carboxy-L-tyrosine anhydride for the incorporation of tyrosine into polypeptide hormones appears to be an effective method for the preparation of these hormones for radioiodination. The technique is simple, gentle, and inexpensive. The only problem encountered with this method has been the formation of insoluble polytyrosyl-relaxin during the incorporation reaction when high molar ratios of *N*-carboxy-L-tyrosine anhydride, to native relaxin are employed. However, a good yield of soluble polytyrosyl-relaxin was obtained when an 8 : 1 molar ratio of *N*-carboxy-L-tyrosine anhydride to native relaxin was used.

D. Radioiodination of Polytyrosyl-Relaxin

Polytyrosyl-relaxin is radioiodinated according to a modification of the method of Hunter and Greenwood (1962). Twenty microliters of 0.5 *M* sodium phosphate, pH 7.5, is added to 2.5 μg polytyrosyl-relaxin dissolved in 5.0 μl 0.5 *M* sodium phosphate at pH 7.5. One millicurie of Na^{125}I is added and the contents are thoroughly mixed. One hundred micrograms of chloramine-T in 25 μl 0.25 *M* sodium phosphate buffer, pH 7.5, is then added and the contents are again thoroughly mixed. After one minute, the reaction is stopped by the addition of 250 μg sodium metabisulfite, which is dissolved in 100 μl 0.05 *M* sodium phosphate buffer at pH 7.5. Following the addition of sodium metabisulfite, 100 μl transfer solution which contains 16% sucrose and 1.0 mg potassium iodide is added. The contents of the reaction vial are immediately layered on a 1.0 × 15 cm column of BioGel P-6 (BioRad Laboratories) equilibrated with 0.05 *M* sodium phosphate at pH 7.5. One hundred microliters of rinse solution containing 8% sucrose and 1.0 mg of potassium iodide is added to the reaction vial and then layered on the column. Twelve-drop aliquots of the column eluate are collected in 12 × 75 mm polystyrene tubes containing 0.5 ml PBS–5% ovalbumin. The radioactivity elution profile is determined by counting 1.0-μl aliquots of each tube in an automatic gamma counter.

Polytyrosyl-relaxin readily incorporates ^{125}I. A typical elution pattern showing the separation of ^{125}I-polytyrosyl-relaxin from free ^{125}I is shown in Figure 2C. The two or three tubes of ^{125}I-polytyrosyl-relaxin containing the highest radioactivity are diluted with PBS–1% ovalbumin so that 100 μl contains 55,000 to 58,000 cpm. The specific radioactivity of ^{125}I-polytyrosyl-relaxin obtained by this procedure ranges from 80–100 μCi/μg. ^{125}I-Polytyrosyl-relaxin is routinely used for three to five weeks without repurification.

E. Assay Procedure

Double antibody relaxin radioimmunoassays are conducted in 12 × 75 mm disposable glass culture tubes. Quantities of standard native relaxin ranging from 8.0 to 2000 pg or unknowns are placed in each tube and sufficient PBS–1% ovalbumin is added to bring the volume to 500 μl. Two hundred microliters of rabbit anti-porcine relaxin antiserum 1082, diluted 1 : 20,000 in 0.05 M EDTA–PBS and containing 1 : 60 male rabbit serum, is added to each tube. The contents are incubated at 4°C for 24 hours. One hundred microliters of ^{125}I-polytyrosyl-relaxin (prepared by diluting the ^{125}I-polytyrosyl-relaxin obtained from the BioGel P-6 column with PBS–1% ovalbumin so that on the day of iodination 100 μl contained 55,000–58,000 cpm) is added to each tube and the contents are again incubated at 4°C for 24 hours. It is estimated that the quantity of radioiodinated ^{125}I-polytryosyl-relaxin added to each tube is approximately 120 pg. Twenty-four hours later, 200 μl sheep anti-rabbit γ-globulin, at a dilution which will enable maximum precipitation of bound ^{125}I-polytyrosyl-relaxin, is added to each tube. The contents are mixed and incubated at 4°C for 72 hours. Three milliliters of cold PBS is then added to each tube and the tubes are centrifuged for 30 minutes at 3000 g at 4°C. The supernatants are decanted and the precipitates are counted in an automatic gamma counter.

Native relaxin standards and unknowns are normally assayed in quadruplicate. Either plasma or serum may be employed with the relaxin radioimmunoassay. Multiple volumes of each unknown ranging from 1.0 μl, when relaxin levels are high, to 500 μl, when relaxin levels are low, are employed with the radioimmunoassay. Logit and log transformation (Rodbard and Lewald, 1970) are used to obtain a linear dose–response curve.

III. RADIOIMMUNOASSAY CHARACTERIZATION

A. Sensitivity

The porcine relaxin radioimmunoassay is approximately 1000 times more sensitive than bioassays for this hormone. The least detectable

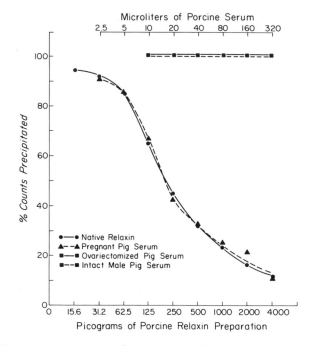

Figure 3. Dose–response curves for porcine native relaxin, pregnant pig serum, ovariectomized female pig serum, and intact male pig serum in the porcine relaxin radioimmunoassay. (Reproduced from Sherwood *et al.*, 1975a, with permission of the publisher.)

dose, as defined by Feldman and Rodbard (1971), which is measured with this radioimmunoassay is 32 pg of native relaxin. A typical standard curve obtained with native relaxin is shown in Figure 3. When logit and log transformations are used, a linear regression is obtained from 32 to 1000 pg.

B. Specificity

1. Hormone Specificity

All experiments which have been conducted indicate that the porcine relaxin radioimmunoassay is specific for relaxin. First, the slope of the dose–response curve obtained with multiple volumes of late pregnancy pig serum does not differ from the dose–response curve obtained with native relaxin (Figure 3). Second, porcine insulin, FSII, LH, and TSH do not react in the assay system in doses up to 1.0 μg. Third, when late pregnancy pig serum spiked with ^{125}I-polytyrosyl-relaxin was filtered through a column of BioGel P-10, the immunoreactive peak coeluted with ^{125}I-polytyrosyl-relaxin, thereby indicating that the immunoreactive substance within late pregnancy pig serum and porcine relaxin are of similar size (Sherwood et al., 1975a).

2. Species Specificity

Apparently, there are limitations in the number of species for which this porcine relaxin radioimmunoassay is valid. No immunoreactive substance has been detected within late pregnancy sera obtained from cows, guinea pigs, monkeys, or human beings. There is some cross-reactivity of the rabbit anti-porcine relaxin sera with rat relaxin, since immunoreactive substance(s) are found in rat sera during late pregnancy. However, rat relaxin seems to have a lower affinity for the anti-porcine relaxin sera than porcine relaxin, since the slopes of the regression lines obtained with several dilutions of pregnant rat sera are much lower than those obtained with pregnant pig sera. This reduced regression, relative to the native relaxin porcine standard, is common for all four rabbit anti-porcine relaxin sera.

C. Precision and Reproducibility

The porcine relaxin radioimmunoassay is much more precise than relaxin bioassay procedures. The intraassay coefficient of variation ranges from approximately 8 to 13%. During late pregnancy, the levels of relaxin are so high in the pig that only 1.0- or 2.0-μl aliquots of plasma are required for the radioimmunoassay. The precision of determinations on these samples is improved if 100-μl aliquots of the late pregnancy pig plasma are diluted 10- to 100-fold with PBS–1% ovalbumin before pipetting them into the reaction tubes.

The reproducibility of the porcine relaxin radioimmunoassay was determined by measuring the relaxin content of a serum sample obtained from a pig during late pregnancy in nine independent radioimmunoassays. The interassay coefficient of variation was 8.1%.

IV. LEVELS OF CIRCULATING RELAXIN

In the pig, gestation ranges from approximately 114 to 117 days. All available evidence indicates that high levels of relaxin are found in porcine plasma only during very late pregnancy. Bioassay and histologic studies with pregnant pig plasma led Belt *et al.* (1971) to conclude that relaxin is discharged from the granulosa luteal cells of the corpora lutea during very late pregnancy. Sherwood *et al.* (1975b) measured relaxin concentrations in the peripheral plasma of the pig throughout pregnancy and at parturition with the porcine relaxin radioimmunoassay. These workers reported that relaxin concentrations remained below 2.0 ng/ml during the first 100 days of pregnancy and then rose gradually to a mean of approximately 12 ng/ml by three

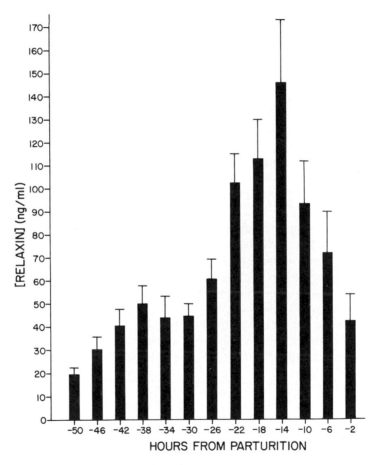

Figure 4. Relaxin concentrations obtained at four-hour intervals from 50 hours to two hours before parturition in the pig. Means of six animals (+ standard error of mean) are shown. (Reproduced from Sherwood *et al.*, 1975b, with permission of the publisher.)

days before parturition. At this time, relaxin levels rose more rapidly and increased to a mean concentration of 44.0 ng/ml by 30 hours before parturition. Relaxin concentrations then increased sharply to a mean of 145.6 ng/ml by 14 hours before parturition (Figure 4). This maximum was followed by a rapid decrease to a mean of 42.4 ng/ml by 2 hours before parturition. At one day following parturition, relaxin levels were less than 1.0 ng/ml. Relaxin was not detected in serum obtained from adult male pigs (Figure 3).

ACKNOWLEDGMENTS

The author is indebted to the contributions of his colleagues whose work provided much of the information presented in this chapter: G. W. BeVier, M. L. Birkhimer, C. C. Chang, P. J. Dziuk, G. L. Jackson, and K. R. Rosentreter. Work supported in part by the National Institute of Child Health and Human Development, NIH, Grant 5 RO1 HDO8700.

REFERENCES

Becker, R. R., and Stahmann, M. A. (1953). Protein modification by reaction with N-carboxyamino acid anhydrides. *J. Biol. Chem.* **204**, 745–752.

Belt, W. D., Anderson, L. L., Cavazos, L. F., and Melampy, R. M. (1971). Cytoplasmic granules and relaxin levels in porcine corpora lutea. *Endocrinology* **89**, 1–10.

Feldman, H., and Rodbard, D. (1971). Mathematical theory of radioimmunoassay. In "Principles of Competitive Protein-Binding Assays" (W. D. Odell and W. H. Daughaday, eds.), pp. 158–203. Lippincott, Philadelphia, Pennsylvania.

Gornall, A. G., Bardawill, C. J., and David, M. M. (1949). Determination of serum proteins by means of the biuret reaction. *J. Biol. Chem.* **177**, 751–766.

Hall, K. (1960). Relaxin. *J. Reprod. Fertil.* **1**, 368–384.

Hunter, W. M., and Greenwood, F. C. (1962). Preparation of Iodine-131 labelled human growth hormone of high specific activity. *Nature (London)* **194**, 495–496.

Marder, S. N., and Money, W. L. (1944). Concentration of relaxin in the blood serum of pregnant and postpartum rabbits. *Endocrinology* **34**, 115–121.

Rodbard, D., and Lewald, J. E. (1970). Computer analysis of radioligand assay and radioimmunoassay data. *Steroid Assay Protein Binding, Karolinska Symp. Res. Methods Reprod. Endocrinol., 2nd*, pp. 79–103.

Sherwood, O. D., and O'Byrne, E. M. (1974). Purification and characterization of porcine relaxin. *Arch. Biochem. Biophys.* **160**, 185–196.

Sherwood, O. D., Rosentreter, K. R., and Birkhimer, M. L. (1975a). Development of a radioimmunoassay for porcine relaxin using ^{125}I-labeled polytyrosyl-relaxin. *Endocrinology* **96**, 1106–1113.

Sherwood, O. D., Chang, C. C., BeVier, G. W., and Dziuk, P. J. (1975b). Radioimmunoassay of plasma relaxin levels throughout pregnancy and at parturition in the pig. *Endocrinology* **97**, 834–837.

Steinetz, B. G., Beach, V. L., and Kroc, R. L. (1969). Bioassay of relaxin. *Methods Horm. Res.* **2**, Part A, 481–513.

Zarrow, M. X. (1947). Relaxin content of blood, urine and other tissues of pregnant and postpartum guinea pigs. *Proc. Soc. Exp. Biol. Med.* **66**, 488–491.

Zarrow, M. X., Holmstrom, E. G., and Salhanick, H. A. (1955). The concentration of relaxin in the blood serum and other tissues of women during pregnancy. *J. Clin. Endocrinol. Metab.* **15**, 22–27.

VASOACTIVE PEPTIDE HORMONES

45

Renin and the Angiotensins

ARTHUR E. FREEDLENDER AND
THEODORE L. GOODFRIEND

I. INTRODUCTION

Renin is a proteolytic enzyme synthesized and secreted by specialized cells in the kidney and probably in other organs, such as uterus and blood vessels. It cleaves a circulating α_2-globulin substrate synthesized in the liver. The products of this cleavage are a large molecule of unknown function, and the decapeptide, angiotensin I. Angiotensin I is subject to hydrolysis by a variety of enzymes, but the dipeptidase known as converting enzyme is physiologically most significant and digests it to angiotensin II. Angiotensin II can then be cleaved to smaller fragments, one of which is now called angiotensin III. The formulas for these peptides are depicted in Table I. The three peptides designated with roman numerals have characteristic pharmacologic properties (Peach, 1977). Each of the peptides and the en-

889

Methods of Hormone Radioimmunoassay, Second Edition
Copyright © 1979 by Academic Press, Inc.

Table I   Angiotensins

1	2	3	4	5	6	7	8	9	10
NH$_2$-Asp	Arg	Val	Tyr	Ile	His	Pro	Phe	His	Leu-COOH

$\longleftarrow$———————————— Angiotensin I ————————————$\longrightarrow$
　　$\longleftarrow$——————— (Des^1)-Angiotensin I ———————$\longrightarrow$
$\longleftarrow$———————— Angiotensin II ————————$\longrightarrow$
　　$\longleftarrow$————————— Angiotensin III —————————$\longrightarrow$
　　　$\longleftarrow$————(Des^{1,2})-Angiotensin II————$\longrightarrow$

zymes that form them are objects of study in clinical and research laboratories. Radioimmunoassays form the basis of the most convenient techniques used in their measurement.

II. METHODS OF RADIOIMMUNOASSAY

A. Source of Hormones

Angiotensins I, II, and III suitable for iodination and immunization may be obtained from Beckman Instruments, Palo Alto, California; Bachem, Inc., Torrance, California; or Peninsula Laboratories, San Carlos, California.

For standards we recommend the use of the following well-characterized materials from the Medical Research Council, Division of Biological Standards, National Institute for Medical Research, Hampstead Laboratories, Holly Hill, London, England.

Angiotensin I—(Asp^1, Ileu^5) Synthetic 71/328
Angiotensin II—Research Standard A (Asp^1, Ileu^5) Synthetic 70/302
Human Renin—Research Standard A 68/356

These angiotensins are identical in amino acid sequence to those found in human plasma, and their use avoids the pitfall of nonidentity of standards and unknowns discussed by Hollemans (1970).

B. Preparation of Immunogen and Immunization Schedule

Although native angiotensins are poor immunogens, antisera to angiotensins are easily produced in rabbits using angiotensin conjugated by carbodiimide condensation to albumin (Goodfriend et al., 1964) or succinylated polylysine (Stason et al., 1967). Alternatively, angiotensin may be adsorbed onto microparticles of carbon black (Boyd and Peart,

1968). Identical techniques are applicable to the generation of antibodies to angiotensin I and II.

Carbodiimide condensation is performed as follows (proportionally smaller amounts of reagents and water may be used):

1. At room temperature, dissolve 25 mg angiotensin I or II and 25 mg rabbit serum albumin in 2.5 ml of distilled water.

2. Add 375 mg dry 1-ethyl-3-(3-dimethylaminopropyl)-carbodiimide hydrochloride (Story Chemical Company, Muskeegon, Michigan) and allow the mixture to remain at room temperature for 24 hours. The carbodiimide should be handled with caution, since it can cross-link skin proteins and, on reexposure, can evoke an inflammatory response.

3. Dialyze the mixture against two liters of 0.15 M NaCl for 24 hours. Change the dialysate four times during this period to remove the toxic carbodiimide.

4. This material may be stored frozen until use. The degree of conjugation of the polypeptide hormone can be determined using tracer amounts of labeled hormone, but there is no information available at present correlating the amount of angiotensin conjugated to the immunogenicity of the complex immunogen.

Prior to immunization, the angiotensin–protein conjugate is emulsified with three volumes of complete Freund's adjuvant containing an additional 10 mg/ml of dried *Mycobacterium butyricum*. Optimal emulsification is most easily accomplished by rapid and repeated transfer between two syringes connected by an 18 gauge luer adaptor.

For primary immunization a total of 2.0 ml of the emulsion containing 2.0 mg of conjugate is injected intramuscularly or into the toe pads or dorsal skin of rabbits, preferably of several strains. The injections are administered at multiple sites. Booster injections are begun after three or more weeks by injection of 0.5 ml of the emulsion intramuscularly or intraperitoneally.

The interval between first and subsequent booster injections can be determined by periodic testing of sera. Some investigators have found better yields of high-affinity antisera by withholding booster injections until the titers fall, rather than using more frequent injections.

Satisfactory antibodies for radioimmunoassay are usually produced within six months, and animals continue to produce antisera for several months following their last booster injections. Animals producing high titer avid antisera may be bled of 35–50 ml at weekly intervals. We believe that better results are obtained by beginning immunization of many rabbits of several strains, then boosting only those with reasonable titers and affinities rather than using a small number of rabbits treated intensively.

Thimerosal (0.1 mg/ml) is added to angiotensin antisera as a preservative and the antisera are then heated to 56°C for 30 minutes to diminish intrinsic enzymatic and complement activity. Antisera may be stored in aliquots at −20° for years without loss of titer or avidity. However, repetitive freezing and thawing may result in a significant loss of activity and should be avoided.

Using the procedures described in this section, one can reasonably expect that at least one out of six immunized animals will produce antisera of sufficient sensitivity to allow the detection of 25 pg angiotensin I or II at a titer of 1 : 10,000.

Antiserum to angiotensin I can be obtained from Arnel Products, Brooklyn, New York; CalBiochem, Los Angeles, California; Endocrine Sciences, Tarzana, California; Monobind, Santa Monica, California; and Sylvana Company, Millburn, New Jersey. Antiserum to angiotensin II can be obtained from New England Nuclear, Boston, Massachusetts; and Sylvana Company, Millburn, New Jersey.

C. Characterization of Antibody

Antisera to angiotensins vary widely in their titer, avidity, and specificity, and no correlation among these three parameters (see Table II) exists. Antisera to angiotensin I are fairly specific with re-

Table II   Specificity of Angiotensin II Antisera[a]

Anti-serum	Dilution	A II detected (mg)	Relative inhibition by unlabeled				
			A II	Des[1]-A II	Des[1,2]-A II	Des[8]-A II	A I
DA-15	1 : 13,000	30	100	217	100	<1	<1
DA-18	1 : 35,000	100	100	95	160	<1	<1
FF-E2	1 : 10,000	10	100	29	6	—	<1
FK-19	1 : 60,000	30	100	164	63	—	<1
GW-1	1 : 10,000	10	100	4	<1	—	<1
HI-25	1 : 15,000	30	100	9	6	—	1
OW-1	1 : 1,600	30	100	14	5	—	2
WA-1	1 : 3,000	30	100	39	<1	—	<1
WA-4	1 : 15,000	10	100	85	79	—	8
SY-44	1 : 22,000	10	100	95	83	—	3

[a] Antisera were diluted to bind approximately 50% of 10 pg of ^{125}I-angiotensin II (A II) using assay conditions described in the text. The amount of unlabeled congener required to reduce initial binding by 50% was used as the standard of comparison. Data are unpublished observations of T. L. Goodfriend and D. L. Ball.

spect to their relative affinities for the decapeptide as compared to the octapeptide (angiotensin I versus II); however, they cross-react to a great extent with the nonapeptide (Des-Asp[1])-angiotensin I. Antisera to angiotensin II cross-react significantly with smaller peptides, as shown in Table II. A possible explanation of the paradoxical affinity of antisera for degradation products is the degradation of the immunizing antigen in the rabbits while they are mounting an immune response. Alternatively, one can postulate that these smaller peptides contain the intact antigenic determinant of the immunogen.

There are no antisera available that have useful selectivity for angiotensin III. A binding factor has been found in some patients' plasmas, particularly those with mental retardation, that can be used in radioimmunoassays for this heptapeptide. Its supply is obviously limited, its titer is low, and its affinity restricts sensitivity to the range of 30 pg/ml or greater (Goodfriend et al., 1976).

D. Preparation and Sources of Radioactive Ligand

Both angiotensin I and II are readily iodinated using ^{125}I. This isotope has significant advantages over ^{131}I (Freedlender, 1969; Hunter, 1966). The method to be described incorporates the principles of Greenwood et al. (1963) and is a modification of the procedure of Nielsen et al. (1971). The reaction is carried out in an ice bath in a glass scintillation vial with continuous magnetic stirring.

1. Add 2.5 ml 0.05 M phosphate buffer, pH 7.5.
2. Add 2.5 mCi ^{125}I.
3. Add 100 μl angiotensin I or II (1 mg/ml in H_2O).
4. Add dropwise 0.5 ml chloramine-T (20 μg/ml) over the course of one minute. The chloramine-T is dissolved immediately prior to use in 0.05 M phosphate buffer, pH 7.5.
5. After ten minutes add 0.7 ml freshly prepared sodium metabisulfite (20 μg/ml in 0.05 M phosphate buffer, pH 7.5).
6. Transfer the reaction mixture to a 1.0×100 cm DEAE-Sephadex A-25 column at 4°C equilibrated with 0.05 M phosphate buffer, pH 7.5, containing 0.1 mg/ml thimerosal and elute at a flow rate of 12 ml/hour. Fractions are collected in 6.0-ml aliquots. Prior to initial use of the column, 5.0 ml 2% crystalline bovine serum albumin is washed through the column. The column may be reused for at least 20 iodinations.
7. The first radioactive peak eluted is ^{125}I-monoiodoangiotensin. This is preserved by diluting to a concentration of less than 25 μCi/ml in a solution of 0.8 M glycine, 0.2 M NaCl, 0.05 M phosphate, pH 7.5,

and 0.25% crystalline bovine serum albumin. The final solution is stored at $-20°C$ and is stable for several months.

Unreacted angiotensin is eluted from the DEAE-Sephadex column before iodinated peaks. Therefore, the ^{125}I-monoiodoangiotensin selected for assay should come from the center or trailing portion of its elution peak to minimize contamination that would lower specific activity.

The methodology described in this section has several advantages. The use of a dilute solution of chloramine-T, added slowly to avoid high local concentrations, results in minimal damage to the polypeptide by the oxidizing agent. The high polypeptide–iodine ratio yields less than 5% diiodoangiotensin (Nielsen et al., 1971), which has only 10% of the immunoreactivity of monoiodoangiotensin (Lin et al., 1970). Ion-exchange chromatography completely separates the monoiodo from the diiodo derivative, and effects nearly complete separation of the unlabeled angiotensin from the mono-iodoangiotensin. The resultant specific activity of the final product, measured by radioimmunoassay is approximately 1000 $\mu Ci/\mu g$. The glycine–NaCl–phosphate–albumin preservative solution prolongs shelf life, presumably by raising the dielectric constant and reducing interactions due to electrostatic forces.

Both monoiodoangiotensin I and II prepared by the above method are available from New England Nuclear, Boston, Massachusetts. Other sources of iodinated angiotensins are: Cambridge Nuclear Corporation, Billerica, Massachusetts; CEA-CEN, Sorin, Italy; E. R. Squibb and Sons, New Brunswick, New Jersey; and Nuclear International Corporation, Waltham, Massachusetts.

E. Preparation of Subjects and Samples

1. Angiotensins

Plasma contains at least two different but unknown substances that can alter the antigen–antibody reaction of angiotensin radioimmunoassays (Goodfriend, 1969; Goodfriend et al., 1976; Page et al., 1971). Since plasma levels of angiotensin I and II are near the sensitivity limits of the radioimmunoassay, dilution of samples to lessen interference is not feasible.

To control interference, two different approaches have been used. Goodfriend et al. (1968) measured angiotensin in undiluted plasma by comparing it to a standard curve made in the same plasma, which had been rendered angiotensin-free by treatment with one-tenth volume of Dowex AG-50W-X4, hydrogen form. The resin had been previously washed in succession with 0.2 M diethylamine in 1.0 M NH$_4$OH, water, 0.2 M NH$_4$Ac, pH 6.0, and water. Boyd and co-workers (1967) extracted angiotensin from plasma with Fuller's Earth, then eluted the angiotensin from the adsorbent and redissolved it for assay. The latter method has the virtue of concentrating the polypeptide. Both methods depend on the specificity of the adsorbent. If interfering substances are adsorbed, falsely elevated values for angiotensin will result.

In addition to control of interfering substances, plasma enzymes that can form and degrade angiotensins must be inhibited. Renin is partially inhibited by mercuric acetate or mercuric iodide, and complete enzyme inhibition can be achieved by boiling (Stockigt *et al.*, 1971) or cold ethanol (Cain *et al.*, 1972). The latter two techniques have the advantage of removing some interfering substances. Converting enzyme and some of the angiotensinase activity are inhibited by 2.6 mM EDTA, 1.6 mM dimercaprol, and 3.4 mM 8-hydroxyquinoline sulfate (Haber *et al.*, 1969). More complete inhibition of angiotensinase activity can be achieved by the addition of 0.5 mg/ml phenylmethylsulfonyl fluoride (PMSF) to the EDTA, dimercaprol, and 8-hydroxyquinoline sulfate. (Kodish and Katz, 1974).

Angiotensins may be extracted from plasma as follows (modified from Boyd *et al.*, 1967).

1. Draw blood into a chilled syringe or Vacutainer containing sufficient EDTA, 8-hydroxyquinoline sulfate, and PMSF to achieve the concentrations stated above.

2. Immediately transfer the blood to cold centrifuge tubes and separate plasma by centrifugation at 4°C. Plasma can be stored at −20°C.

3. Add 10 mg acid-washed Fuller's Earth per milliliter of plasma, mix for five minutes at 4°C, centrifuge at 4°C, and discard supernatant.

4. Wash with an equal volume of distilled water.

5. Wash with an equal volume of distilled water–methanol (1 : 1, v/v).

6. Add 4.0 ml concentrated ammonia in methanol (4 : 6, v/v), mix for five minutes at room temperature, and centrifuge.

7. Transfer three 1.0-ml aliquots of supernatant to disposable radioimmunoassay tubes and take to dryness at 45°C *in vacuo*.

Recovery of angiotensins may be determined by adding tracer amounts of iodinated or tritiated angiotensins to pooled plasma before extraction is begun.

Some investigators have observed variations among samples of Fuller's Earth, despite careful washing with dilute HCl. All tubes and pipettes should be chosen or coated to avoid adsorption of angiotensin and washed to remove detergents which interfere with the antigen–antibody reaction (Goodfriend et al., 1968). The use of Fuller's Earth to extract angiotensin from plasma is simple, convenient, and gives reproducible results (McBride et al., 1971).

To measure the various angiotensins separately, extracts of plasma or other fluids may be fractionated chromatographically. The first such experiments were performed by Cain and Catt (1969). The most recent experiments of this nature were performed by Semple and Morton (1976). Measured amounts of plasma were made up to 10 ml with 0.154 M saline and incubated with 400 mg of Dowex AG 50W-X2 (50–100 mesh, H^+ form) for 60 minutes. The angiotensins were eluted from the resin with ammonia and dried at 37°C in air. After dissolution in 0.1 ml of 30% ammonia–methanol (9 : 1, v/v), angiotensins II and III were separated by paper chromatography on Whatman 3 MM paper in n-butanol–acetic acid–water–pyridine (15 : 3 : 12 : 10), pH 5.2 for 15–16 hours. R_f's of angiotensins II and III were 0.50 and 0.67, respectively. This system did not separate angiotensin I from the other peptides.

2. Renins

Renin is released into the circulation in response to a variety of stimuli (Davis and Freeman, 1976). There is no easy way to prepare animals or humans so that all possible regulators of renin release are controlled. The major factors that can be manipulated are the sodium content of the diet, posture, and drugs (including anesthetics). For studies on humans, dietary constancy to a state of sodium equilibrium is attempted and checked by measuring total urinary excretion of sodium. The subjects are instructed to be either supine or on their feet for 30 to 120 minutes, and drugs affecting renal function or sympathetic nervous system function are withheld when possible. Despite this, measurements are confounded by moment-to-moment changes in renin release that probably result from an endogenous biorhythm or cerebral activity (Weinberger et al., 1972; Horvath et al., 1977).

Renin measurements are very useful for the diagnosis of renal disease, especially unilateral renal artery stenosis. In this situation, the samples are taken from the renal veins of patients, and frequently from other sites. The goal of such a study is the discovery of a lesion that results in excessive renin secretion and which is amenable to surgery. Therefore, the essential data are comparisons among samples from a single subject. Although this eliminates problems introduced by variations among subjects, it still encompasses problems resulting from changes in renin release as a function of time (Horvath *et al.*, 1977). The difference in venous renin concentration between normal and abnormal kidneys may be accentuated by the salt "repletion–depletion" protocol recommended by Strong *et al.* (1971).

Finally, the collection and storage of plasma and tissue samples for measurements of renin must be performed with consideration to the possible activation of prorenin. This process was observed by Lumbers (1971), who catalyzed the conversion by addition of acid. More recently, Sealey *et al.* (1977) found it to be catalyzed by reduced temperature. Thus, samples stored chilled or acidified may display increases in the level of active renin before or during assays. In general, the safest procedure is to draw blood into glass tubes containing sufficient Na$_2$-EDTA to give a final concentration of 1.0 mg/ml, centrifuge the blood quickly at room temperature to sediment cells, then freeze the plasma to at least $-20°C$. Samples with high renin activities may generate considerable amounts of angiotensin I before and during freezing. This will not confuse the assay if angiotensin I is eventually measured before and after the renin enzyme incubation step.

F. Assay Procedures and Separation Techniques

1. Angiotensin Radioimmunoassay

Numerous radioimmunoassays for angiotensins have been reported. The methods do not appear to differ significantly in their essentials. One study of the variables encountered in incubation and separation techniques has been reported by Goodfriend *et al.* (1968). The procedure described below has been selected for its technical facility and reproducibility. It is suitable for the measurement of angiotensin I or II in biologic fluids and for the polypeptides in incubation mixtures designed to assay renin substrate or enzymes that form, convert, or destroy angiotensins. Only the labeled polypeptide and antiserum must be changed to suit the specific goal.

a. The following buffer is used for all dilutions: 0.01 *M* potassium phosphate, pH 7.4, containing 3 m*M* EDTA, 0.15 m*M* 8-hydroxyquinoline sulfate, 0.02% neomycin sulfate, and 2.5 mg/ml crystalline bovine serum albumin. The buffer is heated to 56°C for 30 minutes to destroy angiotensinase activity in albumin and then stored at 4°C. All procedures are performed at 4°C.

b. To each tube containing plasma or dried, extracted angiotensin add sufficient buffer to bring to a final volume of 1.0 ml.

c. Standard curves are prepared in triplicate in 1.0 ml volumes. The range of the curve is determined by the sensitivity of the antisera. Twofold dilutions from 1.0 ng to 2.0 pg are used for sensitive antisera.

d. ^{125}I-Angiotensin (10 pg or approximately 10,000 cpm in 0.1 ml) is added to each tube.

e. Diluted antiserum (0.1 ml) is the final addition. The dilution selected is that which will bind 40–60% of the labeled hormone in the absence of exogenous hormone.

f. Incubate at 4°C for 2 to 24 hours. Although this antigen–antibody reaction does not reach equilibrium in 2 hours, clinical considerations may force a more rapid but less sensitive determination.

g. Add 1.0 ml of a suspension of Norit A neutral charcoal (Fisher) and Dextran T-70 (Pharmacia) in 0.01 M phosphate buffer, pH 7.4. The stock charcoal suspension is 2.5% charcoal with 0.25% dextran, as suggested by Herbert et al. (1965). However, this concentration may adsorb all radioactive angiotensin (Waxman et al., 1967). Therefore dilutions of charcoal usually must be used, and these will vary both with different antisera and different samples. For example, more avid antisera and samples containing protein require more concentrated charcoal. Ideally, the charcoal should bind all of the label in the absence of antibody and none in the presence of excess antibody, but this ideal has never been achieved. If more than 85% of the label appears in the supernatant after charcoal adsorption in the presence of excess antibody, the procedure is satisfactory. With the use of an avid antiserum and a protein concentration of 2.5 mg/ml, a 1 : 5 dilution of the stock charcoal suspension has proved convenient. All samples should be exposed to the charcoal for an *equal* and *brief* period of time (less than ten minutes) and centrifuged and decanted as near to simultaneously as possible.

h. Supernatant (antibody-bound hormone) and charcoal (free hormone) are counted for radioactivity.

i. Amounts of angiotensin in the sample are calculated from standard curves and are corrected for known losses during extraction and dilution.

2. Renin Assays

Renin is synthesized as a proenzyme of high molecular weight and is converted in one or more steps to the smaller, active proteolytic enzyme whose hydrolysis of renin substrate is its best known characteristic. Beginnings have been made in development of a direct immunoassay of the renin enzyme molecule itself, but these experiments are thrown into confusion by the existence of several possible precursors and several possible organ sources that may give rise to immunologic heterogeneity (Michelakis *et al.*, 1974; Malling and Poulsen, 1977; de Senarclens *et al.*, 1977). At the present time, the most practical method for measuring renin is the technique that involves an incubation step to permit generation of angiotensin I, followed by a radioimmunoassay of the angiotensin I generated. Still, the existence of prorenins confuses the assay-based enzymatic activity because storage of samples can allow or even accelerate conversion of circulating precursors into enzymatically active molecules, as noted above (Sealey *et al.*, 1977).

Even when problems introduced by prorenins are disregarded or solved, controversies enliven interpretation of renin measurements. They can be reduced to a question of the investigator's intent to measure the activity of renin and related enzymes in circulating blood or to measure the total amount of renin released into the blood by the kidney and other sources. If the intent is to measure renin-like activity, the blood should be tested with as little tampering as possible. The datum would be called "plasma renin activity" (PRA). If the intent is to determine the amount of renin, the sample should be adjusted to maximize and control the enzyme reaction in ways that are traditional in biochemistry. The datum would be called "plasma renin concentration" (PRC). Both data would be approximations, since the activity of renin in the circulation cannot be tested directly, and the concentration of an enzyme cannot be measured precisely by tests of its activity alone.

a. Plasma Renin Activity (PRA)

1. Add inhibitors to thawed plasma to achieve concentrations as follows: 0.5 mg/ml phenylmethylsulfonyl fluoride, 0.5 mg/ml 8-hydroxyquinoline sulfate, 1.0 mg/ml dimercaprol, and 0.2% neomycin. It is assumed here that the plasma already contains EDTA at a concentration of 1.0 mg/ml. The first three reagents are added from ethanolic stock solutions.

2. Buffer with 0.1 ml 0.5M phosphate, pH 7.4, per milliliter of plasma.

3. Incubate two aliquots of plasma from 0.5 to 18 hours at 37°C, and then chill. Hold a second set of samples at 4°C ("nonincubated plasma"). The duration of incubation will vary with the sensitivity of the angiotensin I antisera used for radioimmunoassay and the level of

renin activity. If the general range of renin activity is unknown, the incubation can be terminated at three hours, aliquots taken, and the remainder frozen. The frozen mixture can be thawed and incubated for longer times if the initial assay reveals very low activity.

4. Assay 50-μl aliquots of incubated plasma and nonincubated plasma for angiotensin I as described above.

5. Calculate renin activity in terms of nanograms of angiotensin I produced per milliliter of plasma per hour of incubation. This calculation will require adjustments for the volume of plasma, the time of incubation, and the amount of angiotensin I found in the incubated sample.

b. Plasma Renin Concentration (PRC)

1. Collect plasma and add inhibitors as described above for plasma renin activity.

2. Add 50 μl plasma to 50 μl sheep substrate (Skinner, 1967) in four tubes. Uniform substrate is purified from heparinized, previously nephrectomized sheep. Plasma is dialyzed for 36 hours at 3°C against 0.3 M citric acid–0.05 M phosphate–0.16 M NaCl, pH 3.9, containing 5 mM EDTA. After heating to 32°C for 45 minutes, the plasma is dialyzed to a final pH of 7.5 against 0.175 M phosphate, 0.075 M NaCl, pH 7.5, and stored at -20°C with 2 mg/ml neomycin sulfate, and 100 U/ml Trasylol.

3. Adjust pH to 7.0 with 0.1 M phosphate buffer.

4. Incubate two tubes for 0.5–17 hours at 37°C, and hold two tubes at 4°C.

5. Assay for angiotensin I and calculate renin as described above.

c. Comment.
In the protocols described above, EDTA inhibits converting enzyme and stops the renin reaction at angiotensin I (Haber *et al.*, 1969). It also inhibits other enzymes that can destroy angiotensins. Phenylmethylsulfonyl fluoride inhibits enzymes that can cleave the generated angiotensin I. It has been shown to result in higher apparent rates of angiotensin generation than occur in its absence (Kodish and Katz, 1974). The other reagents help inhibit proteolysis and bacterial growth. It is advisable to buffer plasma at neutral pH, because loss of carbon dioxide can cause a drift to the alkaline range. Although the reaction of human renin with human substrate is optimum at pH 5.5 to 6.0, this is inappropriate for measurement of plasma renin activity, when the goal is an approximation of the activity of the enzyme in the circulation. Sheep substrate is added to saturate the enzyme for mea-

surement of its concentration. Paradoxically, the optimum pH for the reaction of human renin with sheep substrate is 7.0. Use of a buffer near neutral pII has the additional advantage of lessening the activity of "pseudorenins" and cathepsin D whose optima are in the acid range (Skeggs *et al.*, 1969; Oparil *et al.*, 1974; Day and Reid, 1976).

Another approach to the measurement of renin concentration is the use of added increments of purified renin that enable control of variables, such as activators or inhibitors in the sample (Haas and Goldblatt, 1972).

III. VERIFICATION OF ASSAY RESULTS AND SPECIAL PROBLEMS

Radioimmunoassays are customarily verified by comparing the results of serial dilutions of unknowns with serial dilutions of standards. The curves should be parallel. Nonparallelism indicates that the unknown contains nonspecific immunologically unrelated interfering factors, biologically inactive fragments of the antigen, partially denatured antigen containing the antigenic determinant, fragments of the antigen containing only part of the antigenic determinants, or other compounds which contain regions of homology with the antigenic determinant (Hurn and Landon, 1971).

In the case of angiotensin radioimmunoassays, the customary verification of assay results is complicated by several factors mentioned in preceding sections. The antisera are seldom strictly specific; the samples usually contain the principal cross-reactants, i.e., nonapetide, heptapeptide, and hexapeptide congeners; samples such as plasma may continue to produce and/or destroy antigen during the assay; the samples frequently contain material that affects the assay by interfering with the antigen–antibody reaction or binding of angiotensins itself; and the labeled antigen may contain labeled cross-reacting congeners.

One problem observed by many investigators using radioimmunoassay to measure labile substances has recently returned to plague the angiotensin field, i.e., systems that degrade labeled antigen can masquerade as unlabeled antigen. Morris and Johnston (1977) and Reid *et al.* (1977) showed that substances purported to be immunoreactive angiotensin were, in fact, one or more enzymes that attacked labeled peptides. Proteolysis can reduce the fraction of radioactivity bound to antibody just as unlabeled antigen can. This shows the need to verify immunoassay results with some other analytic tool, such as bioassay, chromatography, or at least a modification of the radioimmunoassay procedure, that permits proof that both bound and free labeled antigens remain intact during the entire assay procedure.

Several approaches have been used to avoid the difficulties enumerated above and others inherent in angiotensin assays. Angiotensin has been extracted from the sample before assay by a variety of procedures to eliminate the problem of interfering substances. This is a more economical method than one that uses a duplicate sample for the standard curve. McBride *et al.* (1971) provided evidence that the best extraction procedure used Fuller's Earth. However, these extractions do not discriminate among the immunoreactive and biologically active congeners, such as des^1-angiotensin II (Dusterdieck and McElwee, 1971). Furthermore, the adsorbent may extract interfering substances other than angiotensins (Katz and Smith, 1972). Cain and Catt (1969), Pernottet and co-workers (1972), and Semple and Morton (1976) described chromatographic procedures for separation and purification of angiotensin congeners. By such a procedure, Pernottet and co-workers (1972) defined the normal arterial plasma level of angiotensin II octapeptide as 11.2 ± 3.4 pg/ml. These values are lower than those reported by others who omitted steps to separate the congeners.

Experience with other radioimmunoassays indicates that the problems resulting from cross-reactivity and interference will diminish as more sensitive and specific antisera are produced (Hunter, 1971). At the present time, several antisera are available that can detect 10 pg of angiotensin I and 3.0 pg of angiotensin II or des^1-angiotensin II heptapeptide. Table II reviewed the range of specificities available in several laboratories. Development of better antisera will not obviate the need for adequate standards and attention to species differences in angiotensins (Hollemans, 1970).

IV. COMMERCIAL KITS AND CONCLUDING COMMENTS

Kits for the measurement of renin are distributed by several companies. All are designed to measure angiotensin I by radioimmunoassay. New England Nuclear, Boston, Massachusetts, produces a kit containing labeled monoiodoangiotensin I prepared by the method of Nielsen *et al.* (1971) and a separation step for terminating the radioimmunoassay by charcoal adsorption. It includes a buffer that fixes the pH of the enzyme incubation step at 6.0. Mallinckrodt Nuclear, St. Louis, Missouri, produces a kit in which the separation step of the radioimmunoassay uses a strip of solid ion-exchange resin. The kit from Clinical Assays, Cambridge, Massachusetts, uses antibody adsorbed to test tubes so that the separation step at the end of the assay is the ultimate in convenience, i.e., simple decantation. Other kit manufacturers are Pharmacia Laboratories, Piscataway, New Jersey; Schwarz-Mann, Orangeburg, New York; and E. R. Squibb, Inc., Princeton, New Jersey.

None of the kits includes reagents necessary to measure renin concentration, i.e., internal renin standard or exogenous substrate. However, all are suitable for clinical renin measurements aimed at screening peripheral blood for very low renin levels, as are found in primary aldosteronism, or relatively high renin levels, as are found in renal venous blood from cases of unilateral renal artery stenosis. Regardless of the source of reagents, variation and deterioration of standards, labeled antigens, and antisera make it imperative to measure renin and angiotensin standards with each group of unknown samples.

A novel approach for the measurement of renin activity has been suggested by Ontjes et al. (1972). A radiolabeled synthetic renin substrate analog was covalently coupled to an insoluble matrix, and renin activity was determined following incubation by measuring the generation of radiolabeled product in the supernatant. The method, however, was not sufficiently sensitive to measure renin activity in plasma. Since that report, two kinds of labeled natural substrate have been used in analogous fashion. Lentz et al. (1976) utilized ^{14}C-carbamyl hog substrate. Campbell and Skinner (1975) iodinated sheep substrate and were able to measure plasma renin levels with it. Renin substrate was purified from heparinized plasma of six-day-nephrectomized sheep. One hundred milliliters of plasma was dialyzed at 4°C for 18 hours against five liters of 0.02 M phosphate buffer, pH 7.5, and was applied to a 2.5 × 100 cm column of DEAE-Sephadex A50 equilibrated with the same buffer. The substrate was eluted in the same buffer with a linear gradient from 0(500 ml) to 0.5 M NaCl (500 ml) and emerged as a single smooth peak between 0.10 M and 0.15 M NaCl. The eluate was concentrated by ultrafiltration, dialyzed at 4°C for 18 hours against five liters of 0.02 M phosphate buffer, pH 7.5, and chromatographed at 4°C over a 2.5 × 100 cm column of Sephadex G-100 in the same buffer. Ten-milliliter fractions were collected, and the sheep substrate appeared in fractions 21–30 and was stored frozen at −10°C.

One milliliter of the purified sheep renin substrate containing 4.5 nmole angiotensin II and 730 mg protein was iodinated by incubation with 1.0 mCi ^{125}I in 0.2 ml water, 0.1 ml 1.0 M Tris–HCl buffer, pH 8.6, and 0.1 ml 61 mM chloramine-T. After agitating for 60 seconds at room temperature, the reaction was terminated by the addition of 0.2 ml 88 mM sodium metabisulfite, followed by 0.3 ml 0.6 M KI and 4.0 ml cold sheep renin substrate. Unreacted iodide was removed by dialysis against six changes of 0.1 M phosphate buffer, pH 7.5, containing 0.075 M NaCl, and 1 mM EDTA for 28 hours at 0°C. The iodinated substrate was further diluted with cold sheep substrate to a specific activity of 2000–5000 counts per second/nmole angiotensin II and frozen at −10°C.

For the measurement of plasma renin concentrations, 0.05 ml ^{125}I-labeled sheep substrate (2000–5000 cps) was incubated for 30 minutes at 37°C with 0.45 ml of either unknown plasmas or renin standards (0–1000 μIU/ml) and rapidly cooled to 0°C. Plasma was previously acidified by dialysis at 32°C to pH 3.3 to activate inactive renin and then dialyzed against 0.1 M phosphate, 0.075 M NaCl, 1.0 mM EDTA, pH 7.5, prior to assay.

Angiotensin II, generated during the incubation, was absorbed by the addition of 2.0 ml coated charcoal at 0°C. The tubes were immediately centrifuged at 1000 g for three minutes, the supernatants discarded, and the charcoal pellets washed twice with 3.0 ml 0.1 M phosphate, 0.075 M NaCl, 1.0 mM EDTA, pH 7.5, and counted. The coated charcoal was prepared by incubating 0.5 gm Norit A charcoal with 100 ml 32 mg/100 ml human γ-globulin for 24 hours. The charcoal suspension was then centrifuged, the supernatant was discarded, and the charcoal was resuspended in 100 ml 10 mg/ml BSA.

The quantity of ^{125}I-angiotensin II generated was shown to be linearly related to renin concentration. This approach, although not currently employed in the authors' laboratories, holds great promise for simplifying renin assays. It would completely eliminate all problems related to radioimmunoassay. Then, the irreducible problems related to patient and sample preparation, prorenins, and renin modulators in plasma would be the only obstacles to an ideal assay.

ACKNOWLEDGMENTS

The authors wish to thank Mr. Dennis Ball for his assistance in preparing this manuscript, and the Medical Research Council, United Kingdom, for supplying us with angiotensin and renin standards. Work supported in part by the Medical Research Services of the Veterans Administration.

REFERENCES

Boyd, G. W., and Peart, W. S., (1968). The production of high-titre antibody against free angiotensin II. *Lancet* **2**, 129–133.

Boyd, G. W., Landon, J., and Peart, W. S. (1967). Radioimmunoassay for determining plasma-levels of angiotensin II in man. *Lancet* **2**, 1002–1005.

Cain, M. D., and Catt, K. J. (1969). Chromatography and radioimmunoassay of angiotensin II and metabolites in blood. *Biochim. Biophys. Acta* **194**, 322–324.

Cain, M. D., Coghlan, J. P., and Catt, K. J. (1972). Measurement of angiotensin II in blood by radioimmunoassay. *Clin. Chim. Acta* **39**, 21–34.

Campbell, D. J., and Skinner, S. L. (1975). Measurement of renin concentration in human plasma using ^{125}I-labelled sheep renin substrate. *Clin. Chim. Acta* **65**, 361–370.

Davis, J. O., and Freeman, R. H. (1976). Mechanisms regulating renin release. *Physiol. Rev.* **56**, 1–44.

Day, R. P., and Reid, I. A. (1976). Renin activity in dog brain: Enzymological similarity to Cathepsin D. *Endocrinology* **99**, 93–100.

Dusterdieck, G., and McElwee, G. (1971). Estimation of angiotensin II concentration in human plasma by radioimmunoassay. Some applications to physiological and clinical states. *Eur. J. Clin. Invest.* **2**, 32–38.

Freedlender, A. E. (1969). Practical and theoretical advantages for the use of ^{125}I in radioimmunoassay. *Proteins Polypeptide Horm., Proc. Int. Symp., 1968* pp. 351–353.

Goodfriend, T. L. (1969). Radioimmunoassay for bradykinin and angiotensin. *Protein Polypeptide Horm., Proc. Int. Symp., 1968* pp. 91–92.

Goodfriend, T. L., Levine, L., and Fasman, G. D. (1964). Antibodies to bradykinin and angiotensin: A use of carbodiimides in immunology. *Science* **144**, 1344–1346.

Goodfriend, T. L., Ball, D. L., and Farley, D. B. (1968). Radioimmunoassay of angiotensin. *J. Lab. Clin. Med.* **72**, 648–662.

Goodfriend, T. L., Sindel, M., Fyhrquist, F., Hong, R., Azen, E., and Stewart, J. M. (1976). Peptide-binding macromolecules in the blood of seriously ill or mentally retarded patients. *J. Lab. Clin. Med.* **87**, 299–319.

Greenwood, F. C., Hunter, W. M., and Glover, J. S. (1963). The preparation of ^{131}I-labelled human growth hormone of high specific activity. *Biochem. J.* **89**, 114–123.

Haas, E., and Goldblatt, H. (1972). Indirect assay of plasma renin. *Lancet* **1**, 1330–1332.

Haber, E., Koerner, T., Page, L. B., Kliman, B., and Purnode, A. (1969). Application of a radioimmunoassay for angiotensin I to the physiologic measurement of plasma renin activity in normal human subjects. *J. Clin. Endocrinol. Metab.* **29**, 1349–1355.

Herbert, V., Lau, K. S., Gottlieb, C. W., and Bleicher, S. J. (1965). Coated charcoal immunoassay of insulin. *J. Clin. Endocrinol. Metab.* **25**, 1375–1384.

Hollemans, H. J. G. (1970). Proposition for an international angiotensin standard for renin measurement in human plasma. *Clin. Chim. Acta* **27**, 99–103.

Horvath, J. S., Baxter, C. R., Sherbon, K., Smee, I., Roche, J., Uther, J. B., and Tiller, D. J. (1977). An analysis of errors found in renal vein sampling for plasma renin activity. *Kidney Int.* **11**, 136–138.

Hunter, W. M. (1966). Iodination of protein compounds. *In* "Radioactive Pharmaceuticals" (G. A. Andrews, R. M. Kniseley, and H. N. Wagner, eds.), pp. 245–264. At. Energy Comm., Oak Ridge, Tennessee.

Hunter, W. M. (1971). The preparation and assessment of iodinated antigens. *In* "Radioimmunoassay Methods" (K. E. Kirkham and W. M. Hunter, eds.), pp. 3–22. Churchill, London.

Hurn, B. A. L., and Landon, J. (1971). Antisera for radioimmunoassay. *In* "Radioimmunoassay Methods" (K. E. Kirkham and W. M. Hunter, eds.), pp. 121–142. Churchill, London.

Katz, F. H., and Smith, J. A. (1972). Radioimmunoassay of angiotensin I: Comparison of two renin activity methods and use for other measurements of the renin system. *Clin. Chem.* **18**, 528–533.

Kodish, M. E., and Katz, F. H. (1974). Plasma renin concentration: Comparison of angiotensinase inhibitors and correlation with plasma renin activity and aldosterone. *J. Lab. Clin. Med.* **83**, 705–715.

Lentz, K. E., Skeggs, L. T., Dorer, F. E., Kahn, J. R., and Levine, M. (1976). A new radiolabeled protein renin substrate. *Anal. Biochem.* **74**, 1–11.

Lin, S., Ellis, H., Weisblum, B., and Goodfriend, T. L. (1970). Preparation and properties of iodinated angiotensins. *Biochem. Pharmacol.* **19**, 651–662.

Lumbers, E. R. (1971). Activation of renin in human amniotic fluid by low pH. *Enzymologia* **40**, 329–336.

McBride, J. W., Overturf, M., and Fitz, A. (1971). Extraction and recovery of angiotensin II from plasma. *Anal. Biochem.* **42**, 29–37.

Malling, C., and Poulsen, K. (1977). A direct radioimmunoassay for plasma renin in mice and its evaluation. *Biochim. Biophys. Acta* **491**, 532–541.

Michelakis, A. M., Yoshida, H., Menzie, J., Murakami, K., and Inagami, T. (1974). A radioimmunoassay for the direct measurement of renin in mice and its application to submaxillary gland and kidney studies. *Endocrinology* **94**, 1101–1105.

Morris, B. J., and Johnston, C. I. (1977). Identification of "angiotensin immunoreactive material" in rat kidney. *Endocrinology* **100**, 1409–1417.

Nielsen, M. D., Jorgensen, M., and Giese, J. (1971). ^{125}I-labelling of angiotensin I and II. *Acta Endocrinol. (Copenhagen)* **67**, 104–116.

Ontjes, D. A., Majstoravich, J., Jr., and Roberts, J. C. (1972). Radiochemical assay for renin using a synthetic insoluble substrate. *Anal. Biochem.* **45**, 374–386.

Oparil, S., Koerner, T. J., and Haber, E. (1974). Effects of pH and enzyme inhibitors on apparent generation of angiotensin I in human plasma. *J. Clin. Endocrinol. Metab.* **39**, 965–968.

Page, L. B., Desaulles, E., Lagg, S., and Haber, E. (1971). Interference with immunoassays of angiotensin I and II by proteins in human plasma. *Clin. Chim. Acta* **34**, 55–62.

Peach, M. (1977). Renin–angiotensin system. *Physiol. Rev.* **57**, 313–370.

Pernottet, M. G., Angels D'Auriac, G., and Meyer, P. (1972). Improved technique for radioimmunoassay of angiotensin II in plasma. *Rev. Eur. Etud. Clin. Biol.* **17**, 111–113.

Reid, I. A., Day, R. P., Moffat, B., and Hughes, H. G. (1977). Apparent angiotensin immunoreactivity in dog brain resulting from angiotensinase. *J. Neurochem.* **28**, 435–438.

Sealey, J. E., Moon, C., Laragh, J. H., and Atlas, S. A. (1977). Plasma prorenin in normal hypertensive, and anephric subjects and its effects on renin measurements. *Circ. Res.* **40**, 41–45.

Semple, P. F., and Morton, J. J. (1976). Angiotensin II and angiotensin III in rat blood. *Circ. Res.* **38**, Suppl. 11, 122–126.

de Senarclens, C. F., Pricam, C. E., Banichaki, F. D., and Vallaton, M. B. (1977). Renin synthesis, storage, and release in the rat: A morphological and biochemical study. *Kidney Int.* **11**, 161–169.

Skeggs, L. T., Lentz, K. E., Kahn, J. R., Dorer, F. E., and Levine, M. (1969). Pseudo-renin—A new angiotensin-forming enzyme. *Circ. Res.* **25**, 451–462.

Skinner, S. L. (1967). Improved assay methods for renin "concentration" and "activity" in human plasma. *Circ. Res.* **20**, 391–402.

Skinner, S. L., Dunn, J. R., Mazzetti, J., Campbell, D. J., and Fidge, N. H. (1975). Purification, properties and kinetics of sheep and human renin substrates. *Aust. J. Exp. Biol. Med. Sci.* **53**, 77–88.

Stason, W. B., Vallotton, M., and Haber, E. (1967). Synthesis of an antigenic copolymer of angiotensin and succinylated poly-L-lysine. *Biochim. Biophys. Acta* **133**, 582–584.

Stockigt, J. R., Collins, R. D., and Biglieri, E. G. (1971). Determination of plasma renin concentration by angiotensin I immunoassay. *Circ. Res.* **28, 29**, Suppl. II, 175–191.

Strong, C. G., Hunt, J. C., Sheps, S. G., Tucker, R. M., and Bernatz, P. E. (1971). Renal venous renin activity: Enhancement of sensitivity of lateralization by sodium depletion. *Am. J. Cardiol.* **27**, 602–611.

Waxman, S., Goodfriend, T. L., and Herbert, V. (1967). Angiotensin assay and assessment of free iodide contamination using dilute coated charcoal. *Clin. Res.* **15**, 457.

Weinberger, M. H., Rosner, D. R., Kem, D. C., Joyner, L., and Foust, G. (1972). Early morning variation in plasma renin activity in normal, recumbent humans. *Adv. Exp. Med. Biol.* **17**, 189–191.

46

Bradykinin

THEODORE L. GOODFRIEND AND
CHARLES E. ODYA

I. INTRODUCTION

Bradykinin is a polypeptide of nine amino acids formed by proteolysis of a circulating globulin. Cleavage of the precursor (kininogen) to produce bradykinin and other small peptides containing bradykinin can be effected by many enzymes, of which the best known is kallikrein. The system of proenzymes, enzymes, precursors, products, and enzyme inhibitors has been the subject of extensive work and speculation occasioned by the extreme potency of bradykinin and related kinins as smooth muscle stimulants and as possible mediators of inflammation (Erdös, 1970; Rocha e Silva, 1970). The polypeptides discussed below are listed in Table I.

Among the features of the kinin system that complicate its radioimmunoassay are (1) the weak immunogenicity of the polypeptides, (2) the absence of an easily labeled residue in the native kinins, necessitating the use of analogs which contain tyrosine or adducts which are

909

Methods of Hormone Radioimmunoassay, Second Edition
Copyright © 1979 by Academic Press, Inc.
All rights of reproduction in any form reserved. ISBN 0-12-379260-6

Table I   Amino Acid Sequences of Bradykinin and Analogs

	Residue No.								
	1	2	3	4	5	6	7	8	9
Bradykinin	NH$_2$-Arg-	Pro-	Pro-	Gly-	Phe-	Ser-	Pro-	Phe-	Arg -COOH
Kallidin	NH$_2$- Lys-	Arg-	Pro-	Pro-	Gly-	Phe-	Ser-	Pro-	Phe- Arg -COOH
Des^9-bradykinin	NH$_2$-Arg-	Pro-	Pro-	Gly-	Phe-	Ser-	Pro-	Phe-	COOH
Tyr^5-bradykinin	NH$_2$-Arg-	Pro-	Pro-	Gly-	Tyr-	Ser-	Pro-	Phe-	Arg -COOH
Tyr^8-bradykinin	NH$_2$-Arg-	Pro-	Pro-	Gly-	Phe-	Ser-	Pro-	Tyr-	Arg -COOH
Desaminotyrosyl-bradykinin	H- Tyr-	Arg-	Pro-	Pro-	Gly-	Phe-	Ser-	Pro-	Phe- Arg -COOH
Tyr^1-kallidin	NH$_2$- Tyr-	Arg-	Pro-	Pro-	Gly-	Phe-	Ser-	Pro-	Phe- Arg -COOH

easily iodinated but antigenically distinct from the endogenous polypeptides, (3) the immunologic similarity of congeners of bradykinin with significant biologic effects, such as the decapeptide kallidin, (4) the immunologic similarity of degradation products with very attenuated biologic activity, such as des^9-bradykinin, (5) the extreme susceptibility of the kinins to degradation by proteolytic enzymes found in biologic fluids, (6) the possible formation of kinins by enzymes acting on precursors in the samples and antisera used as reagents, and (7) the problem common to many biologically active polypeptides—the tendency to adsorb to surfaces presented by test tubes, pipettes, clots, cells, and precipitates.

II. RADIOIMMUNOASSAY METHODOLOGY

A. Preparation of Samples

The goal of methods used to prepare samples is the instantaneous total inhibition of all enzymes which might form or destroy bradykinin or its congeners without permanently sequestering or adsorbing the kinin in the sample. The method chosen will depend on the amount and nature of contaminating enzymes. The most troublesome common sample is blood, which not only contains enzymes and kininogens but also cells that take time to centrifuge at a temperature above 0°C and

protein in a quantity large enough to adsorb polypeptide when precipitating reagents are added. The magnitude of the problem in preparing blood for measurement is indicated by the estimated half-life of
bradykinin in blood—less than one minute. Secretions of digestive
organs may be even more troublesome. Cerebrospinal and synovial
fluids are simpler.

One approach to instantaneous preservation of polypeptide is de-
liberate adsorption by resins or particles from which the compound
can be eluted after enzymes and cells have been washed away. The
kinin is protected from degradation while adsorbed, but this procedure does not prevent simultaneous formation or liberation of new
kinins from precursors in the sample.

Figure 1 presents a flow diagram incorporating many of the suggestions made by investigators who have measured bradykinin. Proce-

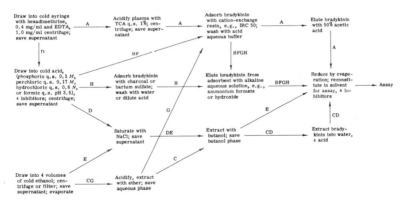

Figure 1. Composite flow diagram of sample preparation for the assay of bradykinin.
The various steps are those used by the authors listed below, and the lettered lines
indicate the sequence of steps each author recommends. For precise directions the
references should be consulted because different authors emphasize certain aspects of
methodology. This diagram indicates no attempt to assess the preferred sequence for a
given sample. As mentioned in the text, we urge that any sequence be controlled by
measurement of recovery and artifactual kinin generation. Reference A exemplifies this
type of approach. Key to references: (A) Talamo *et al.*, 1969; (B) Webster and Gilmore,
1965; (C) Binia *et al.*, 1963; (D) Abe *et al.*, 1966; (E) Brocklehurst and Zeitlin, 1967; (F)
Melmon *et al.*, 1968; (G) Oates *et al.*, 1964; (H) T. L. Goodfriend and S. Palmer, unpublished observations.

dure A has been thoroughly tested, but has the disadvantage of including a centrifugation step to remove blood cells before addition of acid. Drawing blood directly into acid prevents enzyme action during the first centrifugation step, but the acid added to whole blood would be more effective if it dissolved protein instead of precipitating it. Formic acid has this advantage. Otherwise, a gross clot of cells and protein results. We have used charcoal to adsorb bradykinin from formic acid-treated blood, because ion-exchange resins do not retrieve bradykinin as well from formic acid-treated solution. We have occasionally used barium sulfate (Barimex) as an adsorbent because it is commonly administered to humans for gastrointestinal tract radiography and would enable a "chemical biopsy" of digestive fluids at the same time.

The ability of blood precipitates to adsorb bradykinin was clearly demonstrated by Mashford and Roberts (1972), who showed that the simple use of room temperature ethanol instead of chilled ethanol resulted in a precipitate of blood that did not adsorb added bradykinin. By contrast, the precipitate with chilled ethanol adsorbed at least 40% of added polypeptide.

Individual needs will determine the particular path of sample preparation chosen from Figure 1. We recommend editing and selecting from the alternatives presented in the figure. For example, it is clear from the results of Talamo *et al.* (1969) that surface contact with glass or resin can generate large quantities of bradykinin in raw plasma, despite rapid inactivation of enzymes with ethanol. Therefore, the use of ethanol requires measures to prevent activation of kallikrein. Mashford and Roberts (1972) collect blood in a syringe containing 1,10-phenanthroline to prevent kininase activation during subsequent ethanol precipitation. It is also mandatory to use unreactive surfaces, such as siliconized glass or plastic, to prevent enzyme activation in protein-rich solutions and to add proteins to prevent adsorption from protein-poor solutions. Siliconized surfaces may have prevented kallikrein activation in experiments with ethanol by Mashford and Roberts (1972).

It is also advisable to perform pilot experiments to determine recovery under specified circumstances. This need is accentuated by the differences among samples, not only between blood and spinal fluid, for example, but between blood from healthy donors and that from patients with active pancreatitis or other diseases which result in elevated plasma enzymes. The best control of variables in the sample preparation is the routine addition of a trace of labeled bradykinin to the sample before it is handled in any way. The label used to monitor recovery should be distinct from that used in the final assay. For example, tritiated bradykinin could be added to the crude sample without interfering with a radioimmunoassay using [125]I.

Considering all of the problems mentioned above, we recommend the procedure of Mashford and Roberts (1972) for preparation of blood specimens, primarily because it results in the lowest reported normal values for blood bradykinin, and because it includes a short time interval between venesection and complete enzyme inactivation with ethanol. Improved enzyme inhibitors and better antisera may eventually eliminate the extraction step and enable a simple one-step procedure.

Procedure

1. Blood is drawn rapidly through a siliconized Teflon catheter into a chilled plastic syringe containing 0.05 ml 0.5 M 1,10-phenanthroline in 25% ethanol for each 5.0 ml of blood.

2. The syringe containing blood is immediately emptied into four volumes of room temperature ethanol contained in a siliconized centrifuge tube.

3. The blood–ethanol mixture is centrifuged at 2500 g for 15 minutes in a refrigerated centrifuge.

4. The supernatant and two washes of the pellet with 75% ethanol are decanted into a siliconized vessel suitable for evaporation, and the ethanol is removed under vacuum at 40°C. Octanol (0.5 ml) prevents frothing during this procedure.

5. The aqueous residue of approximately 2.0 ml can be cleared of lipid by acidification with 5.0 ml of 0.01 M HCl and washing with ether.

6. The residual aqueous solution is dried for storage, then reconstituted for assay in 0.1 M Tris buffer, pH 7.4, containing 0.2% gelatin, or 0.01% casein, 0.1% neomycin, and 0.01 M EDTA.

B. Antisera

1. Immunogen

Successful immunization of animals to bradykinin has been reported only when the nonapeptide was injected as a complex with a larger carrier protein or in the kininogen form (Webster *et al.*, 1970). Although rabbits, sheep, goats, and monkeys have been immunized with complexes of bradykinin and a variety of carriers, or in the kininogen form, Talamo and co-workers (1969) presented evidence that the best carrier was ovalbumin. On the other hand, Skowsky and

Fisher (1972) suggested the use of thyroglobulin as a carrier for small polypeptides.

Several immunization procedures have been suggested. None appears to be incompatible with the simultaneous use of another. The objective is at least one useful antiserum. Therefore, we recently combined two procedures with good results. We immunized with a mixture of complexes, coupling bradykinin to both ovalbumin and thyroglobulin using two sequential coupling reagents, and obtained satisfactory antisera in eight of ten rabbits. By our definition, a satisfactory antiserum binds 3.0 pg of the 10 pg of labeled kinin added at an antiserum dilution of 1 : 100. The best antiserum we have obtained bound 3.0 pg of ^{125}I-Tyr^5-bradykinin at an antiserum dilution of 1 : 76,000.

The method of coupling was to dissolve 5.0 mg bradykinin and 4.5 mg ovalbumin or 3.5 mg thyroglobulin in 0.5 ml water, then add 50 mg 1-ethyl-3-(3-dimethylaminopropyl)-carbodiimide (Ott Chemical Company), allow to react at room temperature for 16 hours, then add 0.2 ml 4% glutaraldehyde, allow to react for 16 hours, then dialyze against two liters of water with two changes over 48 hours.

2. Schedule and Route of Administration

The dialyzed complexes were combined and emulsified with an equal volume of complete Freund's adjuvant. Some authors reenforce the adjuvant with an additional 10 mg of killed acid-fast bacilli. One milliliter of antigen–adjuvant emulsion, containing approximately 2.0 mg bradykinin–protein complex, was injected subcutaneously into the hind toe pads of rabbits from four different strains. Three weeks later, an equal dose of the same mixture was injected into a different subcutaneous site. When the attained titers began to fall, roughly six weeks later, the booster injections were repeated.

Eisen and Siskind (1964) showed with a model hapten that antibody affinity increased with time after primary immunization, especially when the immunizing dose was small. Fujio and Karush (1966) found that a long delay between the first and subsequent challenges also resulted in higher affinity antibodies. Vaitukaitis and co-workers (1971) showed that injection of relatively small quantities of immunizing antigen into multiple intradermal sites was effective and economical in producing high affinity antisera to haptens. In the light of these suggestions, it may be profitable to use small immunizing doses divided among many subcutaneous sites, then wait longer than three weeks before boosting. It is also our impression that much is to be gained by immunizing many rabbits of diverse strains and holding only the more promising animals after the results of one booster injection are known.

3. Treatment of Antisera

Antibody, the necessary reagent for radioimmunoassay, is delivered by the immunized animal in plasma contaminated with enzymes, bradykinin precursors, and fragments. The same is true of anti-antibody used in double antibody separation steps. Unless it can be diluted adequately, antiserum itself will interfere with radioimmunoassay. We treat the antiserum at 60°C for 30 minutes to reduce enzyme activity and add enzyme inhibitors to the final assay mixture (see below).

C. Labeled Antigen

The usefulness of a radioactive antigen is increased when labeled with an isotope of high specific activity and easy detection, and is decreased when significant structural differences between the labeled and the sample antigens occur. In the case of bradykinin, substitution with ^{14}C or tritium alters the antigen very little, but results in relatively low specific activity. Iodine isotopes have high activity, but a method for iodination of the unmodified polypeptide is not known. All modifications that enable the use of radioactive iodine result in significant alteration of the antigen's structure. We have found it advisable, therefore, to test each promising antiserum with a variety of labeled bradykinin analogs to find the best combination.

Synthesis of a complex containing native bradykinin coupled to an iodinatable residue is readily accomplished (Goodfriend and Ball, 1969). An active ester of deaminotyrosine, the p-nitrophenyl ester of p-hydroxyphenylpyruvic acid (ONP ester, Cyclo Chemical), will couple to the α-amino group of bradykinin. Our procedure has been to add 12 mg of the active ester to 3.0 mg bradykinin in 0.5 ml dimethylformamide. After 18 hours at 40°C, the derivative decapeptide was partly purified by adding 2.0 ml water and extracting unreacted reagents with chloroform–ethyl ether (1:1). The polypeptide was purified further by paper chromatography developed with n-butanol–acetic acid–pyridine–water (135:33:10:22). The product has an R_f of 0.7. The Tyr^8 analog of bradykinin can be obtained commercially, (e.g., Bachem, Inc., Torrance, California). The analogs mentioned in this chapter are listed in Table I.

Derivatives of bradykinin or kallidin that contain tyrosine can be iodinated easily according to standard techniques, such as that using chloramine-T. To 2.0 mCi of ^{125}I is added 2.0 ml of 0.05 M sodium phosphate buffer, pH 7.5, and 100 μg of kinin analog. The mixture is stirred in an ice bath. Chloramine-T, freshly prepared, is added drop-wise, 0.5 ml of a solution containing 50 μg/ml. After ten minutes of stirring, freshly prepared sodium metabisulfite is added, 0.5 ml of a solution containing 50 μg/ml. After ten minutes, the mixture is ready for purification.

The maximum specific activity obtained when one carrier-free ^{125}I atom combines with one mole of polypeptide is 2.0 Ci per μmole. The products of most iodination procedures are unreacted iodide, polypeptide, and monoiodinated and diiodinated polypeptide. Diiodinated analogs of kinin are much less reactive with antibodies than are the monoiodinated derivatives. Therefore, the diiodinated products as well as the unreacted peptide and iodide should be removed from the monoiodinated derivative to maximize the value of the labeled kinin.

Purification of monoiodinated kinin is achieved by column chromatography on a 1.0 × 35 cm column of CM-Sephadex C-25 equilibrated and eluted with 0.05 M ammonium acetate, pH 8.0. The radioactive fractions eluted are free iodide, occasionally some acidic material of unknown composition, diiodinated analog, and finally monoiodinated kinin analog. The unreacted polypeptide elutes after the iodinated derivatives. This elution may consume 750 ml buffer with a column of the stated dimensions.

We have observed rapid deterioration of iodinated Tyr[8]-bradykinin at room temperature. Therefore, the labeled material is divided into aliquots and stored at −70°C. We have also observed that a solution suggested by Freedlender (see Chapter 45) retards deterioration of the labeled polypeptide. It contains 0.8 M glycine, 0.2 M sodium chloride, 0.05 M potassium phosphate, pH 7.5, and 0.25% bovine albumin. This solution is used to dilute stocks of radioactive bradykinin before dividing and freezing aliquots.

D. Incubation Conditions

The procedures described below concern primarily those assays using ^{125}I-labeled derivatives of bradykinin reacting with rabbit antibody. The test tubes that fit radiation counters are most convenient for the assay itself, but frequently are made of plastic that is highly adsorptive of labeled bradykinin (and presumably unlabeled bradykinin). In general, soft plastic, such as cellulose nitrate, is less adsorptive than rigid plastic or glass. The adsorption of labeled bradykinin is sensitive to the presence of polypeptides, including bradykinin itself. It is possible, therefore, to obtain a convincing but false standard curve simply by adding bradykinin in increasing amounts to a constant amount of labeled polypeptide, and incubating in tubes either in the absence of other protein or without prior coating of the tubes.

To prevent adsorption of kinin to test tubes and pipettes, we coat glassware in advance with a solution of 0.1% casein or 0.05% albumin for 16 hours at 4°C. Talamo *et al.* (1969) used 0.1% lysozyme (muramidase). The proteins are seldom supplied free of proteolytic enzymes, so they should be treated at 60°C for 20 minutes (albumin) or autoclaved and filtered (casein) before use. An alternative procedure is the addition of a similar concentration of protein to the incubation buffer itself. Glassware may also be siliconized as an added precaution. Pipettes should be rinsed with the solution to be delivered by filling and emptying a few times before dispensing the first aliquots.

The incubation of labeled antigen, antiserum, and unknown is carried out at 4°C for 2 to 24 hours. In one experiment, we found that the amount of labeled bradykinin bound to antibody after two hours was 80% of the amount that bound in 24 hours, and the standard curves of unlabeled bradykinin were identical at the two times. Considering the problems caused by degradation and adsorption, these results suggest that short incubation times are preferable.

We incubate the assay mixture in a solution of 0.01 M sodium phosphate buffer, pH 7, that contains 0.01% casein and 0.01 M 1,10-phenanthroline. One of our antisera bound more of a trace amount of labeled bradykinin at pH 8.2 than at 7.2, but since other laboratories have used buffers at more neutral pH, we presume the optimum conditions differ among antisera. The effect of pH on nonspecific binding is also considerable and should be tested in each system and each type of tube.

The considerations that dictate addition of enzyme inhibitors to fresh blood also apply to their use in assay mixtures which contain antiserum or active enzymes that remain in the sample. However, it must be established that the inhibitor does not so reduce the antigen–antibody reaction that the assay becomes impractical. Table II lists the enzyme inhibitors recommended for inhibition of plasma kininases and kallikrein and the effects of these on one antigen–antibody reaction we have tested. We now use 0.01 M 1,10-phenanthroline as an additive in our standard buffer. It increases the amount of labeled hormone bound by one antiserum without increasing the nonspecific binding. Others have found it the best inhibitor of kininases. We suspect that the addition of this or superior reagents will become routine

Table II   Inhibitors of Plasma Kininases and Kallikrein

Reagents[a]	Concentration (M)	Effect on one antigen–antibody reaction[b]	Reference
Dimercaprol (BAL)	2×10^{-3}	+++	Ferreira and Rocha e Silva (1962)
1,10-Phenanthroline	10^{-3}	+	Erdös and Sloane (1962)
EDTA	3×10^{-3}	−	Erdös and Sloane (1962)
8-Hydroxyquinoline	3×10^{-3}	−	Ferreira and Rocha e Silva (1962)
8-Hydroxyquinoline sulfonate	3×10^{-4}	n.t.	Erdös and Wohler (1963)
Bothrops polypeptide	2×10^{-6}	+	Ferreira (1965)
Tryspin inhibitor (soy bean)	0.1 mg/ml	−	Back and Steger (1968)
Trasylol	500 U/ml	±	Back and Steger (1968)
Hexadimethrine (polybrene)	1.6×10^{-1}	−	Armstrong and Stewart (1962)
EACA (ϵ-aminocaproic acid)	3×10^{-3}	+	Erdös and Sloane (1962)
Hydrocortisone	2×10^{-4}	n.t.	Dyrud *et al.* (1965)
Heavy metals (Cd, Hg, Mn)	10^{-3}	−	Erdös and Sloane (1962)
Arginine	3×10^{-3}	+	Erdös and Sloane (1962)
Phenylalanylarginine	10^{-2}	n.t.	Yang and Erdös (1967)
NH_2-Phe-Ser-Pro-Phe-Arg-COOH	10^{-4}	−	Garbe (1967)

[a] Kallikrein inhibitors are indicated by the asterisk.

[b] The + symbol indicates that the reagent increased the degree of antigen–antibody reaction, probably by preserving the labeled polypeptide. BAL was unusually effective (+++) in this respect. The − symbol indicates that the reagent decreased reactivity, probably by a direct effect on the antibody. n.t., Not tested.

in the future. It merits repetition that each antiserum and antigen combination may react differently to inhibitors. For example, some antisera have been known to require the presence of divalent cations and be inhibited by EDTA.

Our standard radioimmunoassay tubes contain a final volume of 0.5 ml. All reagents are diluted in 0.01 M sodium phosphate, pH 7, 0.01 M 1,10-phenanthroline, and 0.01% casein. The final mixture includes 0.2 ml of a dilution of labeled kinin containing 10,000 cpm radioactivity, 0.1 ml antiserum diluted 1 : 12,000 (final dilution 1 : 60,000), and 0.2 ml buffer, standard, (0.005–5.0 ng) or unknown. All tubes are repeated in triplicate. A tube containing buffer in place of antiserum is processed to determine the correction caused by coprecipitation or coadsorption.

The selection of labeled antigen is critical. We have found that each antiserum has a spectrum of specificity that cannot be predicted. Despite a common immunogen, some animals produce antibodies more avid for iodo-Tyr^1-kallidin, while others are more avid for iodo-Tyr^5- or iodo-Tyr^8-bradykinin. The antigen bound most avidly results in the best assay combination. This should be determined for each antiserum, if possible.

E. Separation Techniques

Examples of gentle procedures for separating antibody-bound labeled antigen from free antigen are precipitation of the antibody with anti-antibody (the double antibody procedure) or ammonium sulfate, and prior adsorption of antibody on solid phase supports such as the incubation tube itself. More disruptive procedures involve the use of undiluted charcoal suspensions or zirconyl phosphate gel at extremes of pH.

For routine tests of new antisera, new labeled hormone, or protein-poor unknown samples, we separate antibody-bound from free labeled hormone by adding 0.1 ml pooled rabbit serum, followed by a volume of chilled, neutral, saturated ammonium sulfate sufficient to achieve 50% saturation. If the sample is protein-rich, pooled rabbit serum is only added to standard and control tubes. This mixture is shaken briefly, allowed to stand two hours at 4°C, and centrifuged at 1000 g for 15 minutes in a refrigerated centrifuge. The supernatant is aspirated, the pellet resuspended in 2.0 ml cold half-saturated ammonium sulfate, centrifuged, and the precipitate counted in an automatic gamma ray detector.

The technique for double antibody precipitation is straightforward, and involves the addition of nonimmunized rabbit serum to give a total of 10 μl rabbit serum per tube, followed by the appropriate dilution of anti-antibody, such as sheep anti-rabbit γ-globulin. Because this procedure involves addition of two aliquots of serum in addition to the anti-bradykinin antiserum, it may introduce new kinin formation or degradation.

Charcoal suspensions, whether coated or not, can result in total adsorption of the labeled hormone when the hormone is bound weakly by antisera. However, coated charcoal can be made useful for termination of some assays using antisera of low avidity by diluting the charcoal and using very brief times of adsorption. The original suspension formulated by Herbert and co-workers (1965) was 2.5% charcoal coated with 0.25% dextran. The dilution used by Talamo et al. (1969) was 3 : 10, and for one of our antisera it was necessary to dilute the original charcoal 1 : 50.

In our charcoal procedure, a suspension containing the appropriate amount of charcoal is added in a volume five times as large as the original incubation mixture (i.e., 2.5 ml) to assure complete mixing during the addition, and the suspension is centrifuged in a refrigerated centrifuge at 1000 g within five minutes of the charcoal addition. Delays between addition and centrifugation have the same result as the use of excess charcoal, i.e., part of the antibody-bound label is adsorbed. Not only does the appropriate amount of charcoal vary with the specific antiserum but it also varies with the amount of protein in the final assay mixture. Therefore, no specific recommendation is possible.

Zirconyl phosphate gel, prepared according to the procedure of Hansen et al. (1966), can be used to separate bound and free labeled bradykinin. At pH 6.0, it adsorbs antibody and its bound label while leaving unbound bradykinin in solution.

III. VALIDATION AND STANDARDS

Synthetic bradykinin is available commercially (Beckman and Bachem). Standards of possible cross-reacting precursors or products are harder to obtain. It would be very important, however, to establish the degree of cross-reactivity of some of these more likely contaminants before stating assay results in terms of bradykinin nonapeptide. For example, untreated plasma contains far more kininogen than kinin, and kininogen binds to most bradykinin antisera. Even weak cross-reaction by this plentiful globulin would confuse assays for bradykinin. One degradation product, des[9]-bradykinin, reacts at least 5% as well with some antisera as does native bradykinin or kallidin (Fischer et al., 1969). With other antisera, des[9]-bradykinin reacts fully as well as bradykinin (M. E. Webster, personal communication). Yet both kininogen and des[9]-bradykinin are virtually inert biologically. Thus, some radioimmunoassays would overestimate kinin by virtue of inert cross-reactants.

Considering the multiple weak points in radioimmunoassays using antisera of low affinity, the construction of standard curves is subject to many artifacts. For example, it is likely that complex biologic fluids contain compounds that interfere with antigen–antibody reactions, such as cross-reacting polypeptides, detergent bile acids, or salts. In addition, there may be compounds that interfere with separation techniques based on adsorption of bound or free hormone. Macromolecules that bind bradykinin would increase the bound fraction of label, while polypeptides that adsorb to charcoal might decrease the free fraction. We have also observed an interaction of bradykinin with phospholipids such as lecithin. Variations in these materials would mimic variations in bradykinin. Therefore, standard curves in buffer could not be used for samples in plasma. Interfering substances would certainly be present in unextracted plasma or urine and might follow bradykinin through extraction or purification steps.

Validation of radioimmunoassay results is customarily performed by the use of multiple assays of a single sample in serial concentrations. The serial concentration curve should be compared with serial additions of bradykinin. If the two sets of data fall on the same curve, then the assay probably measures bradykinin alone. If the curves are different, then the unknown represents something other than pure bradykinin. For example, an unknown aliquot is estimated to contain 1.0 ng bradykinin, then addition of 1.0 ng pure bradykinin to this sample should have the same effect as the addition of another aliquot of sample. If the doubled unknown inhibits the antigen–antibody reaction more or less than the addition of 1.0 ng bradykinin, the unknown must contain something different from pure bradykinin. In other words, the curve of dilutions of sample and the curve of dilutions of standard should be parallel.

Problems caused by inhibitors of the antigen–antibody reaction will be minimized when more avid, more sensitive, and more specific antisera are available. Until then, the only way to ensure that a radioimmunoassay is measuring bradykinin itself is to confirm the result with bioassays of complementary specificity.

We are able to detect 20–200 pg of bradykinin in a final assay volume of 0.5 ml using antisera prepared in our laboratory and by others, when appropriate analogs labeled with ^{125}I are employed. Mashford and Roberts (1972) report a sensitivity of 25 pg. Our standard curves are most steep in the range between 0.1 and 1.0 ng/ml. This sensitivity is adequate to measure bradykinin if it circulates in a concentration of 0.2 to 3.0 ng/ml, but that concentration is ten times greater than levels of other potent plasma polypeptides, such as angiotensin. Judging by the history of other radioimmunoassays, it is to be anticipated that new antisera will be produced with sufficiently high affinities to enable measurements in lower ranges. Until then, the method is no more sensitive than standard bioassays using smooth muscle contraction and equally prone to interference, albeit from different types of substances (e.g., kininogen).

The constant feature of radioimmunoassay that recommends it for measurement of bradykinin is convenience. It is easy to set up protocols and runs that will measure fifty samples and standard curves in duplicate or triplicate, consuming only two days of one technician's time. The data can be retrieved directly from the radiation counter and transformed automatically by computer into gravimetric equivalents.

ACKNOWLEDGMENTS

The authors acknowledge the experimental data provided by Mr. Dennis Ball and Dr. Susan Palmer, which contributed to the conclusions drawn in the text of this chapter. Antisera were generously supplied by Dr. Marion Webster, National Heart Institute, Dr. Oscar Carretero, Henry Ford Hospital, Dr. Theodore Dalakos, SUNY Upstate Medical Center, and Dr. Rupert Perrin, Calbiochem. Samples of p-hydroxyphenylpyruvic acid ONP ester were supplied by Dr. Herman Plaut, Cyclo Chemical Corp. Bradykinin analogs were the gifts of Dr. Clara Peña, Dr. John Stewart, Dr. Eugen Schnabel, and Dr. Eberhard Schroder. The authors are indebted to Drs. Marion Webster and Richard Talamo for a careful review of the manuscript and many helpful suggestions. Supported by the Medical Research Service of the Veterans Administration, Research Grant No. HL-09922, from the National Heart, Lung and Blood Institute, and a grant from the Upjohn Company.

REFERENCES

Abe, K., Watanabe, N., Kumagai, N., Mouri, T., Seki, T., and Yoshinaga, K. (1966). Estimation of kinin in peripheral blood in man. *Tohoku J. Exp. Med.* **89,** 103–112.

Armstrong, D. A. J., and Stewart, J. W. (1962). Anti-heparin agents as inhibitors of plasma kinin formation. *Nature (London)* **194,** 689.

Back, N., and Steger, R. (1968). Effect of inhibitors on kinin-releasing activity of proteases. *Fed. Proc., Fed. Am. Soc. Exp. Biol.* **27,** 96–99.

Binia, A., Fasciolo, J. C., and Carretero, O. A. (1963). A method for the estimation of bradykinin in blood. *Acta Physiol. Lat. Am.* **13,** 101–109.

Brocklehurst, W. E., and Zeitlin, I. J. (1967). Determination of plasma kinin and kininogen levels in man. *J. Physiol. (London)* **191,** 417–426.

Dyrud, O. K., Rinvik, S. F., and Jensen, K. B. (1964). Effects of inhibitors on the *in vitro* inactivation of bradykinin by various kininases. *Acta Pharmacol. Toxicol.* **23,** 235–249.

Eisen, H. N., and Siskind, G. W. (1964). Variations in affinities of antibodies during the immune response. *Biochemistry* **3,** 996–1008.

Erdös, E. G. (1970). Bradykinin, kallidin, and kallikrein. *In* "Handbook of Experimental Pharmacology," Vol. 25. Springer-Verlag, Berlin.

Erdös, E. G., and Sloane, E. M. (1962). An enzyme in human blood plasma that inactivates bradykinin and kallidins. *Biochem. Pharmacol.* **11,** 585–592.

Erdös, E. G., and Wohler, J. R. (1963). Inhibition *in vivo* of the enzymatic inactivation of bradykinin and kallidin. *Biochem. Pharmacol.* **12,** 1193–1199.

Ferreira, S. H. (1965). A bradykinin-potentiating factor (BPF) present in the venom of *Bothrops jararaca. Br. J. Pharmacol. Chemother.* **24,** 163–169.

Ferreira, S. H., and Rocha e Silva, M. (1962). Potentiation of bradykinin by dimercaptopropanol (BAL) and other inhibitors of its destroying enzyme in plasma. *Biochem. Pharmacol.* **11**, 1123–1128.

Fischer, J., Spragg, J., Talamo, R. C., Pierce, J. V., Suzuki, K., Austen, K. F., and Haber, E. (1969). Structural requirements for binding of bradykinin to antibody. III. The effect of carrier on antibody specificity. *Biochemistry* **8**, 3750–3757.

Fujio, H., and Karush, F. (1966). Antibody affinity. II. Effect of immunization interval on antihapten antibody in the rabbit. *Biochemistry* **5**, 1856–1861.

Garbe, G. (1967). Quantitative kininogenbestimmung in menschlichem plasma. *Naunyn-Schmiedebergs Arch. Pharmakol. Exp. Pathol.* **256**, 112–118.

Goodfriend, T. L., and Ball, D. L. (1969). Radioimmunoassay of bradykinin: Chemical modification to enable use of radioactive iodine. *J. Lab. Clin. Med.* **73**, 501–511.

Hansen, H. J., Miller, O. N., and Tan, C. H. (1966). Assay of the autohumoral antibody that neutralizes the vitamin B_{12} combining site of intrinsic factor in serum from patients with pernicious anemia. *Am. J. Clin. Nutr.* **19**, 10–15.

Herbert, V., Lau, K. S., Gottlieb, C. W., and Bleicher, S. J. (1965). Coated charcoal immunoassay of insulin. *J. Clin. Endocrinol. Metab.* **25**, 1375–1380.

Mashford, M. L., and Roberts, M. L. (1972). Determination of blood kinin levels by radioimmunoassay. *Biochem. Pharmacol.* **21**, 2727–2735.

Melmon, K. L., Cline, M. J., Hughes, T., and Nies, A. S. (1968). Kinins: Possible mediators of neonatal circulatory changes in man. *J. Clin. Invest.* **47**, 1295–1302.

Oates, J. A., Gillespie, L., Mason, D. T., Melmon, K., and Sjoerdsma, A. (1964). Release of a kinin peptide in the carcinoid syndrome. *Lancet* **1**, 514–517.

Rocha e Silva, M. (1970). "Kinin Hormones." Thomas, Springfield, Illinois.

Skowsky, W. R., and Fisher, D. A. (1972). The use of the thyroglobulin to induce antigenicity to small molecules. *J. Lab. Clin. Med.* **80**, 134–144.

Talamo, R. C., Haber, E., and Austen, K. F. (1969). A radioimmunoassay for bradykinin in plasma and synovial fluid. *J. Lab. Clin. Med.* **74**, 816–827.

Vaitukaitis, J., Robbins, J. B., Nieschlag, E., and Ross, G. T. (1971). A method for producing specific antisera with small doses of immunogen. *J. Clin. Endocrinol. Metab.* **33**, 988–991.

Webster, M. E., and Gilmore, J. P. (1965). The estimation of the kallidins in blood and urine. *Biochem. Pharmacol.* **14**, 1161–1163.

Webster, M. E., Pierce, J. V., and Sampaio, M. U. (1970). Studies on antibody to bradykinin. *In* "Bradykinin and Related Kinins: Cardiovascular, Biochemical, and Neural Actions" (F. Sicuteri, M. Rocha e Silva, and N. Back, eds.), pp. 57–64. Plenum, New York.

Yang, H. Y. T., and Erdös, E. G. (1967). Second kininase in human blood plasma. *Nature (London)* **215**, 1402–1403.

GROWTH FACTORS

47

Urogastrone—Epidermal Growth Factor

HARRY GREGORY, JENNIFER E. HOLMES, AND
IAN R. WILLSHIRE

I. INTRODUCTION

The existence of urogastrone was derived from the observation that the incidence of peptic ulceration was low during pregnancy (Sandweiss *et al.*, 1938). Subsequently, it was shown that, in general, extracts of human urine caused inhibition of gastric acid secretion; it was also proposed that these extracts could induce ulcer healing by a direct effect upon gastric epithelium (Sandweiss, 1945). Only recently has highly purified urogastrone been obtained, and the structure has been shown to be that of a 53-residue polypeptide containing three internal disulfide bonds (Gregory, 1975). Part of the product was obtained as a 52-amino acid unit in which a C-terminal arginine was absent. The purified peptide causes inhibition of gastric acid secretion

927

Methods of Hormone Radioimmunoassay, Second Edition
Copyright © 1979 by Academic Press, Inc.
All rights of reproduction in any form reserved. ISBN 0-12-379260-6

Table I Structures of Urogastrone and Mouse Epidermal Growth Factor (mEGF)[a]

		10	20
mEGF	*Asn-Ser*-Tyr-Pro-Gly-*Cys*-Pro-Ser-Ser-Tyr-Asp-Gly-Tyr-*Cys*-Leu-Asn-Gly-Gly-Val-*Cys*-Met-His-Ile-Glu-
Urogastrone	*Asn-Ser*-Asp-Ser-Glu-*Cys*-Pro-Leu-Ser-His-Asp-Gly-Tyr-*Cys*-Leu-His-Asp-Gly-Val-*Cys*-Met-Tyr-Ile-Glu-

		30	40
mEGF	Ser-Leu-Asp-Ser-Tyr-Thr-*Cys*-Asn-*Cys*-Val-Ile-Gly-Tyr-Ser-Gly-Asp-Arg-*Cys*-Gln-Thr-Arg-Asp-Leu-Arg-
Urogastrone	Ala-Leu-Asp-Lys-Tyr-Ala-*Cys*-Asn-*Cys*-Val-Val-Gly-Tyr-Ile-Gly-Glu-Arg-*Cys*-Gln-Tyr-Arg-Asp-Leu-Lys-

		50
mEGF	*Trp-Trp-Glu-Leu-Arg*
Urogastrone	*Trp-Trp-Glu-Leu-Arg*

[a] Residues in italics occupy the same position in mEGF and urogastrone.

at doses of less than 0.25 μg/kg without affecting other secretions or functions, including respiration and blood pressure (Gerring *et al.*, 1974).

Mouse epidermal growth factor (mEGF), obtained from the sub-maxillary glands of male mice, was shown to affect epithelial proliferation in a variety of circumstances; the structure was also that of a 53-residue polypeptide (Savage *et al.*, 1972). In mEGF, which is also a potent inhibitor of gastric acid secretion (Bower *et al.*, 1975), 37 of the residues occupy the same relative positions as in urogastrone (Table I). Urogastrone has corresponding effects upon epidermal growth (Gregory, 1975). Finally the two peptides share a common receptor on human fibroblasts (Hollenberg and Gregory, 1977).

While the biologic actions of urogastrone are well established, its hormonal status as a human epithelial growth agent or a modulator in the control of gastric acid secretion remains uncertain. A radioimmunoassay was developed primarily to investigate further its role and origin in the body. Radioimmunoassay systems have been described for mEGF (Byyny *et al.*, 1972; Ances, 1973), and we also developed a system similar to that for urogastrone both as a control for human studies and to study the extent of cross-reaction in species other than the human or mouse.

II. METHODS OF RADIOIMMUNOASSAY

A. Source of Peptides

There is no simple commercial preparation of these peptides. By a complex process, pure urogastrone can be obtained from human urine in yields of approximately 1.0 mg per 1000 liter (Gregory and Willshire, 1975), and this is the major problem for wider application of the assay. mEGF is present to the extent of over 0.1% of the wet weight of the male mouse submaxillary gland, and a good isolation process has been described (Savage and Cohen, 1972).

The initial step in the purification of urogastrone is acidification of chloroform-saturated male urine with glacial acetic acid (2.0 ml/liter urine). Twenty milliliters of 25% aqueous tannic acid is added, and 60 minutes later, 1.0 gm/liter acid-washed Celite 545 is added and the precipitate is allowed to settle for 12 hours. The supernatant is aspirated and the residue is transferred to a glass funnel and washed successively with water and methanol until colorless. The dried residue is blended to a thick paste using 1% methanol in concentrated HCl, filtered, and washed until colorless. Four volumes of acetone are added; the precipitate is collected by centrifugation, washed twice with acetone, and dried *in vacuo*. This stage should provide 20–30 mg extract per liter of urine. Twenty grams of this extract are dissolved in water, titrated to pH 5–6 with concentrated ammonia, and diluted to two liters. This material is passed down a 2.8 × 35 cm column of De-Acidite G-1P resin, 3–5% DVP, 100–200 mesh (Permutit Co.) The product is eluted with 400 ml 50% aqueous acetic acid, lyophilized, and dissolved in water (pH 7–8). It is purified on a 2.8 × 100 cm column of Sephadex G-50 in 0.1 M NH_4HCO_3, flow rate 40 ml/hour. The eluates between 350 and 500 ml are pooled and lyophilized (1.5 gm). Six grams of extract is differentially extracted in *t*-butanol (150 ml), water (150 ml), and ammonium sulfate (30 gm) 4.0 × 30 ml and in isopropanol (300 ml), water (300 ml), and ammonium sulfate (60 gm) 3.0 × 30 ml. The isopropanol extracts are evaporated and lyophilized. The remaining steps in the purification are summarized in Table II.

mEGF is extracted by homogenizing submaxillary gland tissue in 0.05 M acetic acid (6 ml/gm) at 4°C for three minutes. The supernatant from a 30-minute 100,000 g centrifugation is collected by decanting through glass wool. The pellet is washed twice with 4.0 ml/gm of 0.0005 M acetic acid, and the supernatants are pooled and lyophilized. The residue is dissolved in 7 ml 1.0 N HCl and 18 ml 0.05 N HCl and chromatographed on a 5.0 × 90 cm reverse flow column of BioGel P-10, 200–400 mesh, HCl–NaCl buffer (0.05 N HCl containing 0.15 M NaCl), 5°C, 36-cm head pressure, 45–50 ml/hour. The peak monitored by absorbancy at 280 nm and eluting at 1.6-column volumes is neutralized to pH 5–7 with 1.0 N NaOH, concentrated to 10 ml by ultrafiltration (UM-2), diluted with 250 ml 0.02 M ammonium acetate, pH 5.6, and reconcentrated to 10 ml. This material is added to a 1.5 × 20 cm column of DEAE-cellulose; elution is accomplished using a linear gradient 0.02 M (125 ml) to 0.2 M (125 ml) ammonium acetate, pH 5.6, at a pump flow rate of 12 ml/hour at 5°C, collecting 6.0-ml fractions. The material in the major uv absorbing peak (fractions 31–39) is lyophilized, dissolved in 10 ml 0.05 M acetic acid, and relyophilized. It is quite pure.

B. Production of Antisera

Attempts were made to raise antibodies in both rabbits and guinea pigs using urogastrone conjugates to BSA and to polylysine and with urogastrone self-condensed using carbodiimide, but best results were obtained by the following simple procedure. Two male Dutch rabbits

Table II Purification of Urogastrone

Extract	Column	Fractions saved
1. Dissolved in 35 ml water	3.3 × 100 cm Sephadex G-25 in 0.4 M acetic acid, flow rate 50 ml/hour, 10-ml fractions	43–70
2. Applied as 10 mg/ml in water	3.2 × 24 cm carboxymethyl cellulose in ammonium acetate–acetic acid 0.01 M, pH 4.5, 45 ml/hour, 8.0-ml fractions; after 20 fractions gradient elution 0.01 M, pH 4.5 (500 ml)/0.2 M, pH 6.7 (500 ml)	96–109
3. Dissolved in 2 ml water	1.6 × 120 cm BioGel P-6, 200–400 mesh, 0.1 M acetic acid, 10 ml/hour, 3.0-ml fractions	70–84
4. Applied as 5 mg/ml in water	1.4 × 20 cm carboxymethyl cellulose in acetate, linear gradient elution 0.01 M, pH 5.0 (200 ml)/0.5 M, pH 5.0 (200 ml), 15 ml/hour, 3.0-ml fractions	46–54
5. Dissolved in minimal amount of water	1.5 × 85 cm BioGel P-6, 200–400 mesh, 0.05 M ammonium acetate, 5.0 ml/hour, 2.0-ml fractions	27–42
6. Applied as 5 mg/ml in water	1.0 × 10 cm aminoethyl cellulose in ammonium acetate–acetic acid, 0.01 M, pH 5.5, 4.0 ml/hour, 2.0 ml-fractions; after 10 fractions linear gradient elution 0.01 M (40 ml)/0.30 M (40 ml)	β27–33 γ33–42
7. Applied as 2 mg/ml in water	1.0 × 32 cm carboxymethyl cellulose, acetate pH 4.8 (β) or 5.0 (γ) linear gradient elution 0.01 M (130 ml) 0.5 M (65) ml, 5.0 ml/hour, 2.0-ml fractions	52–56
8. Applied in minimal water	1.0 × 100 cm BioGel P-6, 200–400 mesh, 0.05 M ammonium acetate, 3.0 ml/hour, 1.0-ml fractions	24–31

(about 2.5 kg) were treated with 10% pure urogastrone for the initial immunization. Each rabbit received 1.0 mg of this material in complete Freund's adjuvant given subcutaneously to four sites on each thigh and then they were twice boosted at one-month intervals with 0.2 mg pure urogastrone in incomplete Freund's adjuvant again given subcutaneously. A further boost of 0.2 mg pure material was given intradermally at four sites. The animals were bled from the ear vein about two weeks later. Subsequently, the rabbits were boosted at intervals of three months or more. Serum was collected after two weeks when the response was highest, but the titers did not exceed those found in the earlier samples. Essentially the same procedure was followed with mEGF, but all immunizations were carried out with pure material. Earlier workers (Byyny *et al.*, 1972) produced good antisera by injecting the mEGF immunogen into the foot pad of rabbits. The two rabbits immunized with urogastrone gave almost identical titer and assay sensitivity as did those injected with mEGF. Antibodies to mEGF had higher titer but lower sensitivity. Titers of urogastrone and mEGF antibodies fell quite sharply after three to four weeks, but interestingly, marmosets immunized with either urogastrone or EGF maintained high antibody titers many months after the last injection. The antisera were made up to 0.1% in sodium azide, subdivided into small aliquots, and stored at $-20°C$. The use of globulin fractions isolated from serum by ammonium sulfate precipitation and gel chromatography gave reduced sensitivity in the assay.

C. Preparation of Radioactive Peptides

Iodination of urogastrone has been carried out by a number of methods. Chloramine-T and vapor phase chlorine (Butt, 1972) gave products of erratic quality, although substitution of urogastrone with one atom of chlorine by the latter method resulted in a biologically active product. Lactoperoxidase produced an acceptable product initially, but antibody binding faded quite rapidly. A method involving chlorine water (Redshaw and Lynch, 1974) has been shown to be most consistent, and thus, has been used both for urogastrone and mEGF.

Urogastrone or mEGF (1.0 μg, 0.16 nmole) in 0.5 M phosphate buffer, pH 8.1 (10 μl), is treated with Na^{125}I (500 μCi, 0.25 nmole) in the same buffer (20 μl). A freshly prepared 0.001 M solution of chlorine in 0.05 M phosphate buffer, pH 8.1, is added (10 μl, 10 nmole) and the solution is continuously agitated for 30 seconds at ambient temperature. A solution (250 μl) is added containing 10 mg/ml bovine serum albumin, 10 mg/ml potassium iodide, and 1.0 mg/ml sodium metabisulfite, and the reaction mixture is immediately applied to a 60 $\times$ 0.9 cm column of BioGel P6 (200–400 mesh) prepared and equilibrated in the standard incubation buffer described in Section II,D. The column is run at 4°C and gives a distribution of radioactivity as shown (Figure 1). Although urogastrone and mEGF are of similar size, they elute from the column in characteristically different positions. Separation by this system is preferred to other chromatographic methods, such as carboxymethyl cellulose, because it is rapid, reproducible, all the radioactivity is eluted from the column, and the same column can be used repeatedly to yield good products. Only fractions from the center

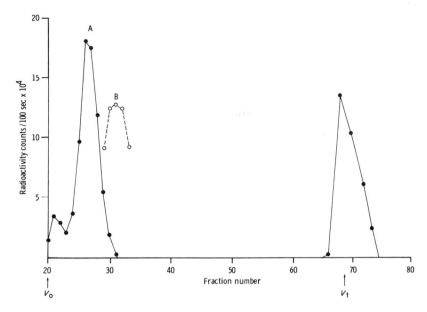

Figure 1.   Purification of ^{125}I-urogastrone (A) or mEGF (B) is carried out on a column (60 × 0.9 cm) of BioGel-P6 using assay buffer (see text, Section II,D) at 4°C. One-milliliter fractions are collected and 1.0 μl samples are counted.

of the peaks are used in the assays; these are combined, stored at 4°C, and diluted immediately prior to use. An aliquot equivalent to 40 pg starting peptide usually results in 15,000 counts per 100 seconds.

The extent to which labeled urogastrone is bound to antibody at different dilutions is illustrated in Figure 2, in which bound and free labeled ligand were separated by charcoal and second antibody methods. Charcoal bound >95% of label, but in the presence of excess antibody, less than 10% was available to the charcoal. In comparison, at a fixed second antibody concentration, excess anti-urogastrone or mEGF bound 75–90% of the ^{125}I-labeled peptides to the level at which precipitation was impaired. In the absence of first antibody replacing it with normal rabbit serum, less than 5% of the radioactivity appeared in the precipitate.

D. Assay Procedure

Although the radioimmunoassays for mEGF and urogastrone are separate and homologous, their methodologies are identical. The standard radioimmunoassay buffer is composed of 0.04 M phosphate

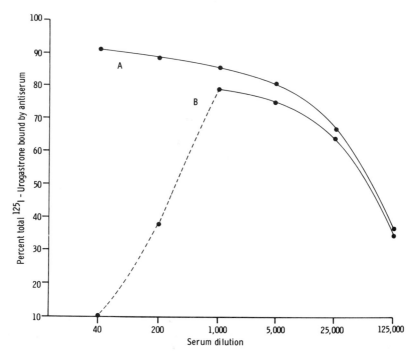

Figure 2. Typical results showing the maximum binding of ^{125}I-urogastrone to antiserum with separation of free material by charcoal (A) or bound material using a second antibody (B). mEGF gave similar results.

buffer, 0.15 M sodium chloride, 0.01 M EDTA, 0.5% bovine serum albumin, and 0.1% sodium azide adjusted to pH 7.2 with 1.0 N sodium hydroxide. Each assay tube is prepared by adding labeled urogastrone (~40 pg) in buffer (250 μl), suitably diluted antiserum (1 : 50,000) in buffer containing 4.0 μl/ml normal rabbit serum of the same strain (250 μl), and standards, urine, or serum samples diluted with buffer (250 μl). Although urogastrone is quite stable in solution at pH 1–11 for prolonged periods, solutions of high dilution occasionally give erratic results. Standards are, therefore, prepared by micropipetting from more concentrated stock solutions ($\geq$ 1.0 ng/ml) which are stored at $-20°$C. Assays are kept at 4°C for a minimum of three days. The separation stage is carried out by adding donkey anti-rabbit precipitating serum (Burroughs Wellcome) in buffer (250 μl) at the appropriate dilution (usually ~1 : 50) and keeping the assay reaction tubes at 4°C for one additional day. The assay tubes are centrifuged at 1250 g for ten minutes, the supernatants are withdrawn, and the precipitates are counted. Alternatively, separation can be effectively achieved by adding 100 μl of dextran-coated charcoal [8% Norit OL and 0.8% dextran (MW 60-900000), in 0.05 M phosphate, pH 7.2, 0.1% sodium azide]. After five minutes of contact, the reaction tubes are centrifuged, the supernatants are withdrawn, and the unbound label is counted in the charcoal residues.

A number of methods of separating the bound and free label, such as differential precipitation with ammonium sulfate or alcohols have been examined, but the two well-known methods gave the best results, and because of slightly greater sensitivity the double antibody method has been used most frequently. Solid-phase and chromatoelectrophoretic systems have been described for mEGF (Byyny et al., 1972). Ances (1973) has described a double antibody method which allows detection of 25 pg of the peptide. With our antiserum only 50 pg mEGF is measurable, but determinations of 5.0 pg urogastrone can be made (Figure 3). Assays are carried out in duplicate, or more rarely, in triplicate, individual determinations agreeing within 5%. In a series of standard curves performed over a period of six months using different labels, precipitating antibody, and buffer, the value for 60% displacement was equivalent to 41, 39, 34, 34, 35, and 31 pg urogastrone, respectively.

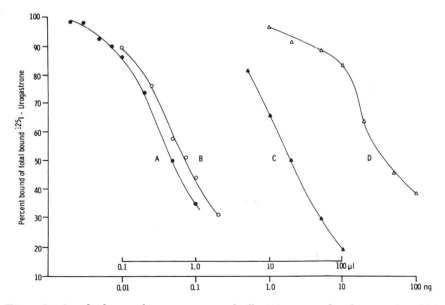

Figure 3. Standard curve for urogastrone in buffer (A) compared to those produced by individual urine (B) or serum samples (C) and also the effect of mEGF (D).

E. Cross-Reactivity

The urogastrone assay is not affected by a range of peptides, such as gastrin, insulin, glucagon, LH, FSH, prolactin, ACTH, LH-RH, or bradykinin, up to 5.0 μg. Some reaction is observed with hCG preparations, but this can be explained by assuming that these contain urogastrone to the extent of one part in 10^5. The only other peptide giving obvious cross-reaction is mEGF (Figure 3), but the sensitivity is reduced by approximately 10^3. This may reflect the fact that, although 37 of the 53 residues are common to both molecules, there are in fact only two common sequences as long as a pentapeptide (Gregory, 1975).

The mEGF assay demonstrates even less cross-reaction with urogastrone. Thus, although the urogastrone assay will measure the amount of urogastrone in <1.0 μl human urine, the mEGF assay cannot be used to measure urinary urogastrone because of the unacceptably large volumes required. On the other hand, the mEGF system shows a good correlation with a simple extract of male mouse submaxillary gland (Figure 4). As shown by earlier workers, mEGF levels exceed >1.0 mg/gm wet weight of salivary gland (Byyny et al., 1972).

Samples of up to 50 μl of animal urines were examined in both assays, and it was found that the urogastrone assay gave positive re-

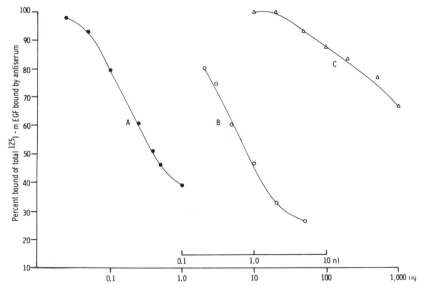

Figure 4. Standard curve for mEGF (A) compared to an extract of mouse submaxillary gland (supernatant from 600 mg of gland and 2.5 ml saline) (B) and urogastrone (C).

sults with human, monkey, and marmoset urines, whereas mouse, rat, and guinea pig urines reacted in the mEGF assay. Neither assay was influenced by urine samples from other animals, such as cow, sheep, pig, dog, cat, although at least some of these contain material capable of inhibiting gastric acid secretion.

III. UROGASTRONE MEASUREMENTS

A. Urine

The reaction curve produced by human urine closely parallels that obtained using pure urogastrone in assay buffer (Figure 3). However, urine has no effect upon the mEGF system used as control under identical conditions. Measurements of pooled human urine samples collected daily as the source of urogastrone yielded levels of 30 μg/liter of immunoreactive material. Calculations based upon the amounts of biologically active isolated material indicated similar quantities (Gregory and Willshire, 1975), thus providing good correlation of bio- and immunoactivity. To extend investigations to the source and physiological role of urogastrone, measurements were made upon 24-hour urine samples collected saturated with chloroform as preservative. As little as 1.0 μl was taken for measurement, and results were expressed as output of urogastrone per day per kilogram body weight. The range among normal controls was rather wide, 120–1200 ng/kg/day. However, in the age range 20–60, similarly expressed results showed a significantly lower output in males, 592 ± 46 ($n = 32$), than females, 805 ± 56 ($n = 23$) $p < 0.005$. There was a trend toward higher levels in children, but sufficient measurements have yet to be made to demonstrate a clear difference. This statement also applies to the many abnormal states currently under investigation.

B. Plasma or Serum

Filtration through charcoal removed urogastrone from human serum. When a standard curve was constructed in charcoal-treated human serum, it caused slight displacement relative to a standard curve in buffer alone. However, the effect of charcoal-absorbed human serum was the same as that produced by dog serum or commercially available horse serum; the latter has been used routinely for standardization in the radioimmunoassay system. No differences have been observed in measuring serum or plasma samples collected with different anticoagulants when up to 100 μl was included in the assay. Smaller volumes were made to 100 μl with filtered horse serum.

Urogastrone and mEGF are stable in blood. Known amounts of each peptide were added to fresh blood samples which were allowed to clot in ice. Serum measurements reflected the added material and the dilution curve was parallel to the assay calibration curve. However, measurements of urogastrone or mEGF following intravenous administration of peptide to dogs showed that the quantity in blood had fallen to undetectable levels by five minutes. Earlier studies reported a half-life of 8.5 minutes for mEGF in mice (Cohen and Savage, 1974).

The dilution curve produced by a human serum sample which produced a high degree of cross-reaction in the urogastrone assay is shown in Figure 3. Since the same sample has a negligible effect in the mEGF system, nonspecific interference is unlikely. Measurements of a series of 17 human sera resulted in a mean value of 500 pg/ml immunoreactive material. When urine samples are subjected to gel chromatography upon columns of Sephadex G-50, the immunoreactivity is located entirely at $2.0 \times V_0$ and is coincident with pure isolated urogastrone. However, with serum samples, only a small proportion is found at that position, and the dominant immunoreactive species is found at V_0 (Gregory et al., 1978). Intravenously administered urogastrone in doses of 250 ng/kg/hr or less are known to produce intense inhibition of gastric acid secretion in man (Elder et al., 1975); since the half-life in blood is of the order of a few minutes, this inhibition should occur at blood levels much lower than those found in many normal subjects. The correlation of biologic activity with the two immunoreactive species remains to be made in many subjects with multiple sampling.

It was reported earlier that a mEGF assay system detected levels of 1.5 ng/ml in pregnancy serum, but no immunoreactive material was noted in normal serum (Ances, 1973). However, using our mEGF assay, we have found no activity in pregnancy serum, but have noted measurable amounts of urogastrone-like material.

REFERENCES

Ances, I. G. (1973). Serum concentrations of epidermal growth factor in human pregnancy. Am. J. Obstet. Gynecol. 115, 357–362.
Bower, J. M., Camble, R., Gregory, H., Gerring, E. L., and Willshire, I. R. (1975). The inhibition of gastric acid secretion by epidermal growth factor. Experientia 31, 825–826.

Butt, W. R. (1972). The iodination of follicle stimulating and other hormones for radioimmunoassay. *J. Endocrinol.* **55**, 453–454.

Byyny, R. L., Orth, D. N., and Cohen, S. (1972). Radioimmunoassay of epidermal growth factor. *Endocrinology* **90**, 1261–1266.

Cohen, S., and Savage, C. R., Jr. (1974). Recent studies on the chemistry and biology of epidermal growth factor. *Recent Prog. Horm. Res.* **30**, 551–574.

Elder, J. B., Ganguli, P. C., Gillespie, I. E., Gerring, E. L., and Gregory, H. (1975). Effect of urogastrone upon gastric secretion and plasma gastrin in normal subjects. *Gut* **16**, 887–893.

Gerring, E. L., Bower, J. M., and Gregory, H. (1974). Urogastrone: A potential drug in the treatment of duodenal ulcer. *In* "Chronic Duodenal Ulcer" (C. Wastell, ed.), pp. 171–179. Butterworth, London.

Gregory, H. (1975). Isolation and structure of urogastrone and its relationship to epidermal growth factor. *Nature (London)* **257**, 325–327.

Gregory, H., and Willshire, I. R. (1975). The isolation of the urogastrones—inhibitors of gastric acid secretion—from human urine. *Hoppe-Seyler's Z. Physiol. Chem.* **356**, 1765–1774.

Gregory, H., Bower, J. M., and Willshire, I. R. (1978). Urogastrone and epidermal growth factor. *In* "Growth Factors" (K. W. Kastrup and J. H. Nielsen, eds.), pp. 75–84. Pergamon, Oxford.

Redshaw, M. R., and Lynch, S. S. (1974). An improved method for the preparation of iodinated antigens for radioimmunoassay. *J. Endocrinol.* **60**, 527–528.

Sandweiss, D. J. (1945). Enterogastrone, anthelone and urogastrone. *Gastroenterology* **5**, 404–415.

Sandweiss, D. J., Salzstein, H. C., and Farbman, A. (1938). The prevention or healing of experimental peptic ulcer in Mann-Williamson dogs with anterior pituitary-like hormone (Antuitrin-S). *Am. J. Dig. Dis.* **5**, 24–30.

Savage, C. R., Jr., and Cohen, S. (1972). Epidermal growth factor and a new derivative. *J. Biol. Chem.* **247**, 7609–7611.

Savage, C. R., Jr., Inagami, T., and Cohen, S. (1972). The primary structure of epidermal growth factor. *J. Biol. Chem.* **247**, 7612–7621.

48

Nerve Growth Factor: Radioimmunoassay and Bacteriophage Immunoassay

MICHAEL YOUNG, MURIEL H. BLANCHARD,
AND JUDITH D. SAIDE

I. BACKGROUND INFORMATION

A. Historical Aspects

Nerve growth factor (NGF) is a protein, discovered nearly 30 years ago, whose physiologic function *in vivo* remains unclear. In an attempt

941

Methods of Hormone Radioimmunoassay, Second Edition
Copyright © 1979 by Academic Press, Inc.
All rights of reproduction in any form reserved. IS BN 0-12-379260-6

to place the current status of NGF research in perspective, we briefly summarize here certain pertinent historical features of the factor and its discovery.

Nerve growth factor was first discovered by Levi-Montalcini and Hamburger (1951, 1953) as a soluble and diffusible factor released by two mouse sarcomas, called 180 and 37. They observed that implantation of these sarcomas into chick embryos resulted in a profound growth of sensory and sympathetic nerves into the tumors. The nature of these tumors is not precisely known, since a survey of the older literature (ca. 1914) reveals that they both originated as carcinomas, not sarcomas (see Oger *et al.*, 1974).

Sympathetic ganglia of mice of all ages are responsive to the nerve growth-promoting effects of NGF. Sensory ganglia are sensitive to the factor only during a limited time span of embryonic development (Levi-Montalcini and Angeletti, 1968). Moreover, injection of an antiserum to NGF into newborn mice results in destruction of sympathetic nerve cells (Levi-Montalcini and Angeletti, 1968).

A sensitive, *in vitro*, qualitative biologic assay for NGF (or NGF-producing tissues) has been developed. For example, when chick sympathetic or embryonic sensory ganglia in culture are treated with very low concentrations (~ 1.0 ng/ml) of the growth factor, a dense fibrillar halo of neurites is produced after about 18–24 hours (Levi-Montalcini and Angeletti, 1968). In addition, nerve growth factor activity can be detected in a variety of tissue extracts, as well as in serum.

On the basis of the above findings, many investigators believe that NGF somehow plays a role in the development or maintenance, or both, of the sensory and sympathetic nervous systems. So far, the validity of this hypothesis has not been firmly established.

References to the early NGF literature may be found in several detailed reviews (Levi-Montalcini and Angeletti, 1968, 1961; Levi-Montalcini, 1966).

B. Glandular and Cellular Sources of NGF

For unknown reasons, NGF is present in high concentrations in the submandibular glands of mice. Adult male glands contain higher levels than female glands, and newborn mice of both sexes possess only small amounts of the factor (Levi-Montalcini and Angeletti, 1968; Hendry, 1972).

The submandibular glands of mice are known to be sexually dimorphic. Castration of adult animals produces a marked decrease in gland levels of NGF, and administration of testosterone reverses this effect (Hendry and Iversen, 1973; Levi-Montalcini and Angeletti, 1968).

The mouse submandibular gland is not an endocrine organ for secretion of NGF. Rather, it is an exocrine gland for the factor. For example, bilateral sialoadenectomy has no effect upon circulating serum levels of NGF, and adult male and female sera contain comparable concentrations of the factor. In contrast, extremely high concentrations of NGF are continuously secreted into submandibular gland saliva, concentrations which are several orders of magnitude higher than those required to display biologic activity in the *in vitro* ganglion assay system. Furthermore, saliva concentrations in males and females reflect closely the sexual dimorphism of the glands. The reason for such high NGF levels in saliva is not known, but it has been suggested that the growth factor may play some hitherto unsuspected role in this secretion (Murphy *et al.*, 1977a).

High concentrations of NGF are also present in the venoms of certain poisonous snakes (e.g., *Crotalidae, Elapidae,* and *Viperidae*) (Levi-Montalcini and Angeletti, 1968). The reason for this is not known, and, furthermore, it is not clear what the embryological relationship is (if any) of snake venom glands to the mouse submandibular gland (Gans and Elliott, 1968).

In addition to the glandular production and secretion of NGF discussed above, recent studies reveal that a variety of both transformed and primary cells in culture synthesize a nerve growth factor which is biologically and immunologically indistinguishable from mouse submandibular gland NGF. Table I presents a list of cells which have so far been examined, together with references to the original papers. It is not known why so many different kinds of cells secrete NGF, but it

Table I   Cells Which Secrete NGF in Culture

Cell type	Source	Reference
L cells	Mouse	Oger *et al.* (1974)
3T3 cells	Mouse	Oger *et al.* (1974)
SV40 3T3 cells	Mouse	Oger *et al.* (1975)
Neuroblastoma	Mouse	Murphy *et al.* (1975)
Melanoma	Mouse	Young *et al.* (1976a)
Primary myoblasts	Rat	Murphy *et al.* (1977b)
Lg myoblasts	Rat	Murphy *et al.* (1977b)
C-6 glioma	Rat	Murphy *et al.* (1977c)
Primary fibroblasts	Chick	Young *et al.* (1975)
Primary fibroblasts	Human	Saide *et al.* (1975)

has been suggested that serum NGF arises from *in vivo* multifocal cellular secretion of the factor (Murphy *et al.*, 1977a).

C. Chemical Properties of NGF

The biologically active form of NGF has been completely purified from mouse submandibular glands (Bocchini and Angeletti, 1969). The molecular weight of the protein is 26,500 gm/mole, and it consists of two identical and noncovalently joined subunits (Angeletti *et al.*, 1973). Each of the constituent polypeptide chains contains three intrachain disulfide bonds, and sequence studies indicate that mouse gland NGF bears certain similarities to the amino acid sequence of insulin (Frazier *et al.*, 1972). Moreover, sequence studies of cobra (*Naja naja*) venom NGF indicate that this molecule is highly homologous to the structure of mouse gland NGF (Hogue-Angeletti *et al.*, 1976). Thus, the primary structure of NGF appears to be conserved over a wide range of the evolutionary spectrum.

NGF in aqueous solution at neutral pH comprises a rapidly reversible monomer–dimer equilibrium system, and estimates of the association constant for this reaction indicate that monomer (13,000 MW, 118 amino acid residues (Table II) is the predominant species at concentrations (~1.0 ng/ml or less) commonly employed in the ganglion bioassay system. Consequently, it is the individual subunits of NGF that are the biologically active species, at least *in vitro* (Young *et al.*, 1976b).

In contrast to the size of the biologically active form of mouse submandibular gland NGF, recent studies have shown that the NGF secreted by both L cells and muscle cells in culture is a much larger, highly stable macromolecule of molecular weight between 140,000 and 160,000 gm/mole (Pantazis *et al.*, 1977a; Murphy *et al.*, 1977b).

Table II   Structure of Mouse Submandibular Gland Nerve Growth Factor

1   10   20

NH$_2$- Ser -Ser-Thr-His-Pro-Val-Phe-His-Met- Gly -Glu-Phe-Ser-Val-Cys-Asp-Ser-Val-Ser- Val -Trp-

           30   40

Val-Gly-Asp-Lys-Thr-Thr-Ala-Thr- Asn -Ile-Lys-Gly-Lys-Glu-Val-Thr-Val-Leu- Ala -Glu-Val-Asn-

         50   60

Ile-Asn-Asn-Ser-Val-Phe- Arg -Gln-Tyr-Phe-Phe-Glu-Thr-Lys-Cys-Arg- Ala -Ser-Asn-Pro-Val-Glu-

        70   80

Ser-Gly-Cys-Arg- Gly -Ile-Asp-Ser-Lys-His-Trp-Asn-Ser-Tyr- Cys -Thr-Thr-Thr-His-Thr-Phe-Val-

      90   100

Lys-Ala- Leu -Thr-Thr-Asp-Glu-Lys-Gln-Ala-Ala-Trp- Arg -Phe-Ile-Arg-Ile-Asp-Thr-Ala-Cys-Val-

110   118

Cys -Val-Leu-Ser-Arg-Lys-Ala-Thr- Arg-COOH

Moreover, L cell NGF contains as part of its structure a molecule which is electrophoretically, biologically, and immunologically indistinguishable from mouse gland NGF. At the present time, it is not clear why cell-secreted NGF and purified gland NGF differ so significantly in molecular weight, since both are mouse-derived proteins. Perhaps they serve different functions as yet undiscovered. Alternatively, it may be that modifications (enzymic or otherwise) which occur during isolation of the smaller (gland) NGF render it considerably less stable (Pantazis *et al.*, 1977a,b).

Finally, it should be noted that several studies have appeared on the interaction of mouse gland NGF with its nervous system receptors. For a comprehensive review of this work, the reader is referred to the paper of Bradshaw *et al.* (1976).

Against this background, we now turn to procedures for the quantitative measurement of NGF both by radioimmunoassay and by bacteriophage immunoassay. The reader is also referred to the paper of Hendry (1972) where a different radioimmunoassay method is described.

II. RADIOIMMUNOASSAY

A. Reagents

Nerve growth factor is prepared from adult male mouse submandibular glands by the method of Bocchini and Angeletti (1969). These preparations have repeatedly been shown to be electrophoretically homogeneous in three different solvent systems and to yield single precipitin arcs upon immunoelectrophoresis against crude submandibular gland extracts (Oger *et al.*, 1974).

For purification, NGF is extracted from 40–50 gm of mouse salivary glands by adding three volumes ice-cold water and homogenizing for two minutes in a Waring blender and one minute in a Potter homogenizer. The homogenate is centrifuged at 13,000 rpm for 30 minutes, and 0.5 ml cold water and one volume of $0.2\,M$ streptomycin sulfate (Squibb) in $0.1\,M$ Tris–HCl, pH 7.5, are added to nine volumes of supernate. The mixture is maintained at 2°C for 30 minutes, centrifuged as above, and the supernate is lyophilized. The extract is dissolved in 6.0 ml $0.05\,M$ Tris–HCl buffer, pH 7.5, containing $5.0 \times 10^{-4}\,M$ EDTA, applied to a 2.7×143 cm column of Sephadex G-100, and eluted with the same buffer at 1.5 ml/cm²/hour collecting 7.0–8.0-ml fractions. Fractions 35–45 are pooled and dialyzed overnight against 0.05 M acetate, pH 5.0. After spinning off any precipitate formed, the partially purified NGF is applied to a 1.5 × 8 cm column of CM52 in 0.05 M acetate. The purified NGF is eluted using a linear elution gradient, 0–1.0 M NaCl (total volume 750 ml), collecting 3.0 ml fractions. The desired product is eluted in fractions 210–270 at 0.5 M NaCl in the gradient, concentrated, and stored at 0°C.

Glass double distilled H_2O is used for all solutions, and all buffer salts are reagent grade. $Na^{125}I$ (carrier-free) is obtained from New England Nuclear, chloramine-T from Eastman, bovine serum albumin (recrystallized) from Sigma Chemical Co., Sephadex from Pharmacia; 2-mercaptoethanol from Sigma and anion exchange resin AG-1X8, 200–400 mesh, from Bio-Rad Laboratories. Rabbit γ-globulin fraction II is obtained from ICN Pharmaceuticals, Inc., and lyophilized goat antisera directed against rabbit IgG, from Miles-Yeda, Ltd.

B. Preparation of Antibodies Monospecific for NGF

Rabbits are immunized by foot pad injection of 0.2 mg NGF in 0.2 ml 0.1 M phosphate, pH 7, and 0.2 ml complete Freund's adjuvant. An intravenous booster injection of 0.1 mg NGF is given seven weeks later, and the animals are bled the following week. Antisera are stored at −15°C until used.

To determine the optimal concentrations of rabbit IgG and goat anti-rabbit IgG antiserum to be used in the immunoassay, precipitin curves are constructed, and the Lowry procedure is used to determine protein concentrations.

C. Iodination of NGF

To 2.0 mCi of $Na^{125}I$ in the manufacturer's V vial are added the following reagents, in the following order, at room temperature.

1. 100 μl 1.0 M potassium phosphate, pH 7.0
2. 200 μl 0.1 M potassium phosphate, pH 7.0
3. 25 μl NGF, 200 μg/ml
4. 10 μl of a 1.0 mg/ml solution of chloramine-T (freshly prepared) in H_2O. Reaction is allowed to proceed for exactly 30 seconds.
5. 10 μl of a 1:400 dilution (freshly prepared) of 2-mercaptoethanol in H_2O.

The iodinated protein solution is then applied to a 1.0 × 1.0 cm plastic column of Bio-Rad AG-1X8 resin, 200–400 mesh that has been thoroughly equilibrated with 0.1 M potassium phosphate, pH 7.0, con-

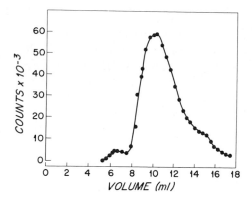

Figure 1. Sephadex G-75 chromatographic profile of ^{125}I-NGF. NGF was iodinated as described in the text using 2-mercaptoethanol to terminate the reaction. Column: 1 × 23 cm equilibrated with 0.1 M potassium phosphate, 1.0 mg/ml bovine serum albumin, pH 7.0.

taining 1.0 mg/ml bovine serum albumin. Ten 200-μl fractions are collected in plastic test tubes (Falcon), and the peak fractions, representing a total of about 6×10^8 cpm, are pooled and stored at 4°C until used. This procedure routinely yields ^{125}I-NGF preparations containing 0.6 gm-atom iodine per mole of protein.

Figure 1 illustrates a typical Sephadex G-75 gel filtration profile of freshly prepared solutions of ^{125}I-NGF. One major zone is present plus two minor peaks. The major peak has a partition coefficient which is identical to that of unlabeled NGF, and, as shown in Figure 2, this fraction migrates electrophoretically with a mobility indistinguishable

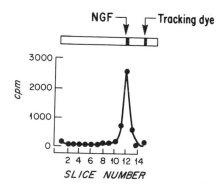

Figure 2. Polyacrylamide gel electrophoretic pattern of the major ^{125}I-NGF fraction shown in Figure 1. Solvent is 0.9 M acetic acid and 6.0 M urea. Figure also illustrates the electrophoretic pattern of unlabeled NGF.

from that of unlabeled protein. Both of the minor components depicted in Figure 1 migrate electrophoretically with the tracking dye, even though the largest fraction shown in Figure 1 moves near the void volume of the column. Consequently, this component(s) is probably an aggregate of NGF fragments. Alternatively, it could represent ^{125}I-NGF noncovalently bound to serum albumin. Fractions corresponding to the major peak (Figure 1) are pooled and used for radioimmunoassay. ^{125}I-NGF prepared in this way is quantitatively bound by antibody, although the degree of binding slowly declines to about 50% of initial values in three weeks. After this time, ^{125}I-NGF preparations are discarded.

The use of sodium metabisulfite (for reduction of I_2 to I^- to stop the chloramine-T reaction) should be avoided. Although this reagent has been used successfully in many protein iodination systems, it causes severe damage to the structure of NGF. Figure 3 presents a Sephadex G-75 gel filtration profile of a solution of ^{125}I-NGF in which the oxidation reaction was terminated with sodium metabisulfite. It will be seen that the chromatogram displays gross heterogeneity. Since NGF contains several disulfide bonds, it is likely that —S—S— bond reduction is, in part, responsible for this effect. The use of 2-mercaptoethanol routinely eliminates this problem.

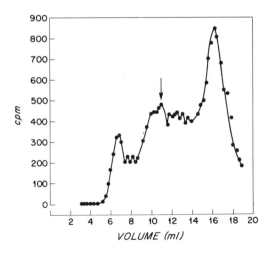

Figure 3. Sephadex G-75 chromatographic profile of ^{125}I-NGF. NGF was iodinated exactly as described in the text except that 100 μl sodium metabisulfite (0.63 mg/ml) was substituted for 10 μl of a 1 : 400 dilution of 2-mercaptoethanol in H_2O. The arrow marks the elution position of native unlabeled NGF (cf. Figure 1).

D. The Immunoassay Procedure

The radioimmunoassay is carried out in a total solution volume of 1.0 ml. Reagents are added to plastic tubes (Falcon, 12 × 75 mm) in the following order.

1. 0.6 ml 0.1 M potassium phosphate, pH 7.0.

2. 100 μl of unknown solution or standard solution. Ten standard dilutions of unlabeled NGF are prepared with a solvent consisting of 0.1 M potassium phosphate, 1.0 mg/ml bovine serum albumin, and 0.02% sodium azide, pH 7.0. Standards are prepared in such a way that they contain concentrations evenly spaced over the range 5.0–250 ng/ml of NGF. Thus, the final concentrations of standards in the assay solutions are between 0.5–25 ng/ml.

3. 100 μl of a ^{125}I-NGF solution. The stock ^{125}I-NGF solution is diluted with 0.1 M potassium phosphate containing 10 mg/ml serum albumin, 0.1 M ethylenediaminetetraacetic acid (EDTA), and 0.15 mg/ml rabbit γ-globulin, pH 7.0. This solution is prepared so that 100 μl will contain approximately 2×10^5 cpm.

4. 100 μl NGF antiserum, diluted with 0.1 M potassium phosphate, pH 7.0, to a degree that will yield 50% binding of ^{125}I-NGF (in our system, 1 : 40,000). The appropriate dilution of each individual antiserum to achieve 50% binding is determined titrimetrically.

5. Control tubes are also prepared which contain either no NGF antiserum or no NGF. In these cases, 100 μl 0.1 M potassium phosphate, pH 7.0, is substituted.

6. The assay solutions are incubated for 16 hours at 4°C, at which time 100 μl of a solution of goat anti-rabbit IgG antiserum is added after reconstituting the lyophilized antiserum with H_2O. With each batch of antiserum we determine the concentration required to give 50% binding of ^{125}I-NGF.

7. Tubes are centrifuged at 4° for 30 minutes at 400 g, and 200 μl of the supernatant solutions is removed for counting. Standard curves are constructed from a plot of ln[^{125}I-NGF bound]/[^{125}I-NGF unbound] versus ln [NGF].

III. BACTERIOPHAGE IMMUNOASSAY

A. Principle of the Method

The bacteriophage immunoassay serves a valuable purpose in that it is based upon the use of a totally different kind of tracer than that used in radioimmunoassay and is a useful second method for checking the results of the isotopic assay.

It has long been known that treatment of bacteriophages with anti-phage antiserum renders these viruses noninfective for their host bacterium. This finding led to the idea that if antigens were covalently coupled to bacteriophages, then antibody to the coupled antigen might block infectivity. This proved to be the case, and several antigens have been linked to phage. The principle of the assay method is that phage–antigen conjugates are rendered noninfective for bacteria by antisera to the coupled antigen, and free antigen competes for antibody in this reaction. The higher the concentration of free antigen, the fewer phage–antigen particles will be inactivated by antibody. Thus, by quantitating the number of viable phage, it is possible to measure the concentration of free uncoupled antigen. A successful phage immunoassay for NGF has already been developed (Oger *et al.*, 1974). For an account of phage biology and immunology, the reader is referred to the book by Adams (1959), and for a comprehensive review of phage immunoassays, in general, the work of Haimovich and Sela (1977) should be consulted.

The basic features of the phage assay procedure are as follows. Phage–antigen conjugates are prepared and purified. These conjugates are then treated with antibody to the antigen in the presence of various concentrations of the antigen. After a suitable time period, a second antibody (directed against the first) is added and an aliquot of the mixture is plated with the host bacterium (usually *E. coli*) onto agar in a petri dish. Phage infectivity is reflected by the formation of plaques upon the agar surface, and a simple count of plaques is sufficient to determine the number of infective phage. This value is then related to the concentration of free antigen, and a standard curve is constructed. The details are given below.

B. Reagents

For a detailed account of phage physiology, assay methods, and host specificity, Adams' book (1959) should be studied. For a description of the agar plating technique for phage analyses, see the Appendix to the same treatise.

The following reagents are needed for the plaque-assay technique.

    1. Medium-21 (M-21)
       2.5 gm Bactopeptone (Difco)
       0.5 gm glucose

2.5 gm NaCl
4.0 gm nutrient broth (Difco)
500 ml H$_2$O

This solution is adjusted to pH 7.0 with 1.0 N NaOH and autoclaved.

2. Bottom layer agar for petri dishes
   5.5 gm Bactoagar (Difco)
   5.0 gm Bactotryptone (Difco)
   4.0 gm NaCl
   0.5 gm glucose
   500 ml H$_2$O

Mix thoroughly and adjust to pH 7.0 with 1.0 N NaOH. Then heat gently while stirring to dissolve all reagents. Autoclave. While still hot, deliver 20 ml each of the melted agar into 100 × 15 mm petri dishes. Let cool and store dishes inverted at 4°C.

3. Upper layer agar
   1.4 gm Bactoagar
   2.0 gm Bactotryptone
   1.6 gm NaCl
   0.2 gm glucose
   200 ml H$_2$O

Adjust to pH 7.0 with 1.0 N NaOH, heat to dissolve as above, and deliver 2.5 ml each of melted agar into a series of glass test tubes (18 × 150 mm). Autoclave, and store covered tubes at 4°C.

4. All other reagents, antisera, etc., are the same as described for the radioimmunoassay.

C. Preparation of NGF–Phage Conjugates

For conjugation of NGF, we have chosen the wild-type strain of bacteriophage T4 (T4 Dr$^+$), which may be obtained from the American Type Culture Collection. To prepare a high-titer phage stock (10^{13} phage/ml), an overnight culture of *E. coli* B in M-21 is prepared by inoculating 5.0 ml of medium with *E. coli*. The following morning the culture is added to 500 ml of M-21 at 37°C on a shaker bath; the flask is aerated for 2½ hours, at which time the *E. coli* should be in mid-log phase. The culture is infected by addition of 0.11 ml of a phage solution of 10^{10}/ml (American Type Culture) to the 500-ml flask. After four hours of aeration and shaking (using Dow Corning B Antifoam agent to minimize foaming as the bacteria lyse), 5.0 ml chloroform and 1.0 mg each RNAse and DNase I are added. The mixtures are shaken vigorously intermittently over 60 minutes, centrifuged at 7000 rpm for five minutes to remove bacteria and debris, and the supernatant is stored at 4°C overnight. To pellet the phage, the supernatant is centrifuged at 40,000 g for one hour. The pellet is resuspended in 10 ml solvent M-9, which consists of: 1.0 gm NH_4Cl, 0.13 gm $MgSO_4$, 3.0 gm KH_2PO_4, 6.0 gm NaH_2PO_4, and 1.0 liter H_2O. Adjust to pH 6.8 with 1.0 N NaOH. Repeat the 7000 rpm spin (five minutes) and 40,000 g spin (60 minutes) sequentially twice each, resuspending initially in 2.0 ml and finally in 1.0 ml M-9. An approximate phage count can be made by reading absorbancy at 260 nm; OD_{260} of a solution of 10^{12} phage particles per milliliter is 7.3. The definitive phage count can be determined by plating high dilutions of stock upon bottom agar in Petri dishes as described by Adams (1959).

For conjugation of NGF, 50 μl of a 10 mg/ml solution of NGF (solvent: 0.05 M sodium acetate, pH 5.0) is added to 50 μl phage ($\sim 10^{13}$ phage/ml) dissolved in M-9 medium. This mixture is treated with 25 μl of $in~vacuo$ redistilled glutaraldehyde (0.05% solution in H_2O) for 30 minutes at room temperature. To stop the reaction, 1.0 ml M-21 is added, and the resulting solution is centrifuged at 33,000 g for one hour to pellet the conjugate. The pellet is resuspended in 1.0 ml M-9, and the entire centrifugation and resuspension procedure is repeated three more times. The final pellet is resuspended in 1.0 ml of M-9 and stored at 4°C. This coupling procedure results in about 50% inactivation of the phage particles, as measured by plaque count assays. Such phage–NGF conjugates are completely stable for at least four years at 4°C. Neither infectivity nor immunoreactivity is diminished over this time period. Thus, unlike iodinated-NGF, phage–NGF preparations are highly stable for long periods of time.

D. The Immunoassay Procedure

1. Immunologic Aspects

The following reagents are added to 12 × 75 mm plastic Falcon tubes.

a. 100 μl of unknown solution or NGF standard solution. Standards containing 5–500 ng/ml are prepared with M-21 as solvent.

b. 100 μl phage–NGF solution containing 1600–2000 infective phage particles, as determined by prior plaque assays.

c. 100 μl of a 1 : 10^3 dilution of anti-NGF antiserum diluted with

M-21. The optimal concentration will need to be determined for each antiserum.

d. Control tubes are also prepared in which $100 \mu l$ M-21 is substituted for antiserum and also in which $100 \mu l$ M-21 is substituted for free NGF.

e. These solutions are incubated at 4°C for 12–16 hours.

f. $100 \mu l$ of goat anti-rabbit IgG antiserum is added. The lyophilized second antiserum is reconstituted with M-21. To determine the appropriate concentration of goat antiserum to be used, serial dilutions are incubated with phage–NGF plus first antibody as described above, and the highest dilution which yields maximum inactivation of phage is determined by the plating assays described below. With optimum concentrations of both first and second antibodies, 80–90% inactivation should be achieved in the absence of free NGF.

2. The Plating Assay for Phage

For optimum infectivity of the host bacteria, a mid-log growth phage culture is required.

a. Inoculate 10 ml M-21 with *E. coli* B (American Type Culture Collection, Rockville, Maryland). Incubate overnight at 37°C. This culture must be prepared the day before the plating assay is carried out.

b. The next day, add 1.0 ml of this culture to 50 ml M-21 and shake vigorously with an incubator–shaker apparatus at 37°C for two hours. Remove 25 ml of this culture and centrifuge five minutes at $6000\,g$ to pellet the bacteria. Resuspend bacterial precipitate in 5.0 ml M-21.

c. For plating, melt upper-layer agar-containing test tubes (see Section III,B, above) in a boiling H_2O bath. Once melted, transfer tubes to a 45°C water bath. (The temperature here is critical.) To these tubes, add 0.1 ml of the *E. coli* suspension described in (b). Then add $100 \mu l$ of solution from the assay tubes (prepared as described in Section III,D,1). Mix and rapidly pour the melted agar evenly onto bottom agar in petri dishes. After agar has hardened, incubate plates inverted overnight at 37°C.

d. Plaques are readily counted the following day, and several commercially available plaque-counting instruments are available for this purpose. A standard curve is then constructed from plaque counts for the standard NGF-containing samples and the NGF concentrations (Figure 4). Values for unknown NGF samples are readily interpolated from such a plot.

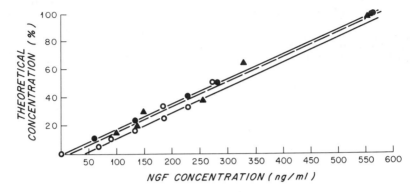

Figure 4. Serial dilution curves of human NGF obtained from phage and radioimmunoassays of Cohn fraction III for comparison with the dilution curve of pure mouse submandibular gland NGF. Samples were diluted as shown on the ordinate, and the resulting experimentally measured concentrations are given on the abscissa. O—O, Radioimmunoassay of human NGF; ●—●, radioimmunoassay of mouse NGF; ▲—▲, phage immunoassay of human NGF.

IV. MEASUREMENT OF NGF IN CELLS AND BIOLOGIC FLUIDS

The sensitivity of the NGF radioimmunoassay presented here is 0.5 ng/ml, and that of the phage assay is no better than 1.0 ng/ml. It will be appreciated from the foregoing that the phage assay is more cumbersome and time-consuming than the isotopic assay, but it provides a valuable check upon results obtained from the latter procedure.

Both phage and radioimmunoassay methods have been used successfully to measure NGF concentrations in tissue culture media and in serum. NGF levels arising from the cell types listed in Table I were measured by both assays and the results were quite similar. Moreover, both methods yielded values which were consistent with results of semiqualitative biologic assays for NGF. Further, we have found little, if any, variation among different assays, ^{125}I-NGF or phage–NGF preparations, or antisera employed.

Recently, there has been considerable interest in measurements of NGF concentrations in serum including human serum (see, e.g., Young *et al.*, 1976a; Siggers *et al.* 1976). Although immunoreactive NGF has been identified in human sera (6.0–10 ng/ml), it cannot be overemphasized that all of these studies have utilized mouse NGF as standards and antibodies to mouse NGF. Consequently, much caution must be exercised when interpreting NGF levels in biologic fluids of nonmouse origin. It is essential in these cases that as many different types of assays as possible be employed in order to minimize artifacts. Even then, interpretation of results (e.g., changes in NGF concentrations in certain disease states, as in cell proliferative states including Paget's disease and healing burns) can be complicated.

Figure 5 illustrates a comparison of dilution curves for pure mouse NGF and human serum NGF by both bacteriophage and radioimmunoassays. This figure was constructed from studies on Cohn fraction III of human serum, a fraction which has previously been shown to contain the highest concentration of a substance which reacts with antibody to NGF (Young *et al.*, 1976a). What is plotted here is the concentration of NGF measured by immunoassay (x axis) versus the concentration which would be expected based simply upon serial volumetric dilutions. Examination of this figure reveals that the dilution curves are reasonably well-behaved and that both phage and radioimmunoassays yield comparable results. Yet this result does not mean that the antiserum used necessarily recognizes a molecular structure which is closely similar to that of mouse NGF. Moreover, it will be appreciated that the radioimmunoassay curve for human serum does not intersect the y axis at zero NGF concentration. Thus, it must be assumed that some type of nonspecific, or interfering, reaction is operative in this assay.

Figure 6 illustrates that when mouse NGF is added to human

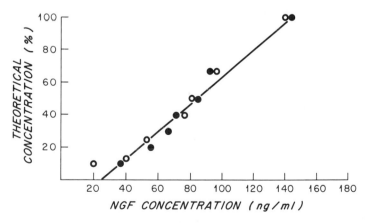

Figure 5. Radioimmunoassays of human serum to which pure mouse NGF has been added. O—O, Serial dilutions of freshly prepared human serum; ●—●, assays of the same dilutions of serum to each of which was added 5.0 ng pure mouse submandibular gland NGF. The resulting plot was obtained after subtraction of 5.0 ng from each of the measured values (i.e., the value for serum NGF plus mouse NGF).

INHIBITION OF INACTIVATION OF
T₄-NGF WITH ANTI-NGF BY NGF

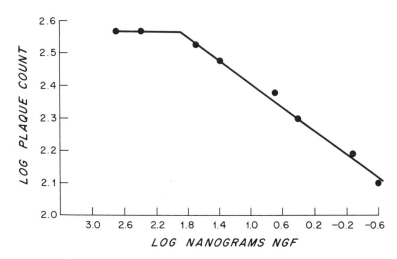

Figure 6. Calibration curve for measurement of NGF using the bacteriophage T4 immunoassay. (Reproduced from Oger *et al.*, 1974, with permission of the publisher.)

serum, it can be quantitatively recovered. A constant amount of mouse NGF was added to a series of human serum dilutions. Following radioimmunoassay, this number was subtracted from the measured values, and the resulting NGF concentrations were compared to those to which no mouse NGF was added. Within experimental error, the two sets of dilution values were superimposable. Yet again, the line did not intersect the ordinate properly.

We present the above data to call attention to the pitfalls that can accompany NGF assays of nonmouse species and to illustrate a comparison of the phage and radioimmunoassays.

V. SUMMARY

As noted under Background Information, the *in vivo* role of NGF is not yet clear. In the usual sense, this growth factor cannot be called a hormone, since no gland has been shown to be responsible for its secretion into the circulation. Furthermore, many different kinds of cells have the capacity to secrete NGF in culture. Before the physiologic role of NGF is clearly understood, the meaning of its presence in saliva and in snake venom and its secretion by cells will have to be explained in a satisfactory and unified fashion. The combined use of both of the immunoassays described here should be helpful in achieving this goal.

REFERENCES

Adams, M. H. (1959). "Bacteriophages." Wiley (Interscience), New York.

Angeletti, R. H., Hermodson, M. A., and Bradshaw, R. A. (1973). Amino acid sequence of mouse 2.5 S nerve growth factor. II. Isolation and characterization of the thermolytic and peptic peptides and the complete covalent structure. *Biochemistry* **12**, 100–115.

Bocchini, V., and Angeletti, P. U. (1969). The nerve growth factor: Purification as a 30,000-molecular weight protein. *Proc. Natl. Acad. Sci. U.S.A.* **64**, 787–794.

Bradshaw, R. A., Pulliam, M. W., Jeng, I. M., Andres, R. Y., Szutowicz, A., Frazier, W. A., Hogue-Angeletti, R. A., and Silverman, R. E. (1976). Specific interaction of nerve growth factor with receptors in the central and peripheral nervous systems. *In* "Surface Membrane Receptors" (R. A. Bradshaw *et al.*, eds.), pp. 227–246. Plenum, New York.

Frazier, W. A., Hogue-Angeletti, R. A., and Bradshaw, R. A. (1972). Nerve growth factor and insulin. *Science* **176**, 482–488.

Gans, C., and Elliott, W. B. (1968). Snake venoms: Production, injection, action. *Adv. Oral Biol.* **3**, 45–81.

Haimovich, J., and Sela, M. (1977). Antibody reactions with chemically modified bacteriophages. *Methods Immunol. Immunochem.* **4**, 386–398.

Hendry, I. A. (1972). Developmental changes in tissue and plasma concentrations of the biologically active species of nerve growth factor in the mouse, by using a two-site radioimmunoassay. *Biochem. J.* **128**, 1265–1272.

Hendry, I. A., and Iversen, L. L. (1973). Reduction in the concentration of nerve growth factor in mice after sialectomy and castration. *Nature (London)* **243**, 500–504.

Hogue-Angeletti, R. A., Frazier, W. A., Jacobs, J. W., Niall, H. D., and Bradshaw, R. A. (1976). Purification, characterization, and partial amino acid sequence of nerve growth factor from cobra venom. *Biochemistry* **15**, 26–34.

Levi-Montalcini, R. (1966). The nerve growth factor: Its mode of action in sensory and sympathetic nerve cells. *Harvey Lect.* **60**, 217–259.

Levi-Montalcini, R., and Angeletti, P. U. (1961). Biological properties of a nerve-growth promoting protein and its antiserum. *In* "Regional Neurochemistry" (S. Kety and J. Elkes, eds.), pp. 362–376. Pergamon, Oxford.

Levi-Montalcini, R., and Angeletti, P. U. (1968). Nerve growth factor. *Physiol. Rev.* **48**, 534–569.

Levi-Montalcini, R., and Hamburger, V. (1951). Selective growth-stimulating effects of mouse sarcoma on the sensory and sympathetic nervous system of the chick embryo. *J. Exp. Zool.* **116**, 321–362.

Levi-Montalcini, R., and Hamburger, V. (1953). A diffusible agent of mouse sarcoma producing hyperplasia of sympathetic ganglia and hyperneurotization of the chick embryo. *J. Exp. Zool.* **123**, 233–288.

Murphy, R. A., Pantazis, N. J., Arnason, B. G. W., and Young, M. (1975). Secretion of a nerve growth factor by mouse neuroblastoma cells in culture. *Proc. Natl. Acad. Sci. U.S.A.* **72**, 1895–1898.

Murphy, R. A., Saide, J. D., Blanchard, M. H., and Young, M. (1977a). Nerve growth factor in mouse serum and saliva. Role of the submandibular gland. *Proc. Natl. Acad. Sci. U.S.A.* **74**, 2330.

Murphy, R. A., Singer, R. H., Saide, J. D., Pantazis, N. J., Blanchard, M. H., Byron, R. S., Arnason, B. G. W., and Young, M. (1977b). Synthesis and secretion of a high molecular weight form of nerve growth factor by skeletal muscle cells in culture. *Proc. Natl. Acad. Sci. U.S.A.* (in press).

Murphy, R. A., Oger, J., Saide, J. D., Blanchard, M. H., Arnason, B. G. W., Hogan, C., Pantazis, N. J., and Young, M. (1977c). Secretion of nerve growth factor by central nervous system glioma cells in culture. *J. Cell Biol.* **72**, 769.

Oger, J., Arnason, B. G. W., Pantazis, N., Lehrich, J., and Young, M. (1974). Synthesis of nerve growth factor by L and 3T3 cells in culture. *Proc. Natl. Acad. Sci. U.S.A.* **11**, 1554–1558.

Pantazis, N. J., Blanchard, M. H., Arnason, B. G. W., and Young, M. (1977a). Molecular properties of the nerve growth factor secreted by L cells. *Proc. Natl. Acad. Sci. U.S.A.* **74**, 1492.

Pantazis, N. J., Murphy, R. A., Saide, J. D., Blanchard, M. H., and Young, M. (1977b). Dissociation of the 7 S–nerve growth factor complex in solution. *Biochemistry* **7**, 1525.

Saide, J. D., Murphy, R. A., Canfield, R. E., Skinner, J., Robinson, D. R., Arnason, B. G. W., and Young, M. (1975). Nerve growth factor in human serum and its secretion by human cells in culture. *J. Cell Biol.* **67**, 376a (Abstract).

Siggers, D. C., Rogers, J. G., Boyer, S. H., Margolet, L., Dokin, H., Banerjee, S. P., and Shooter, E. M. (1976). Increased nerve-growth-factor β-chain cross-reacting material in familial dysautonomia. *N. Engl. J. Med.* **295**, 629–634.

Young, M., Oger, J., Blanchard, M. H., Asdourian, H., Amos, H., and Arnason, B. G. W. (1975). Secretion of a nerve growth factor by primary chick fibroblasts. *Science* **187**, 361–362.

Young, M., Murphy, R. A., Saide, J. D., Pantazis, N. J., Blanchard, M. H., and Arnason, B. G. W. (1976a). Studies on the molecular properties of nerve growth factor and its cellular biosynthesis and secretion. *In* "Surface Membrane Receptors" (R. A. Bradshaw *et al.*, eds.), pp. 247–267. Plenum, New York.

Young, M., Saide, J. D., Murphy, R. A., and Arnason, B. G. W. (1976b). Molecular size of nerve growth factor in dilute solution. *J. Biol. Chem.* **251**, 459–464.

49

Somatomedin A, Somatomedin C, and NSILA-s

RONALD H. CHOCHINOV AND
WILLIAM H. DAUGHADAY

959

Methods of Hormone Radioimmunoassay, Second Edition
Copyright © 1979 by Academic Press, Inc.
All rights of reproduction in any form reserved. ISBN 0-12-379260-6

I. INTRODUCTION

It was originally thought that somatotropin acted directly on cartilage to cause growth. However, Salmon and Daughaday (1957) discovered that growth hormone acts through the formation of a substance(s)
operationally termed sulfation factor which acts directly on cartilage.
This factor(s) was later shown to have a larger number of biologic
effects so that the name was changed to somatomedin (Daughaday *et
al.*, 1972). "Somato" relates to somatotropin and "medin" to indicate it
mediates the action of somatotropin.

The standard method of measuring somatomedin activity has been
by bioassay. This technique involves measuring the $^{35}SO_4$ uptake into
rat, porcine, or chick embryo cartilage and is rather a long (three to
four days) and imprecise procedure.

However, in the last five years, several substances with
somatomedin-like properties (which include insulin-like metabolic
activity and growth-promoting activity) have been isolated. Three of
these growth factors, somatomedin A (SmA) (Hall *et al.*, 1975),
somatomedin C (SmC) (Van Wyk *et al.*, 1975), and NSILA-s (nonsuppressible insulin-like activity—soluble in acid ethanol) (Froesch *et al.*,
1975), have been purified from outdated human sera. Their levels in
biologic fluids are now measurable by radioreceptor assay utilizing
human placental membranes as receptors for somatomedins A and C
and rat liver plasma membrane as receptors for NSILA-s. An acidic
peptide also purified from human sera, somatomedin B (SmB), does
not have similar biologic properties compared to the above-mentioned
growth factors. It has only limited growth-promoting activity and,
therefore, will not be discussed in detail. A radioimmunoassay for this
substance has been established by Yalow *et al.* (1975), and interested
readers are referred to this article for technical details.

II. PREPARATION OF BUFFERS AND COLUMNS FOR THE
SOMATOMEDIN A AND C ASSAYS

Since the somatomedin A and C radioreceptor assays are done in a
similar manner, they will be discussed together.

A radioreceptor assay using insulin as the tracer and standard can be done in an identical manner to the somatomedin A and C radioreceptor assay. Therefore, since insulin is in much greater supply, any person wishing to learn the techniques of this radioreceptor assay are urged to start with insulin as the initial substance.

A. Preparation of Buffers

1. Phosphate Buffer (0.25 M)

> 3.5 gm $NaH_2PO_4 \cdot H_2O$ in 100 ml
> 3.6 gm Na_2HPO_4 in 100 ml

Add one part of the monobasic to nine parts of the dibasic buffer; final pH 7.6.

2. Phosphate Buffer (0.05 M)

The above buffer is diluted fivefold with distilled water.

3. 1% Bovine Serum Albumin (BSA)–0.05 M Phosphate Buffer

Add 100 mg commercially available 96–99% pure fraction V BSA to 10 ml 0.05 M phosphate buffer. Store at 4°C.

4. 0.1% BSA–0.05 M Phosphate Buffer

Add 100 mg commercially available 96–99% pure fraction V BSA to 100 ml 0.05 M phosphate buffer. Store at 4°C.

5. Tris-HCl Buffer (0.05 M, pH 7.97, at 4°C)

Add 6.61 gm Tris-HCl and 0.97 gm Tris-base to 1.0 liter distilled water. Store at 4°C.

6. 2% BSA–Tris-HCl Buffer (0.05 M, pH 7.97, at 4°C)

Add 2 gm of radioimmunoassay grade fraction V BSA to 100 ml of the Tris buffer. Store at 4°C.

7. Barbital Buffer (0.1 M)

> 49.44 gm sodium barbital
> 5.54 gm barbituric acid
> 0.48 gm sodium azide

Final pH should be 8.6. Final volume 2.4 liters. This buffer is stored at 4°C and is diluted with an equal volume of distilled water prior to use.

B. Preparation of Sephadex Column

1. Sephadex Column for Initial Purification of Labeled Hormone

Sephadex G-50 (coarse) is placed in $0.05\,M$ barbital buffer or $0.05\,M$ Tris-HCl, pH 7.4, at 25°C and is allowed to swell at room temperature for at least three hours. The slurry is then poured into a 1.5×30 cm or similar size column that has either a mesh guard or plug of glass wool at the bottom. The column is packed to a height of 26 cm. Then 500 μl 1% BSA–$0.05\,M$ phosphate buffer is added to the column to coat the glass and help prevent sticking of iodinated protein that will subsequently be passed through it. The unreacted albumin is eluted from the column with two bed volumes of barbital or Tris buffer and is now ready for use. With careful attention and washout between iodination procedures, this same column can be used for periods of three to six months.

2. Sephadex Column for Repurification of Labeled Somatomedin

Sephadex G-50 (fine) or Sephadex 100 is placed in $0.05\,M$ Tris-HCl buffer and swollen three hours for G-50 and three days for G-100 at room temperature (G-100 can be swollen in five hours by boiling). The Sephadex is packed into a 1.5×30 cm column to a height of 26–28 cm. Again, a small amount of 2% BSA–Tris is filtered on the column to prevent nonspecific adsorption of labeled somatomedin to glass. This albumin is washed out by eluting the column with two bed volumes of buffer. Eluates are collected in 1.0-ml fractions by an automated fraction collector. Most columns last one to two months depending on use.

III. PREPARATION OF PLACENTAL MEMBRANES

The method of preparing the placental membranes is based on the procedure of Cuatrecasas (1972) as modified by Marshall *et al.* (1974). One or two fresh term placentas may be stored in $0.25\,M$ sucrose (85.5 gm/liter) at 4°C for up to 12 hours before use. The whole placentas are washed in ice-cold $0.25\,M$ sucrose to remove as much blood as possible. After the amnionic and chorionic membranes are trimmed, remaining placentas are cut into small pieces, approximately two to three cm^3, trying to remove as much connective tissue as possible, and washed in fresh ice-cold $0.25\,M$ sucrose, removing as much liquid as possible by blotting. The pieces are weighed, and a portion, about 150 gm, is suspended in an equal volume of ice-cold 0.25 M sucrose. They are homogenized in an Omnimixer (Sorvall) for 15 seconds at setting 5, 30 seconds at 7, and 15 seconds at 9, repeating this procedure for the remaining placental pieces. The homogenates are pooled, divided into 100-ml portions for the Polytron PT-10 (Brinkman), and dissociated twice at a setting of 5 for 30 seconds. The ultrasound-treated homogenates are pooled, divided into large Sorvall centrifuge bottles (250 ml), and spun at 600 g for ten minutes at 4°C. The supernatants are saved. The precipitates are resuspended in approximately 100 ml of ice-cold 0.25 M sucrose and recentrifuged at 600 g for 10 minutes at 4°C. The pooled supernatants from the 600 g spin are divided into 250-ml centrifuge bottles and spun at 12,000 g for 30 minutes at 4°C. The supernatants are saved. If the volume is less than 350 ml, the precipitates are suspended in about 100 ml of ice-cold 0.25 M sucrose and the 12,000 g spin is repeated. The total supernatant volume is measured, and NaCl is added to a final concentration of 0.1 M (2.0 gm/350 ml) and MgSO$_4$ to a final concentration of 0.001 M (42 mg/350 ml), stirring for 10–15 minutes at room temperature. The suspension is divided into 50-ml plastic centrifuge tubes and spun at 40,000 g (18,250 rpm using the small head of Sorvall) for 40 minutes at 4°C. The supernatants are discarded. The combined pellets are resuspended in 80 ml 0.05 M Tris-HCl buffer, pH 7.4, at 25°C and spun at 40,000 g for 40 minutes at 4°C. This last step is repeated for a second wash. The pellet is resuspended in 2 volumes using the 0.05 M Tris-HCl buffer and homogenized with seven strokes in a glass homogenizer. The protein content is measured by the method of Lowry et al. (1951), and the preparation is stored in 1.0-ml aliquots at −17°C.

IV. TECHNIQUE OF RADIORECEPTOR ASSAY FOR SOMATOMEDINS A AND C

A. Procurement of Purified Protein for Radioreceptor Assay

Unfortunately purified human somatomedin A and C are difficult for most investigators to obtain. Small amounts of somatomedin A were isolated in Sweden (Hall et al., 1975) and somatomedin C by Van Wyk et al. (1975) of The University of North Carolina, Chapel Hill. Less pure material can be used for standards. If necessary, diluted normal human serum can be used as standard.

In Hall's preparation (Hall, 1972), frozen Cohn fraction IV-1 was dissolved in water and extracted at 40°C with three volumes of 96% ethanol and one-tenth volume of concentrated HCl for 60 minutes. The pH was raised to 8.4 with 4 M NaOH, and the suspension was stirred for an additional 45 minutes and then centrifuged. The supernatant was mixed with four volumes of cold acetone–ethanol, (5 : 3, v/v) at -16°C, collected by centrifugation, and dried *in vacuo*. Seventy-five grams of the extract was extracted twice with 150 ml of 20% formic acid, and the combined supernatants were applied to a 10 × 100 cm column of Sephadex G-75 equilibrated with 1% formic acid containing 0.01 M 2-mercaptoethanol. The biologically active material was recovered from fractions with K_d values of 0.68 to 0.77. The pooled fractions were applied to a 2.5 × 45 cm column of Dowex 50W-X2 (H$^+$) equilibrated in 0.1 M ammonium acetate, pH 5.6. After washing with two volumes of 0.1 M ammonium acetate, the column was eluted successively with 400 ml 0.01 M and then 400 ml 0.1 M diethylamine and 400 ml 0.2 M ammonia. The SmA eluted at 0.1 M diethylamine, was further purified by high voltage electrophoresis in pyridine–acetate buffer at pH 6.5 (60 V/cm), pH 3.6 (10V/cm for three hours) and pH 2.0 (10 V/cm for five hours). The resulting peptide had an activity of 700 U/mg.

Van Wyk *et al.* (1974) purified SmC from acid-ethanol extracts of Cohn fraction IV of human plasma. The first step was gel filtration on a 10 × 95 cm column of Sephadex G-75, eluting with 1% formic acid. Active material, eluted at a K_d of 0.72, was purified by isoelectric focusing between pH 3.5 and 10 in a 440 ml LkB Ampholine column with a 2% ampholyte mixture containing 6.0 M urea for 87 hours at 5°C at 300 V. The anode buffer was 0.13 M H$_3$PO$_4$ in sucrose, and the cathode buffer was 0.3 M ethylenediamine in water. The SmC segregated into the more basic peak (pH 8.4–9.2). A narrow range (pH 8–10) refocusing was performed in 4 M urea. The active fractions (pH 8.6–9.4) were separated from urea and sucrose by chromatography on SP-Sephadex. The SmC was eluted using 0.2 M NH$_4$OH and lyophilized. The ampholyte was removed by gel filtration on a 2.5 × 175 cm column of Sephadex G-50, eluting with 1% formic acid. Fraction 4 was subjected to preparative electrophoresis on 15% polyacrylamide gel containing 4 M urea at pH 2.3. The active fractions, $R_f = 0.4$–0.5, were desalted on Sephadex G-50 as above for use in biologic procedures (Van Wyk *et al.*, 1975). Alternative sources of receptor membranes include human fibroblasts (Rechler *et al.*, 1977) and human mononuclear cells (Thorsson and Hintz, 1977).

B. Radioiodination Technique

Iodination is achieved by the use of very small increments of chloramine-T. The iodination is monitored by trichloroacetic acid (TCA) precipitation.

1. Iodination

In a 10×75 mm plastic tube containing $50-100 \, \mu l$ $0.25 M$ phosphate buffer, $3.0-5.0 \, \mu l$ of a 1.0 mg/ml solution of peptide is added in $0.5 M$ phosphate buffer. (Insulin should be dissolved first in a small amount of $0.01 \, N$ HCl before adding the buffer.) The tube is gently agitated and placed in ice water; $1.0-1.5$ mCi carrier-free ^{125}I of high specific activity (exceeding 200 mCi/ml) is added. Five micrograms of chloramine-T is added in $30 \, \mu l$ buffer solution, and the mixture is shaken gently for three minutes. After three minutes, one or two microliters of the reaction mixture is withdrawn and diluted in 1.0 ml of distilled water. The remainder of the reaction mixture is kept on ice. The diluted tracer is used to check the amount of iodine taken up by the peptide by TCA precipitation.

2. TCA Precipitation

Several 10×75 mm glass tubes are prepared with $800 \, \mu l$ 0.1% BSA–$0.05 \, M$ phosphate buffer. Two to five microliters of diluted labeled protein is added to each of the tubes with mixing. Two hundred microliters of 100% TCA is then added to each tube with shaking. The mixtures are spun at 2000–3000 rpm for five minutes. Each tube is counted before and after aspiration of the supernatant. Ideally, 35–50% of the counts should be retained in the pellet. If this number is $<35\%$, $10-25 \, \mu l$ more of the chloramine-T solution is added to the remaining reaction mixture, and after waiting three minutes, the TCA precipitation procedure is repeated.

When the reaction mixture has achieved the desired TCA precipitability, $200 \, \mu l$ of 1% BSA–$0.05 \, M$ phosphate buffer is added to the reaction tube. After agitation, gel filtration is performed on the G-50 column, eluting with $0.05 \, M$ barbital buffer or $0.03 \, M$ Tris buffer. One-milliliter fractions are collected in siliconized tubes and counts checked are with a Geiger counter. All the tubes with significant activity that appear at the appropriate elution volume for somatomedin A or C (MW $\simeq 7600$, $K_d \simeq 0.5$ on G-50) are saved.

C. Determination of Quality of Labeled Somatomedin

This step is necessary to decide which tubes from the original iodination are to be pooled and stored for future use as tracer in the receptor assay. Ten microliters from each tube is counted and diluted to a final reading of about 20,000 cpm/100 μl.

For each potentially useful tracer tube, six plastic microfuge tubes for Beckman Type B Microfuge are needed. The order of addition is as follows: (1) buffer, (2) tracer, and (3) membrane. The membrane is added last and is prepared in the following manner. An aliquot of frozen membrane is thawed and rehomogenized in a tissue grinder with cold 0.05 M Tris-HCl buffer and diluted to give a final concentration of 100–200 μg membrane protein per 100 μl. When the diluted membrane suspension is added, the reaction tubes are vortexed to ensure a homogeneous suspension.

The first two tubes contain 400 μl 2% BSA–0.05 M Tris-HCl buffer and 100 μl diluted tracer. This is a check of nonspecific sticking to the plastic. The next two tubes (0 standard) contain 300 μl of the 2% BSA–0.05 M Tris-HCl buffer, 100 μl tracer, and 100 μl membrane mixture. The next two tubes contain 100 μl 2% BSA–0.05 M Tris-HCl buffer, 200 μl normal human adult serum (diluted 1 : 10 in 2% BSA–0.05 M Tris-HCl buffer), 100 μl tracer, and 100 μl membrane. This procedure is repeated for each potentially useful tracer tube. After membrane has been added to all the microfuge tubes, each of the tubes should be gently agitated. After 90 minutes at room temperature, the tubes are spun for ten minutes in the Beckman Type B Microfuge in a cold room. After spinning, the supernatant is aspirated and the tubes are counted. The tubes which give >5% binding and at least 50% displacement by the added serum standard are pooled and stored in 400–500-μl aliquots at −10°C. They may last three to six weeks.

D. Technique for Radioreceptor Assay

1. Standards

Somatomedin C standards may be purified SmC (750–1250 U/mg) in concentrations of 2.0–1000 ng/tube or a less pure preparation such as the E-3 standard (Marshall et al., 1974; potency of 15–25 U/mg) in concentrations of 50–5000 ng/tube or a pool of normal human serum which is initially diluted 1 : 10 in 2% BSA–0.05 M Tris HCl buffer in aliquots of 5–200 μl/tube. SmA standard may be purified SmA (200 U/mg) in concentrations of 10–2500 ng/tube or a pool of normal adult human serum diluted 1 : 5, 10–200 µl/tube.

2. Tracer

Prior to each assay, one to two aliquots of 0.4 ml of stored tracer are repurified by gel filtration on Sephadex. The buffer used to elute the column is 0.05 M Tris-HCl without BSA. We have found that by using 0.25% BSA–0.05 M Tris-HCl as elution buffer, 20–25% of the total tracer counts may be bound to protein; 1.0–1.5-ml fractions are collected and counted. The peak tubes that occur at the appropriate MW (7600) (K_d = 0.5 on G-50, K_d = 0.65 on G-100) are pooled, diluted with 2% BSA–0.05 M Tris-HCl to 10,000–20,000 cpm/100 µl and used as tracer in the assay. Although a large amount of aggregation or deiodination may take place over the ensuing weeks, if one selects the tubes with the proper K_d after repurification by gel filtration, useful tracer can be obtained up to six weeks after the original iodination.

3. Samples

Unknowns may consist of serum or other biologic fluids. Serum need only be diluted 1 : 10 in the assay buffer. If other unknown solutions are diluted at least 1 : 10 by the assay buffer, no dialysis is necessary. If the biologic fluid cannot be diluted, then it may be dialyzed against 0.05 M Tris-HCl, pH 7.4, using the Spectropor (molecular weight cutoff 3500) membrane. Dialysis should be carried out against the assay buffer for at least 12 hours. If the sample needs to be concentrated to be measured in the radioreceptor assay, the sample should be lyophilized and then dialyzed with several changes of buffer to remove excess salts.

4. Assay Procedure

The assay is again carried out in the 1.5-ml Beckman microfuge tubes. The total reaction volume is 500 µl. The assay consists of the following tubes: Nos. 1–3, no membrane controls (400 µl buffer, 100 µl tracer); Nos. 3–6, 0 standard (300 µl buffer, 100 µl tracer, 100 µl membrane); Nos. 7–9, 10–12, etc., standards (100–295 µl buffer, 5–200 µl standard, 100 µl tracer, 100 µl membrane); Nos. 13–15, 16–18, etc., unknown samples (100–295 µl buffer, 5–200 µl unknown, 100 µl tracer, 100 µl membrane).

The buffer, standard, unknown, and tracer are again all added to the microfuge tubes before membrane is taken out of freezer. Since the reaction is carried out at 4°C, the rack holding the microfuge tubes should now be immersed in ice water. The membrane is now thawed, rehomogenized in a tissue grinder, and diluted with 0.05 M Tris-HCl buffer so that the final protein concentration is 200–300 μg per 100 μl, and then well agitated. The membrane mixture should be kept at 4°C and vortexed often to ensure homogeneous suspension. After membrane has been added to the last tube, each of the assay tubes should be gently agitated.

These tubes are kept at 4°C for 16–20 hours and then spun for five minutes in the Beckman type B Microfuge. The supernatant is aspirated and the pellets are counted. The counting should be done to ensure that the tube used to check nonspecific binding (i.e., the tube that causes maximal displacement) has at least 600–1000 cpm per minimal time period.

E. Calculation of Results

For small assays, the data can be handdrawn on semilog paper with B/B_0 expressed as percent on the ordinate and the log of the standard concentration at the abscissa. The line of best fit can be estimated by "eye-of-faith." For large assays or assays where more exact answers are necessary, the data are best handled by the logit transformation to allow computer calculation and reporting of the data (Midgley et al., 1969).

F. Quality Control Checks

A flat standard curve with little displacement of label generally indicates a damaged labeled peptide. We have found that whenever a new batch of iodinated peptide or placental membrane is made, it is helpful to check optimal binding and displacement curves for each component. This is most easily done by keeping the final tracer dilution between 10,000–20,000 cpm per 100 μl, varying the membrane concentration starting at 100 μg per 100 μl, and going up by increments of 50 μg to a maximum of 250 μg per 100 μl. The procedure to be followed is the same as that used for checking the tracer as outlined earlier in this chapter (Section IV,C).

It is very helpful to have a sample or standard diluted so that 100 μl of each dilution will give a low, intermediate, and high answer on the assay curve so that intra- and interassay can be more easily monitored. However, these assays are relatively new, and no good figures for inter- or intraassay variability have been published. In our hands, intraassay variability is 6% and interassay variability of standards is 14%.

V. PREPARATION OF BUFFER AND COLUMN FOR THE NSILA-s ASSAY

A. Preparation of Buffers

1. Phosphate Buffer (0.3 M)

 a. 4.14 gm $NaH_2PO_4 \cdot H_2O$ in 100 ml
 b. 5.34 gm $Na_2HPO_4 \cdot 2H_2O$ in 100 ml
Add 9.5 ml of the solution (a) to 40.5 ml solution (b), final pH 7.4. Store at 4°C.

2. 1% BSA–Phosphate buffer (0.3 M)

Add 1.0 gm commercially available 96–99% pure fraction V BSA to 100 ml 0.3 M phosphate buffer. Store at 4°C.

3. Phosphate Buffer (0.03 M)

Add 100 ml 0.3 M phosphate buffer to 900 ml distilled water. Store at 4°C.

4. 0.5% BSA–Phosphate Buffer (0.03 M)

To 100 ml buffer add 0.5 gm commercially available 96–99% pure fraction V BSA. Store at 4°C.

5. 1% BSA–Krebs–Ringer Phosphate Buffer, pH 7.4

Krebs–Ringer phosphate buffer may be prepared by the method described by Dawson *et al.* (1969). To 100 ml of this buffer add 1.0 gm radioimmunoassay grade BSA. Store at 4°C.

B. Preparation of Columns

These columns are prepared as described previously, except the gels are swollen in 0.03 M phosphate buffer; 0.5% BSA–0.03 M phosphate buffer is then used to equilibrate and to elute the columns.

C. Preparation of Rat Liver Plasma Membranes

The technique described below is that of Neville (1968). Sucrose concentrations are give as percent (w/w) at 20°C and checked by an Abbe refractometer. All steps are carried out between 0° and 4°C. Media refers to 0.001 M $NaHCO_3$ (84 mg of $NaHCO_3$ is added to one liter of distilled water).

Eight 100-gm rats (male or female Wistar Furth or Sprague-Dawley) are decapitated, and the livers are quickly excised, trimed free from connective tissue, placed in an ice-cold beaker, and minced with scissors.

Ten grams of minced liver is placed in a large Dounce homogenizer (available from Blaessig Glass Spec. Co., Rochester, New York); 25 ml media is added, and the tissue is homogenized at 4°C with eight vigorous strokes of the loose pestle. This is repeated once. The pooled homogenates are added to 500 ml of media at 4°C, stirred for three minutes, then filtered first through two layers of No. 90 cheesecloth and then four layers of No. 120 cheesecloth. This removes precipitated nuclear protein and connective tissue. The filtered homogenate is equally distributed between four 250-ml glass centrifuge bottles (the bottles are not prechilled) and spun at 1500 g for ten minutes. The supernatant is carefully poured off, and while the tube is upside down, absorbent paper is inserted into the neck to remove excess supernatant. The pellets are poured off into a large Dounce homogenizer and resuspended in 25 ml of media. The above procedure is repeated and the pellets are homogenized with three gentle strokes of the loose pestle.

The stock sucrose solution (69 gm sucrose in 100 ml distilled water) is adjusted to 69 ± 0.1% using a refractometer, and 34 ml is placed in a 100-ml cylinder and cooled in an ice bucket. The homogenate is poured in, and water is added to make a total volume of 60 ml. The solution is mixed vigorously with a rod and checked in a refractometer. With water or 69% sucrose, the sucrose homogenate is adjusted to 44.0 ± 0.1%. Twenty milliliters is poured into each of three S-25 tubes and carefully overlaid with 10 ml 42.3 ± 0.1% sucrose (checked by refractometer). All three tubes are balanced within ±0.05 gm by adding 42.3% sucrose.

Tubes are loaded into a prechilled S-25 rotor (40°C) and spun at 25,000 rpm (90,000 g) for two hours. Tubes are handled carefully to preserve the density interface, removing float with a spatula. Eight milliliters of media is added, and the mixtures are spun to pack the sediment 25,000 g for ten minutes. Four milliliters of media is added and resuspended by squirting one through a No. 22 needle.

A cushion of 4.1 ml 50 ± 1% sucrose is placed in the bottom of two siliconized S-25 tubes. Over each, a linear sucrose gradient is formed from 37 to 3%. The gradients are overlaid with 2.0 ml of resuspended homogenate and spun 2000 rpm (55 g) for one hour. Using a syringe and long blunt No. 20 needle, material is removed at the cushion interface. The material is examined in a phase microscope;

the ratio of vesicles per membrane should not exceed one. Membrane is then aliquoted and stored as described for the somatomedin assay. The plasma membranes isolated by the above technique have been used extensively in NSILA-s binding studies (Megyesi *et al.*, 1974, 1975).

VI. TECHNIQUE OF RADIORECEPTOR ASSAY FOR NSILA-s

A. Procurement of Purified Protein for Radioreceptor Assay

The only source for purified NSILA-s at the present time is from Dr. E. R. Froesch of the Department of Medicine and Biochemistry, University of Zurich, Zurich, Switzerland. However, details on the purification of NSILA-s have been published (Froesch *et al.*, 1975). Less pure preparations may be used as standards.

For those who wish to purify the material, the first step is an acid–alcohol extraction of Cohn fraction II. The extract is chromatographed on Sephadex G-75, eluting with 5.0 M acetic acid–0.15 M NaCl. The active material elutes with K_d of 0.5, and can be further purified on 2.5 × 30 cm columns of carboxymethyl cellulose. NSILA-s is eluted using a gradient of ammonium acetate from 0.05 M, pH 5.0, to 0.3 M, pH 6.8. The pooled active fractions can be chromatographed on a 0.9 × 30 cm of DEAE-Sephadex, eluting with a linear gradient of Tris-HCl from 0.05 M, pH 8.6, to 0.25 M, pH 7.6. Gel filtration on a 0.9 × 150 cm column of Sephadex G-50, eluting with 1.0 M acetic acid, and ion-exchange chromatography on 90.9 × 20 cm column of carboxymethyl cellulose (eluting with a linear gradient of ammonium acetate from 0.05 M, pH 5.0, to 0.2 M, pH 6.8) are the final steps (Humbel *et al.*, 1971).

B. Radioiodination Procedure

This is similar to the technique used for somatomedins A and C. The reaction can be carried out in 10 × 75 cm glass or plastic tube. Thirty microliters of 0.3 M phosphate buffer, pH 7.4, is added to the tube. Then, 10 μl of NSILA-s (1.0 mg/ml dissolved in 0.01 N HCl) and 1.0–2.0 mCi of ^{125}I is added. The tube is gently shaken to mix the reactants. Three to five microliters of a 60 μg/ml solution of chloramine-T is added. If the reaction is carried out on ice, three minutes are needed for the reaction to go to completion, and the material is checked for TCA precipitability as previously described.

If the reaction is carried out at room temperature, after one minute, a small amount of sodium metabisulfite is added. Roth (1973) recommends adding twice the amount of sodium metabisulfite as chloramine-T. Therefore, if 5 μl of a 500 μg/ml solution of chloramine-T was added, 5 μl of a 120 μg/ml solution of sodium metabisulfite is added. This will keep the total reaction volume low. The TCA precipitability is checked as described for the somatomedin A and C assay (Section IV,B), aiming for 30–50% incorporation. If the percent incorporation is insufficient after the first addition of chloramine-T (this is usually the case), 5.0–10 μl more of chloramine-T, depending on the answer obtained from the previous TCA precipitation, is added. When a sufficient iodination is obtained, 1.0 ml of 1% BSA–0.3 M phosphate buffer is added to the reactants, and the mixture is filtered on the G-50 Sephadex (coarse or fine) column.

The peak tubes that elute at the appropriate (K_d of about 0.5) are saved. Each tube is checked to see which ones contain useful tracer.

C. Technique for Radioreceptor Assay

The procedure described is different from the somatomedin radioreceptor assay. The total reaction volume is 150 μl. Incubation is for 90 minutes at room temperature (20°C). All reactants are kept at 20°C. The reaction is carried out in the 400-μl plastic Beckman microfuge tubes.

1. Buffer

1% BSA–Krebs–Ringer phosphate, pH 7.5.

2. Standard

Purified or partially purified NSILA-s.

3. Sample

Sample preparation of serum is necessary in order to obtain an accurate estimate of serum NSILA-s activity. At neutral pH, the majority of NSILA-s in plasma is apparently bound to molecules of high molecular weight. However, purified NSILA-s has a molecular weight of 7500 daltons. Therefore, for the assay of NSILA-s, 0.5 ml plasma is mixed with 0.5 ml 1.0 M acetic acid and filtered on a 0.9 × 55 cm column of Sephadex G-50 fine that is equilibrated with 1.0 M acetic acid. Fractions of 1.0 ml are collected. The fractions that coelute with

^{125}I-NSILA-s marker are lyophilized twice and reconstituted in 1.0 ml of Krebs–Ringer phosphate buffer. It has been shown that this NSILA-s activity from plasma dilutes in parallel with the NSILA-s standard (Megyesi *et al.*, 1974).

4. Tracer

The tracer used is 10,000–20,000 rpm of ^{125}I-NSILA-s. The stored tracer should be filtered on a G-100 or G-50 column equilibrated with 0.5% BSA–0.03 M phosphate buffer before use in the assay. Only the peak tubes that elute at the appropriate molecular weight (7500) are used.

5. Membrane

Membrane suspension is prepared as previously described for the somatomedin assay except that Krebs–Ringer phosphate buffer is used. The final protein concentration should be 200–400 μg/ml.

6. Assay Procedure

The assay is set up as follows: The first three tubes contain 100 μl buffer and 50 μl tracer. The next three tubes (0 standard) contain 50 μl buffer, 50 μl tracer, and 50 μl buffer. The next two or three tubes, depending on the desirability of duplicate versus triplicate standards, contain 25 μl buffer, 25 μl standard, 50 μl tracer, and 50 μl membrane. Standards include 1.0–5000 ng/ml NSILA-s (70 mU/mg). More purified standards will necessitate lesser amounts, and less pure standards will need higher amounts added to the assay tubes.

Unknown tubes will contain 5.0–45 μl sample, 5.0–45 μl buffer, and 50 μl membrane. After the membrane has been added, the tubes are gently agitated, allowed to sit at 20°C for 90 minutes, then spun in the Beckman Type B microfuge for one minute. The supernatants are aspirated and the pellets are counted.

D. Calculation of Results and Quality Control Checks

Calculation of results is similar to that reported for the somatomedin assay. Inter- and intraassay variability is reported to range from 10 to 20% (Megyesi *et al.*, 1974).

VII. CROSS-REACTIVITY WITH OTHER GROWTH FACTORS

A. Somatomedin A Radioreceptor Assay

In the SmA radioreceptor assay, SmC competes in an identical manner. Multiplication stimulating activity (MSA) competes one-quarter as well as SmA. Insulin competes for the receptor but at much higher (100-fold) concentrations. SmB does not compete at all. No information is available on the cross-reactivity of NSILA-s in this assay (Takano *et al.*, 1975; Rechler *et al.*, 1976).

B. Somatomedin C Radioreceptor Assay

In the SmC radioreceptor assay, SmA competes as well as SmC for the receptor (Van Wyk *et al.*, 1975). MSA competes in parallel for the receptor and, in our hands, an impure preparation of NSILA-s (7.0 mU/mg) also competes in parallel for the receptor.

Insulin competes for the receptor, but again, very much higher concentrations are needed (10,000 ng). Proinsulin competes somewhat better for the receptor than does insulin. Rat somatomedin also competes in parallel for the SmC receptor (Chochinov *et al.*, 1977a).

We have purified a large molecular weight protein from midterm human amniotic fluids that will also cause parallel displacement of ^{125}I-SmC from its receptor (Chochinov *et al.*, 1977b). This substance appears to have no intrinsic somatomedin bioactivity, but appears to bind somatomedin C.

Nerve growth factor (NGF), epidermal growth factor (EGF), fibroblast growth factor (FGF), and SmB do not displace the tracer (Van Wyk *et al.*, 1975).

C. NSILA-s Radioreceptor Assay

In the NSILA-s assay, using rat liver plasma membranes, pure NSILA-s and pure MSA compete in an identical manner. Less pure preparations of NSILA-s compete in order of their biologic potencies.

In one study, SmA and SmC competed for the NSILA-s receptor to a lesser degree than did MSA or NSILA-s (Megyesi *et al.*, 1975). Insulin competes poorly for the receptor and only at very high concentrations (10,000–20,000 ng/ml). Proinsulin competes 300 times better than does insulin on a weight basis. SmB, NGF, and FGF show nonparallel minor displacement, while FGF has no effect (Megyesi *et al.*, 1975).

Recently, another assay for NSILA-s has been developed (Zapf *et al.* (1977). This is a highly sensitive and specific protein-binding assay. A partially purified NSILA-s carrier protein derived from human serum is used as the binding protein or receptor. Iodination of NSILA-s is done as described previously. Plasma samples are prepared as described for the radioreceptor assay. In essence the assay is performed as follows.

Partially purified NSILA-s binding protein is obtained by chromatography of powdered acetone-extracted human sera on Sephadex G-200 equilibrated with 1.0 M acetic acid. Approximately two grams of powder is suspended in 60 ml 1.0 M acetic acid, allowed to stir overnight at 4°C, centrifuged, and the supernate is applied to the column. The fraction between 60 and 80% of bed volume contains binding activity stripped of endogenous NSILA-s. These fractions are pooled, concentrated by ultrafiltration, and dialyzed against phosphate buffer, pH 7.0. The binding protein is then diluted in 0.2% BSA–0.1 M phosphate buffer, pH 7.0, so that 0.2 ml yields total binding of tracer of 25–30%. The assay consists of 0.2 ml diluted protein, 0.1 ml [125]-I-NSILA-s (150,000–300,000 cpm), and 0.1 ml of the diluted sample or the NSILA-s standard. All incubations are for two hours at room temperature. Then, 0.5 ml of a suspension of 2.0 gm of activated neutralized charcoal in 100 ml 0.2% BSA–0.1 M PO_4 buffer, pH 7 is added, and the incubation is continued i n ice bath for 20 minutes. After centrifugation, 0.5 ml of the supernate is counted for radioactivity in a gamma counter. Total binding is 25–35%. Specific binding is 15–20%. Sensitivity is 0.5 mU/liter or 1.25 ng/ml. Half-maximal binding is at 5.0–10 ng/ml. Intraassay variation was reported as 7.5 ± 3.9%, while interassay variation is 11.7 ± 2.6%. In this assay hypopituitary sera gave values of 183 ± 27 (SD) mU/liter, normal sera 350 ± 66 mU/liter, and acromegalic sera 486 ± 88 mU liter.

VIII. MEASUREMENT OF SOMATOMEDINS A AND C AND NSILA-s IN BLOOD

The radioreceptor assays for SmA, SmC, and NSILA-s have only recently been developed. They have been utilized for research and not for routine clinical studies. These assays have greatly aided in following the purification of somatomedins.

Clinically, assays can distinguish between hypophysectomized, normal, and acromegalic sera. Sera from hypopituitary patients give low somatomedin values, and acromegalic sera give high values.

Hypopituitary children treated with growth hormone show rises in their radioreceptor assayable somatomedin A, C, and NSILA-s levels in serum. Using the NSILA-s radioreceptor assay, Megyesi *et al.* (1974) have been able to identify a group of subjects with hypoglycemia, extrapancreatic tumors, and markedly elevated NSILA-s levels (normal 1200–2200 ng/ml). These assays will be of great help in further studies on normal and abnormal growth and development.

Radioimmunoassays for the somatomedin peptides will soon be available. A radioimmunoassay for SmC has recently been described (Furlanetto *et al.*, 1977). As expected, with this assay, SmC levels were low in hypopituitary patients and high in acromegalic patients. However, in contrast to the radioreceptor assay for SmC where SmC and SmA compete in almost identical fashion, in the radioimmunoassay, SmA shows only 1% the potency of SmC, indicating that their two substances have immunological differences.

REFERENCES

Chochinov, R. H., Mariz, I. K., and Daughaday, W. H. (1977a) Purification of a Somatomedin from plasma of rats bearing GH producing tissues. *Endocrinology* **100**, 549–556.

Chochinov, R. H., Mariz, I. K., and Daughaday, W. H. (1977b). Characterization of a protein in mid-term human amniotic fluid which reacts in the Somatomedin C radio receptor assay. *J. Clin. Endocrinol. Metab.* **44**, 902–908.

Cuatrecasas, P. (1972). Isolation of the insulin receptor of liver and fat-cell membranes. *Proc. Natl. Acad. Sci. U.S.A.* **69**, 318–322.

Daughaday, W. H., Hall, K., Raben, M. S., Salmon, W. D., Van den Brande, J. L., and Van Wyk, J. J. (1972). Somatomedin: A proposed designation for the "sulfation factor." *Nature (London)* **235**, 107.

Dawson, R. M. C., Elliot, D. C., Elliot, W. H., and Jones, K. M. (1969). pH buffers and physiological media. *In* "Data for Biomedical Research" (R. M. Dawson *et al.*, eds.), Chapter 20, pp. 475–508. Oxford Univ. Press (Clarendon), London and New York.

Froesch, E. R., Schlumf, V., Heimann, R., Zapf, J., Humbel, R. E., and Ritschard, W. J. (1975). Purification procedures for NSILA-s. *Adv. Metab. Disord.* **8**, 203–210.

Furlanetto, R. W., Underwood, L. E., Van Wyk, J. J., and A. Joseph D'Ecole (1977). Estimation of Somatomedin-C levels in normals and patients with pituitary disease by radioimmunoassay. *J. Clin. Invest.* **60**, 648–657.

Hall, K. (1972) Purification of human somatomedin. *Acta Endocrinol. (Copenhagen)*, Suppl. **63**, 29—38.

Hall, K., Takano, K., Fryklund, L., and Sievertsson, H. (1975). Somatomedins. *Adv. Metab. Disord.* **8**, 19–46.

Humbel, R. E., Bunzli, H., Mulhy, K., Oelz, O., Frosch, E. R., and Ritschard, W. J. (1971). Insulin-like substance: the insulin dimer, and non-suppressible insulin-

49. Somatomedin A, Somatomedin C, and NSILA-s 977

like activity. *In* "Diabetes" (R. R. Rodriquez and J. Vallance-Owen, eds.), pp. 306–317. Exerpta Med. Found., Amsterdam.
Lowry, O. W., Rosebrough, N. J., Farr, A. L., and Randall, R. J. (1951). Protein measurement with the Folin phenol reagent. *J. Biol. Chem.* **193**, 265–275.
Marshall, R. N., Underwood, L. E., Viona, S. J., Foushee, D. B., and Van Wyk, J. J. (1974). Characterization of the insulin and Somatomedin C receptors in human placental cell membranes. *J. Clin. Endocrinol. Metab.* **39**, 283–292.
Megyesi, K., Kahn, C. R., Roth, J., and Gorden, P. (1974). Hypoglycemia in association with extrapancreatic tumors: Demonstration of elevated plasma NSILA-s by a new radio-receptor assay. *J. Clin. Endocrinol. Metab.* **38**, 931–934.
Megyesi, K., Kahn, C. R., Roth, J., Neville, D. M., Jr., Nissley, S. P., Humbel, R. E., and Froesch, E. R. (1975). The NSILA-s receptor in liver plasma membranes. Characterization and comparison with the insulin receptor. *J. Biol. Chem.* **250**, 8990–8996.
Midgley, A. R., Niswender, G. D., and Rebar, R. W. (1969). Principles for the assessment of the reliability of radioimmunoassay methods. *Acta Endocrinol. (Copenhagen)*, Suppl. **142**, 163–184.
Neville, D. M., Jr. (1968). Isolation of an organ specific protein antigen from cell-surface membrane of rat liver. *Biochim. Biophys. Acta* **154**, 522–540.
Rechler, M. M., Fryklund, L., Nissley, S. P., Hall, K., Podskalny, J. M., Skottner, A., and Moses, A. C. (1976). Comparison of purified Somatomedin A (Sm-A) and multiplication stimulating activity (MSA) by radio-receptor and biological assays. *Proc. 58th Annu. Meet. Endocr. Soc.* p. 222.
Rechler, M. M., Nissley, S. P., Podskalny, J. M., Moses, A. C., and Fryklund, L. (1977). Identification of a receptor for somatomedin-like polypeptides in human fibroblasts. *J. Clin. Endocrinol. Metab.* **44**, 820–831.
Roth, J. (1973). Peptide hormone binding to receptors: A review of direct studies in vitro. *Metab., Clin. Exp.* **22**, 1054–1073.
Salmon, W. D., and Daughaday, W. H. (1957). A hormonally controlled serum factor which stimulates sulfate incorporation by cartilage in vitro. *J. Lab. Clin. Med.* **49**, 825–836.
Takano, K., Hall, K., Fryklund, L., Holmgren, A., Sievertsson, H., and Uthne, T. (1975). The binding of insulin and Somatomedin A to human placental membrane. *Acta Endocrinol. (Copenhagen)* **80**, 14–31.
Thorsson, A. V., and Hintz, R. L. (1977). Specific ^{125}I-somatomedin receptor on circulating human mononuclear cells. *Biochem. Biophys. Res. Commun.* **74**, 1566–1573.
Van Wyk, J. J., Underwood, L. E., Hintz, R. L., Clemmons, D. R., Voina, S. J., and Weaver, R. P. (1974). The somatomedins: A family of insulin like hormones under growth hormone control. *Recent Prog. Horm. Res.* **30**, 259–318.
Van Wyk, J. J., Underwood, L. E., Baseman, J. B., Hintz, R. L., Clemmons, D. R., and Marshall, R. N. (1975). Explorations of the insulin-like and growth-promoting properties of Somatomedin C by membrane receptor assays. *Adv. Metab. Disord.* **8**, 128–150.
Yalow, R. S., Hall, K., and Luft, R. (1975). Radioimmunoassay of somatomedin B: Application to clinical and physiologic studies. *J. Clin. Invest.* **55**, 127–137.
Zapf, J., Kaufmann, V., Eigenmann, E. J., and Froesch, E. R. (1977). Determination of nonsuppressible insulin-like activity in human serum by a sensitive protein binding assay. *Clin. Chem.* **23**, 677–682.

APPENDIXES

APPENDIX 1   Summary of Radioimmunoassay Methodology

Hormone	Immunogen	Species immunized	Labeled hormone	Separation	Sample preparation	Sensitivity
1. Cyclic AMP (cAMP)	2′-O-succinyl-cAMP–albumin–EDC carbodiimide	Rabbits SQ Goats SQ	^{125}I-Tyrosine methyl ester-2′-O-succinyl cAMP	Sephadex G-10	Tissue—trichloroacetic acid precipitation; ether extraction; Plasma–perchloric acid + Dowex chromatography	5 fmole
Cyclic GMP (cGMP)	2′-O-succinyl-cGMP-keyhole limpet hemocyanin-EDC carbodiimide	Rabbits SQ Goats SQ	^{125}I-Tyrosine methyl ester-2′-O-succinyl cGMP	Sephadex G-10	Plasma and tissue—trichloroacetic acid precipitation; ether extraction	5 fmole
2. Prostaglandins PGE	PGE–KLH–ethyl chloroformate	Rabbits SQ	^{3}H-PGE$_1$	Dextran charcoal	Plasma and tissue—ethyl acetate : isopropanol extraction + silicic acid chromatography—benzene : ethyl acetate : methanol	1.0 pg
PGA	PGA$_1$–HSA–EDC carbodiimide	Rabbits SQ	^{3}H-PGA$_1$	Dextran charcoal	Plasma and tissue—ethyl acetate : isopropanol extraction + silicic acid chromatography—benzene : ethyl acetate : methanol	1.0 pg
PGF	PGF$_{2\alpha}$–BSA–EDC carbodiimide	Rabbits SQ	^{3}H-PGF$_{1\alpha}$	Dextran charcoal	Plasma and tissue—ethyl acetate : isopropanol extraction + silicic acid chromatography—benzene : ethyl acetate : methanol	1.0 pg
Prostaglandin metabolites 15-Keto-PGF$_{2\alpha}$	15-Keto-PGE$_{2\alpha}$–poly-L-lysine–EDC carbodiimide	Rabbits SQ	^{3}H-15-Keto-PGF$_{2\alpha}$	Double antibody	Plasma directly	500 pg
13,14-Dihydro-15-keto-PGF$_{2\alpha}$	13,14-Dihydro-15-keto-PGF$_{2\alpha}$–BSA–EDC carbodiimide	Rabbits SQ	^{3}H-13,14-Dihydro-15-keto-PGF$_{2\alpha}$	Double antibody	Plasma directly	50 pg
15-Keto-PGE$_2$	15-Keto-PGE$_2$–BSA–DCC carbodiimide	Sheep IM	^{3}H-15-Keto-PGE$_2$	Ammonium sulfate	Plasma directly	2 pg
13,14-Dihydro-15-keto-PGE$_2$	13,14-Dihydro-15-keto-PGE$_2$–HSA–DCC carbodiimide	Rabbits SQ	^{3}H-13,14-Dihydro-15-keto-PGE$_2$	Double antibody	Plasma directly	10 pg
Thromboxane B$_2$ (TXB$_2$)	TXB$_2$–HSA-carbonyldiimidazole	Rabbits SQ	^{3}H-TXB$_2$	Polyethylene glycol	Plasma directly	10 pg
3. Thyrotropin-releasing hormone (TRH)	TRH–BSA-bisdiazotized benzidine	Rabbits SQ	^{125}I-TRH	Double antibody	Affinity chromatography	5 pg

(Continued)

APPENDIX 1 (Continued)

Hormone	Immunogen	Species immunized	Labeled hormone	Separation	Sample preparation	Sensitivity
4. Gonadotropin-releasing hormone (GnRH)	GnRH–BSA–bisdiazotized benzidine	Rabbits SQ	^{125}I-GnRH	Double antibody	Methanol extraction	5 pg
5. Somatostatin (SRIF)	Somatostatin–bovine thryoglobulin–CMC carbodiimide	Rabbits SQ	^{125}I-Tyr^1-SRIF	Double antibody	Acetic acid extraction + boiling	1.6 pg
6. Melatonin (MT)	MT–BSA–formaldehyde condensation or diatization + mixed anhydride	Rabbits SQ	^{3}H-MT	Ammonium sulfate	Chloroform extraction	50 pg
	N-succinyl-5-methoxy-tryptophan–BSA–mixed anhydride	Rabbits SQ	^{125}I-N-3-(4-hydroxy-phenyl)-propionyl-5-methoxytryptamine	Double antibody	Chloroform extraction, bicarbonate (pH 10.25), wash	2.3 pg
	N-acetyl-5-methoxy-tryptophan–BSA or TG (thyroglobulin)–carbodiimide	Rabbits SQ	^{3}H-MT	Ammonium sulfate	Chloroform extraction pH 10, then petroleum ether extraction	5 pg
	Indomethacin–HSA–carbodiimide	Rabbits SQ	^{3}H-MT	Double antibody	Chloroform extraction Amberlite XA D$_2$ chromatography, TLC Homogenization (pineal)	23 pg
	MT-p-aminobenzoic acid	Rabbits SQ	^{3}H-MT	Ammonium sulfate		50 pg
	N-acetylserotonin–BSA	Rabbits SQ	^{3}H-MT	Ammonium sulfate	Chloroform extraction pH 10, then Lipidex separation	30 pg
7. Substance P	Substance P–bovine gamma globulin or succinylated thyroglobulin–EDC carbodiimide	Rabbits SQ	^{125}I-Tyr^8-substance P	Dextran charcoal	Acid–acetone or 2 N acetic acid extraction	0.5–1.0 fmol
8. Neurotensin (NT)	NT-succinylated thyroglobulin or keyhole limpet hemocyanin-EDC carbodiimide	Rabbits SQ	^{125}I-NT	Dextran charcoal	Acid–acetone, 2 N acetic acid extraction	1–3 fmol
9. Pituitary gonadotropins	FSH and LH directly	Rabbits SQ Monkeys SQ	^{125}I-FSH–lacto-peroxidase ^{125}I-LH-chloramine-T	Double antibody, antibody polymer, or isopropanol	Plasma or serum directly	100 pg
10. Prolactin	Human prolactin directly	Rabbits SQ	^{125}I-Human prolactin	Double antibody	Serum or plasma directly Tissue—homogenization with ammonium bicarbonate or sodium hydroxide at pH 9.5 or above.	50–150 pg
11. Growth hormone	Human growth hormone directly	Guinea pigs SQ	^{125}I-Human growth hormone	Double antibody	Plasma—directly Tissue—homogenized and extracted with buffered saline	78 pg

	Immunogen	Species	Label	Separation	Extraction	Sensitivity
12. ACTH	Synthetic α¹⁻²⁴ACTH–rabbit serum albumin–EDC carbodiimide	Rabbits SQ	^{125}I-Synthetic hACTH	Double antibody	Silicic acid extraction	1.0 pg
	Commercial zinc porcine ACTH	Guinea pigs SQ				1.0 pg
	Synthetic α¹⁻²⁴ACTH–bovine serum albumin–EDC carbodiimide	Sheep				1–3 pg
	Partially purified human ACTH	Rabbits SQ				10 pg
13. α-MSH	Synthetic α-MSH–rabbit serum albumin–EDC carbodiimide	Rabbits SQ	^{125}I-Synthetic α-MSH	Chromatoelectrophoresis	Cationic exchange (Amberlite CG-50)	50 pg
"β-MSH" (β-LPH, γ-LPH)	Commercial zinc porcine ACTH contaminated with MSH and LPH peptides directly	Guinea pigs SQ	^{125}I-Synthetic "hβMSH"	Chromatoelectrophoresis	Cationic exchange (Amberlite CG-50)	1–5 pg
	Synthetic "hβMSH"–bovine serum albumin–EDC carbodiimide	Rabbits SQ		QUSO–Plasma adsorption	Silicic acid extraction	
14. Thyrotropin (hTSH)	Human thyrotropin directly	Rabbits SQ	^{125}I-hTSH	Double antibody	Serum or plasma directly	0.1–0.3 µU
15. Oxytocin	Oxytocin–BSA–glutaraldehyde	Rabbits SQ	^{125}I- or ^{131}I-oxytocin	Double antibody	Plasma (drawn into phenanthroline) extraction with acetone + petroleum ether	<1.0 pg
16. Vasopressin	Arginine vasopressin–BSA–gluteraldehyde	Rabbits SQ	^{125}I- or ^{131}I-Vasopressin	Polyethylene glycol	Plasma extraction with acetone + petroleum ether Urine—directly	0.1 pg
17. Calcitonin	Synthetic calcitonin directly	Rabbits SQ Guinea pigs SQ	^{125}I- or ^{131}I-Calcitonin	Dextran charcoal, antibody, or polyethylene glycol	Affinity chromatography	5 pg/ml
18. Thyroxine (T4)	T4–BSA–EDC carbodiimide	Rabbits SQ	^{131}I-T4	Dextran charcoal	Serum	100 pg
Triiodothyronine (T3)	T3–BSA–EDC carbodiimide	Rabbits SQ	^{125}I-T3	Dextran charcoal	Serum	125 pg
Reverse triiodothyronine (rT3)	rT3–HSA–CMC carbodiimide	Rabbits SQ	^{125}I-rT3	Double antibody	Serum—ethanol extraction	10 pg
Diiodothyronine (T2)	T2–HSA–CMC carbodiimide	Rabbits SQ	^{125}I-T2	Double antibody	Serum—ethanol extraction	10 pg
19. Parathyroid hormone (PTH)	Partially purified bovine PTH directly	Guinea pigs SQ Rabbits SQ Chickens IV	^{125}I-Bovine PTH	Dextran charcoal	Plasma	4 pg
20. Erythropoietin	Human urinary erythropoietin directly	Rabbits SQ	^{125}I-Erythropoietin	Double antibody	Plasma or serum	1.0 mU/ml

(Continued)

APPENDIX 1 (Continued)

Hormone	Immunogen	Species immunized	Labeled hormone	Separation	Sample preparation	Sensitivity
21. Vitamin D metabolites						
25-Hydroxy-vitamin D (25-OHD)	Radioassay—serum binding protein	—	^{3}H-25-OHD	Dextran charcoal	Serum—ether extraction + silicic acid chromatography	250 pg
1,25-Dihydroxy-vitamin D (1,25-(OH)$_2$D)	Radioassay—avian small intestine cytosol preparation	—	^{3}H-1,2-(OH)$_2$D	Polyethylene glycol	Serum—extraction with chloroform:methanol + LH-20 column chromatography + high pressure liquid chromatography	20 pg
24,25-Dihydroxy-vitamin D (24,25-(OH)$_2$D)	Radioassay—serum binding protein	—	^{3}H-25 OHD$_3$	Dextran charcoal	Serum—ether extraction + LH-20 chromatography	250 pg
22. Gastrin	Human gastrin-2-17-BSA–EDC carbodiimide	Rabbits SQ	^{125}I-Human gastrin I	Double antibody	Serum	1.0 pg
	Crude porcine gastrin I directly	Guinea pigs SQ	^{125}I-Porcine gastrin I	Anion-exchange resin	Plasma	10 pg
23. Secretin	Purified porcine secretin–BSA–EDC carbodiimide	Rabbits SQ	^{125}I-Synthetic secretin	Dextran charcoal	Serum extracted with methanol	8 pg/ml
24. Cholecystokinin-pancreozymin (CCK-PZ)	Partially purified CCK-PZ directly	Rabbits SQ	^{125}I- or ^{131}I-CCK-PZ	Double antibody	Serum heated to 100°C for 5–10 minutes	5 pg/ml
25. Serotonin (5-HT)	5-HT diazotized to BSA–aminophenylalanine–EDC carbodiimide	Rabbits SQ	^{3}H-5-HT	Ammonium sulfate	Whole blood lysed with water + Zn(OH)$_2$	100 pg
26. Gastric inhibitory polypeptide (GIP)	Porcine GIP-BSA-EDC carbodiimide	Rabbits SQ Guinea pigs SQ	^{125}I-Porcine GIP	Dextran charcoal	Serum directly	125 pg/ml
27. Vasoactive intestinal polypeptide (VIP)	Porcine VIP-BSA-EDC carbodiimide	Rabbits SQ	^{125}I-Porcine VIP	Charcoal	Trasylol plasma directly	1 pmol/liter
28. Motilin	Porcine motilin–BSA–EDC carbodiimide	Rabbits SQ Guinea pigs SQ	^{125}I-Porcine motilin	Dextran charcoal	Serum directly	125 pg/ml
29. Bombesin	Bombesin or its C-terminal nonapeptide-BSA-EDC carbodiimide	Rabbits SQ	^{125}I-Tyrosinated bombesin C-terminal nonapeptide	Dextran charcoal	Tissue—acetic acid extraction of boiled tissue	20 pmol/liter
30. Bile acids						
Cholylglycine	Glycylcholate–BSA–EDC carbodiimide	Rabbits SQ	^{3}H-Glycocholic ^{125}I-Cholylglycyl histamine	Ammonium sulfate, polyethylene glycol	Serum directly	5 pmol
Chenodeoxycholyl-glycine	Glycylchenodeoxycholate–BSA–EDC carbodiimide	Rabbits SQ	^{3}H-Glycochenodeoxycholic acid	Ammonium sulfate, polyethylene glycol	Serum directly	5 pmol
Deoxycholylglycine	Glycyldeoxycholate-BSA–EDC carbodiimide	Rabbits SQ	^{3}H-Glycodeoxycholic acid	Ammonium sulfate, polyethylene glycol	Serum directly	5 pmol

Antigen	Immunogen	Animal	Label	Separation	Sample preparation	Sensitivity
Sulfolithocholyl-glycine	Glycylsulfolithocholate–BSA–EDC carbodiimide	Rabbits SQ	³H-Glycolithocholic sulfate; ¹²⁵I-Sulfolithocholyl-glycyl-histamine	Ammonium sulfate, polyethylene glycol	Serum directly	5 pmol
31. Insulin	Porcine insulin directly	Guinea pigs SQ	¹²⁵I-Porcine insulin	Double antibody	Serum or plasma—separation of insulin and proinsulin on Bio-Gel P-30 or Sephadex G-50; Urine—directly at pH 7	1.0 μU
Proinsulin	Porcine insulin directly	Guinea pigs SQ	¹²⁵I-Porcine insulin	Double antibody	Serum—treated with polyethylene glycol; Urine—directly	100 pg
C-peptide	C-peptide–RSA–EDC carbodiimide	Rabbits SQ	¹²⁵I-Tyrosinated C-peptide	Double antibody		75 pg
32. Glucagon	Glucagon absorbed to polyvinylpyrrolidone	Rabbits SQ	¹²⁵I-Glucagon	Dextran charcoal	Plasma containing Trasylol 500 U/ml directly	5 pg
33. Human pancreatic polypeptide (hPP)	Human PP directly	Rabbits SQ	¹²⁵I-HPP or ¹²⁵I-BPP	Double antibody	Plasma or serum directly	2–5 pg
Bovine pancreatic polypeptide (bPP)	Bovine PP directly	Rabbits SQ	¹²⁵I-BPP	Double antibody	Plasma or serum directly	2–5 pg
34. Estrogens — Estradiol	17β-Estradiol hemisuccinate–BSA	Sheep SQ	³H-17β-Estradiol	Dextran charcoal	Plasma—ether extraction + LH-20 chromatography with isooctane : benzene : methanol	25 pg/ml
Estriol	17β-Estradiol hemisuccinate–BSA	Sheep SQ	³H-Estriol	Dextran charcoal	Plasma—ether extraction + LH-20 chromatography with isooctane : benzene : methanol	25 pg/ml
Estrone	17β-Estradiol hemisuccinate–BSA	Sheep SQ	³H-Estrone	Dextran charcoal	Plasma—ether extraction + LH-20 chromatography with isooctane : benzene : methanol	25 pg/ml
Urinary estriol glucuronide	Estriol-16α(β-D-glucuronide)–keyhole limpet hemocyanin–isobutylchlorocarbonate; Estriol-16α(β-D-glucuronide)–BSA–isobutylchlorocarbonate	Sheep SQ; Rabbits SQ	³H-Estriol-16α(β-D-glucuronide)	Dextran charcoal	Urine directly	230 pg
35. Progesterones — Progesterone	11α-Hydroxyprogesterone–BSA–active ester	Rabbits SQ, ID	³H-Progesterone	Dextran charcoal	Serum—petroleum ether extraction + LH-20 chromatography with benzene : methanol	200 pg/ml
20α-dihydroprogesterone	20α-Dihydroprogesterone–BSA–active ester	Rabbits SQ, ID	³H-20α-Dihydroprogesterone	Dextran charcoal	Serum—petroleum ether extraction + LH-20 chromatography with benzene : methanol	100 pg/ml
36. Androgens — Testosterone	Testosterone-3-oxime–BSA	Rabbits SQ	³H-Testosterone	Dextran charcoal	Plasma—ether extraction + LH-20 chromatography with isooctane : benzene : methanol	10 pg

(Continued)

APPENDIX 1 (Continued)

Hormone	Immunogen	Species immunized	Labeled hormone	Separation	Sample preparation	Sensitivity
Dihydrotestosterone	Testosterone-3-oxime–BSA	Rabbits SQ	³H-Testosterone	Dextran charcoal	Plasma—ether extraction + LH-20 chromatography with isooctane : benzene : methanol	10 pg
38. Mineralocorticoids						
Aldosterone	Aldosterone-18,21-di-hemisuccinate–BSA	Sheep ID	³H-Aldosterone	Dextran charcoal	Plasma—alkaline methylene chloride extraction + paper chromatography aldosterone benzene : methanol : water Urine—acid hydrolysis + extraction with methylene chloride + paper chromatography using benzene : methanol : water Tissue—(aldosterone) + 18-OH DOC (plasma) + 18-OH-B (plasma) extraction + lactonization + saponification + paper chromatography	2–3 pg
Aldolactone	Aldolactone-3-oxime-BSA	Sheep ID	³H-Aldosterone γ-etiolactone	Dextran charcoal	Plasma—alkaline methylene chloride extraction + paper chromatography aldosterone-benzene : methanol : water Urine—acid hydrolysis + extraction with methylene chloride + paper chromatography using benzene : methanol : water Tissue—(aldosterone) + 18-OH DOC (plasma) + 18-OH B (plasma) extraction + lactonization + saponification + paper chromatography	6 pg
DOC	17-Hydroxyprogesterone-3-oxime-BSA	Sheep ID	³H-Deoxycorticosterone	Dextran charcoal	Plasma—alkaline methylene chloride extraction + paper chromatography aldosterone-benzene : methanol : water Urine—acid hydrolysis + extraction with methylene chloride + paper chromatography using benzene : methanol : water	4 pg

18-OH-DOC	18-OH-DOC-3-oxime-BSA	Sheep ID	³H-18-OH-DOC	Dextran charcoal	Tissue—(aldosterone) + 18-OH DOC (plasma) + 18-OH-B (plasma) extraction + lactonization + saponification + paper chromatography	2 pg
					Plasma—alkaline methylene chloride extraction + paper chromatography aldosterone-benzene : methanol : water	
					Urine—acid hydrolysis + extraction with methylene chloride + paper chromatography using benzene : methanol : water	
					Tissue—(aldosterone) + 18-OH DOC (plasma) + 18-OH-B (plasma) extraction + lactonization + saponification + paper chromatography	
39. Glucocorticoids and their metabolites						
Cortisol	21-Hemisuccinate–BSA or thyroglobulin	Rabbits IM or ID	³H-Cortisol	Dextran charcoal; solid phase, ammonium sulfate	Plasma—ethanol extraction, dichloromethane extraction, thermodestruction of CBG; simple dilution	5–30 pg
	3-Oxime-21-acetate-BSA	Sheep IM				
	3-oxime-BSA			Double antibody	Urine—dichloromethane extraction with and without chromatography	
	3-20-dioxime-BSA					
	6α- or 6β-hemisuccinoxy-BSA					
Corticosterone	21-Hemisuccinate–BSA	Rabbits IM	³H-Corticosterone	Dextran charcoal	Plasma—benzene extraction or thermodestruction	5–30 pg
	3-oxime–BSA	Sheep IM		Ammonium sulfate		
	3,20-dioxime–BSA			Double antibody		
Compound S	21-Hemisuccinate–BSA	Rabbits IM	³H-17-Hydroxydeoxy-corticosterone	Dextran charcoal	Plasma—dichloromethane extraction with and without chromatography, chloroform extraction	5–30 pg
	3-oxime–BSA	Sheep IM		Double antibody		
	6α- or 6β-hemisuccinoxy-BSA					
Tetrahydrocortisol (THF)	20-oxime-BSA	Rabbits IM	³H-Tetrahydrocortisol	Dextran charcoal	Urine—β-glucuronidase treatment + dichloromethane extraction	20–30 pg
	21-Hemisuccinate–BSA					
Tetrahydrocortisone (THE)	20-oxime-BSA	Rabbits IM	³H-Tetrahydrocortisone	Dextran charcoal	Urine—β-glucuronidase treatment + chloromethane extraction	20–30 pg
	21-Hemisuccinate–BSA					
Tetrahydrocorti-costerone (THB)	20-Oxime-BSA	Rabbits IM	³H-Tetrahydrocorti-costerone	Dextran charcoal	Urine—β-glucuronidase treatment + dichloromethane extraction and paper chromatography	20–30 pg
Tetrahydro-compound S (THS)	20-Oxime-BSA	Rabbits IM	³H-Tetrahydro-17-hydroxycorticosterone	Dextran charcoal	Urine—β-glucuronidase treatment + dichloromethane extraction and paper chromatography	20–30 pg

(Continued)

APPENDIX 1 (Continued)

Hormone	Immunogen	Species immunized	Labeled hormone	Separation	Sample preparation	Sensitivity
40. Arthropod molting hormones						
β-Ecdysone	β-Ecdysone-6-carbomethyloxime-BSA	Rabbits SQ	³H-β-Ecdysone	Ammonium sulfate	Tissue—methanol extraction	2.5 pmol
	Mixture of 2,3,22-N-hydroxysuccinimide esters of β-ecdysone-HSA	Rabbits SQ	H-β-Ecdysone	Ammonium sulfate	Tissue—methanol extraction	4.6 pmol
	Succinic acid esters of β-ecdysone—HSA	Rabbits SQ	¹²⁵I-Succinyl-β-ecdysone-tyrosine methylester	Equilibrium dialysis	Tissue—methanol extraction	3.2 pmol
	β-Ecdysone-6-carboxymethyl-oxime-BSA	Rabbits SQ	¹²⁵I-β-Ecdysone-carboxymethyl oxime—tyramine	Dextran charcoal	Tissue—methanol extraction	0.15 pmol
α-Ecdysone	α-Ecdysone-22-hemisuccinate—bovine thyroglobulin	Rabbits SQ	³H-α-Ecdysone	Ammonium sulfate	Tissue—aqueous extraction	0.15 pmol
41. Human chorionic gonadotropin (hCG)	hCG-β subunit directly	Rabbits ID	¹²⁵I-hCG-β-subunit or ¹²⁵I-hCG	Double antibody	Serum directly	50 pg
42. Placental lactogen	Placental lactogen directly	Rabbits SQ Guinea pigs SQ	¹²⁵I-Human placental lactogen	Double antibody, Solid phase	Plasma or serum directly	50 pg
43. Human chorionic thyrotropin (hCT)	Bovine TSH directly	Rabbits SQ	¹²⁵I-Bovine TSH	Double antibody	Serum directly	0.5 µU/ml
44. Relaxin	Porcine relaxin directly	Rabbits ID	¹²⁵I-Polytyrosylrelaxin	Double antibody	Plasma or serum directly	32 pg
45. Renin	Angiotensin I-RSA-EDC carbodiimide	Rabbits SQ	¹²⁵I-Angiotensin I	Dextran charcoal	Blood drawn into EDTA, 8-hydroxyquinoline sulfate, phenylmethylsulfonyl fluoride, dimercaprol, and neomycin. Renin is measured by evaluating angiotensin I generation in unextracted plasma.	10 pg
Angiotensin II	Angiotensin II-RSA-EDC carbodiimide	Rabbits SQ	¹²⁵I-Angiotensin II	Dextran charcoal	For direct determination in plasma, angiotensins adsorbed to Fuller's earth and removed with ammonia in methanol	10 pg
46. Bradykinin	Bradykinin—ovalbumin or thyroglobulin—EDC carbodiimide	Rabbits SQ	¹²⁵I-Tyrosine-8 bradykinin, ¹²⁵I-tyrosine-5-bradykinin, or ¹²⁵I-p-nitrophenyl ester of p-hydroxyphenyl-pyruvate-bradykinin	Ammonium sulfate	Blood drawn into 0.5 M 1,10-phenanthroline in ethanol + ethanol extraction + acidification + evaporation + dissolution in buffer	20 pg

47. Epidermal growth factor (EGF) Urogastrone	Mouse EGF directly	Rabbits SQ	^{125}I-EGF	Double antibody or dextran charcoal	Serum or urine directly	50 pg
	Human urogastrone directly	Rabbits SQ	^{125}I-Urogastrone	Double antibody or dextran charcoal	Serum or urine directly	5 pg
48. Nerve growth factor (NGF)	NGF directly	Rabbits SQ	^{125}I-NGF	Double antibody	Serum or tissue culture medium directly	0.5 ng/ml
49. Somatomedins NSILA-s	Radioassay—rat liver membranes	—	^{125}I-NSILA-s	Centrifugation	Serum—acetic acid extraction + Sephadex G-50 chromatography	Depends on purity of standards
Somatomedin A	Radioassay—placental membranes	—	^{125}I-Human somatomedin A	Centrifugation	Serum directly	0.1 U/ml
Somatomedin C	Radioassay—placental membranes	—	^{125}I-Human somatomedin C	Centrifugation	Serum directly	0.05 U/ml
	14% Pure somatomedin directly	Rabbits SQ				0.5 mU/ml

APPENDIX 2 Commercial Sources of Radioimmunoassay Components[a,b]

Hormone	Antibody		Hormone for			Labeled hormone	Immunoassay kits
	Immunogen	Antiserum	Immunization	Standard	Labeling		
1. Cyclic AMP		Collaborative Research[1] Schwarz/Mann[2] New England Nuclear[3]	Sigma[4]	Sigma	Sigma	Collaborative Research	Collaborative Research Schwarz/Mann Amersham-Searle[5] Diagnostic Products[6] New England Nuclear
2. Cyclic GMP		Collaborative Research Schwarz/Mann New England Nuclear	Sigma	Sigma	Sigma	Collaborative Research	Collaborative Research Schwarz/Mann Amersham-Searle New England Nuclear
3. Prostaglandins E, A, and F		Calbiochem[7]	Upjohn[8]	Upjohn	New England Nuclear Amersham-Searle	New England Nuclear Amersham-Searle	Clinical Assays[9] Calbiochem
4. Thyrotropin-releasing hormone (TRH)			Abbott[10] Beckman[11]	Abbott Beckman	Abbott Beckman	New England Nuclear	
5. Gonadotropin-releasing hormone	Ayerst[12]		Ayerst Beckman	Ayerst Beckman	Ayerst Beckman		

(Continued)

APPENDIX 2 (Continued)

| Hormone | Antibody | | | Hormone for | | Labeled hormone | Immunoassay kits |
	Immunogen	Antiserum	Immunization	Standard	Labeling		
6. Somatostatin		Immuno Nuclear[13]	Beckman Bachem Fine Chemicals[14]	Immuno Nuclear		Immuno Nuclear	Immuno Nuclear
7. Melatonin		AB Kabi[15] Guildhay Antisera[16]		Sigma Calbiochem Koch-Light[17] Fluka[18]		New England Nuclear	AB Kabi
8. Substance P		Immuno Nuclear	Beckman Peninsula[19] Sigma	Immuno Nuclear	Beckman Peninsula	Immuno Nuclear	Immuno Nuclear
9. Neurotensin (NT)			Beckman Peninsula Bachem Fine Chemicals UCB Bio-products[20]	Beckman Peninsula	Beckman Peninsula		
10. Pituitary gonado-tropins (LH and FSH)	NIAMDD[21]	Calbiochem NIAMDD	NIAMDD	NIAMDD	NIAMDD		Radioassay Systems[22] Serono[23] Calbiochem

Hormone						
11. Prolactin	NIAMDD	NIAMDD Immuno Nuclear Calbiochem	MRC[24] NIAMDD Immuno Nuclear	NIAMDD	Immuno Nuclear	Calbiochem Radioassay Systems Serono
12. Growth hormone	Antibodies for Research[25] Collaborative Research Gateway[26] Calbiochem	NIAMDD Calbiochem	NIAMDD Calbiochem	NIAMDD Calbiochem	New England Nuclear Abbott Cambridge Nuclear[27]	Immuno Nuclear Abbott Serono Calbiochem Curtis[28] Schwarz/Mann Amersham-Searle
13. Adrenocorticotropic hormone (ACTH)	Organon[29]	Organon	Organon	Organon		
14. Melanocyte-stimulating hormones (MSH's)	Ciba-Geigy Parke-Davis[32]		NPA[30] Ciba-Geigy[31] Schwarz/Mann Calbiochem Ciba-Geigy	NPA Ciba-Geigy Schwarz/Mann Calbiochem Ciba-Geigy		
15. Lipotropic hormones (LPH's)	Beckman					

(Continued)

APPENDIX 2 (Continued)

Hormone	Antibody		Hormone for			Labeled hormone	Immunoassay kits
	Immunogen	Antiserum	Immunization	Standard	Labeling		
16. Thyrotropin (human) (hTSH)		Calbiochem Diagnostic Bio-chemistry[33] Nuclear Medical Systems[34]		Calbiochem	Calbiochem	Radioassay Systems Diagnostic Bio-chemistry New England Nuclear Amersham-Searle	Pharmacia[35] Beckman Schwarz/Mann Radioassay Systems Bio-RIA[36] Nuclear Medical Systems Pontex[37] Calbiochem
17. Oxytocin		Calbiochem	Parke-Davis Chemalog[38]	Parke-Davis Chemalog	Parke-Davis Chemalog		
18. (Avp) Vasopressin		Calbiochem	Spectrum Industries[39] Calbiochem Chemalog Hoechst	Spectrum Industries Calbiochem Chemalog	Spectrum Industries Calbiochem Chemalog		
19. Calcitonin (human)	Beckman	Calbiochem	Beckman	Beckman	Beckman	Immuno Nuclear	Immuno Nuclear

20. Thyroxine	Immuno Nuclear	Ciba-Geigy	Ciba-Geigy	Ciba-Geigy	Sigma	Abbott	Clinical Assays Radioassay Systems
21. Triiodothyronine	Calbiochem	Organon	Organon	MRC Immuno Nuclear	Sigma	Abbott	Clinical Assays Radioassay Systems
22. Parathyroid hormone (PTH)	Immuno Nuclear, Nichols' Institute[40], Cambridge Nuclear, CIS Radio-Pharmaceuticals[41], Burroughs Wellcome Research[42], Scantibodies Lab[43], Calbiochem[44], Inolex, Wilson Labs[45]	Inolex	Inolex, Wilson Labs, Calbiochem	Inolex, Wilson Labs, Calbiochem, Immuno Nuclear		Immuno Nuclear, Nichols' Institute, Cambridge Nuclear, CIS Radio-Pharmaceuticals	Immuno Nuclear, Nichols' Institute, Cambridge Nuclear
23. Erythropoietin							
24. Vitamin D metabolites				Calbiochem			

(Continued)

APPENDIX 2 (Continued)

Hormone	Antibody		Immunization	Hormone for		Labeled hormone	Immunoassay kits
	Immunogen	Antiserum		Standard	Labeling		
25. Gastrin and related peptides		Wilson Labs / Radioassay Systems	ICI[46]	ICI (human) / MRC (porcine)	ICI / MRC	Cambridge Nuclear	Squibb / Radioassay Systems
26. Cholecystokinin-pancreozymin (CCK-PZ)			GIH[47] Squibb	GIH Squibb	GIH Squibb		
27. Gastrin tetrapeptide		Schwarz/Mann					
28. Secretin			GIH Sigma	GIH	GIH		
29. Serotonin						New England Nuclear	
30. Gastric inhibitory polypeptide (GIP)			GIH	GIH	GIH		
31. Vasoactive intestinal peptide (VIP)		UCB	GIH	GIH	GIH		
32. Motilin							
33. Bombesin-like peptides			Farmitalia[49] Calbiochem		Farmitalia		

34. Bile acids	Abbott		Calbiochem, Mann Research Labs[50], Sterloids[51], Sigma, Supelco[52]		Abbott, New England Nuclear	Abbott
35. Insulin	Immuno Nuclear	Lilly, Novo[53]	Immuno Nuclear	Lilly, Novo	Cambridge Nuclear, Amersham-Searle, New England Nuclear, Immuno Nuclear	Amersham-Searle Serono, Calbiochem, Curtis, Pharmacia, Schwarz/Mann, Immuno Nuclear
36. C-peptide		Calbiochem, Cambridge Nuclear, Novo		Calbiochem		
37. Glucagon	Lilly[54], Novo	Cambridge Nuclear, Novo	Lilly, Novo, Sigma, Lilly	Lilly, Novo, Sigma, Lilly	Calbiochem, Nuclear Med Lab, Cambridge Nuclear, New England Nuclear	Calbiochem, Cambridge Nuclear, Radioassay Systems
38. Human pancreatic polypeptide (HPP)	Lilly	Lilly	Lilly			

(Continued)

APPENDIX 2 (Continued)

Hormone	Antibody		Hormone for			Labeled hormone	Immunoassay kits
	Immunogen	Antiserum	Immunization	Standard	Labeling		
39. Bovine pancreatic polypeptide (BPP)	Lilly	Lilly	Lilly	Lilly	Lilly		
40. Plasma estradiol		Calbiochem, New England Nuclear		Sigma		New England Nuclear, Amersham-Searle	New England Nuclear
41. Estrone		Calbiochem, New England Nuclear		Sigma		New England Nuclear, Amersham-Searle	New England Nuclear
42. Estriol		Calbiochem, New England Nuclear		Sigma		New England Nuclear	Schwarz/Mann
43. Urinary estriol glucoronide		Calbiochem		Sigma		Amersham-Searle	Schwarz/Mann
44. Progesterone	Steroloids	Endocrine, Calbiochem		Sigma		New England Nuclear, Amersham-Searle	New England Nuclear
45. 20α-Dihydroprogesterone				Sigma		New England Nuclear	

46. Androgens (testosterone and dihydrotestosterone)	Steroloids	Calbiochem	Sigma		New England Nuclear Amersham-Searle	Serono New England Nuclear
47. Radioiodinated steroid hormones						New England Nuclear
48. Mineralocorticoids	NIAMDD Antibodies Endocrine Medical Diagnostic	Steroloids Ikapharm[55]	Steroloids Ikapharm	Steroloids Ikapharm New England Nuclear Amersham-Searle	New England Nuclear Amersham-Searle	CIS New England Nuclear
49. Glucocorticoids	Steroloids Makor Chemicals[56] New England Nuclear Isopac[57] Miles[58] Radioassay Systems Inter Science[59]	Sigma Merck[60] Makor Chemicals	Sigma Merck Makor Chemicals	Sigma Merck Makor Chemicals	Amersham-Searle New England Nuclear	New England Nuclear Schwarz/Mann Serono Bio RIA CIS[61] Diagnostic Products Radioassay Systems Clinical Assays Diagnostics Biochem ICN Medical Diagnostic

(Continued)

APPENDIX 2 (Continued)

Hormone	Antibody		Hormone for			Labeled hormone	Immunoassay kits
	Immunogen	Antiserum	Immunization	Standard	Labeling		
50. Gluco-corticoid metabolites (THE, THF, THB, THS)			Sigma; Merck Makor Chemicals	Sigma; Merck Makor Chemicals	Sigma; Merck Makor Chemicals	New England Nuclear; CIS	Pantex[62]
51. Arthropod molting hormones β-Ecdysone				Simes[63]; Calbiochem Simes		New England Nuclear	
α-Ecdysone							
52. Human chorionic gonadotropin assay				Organon; Ayerst		New England Nuclear	Bio-RIA; Radioassay Systems; Serono
53. Placental lactogens		NIAMDD; Collaborative Research	NIAMDD	NIAMDD; NIAMDD	NIAMDD		New England Nuclear; Bio-Lab SA; Schwarz/Mann Pharmacia Amersham-Searle

54. Human chorionic thyrotropin		NIAMDD / Beckman / Schwarz/Mann	NIAMDD / MRC	NIAMDD / Schwarz/Mann / Beckman		NIAMDD / Squibb / Schwarz/Mann / Clinical Assays / New England Nuclear
55. Relaxin						
56. Renin and the angiotensins	Sylvana[64] / Schwarz/Mann / Squibb / New England Nuclear				NIAMDD / Squibb / Schwarz/Mann / CEA-CEN[65] / New England Nuclear / Cambridge Nuclear / New England Nuclear	
57. Bradykinin			Schwarz/Mann	Schwarz/Mann		
58. Urogastrone-epidermal growth factor						
59. Nerve growth factor: radioimmunoassay and bacteriophage immunoassay						
60. Somatomedin A, C, and NSILA-s						

FOOTNOTES TO APPENDIX 2

[a] Addresses of sources of radioimmunoassay components are as follows (indicated by superscript number in table):

1. Collaborative Research, 1365 Main Street, Waltham, Massachusetts 02154.
2. Schwarz/Mann Labs, Mountain View Avenue, Orangeburg, New York 10962.
3. New England Nuclear Corp., 575 Albany Street, Boston, Massachusetts 02118.
4. Sigma Chemical Company, 3500 De Kalb Street, St. Louis, Missouri 63178.
5. Amersham-Searle, 2636 S. Clearbrook Drive, Arlington Heights, Illinois 60005.
6. Diagnostic Products, 12306 Exposition Blvd., Los Angeles, California 90064.
7. Calbiochem, P.O. Box 12087, San Diego, California 92212.
8. The Upjohn Company, Kalamazoo, Michigan 49001.
9. Clinical Assays Inc., 237 Binney Street, Cambridge, Massachusetts 02142.
10. Abbott Laboratories, Abbott Park, North Chicago, Illinois 60064.
11. Beckman Instruments Inc., Spinco Div., Bioproducts Dept., 117 California Avenue, Palo Alto, California 94301.
12. Ayerst Laboratories, 685 Third Avenue, New York, New York 10017.
13. Immuno Nuclear, Stillwater, Minnesota 55082.
14. Bachem Fire Chemicals, Marina del Rey, California 90291.
15. AB Kabi, Stockholm, Sweden.
16. Guildhay Antisera, England.
17. Koch-Light, Colburn, Bucks., England.
18. Fluka, Buchs SG, Switzerland.
19. Peninsula Laboratories, 611 Taylor Way, Belmont, California 94002.
20. UCB Bioproducts, Brussels, Belgium.
21. NIAMDD—National Institute of Arthritis, Metabolism, and Digestive Diseases, Bethesda, Maryland 20014.
22. Radioassay Systems Laboratories, RIA Products Division, 1511 E. Del Amo. Blvd., Carson, California 90746.
23. Serono Immunochemicals, 607 Boylston Street, Boston, Massachusetts 02116.
24. MRC—Medical Research Council of Great Britain, London, England.
25. Antibodies for Research, P.O. Box 14275, Albuquerque, New Mexico 87111.
26. Gateway Immunoserum, P.O. Box 1735, Cahokia, Illinois 62206.
27. Cambridge Nuclear Corp., 575 Middlesex Turnpike, Billerica, Massachusetts 01821.
28. Curtis Nuclear Corp., 1948 East 46 Street, Los Angeles, California 90058.
29. Organon, Inc., 375 Mt. Pleasant Ave., West Orange, New Jersey 07052.
30. NPA—National Pituitary Agency, Baltimore, Maryland.
31. Ciba-Geigy AG, Basel, Switzerland.
32. Parke-Davis & Company, Detroit, Michigan 48232.
33. Diagnostic Biochemistry, San Diego, California 92212.
34. Nuclear Medical Systems, 515 Superior Avenue, Newport Beach, California 92660.
35. Pharmacia Laboratories, Inc., 800 Centennial Ave., Piscataway, New Jersey 08854.
36. Bio-RIA, Louisville, Kentucky.
37. Pontex.
38. Chemalog Dinamics Corp., South Plainfield, New Jersey 07080.
39. Spectrum Medical Industries Inc., 60916 Terminal Annex, Los Angeles, California 90054.

*Footnotes to Appendix 2 (**Continued**)*

40. Nichols' Institute, San Pedro, California.
41. CIS(IRE), l'Institut des Radioelements, c/o CEN-SCK, Bueretanct, 200, 2400 Mol, Belgium.
42. Burroughs Wellcome Co., 1 Scarsdale Road, Tuckahoe, New York 10707.
43. Scantibodies Laboratory, Lakeside, California 92040.
44. Inolex Corp., Glenwood, Illinois 60425.
45. Wilson Laboratories, 2600 Bond Street, Park Forest, Illinois 60466.
46. ICI-Imperial Chemical Industries, Alderley Park, England.
47. GIH Research Laboratories, Karolinska Institute, Stockholm, Sweden.
48. E. R. Squibb & Sons, P.O. Box 4000, Princeton, New Jersey 08540.
49. Farmatalia, Milan, Italy.
50. Mann Research Laboratories (now Schwarz/Mann Labs).
51. Steroloids Inc., Wilton, New Hampshire 03086.
52. Supelco, Supelco Park, Bellefonte, Pennsylvania 16823.
53. Novo Company, Copenhagen, Denmark.
54. Eli Lilly and Co., 307 E. McCarthy Street, Indianapolis, Indiana 46206.
55. Ikapharm, Ramat-Gan, Israel.
56. Makor Chemicals.
57. Isopac.
58. Miles Laboratories, 195 West Birch St., Kankakee, Illinois 60901.
59. InterScience, 2000 Cotner Avenue, Los Angeles, California 90025.
60. Merck, Sharp & Dohme, Division of Merck & Co., Inc., West Point, Pennsylvania 19486.
61. ICN Medical Diagnosis, ICN Pharmaceuticals, Inc., 2727 Campus Drive, Irvine, California 92664.
62. Pantex.
63. Simes, Milan, Italy.
64. Sylvana Co., 22 East Willow St., Millburn, New Jersey 07041.
65. CEA-CEN, Sorin, Italy.

[b] List of recommended products known to be available at the time of submission of the text.

APPENDIX 3 Normal Values As Determined by Radioimmunoassay

Hormone	Blood	Tissue	Other biologic fluid
1. cAMP and cGMP			
cAMP	15 ± 3 nM	Liver (rat), 960 ± 98 pmole/gm Kidney, 980 ± 92 Muscle, 360 ± 52 Lung, 1250 ± 110 Jejunum, 1010 ± 97 Pituitary, 880 ± 105	Urine—2.50 ± 0.13 μmole/gm creatine/day CSF—23 ± 4 nM
cGMP	5.1 ± 7 nM	Liver (rat), 15 ± 2 pmole/gm Kidney, 38 ± 4 Muscle, 18 ± 1.6 Lung, 56 ± 6 Jejunum, 120 ± 11 Pituitary, 9.0 ± 1.1	Urine—0.55 ± 0.08 μmole/gm creatinine/day CSF—1.9 ± 0.6 nm
2. Prostaglandins			
PGE	385 ± 30 pg/ml	Pancreas 3.5 ng/gm (human) 7.5 ± 2.5 (dog)	Urine—76–281 ng/day
PGF	141 ± 15 pg/ml	Kidney 1.35 ± 0.25 (rat) Pancreas 7.6 ng/gm (human) 8.6 ± 2.6 (dog)	Urine—422–871 ng/day
15-keto-PGF$_2\alpha$	0.5 ng/ml		
13,14-dihydro-15-keto-PGF$_2\alpha$	63–240 pg/ml		
15-keto-PGE$_2$	<50 pg/ml		
13,14-dihydro-15-keto-PGE$_2$	28 pg/ml		
Urinary tetranor metabolites of PGF			Urine—5–14 μg/day, females; 11–53 μg/day, males
3. TRH	7–30 pg/ml (rat)		

(Continued)

APPENDIX 3 (Continued)

Hormone	Blood		Tissue	Other biologic fluid
4. GnRH	1–80 pg/ml (human)			
	2–150 (rat)			
	5–350 (sheep)			
5. Somatostatin			Hypothalamus (rat), 13.4 ± 2 μg/gm	CSF—15–55 pg/ml
			Stalk median eminence, 248 ± 26	
			Ventromedial nucleus, 17.5 ± 2.5	
			Spinal cord, 10.4 ± 1.9	
			Cerebral cortex, 6.7 ± 1.7	
			Posterior pituitary, 5.6 ± 1.9	
			Pancreatic islets, 786 ± 85	
			Pyloric antrum, 6.4 ± 0.9	
	Day	Night		
6. Melatonin				
Human	13.9 ± 0.55 pg/ml	66.1 ± 5.3 pg/ml	Pineal—0.5–7.1 ng/gland	Human urine—0.5–10 ng/4 hours
				Human CSF
Rat	10 ± 2 pg/ml	45 ± 17 pg/ml	Pineal—0.2 ± 0.03 ng/gland (day)	59 ± 33 pg/ml (male)
			1.3 ± 0.3 ng/gland (night)	57 ± 28 pg/ml (female)
Chicken		340 ± 50 pg/ml	Pineal— 3.8 (day)	Urine—0.1–2 ng/12 hours
Calf	19 ± 4 pg/ml	121 ± 24 pg/ml	7.5 ± 0.5 (night)	
7. Substance P	9.0 ± 2.0 fmole/ml (rat)		Hypothalamus (rat), 200 pmole/gm	CSF 28 ± 8 pg/ml (day)
	18.0 ± 5.4 (calf)		Cerebellum, 2	637 ± 133 pg/ml (night)
				8 pmole/liter
8. Neurotensin	40–60 fmole/ml rat		Hypothalamus (rat), 60 pmole/gm	
	20–40 rabbit sheep		Jejunoileum, 40	

9. Gonadotropins

Human FSH		
Children	5 mIU/ml	
Men	10–15	
Women		
Midcycle	20–30	
Rest of cycle	10–20	
Rat FSH		
Proestrus	2000 ng/ml	
Estrus	<100	
Diestrus	<100	
Pseudopregnancy	100	
Human LH		
Children	2–4 mIU/ml	
Men	10–12	
Women		
Midcycle	80	
Rest of cycle	10–30	
Rat LH		
Proestrus	400 ng/ml	
Estrus	400	
Diestrus	200	

10. Prolactin — Up to 25 ng/ml serum — Pituitary, 0.2–1.0 μg/ml wet weight

11. Growth hormone — Less than 5 mg/ml during GTT; rise to >10 ng/ml during insulin and arginine tests — Pituitary, 60 ± 9 μg/ml; Other tissues, none detected

12. ACTH — 6 AM: <120 pg/ml; mean: 55 pg/ml; 6 PM: <75 pg/ml; mean: 35 pg/ml; In hospitalized normal volunteers 6 AM: 39 ± 3 pg/ml; 12 mid: 20 ± 1 pg/ml — Pituitary, 60–250 μg/g — Amniotic fluid—up to 24 weeks, 1–10 μg/ml; term, 0.1–1.0 μg/ml; Urine—fragments detected; values vary widely depending on antiserum used

(Continued)

APPENDIX 3 (Continued)

Hormone	Blood	Tissue	Other biologic fluid
13. α-MSH	Not detectable		
hβMSH (hβLPH + hγLPH)	6 AM: 58 ± 6 pg/ml 12 mid: 15 ± 2 pg/ml		
14. TSH	<0.5–10 μU/ml		
15. Oxytocin			
Chard			
Men	<1.5 pg/ml		
Women	<1.5		
Pregnant women	<1.5		
Kumaresan			
Men	2 pg/ml		
Women (nl)	2		
Pregnant women	40 ± 8 (33–40 weeks)		
16. Vasopressin			
Hydrated	0.45 pg/ml		
Dehydrated	3.7		
17. Calcitonin	<100 pg/ml	Thyroid, central zone, 30–500 ng/gm	Urine, <1.0 ng/ml
18. T3 and T4			
T3			
Normal range	100–170 ng/100 ml		
Mean	138		
Hypo mean	67		
Hyper mean	486		
T4			
Normal range	3.9–9.8 μg/100 ml		
Mean	7.4		
Hypo mean	1.3		
Hyper mean	16.2		

rT3	450 ± 200 pg/ml			
T$_2$				
Normal mean	7.6 ± 2.4 ng/100 ml			
Hyper mean	20.2 ± 7.5			
19. PTH	200–400 pg/ml			
20. Erythropoietin	4.9 ± 0.2 mU/ml (male)			
	4.3 ± 0.2 (female)			
21. Vitamin D metabolites				
25-OHD	4–55 ng/ml			
1,25-(OH)$_2$D	33 ± 6 pg/ml			
24,25-(OH)$_2$D	1–5 ng/ml			
22. Gastrin	<120 pg/ml; mean, 70 pg/ml	Antrum	Corpus	Duodenum
		20.7 ± 4.0 ng/gm		0.6 ng/gm (human)
		2.2 ± 1.2	0.005 ng/gm	(dog)
		5.0 ± 1.9	0.007	(pig)
		1.6 ± 0.8	0.02	(cat)
23. Secretin	37 ± 8 pg/ml			
24. CCK-PZ	60.4 pg/ml; 25% <5 pg/ml	Duodenum (dog), 15.4 ng/gm		
		Stomach, 3.4 ng/gm		
		Jejunum, 6.8 ng/gm		
		Ileum, 9.7 ng/gm		
25. Serotonin	168 ± 13 ng/ml whole blood			
	341 ng/10^9 platelets			
26. GIP	<125–400 pg/ml			
27. VIP	4.5 ± 2 pmole/liter	Colon (human), 136 ± 27		
	(range, <1–20)	pmole/gm		
		Cortex, 25 ± 10 pmole/gm		
28. Motilin	<125–400 pg/ml			
29. Bombesin		Stomach (human, dog), 1–10		
		pmole/gm		
30. Bile acids				
Cholylglycine	0.05–1.0 μM/liter			
Chenodeoxycholylglycine	0.04–1.0			
Deoxycholylglycine	0.02–0.3			
Sulfolithocholylglycine	0.07–0.8			

(Continued)

APPENDIX 3 (Continued)

Hormone	Blood	Tissue	Other biologic fluid
31. Insulin	Fasting: 1–25 μU/ml; mean, 8.44 ± 0.35		
Proinsulin	Fasting: 0.05–0.5 ng/ml; mean, 0.156 ± 0.014		
C-peptide	Fasting: 0.5–2.0 ng/ml		
32. Glucagon	50–150 pg/ml; mean, 75 ± 4	Pancreas 1–2 ng 3–6 μg/gm	
33. Pancreatic polypeptide	50–200 pg/ml (human) 100–200 pg/ml (dog)	3–6 μg/gm pancreas (human); 3–10 μg/gm pancreas (bovine); regionally distributed pancreas (dog)—uncinate process, 120 μg/gm; body, 18 μg/gm; tail, 14 μg/gm	
34. Estrogens			
Estradiol			
Menstrual cycle			
1–10 days	50 pg/ml		
10–12 days	100–150 pg/ml		
12–14 days	350–600 pg/ml		
14–28 days	200–400 pg/ml		
Estriol			
Weeks of pregnancy			
22–30	3–5 ng/ml		
32–37	6–11 ng/ml		
38–41	15–17 ng/ml		

Estrone
Weeks of pregnancy
22–30   3–5 ng/ml
32–37 weeks   5–6 ng/ml
38–41 weeks   7–10 ng/ml
Estriol-16α(β-D-glucuronide)   Urine—12–80 mg/day during pregnancy; 40–100 μg/day during Pergonal treatment

35. Progesterone
Menstrual
Follicular   0.4–0.6 ng/ml
Midluteal   7.7–12.1
Pregnancy
16–18 weeks   48.4 ± 18 ng/ml
28–30 weeks   98 ± 28
38–40 weeks   178.5 ± 48

36. Androgens
Testosterone
Males   4.0–12.0 ng/ml
Females   0.3–1.0
DHT
Males   3.0–8.0 ng/ml
Females   0.1–1.0

38. Mineralocorticoids
Aldosterone   Plasma *ad lib* salt—7 ng/100 ml 10 mEq Na/100 mEq K diet—64 ng/100 ml   Urine aldosterone secretion rate: *ad lib* salt—200 μg/24 hour; 10 mEq Na/100 mEq K diet—812 μg/24 hour
DOC   5 ng/100 ml *ad lib* diet
18-OHDOC   5 ng/100 ml *ad lib* diet; 90 ng/100 ml, 10 mEq Na diet

(Continued)

APPENDIX 3 (Continued)

Hormone	Blood	Tissue	Other biologic fluid
39. Glucocorticoids			
Cortisol	5–20 μg/100		Urine—30–150 μg/24 hr
Corticosterone	0.4–2 μg/100 ml		
Compound S	0.1–0.3 μg/100 ml		
	After metyrapone: 5.0–15.0 μg/100 ml		
Tetrahydrocortisol (THF)			Urine—3.8 ± 1.5 mg/24 hr
Tetrahydrocortisone (THE)			Urine—3.9 ± 1.6 mg/24 hr
Tetrahydrocorticosterone (THB)			Urine—22–178 μg/24 hr
Tetrahydro-Compound S			Urine—280 ± 25 μg/24 hr
40. Ecdysteroids			
Species		Hematopancreas, 406 ng/ml	
		Gill, 154 ng/ml	
		Muscle, 145 ng/ml	
Pachygrapsus crassipes	Premolt serum, 450 ng/ml	Testis, 470 ng/ml	
Gecarcinus lateralis	275 ng/ml	Medial vas deferens, 332 ng/ml	
		Ventral nerve cord, 294 ng/ml	
Carcinus moenas	15 μg/ml	Heart, 294 ng/ml	
Philosamia cynthia (4th larval instar)	125 ng/ml	Y-organ, 550 pg/gland	
Bombyx mori pupae	6.0 μg/ml		
		Whole-animal extracts	
		Drosophila melanogaster purpuria, 408 ng/gm	
		Manduexta 5th instar larvae, 850 ng/gm	

Leucophaea maderae late last
instar, 378 ng/gm
Aedes egypti-fed females,
275 ng/gm
Macrotermes bellicosus
Queens, 1.5 µg/gm
Workers, 50 ng/gm
Queen ovaries, 2.15 µg/gm
Hemolymph, 65 ng/gm
Integument, 25 ng/gm
Fat body, 50 ng/gm
Digestive tract, 110 ng/gm
Head and thorax, 44 ng/gm
Locusta migratoria adult
females
Ovary, 29 µg/gm
Fat body, 103 µg/gm
Hemolymph, 224 µg/gm
Carcass, 426 µg/gm

41. HCG

Human pregnancy
Primary peak (1st trimester),
163,000 mIU/ml
Nadir (2nd trimester), 12,000
Secondary peak (3rd trimester),
63,000

42. PL

4.9 µg/ml (human)
10.15 µg/ml (monkey)
0.5–1.6 (ovine)

43. HCT   <1 µU/ml
44. Relaxin   Before day 100 gestation (pig)
<2 ng/ml
Day 100 until 2 days preceding
parturition 5–40
Day preceding parturition 100–200
Day following parturition <2

300 µg/gm
70 µg/gm
100 µg/gm

(Continued)

APPENDIX 3 (Continued)

Hormone	Blood	Tissue	Other biologic fluid
45. Bradykinin	70 pg/ml		
46. Renin			
Angiotensin II	11.2 ± 3.4 pg/ml		
PRA	0.5–2.5 ng AI/ml/hr		
PRC	15–75 micro Goldblatt units/ml		
47. EGF	Up to 10 pg/ml (mouse)	Male mouse submaxillary gland, 1.5 µg/ml	Urine—up to 1 µg/ml
Urogastrone	Up to 1.0 ng/ml total immunoreactivity (human)		Urine—120–1200 ng/kg/24 hours
48. NGF	6–10 ng NGF immunoreactivity/ml		
49. NSILA-s	350 ± 66 mU/liter		
Somatomedin A	1.00 ± 0.23 U/ml		
Somatomedin C	1.49 ± 0.25 U/ml		

INDEX

A
B
C 9
D 0
E 1
F 2
G 3
H 4
I 5
J 6